Drug Facts and Comparisons®

2003

Pocket Version

Drug Facts and Comparisons® Pocket Version, Seventh Edition, 2003

Adapted from *Drug Facts and Comparisons®* loose-leaf drug information service through the February 2002 update. Previous copyrights 1947-2002 by Facts and Comparisons.

ISBN 1-57439-136-4

Printed in the United States of America

The information contained in *Drug Facts and Comparisons®* pocket version is available for licensing as source data. For more information on data licensing, please call 1-800-223-0554

Published by
Facts and Comparisons®
111 West Port Plaza, Suite 300
St. Louis, Missouri 63146-3098
www.drugfacts.com
314/216-2100 • 800/223-0554

FACTS AND COMPARISONS® PUBLISHING GROUP

Steven K. Hebel, RPh
President and CEO

Kenneth H. Killion
Publisher

Teri H. Burnham
Senior Managing Editor

Renée M. Wickersham
Managing Editor

Sara L. Schweain
Associate Editor

Lindsay D. Harmon
Associate Editor

Linda M. Jones
SGML Specialist

Jennifer K. Walsh
Senior Composition Specialist

Kim S. Spitzmiller, PharmD
Senior Drug Information Specialist

Lori A. Buss, PharmD
Drug Information Specialist

Cathy A. Connolly, PharmD
Drug Information Specialist

Cindy A. Meilink
Marketing Manager

Robert Brown
Director, Marketing and Sales

Laura J. Zyk
Product and Market Analyst

DRUG FACTS AND COMPARISONS® POCKET VERSION REVIEWERS

Kate Farthing, PharmD
Drug Information Coordinator
Oregon Health and Science University
  Drug Information Service
OHSU Hospitals and Clinics
Portland, Oregon

Mary J. Ferrill, PharmD, FASHP
Associate Dean and Professor
Palm Beach Atlantic College
School of Pharmacy
West Palm Beach, Florida

Joyce A. Generali, MS, FASHP
Director, Drug Information Center
Clinical Associate Professor
Kansas University Medical Center
Kansas City, Kansas

Beth Jones, PharmD
Clinical Pharmacist
Missouri Baptist Medical Center
St. Louis, Missouri

Burgunda V. Sweet, PharmD
Director, Drug Information and
  Investigational Drug Services
Clinical Associate Professor of
  Pharmacy
University of Michigan Health System
  and College of Pharmacy
Ann Arbor, Michigan

iii

v

Edward A. Hartshorn, PhD
Clinical Professor
University of Texas at
  Austin, College of
  Pharmacy
University of Texas
Medical Branch at
  Galveston
Galveston, Texas

Tina C. Hussey, PharmD
Drug Information Clinical
  Specialist
University of North Carolina
  Healthcare System

Siret D. Jaanus, PhD
Professor of Pharmacology
Southern California College
  of Optometry
Fullerton, California

**Robert E. Kates, PharmD,
  PhD**
President
Analytical Solutions, Inc.
Sunnyvale, California

Julio R. Lopez, PharmD
Assistant Professor, School
  of Pharmacy, University
  of the Pacific
Assistant Clinical Professor,
  School of Pharmacy,
  University of California,
  San Francisco
Director, Drug Information
  Center, VA Medical
  Center
Martinez, California

Susan O'Donoghue, MD
Associate Director, Cardiac
  Arrhythmia Center
Washington Hospital Center
Washington, DC

**Richard M. Oksas, PharmD,
  MPh**
Pharmaceutical Consultant
Medication Information
  Service
Torrance, California

Edward V. Platia, MD
Director, Cardiac
  Arrhythmia Center
Washington Hospital Center
Professor of Medicine
George Washington
  University School of
  Medicine

Michael T. Reed, PharmD
Associate Professor of
  Clinical Pharmacy
Arnold and Marie Schwartz
  College of Pharmacy and
  Health Sciences of Long
  Island University
Brooklyn, New York
The Mount Sinai Medical
  Center
New York, New York

J. James Rowsey, MD
St. Luke's Cataract and Laser
  Institute
Tarpon Springs, Florida

Frederick L. Ruben, MD
Infectious Disease Division
Montefiore University
  Hospital
University of Pittsburgh
Pittsburgh, Pennsylvania

Mary Beth Shirk, PharmD
Specialty Practice
  Pharmacist
Critical Care Medicine
Clinical Assistant Professor
The Ohio State University
  Medical Center
Columbus, OH

**Burgunda V. Sweet,
  PharmD**
Director, Drug Information
  and Investigational Drug
  Services
Clinical Associate Professor
  of Pharmacy
University of Michigan
  Health System and College
  of Pharmacy
Ann Arbor, Michigan

**Udho Thadani, MBBS,
  FRCP(C), FACC**
Professor of Medicine
Vice Chief of Cardiology and
  Director of Clinical
  Research
University of Oklahoma
  Health Sciences Center
Oklahoma City, Oklahoma

Robert A. Wild, MD
Chief, Section of Research
  & Education in Women's
  Health
Department of Obstetrics
  and Gynecology
University of Oklahoma
  Health Sciences Center
Oklahoma City, Oklahoma

**Thom J. Zimmerman, MD,
  PhD**
Chairman of Department of
  Ophthalmology and Visual
  Sciences
Professor of Pharmacology
  & Toxicology
University of Louisville
Louisville, Kentucky

Table of Contents

How-to-Use viii

Preface x

Nutrients and Nutritional Agents. 1

Hematological Agents. 25

Endocrine and Metabolic Agents 89

Cardiovascular Agents 195

Renal and Genitourinary Agents 315

Respiratory Agents 351

Central Nervous System Agents. 415

Gastrointestinal Agents 663

Systemic Anti-Infective Agents 717

Biologic and Immunologic Agents. 981

Dermatological Agents 1035

Ophthalmic and Otic Agents 1057

Antineoplastic Agents 1087

Appendix 1105

Index 1121

Drug monographs in *Drug Facts and Comparisons®*, *Pocket Version* are arranged by use. Drugs with similar therapeutic or pharmacologic characteristics have been grouped together to allow the health care provider to compare these drugs easily and determine the most appropriate drug therapy. Standard sections within the monographs occur in a consistent format. Once the user is familiar with the organization of the data, the desired information can be located quickly.

Monograph Organization

1 *Therapeutic class:* Drugs that share the same therapeutic class will share a common title that appears on the right-hand pages. The monograph title appears on the left-hand pages. If there is no shared class, the monograph title will repeat on the right-hand page.

2 *Drug name:* Generic names and any common synonyms appear in a horizontal bar that introduces a new monograph. Synonyms follow the generic name in parentheses and are separated by semicolons.

3 *Product table:* Doseforms and strengths of generic drugs are listed in the left column with their schedules (eg, *Rx, otc, c-ii*). If more than one generic entity is included in the monograph (eg, beta blockers), the drugs appear in all caps with specific information below. The more common trade names, with their specific manufacturers/distributors, are listed in the right-hand column. If the drug is available generically, the word "Various" appears at the beginning of the trade name listing.

4 *Warning box:* Potentially life-threatening reactions specified in the product labeling will appear in a box. *Not included in sample.*

5 *Indications:* All FDA-approved indications are included. In addition, off-label uses with substantial documentation may appear under the term "Unlabeled uses."

6 *Administration and Dosage:* Appropriate dosage, dosage range, etc is included. When available, specific information for administration in situations such as renal impairment, elderly patients, etc. is included.

7 *Actions:* A brief discussion of significant pharmacologic and pharmacokinetic information.

8 *Contraindications:* All known contraindications are included.

9 *Warnings:* A brief description of major warnings associated with the drug. Standard sections (eg, Pregnancy, Lactation, Children) appear at the end of this section. The Pregnancy section generally only lists the Standard Pregnancy Category (A, B, C, D, or X). A description of these categories can be found in the Appendix.

10 *Precautions:* Potential conditions for which the patient should be cautioned (eg, photosensitivity) are included, as well as other significant situations where caution is warranted.

11 *Drug Interactions:* Drugs that may interact (affect or be affected by the interacting agent) are listed. Lab test and drug/food interactions are also included.

12 *Adverse Reactions:* Where possible, reactions that occur in 3% or more of patients have been listed. When percentages were not available, significant reactions not discussed in Warnings or Precautions are included.

❷ CYCLOBENZAPRINE HCl

Tablets: 10 mg (*Rx*)	Various, *Flexeril* (Merck)

❺ Indications
Musculoskeletal conditions: Adjunct to rest and physical therapy for relief of muscle spasm associated with acute painful musculoskeletal conditions.

Unlabeled uses: Cyclobenzaprine (10 to 40 mg/day) appears to be a useful adjunct in the management of the fibrositis syndrome.

❻ Administration and Dosage
Give 10 mg 3 times daily (range, 20 to 40 mg daily in divided doses). Do not exceed 60 mg/day. Do not use longer than 2 or 3 weeks.

❼ Actions
Pharmacology: Cyclobenzaprine, structurally related to the tricyclic antidepressants (TCAs), relieves skeletal muscle spasm of local origin without interfering with muscle function. It is ineffective in muscle spasm due to CNS disease. The net effect is a reduction of tonic somatic motor activity, influencing both gamma and alpha motor systems.

Pharmacokinetics: Cyclobenzaprine is well absorbed after oral administration, but there is a large intersubject variation in plasma levels. Peak plasma levels are reached in 4 to 6 hours. The onset of action occurs in 1 hour with a duration of 12 to 24 hours. It is highly bound to plasma proteins, extensively metabolized primarily to glucuronide-like conjugates and excreted primarily via the kidneys. Elimination half-life is 1 to 3 days.

❽ Contraindications
Hypersensitivity to cyclobenzaprine; concomitant use of monoamine oxidase (MAO) inhibitors or within 14 days after their discontinuation; acute recovery phase of MI and in patients with arrhythmias, heart block, or conduction disturbances or CHF; hyperthyroidism.

❾ Warnings
Spasticity: Cyclobenzaprine is not effective in the treatment of spasticity associated with cerebral or spinal cord disease, or in children with cerebral palsy.

Duration: Use only for short periods (up to 2 or 3 weeks); effectiveness for more prolonged use is not proven.

Similarity to TCAs: Cyclobenzaprine is closely related to the TCAs. In short-term studies for indications other than muscle spasm associated with acute musculoskeletal conditions, and usually at doses greater than those recommended, some of the more serious CNS reactions noted with the TCAs have occurred.

Pregnancy: Category B.

Lactation: It is not known whether cyclobenzaprine is excreted in breast milk.

Children: Safety and efficacy in children < 15 years of age have not been established.

❿ Precautions
Anticholinergic effects: Because of its anticholinergic action, use with caution in patients with a history of urinary retention, angle-closure glaucoma, and increased intraocular pressure.

Hazardous tasks: May impair mental or physical abilities required for performance of hazardous tasks; patients should observe caution while driving or performing other tasks requiring alertness, coordination, and physical dexterity.

⓫ Drug Interactions
Drugs that may interact with cyclobenzaprine HCl include MAO inhibitors and TCAs.

⓬ Adverse Reactions
Adverse reactions occurring in ≥ 3% of patients include drowsiness, dizziness, fatigue, tiredness, asthenia, blurred vision, headache, nervousness, confusion, dry mouth, nausea, constipation, dyspepsia, unpleasant taste, purpura, bone marrow depression, leukopenia, eosinophilia, thrombocytopenia, elevation and lowering of blood sugar levels, and weight gain or loss.

PREFACE

The Pocket Version of *Drug Facts and Comparisons®* (DFC) is an abridged version of the full *DFC* publication designed for quick reference by the health care professional. The purpose of *DFC Pocket Version* is to provide an easy-to-use, concise, portable version that can be utilized in daily practice. It is not intended to replace the complete information found in *DFC*; however, it provides the same reliable source of drug information.

In addition to the extensive review panel for *DFC*, a separate panel of drug information specialists and hospital pharmacists was established to determine which drug monographs would be most valuable to you along with the data for each drug you need most. The book is arranged therapeutically in 13 chapters in a consistent format. Single-agent monographs have been pared down to provide the essential information that a health care provider needs to aid in drug therapy decisions. Product tables that list trade names, doseforms, strengths, and manufacturers are included at the beginning of each monograph. Group monographs contain product information and dosing instructions for each of the drugs in a specific class (eg, beta blockers). Indications, administration and dosage, actions, contraindications, warnings, drug interactions, and significant adverse reactions (those occurring in ≥ 3% of patients) are also included for all monographs. The useful tables that are so common to *DFC* have, for the most part, been retained in the Pocket Version.

Appendix material (eg, Management of Overdosage, FDA Pregnancy Categories) is also available for reference. A comprehensive index will help you reach the desired information quickly and easily.

Facts and Comparisons® hopes you find *Drug Facts and Comparisons® Pocket Version* a valuable tool in daily practice. As always, your comments and suggestions are appreciated.

Steven K. Hebel, RPh
President and CEO

Chapter 1
NUTRIENTS AND NUTRITIONAL AGENTS

Recommended Dietary Allowances, 3
Vitamins, 7
    Vitamin C, 7
Minerals and Electrolytes, 9
    Calcium, 9
    Magnesium, 13
    Potassium Replacement Products, 15
Nutritional Therapy, 20
    Sodium Chloride, 20
    Sodium Bicarbonate, 22

RECOMMENDED DIETARY ALLOWANCES OF VITAMINS AND MINERALS

Recommended Dietary Allowances (RDA) are published by the Food and Nutrition Board, National Research Council-National Academy of Sciences, as a guide for nutritional problems and to provide standards of good nutrition for different age groups. They are revised periodically.

The RDA values are *not requirements*; they are *recommended* daily intakes of certain essential nutrients. Based on available scientific knowledge, they are believed to be adequate for known nutritional needs for most *healthy* people under usual environmental stresses. The recommended allowances vary for age and sex, with extra allowances for women during pregnancy and lactation. The most commonly used RDA values (the "reference male" and "reference female") are those of adults 23 to 50 years of age. With the exception of energy (kilocalories), the RDA provide for individual requirement variations and prevent symptoms of clinical deficiency of 97% of the population.

RDA have been established for many essential nutrients; however, present knowledge of human nutritional needs of pantothenic acid and biotin is incomplete. Therefore, to ensure adequate nutrient intake, obtain the recommended allowances from as varied a selection of foods as possible. Nutritionists suggest that dietary planning include regular intake of each of the four basic food groups:

1.) Milk, cheese, dairy products – Minimum 2 servings/day.
2.) Meat, poultry, fish, beans – Minimum 2 servings/day.
3.) Vegetables, fruit – Minimum 4 servings/day.
4.) Bread, cereal (whole-grain and enriched or fortified) – Minimum 4 servings/day.

Such a balance, in sufficient quantities will provide about 1200 kcal, enough protein, and most of the vitamins and minerals required daily. A person may increase nutrient and energy intake by consuming larger quantities (or more servings/day) of the 4 basic food groups. Nutrient and energy intake may also be increased by selecting food from the fifth group, fats-sweets-alcohol, which provides mainly energy.

RDA quantities apply only to healthy people and are not intended to cover therapeutic nutritional requirements in disease or other abnormal states (ie, metabolic disorders, weight reduction, chronic disease, drug therapy). Although certain single nutrients in larger quantities may have pharmacologic actions, these are unrelated to nutritional functions. There is no convincing evidence that consuming excessive quantities of single nutrients will cure or prevent nonnutritional diseases.

The "official" listings of United States Recommended Daily Allowances (US-RDAs) should not be confused with the RDA values. US-RDA are derived from the 1968 RDA and serve as legal standards for nutritional labeling of food and dietary food and dietary supplement products controlled by the FDA. Generally, they represent the higher value of the male or female RDA and are grouped into only 3 age brackets plus 1 category for pregnant or lactating women. Prior to 1972, these allowances were erroneously listed as minimum daily requirements (MDR). A second fallacy perpetuated by US-RDA labeling of foods is the implication that a food is defective if it does not contain all the officially established nutrients in their full US-RDA quantities. No individual food is nutritionally complete, but several foods together should complement each other to provide maximal nutrient balance and to minimize naturally occurring toxic principles consumed from any individual foodstuff.

The RDA for adult males and adult females are included in each individual vitamin monograph. The table on the following page presents the listing of vitamin and mineral RDA values for all age groups as published in *Recommended Dietary Allowances*, 10th Edition, National Academy of Sciences, Washington, DC, 1989.

RECOMMENDED DIETARY ALLOWANCES [1]

	Patient parameters					Fat-soluble vitamins					Water-soluble vitamins						Minerals						
Age (years) or Condition	Weight[2] (kg)	(lb)	Height[2] (cm)	(in)	Protein (g)	Vitamin A (µg RE[3])	Vitamin D (IU[4])	Vitamin E (IU[5])	Vitamin K (µg)	Ascorbic acid (C) (mg)	Thiamine (B_1) (mg)	Riboflavin (B_2) (mg)	Niacin (B_3) (mg)	Pyridoxine (B_6) (mg)	Folate (µg)	Cyanocobalamin (B_{12}) (µg)	Calcium (mg)	Phosphorus (mg)	Magnesium (mg)	Iron (mg)	Zinc (mg)	Iodine (µg)	Selenium (µg)
Infants																							
0.0-0.5	6	13	60	24	13	375	300	4	5	30	0.3	0.4	5	0.3	25	0.3	400	300	40	6	5	40	10
0.5-1	9	20	71	28	14	375	400	6	10	35	0.4	0.5	6	0.6	35	0.5	600	500	60	10	5	50	15
Children																							
1-3	13	29	90	35	16	400	400	9	15	40	0.7	0.8	9	1	50	0.7	800	800	80	10	10	70	20
4-6	20	44	112	44	24	500	400	10	20	45	0.9	1.1	12	1.1	75	1	800	800	120	10	10	90	20
7-10	28	62	132	52	28	700	400	10	30	45	1	1.2	13	1.4	100	1.4	800	800	170	10	10	120	30
Males																							
11-14	45	99	157	62	45	1000	400	15	45	50	1.3	1.5	17	1.7	150	2	1200	1200	270	12	15	150	40
15-18	66	145	176	69	59	1000	400	15	65	60	1.5	1.8	20	2	200	2	1200	1200	400	12	15	150	50
19-24	72	160	177	70	58	1000	400	15	70	60	1.5	1.7	19	2	200	2	1200	1200	350	10	15	150	70
25-50	79	174	176	70	63	1000	200	15	80	60	1.5	1.7	19	2	200	2	800	800	350	10	15	150	70
51+	77	170	173	68	63	1000	200	15	80	60	1.2	1.4	15	2	200	2	800	800	350	10	15	150	70
Females																							
11-14	46	101	157	62	46	800	400	12	45	50	1.1	1.3	15	1.4	150	2	1200	1200	280	15	12	150	45
15-18	55	120	163	64	44	800	400	12	55	60	1.1	1.3	15	1.5	180	2	1200	1200	300	15	12	150	50
19-24	58	128	164	65	46	800	400	12	60	60	1.1	1.3	15	1.6	180	2	1200	1200	280	15	12	150	55
25-50	63	138	163	64	50	800	200	12	65	60	1.1	1.3	15	1.6	180	2	800	800	280	15	12	150	55
51+	65	143	160	63	50	800	200	12	65	60	1	1.2	13	1.6	180	2	800	800	280	10	12	150	55
Pregnant					60	800	400	15	65	70	1.5	1.6	17	2.2	400	2.2	1200	1200	320	30	15	175	65
Lactating – 1st 6 mo.					65	1300	400	18	65	95	1.6	1.8	20	2.1	280	2.6	1200	1200	355	15	19	200	75
2nd 6 mo.					62	1200	400	16	65	90	1.6	1.7	20	2.1	260	2.6	1200	1200	340	15	16	200	75

Reproduced from: *Recommended Dietary Allowances*, 10th edition, 1989, National Academy of Sciences, National Academy Press, Washington, DC.

[1] The allowances, expressed as average daily intakes over time, are intended to provide for individual variations among most normal people as they live in the US under usual environmental stresses. Diets should be based on a variety of common foods in order to provide other nutrients for which human requirements have been less well defined.

[2] Weights and heights of Reference Adults are actual medians for the US population of the designated age, as reported by NHANES II. The median weights and heights of those < 19 years of age were taken from Hamill PV, et al. *Am J Clin Nutr.* 1979;32:607-629. The use of these figures does not imply that the height-to-weight ratios are ideal.

[3] Retinol equivalents. 1 retinol equivalent = 1 mcg retinol or 6 mcg β-carotene.

[4] As cholecalciferol. 10 mcg cholecalciferol = 400 IU of vitamin D.

[5] α-Tocopherol equivalents. 1 mg d-α-tocopherol = α-TE = 1.49 IU.

Dietary Reference Intakes (DRIs) refer to nutrient intake values estimated to be adequate for 50% of age- and gender-specific groups. As seen in the table below, DRIs are comprised of RDAs in bold type and Adequate Intakes (AIs) in ordinary type followed by asterisk (*). These values may be used as goals for individual intake. RDAs are estimated to meet the needs of most individuals (97% to 98%). For healthy breastfed infants, the AI represents mean intake. For all other life-stage groups, the AI is believed to cover the needs of all individuals, but a lack of data or uncertainty in the data prevent specifying with confidence what percentage of individuals covered by this intake.

Food and Nutrition Board, Institute of Medicine – National Academy of Science Dietary Reference Intakes: Recommended Intakes for Individuals

Life-stage group	Calcium (mg/d)	Phosphorus (mg/d)	Magnesium (mg/d)	Vitamin D (mcg/d)[a,b]	Fluoride (mg/d)	Thiamine (mg/d)	Riboflavin (mg/d)	Niacin (mg/d)[c]	Vitamin B_6 (mg/d)	Folate (mcg/d)[d]	Vitamin B_{12} (mcg/d)	Pantothenic acid (mg/d)	Biotin (mcg/d)	Choline[e] (mg/d)
Infants														
0-6 mo.	210*	100*	30*	5*	0.01*	0.2*	0.3*	2*	0.1*	65*	0.4*	1.7*	5*	125*
7-12 mo	270*	275*	75*	5*	0.5*	0.3*	0.4*	4*	0.3*	80*	0.5*	1.8*	6*	150*
Children														
1-3 yr	500*	460	80	5*	0.7*	0.5	0.5	6	0.5	150	0.9	2*	8*	200*
4-8 yr	800*	500	130	5*	1*	0.6	0.6	8	0.6	200	1.2	3*	12*	250*
Males														
9-13 yr	1300*	1250	240	5*	2*	0.9	0.9	12	1.0	300	1.8	4*	20*	375*
14-18 yr	1300*	1250	410	5*	3*	1.2	1.3	16	1.3	400	2.4	5*	25*	550*
19-30 yr	1000*	700	400	5*	4*	1.2	1.3	16	1.3	400	2.4	5*	30*	550*
31-50 yr	1000*	700	420	5*	4*	1.2	1.3	16	1.3	400	2.4	5*	30*	550*
51-70 yr	1200*	700	420	10*	4*	1.2	1.3	16	1.7	400	2.4[f]	5*	30*	550*
>70 yr	1200*	700	420	15*	4*	1.2	1.3	16	1.7	400	2.4[f]	5*	30*	550*
Females														
9-13 yr	1300*	1250	240	5*	2*	0.9	0.9	12	1.0	300	1.8	4*	20*	375*
14-18 yr	1300*	1250	360	5*	3*	1	1	14	1.2	400[g]	2.4	5*	25*	400*
19-30 yr	1000*	700	310	5*	3*	1.1	1.1	14	1.3	400[g]	2.4	5*	30*	425*
31-50 yr	1000*	700	320	5*	3*	1.1	1.1	14	1.3	400[g]	2.4	5*	30*	425*
51-70 yr	1200*	700	320	10*	3*	1.1	1.1	14	1.5	400	2.4[f]	5*	30*	425*
>70 yr	1200*	700	320	15*	3*	1.1	1.1	14	1.5	400	2.4[f]	5*	30*	425*
Pregnancy														
≤18 yr	1300*	1250	400	5*	3*	1.4	1.4	18	1.9	600[h]	2.6	6*	30*	450*
19-30 yr	1000*	700	350	5*	3*	1.4	1.4	18	1.9	600[h]	2.6	6*	30*	450*
31-50 yr	1000*	700	360	5*	3*	1.4	1.4	18	1.9	600[f]	2.6	6*	30*	450*

Food and Nutrition Board, Institute of Medicine – National Academy of Science Dietary Reference Intakes: Recommended Intakes for Individuals

Life-stage group	Calcium (mg/d)	Phosphorus (mg/d)	Magnesium (mg/d)	Vitamin D (mcg/d)[a,b]	Fluoride (mg/d)	Thiamine (mg/d)	Riboflavin (mg/d)	Niacin (mg/d)[c]	Vitamin B6 (mg/d)	Folate (mcg/d)[d]	Vitamin B12 (mcg/d)	Pantothenic acid (mg/d)	Biotin (mcg/d)	Choline[e] (mg/d)
Lactation														
≤18 yr	1300*	1250	360	5*	3*	1.5	1.6	17	2	500	2.8	7*	35*	550*
19-30 yr	1000*	700	310	5*	3*	1.5	1.6	17	2	500	2.8	7*	35*	550*
31-50 yr	1000*	700	320	5*	3*	1.5	1.6	17	2	500	2.8	7*	35*	550*

[a] As cholecalciferol. 1 mcg cholecalciferol = 40 IU vitamin D.

[b] In the absence of adequate exposure to sunlight.

[c] As niacin equivalents (NE). 1 mg of niacin = 60 mg of tryptophan; 0 to 6 months = preformed niacin (not NE).

[d] As dietary folate equivalents (DFE). 1 DFE = 1 mcg food folate = 0.6 mcg of folic acid (from fortified food or supplement) consumed with food = 0.5 mcg of synthetic (supplemental) folic acid taken on an empty stomach.

[e] Although AIs have been set for choline, there are few data to assess whether a dietary supply of choline is needed at all stages of the life-cycle, and it may be that the choline requirement can be met by endogenous synthesis at some of these stages.

[f] Because 10% to 30% of older people may malabsorb food-bound B_{12}, it is advisable for those > 50 years to meet their RDA mainly by consuming foods fortified with B_{12} or a supplement containing B_{12}.

[g] In view of evidence linking folate intake with neural tube defects in the fetus, it is recommended that all women capable of becoming pregnant consume 400 mcg of synthetic folic acid from fortified foods and/or supplements in addition to intake of food folate from a varied diet.

[h] It is assumed that women will continue consuming 400 mcg of folic acid until their pregnancy is confirmed and they enter prenatal care, which ordinarily occurs after the end of the periconceptional period – the critical time for formation of the neural tube.

VITAMIN C (Ascorbic Acid)

ASCORBIC ACID

Tablets: 25, 50, 100, 250, 500, and 1000 mg (*otc*)	Various, *One A Day Extras Vitamin C* (Miles)
Tablets, chewable: 60, 100, 250, and 500 mg (*otc*)	Various
Tablets and caplets, timed release: 500, 1000, and 1500 mg (*otc*)	Various
Caplets: 500 mg (*otc*)	*SunKist Vitamin C* (Ciba)
Capsules, timed-release: 500 mg (*otc*)	Various, *Ascorbicap* (ICN), *Cevi-Bid* (Geriatric)
Lozenges: 60 mg (*otc*)	*N'ice Vitamin C Drops* (SmithKline Beecham Consumer)
Crystals: 4 g/teaspoonful (*otc*)	*Vita-C* (Freeda)
Powder: 4 g/teaspoonful (*otc*)	*Dull-C* (Freeda)
Liquid: 35 mg/0.6 mL (*otc*)	*Ce-Vi-Sol* (Mead Johnson Nutritional)
Solution: 100 mg/mL (*otc*)	*Cecon* (Abbott)
Syrup: 500 mg/5 mL (*otc*)	Various
Injection: 250 and 500 mg/mL (*Rx*)	Various

CALCIUM ASCORBATE

Tablets: 610 mg (equiv. to 500 mg ascorbic acid)	Various
Powder: 1 g (equiv. to 826 mg ascorbic acid)/ ¼ teaspoonful	Various

SODIUM ASCORBATE

Tablets: 585 mg (equiv. to 500 mg ascorbic acid) (*otc*)	Various
Crystals: 1020 mg (equiv. to 900 mg ascorbic acid)/ ¼ teaspoonful (*otc*)	Various
Injection: 250 mg/mL (equiv. to 222 mg/mL ascorbic acid) (*Rx*)	Various
562.5 mg/mL (equiv. to 500 mg/mL ascorbic acid) (*Rx*)	*Cenolate* (Abbott)

Indications

Prevention and treatment of scurvy. Parenteral administration is desirable in an acute deficiency or when absorption of oral ascorbic acid is uncertain.

Unlabeled uses: Vitamin C ($\geq$ 2 g/day) may be used as a urinary acidifier in conjunction with methenamine therapy.

Vitamin C in doses of $\geq$ 150 mg has been used to control idiopathic methemoglobinemia (less effective than methylene blue).

Administration and Dosage

Parenteral: Administer IV, IM, or SC. Avoid too rapid IV injection. Absorption and utilization are somewhat more efficient with the IM route, which is usually preferred.

Infants: Average daily protective requirement is 30 mg. The usual curative dose is 100 to 300 mg daily, continued as long as clinical symptoms persist or until saturation, as indicated by excretion tests, has been attained.

Premature infants: May require 75 to 100 mg/day.

Adults: The average protective dose is 70 to 150 mg/day. For scurvy, 300 mg to 1 g daily is recommended. However, up to 6 g/day has been administered parenterally to normal adults without evidence of toxicity.

Enhanced wound healing – Doses of 300 to 500 mg daily for 7 to 10 days both preoperatively and postoperatively are adequate, although considerably larger amounts have been recommended.

Burns – For severe burns, daily doses of 1 to 2 g are recommended.

In other conditions in which the need for vitamin C is increased, 3 to 5 times the daily optimum allowances appears adequate.

Actions

Pharmacology: Vitamin C, a water-soluble vitamin, is an essential vitamin in man; however, its exact biological functions are not fully understood. It is essential for the formation and the maintenance of intercellular ground substance and collagen, for catecholamine biosynthesis, for synthesis of carnitine and steroids, for conversion of folic acid to folinic acid and for tyrosine metabolism.

The deficiency state *scurvy* is characterized by degenerative changes in the capillaries, bone, and connective tissues. Mild vitamin C deficiency symptoms may include faulty bone and tooth development, gingivitis, bleeding gums, and loosened teeth.

Absorption of dietary ascorbate from the intestines is nearly complete. Vitamin C is readily available in citrus fruit, tomatoes, potatoes, and leafy vegetables.

Warnings

Excessive vitamin C doses: Diabetics, patients prone to recurrent renal calculi, those undergoing stool occult blood tests and those on sodium restricted diets or anticoagulant therapy should not take excessive doses of vitamin C over an extended time period.

Pregnancy: Category C. Do not administer ascorbic acid to pregnant women in excess of the amount needed for treatment. The possibility of the fetus adapting to high levels of the vitamin could result in a scorbutic condition after birth when the intake drops to normal levels. This action is controversial.

Lactation: Ascorbic acid is excreted in breast milk.

Drug Interactions

Contraceptives (oral) and estrogens: Ascorbic acid increases serum levels of estrogen and estrogen contained in oral contraceptives, possibly resulting in adverse reactions.

Warfarin: The anticoagulant action of warfarin may be reduced.

Drug/Lab test interactions: Large doses (> 500 mg) of vitamin C may cause false-negative urine glucose determinations.

No exogenous vitamin C should be ingested for 48 to 72 hours before amine-dependent stool occult blood tests are conducted because possible false-negative results may occur.

Adverse Reactions

Large doses may cause diarrhea and precipitation of cystine, oxalate, or urate renal stones if the urine becomes acidic during therapy.

Transient mild soreness may occur at the site of IM or SC injection. Too rapid IV administration may cause temporary faintness or dizziness.

CALCIUM

CALCIUM ACETATE

Tablets: 667 mg (169 mg calcium) (*Rx*)	*Calphron* (Nepro-Tech), *PhosLo* (Branitree)

CALCIUM CARBONATE

Tablets: 650 and 667 mg, and 1.25 and 1.5 g (260 mg calcium) (*otc*)	Various, *Cal-Plus* (Geriatric Pharm.), *Caltrate 600* (Lederle), *Os-Cal 500* (SmithKline Beecham), *Oyster Shell Calcium-500* (Vangard)
Tablets, chewable: 750 mg and 1.25 g (*otc*)	*Calci-Chew* (R & D), *Caltrate, Jr.* (Lederle), *Os-Cal 500*, *Tums 500* (SmithKline Beecham)
Capsules: 125 mg (50 mg calcium) (*otc*)	*Cal-Guard Softgels* (Rugby)
1250 mg powdered calcium carbonate (500 mg calcium) (*otc*)	*Calci-Mix* (R & D)
Oral Suspension: 1.25 g (500 mg calcium) per 5 mL (*otc*)	Various
Powder: 6.5 g (2400 mg calcium) per packet (*otc*)	*Cal Carb-HD* (Konsyl Pharm.)

CALCIUM CHLORIDE

Injection: 10% (*Rx*)	Various

CALCIUM CITRATE

Tablets: 950 mg (200 mg calcium) (*otc*)	*Citracal* (Mission)
Tablets, effervescent: 2376 mg (500 mg calcium) (*otc*)	*Citracal Liquitab* (Mission)

CALCIUM GLUBIONATE

Syrup: 1.8 mg calcium glubionate (115 mg calcium) per 5 mL (*otc*)	*Neo-Calglucon* (Sandoz)

CALCIUM GLUCEPTATE

Injection: 1.1 g/5 mL (*Rx*)	Various

CALCIUM GLUCONATE

Tablets: 500 mg (45 mg calcium), 650 mg (58.5 mg calcium), 975 mg (87.75 mg calcium), 1 g (90 mg calcium) (*otc*)	Various
Injection: 10% (*Rx*)	Various

CALCIUM LACTATE

Tablets: 325 mg (42.25 mg calcium), 650 mg (84.5 mg calcium) (*otc*)	Various

CALCIUM SALT COMBINATIONS

Injection: 50 mg calcium glycerophosphate and 50 mg calcium lactate per 10 mL in sodium chloride solution (0.08 mEq Ca/mL) (*Rx*)	*Calphosan* (Glenwood)

TRICALCIUM PHOSPHATE

Tablets: 1565.2 mg (600 mg calcium) (*otc*)	*Posture* (Whitehall)

Indications

Oral: As a dietary supplement when calcium intake may be inadequate.

In the treatment of calcium deficiency states that may occur in diseases such as: Tetany of newborn; end-stage renal disease, mild to moderate renal insufficiency; renal osteodystrophy; acute and chronic hypoparathyroidism; pseudohypoparathyroidism; postmenopausal and senile osteoporosis; rickets and osteomalacia. Some studies have suggested that the use of calcium citrate is more effective than calcium carbonate in the treatment of postmenopausal osteoporosis.

Calcium acetate (PhosLo) – Control of hyperphosphatemia in end-stage renal failure; does not promote aluminum absorption.

Parenteral:

Hypocalcemia – For a prompt increase in plasma calcium levels (eg, neonatal tetany and tetany due to parathyroid deficiency, vitamin D deficiency, alkalosis); prevention of hypocalcemia during exchange transfusions; conditions associated with intestinal malabsorption.

Calcium chloride and gluconate – Adjunctive therapy in the treatment of insect bites or stings, such as Black Widow spider bites to relieve muscle cramping; sensitivity reactions, particularly when characterized by urticaria; depression due to overdosage of magnesium sulfate; acute symptoms of lead colic; rickets; osteomalacia.

Calcium chloride – To combat the deleterious effects of severe hyperkalemia as measured by ECG, pending correction of increased potassium in the extracellular fluid.

Cardiac resuscitation: Particularly after open heart surgery, when epinephrine fails to improve weak or ineffective myocardial contractions.

Calcium gluconate – To decrease capillary permeability in allergic conditions, non-thrombocytopenic purpura and exudative dermatoses such as dermatitis herpetiformis; for pruritus of eruptions caused by certain drugs; in hyperkalemia, calcium gluconate may aid in antagonizing the cardiac toxicity, provided the patient is not receiving digitalis therapy.

Unlabeled uses:

Oral – Calcium supplementation may lower blood pressure in some hypertensive patients with indices suggesting calcium "deficiency." However, other hypertensives may experience a pressor response.

In one study, calcium administration significantly reduced premenstrual symptoms of fluid retention, pain, and negative affect.

Parenteral – Calcium salts have been used to treat verapamil overdose, treat acute hypotension from verapamil, and prevent initial hypotension in patients requiring verapamil for whom decreases in blood pressure could be detrimental.

Administration and Dosage

Oral: Calcium must be in a soluble, ionized form to be absorbed. Solubility (except calcium lactate) is increased by acidic pH. Give with meals to maximize acidity and solubility.

Dietary supplement – The usual daily dose is 500 mg to 2 g, 2 to 4 times/day.

An NIH Consensus Development conference recommends a calcium intake for adults of 1000 to 1500 mg/day to reduce bone loss associated with aging.

PhosLo – 2 tablets with each meal. The dosage may be increased to bring the serum phosphate value < 6 mg/dL, as long as hypercalcemia does not develop. Most patients require 3 to 4 tablets with each meal.

Parenteral: Calcium gluconate is generally preferred over calcium chloride as it is less irritating.

IV – Warm solutions to body temperature and give slowly (0.5 to 2 mL/min); stop if patient complains of discomfort. Resume when symptoms disappear. Following injection, patient should remain recumbent for a short time. Repeated injections may be needed because of the rapid calcium excretion. Inject **calcium chloride** and **gluconate** through a small needle into a large vein to minimize venous irritation.

IM administration – IM administration of **calcium gluceptate** and **gluconate** may be tolerated; however, reserve this route for emergencies when technical difficulty makes IV injection impossible. Administer **calcium gluconate** only by the IV route and **calcium chloride** by the IV or intraventricular route.

CALCIUM CHLORIDE –

For IV use only: Injection is irritating to veins and must not be injected into tissues, because severe necrosis and sloughing may occur. Avoid extravasation. Administer slowly (not to exceed 0.5 to 1 mL/min).

Intraventricular administration – In cardiac resuscitation, injection may be made into the ventricular cavity; do not inject into the myocardium. Intraventricular injection may be administered by personnel who are well trained in the technique and familiar with possible complications. Break off the IV needle supplied with the syringe and replace with a suitable intracardiac needle by affixing it firmly to the Luer taper provided on the syringe. After the injection has been completed, remove the needle/syringe assembly from the injection site by grasping the needle at the Luer fitting.

The intraventricular dose usually ranges from 200 to 800 mg (2 to 8 mL).

Hypocalcemic disorders:

Adults – 500 mg to 1 g at intervals of 1 to 3 days, depending on response of patient or serum calcium determinations. Repeated injections may be required.

Children – 0.2 mL/kg up to 1 to 10 mL/day.

Magnesium intoxication: Give 500 mg promptly; observe patient for signs of recovery before further doses are given.

Hyperkalemic ECG disturbances of cardiac function: Adjust dosage by constant monitoring of ECG changes during administration.

Cardiac resuscitation:

Adults – Dose ranges from 500 mg to 1 g IV or 200 to 800 mg injected into the ventricular cavity.

Children – 0.2 mL/kg

CALCIUM GLUCEPTATE –

IM: 2 to 5 mL (0.44 to 1.1 g). Inject 5 mL (1.1 g) doses in the gluteal region or, in infants, in the lateral thigh.

IV: 5 to 20 mL (1.1 to 4.4 g). Warm solution to body temperature and administer slowly ($\leq$ 2 mL/min).

Exchange transfusions in newborns: 0.5 mL (0.11 g) after every 100 mL of blood exchanged.

CALCIUM GLUCONATE – For IV use only, either directly or by infusion; SC or IM injection may cause severe necrosis and sloughing. Do not exceed a rate of 0.5 to 2 mL/min. Calcium gluconate may also be administered by intermittent infusion at a rate not exceeding 200 mg/min, or by continuous infusion. Discontinue injection if the patient complains of discomfort. Do not use IM, as abscess formation and local necrosis may occur.

Adults: 2.3 to 9.3 mEq (5 to 20 mL) as required. Dosage range is 4.65 to 70 mEq/day.

Children: 2.3 mEq/kg/day or 56 mEq/m^2/day, well diluted; give slowly in divided doses.

Infants: Not more than 0.93 mEq (2 mL).

Emergency elevation of serum calcium:

Adults – 7 to 14 mEq (15 to 30.1 mL) IV.

Children – 1 to 7 mEq (2.2 to 15 mL).

Infants – < 1 mEq (2.2 mL). Depending on patient response, these doses can be repeated every 1 to 3 days.

Hypocalcemic tetany:

Adults – 4.5 to 16 mEq of calcium (9.7 to 34.4 mL) may be given IM until therapeutic response occurs.

Children – 0.5 to 0.7 mEq/kg (1.1 to 1.5 mL/kg) IV 3 or 4 times/day or until tetany is controlled.

Neonates – 2.4 mEq/kg/day (5.2 mL/kg/day) in divided doses.

Hyperkalemia with secondary cardiac toxicity: Administer IV to provide 2.25 to 14 mEq (4.8 to 30.1 mL) while monitoring ECG. If necessary, repeat doses after 1 to 2 minutes.

Magnesium intoxication:

Adults – Initial dose is 4.5 to 9 mEq (9.7 to 19.4 mL) IV. Adjust subsequent doses to patient response. If IV use is not possible, give 2 to 5 mEq (4.3 to 10.8 mL) IM.

Exchange transfusion:

Adults – Approximately 1.35 mEq (2.9 mL) IV concurrent with each 100 mL of citrated blood.

Neonates – Administer IV at a dosage of 0.45 mEq (1 mL)/100 mL of exchanged citrated blood.

Admixture incompatibilities: Calcium salts should not generally be mixed with **carbonates, phosphates, sulfates,** or **tartrates** in parenteral admixtures; they are conditionally compatible with potassium phosphates, depending on concentration. Calcium ions will chelate **tetracycline.**

Actions

Pharmacology: Calcium is essential for the functional integrity of the nervous and muscular systems, for normal cardiac contractility and the coagulation of blood. It also functions as an enzyme cofactor and affects the secretory activity of endocrine and exocrine glands. Normal levels are 8.5 to 10.5 mg/dL.

Hypocalcemia –

Symptoms: Tetany; paresthesias; laryngospasm; muscle spasms; seizures (usually grand mal); irritability; depression; psychosis; prolonged QT interval; intestinal cramps and malabsorption; respiratory arrest. Prolonged hypocalcemia may be associated with ectodermal defects including the nails, skin, and teeth.

Pharmacokinetics: Differences in absorption and bioavailability between various calcium salts appear to exist, as well as between different preparations of the same salt.

Approximately 80% of body calcium is excreted in the feces as insoluble salts; urinary excretion accounts for the remaining 20%.

Elemental Calcium Content of Calcium Salts		
Calcium salt	% Calcium	mEq Ca^{++}/g
Calcium glubionate	6.5	3.3
Calcium gluconate	9.3	4.6
Calcium lactate	13	9.2
Calcium citrate	21	12
Calcium acetate	25	12.6
Tricalcium phosphate	39	19.3
Calcium carbonate	40	20
Calcium chloride	27.3	13.6
Calcium gluceptate	8.2	4.1

Contraindications

Oral: Renal calculi; hypophosphatemia; hypercalcemia.

Parenteral: Hypercalcemia; ventricular fibrillation; digitalized patients.

Warnings

Extravasation: **Calcium chloride** and **gluconate** can cause severe necrosis, sloughing, and abscess formation with IM or SC administration.

PhosLo: End-stage renal failure patients may develop hypercalcemia when given calcium with meals. Do not give other calcium supplements concurrently with *PhosLo.* Monitor serum calcium levels twice weekly during the early dose adjustment period. Do not allow serum calcium times phosphate product to exceed 66.

Pregnancy: Category C. (*PhosLo* and parenteral).

Precautions

Oral:

Hypercalcemia/hypercalciuria – Hypercalcemia/hypercalciuria may result when therapeutic amounts are given for prolonged periods. Avoid by frequent monitoring of plasma and urine calcium levels.

Parenteral:

Cardiovascular effects – Prevent a high concentration of calcium from reaching the heart because of the danger of cardiac syncope.

Drug Interactions

Calcium citrate: Avoid concurrent aluminum-containing antacids.

Drugs that may affect calcium include thiazide diuretics.

Drugs that may be affected by calcium include atenolol, sodium polystyrene sulfonate, tetracyclines, and verapamil. *Oral only:* Iron salts, quinolones; *parenteral only:* Digitalis glycosides.

Drug/Lab test interactions: Transient elevations of plasma 11-hydroxy-corticosteroid levels (Glenn-Nelson technique) may occur when IV calcium is administered, but levels return to control values after 1 hour. In addition, IV calcium gluconate can produce false-negative values for serum and urinary magnesium.

Drug/Food interactions: Diets high in dietary fiber have been shown to decrease absorption of calcium due to decreased transit time in the GI tract and complexing of fiber with the calcium.

Calcium acetate, when taken with meals, combines with dietary phosphate to form insoluble calcium phosphate which is excreted in the feces.

Adverse Reactions

Oral – GI disturbances are rare. Mild hypercalcemia (Ca^{++} > 10.5 mg/dL) may be asymptomatic or manifest itself as: Anorexia; nausea; vomiting; constipation; abdominal pain; dry mouth; thirst; polyuria. More severe hypercalcemia (Ca^{++} 12 mg/dL) is associated with confusion, delirium, stupor, and coma.

The risk of hypercalcemia with calcium acetate may be less than that of calcium carbonate and calcium citrate.

IM administration – Mild local reactions may occur (calcium glucepate). Local necrosis and abscess formation may occur with **calcium gluconate,** and severe necrosis and sloughing may occur with IM or SC administration of **calcium chloride.**

IV administration – Rapid IV administration may cause bradycardia, sense of oppression, tingling, metallic, calcium, or chalky taste, or "heat waves". Rapid IV **calcium gluconate** may cause vasodilation, decreased blood pressure, cardiac arrhythmias, syncope, and cardiac arrest. **Calcium chloride** injections cause peripheral vasodilation and a local burning sensation; blood pressure may fall moderately.

MAGNESIUM

Tablets: 400 mg magnesium (oxide) (*otc*)	Mag-200 (Optimox)
400 mg magnesium oxide (241.3 mg magnesium) (*otc*)	Mag-Ox 400 (Blaine)
500 mg magnesium gluconate (27 mg magnesium) (*otc*)	Almora (Forest), Magonate (Fleming)
500 mg magnesium gluconate (29 mg magnesium) (*otc*)	Magtrate (Mission)
500 mg magnesium amino acids chelate (100 mg magnesium) (*otc*)	Chelated Magnesium (Freeda)
Tablets, sustained release: 535 mg magnesium chloride hexahydrate (64 mg magnesium) (*otc*)	Slow-Mag (Searle)
Caplets, sustained release: 84 mg magnesium (as lactate) (*otc*)	Mag-Tab SR (Niche)
Capsules: 140 mg magnesium oxide (84.5 mg magnesium) (*otc*)	Uro-Mag (Blaine)
Liquid: 54 mg/5 mL magnesium (as gluconate) (*otc*)	Magonate (Fleming)
Injection: 20% magnesium chloride (1.97 mEq/mL) (*Rx*)	Various
Injection: Magnesium sulfate. 10% (0.8 mEq/mL), 12.5% (1 mEq/mL) and 50% (4 mEq/mL) (*Rx*)	Various

Indications

Oral: As a dietary supplement.

Parenteral:

Hypomagnesemia – Magnesium sulfate is used as replacement therapy in magnesium deficiency especially in acute hypomagnesemia accompanied by signs of tetany similar to those observed in hypocalcemia. In such cases, the serum magnesium (Mg++) level is usually below the lower limit of normal (1.5 to 2.5 or 3 mEq/L) and the serum calcium (Ca++) level is normal (4.3 to 5.3 mEq/L) or elevated.

Total parenteral nutrition: Total parenteral nutrition patients may develop hypomagnesemia (<1.5 mEq/L) without supplementation. Magnesium is added to correct or prevent hypomagnesemia.

Preeclampsia/eclampsia/nephritis (magnesium sulfate) – Prevention and control of convulsions of severe preeclampsia and eclampsia and for control of hypertension, encephalopathy, and convulsions associated with acute nephritis in children.

Administration and Dosage

Oral: 1 g magnesium = 83.3 mEq (41.1 mmol).

Dietary supplement – 54 to 483 mg/day in divided doses. Refer to product labeling. Magnesium-containing antacids may also be used.

Parenteral:

IV administration – Do not exceed 1.5 mL/min of a 10% concentration (or its equivalent), except in cases of severe eclampsia with seizures. Dilute IV infusion solutions to a concentration of ≤ 20% prior to IV administration. The most commonly used diluents are 5% Dextrose Injection and 0.9% Sodium Chloride Injection.

IM administration – Deep IM injection of the undiluted (50%) solution is appropriate for adults, but dilute to ≤ 20% concentration prior to IM injection in children.

Admixture incompatibilities – Magnesium sulfate in solution may result in a precipitate formation when mixed with solutions containing: Alcohol (in high concentrations); alkali carbonates and bicarbonates; alkali hydroxides; arsenates; barium; calcium; clindamycin phosphate; heavy metals; hydrocortisone sodium succinate; phosphates; polymyxin B sulfate; procaine HCl; salicylates; strontium; tartrates.

Hyperalimentation – Maintenance requirements are not precisely known. Maintenance dose range:

> *Adults:* 8 to 24 mEq/day.
>
> *Infants:* 2 to 10 mEq/day.

Mild magnesium deficiency –

> *Adults:* 1 g (8.12 mEq; 2 mL of 50% solution) IM every 6 hours for 4 doses (total of 32.5 mEq/24 hours).

Severe hypomagnesemia –

> *IM:* As much as 2 mEq/kg (0.5 mL of 50% solution) within 4 hours if necessary.
>
> *IV:* 5 g (≈ 40 mEq)/L of 5% Dextrose Injection or 0.9% Sodium Chloride solution, infused over 3 hours. In treatment of deficiency states, observe caution to prevent exceeding renal excretory capacity.

Seizures associated with preeclampsia/eclampsia/nephritis – Refer to Anticonvulsants, Miscellaneous for complete dosing information.

Actions

Pharmacology: Magnesium is an electrolyte that is necessary in a number of enzyme systems, phosphate transfer, muscular contraction, and nerve conduction. While there are large stores of magnesium present intracellularly and in bone in adults, these stores often are not mobilized sufficiently to maintain plasma levels; therefore, serum levels may not reflect total magnesium stores.

Magnesium prevents or controls convulsions by blocking neuromuscular transmission and decreasing the amount of acetylcholine liberated at the end plate by the motor nerve impulse. Normal plasma magnesium levels range from 1.5 to 2.5 mEq.

Magnesium acts peripherally to produce vasodilation. With low doses, only flushing and sweating occur; larger doses cause a lowering of blood pressure and CNS depression.

Pharmacokinetics: IM injection results in therapeutic plasma levels within 60 minutes and persists for 3 to 4 hours. IV doses provide immediate effects that last for 30 minutes. Effective anticonvulsant serum levels range from 2.5 to 7.5 mEq/L. Magnesium is excreted by the kidneys at a rate proportional to the plasma concentration and glomerular filtration.

Contraindications

Magnesium sulfate: Heart block or myocardial damage; IV magnesium to patients with preeclampsia during the 2 hours preceding delivery.

Magnesium chloride: Renal impairment; marked myocardial disease; coma.

Warnings

Renal function impairment: Use with caution. Parenteral use in the presence of renal insufficiency may lead to magnesium intoxication.

Elderly: Geriatric patients often require reduced dosage because of impaired renal function. In patients with severe impairment, dosage should not exceed 20 g in 48 hours. Monitor serum magnesium in such patients.

Pregnancy: Category A.

Lactation: Magnesium is distributed into milk during parenteral magnesium sulfate administration.

Children: Safety and efficacy in children have not been established.

Precautions

Monitoring: Maintain urine output at a level of ≥ 100 mL every 4 hours. Monitor serum magnesium levels and clinical status to avoid overdosage in preeclampsia.

Serum magnesium levels usually sufficient to control convulsions range from 3 to 6 mg/dL (2.5 to 5 mEq/L). Keep an injectable calcium salt immediately available to counteract potential hazards of magnesium intoxication in eclampsia.

Flushing/Sweating: Administer with caution if flushing or sweating occurs.

Renal disease: Do not use without physician supervision because of potential accumulation.

Excessive dosage: Excessive dosage may cause diarrhea and GI irritation.

Drug Interactions

Drugs that may be affected by magnesium salts include aminoquinolines, digoxin, nitrofurantoin, penicillamine, and tetracyclines.

Effects of nondepolarizing neuromuscular blocking agents may be increased by concurrent magnesium sulfate.

Adverse Reactions

Adverse effects are usually the result of magnesium intoxication and include flushing; sweating; hypotension; stupor; depressed reflexes; flaccid paralysis; hypothermia; circulatory collapse; cardiac and CNS depression proceeding to respiratory paralysis (the most life-threatening effect).

Hypocalcemia with signs of tetany secondary to magnesium sulfate therapy for eclampsia has occurred.

POTASSIUM REPLACEMENT PRODUCTS

POTASSIUM REPLACEMENT PRODUCTS

Tablets, controlled release: 6.7 mEq (500 mg) potassium chloride in a wax matrix (*Rx*)	*Kaon-Cl* (Adria)
8 and 10 mEq (600 and 750 mg) potassium chloride in a wax matrix (*Rx*)	Various, *Klor-Con 8* (Upsher-Smith), *Slow-K* (Summit), *Kaon Cl-10* (Adria), *Klor-Con 10* (Upsher-Smith), *Klotrix* (Bristol), *K-Tab* (Abbott)
Tablets, extended release: 750 mg potassium chloride equivalent to 10 mEq potassium in a wax matrix (*Rx*)	Various
Tablets, controlled release: 750 mg microcapsulated potassium chloride equivalent to 10 mEq potassium (*Rx*)	*K-Dur 10* (Key), *Ten-K* (Summit)
1500 mg microcapsulated potassium chloride equivalent to 20 mEq potassium (*Rx*)	*K-Dur 20* (Key)
Tablets: 500 mg potassium gluconate (83.45 mg potassium) (*Rx*)	Various
595 mg potassium gluconate (99 mg potassium) (*Rx*)	Various
Tablets, effervescent: 20 mEq potassium (from potassium bicarbonate) (*Rx*)	*K + Care ET* (Alra)
20 mEq potassium (from potassium chloride and bicarbonate and lysine HCl) (*Rx*)	*Klorvess* (Sandoz)
25 mEq potassium (from potassium chloride and bicarbonate and lysine HCl) (*Rx*)	*K•Lyte/Cl* (Bristol)
50 mEq potassium (from potassium Cl and bicarbonate, lysine monohydrochloride and citric acid) (*Rx*)	*K•Lyte/Cl 50* (Bristol)
25 mEq potassium (from potassium bicarbonate) (*Rx*)	*K + Care ET* (Alra)
25 mEq potassium (as bicarbonate and citrate) (*Rx*)	Various, *Effer-K* (Nomax), *Klor-Con/EF* (Upsher-Smith), *K•Lyte* (Bristol)
50 mEq potassium (from potassium bicarbonate and citrate and citric acid) (*Rx*)	*K•Lyte DS* (Bristol)
Capsules, controlled release: 600 mg potassium chloride equivalent to 8 mEq potassium. Microencapsulated particles (*Rx*)	*Micro-K Extencaps* (Robins)
10 mEq (750 mg) potassium chloride. Microencapsulated particles (*Rx*)	Various, *K-Lease* (Adria), *K-Norm* (Fisons), *Micro-K 10 Extencaps* (Robins)
Liquid: 20 mEq/15 mL potassium and chloride (10% KCl) (*Rx*)	Various, *Cena-K* (Century), *Kaochlor 10% and S-F* (Adria), *Kay Ciel* (Forest), *Klorvess* (Sandoz)
30 mEq/15 mL potassium and chloride (15% KCl) (*Rx*)	*Rum-K* (Fleming)

40 mEq/15 mL potassium and chloride (20% KCl) (*Rx*)	Various, *Cena-K* (Century), *Kaon-Cl 20%* (Adria)
20 mEq/15 mL potassium (as potassium gluconate) (*Rx*)	Various, *Kaon* (Adria), *K-G Elixir* (Geneva)
45 mEq/15 mL potassium (from potassium acetate, potassium bicarbonate and potassium citrate) (*Rx*)	*Tri-K* (Century)
20 mEq/15 mL potassium (as potassium gluconate & potassium citrate) (*Rx*)	*Twin-K* (Boots)
20 mEq potassium and 3.4 mEq chloride/15 mL (from potassium gluconate and potassium chloride (*Rx*)	*Kolyum* (Fisons)
Powder: 15 mEq potassium chloride per packet (*Rx*)	*K + Care* (Alra)
20 mEq potassium chloride per packet (*Rx*)	Various, *Gen-K* (Goldline), *Kay Ciel* (Forest), *K + Care* (Alta), *K-Lor* (Abbott), *Klor-Con* (Upsher-Smith), *Micro-K LS* (Robins)
25 mEq potassium chloride per dose (*Rx*)	*K•Lyte/Cl* (Mead-J)
20 mEq each potassium and chloride (potassium chloride, bicarbonate and citrate and lysine HCl)/packet (*Rx*)	*Klorvess Effervescent Granules* (Sandoz)
POTASSIUM ACETATE	
Injection: 2 and 4 mEq/mL (*Rx*)	Various
POTASSIUM CHLORIDE CONCENTRATE	
Injection: 2 mEq/mL and 10, 20, 30, 40, 60, and 90 mEq (*Rx*)	Various

Indications

Oral: Treatment of hypokalemia in the following conditions: With or without metabolic alkalosis; digitalis intoxication; familial periodic paralysis; diabetic acidosis; diarrhea and vomiting; surgical conditions accompanied by nitrogen loss, vomiting, suction drainage, diarrhea, and increased urinary excretion of potassium; certain cases of uremia; hyperadrenalism; starvation and debilitation; corticosteroid or diuretic therapy.

Prevention of potassium depletion when dietary intake is inadequate in the following conditions: Patients receiving digitalis and diuretics for CHF; significant cardiac arrhythmias; hepatic cirrhosis with ascites; states of aldosterone excess with normal renal function; potassium-losing nephropathy; certain diarrheal states.

When hypokalemia is associated with alkalosis, use potassium chloride. When acidosis is present, use the bicarbonate, citrate, acetate, or gluconate potassium salts.

IV:

Potassium acetate – Potassium acetate is useful as an additive for preparing specific IV fluid formulas when patient needs cannot be met by standard electrolyte or nutrient solutions.

Also indicated for marked loss of GI secretions by vomiting, diarrhea, GI intubation, or fistulas; prolonged diuresis; prolonged parenteral use of potassium-free fluids; diabetic acidosis, especially during vigorous insulin and dextrose treatment; metabolic alkalosis; attacks of hereditary or familial periodic paralysis; hyperadrenocorticism; primary aldosteronism; overmedication with adrenocortical steroids, testosterone, or corticotropin; healing phase of scalds or burns; cardiac arrhythmias, especially due to digitalis glycosides.

Administration and Dosage

Oral: The usual dietary intake of potassium ranges between 40 to 150 mEq/day.

Individualize dosage. Usual range is 16 to 24 mEq/day for the prevention of hypokalemia to 40 to 100 mEq/day or more for the treatment of potassium depletion.

Reserve slow release potassium chloride preparations for patients who cannot tolerate liquids or effervescent potassium preparations, or for patients in whom there is a problem of compliance with these preparations.

Some studies suggest the "microencapsulated" preparations are less likely to cause GI damage; however, evidence conflicts and a specific recommendation of one solid oral product over another cannot be made. Avoid enteric coated products.

Potassium intoxication may result from any therapeutic dosage.

IV:

Do not administer undiluted potassium – Potassium preparations must be diluted with suitable large volume parenteral solutions, mixed well and given by slow IV infusion.

Too rapid infusion of hypertonic solutions may cause local pain and, rarely, vein irritation. Adjust rate of administration according to tolerance. Use of the largest peripheral vein and a small bore needle is recommended.

The usual additive dilution of potassium chloride is 40 mEq/L of IV fluid. The maximum desirable concentration is 80 mEq/L, although extreme emergencies may dictate greater concentrations.

In critical states, potassium chloride may be administered in saline (unless saline is contraindicated) because dextrose may lower serum potassium levels by producing an intracellular shift.

Avoid "layering" of potassium by proper agitation of the prepared IV solution. Do not add potassium to an IV bottle in the hanging position.

Individualize dosage. Guide dosage and rate of infusion by ECG and serum electrolyte determinations. The following may be used as a guide:

Potassium Dosage/Rate of Infusion Guidelines			
Serum K+	Maximum infusion rate	Maximum concentration	Maximum 24 hour dose
> 2.5 mEq/L	10 mEq/hr	40 mEq/L	200 mEq
< 2 mEq/L	40 mEq/hr	80 mEq/L	400 mEq

Add electrolytes to the mixed solutions only after considering electrolytes already present and potential incompatibilities such as calcium and phosphate or sulfate.

Children – IV infusion up to 3 mEq/kg or 40 mEq/m^2/day. Adjust volume of administered fluids to body size.

Actions

Pharmacology: Potassium participates in a number of essential physiological processes, such as maintenance of intracellular tonicity and a proper relationship with sodium across cell membranes, cellular metabolism, transmission of nerve impulses, contraction of cardiac, skeletal, and smooth muscle, acid-base balance, and maintenance of normal renal function. Normal potassium serum levels range from 3.5 to 5 mEq/L.

mEq/g of Various Potassium Salts	
Potassium salt	mEq/g
Potassium gluconate	4.3
Potassium citrate	9.8
Potassium bicarbonate	10
Potassium acetate	10.2
Potassium chloride	13.4
Dibasic potassium phosphate[1]	11.5
Monobasic potassium phosphate[1]	7.3

[1] Commercial preparations of potassium phosphate injection contain a mixture of both mono- and dibasic salts.

Potassium participates in carbohydrate utilization and protein synthesis and is critical in regulating nerve conduction and muscle contraction, particularly in the heart.

Pharmacokinetics: Normally about 80% to 90% of potassium intake is excreted in urine with the remainder voided in stool and, to a small extent, in perspiration. Kidneys do not conserve potassium well; during fasting or in patients on a potassium-free diet, potassium loss from the body continues, resulting in potassium depletion. A deficiency of either potassium or chloride will lead to a deficit of the other.

Contraindications

Oral: Severe renal impairment with oliguria or azotemia; untreated Addison's disease; hyperkalemia from any cause; adynamia episodica hereditaria; acute dehydration; heat cramps; patients receiving potassium-sparing diuretics or aldosterone-inhibiting agents.

IV: Diseases where high potassium levels may be encountered; hyperkalemia; renal failure and conditions in which potassium retention is present; oliguria or azotemia; anuria; crush syndrome; severe hemolytic reactions; adrenocortical insufficiency (untreated Addison's disease); adynamica episodica hereditaria; acute dehydration; heat cramps; hyperkalemia from any cause; early postoperative oliguria except during GI drainage.

Warnings

Hyperkalemia: This occurs most commonly in patients given IV potassium, but also may occur in patients given oral potassium. Potentially fatal hyperkalemia can develop rapidly and may be asymptomatic.

GI lesions: Potassium chloride tablets have caused stenotic or ulcerative lesions of the small bowel and death. These lesions are caused by a concentration of potassium ion in the region of a rapidly dissolving tablet, which injures the bowel wall and produces obstruction, hemorrhage, or perforation. The reported frequency of small bowel lesions is much less with wax matrix tablets and microencapsulated tablets than with enteric coated tablets. Immediately discontinue either type of tablet and consider the possibility of bowel obstruction or perforation if severe vomiting, abdominal pain or distention, or GI bleeding occurs.

Patients at greatest risk for developing potassium chloride-induced GI lesions include: The elderly, the immobile and those with scleroderma, diabetes mellitus, mitral valve replacement, cardiomegaly, or esophageal stricture/compression.

Metabolic acidosis and hyperchloremia: Potassium depletion is rarely associated with metabolic acidosis and hyperchloremia. Replace with potassium bicarbonate, citrate, acetate, or gluconate.

Potassium intoxication: Do not infuse rapidly. High plasma concentrations of potassium may cause death through cardiac depression, arrhythmias, or arrest. Monitor potassium replacement therapy whenever possible by continuous or serial ECG. In addition to ECG effects, local pain, and phlebitis may result when a > 40 mEq/L concentration is infused.

Renal impairment or adrenal insufficiency – Renal impairment or adrenal insufficiency may cause potassium intoxication. Potassium salts can produce hyperkalemia and cardiac arrest. Potentially fatal hyperkalemia can develop rapidly and be asymptomatic. Use with great caution, if at all.

Concentrated: Concentrated potassium solutions are for IV admixtures only; do not use undiluted. Direct injection may be instantaneously fatal.

Metabolic alkalosis: Potassium depletion is usually accompanied by an obligatory loss of chloride resulting in hypochloremic metabolic alkalosis. Treat the underlying cause of potassium depletion and administer IV potassium chloride.

Use solutions containing acetate ion carefully in metabolic or respiratory alkalosis, and when there is an increased level or impairment of utilization of this ion.

Musculoskeletal/Cardiac effects: When serum sodium or calcium concentration is reduced, moderate elevation of serum potassium may cause toxic effects on the heart and skeletal muscle. Weakness and later paralysis of voluntary muscles, with consequent respiratory distress and dysphagia, are generally late signs, sometimes significantly preceding dangerous or fatal cardiac toxicity.

Renal function impairment: Renal function impairment requires careful monitoring of the serum potassium concentration and appropriate dosage adjustment.

Pregnancy: Category C.

Children: Safety and efficacy for use in children have not been established.

Precautions

Monitoring: Close medical supervision with frequent ECGs and serum potassium determinations. Plasma levels are not necessarily indicative of tissue levels.

Fluid/Solute overload: IV administration can cause fluid or solute overloading resulting in dilution of serum electrolyte concentrations, overhydration, congested states, or pulmonary edema.

Special risk: Use with caution in the presence of cardiac disease, particularly in digitalized patients or in the presence of renal disease, metabolic acidosis, Addison's disease, acute dehydration, prolonged or severe diarrhea, familial periodic paralysis, hypoadrenalism, hyperkalemia, hyponatremia, and myotonia congenita.

Drug Interactions

Drugs that may interact include ACE inhibitors, potassium-sparing diuretics, digitalis, and potassium-containing salt substitutes.

Adverse Reactions

Oral: Adverse reactions may include nausea, vomiting, diarrhea, flatulence, and abdominal discomfort due to GI irritation. They are best managed by diluting the preparation further, by taking with meals, or by dose reduction. Severe reactions may include hyperkalemia; GI obstruction, bleeding, ulceration, or perforation.

Parenteral: Hyperkalemia — Adverse reactions involve the possibility of potassium intoxication. Signs and symptoms include paresthesias of extremities; flaccid paralysis; muscle or respiratory paralysis; areflexia; weakness; listlessness; mental confusion; weakness and heaviness of legs; hypotension; cardiac arrhythmias; heart block; ECG abnormalities such as disappearance of P waves, spreading and slurring of the QRS complex with development of a biphasic curve and cardiac arrest.

SODIUM CHLORIDE

Solution: 0.45% (77 mEq/L sodium, 77 mEq/L chloride) (*Rx*)	Various
0.9% (154 mEq/L sodium, 154 mEq/L chloride) (*Rx*)	Various
3% (513 mEq/L sodium, 513 mEq/L chloride) (*Rx*)	Various
5% (855 mEq/L sodium, 855 mEq/L chloride) (*Rx*)	Various
Solution: 0.9% sodium chloride (as Bacteriostatic Sodium Chloride Inj) (*Rx*)	Various
Concentrated Solution: 14.6% and 23.4% sodium chloride (*Rx*)	Various
Tablets: 650 mg, 1 and 2.25 g (*otc*)	Various
Tablets, slow release: 410 mg sodium chloride and 150 mg potassium chloride in wax matrix (*otc*)	*Slo-Salt-K*(Mission)

Indications

IV:

Hyponatremia – For parenteral restoration of sodium ion in patients with restricted oral intake. Sodium replacement is specifically indicated in patients with hyponatremia or low salt syndrome. Sodium Chloride may also be added to compatible carbohydrate solutions such as Dextrose in Water to provide electrolytes.

Diluents – Sodium Chloride Injections are also indicated as pharmaceutic aids and diluents for the infusion of compatible drug additives.

0.9% Sodium Chloride (Normal Saline) – 0.9% Sodium Chloride (Normal Saline), which is isotonic, restores both water and sodium chloride losses. Other indications for parenteral 0.9% saline include: Diluting or dissolving drugs for IV, IM, or SC injection; flushing of IV catheters; extracellular fluid replacement; treatment of metabolic alkalosis in the presence of fluid loss and mild sodium depletion; as a priming solution in hemodialysis procedures and to initiate and terminate blood transfusions without hemolyzing red blood cells.

0.45% Sodium Chloride (Hypotonic) – 0.45% Sodium Chloride (Hypotonic) is primarily a hydrating solution and may be used to assess the status of the kidneys, because more water is provided than is required for salt excretion. It also may be used in the treatment of hyperosmolar diabetes where the use of dextrose is inadvisable and there is a need for large amounts of fluid without an excess of sodium ions.

3% or 5% Sodium Chloride (Hypertonic) – 3% or 5% Sodium Chloride (Hypertonic) is used in hyponatremia and hypochloremia due to electrolyte and fluid loss replaced with sodium-free fluids; drastic dilution of body water following excessive water intake; emergency treatment of severe salt depletion.

Bacteriostatic Sodium Chloride – Only for diluting or dissolving drugs for IV, IM, or SC injection.

Concentrated Sodium Chloride – As an additive in parenteral fluid therapy for use in patients who have special problems of sodium electrolyte intake or excretion. It is intended to meet the specific requirements of the patient with unusual fluid and electrolyte needs. After available clinical and laboratory information is considered and correlated, determine the appropriate number of milliequivalents of Concentrated Sodium Chloride Injection, USP and dilute for use.

Oral: Prevention or treatment of extracellular volume depletion, dehydration, or sodium depletion; aid in the prevention of heat prostration.

Administration and Dosage

IV: In the average adult, daily requirements of sodium and chloride are met by the infusion of 1 L of 0.9% Sodium Chloride (154 mEq each of sodium and chloride). Base fluid administration on calculated maintenance or replacement fluid requirements.

IV catheters – Prior to and after administration of the medication, entirely flush the catheter with preservative free 0.9% Sodium Chloride for Injection.

Calculation of sodium deficit – To calculate the amount of sodium that must be administered to raise serum sodium to the desired level, use the following equation (TBW = total body water): Na deficit (mEq) = TBW (desired – observed plasma Na).

Base the repletion rate on the degree of urgency in the patient. Use of hypertonic saline (eg, 3% or 5%) will correct the deficit more rapidly.

Concentrated Sodium Chloride – Not for direct infusion. Must be diluted before use.

The dosage as an additive in parenteral fluid therapy is predicated on specific requirements of the patient. The appropriate volume is then withdrawn for proper dilution. Having determined the mEq of sodium chloride to be added, divide by 4 to calculate the number of mL to be used. Withdraw this volume and transfer into appropriate IV solutions, such as 5% Dextrose Injection. The properly diluted solution may be given IV.

Admixture incompatibilities – Some additives may be incompatible. Consult a pharmacist.

To minimize the risk of possible incompatibilities arising from mixing this solution with other additives that may be prescribed, inspect the final infusate for cloudiness or precipitation immediately after mixing, prior to administration and periodically during administration. Do not store.

Oral: Refer to specific product labeling for dosage guidelines.

Actions

Pharmacology: Normal osmolarity of the extracellular fluid ranges between 280 to 300 mOsm/L; it is primarily a function of sodium and its accompanying ions, chloride, and bicarbonate. Sodium chloride is the principal salt involved in maintenance of plasma tonicity. One gram of sodium chloride provides 17.1 mEq sodium and 17.1 mEq chloride.

Contraindications

Hypernatremia; fluid retention; when the administration of sodium or chloride could be clinically detrimental.

3% and 5% sodium chloride solutions: Elevated, normal, or only slightly decreased plasma sodium and chloride concentrations.

Bacteriostatic sodium chloride: Newborns; for fluid or sodium chloride replacement.

Warnings

Fluid/Solute overload: Excessive amounts of sodium chloride by any route may cause hypokalemia and acidosis. Administration of IV solutions can cause fluid or solute overload resulting in dilution of serum electrolyte concentrations, CHF, overhydration, congested states, or acute pulmonary edema, especially in patients with cardiovascular disease and in patients receiving corticosteroids or corticotropin or drugs that may give rise to sodium retention.

Infusion of > 1 L of isotonic (0.9%) sodium chloride may supply more sodium and chloride than normally found in serum, resulting in hypernatremia; this may cause a loss of bicarbonate ions, resulting in an acidifying effect.

Bacteriostatic Sodium Chloride: Do not use in newborns. Benzyl alcohol as a preservative in Bacteriostatic Sodium Chloride Injection has been associated with toxicity in newborns. These solutions have not been reported to cause problems in older infants, children, and adults.

Concentrated Sodium Chloride Injection: Inadvertent direct injection or absorption of concentrated Sodium Chloride Injection may give rise to sudden hypernatremia and such complications as cardiovascular shock, CNS disorders, extensive hemolysis, cortical necrosis of the kidneys, and severe local tissue necrosis (if administered extravascularly). Do not use unless solution is clear. When administered peripherally, slowly infuse through a small bore needle placed well within the lumen of a large vein to minimize venous irritation. Carefully avoid infiltration.

Surgical patients: Surgical patients should seldom receive salt-containing solutions immediately following surgery unless factors producing salt depletion are present. Because of renal retention of salt during surgery, additional electrolytes given IV may result in fluid retention, edema, and overloading of the circulation.

Renal function impairment: Infusions of sodium ions may result in excessive sodium retention; administer with care.

Pregnancy: Category C.

Children: Safety and efficacy have not been established.

Precautions

Monitoring: Monitor changes in fluid balance, electrolyte concentrations, and acid-base balance during prolonged parenteral therapy or whenever the condition of the patient warrants such evaluation. Significant deviations from normal concentrations may require tailoring of the electrolyte pattern.

Hypokalemia: Hypokalemia may result from excessive administration of potassium-free solutions.

Special risk patients: Administer cautiously to patients with decompensated cardiovascular, cirrhotic, and nephrotic disease; circulatory insufficiency; hypoproteinemia; hypervolemia; urinary tract obstruction; CHF; and to patients with concurrent edema and sodium retention; those receiving corticosteroids or corticotropin; and those retaining salt.

Elderly or postoperative patients: Exercise care in administering sodium-containing solutions in renal or cardiovascular insufficiency, with or without CHF.

3% and 5% sodium chloride solutions: Infuse very slowly and use with caution to avoid pulmonary edema; observe patients constantly.

SODIUM BICARBONATE

Injection: 4.2% (0.5 mEq/mL), 5% (0.6 mEq/mL), 7.5% (0.9 mEq/mL), 8.4% (1 mEq/mL) (*Rx*)	Various
Neutralizing Additive Solution: 4% (0.48 mEq/mL) (*Rx*)	*Neut* (Abbott)
4.2% (0.5 mEq/mL) (*Rx*)	Various

Indications

Metabolic acidosis: In severe renal disease; uncontrolled diabetes; circulatory insufficiency due to shock, anoxia, or severe dehydration; extracorporeal circulation of blood; cardiac arrest; and severe primary lactic acidosis where a rapid increase in plasma total CO_2 content is crucial. Treat metabolic acidosis in addition to measures designed to control the cause of the acidosis. Because an appreciable time interval may elapse before all ancillary effects occur, bicarbonate therapy is indicated to minimize risks inherent to acidosis itself.

At one time it was suggested to administer bicarbonate during cardiopulmonary resuscitation following cardiac arrest; however, recent evidence suggests that little benefit is provided and its use may be detrimental. For treatment of acidosis in this clinical situation, concentrate efforts on restoring ventilation and blood flow. According to the American Heart Association guidelines, use as a last resort after other standard measures have been utilized.

Urinary alkalinization: In the treatment of certain drug intoxications (eg, salicylates, lithium) and in hemolytic reactions requiring alkalinization of the urine to diminish nephrotoxicity of blood pigments.

Severe diarrhea: Severe diarrhea that is often accompanied by a significant loss of bicarbonate.

Neutralizing additive solution: To reduce the incidence of chemical phlebitis and patient discomfort due to vein irritation at or near the infusion site by raising the pH of IV acid solutions.

Administration and Dosage

One g sodium bicarbonate provides 11.9 mEq each of sodium and bicarbonate.

Cardiac arrest: Bicarbonate administration in this situation may be detrimental. Administer according to results of arterial blood pH and $PaCO_2$ and calculation of base deficit. Flush IV lines before and after use.

Adults – A rapid IV dose of 200 to 300 mEq of bicarbonate, given as a 7.5% or 8.4% solution.

Infants (≤ 2 years of age) – 4.2% solution for IV administration at a rate not to exceed 8 mEq/kg/day to guard against the possibility of producing hypernatremia, decreasing CSF pressure, and inducing intracranial hemorrhage.

Initial dose – 1 to 2 mEq/kg/min given over 1 to 2 minutes followed by 1 mEq/kg every 10 minutes of arrest. If base deficit is known, give calculated dose of 0.3 × kg × base deficit. If only 7.5% or 8.4% sodium bicarbonate is available, dilute 1:1 with 5% Dextrose in Water before administration.

Severe metabolic acidosis – Administer 90 to 180 mEq/L ($\approx$ 7.5 to 15 g) at a rate of 1 to 1.5 L during the first hour. Adjust to patient's needs for further management.

Less urgent forms of metabolic acidosis – Sodium Bicarbonate Injection may be added to other IV fluids. The amount of bicarbonate to be given to older children and adults over a 4- to 8-hour period is $\approx$ 2 to 5 mEq/kg, depending on the severity of the acidosis as judged by the lowering of total CO_2 content, blood pH, and clinical condition. Initially, an infusion of 2 to 5 mEq/kg over 4 to 8 hours will produce improvement in the acid-base status of the blood.

Alternatively, estimates of the initial dose of sodium bicarbonate may be based on the following equation:

$$0.5 \text{ (L/kg)} \times \text{body weight (kg)} \times \text{desired increase in serum } HCO_3- \text{ (mEq/L)} = \text{bicarbonate dose (mEq)}$$

or

$$0.5 \text{ (L/kg)} \times \text{body weight (kg)} \times \text{base deficit (mEq/L)} = \text{bicarbonate dose (mEq)}.$$

The next step of therapy is dependent on the clinical response of the patient. If severe symptoms have abated, reduce frequency of administration and dose.

If the CO_2 plasma content is unknown, a safe average dose of sodium bicarbonate is 5 mEq (420 mg)/kg.

It is unwise to attempt full correction of a low total CO_2 content during the first 24 hours, because this may accompany an unrecognized alkalosis due to delayed readjustment of ventilation to normal. Thus, achieving total CO_2 content of about 20 mEq/L at the end of the first day will usually be associated with a normal blood pH.

Neutralizing additive solution – One vial of neutralizing additive solution added to 1 L of any of the commonly used parenteral solutions including Dextrose, Sodium Chloride, Ringer's, etc, will increase the pH to a more physiologic range (specific pH may vary slightly).

Note – Some products such as amino acid solutions and multiple electrolyte solutions containing dextrose will not be brought to near physiologic pH by the addition of sodium bicarbonate neutralizing additive solution. This is due to the relatively high buffer capacity of these fluids.

Admixture incompatibilities – Avoid adding sodium bicarbonate to parenteral solutions containing **calcium**, except where compatibility is established; precipitation or haze may result. **Norepinephrine**, **dopamine**, and **dobutamine** are incompatible.

Actions

Pharmacology: Increases plasma bicarbonate; buffers excess hydrogen ion concentration; raises blood pH; reverses the clinical manifestations of acidosis.

Pharmacokinetics: Sodium bicarbonate in water dissociates to provide sodium and bicarbonate ions. Sodium is the principal cation of extracellular fluid. Bicarbonate is a normal constituent of body fluids and normal plasma level ranges from 24 to 31 mEq/L. Plasma concentration is regulated by the kidney. Bicarbonate anion is considered "labile" because, at a proper concentration of hydrogen ion, it may be converted to carbonic acid, then to its volatile form, carbon dioxide, excreted by lungs. Normally, a ratio of 1:20 (carbonic acid: bicarbonate) is present in extracellular fluid. In a healthy adult with normal kidney function, almost all the glomerular filtered bicarbonate ion is reabsorbed; < 1% is excreted in urine.

Contraindications

Losing chloride by vomiting or from continuous GI suction; receiving diuretics known to produce a hypochloremic alkalosis; metabolic and respiratory alkalosis; hypocalcemia in which alkalosis may produce tetany, hypertension, convulsions, or congestive heart failure (CHF); when sodium use could be clinically detrimental.

Neutralizing additive solution: Do not use as a systemic alkalinizer.

Warnings
Cardiac effects:

Cardiac arrest – The risk of rapid infusion must be weighed against the potential for fatality due to acidosis.

CHF – Because sodium accompanies bicarbonate, use cautiously in patients with CHF or other edematous or sodium-retaining states.

Fluid/Solute overload: IV administration can cause fluid or solute overloading resulting in dilution of serum electrolyte concentrations, overhydration, congested states, or pulmonary edema.

Extravasation: Extravasation of IV hypertonic solutions of sodium bicarbonate may cause chemical cellulitis (because of their alkalinity), with tissue necrosis, ulceration, or sloughing at the site of infiltration. Prompt elevation of the part, warmth, and local injection of lidocaine or hyaluronidase are recommended to prevent sloughing.

Too rapid infusion: Too rapid infusion of hypertonic solutions may cause local pain and venous irritation. Adjust the rate of administration according to tolerance. Use of the largest peripheral vein and a well placed small bore needle is recommended.

Too rapid or excessive administration may result in hypernatremia and alkalosis accompanied by hyperirritability or tetany. Hypernatremia may be associated with edema and exacerbation of CHF due to the retention of water, resulting in an expanded extracellular fluid volume.

Renal function impairment: Administration of solutions containing sodium ions may result in sodium retention. Use with caution. Also use cautiously in oliguria or anuria.

Elderly: Exercise particular care when administering sodium-containing solutions to elderly or postoperative patients with renal or cardiovascular insufficiency, with or without CHF.

Pregnancy: Category C.

Children:

Neonates and children (< 2 years of age) – Rapid injection (10 mL/min) of hypertonic sodium bicarbonate solutions may produce hypernatremia, a decrease in cerebrospinal fluid pressure and possible intracranial hemorrhage. Do not administer > 8 mEq/kg/day. A 4.2% solution is preferred for such slow administration.

Precautions
Monitoring: Adverse reactions may result from an excess or deficit of one or more of the ions in the solution; frequent monitoring of electrolyte levels is essential.

Avoid overdosage and alkalosis: Avoid overdosage and alkalosis by giving repeated small doses and periodic monitoring by appropriate laboratory tests.

Potassium depletion: Potassium depletion may predispose to metabolic alkalosis, and coexistent hypocalcemia may be associated with carpopedal spasm as the plasma pH rises. Minimize by treating electrolyte imbalances prior to or concomitantly with bicarbonate.

Chloride loss: Patients losing chloride by vomiting or GI intubation are more susceptible to developing severe alkalosis if given alkalinizing agents.

Neutralizing additive solution: Administer this solution promptly. When introducing additives, mix thoroughly, and do not store. Raising pH of IV fluids with neutralizing additive solution will reduce incidence of chemical irritation caused by infusate.

Drug Interactions
Drugs that may interact include chlorpropamide, lithium, methotrexate, salicylates, tetracyclines, anorexiants, flecainide, mecamylamide, quinidine, and sympathomimetics.

Adverse Reactions
Adverse reactions may include extravasation; local pain; venous irritation; hypernatremia; alkalosis.

Chapter 2
HEMATOLOGICAL AGENTS

Iron-Containing Products, 27
  Oral, 27
  Parenteral, 30
Folic Acid Derivatives, 35
  Leucovorin Calcium, 36
Vitamin B_{12}, 39
Vitamin K (Phytonadione), 42
Recombinant Human Erythropoietin, 45
  Epoetin Alfa, 45
  Darbepoetin Alfa, 49
Antiplatelet Agents, 53
  Dipyridamole, 53
  Dipyridamole and Aspirin, 54
  Ticlopidine, 56
  Clopidogrel, 59
Anticoagulants, 61
  Low Molecular Weight Heparins, 63
  Heparin, 69
  Coumarin and Indandione Derivatives, 73
  Lepirudin, 78
  Argatroban, 82
  Bivalirudin, 84

IRON-CONTAINING PRODUCTS, ORAL

FERROUS SULFATE

Tablets: 324 and 325 mg (otc)	Various
Syrup: 90 mg/5 mL (otc)	Fer-In-Sol (Mead Johnson)
Elixir: 220 mg/5 mL (otc)	Various, Feosol (SmithKline Beecham)
Drops: 75 mg/0.6 mL (otc)	Various, Fer-In-Sol (Mead Johnson), Fer-gen-sol (Zenith Goldline), Fer-Iron (Rugby)

FERROUS SULFATE EXSICCATED

Tablets: 187 and 200 mg (otc)	Feosol (SmithKline Beecham), Feratab (Upsher-Smith)
Tablets, slow release: 160 mg (otc)	Slow FE (Novartis)
Capsules, extended release: 160 mg (otc)	Fe⁵⁰ (UCB Pharma)

FERROUS GLUCONATE

Tablets: 240 and 325 mg (otc)	Various, Fergon (Bayer)

FERROUS FUMARATE

Tablets: 63, 200, 324, 325, and 350 mg (otc)	Various, Femiron (Menley & James), Hemocyte (U.S. Pharm.), Ircon (Kenwood), Nephro-Fer (R & D Labs)
Tablets, chewable: 100 mg (otc)	Feostat (Forest)
Suspension: 100 mg/5 mL (otc)	Feostat (Forest)
Drops: 45 mg/0.6 mL (otc)	Feostat (Forest)

CARBONYL IRON

Caplets: 50 mg (otc)	Feosol (SmithKline Beecham)
Suspension: 15 mg carbonyl iron/1.25 mL (otc)	Icar (Hawthorn)

POLYSACCHARIDE-IRON COMPLEX

Tablets: 50 mg (otc)	Niferex (Schwarz Pharma)
Capsules: 150 mg (otc)	Hytinic (Hyrex), Ferrex 150 (Breckenridge), Niferex-150 (Schwarz Pharma), Nu-Iron 150 (Merz)
Elixir: 100 mg iron/5 mL (otc)	Niferex (Schwarz Pharma), Nu-Iron (Merz), Hytinic (Hyrex)

MODIFIED IRON PRODUCTS

Tablets, timed release: Ferrous fumarate equivalent to 50 mg iron (otc)	Ferro-Sequels (Self-Care)

IRON WITH VITAMIN C

Tablets, timed-release: 65 mg Fe, 150 mg ascorbic acid (otc)	Irospan (Fielding)
105 mg Fe, 500 mg sodium ascorbate (otc)	Fero-Grad-500 (Abbott)
110 mg Fe, 200 mg ascorbic acid (otc)	Hemaspan (Bock)
Capsules, timed-release: 20 mg Fe, 300 mg ascorbic acid (Rx)	Cevi-Fer (Roberts)
65 mg Fe, 150 mg ascorbic acid (otc)	Irospan (Fielding)

Indications

Iron deficiency: For the prevention and treatment of iron deficiency anemias.

Iron supplement: As a dietary supplement for iron.

Unlabeled uses: Iron supplementation may be required by most patients receiving epoetin therapy. Failure to administer iron supplements (oral or IV) during epoetin therapy can impair the hematologic response to epoetin.

Administration and Dosage

Iron replacement therapy in deficiency states:

Adults – 100 to 200 mg (2 to 3 mg/kg) elemental iron daily in 3 divided doses is the usual therapeutic dose.

Children 2 to 12 years of age (15 to 30 kg) – 50 to 100 mg (1 to 1.5 mg/kg) in 3 to 4 divided doses.

Children 6 months to 2 years of age – Up to 6 mg/kg/day in 3 to 4 divided doses.

Infants – 10 to 25 mg/day in 3 to 4 divided doses.

The length of iron therapy depends upon the cause and severity of the iron deficiency. In general, ≈ 4 to 6 months of oral iron therapy is required to reverse uncomplicated iron deficiency anemias.

Iron supplementation: Consider only in individuals with documented risk factors for iron deficiency.

Recommended Dietary Allowances (RDAs) – Adult males (≥ 19 years of age) – 10 mg; adult females (11 to 50 years of age) – 15 mg, (≥ 51 years of age) – 10 mg; pregnancy – 30 mg; lactation – 15 mg.

For a complete listing of RDAs by age and sex, refer to the RDA table in the Nutritionals chapter.

Pregnancy – 15 to 30 mg elemental iron daily (not taken with meals) should be adequate to meet the daily requirement of the last 2 trimesters.

Actions

Pharmacology: Iron, an essential mineral, is a component of hemoglobin, myoglobin, and a number of enzymes. Approximately two-thirds of total body iron is in the circulating red blood cell mass in hemoglobin, the major factor in oxygen transport.

Pharmacokinetics:

Absorption/Distribution – The average dietary intake of iron is 12 to 20 mg/day for males and 8 to 15 mg/day for females; however, only ≈ 10% of this iron is absorbed (1 to 2 mg/day) in individuals with adequate iron stores. Absorption is enhanced (20% to 30%) when storage iron is depleted or when erythropoiesis occurs at an increased rate. Sustained-release or enteric-coated preparations reduce the amount of available iron; absorption from these doseforms is reduced because iron is transported beyond the duodenum. Dose also influences the amount of iron absorbed. The amount of iron absorbed increases progressively with larger doses; however, the percentage decreases. Food can decrease the absorption of iron by 40% to 66%; however, gastric intolerance may often necessitate administering the drug with food.

Excretion: The daily loss of iron from urine, sweat, and sloughing of intestinal mucosal cells amounts to ≈ 0.5 to 1 mg in healthy men. In menstruating women, ≈ 1 to 2 mg is the normal daily loss.

Elemental Iron Content of Iron Salts	
Iron salt	% Iron
Ferrous sulfate	≈ 20
Ferrous sulfate, exsiccated	≈ 30
Ferrous gluconate	≈ 12
Ferrous fumarate	≈ 33

Contraindications

Hemochromatosis; hemosiderosis; hemolytic anemias; known hypersensitivity to any ingredients.

Warnings

Chronic iron intake: Individuals with normal iron balance should not take iron chronically.

Accidental overdose: Accidental overdose of iron-containing products is a leading cause of fatal poisonong in children < 6 years of age. Keep this product out of reach of children.

Precautions

Intolerance: Discontinue use if symptoms of intolerance appear.

GI effects: Occasional GI discomfort, such as nausea, may be minimized by taking with meals and by slowly increasing to the recommended dosage.

Drug Interactions

Iron salts may be affected by the following agents: Antacids, ascorbic acid, chloramphenicol, cimetidine, and tetracyclines.

Agents that may be affected by iron salts include: Levodopa, levothyroxine, methyldopa, penicillamine, quinolones, and tetracyclines.

Drug/Food interactions: Eggs and milk inhibit iron absorption. Coffee and tea consumed with a meal or 1 hour after a meal may significantly inhibit the absorption of dietary iron; clinical significance has not been determined. Administration of calcium and iron supplements with food can reduce ferrous sulfate absorption by 33%. If combined iron and calcium supplementation is required, iron absorption is not decreased if calcium carbonate is used and the supplements are taken between meals.

Adverse Reactions

GI irritation; anorexia; nausea; vomiting; constipation; diarrhea. Stools may appear darker in color. Iron-containing liquids may cause temporary staining of the teeth.

IRON DEXTRAN

Injection: 50 mg iron/mL (as dextran) (*Rx*)   *InFeD* (Schein), *DexFerrum* (American Regent)

> **Warning:**
> The parenteral use of complexes of iron and carbohydrates has resulted in fatal ana-
> phylactic-type reactions. Deaths associated with such administration have been
> reported; therefore, use iron dextran injection only in those patients in whom
> the indications have been clearly established and laboratory investigations con-
> firm an iron deficient state not amenable to oral iron therapy.

Indications

For treatment of patients with documented iron deficiency in whom oral administration is unsatisfactory or impossible.

Unlabeled uses: Iron supplementation may be required by most patients receiving epoetin therapy. Failure to administer iron supplements (oral or IV) during epoetin
therapy can impair the hematologic response to epoetin.

Administration and Dosage

Maximum dose: 2 mL of undiluted iron dextran daily.

Iron deficiency anemia: The accompanying formula and table are applicable for dosage
determinations only in patients with iron deficiency anemia; they are not to be
used for dosage determinations in patients requiring iron replacement for blood loss.

The total amount of iron (in mL) required to restore hemoglobin to normal levels and to replenish iron stores may be approximated from the following formula:

Dose (mL) = 0.0442 (desired Hb − observed Hb) × Weight* + (0.26 × Weight*)

*For adults and children > 15 kg (33 lbs), use the lesser of lean body weight or
actual body weight in kilograms. Lean body weight is 50 kg (for males) or 45.5 kg
(for females) plus 2.3 kg for each inch over 5 feet. For children 5 to 15 kg (11 to
33 lbs), use actual weight in kilograms.

Total Amount of Iron Dextran Required (to the nearest mL) for Hemoglobin and Iron Stores Replacement[1]								
Lean body weight[2]		Amount required (mL) based on observed hemoglobin						
kg	lb	3 g/dL	4 g/dL	5 g/dL	6 g/dL	7 g/dL	8 g/dL	9 g/dL	10 g/dL
5	11	3	3	3	3	2	2	2	2
10	22	7	6	6	5	5	4	4	3
15	33	10	9	9	8	7	7	6	5
20	44	16	15	14	13	12	11	10	9
25	55	20	18	17	16	15	14	13	12
30	66	23	22	21	19	18	17	15	14
35	77	27	26	24	23	21	20	18	17
40	88	31	29	28	26	24	22	21	19
45	99	35	33	31	29	27	25	23	21
50	110	39	37	35	32	30	28	26	24
55	121	43	41	38	36	33	31	28	26
60	132	47	44	42	39	36	34	31	28
65	143	51	48	45	42	39	36	34	31
70	154	55	52	49	45	42	39	36	33
75	165	59	55	52	49	45	42	39	35
80	176	63	59	55	52	48	45	41	38
85	187	66	63	59	55	51	48	44	40
90	198	70	66	62	58	54	50	46	42
95	209	74	70	66	62	57	53	49	45
100	220	78	74	69	65	60	56	52	47
105	231	82	77	73	68	63	59	54	50
110	242	86	81	76	71	67	62	57	52

Total Amount of Iron Dextran Required (to the nearest mL) for Hemoglobin and Iron Stores Replacement[1]									
Lean body weight[2]		Amount required (mL) based on observed hemoglobin							
kg	lb	3 g/dL	4 g/dL	5 g/dL	6 g/dL	7 g/dL	8 g/dL	9 g/dL	10 g/dL
115	253	90	85	80	75	70	65	59	54
120	264	94	88	83	78	73	67	62	57

[1] Table values were calculated based on a normal adult hemoglobin of 14.8 g/dL for weights > 15 kg (33 lbs) and a hemoglobin of 12 g/dL for weights ≤ 15 kg (33 lbs).
[2] For adults and children > 15 kg (33 lbs), use the lesser of lean body weight or actual body weight in kilograms. See above equation.

Test dose – Prior to administering the first therapeutic dose, give all patients an IV test dose of 0.5 mL. Administer the test dose at a gradual rate over ≥ 30 seconds (*InFeD*) or ≥ 5 minutes (*DexFerrum*). Although anaphylactic reactions known to occur following administration are usually evident within a few minutes or sooner, it is recommended that a period of ≥ 1 hour elapse before the remainder of the initial therapeutic dose is given.

Individual doses of ≤ 2 mL may be given on a daily basis until the calculated total amount required has been reached.

Give undiluted and slowly, ≤ 50 mg/min (≤ 1 mL/min).

IV injection – Individual doses of ≤ 2 mL may be given on a daily basis until the calculated total amount required has been reached.

Give undiluted and slowly (≤ 1 mL/min).

IM injection – If no adverse reactions are observed, the injection can be given according to the following schedule until the calculated total amount required has been reached. Each day's dose should ordinarily not exceed 0.5 mL (25 mg iron) for infants < 11 lb, 1 mL (50 mg iron) for children < 22 lb and 2 mL (100 mg iron) for other patients.

Inject only into the muscle mass of the upper outer quadrant of the buttock (never into the arm or other exposed areas) and inject deeply with a 2- or 3-inch 19- or 20-gauge needle. If the patient is standing, have them bear their weight on the leg opposite the injection site, or if in bed, have them in a lateral position with injection site uppermost. To avoid injection or leakage into the subcutaneous tissue, a Z-track technique (displacement of the skin laterally prior to injection) is recommended.

Iron replacement for blood loss – Direct iron therapy in these patients toward replacement of the equivalent amount of iron represented in the blood loss. The table and formula described under *Iron deficiency anemia* are not applicable for simple iron replacement values.

The following formula is based on the approximation that 1 mL of normocytic, normochromic red cells contains 1 mg elemental iron:

Replacement iron (in mg) = Blood loss (in mL) x hematocrit

Actions

Pharmacology: Iron dextran, a hematinic agent, is a complex of ferric hydroxide and dextran for IM or IV use. The iron dextran complex is dissociated by the reticuloendothelial system, and the ferric iron is transported by transferrin and incorporated into hemoglobin and storage sites.

Pharmacokinetics: The major portion of IM injections of iron dextran is absorbed within 72 hours; most of the remaining iron is absorbed over the ensuing 3 to 4 weeks. Various studies have yielded half-life values ranging from 5 hours (circulating iron dextran) to > 20 hours (total iron, both circulating and bound).

Contraindications

Hypersensitivity to the product; all anemias not associated with iron deficiency; acute phase of infectious kidney disease.

Warnings

Maximum dose: 2 mL of undiluted iron dextran is the maximum recommended daily dose.

Accidental overdose: Accidental overdose of iron-containing products is a leading cause of fatal poisoning in children < 6 years of age. Keep this product out of reach of children.

Hepatic function impairment: Use this preparation with extreme caution in the presence of serious impairment of liver function.

Pregnancy: Category C.

Lactation: Traces of unmetabolized iron dextran are excreted in breast milk. Exercise caution when administering to a nursing woman.

Children: Not recommended for use in infants < 4 months of age.

Precautions

Monitoring: Serum iron determinations (especially by colorimetric assays) may not be meaningful for 3 weeks; serum ferritin peaks after ≈ 7 to 9 days and slowly returns to baseline after ≈ 3 weeks.

Iron overload: Unwarranted therapy with parenteral iron will cause excess storage of iron with the consequent possibility of exogenous hemosiderosis.

Cardiovascular disease: Adverse reactions of iron dextran may exacerbate cardiovascular complications in patients with preexisting cardiovascular disease.

Allergies/Asthma: Use with caution in patients with history of significant allergies/asthma.

Arthritis: Patients with rheumatoid arthritis may have an acute exacerbation of joint pain and swelling following administration of iron dextran.

Drug Interactions

Chloramphenicol: Serum iron levels may be increased because of decreased iron clearance and erythropoiesis due to direct bone marrow toxicity from chloramphenicol.

Drug/Lab test interactions: Large doses of iron dextran (≥ 5 mL) give a brown color to serum from a blood sample drawn 4 hours after administration; they may cause falsely elevated values of serum bilirubin and falsely decreased values of serum calcium.

Adverse Reactions

Anaphylactic reactions including fatal anaphylaxis; other hypersensitivity reactions including dyspnea, urticaria, other rashes, and febrile episodes; inflammation at or near injection site, including sterile abscesses (IM); brown skin discoloration at injection site (IM); flushing and hypotension with overly rapid IV administration; hypotensive reaction; arthralgia.

The following pattern of signs/symptoms has been reported as a delayed (1 to 2 days) reaction at recommended doses: Fever; chills; backache; headache; myalgia; malaise; nausea; vomiting; dizziness.

IRON SUCROSE

Injection: 20 mg elemental iron/mL (*Rx*)   Venofer[1] (American Regent Labs)

[1] Preservative free.

Indications
Iron deficiency anemia: For the treatment of iron deficiency anemia in patients undergoing chronic hemodialysis who are receiving supplemental erythropoietin therapy.

Unlabeled uses: Anemia in peritoneal dialysis patients; anemia in predialysis patients; bloodless surgery; autologous blood donation.

Administration and Dosage
The dosage of iron sucrose is expressed in terms of milligrams of elemental iron. Each 5 mL vial contains 100 mg of elemental iron (20 mg/mL).

Iron deficiency anemia: The recommended dosage of iron sucrose for the repletion treatment of iron deficiency in hemodialysis patients is 5 mL of iron sucrose (100 mg of elemental iron) delivered IV during the dialysis session. Most patients will require a minimum cumulative dose of 1000 mg of elemental iron, administered over 10 sequential dialysis sessions, to achieve a favorable hemoglobin or hematocrit response. Patients may continue to require therapy with iron sucrose or other IV iron preparations at the lowest dose necessary to maintain target levels of hemoglobin, hematocrit, and laboratory parameters of iron storage within acceptable limits.

Iron sucrose must be only administered IV (directly into the dialysis line) either by slow injection or by infusion.

Slow IV injection: In chronic renal failure patients, iron sucrose may be administered by slow IV injection into the dialysis line at a rate of 1 mL (20 mg iron) undiluted solution per minute (ie, 5 min/vial) not exceeding 1 vial of iron sucrose (100 mg elemental iron) per injection. Discard any unused portion.

Infusion: Iron sucrose may be also administered by infusion (into the dialysis line for hemodialysis patients). This may reduce the risk of hypotensive episodes. The content of each vial must be diluted exclusively in a maximum of 100 mL of 0.9% NaCl, immediately prior to infusion. Infuse the solution at a rate of 100 mg of iron over a period of ≥ 15 minutes. Discard unused diluted solution.

IV incompatibility: Do not mix iron sucrose with other medications or add to parenteral nutrition solutions for IV infusion.

Adults: 100 mg iron administered 1 to 3 times/week to a total dose of 1000 mg in 10 doses, repeat if needed. Frequency of dosing should be ≤ 3 times/week.

Actions
Pharmacology: Iron is essential to the synthesis of hemoglobin to maintain oxygen transport and to the function and formation of other physiologically important heme and nonheme compounds.

Pharmacokinetics: In healthy adults treated with IV doses of iron sucrose, its iron component exhibits first order kinetics with an elimination half-life of 6 hours, total clearance of 1.2 L/hr, non-steady state apparent volume of distribution of 10 L, and steady-state apparent volume of distribution of 7.9 L.

Following IV administration of iron sucrose, it is dissociated into iron and sucrose by the reticuloendothelial system. The sucrose component is eliminated mainly by urinary excretion. Some iron also is eliminated in the urine.

Contraindications
Evidence of iron overload; known hypersensitivity to iron sucrose or any of its inactive components; anemia not caused by iron deficiency.

Warnings
Hypotension: Hypotension has been reported frequently in patients receiving IV iron. Hypotension following administration of iron sucrose may be related to rate of administration and total dose administered. Take caution to administer iron sucrose according to recommended guidelines.

Hypersensitivity reactions: Potentially fatal hypersensitivity reactions characterized by ana-phylactic shock, loss of consciousness, collapse, hypotension, dyspnea, or convul-sion have been reported rarely in patients receiving iron sucrose.

Elderly: In general, dose selection for an elderly patient should be cautious, usually start-ing at the low end of the dosing range, reflecting the greater frequency of decreased hepatic, renal, or cardiac function, and of concomitant disease or other drug therapy.

Pregnancy: Category B.

Lactation: It is not known whether this drug is excreted in human breast milk.

Children: Safety and efficacy of iron sucrose in pediatric patients have not been estab-lished.

Precautions

Monitoring: Exercise caution to withhold iron administration in the presence of evi-dence of tissue iron overload. Periodically monitor hematologic and hematinic parameters (hemoglobin, hematocrit, serum ferritin, and transferrin saturation). Withhold iron therapy in patients with evidence of iron overload. Transferrin satu-ration values increase rapidly after IV administration of iron sucrose; thus, serum iron values may be reliably obtained 48 hours after IV dosing.

Drug Interactions

Drug interactions involving iron sucrose have not been studied. However, like other parenteral iron preparations, iron sucrose may be expected to reduce the absorp-tion of concomitantly administered oral iron preparations. Do not administer con-comitantly with oral iron preparations.

Adverse Reactions Adverse events whether or not related to iron sucrose administration reported by > 5% of treated patients are as follows: Hypotension (36%); cramps/leg cramps (23%); nausea, headache, vomiting, and diarrhea.

Hypersensitivity: In clinical trials, several patients experienced pruritus and 1 patient experienced a facial rash. From the spontaneous reporting system, 27 patients reported anaphylactoid reactions including 8 patients who experienced serious or life-threatening reactions (anaphylactic shock, loss of consciousness, collapse, hypo-tension, dyspnea, or convulsion) associated with iron sucrose administration in the estimated > 450,000 patients exposed to iron sucrose between 1992 and 1999.

FOLIC ACID (Folacin; Pteroylglutamic Acid; Folate)

Tablets: 0.4 mg, 0.8 mg, 1 mg (*Rx*[1]) Various
Injection: 5 mg/mL (*Rx*) Various, *Folvite* (Lederle)

[1] Although most folic acid products carry the *Rx* legend, products that provide ≤ 0.4 mg (or 0.8 mg for pregnant or lactating women) may be *otc* items.

Indications
Megaloblastic anemia: Treatment of megaloblastic anemias due to a deficiency of folic acid as seen in tropical or nontropical sprue, anemias of nutritional origin, pregnancy, infancy, or childhood.

Administration and Dosage
Give orally, except in severe intestinal malabsorption. Although most patients with malabsorption cannot absorb food folates, they are able to absorb folic acid given orally.

Parenteral administration is not advocated but may be necessary in some individuals (eg, patients receiving parenteral or enteral alimentation). Give IM, IV, or SC if disease is very severe or GI absorption is very severely impaired. Doses > 0.1 mg should not be used unless anemia due to vitamin B_{12} deficiency has been ruled out or is being adequately treated with cobalamin.

Usual therapeutic dosage: Up to 1 mg daily. Resistant cases may require larger doses.

Maintenance: When clinical symptoms have subsided and the blood picture has normalized, use the dosage below. Never give < 0.1 mg/day. Keep patients under close supervision and adjust maintenance dose if relapse appears imminent. In the presence of alcoholism, hemolytic anemia, anticonvulsant therapy, or chronic infection, the maintenance level may need to be increased.

   Infants – 0.1 mg/day.
   Children (< 4 years of age) – Up to 0.3 mg/day.
   Adults and children (> 4 years of age) – 0.4 mg/day.
   Pregnant and lactating women – 0.8 mg/day.

Recommended Dietary Allowances (RDAs): Adult males, 0.15 to 0.2 mg/day; females, 0.15 to 0.18 mg/day.

For a complete listing of RDAs by age and sex, refer to the RDA table in the Nutritionals chapter.

Actions
Pharmacology: Exogenous folate is required for nucleoprotein synthesis and maintenance of normal erythropoiesis. Folic acid stimulates production of red and white blood cells and platelets in certain megaloblastic anemias.

Pharmacokinetics: Oral synthetic folic acid is a monoglutamate and is completely absorbed following administration, even in the presence of malabsorption syndromes.

Folic acid appears in the plasma ≈ 15 to 30 minutes after an oral dose; peak levels are generally reached within 1 hour. After IV administration, the drug is rapidly cleared from the plasma. Folic acid is metabolized in the liver. Normal serum levels of total folate have been reported to be 5 to 15 ng/mL; normal CSF levels are ≈ 16 to 21 ng/mL. In general, folate serum levels < 5 ng/mL indicate folate deficiency, and levels < 2 ng/mL usually result in megaloblastic anemia. A majority of the metabolic products appeared in the urine after 6 hours; excretion was generally complete within 24 hours.

Contraindications
Treatment of pernicious anemia and other megaloblastic anemias where vitamin B_{12} is deficient (not effective).

Warnings
Pernicious anemia: Folic acid in doses > 0.1 mg/day may obscure pernicious anemia in that hematologic remission can occur while neurologic manifestations remain progressive.

Except during pregnancy and lactation, do not give folic acid in therapeutic doses > 0.4 mg/day until pernicious anemia has been ruled out. Do not include daily doses exceeding the Recommended Dietary Allowance in multivitamin preparations; if therapeutic amounts are necessary, give folic acid separately.

Elderly: It may be prudent to consider the status of folate in people > 65 years of age.

Pregnancy: Category A.

Lactation: Folic acid is excreted in breast milk.

Drug Interactions

Drugs that may interact with folic acid include aminosalicylic acid, oral contraceptives, dihydrofolate reductase inhibitors (eg, methotrexate, trimethoprim), sulfasalazine, hydantoins.

Adverse Reactions

Adverse reactions may include erythema, skin rash, nausea, abdominal distention, altered sleep patterns, irritability, mental depression, confusion, and impaired judgement.

LEUCOVORIN CALCIUM (Folinic Acid; Citrovorum Factor)

Tablets: 5, 15, and 25 mg (*Rx*)	Various
Injection: 3 mg/mL (*Rx*)	Various
Powder for Injection: 50, 100, and 350 mg/vial (*Rx*)	Various

Indications

Oral and parenteral: Leucovorin "rescue" after high-dose methotrexate therapy in osteosarcoma.

Parenteral: Treatment of megaloblastic anemias due to folic acid deficiency when oral therapy is not feasible.

In combination with 5-fluorouracil (5-FU) to prolong survival in the palliative treatment of patients with advanced colorectal cancer.

Administration and Dosage

Oral administration of doses > 25 mg is not recommended.

Advanced colorectal cancer: Either of the following 2 regimens is recommended:

1.) Leucovorin 200 mg/m^2 by slow IV injection over a minimum of 3 minutes, followed by 5-FU 370 mg/m^2 by IV injection.

2.) Leucovorin 20 mg/m^2 by IV injection followed by 5-FU 425 mg/m^2 by IV injection.

Treatment is repeated daily for 5 days. This 5-day treatment course may be repeated at 4-week (28-day) intervals for 2 courses and then repeated at 4- to 5-week (28- to 35-day) intervals provided that the patient has completely recovered from the toxic effects of the prior treatment course.

Institute dosage modifications of 5-FU as follows, based on the most severe toxicities: If diarrhea or stomatitis are moderate, WBC/mm^3 nadir is 1000 to 1900 or platelets/mm^3 are 25,000 to 75,000, reduce the 5-FU dose by 20%; if diarrhea or stomatitis are severe, WBC/mm^3 nadir is < 1000, or platelets/mm^3 are < 25,000, reduce the 5-FU dose by 30%.

If no toxicity occurs, the 5-FU dose may increase 10%.

Defer treatment until WBCs are 4000/mm^3 and platelets are 130,000/mm^3. If blood counts do not reach these levels within 2 weeks, discontinue treatment.

Leucovorin rescue after high-dose MTX therapy: The recommendations for leucovorin rescue are based on an MTX dose of 12 to 15 g/m^2 administered by IV infusion over 4 hours. Leucovorin rescue at a dose of 15 mg ($\approx$ 10 mg/m^2) every 6 hours for 10 doses starts 24 hours after the beginning of the MTX infusion. In the presence of GI toxicity, nausea, or vomiting, administer leucovorin parenterally.

Determine serum creatinine and MTX levels at least once daily. Continue leucovorin administration, hydration, and urinary alkalinization (pH of ≥ 7) until the MTX level is $< 5 \times 10^{-8}$M (0.05 mcM).

If significant clinical toxicity is observed, extend leucovorin rescue for an additional 24 hours (total of 14 doses over 84 hours) in subsequent courses of therapy.

Impaired MTX elimination or inadvertent overdosage: Begin leucovorin rescue as soon as possible after an inadvertent overdosage and within 24 hours of MTX administration when there is delayed excretion (see Warnings). Administer leucovorin 10 mg/m^2 IV, IM, or orally every 6 hours until the serum MTX level is $< 10^{-8}$M. In the presence of GI toxicity, nausea, or vomiting, administer leucovorin parenterally.

Determine serum creatinine and MTX levels at 24-hour intervals. If the 24-hour serum creatinine has increased 50% over baseline or if the 24 or 48 hour MTX level is $> 5 \times 10^{-6}$M or $> 9 \times 10^{-7}$M, respectively, increase the dose of leucovorin to 100 mg/m^2 IV every 3 hours until the MTX level is $< 10^{-8}$M.

Megaloblastic anemia due to folic acid deficiency: ≤ 1 mg leucovorin/day. There is no evidence that doses > 1 mg/day have greater efficacy than 1 mg doses.

Actions

Pharmacology: Leucovorin is one of several active, chemically reduced derivatives of folic acid. It is useful as an antidote to drugs that act as folic acid antagonists. Administration of leucovorin can counteract the therapeutic and toxic effects of folic acid antagonists such as methotrexate (MTX), which act by inhibiting dihydrofolate reductase.

Pharmacokinetics:

Leucovorin Pharmacokinetics[1]			
Parameter	IV	IM	Oral
Total reduced folates:			
Mean peak conc. (ng/mL)	1259 (range, 897-1625)	436 (range, 240 to 725)	393 (range, 160 to 550)
Mean time to peak	10 min	52 min	2.3 hrs
Terminal half-life	6.2 hrs	6.2 hrs	5.7 hrs
5-Methyl-THF[2]			
Mean peak conc. (ng/mL)	258	226	367
Mean time to peak	1.3 hrs	2.8 hrs	2.4 hrs
5-Formyl-THF[3]			
Mean peak conc. (ng/mL)	1206	360	51
Mean time to peak	10 min	28 min	1.2 hrs

[1] Following administration of a 25 mg dose.
[2] The major metabolite to which leucovorin is primarily converted in the intestinal mucosa and which becomes the predominant circulating form of the drug.
[3] The parent compound.

Following oral administration leucovorin is rapidly absorbed and expands the serum pool of reduced folates. Oral absorption of leucovorin is saturable at doses > 25 mg. The apparent bioavailability of leucovorin was 97% for 25 mg, 75% for 50 mg, and 37% for 100 mg.

Contraindications

Pernicious anemia and other megaloblastic anemias secondary to the lack of vitamin B_{12}.

Warnings

Anemias: Leucovorin is improper therapy for pernicious anemia and other megaloblastic anemias secondary to the lack of vitamin B_{12}.

5-Fluorouracil dosage/toxicity: Leucovorin enhances the toxicity of 5-FU.

Therapy with leucovorin/5-FU must not be initiated or continued in patients who have symptoms of GI toxicity of any severity, until those symptoms have completely resolved. Patients with diarrhea must be monitored with particular care until the diarrhea has resolved, as rapid clinical deterioration leading to death can occur.

Methotrexate concentrations: Monitoring of the serum MTX concentration is essential in determining the optimal dose and duration of treatment with leucovorin. Delayed MTX excretion may be caused by a third space fluid accumulation, renal insufficiency, or inadequate hydration. Under such circumstances, higher doses of leucovorin or prolonged administration may be indicated. Doses higher than those recommended for oral use must be given IV.

Calcium content: Because of the calcium content of the leucovorin solution, inject no more than 160 mg/min IV.

Folic acid antagonist overdosage: In the treatment of accidental overdosages of folic acid antagonists, administer leucovorin as promptly as possible. As the time interval between antifolate administration (eg, MTX) and leucovorin rescue increases, leucovorin's effectiveness in counteracting toxicity decreases.

Elderly: Take particular care in the treatment of elderly or debilitated colorectal cancer patients, as these patients may be at increased risk of severe toxicity.

Pregnancy: Category C.

Lactation: It is not known whether this drug is excreted in breast milk.

Drug Interactions
Drugs that may be affected by leucovorin include anticonvulsants.

Adverse Reactions
Allergic sensitization, including anaphylactoid reactions and urticaria, following administration of both oral and parenteral leucovorin.

The following adverse events occurred when leucovorin was administered at both high (200 mg/m^2) and low (20 mg/m^2) doses in combination with 5-FU: Leukopenia, thrombocytopenia, infection, nausea, vomiting, diarrhea, stomatitis, constipation, lethargy/malaise/fatigue, alopecia, dermatitis, anorexia.

VITAMIN B$_{12}$

CYANOCOBALAMIN	
Tablets: 500 and 1000 mcg (otc)	Various
Injection: 100 and 1000 mcg/mL (Rx)	Various, Crysti 1000 (Roberts Hauck), Cyanoject (Mayrand)
HYDROXOCOBALAMIN	
Injection: 1000 mcg/mL (Rx)	Various, LA-12 (Hyrex), Hydro-Crysti-12 (Roberts Hauck)

Indications
Vitamin B$_{12}$ deficiency: Vitamin B$_{12}$ deficiency due to malabsorption syndrome as seen in pernicious anemia; GI pathology, dysfunction or surgery; fish tapeworm infestation; malignancy of pancreas or bowel; gluten enteropathy; sprue; small bowel bacterial overgrowth; total or partial gastrectomy; accompanying folic acid deficiency.

Increased vitamin B$_{12}$ requirements: Increased vitamin B$_{12}$ requirements associated with pregnancy, thyrotoxicosis, hemolytic anemia, hemorrhage, malignancy, and hepatic and renal disease.

Vitamin B$_{12}$ absorption test: Vitamin B$_{12}$ absorption test (Schilling test).

Administration and Dosage
CYANOCOBALAMIN, CRYSTALLINE:

Addisonian pernicious anemia – Parenteral therapy is required for life; oral therapy is not dependable. Administer 100 mcg daily for 6 or 7 days by IM or deep SC injection. If there is clinical improvement and a reticulocyte response, give the same amount on alternate days for 7 doses, then every 3 to 4 days for another 2 to 3 weeks. By this time, hematologic values should have become normal. Follow this regimen with 100 mcg monthly for life. Administer folic acid concomitantly if needed.

Other patients with vitamin B$_{12}$ deficiency – In seriously ill patients, administer both vitamin B$_{12}$ and folic acid. It is not necessary to withhold therapy until the precise cause of B$_{12}$ deficiency is established. For hematologic signs, children may be given 10 to 50 mcg/day for 5 to 10 days followed by 100 to 250 mcg/dose every 2 to 4 weeks; for neurologic signs, 100 mcg/day for 10 to 15 days, then once or twice weekly for several months, possibly tapering to 250 to 1000 mcg/month by 1 year.

Oral – Up to 1000 mcg/day. Oral vitamin B$_{12}$ therapy is not usually recommended for vitamin B$_{12}$ deficiency. The maximum amount of vitamin B$_{12}$ that can be absorbed from a single oral dose is 1 to 5 mcg. The percent absorbed decreases with increasing doses.

IM or SC – 30 mcg/day for 5 to 10 days followed by 100 to 200 mcg/month. Larger doses (eg, 1000 mcg) have been recommended, even though a larger amount is lost through excretion. However, it is possible that a greater amount is retained, allowing for fewer injections.

HYDROXOCOBALAMIN, CRYSTALLINE: Administer IM only. The recommended dosage is 30 mcg/day for 5 to 10 days, followed by 100 to 200 mcg/month. Children may be given a total of 1 to 5 mg over ≥ 2 weeks in doses of 100 mcg, then 30 to 50 mcg every 4 weeks for maintenance. Institute concurrent folic acid therapy at the beginning of treatment if needed.

Schilling test: The flushing dose is 1000 mcg IM.

Actions
Pharmacology: Vitamin B$_{12}$ is essential to growth, cell reproduction, hematopoiesis, and nucleoprotein and myelin synthesis. Its physiologic role is associated with methylation, participating in nucleic acid and protein synthesis. Cyanocobalamin participates in red blood cell formation through activation of folic acid coenzymes. Hydroxocobalamin (vitamin B$_{12a}$) functions the same as cyanocobalamin.

Pharmacokinetics: Absorption of vitamin B$_{12}$ depends on the presence of sufficient intrinsic factor and calcium. In general, absorption of oral B$_{12}$ is inadequate in malabsorptive states and in pernicious anemia (unless intrinsic factor is simultaneously administered).

Cyanocobalamin – Cyanocobalamin is rapidly absorbed from IM and SC injection sites; the plasma level peaks within 1 hour. Once absorbed, it is bound to plasma proteins, stored mainly in the liver and is slowly released when needed to carry out normal cellular metabolic functions. Within 48 hours after injection of 100 to 1000 mcg of vitamin B$_{12}$, 50% to 98% of the dose appears in the urine. The major portion is excreted within the first 8 hours. More rapid excretion occurs with IV administration; there is little opportunity for liver storage.

Hydroxocobalamin – Hydroxocobalamin (vitamin B$_{12a}$) is more highly protein bound and is retained in the body longer than cyanocobalamin. However, it has no advantage over cyanocobalamin.

Contraindications

Hypersensitivity to cobalt, vitamin B$_{12}$, or any component of these products.

Warnings

Inadequate response: A blunted or impeded therapeutic response may be due to infection, uremia, bone marrow suppressant drugs, concurrent iron or folic acid deficiency, or misdiagnosis.

Vitamin B$_{12}$ deficiency: Vitamin B$_{12}$ deficiency allowed to progress for > 3 months may produce permanent degenerative lesions of the spinal cord.

Optic nerve atrophy: Patients with early Leber's disease (hereditary optic nerve atrophy) treated with cyanocobalamin suffer severe and swift optic atrophy.

Hypokalemia: Hypokalemia and sudden death may occur in severe megaloblastic anemia which is treated intensely.

Pregnancy: Category C (parenteral).

Lactation: Vitamin B$_{12}$ is excreted in breast milk in concentrations that approximate the mother's vitamin B$_{12}$ blood level. Amounts of B$_{12}$ recommended by the Food and Nutrition Board, National Academy of Sciences-National Research Council (2.6 mcg/day) should be consumed during lactation.

Children: The Food and Nutrition Board, National Academy of Sciences-National Research Council recommends a daily intake of 0.3 to 0.5 mcg/day for infants < 1 year of age and 0.7 to 1.4 mcg/day for children 1 to 10 years of age.

Precautions

Monitoring: During treatment of severe megaloblastic anemia, monitor serum potassium levels closely for the first 48 hours and replace potassium if necessary. Obtain reticulocyte counts, hematocrit and vitamin B$_{12}$, iron and folic acid plasma levels prior to treatment and between the fifth and seventh days of therapy, and then frequently until the hematocrit is normal. If folate levels are low, also administer folic acid.

Test dose: Anaphylactic shock and death have occurred after parenteral vitamin B$_{12}$ administration. Give an intradermal test dose in patients sensitive to the cobalamins.

Folate: Doses > 10 mcg/day may produce hematologic response in patients with folate deficiency. Indiscriminate use may mask the true diagnosis of pernicious anemia.

Doses of folic acid > 0.1 mg/day may result in hematologic remission in patients with vitamin B$_{12}$ deficiency. Neurologic manifestations will not be prevented with folic acid, and if not treated with vitamin B$_{12}$, irreversible damage will result.

Polycythemia vera: Vitamin B$_{12}$ deficiency may suppress the signs of polycythemia vera.

Vegetarian diets: Vegetarian diets containing no animal products (including milk products or eggs) do not supply any vitamin B$_{12}$.

Immunodeficient patients: Vitamin B$_{12}$ malabsorption may occur in patients with AIDS or HIV infection. Consider monitoring levels.

Drug Interactions

Drugs that may affect vitamin B$_{12}$ include aminosalicylic acid, chloramphenicol, colchicine, and alcohol.

Drug/Lab test interactions: Methotrexate, pyrimethamine, and most antibiotics invalidate folic acid and vitamin B_{12} diagnostic microbiological blood assays.

Adverse Reactions

The following reactions are associated with parenteral vitamin B_{12}: Anaphylactic shock, death, pulmonary edema, congestive heart failure early in treatment, severe and swift optic nerve atrophy.

PHYTONADIONE (K₁, Phylloquinone, Methylphytyl Naphthoquinone)

Tablets: 5 mg (*Rx*)
Injection (aqueous colloidal solution): 2 mg/mL (*Rx*)

Injection (aqueous dispersion): 10 mg/mL (*Rx*)

Mephyton (Merck)
Various, *AquaMEPHYTON* (Merck), *Konakion* (Roche)
AquaMEPHYTON (Merck), *Konakion* (Roche)

> **Warning:**
>
> *IV use:* Severe reactions, including fatalities, have occurred during and immediately after IV injection, even with precautions to dilute the injection and to avoid rapid infusion. These severe reactions resemble hypersensitivity or anaphylaxis, including shock and cardiac or respiratory arrest. Some patients exhibit these severe reactions on receiving vitamin K for the first time. Therefore, restrict the IV route to those situations where other routes are not feasible and the serious risk involved is justified.

Indications

Coagulation disorders: Coagulation disorders due to faulty formation of factors II, VII, IX, and X when caused by vitamin K deficiency or interference with vitamin K activity.

Oral: Anticoagulant-induced prothrombin deficiency (see Warnings); hypoprothrombinemia secondary to salicylates or antibacterial therapy; hypoprothrombinemia secondary to obstructive jaundice and biliary fistulas, but only if bile salts are administered concomitantly with phytonadione.

Parenteral: Anticoagulant-induced prothrombin deficiency; hypoprothrombinemia secondary to conditions limiting absorption or synthesis of vitamin K (eg, obstructive jaundice, biliary fistula, sprue, ulcerative colitis, celiac disease, intestinal resection, cystic fibrosis of the pancreas, regional enteritis); drug-induced hypoprothrombinemias due to interference with vitamin K metabolism (eg, antibiotics, salicylates); prophylaxis and therapy of hemorrhagic disease of the newborn.

Administration and Dosage

If possible, discontinue or reduce the dosage of drugs interfering with coagulation mechanisms (eg, salicylates, antibiotics) as an alternative to phytonadione. The severity of the coagulation disorder should determine whether the immediate administration of phytonadione is required in addition to discontinuation or reduction of interfering drugs.

Inject SC or IM when possible. In older children and adults, inject IM in the upper outer quadrant of the buttocks. In infants and young children, the anterolateral aspect of the thigh or the deltoid region is preferred. When IV administration is unavoidable, inject very slowly, not exceeding 1 mg/min.

Anticoagulant-induced prothrombin deficiency in adults: 2.5 to 10 mg or up to 25 mg (rarely, 50 mg) initially. Determine subsequent doses by prothrombin time (PT) response or clinical condition. If in 6 to 8 hours after parenteral administration (or 12 to 48 hours after oral administration), the PT has not been shortened satisfactorily, repeat dose. If shock or excessive blood loss occurs, transfusion of blood or fresh frozen plasma may be required.

Hemorrhagic disease of the newborn:

Prophylaxis – Single IM dose of 0.5 to 1 mg within 1 hour after birth. This may be repeated after 2 to 3 weeks if the mother has received anticoagulant, anticonvulsant, antituberculous, or recent antibiotic therapy during her pregnancy. Twelve to 24 hours before delivery, 1 to 5 mg may be given to the mother.

Oral doses of 2 mg have been shown to be adequate for prophylaxis.

Treatment – 1 mg SC or IM. Higher doses may be necessary if the mother has been receiving oral anticoagulants. Empiric administration of vitamin K₁ should not replace proper laboratory evaluation. A prompt response (shortening of the PT in 2 to 4 hours) is usually diagnostic of hemorrhagic disease of the newborn; failure to respond indicates another diagnosis or coagulation disorder. Give blood or blood products such as fresh frozen plasma if bleeding is excessive. However, this therapy does not correct the underlying disorder; give phytonadione concurrently.

Hypoprothrombinemia due to other causes in adults: 2.5 to 25 mg (rarely, up to 50 mg); amount and route of administration depends on severity of condition and response obtained. Avoid oral route when clinical disorder would prevent proper absorption. Give bile salts with tablets when endogenous supply of bile to GI tract is deficient.

Actions

Pharmacology: Vitamin K promotes the hepatic synthesis of active prothrombin (factor II), proconvertin (factor VII), plasma thromboplastin component (factor IX), and Stuart factor (factor X). The mechanism by which vitamin K promotes formation of these clotting factors involves the hepatic post-translational carboxylation of specific glutamate residues to gamma-carboxylglutamate residues in proteins involved in coagulation, thus leading to their activation.

Phytonadione (vitamin K₁) is a lipid-soluble synthetic analog of vitamin K. Phytonadione possesses essentially the same type and degree of activity as the naturally occurring vitamin K.

Pharmacokinetics: Phytonadione is only absorbed from the GI tract via intestinal lymphatics in the presence of bile salts. Although initially concentrated in the liver, vitamin K is rapidly metabolized, and very little tissue accumulation occurs.

Parenteral phytonadione is generally detectable within 1 to 2 hours. Phytonadione usually controls hemorrhage within 3 to 6 hours. A normal prothrombin level may be obtained in 12 to 14 hours. Oral phytonadione exerts its effect in 6 to 10 hours.

The US daily allowances – The US daily allowances for vitamin K have not been officially established, but have been estimated to be 10 to 20 mcg for infants, 15 to 100 mcg for children and adolescents, and 70 to 140 mcg for adults. Usually, dietary vitamin K will satisfy these requirements, except during the first 5 to 8 days of the neonatal period.

Recommended Dietary Allowances as published by the National Academy of Sciences are as follows: Adult males, 45 to 80 mcg/day; adult females, 45 to 65 mcg/day.

Contraindications

Hypersensitivity to any component of the product.

Warnings

Oral anticoagulant-induced hypoprothrombinemia: Vitamin K will not counteract the anticoagulant action of heparin.

Immediate coagulant effect should not be expected. It takes a minimum of 1 to 2 hours for a measurable improvement in the PT.

The prothrombin test is sensitive to the levels of factors II, VII, and X. Fresh plasma or blood transfusions may be required for severe blood loss or lack of response to vitamin K.

With phytonadione use and anticoagulant therapy indicated, the patient is faced with the same clotting hazards prior to starting anticoagulant therapy. Phytonadione is not a clotting agent, but overzealous therapy may restore original thromboembolic phenomena conditions. Keep dosage as low as possible and check PT regularly.

Hepatic function impairment: Hypoprothrombinemia due to hepatocellular damage is not corrected by administration of vitamin K. Repeated large doses of vitamin K are not warranted in liver disease if the initial response is unsatisfactory (Koller test). Failure to respond to vitamin K may indicate a coagulation defect or a condition unresponsive to vitamin K. In hepatic disease, large doses may further depress liver function.

Paradoxically, giving excessive doses of vitamin K or its analogs in an attempt to correct hypoprothrombinemia associated with severe hepatitis or cirrhosis may actually result in further depression of the prothrombin concentration.

Pregnancy: Category C.

Lactation: Vitamin K is excreted in breast milk.

Children: Safety and efficacy in children have not been established. Hemolysis, jaundice, and hyperbilirubinemia in newborns, particularly in premature infants, have been reported with vitamin K. These effects may be dose-related. Therefore, do not exceed recommended dose.

Drug Interactions

Drugs that may interact include anticoagulants and mineral oil.

Adverse Reactions

Adverse reactions from parenteral administration may include transient "flushing sensations" and "peculiar" sensations of taste. Deaths have occurred after IV administration. Hyperbilirubinemia has been observed in the newborn following administration of phytonadione. Anaphylactoid reactions may occur with either doseform.

EPOETIN ALFA (Erythropoietin; EPO)

Injection: 2000, 3000, 4000, 10,000 and 20,000 units per mL (*Rx*)   *Epogen* (Amgen), *Procrit* (Ortho Biotech)

Indications

Treatment of anemia associated with chronic renal failure (CRF): Treatment of anemia associated with CRF, including patients on dialysis (end-stage renal disease) and patients not on dialysis, to elevate or maintain the red blood cell level (as manifested by the hematocrit or hemoglobin determinations) and to decrease the need for transfusions.

Treatment of anemia related to zidovudine therapy in HIV-infected patients: To elevate or maintain the red blood cell level (as manifested by the hematocrit or hemoglobin determinations) and to decrease the need for transfusions in these patients when the endogenous erythropoietin level is $\leq$ 500 mU/mL and the dose of zidovudine is $\leq$ 4200 mg/week.

Treatment of anemia in cancer patients on chemotherapy: Treatment of anemia in patients with non-myeloid malignancies where anemia is due to the effect of concomitantly administered chemotherapy. It is intended to decrease the need for transfusions in patients who will be receiving chemotherapy for a minimum of 2 months.

Reduction of allogeneic transfusion in surgery patients: For the treatment of anemic patients (hemoglobin > 10 to $\leq$ 13 g/dL) scheduled to undergo elective, noncardiac, nonvascular surgery to reduce the need for allogeneic blood transfusions. Epoetin alfa is indicated for patients at high risk for perioperative transfusions with significant, anticipated blood loss.

Administration and Dosage

CRF patients:

Epoetin Alfa: General Therapeutic Guidelines in CRF Patients	
Starting dose	50 to 100 U/kg 3 times/week IV or SC
Reduce dose when:	1) Hematocrit approaches 36% or 2) Hematocrit increases > 4 points in any 2-week period.
Increase dose if:	Hematocrit does not increase by 5 to 6 points after 8 weeks of therapy, and hematocrit is below suggested target range.
Maintenance dose	Individualize.
Suggested target hematocrit range	30% to 36%

Starting doses over the range of 50 to 100 U/kg 3 times/week are safe and effective in increasing hematocrit and eliminating transfusion dependency in patients with CRF. Reduce the dose as the hematocrit approaches 36% or increases by > 4 points in any 2-week period. At the physician's discretion, the suggested target hematocrit range may be expanded to achieve maximal patient benefit.

Epoetin alfa may be given either as an IV or SC injection. In patients on hemodialysis, epoetin alfa usually has been administered as an IV bolus 3 times/week. While the administration is independent of the dialysis procedure, epoetin alfa may be administered into the venous line at the end of the dialysis procedure to obviate the need for additional venous access.

Dose adjustment – The time required to elicit a clinically significant change in hematocrit (increase or decrease) following any dose adjustment may be 2 to 6 weeks. Dose adjustment should not be made more frequently than once a month, unless clinically indicated. After any dose adjustment, determine the hematocrit twice weekly for at least 2 to 6 weeks.

- If the hematocrit is increasing and approaching 36%, reduce the dose to maintain the suggested target hematocrit range. If the reduced dose does not stop the rise in hematocrit and it exceeds 36%, temporarily withhold doses until the hematocrit begins to decrease, then reinitiate at a lower dose.
- At any time, if the hematocrit increases by > 4 points in a 2-week period,

immediately decrease the dose. After the dose reduction, monitor the hematocrit twice weekly for 2 to 6 weeks and make further dose adjustments as outlined in the maintenance dose section.

- If a hematocrit increase of 5 to 6 points is not achieved after an 8-week period and iron stores are adequate, the dose may be incrementally increased. Further increases may be made at 4- to 6-week intervals until the desired response is attained.

Maintenance –

Dialysis patients: Median dose is 75 U/kg 3 times/week (range, 12.5 to 525 U/kg 3 times/week).

Nondialysis CRF patients: Dose of 75 to 150 U/kg/week has maintained hematocrits of 36% to 38% for up to 6 months.

Delayed or diminished response – Over 95% of patients with CRF responded with clinically significant increases in hematocrit, and virtually all patients were transfusion-independent within ≈ 2 months of initiation of therapy.

If a patient fails to respond or maintain a response, consider other etiologies and evaluate as clinically indicated.

Zidovudine-treated, HIV-infected patients: Available evidence suggests that patients receiving zidovudine with endogenous serum erythropoietin levels > 500 mU/mL are unlikely to respond to therapy.

Initial dose – For patients with serum erythropoietin levels ≤ 500 mU/mL who are receiving a dose of zidovudine ≤ 4200 mg/week, the recommended starting dose is 100 U/kg as an IV or SC injection 3 times/week for 8 weeks.

If the response is not satisfactory in terms of reducing transfusion requirements or increasing hematocrit after 8 weeks of therapy, the dose can be increased by 50 to 100 U/kg 3 times/week. Evaluate response every 4 to 8 weeks thereafter and adjust the dose accordingly by 50 to 100 U/kg increments 3 times/week. If patients have not responded satisfactorily to a 300 U/kg dose 3 times/week, it is unlikely that they will respond to higher doses.

Maintenance dose – When the desired response is attained, titrate the dose to maintain the response based on factors such as variations in zidovudine dose and the presence of intercurrent infectious or inflammatory episodes. If the hematocrit exceeds 40%, stop the dose until the hematocrit drops to 36%. When resuming treatment, reduce the dose by 25%, then titrate to maintain the desired hematocrit.

Cancer patients on chemotherapy:

Starting dose – 150 units/kg SC 3 times/week. In general, patients with lower baseline serum erythropoietin levels responded more vigorously to epoetin alfa. Treatment of patients with grossly elevated erythropoietin levels (eg, > 200 mU/mL) is not recommended. Monitor hematocrit on a weekly basis until hematocrit becomes stable.

Dose adjustment – If response is not satisfactory in terms of reducing transfusion requirement or increasing hematocrit after 8 weeks of therapy, the dose may be increased up to 300 units/kg 3 times/week. If patients do not respond, it is unlikely that they will respond to higher doses. If hematocrit exceeds 40%, hold the dose until it falls to 36%. Reduce dose by 25% when treatment is resumed and titrate to maintain desired hematocrit. If initial dose includes a very rapid hematocrit response (eg, increase of > 4 percentage points in any 2-week period), reduce dose.

Surgery – Prior to initiating treatment with epoetin alfa, obtain a hemoglobin to establish that it is > 10 to ≤ 13 g/dL. The recommended dose is 300 U/kg/day SC for 10 days before surgery, on the day of surgery and for 4 days after surgery.

An alternate dose schedule is 600 U/kg SC in once-weekly doses (21, 14, and 7 days before surgery) plus a fourth dose on the day of surgery.

All patients should receive adequate iron supplementation. Initiate iron supplementation no later than the beginning of treatment with epoetin alfa and continue throughout the course of therapy.

Actions

Pharmacology: Erythropoietin is a glycoprotein that stimulates red blood cell production. It is produced in the kidney and stimulates the division and differentiation of erythroid progenitors in bone marrow. Hypoxia and anemia generally increase the production of erythropoietin, which in turn stimulates erythropoiesis. In patients with CRF, erythropoietin production is impaired; this deficiency is the primary cause of their anemia. Epoetin alfa stimulates erythropoiesis in anemic patients on dialysis and those who do not require regular dialysis.

Pharmacokinetics: Epoetin alfa IV is eliminated via first-order kinetics with a circulating half-life of 4 to 13 hours in patients with CRF. Within the therapeutic dosage range, detectable levels of plasma erythropoietin are maintained for at least 24 hours. After SC administration of epoetin alfa to patients with CRF, peak serum levels are achieved within 5 to 24 hours after administration and decline slowly thereafter. The half-life in healthy volunteers is ≈ 20% shorter than in CRF patients.

Contraindications

Uncontrolled hypertension; hypersensitivity to mammalian cell-derived products or to human albumin.

Warnings

Anemia: Not intended for CRF patients who require correction of severe anemia; epoetin alfa may obviate the need for maintenance transfusions but is not a substitute for emergency transfusion. Not indicated for treatment of anemia in HIV-infected patients or cancer patients due to other factors such as iron or folate deficiencies, hemolysis, or GI bleeding, which should be managed appropriately.

Hypertension: Up to 80% of patients with CRF have a history of hypertension. Do not treat patients with uncontrolled hypertension; monitor blood pressure adequately before initiation of therapy. Although there does not appear to be any direct pressor effects of epoetin, blood pressure may rise during therapy. During the early phase of treatment when the hematocrit is increasing, ≈ 25% of patients on dialysis may require initiation of, or increases in, antihypertensive therapy. Hypertensive encephalopathy and seizures have occurred in patients with CRF treated with epoetin.

It is recommended that the epoetin dose be decreased if the hematocrit increase exceeds 4 points in any 2-week period because of the possible association of excessive rate of rise of hematocrit with an exacerbation of hypertension.

Seizures: Because the relationship between seizures and the rate of rise of hematocrit is uncertain, decrease the dose of epoetin alfa if the hematocrit increase exceeds 4 points in any 2-week period. In patients on dialysis, there appeared to be a higher incidence of seizures during the first 90 days of therapy when compared with subsequent 90-day periods.

Thrombotic events: During hemodialysis, patients treated with epoetin alfa may require increased anticoagulation with heparin to prevent clotting of the artificial kidney. Overall, for patients with CRF (whether on dialysis or not), other thrombotic events have occurred at an annualized rate of < 0.04 events per patient-year of epoetin alfa.

Heart disease/congestive heart failure (CHF): In chronic renal failure patients on hemodialysis with clinically evident ischemic heart disease or CHF, manage the hematocrit carefully, not to exceed 36%.

Allergic reactions: Skin rashes and urticaria are rare, mild, and transient. If an anaphylactoid reaction occurs, immediately discontinue the drug and initiate appropriate therapy. Refer to Management of Acute Hypersensitivity Reactions.

Pregnancy: Category C.

Lactation: It is not known whether epoetin alfa is excreted in breast milk.

Children: Safety and efficacy have not been established.

Precautions

Monitoring:

Patients with CRF not requiring dialysis – Monitor blood pressure and hematocrit no less frequently than for patients maintained on dialysis. Closely monitor renal function and fluid and electrolyte balance, as an improved sense of well-being may obscure the need to initiate dialysis in some patients.

Determine the hematocrit twice a week until it has stabilized in the target range and the maintenance dose has been established. After any dose adjustment, determine the hematocrit twice weekly for at least 2 to 6 weeks until the hematocrit has stabilized; then monitor at regular intervals.

Perform complete blood count with differential and platelet counts regularly. Modest increases have occurred in platelets and white blood cell counts, but values remained within normal ranges.

Monitor serum chemistry values (including blood urea nitrogen [BUN], uric acid, creatinine, phosphorus, and potassium) regularly.

Zidovudine-treated, HIV-infected patients – Measure hematocrit once a week until it is stabilized; measure periodically thereafter.

Iron evaluation – During therapy, absolute or functional iron deficiency may develop. Transferrin saturation should be at least 20%, and ferritin should be at least 100 ng/mL. Prior to and during therapy, evaluate the patient's iron status, including transferrin saturation (serum iron divided by iron binding capacity) and serum ferritin. Virtually all patients will eventually require supplemental iron to increase or maintain transferrin saturation to levels that will adequately support epoetin alfa-stimulated erythropoiesis.

Hematology: The elevated bleeding time characteristic of CRF decreases toward normal after correction of anemia in epoetin alfa-treated patients. Reduction of bleeding time also occurs after correction of anemia by transfusion. Allow sufficient time to determine a patient's responsiveness before adjusting the dose. An interval of 2 to 6 weeks may occur between the time of a dose adjustment and a significant change in hematocrit.

Porphyria – Porphyria exacerbation has been observed rarely in epoetin alfa-treated patients with CRF. Use with caution in patients with known porphyria.

Bone marrow fibrosis: Bone marrow fibrosis is a complication of CRF and may be related to secondary hyperparathyroidism or unknown factors.

Delayed or diminished response: If the patient fails to respond or to maintain a response to doses within the recommended range, consider and evaluate the following etiologies:

1.) Functional iron deficiency may develop with normal ferritin levels but low transferrin saturation (< 20%), presumably due to the inability to mobilize iron stores rapidly enough to support increased erythropoiesis.
2.) Underlying infectious, inflammatory, or malignant processes.
3.) Occult blood loss.
4.) Underlying hematologic diseases.
5.) Vitamin deficiencies: Folic acid or vitamin B_{12}.
6.) Hemolysis.
7.) Aluminum intoxication.
8.) Osteitis fibrosa cystica.
9.) Increase in zidovudine dosage.

Diet: As the hematocrit increases and patients experience an improved sense of well-being, reinforce the importance of compliance with dietary guidelines and frequency of dialysis.

Hyperkalemia – Hyperkalemia is not uncommon in patients with CRF.

Dialysis management: Therapy with epoetin alfa results in an increase in hematocrit and a decrease in plasma volume that could affect dialysis efficiency.

Adverse Reactions

CRF patients – Epoetin alfa is generally well tolerated. The following adverse reactions are frequent (> 3%) sequelae of CRF and are not necessarily due to epoetin alfa therapy: Hypertension, headache, arthralgia, nausea, edema, fatigue, diarrhea, vomiting, chest pain, asthenia, dizziness, and clotted vascular access.

Zidovudine-treated HIV-infected patients – Adverse experiences > 3% were consistent with the progression of HIV infection: Pyrexia, fatigue, headache, cough, diarrhea, rash, nausea, respiratory congestion, shortness of breath, asthenia, and dizziness.

Surgery patients – Adverse reactions ≥ 3% include pyrexia; nausea; constipation; skin reactions at injection site; vomiting; itching; insomnia; headache; dizziness; urinary tract infection; hypertension; anxiety; diarrhea; dyspepsia; edema.

Cancer patients in chemotherapy – Adverse reactions > 3% were consistent with the underlying disease state: Pyrexia, diarrhea, nausea, vomiting, edema, asthenia, fatigue, shortness of breath, paresthesia, upper respiratory infection, dizziness, and trunk pain.

DARBEPOETIN ALFA

Solution:[1] 25, 40, 60, 100, 200 mcg/mL (*Rx*)   *Aranesp* (Amgen)

[1] In polysorbate or albumin solution. The polysorbate solution contains 8.18 mg sodium chloride. The albumin solution contains 2.5 mg albumin (human) and 8.18 mg sodium chloride.

Indications

Anemia: Anemia associated with chronic renal failure, including patients on and not on dialysis.

Administration and Dosage

Administer IV or SC as a single weekly injection. Start and slowly adjust the dose as described below based on hemoglobin levels. If a patient fails to respond or maintain a response, consider and evaluate other etiologies. When darbepoetin therapy is initiated or adjusted, follow the hemoglobin level weekly until stabilized, and monitor at least monthly thereafter.

For patients who respond to darbepoetin with a rapid increase in hemoglobin (eg, > 1 g/dL in any 2-week period), reduce the dose of darbepoetin because of the association of excessive rate of rise of hemoglobin with adverse events.

Correction of anemia: The recommended starting dose of darbepoetin for the correction of anemia in chronic renal failure (CRF) patients is 0.45 mcg/kg body weight, administered as a single IV or SC injection once weekly. Titrate doses to not exceed a target hemoglobin concentration of 12 g/dL. For many patients, the appropriate maintenance dose will be lower than this starting dose. Predialysis patients, in particular, may require lower maintenance doses. Also, some patients have been treated successfully with SC darbepoetin administered once every 2 weeks.

Conversion from epoetin alfa to darbepoetin: Estimate the starting weekly dose of darbepoetin based on the weekly epoetin alfa dose at the time of substitution. Titrate doses to maintain the target hemoglobin. Due to the longer serum half-life, administer darbepoetin less frequently than epoetin alfa. Administer once a week if patient was receiving epoetin alfa 2 to 3 times/week. Administer darbepoetin once every 2 weeks if the patient was receiving epoetin alfa once per week. Maintain the route of administration (IV or SC).

| Estimated Darbepoetin Starting Doses (mcg/week) Based on Previous Epoetin Alfa Dose (units/week) ||
Previous weekly epoetin alfa dose (units/week)	Weekly darbepoetin dose (mcg/week)
< 2500	6.25
2500 to 4999	12.5
5000 to 10,999	25
11,000 to 17,999	40
18,000 to 33,999	60
34,000 to 89,999	100
≥ 90,000	200

Dose adjustment: Do not increase doses more frequently than once a month. If the hemoglobin is increasing and approaching 12 g/dL, reduce the dose by ≈ 25%. If the hemoglobin continues to increase, withhold doses temporarily until the hemoglobin begins to decrease, at which point therapy should be reinitiated at a dose ≈ 25% below the previous dose. If the hemoglobin increases by > 1 g/dL in a 2-week period, decrease the dose by ≈ 25%.

If the increase in hemoglobin is < 1 g/dL over 4 weeks and iron stores are adequate, the dose of darbepoetin may be increased by ≈ 25% of the previous dose. Further increases may be made at 4-week intervals until the specified hemoglobin is obtained.

Maintenance dose: Adjust darbepoetin dosage to maintain a target hemoglobin not to exceed 12 g/dL. If the hemoglobin exceeds 12 g/dL, the dose may be adjusted as described above. Doses must be individualized to ensure that hemoglobin is maintained at an appropriate level for each patient.

Preparation: Do not shake. Vigorous shaking may denature darbepoetin, rendering it biologically inactive. Do not dilute. Do not administer darbepoetin in conjunction with other drug solutions. Darbepoetin is packaged in single-use vials and contains no preservatives. Discard any unused portion. Do not pool unused portions.

Actions

Pharmacology: Darbepoetin alfa is an erythropoiesis-stimulating protein produced in Chinese hamster ovary (CHO) cells by recombinant DNA technology. Darbepoetin stimulates erythropoiesis by the same mechanism as endogenous erythropoietin. Erythropoietin is produced in the kidney and released into the bloodstream in response to hypoxia. In responding to hypoxia, erythropoietin interacts with progenitor stem cells to increase red cell production. Production of endogenous erythropoietin is impaired in patients with CRF, and erythropoietin deficiency is the primary cause of their anemia. Increased hemoglobin levels are not generally observed until 2 to 6 weeks after initiating treatment with darbepoetin.

Pharmacokinetics:

Absorption – Darbepoetin has an ≈ 3-fold longer terminal half-life than epoetin alfa when administered by either the IV or SC route.

Following IV administration to adult CRF patients, darbepoetin serum concentration time profiles are biphasic, with a distribution half-life of ≈ 1.4 hours and mean terminal half-life of ≈ 21 hours.

Following SC administration, the absorption is slow and rate-limiting and the terminal half-life is 49 hours (range, 27 to 89 hours), which reflects the absorption half-life. The peak concentration occurs at 34 hours (range, 24 to 72 hours) post-SC administration in adult CRF patients, and bioavailability is ≈ 37% (range, 30% to 50%).

Distribution – The distribution of darbepoetin in adult CRF patients is predominantly confined to the vascular space (≈ 60 mL/kg). The pharmacokinetic parameters indicate dose-linearity over the therapeutic dose range. With once-weekly dosing, steady-state serum levels are achieved within 4 weeks with a < 2-fold increase in peak concentration when compared with the initial dose. Accumulation was negligible following IV and SC dosing over 1 year of treatment.

Contraindications

Uncontrolled hypertension; known hypersensitivity to the active substance or any of the excipients.

Warnings

Cardiovascular events, hemoglobin, and rate of rise of hemoglobin: Darbepoetin and other erythropoietic therapies may increase the risk of cardiovascular events, including death, in patients with CRF. The higher risk of cardiovascular events may be associated with higher hemoglobin or higher rates of rise of hemoglobin.

In patients treated with darbepoetin or other recombinant erythropoietins in darbepoetin clinical trials, increases in hemoglobin greater than ≈ 1 g/dL during any 2-week period were associated with increased incidence of cardiac arrest, neurologic events (including seizures and stroke), exacerbations of hypertension, CHF, vascular thrombosis/ischemia, infarction, acute MI, and fluid overload/edema. It is recommended that the dose of darbepoetin be decreased if the hemoglobin increase exceeds 1 g/dL in any 2-week period because of the association of excessive rate of rise of hemoglobin with these events.

Hypertension: Do not treat patients with uncontrolled hypertension with darbepoetin; adequately control blood pressure before initiation of therapy. Blood pressure may rise during treatment of anemia with darbepoetin or epoetin alfa. Hypertensive encephalopathy and seizures have been observed in patients with CRF treated with darbepoetin or epoetin alfa.

Take special care to closely monitor and control blood pressure in patients treated with darbepoetin. Advise patients of the importance of compliance with antihypertensive therapy and dietary restrictions. If blood pressure is difficult to control by pharmacologic or dietary measures, reduce or withhold the dose of darbepoetin. A clinically significant decrease in hemoglobin may not be observed for several weeks.

Seizures: Seizures have occurred in patients with CRF participating in clinical trials of darbepoetin and epoetin alfa. During the first several months of therapy, closely monitor blood presssure and the presence of premonitory neurologic symptoms. While the relationship between seizures and the rate of rise of hemoglobin is uncertain, it is recommended that the dose of darbepoetin be decreased if the hemoglobin increase exceeds 1 g/dL in any 2-week period.

Albumin (human): Darbepoetin is supplied in 2 formulations with different excipients, 1 containing polysorbate 80 and another containing albumin (human), a derivative of human blood.

Fertility impairment: When administered IV to male and female rats prior to and during mating, an increase in postimplantation fetal loss was seen at doses ≥ 0.5 mcg/kg/dose, administered 3 times/week (3-fold higher than the recommended weekly starting dose in humans).

Elderly: No overall differences in safety and efficacy were observed between older patients and younger patients, but greater sensitivity of some older individuals cannot be ruled out.

Pregnancy: Category C.

Lactation: It is not known whether darbepoetin is excreted in human milk.

Children: The safety and efficacy of darbepoetin in pediatric patients have not been established.

Precautions

Monitoring: After initiating therapy, determine the hemoglobin weekly until it has stabilized and the maintenance dose has been established. After a dose adjustment, determine the hemoglobin weekly for ≥ 4 weeks until it has been determined that the hemoglobin has stabilized in response to the dose change. Then monitor the hemoglobin at regular intervals.

Evaluate iron status for all patients before and during treatment. Supplemental iron therapy is recommended for all patients whose serum ferritin is < 100 mcg/L or whose serum transferrin saturation is < 20%.

Compromised erythropoietic response: A lack of response or failure to maintain a hemoglobin response with darbepoetin doses within the recommended dosing range should prompt a search for causative factors. Deficiencies of folic acid or vitamin B_{12} should be excluded or corrected.

The safety and efficacy of darbepoetin therapy have not been established in patients with underlying hematologic diseases (eg, hemolytic anemia, sickle cell anemia, thalassemia, porphyria).

Hematology: Allow sufficient time to determine a patient's responsiveness to a dosage of darbepoetin before adjusting the dose. Because of the time required for erythropoiesis and the red cell half-life, an interval of 2 to 6 weeks may occur between the time of a dose adjustment (initiation, increase, decrease, or discontinuation) and a significant change in hemoglobin.

Patients with CRF not requiring dialysis: Patients with CRF not yet requiring dialysis may require lower maintenance doses of darbepoetin than patients receiving dialysis. Predialysis patients may be more responsive to the effects of darbepoetin, and require judicious monitoring of blood pressure and hemoglobin. Also closely monitor renal function and fluid and electrolyte balance.

Dialysis management: Therapy with darbepoetin results in an increase in red blood cells and a decrease in plasma volume, which could reduce dialysis efficiency; patients who are marginally dialyzed may require adjustments in their dialysis prescription.

Adverse Reactions

The most frequently reported serious adverse reactions with darbepoetin were vascular access thrombosis, CHF, sepsis, and cardiac arrhythmia. The most commonly reported adverse reactions were infection, hypertension, hypotension, myalgia, headache, and diarrhea. The most frequently reported adverse reactions resulting in clinical intervention (eg, discontinuation of darbepoetin, adjustment in dosage, the need for comedication to treat an adverse reaction symptom) were hypotension, hypertension, fever, myalgia, nausea, and chest pain.

Adverse reactions occurring in ≥ 3% of patients include the following: Hypertension, hypotension, cardiac arrhythmias/cardiac arrest, angina pectoris/cardiac chest pain, pruritus, thrombosis vascular access, CHF, headache, dizziness, diarrhea, vomiting, nausea, abdominal pain, constipation, myalgia, arthralgia, limb pain, back pain, upper respiratory tract infection, dyspnea, cough, bronchitis, infection (eg, sepsis, bacteremia, pneumonia, pertitonitis, abscess), peripheral edema, fatigue, fever, death, injection site pain, unspecified chest pain, fluid overload, access infection influenza-like symptoms, access hemorrhage, asthenia.

DIPYRIDAMOLE

Tablets: 25, 50, and 75 mg (Rx)   Various, *Persantine* (Boehringer Ingelheim)

Indications

Thromboembolic complications: Adjunct to coumarin anticoagulants in the prevention of postoperative thromboembolic complications of cardiac valve replacement.

Administration and Dosage

Adjunctive use in prophylaxis of thromboembolism after cardiac valve replacement: The recommended dose is 75 to 100 mg 4 times/day as an adjunct to the usual warfarin therapy.

Actions

Pharmacology: Dipyridamole lengthens abnormally shortened platelet survival time in a dose-dependent manner.

Dipyridamole is a platelet adhesion inhibitor, although the mechanism of action has not been fully elucidated. The mechanism may relate to: 1) Inhibition of red blood cell uptake of adenosine, itself an inhibitor of platelet reactivity, 2) phosphodiesterase inhibition leading to increased cyclic-3', 5'-adenosine monophosphate within platelets and, 3) inhibition of thromboxane A_2 formation, which is a potent stimulator of platelet activation.

Pharmacokinetics:

  Metabolism – Following an oral dose of dipyridamole, the average time to peak concentration is $\approx$ 75 minutes. The decline in plasma concentration fits a two-compartment model. The α half-life (the initial decline following peak concentration) is $\approx$ 40 minutes. The β half-life (the terminal decline in plasma concentration) is $\approx$ 10 hours. Dipyridamole is highly bound to plasma proteins. It is metabolized in the liver where it is conjugated as a glucuronide and excreted with the bile.

Warnings

Fertility impairment: A significant reduction in number of corpora lutea with consequent reduction in implantations and live fetuses was observed at 155 times the maximum recommended human dose.

Pregnancy: Category B.

Lactation: Dipyridamole is excreted in breast milk.

Children: Safety and efficacy in children < 12 years of age have not been established.

Precautions

Hypotension: Use with caution in patients with hypotension because it can produce peripheral vasodilation.

Adverse Reactions

Adverse reactions at therapeutic doses are usually minimal and transient. With long-term use, initial side effects usually disappear. The following reactions were reported in 2 heart valve replacement trials comparing dipyridamole and warfarin therapy to either warfarin alone or warfarin and placebo: Dizziness, abdominal distress, headache, and rash.

On those uncommon occasions when adverse reactions have been persistent or intolerable, they have ceased on withdrawal of the medication.

DIPYRIDAMOLE AND ASPIRIN

Capsules: 200 mg extended-release dipyridamole/25 mg aspirin (*Rx*)   Aggrenox (Boehringer Ingelheim)

Indications
Stroke: To reduce the risk of stroke in patients who have had transient ischemia of the brain or complete ischemic stroke due to thrombosis.

Administration and Dosage
The recommended dose of dipyridamole and aspirin combination therapy is 1 capsule given orally twice daily, 1 in the morning and 1 in the evening. Swallow whole; do not crush or chew.

Do not interchange with individual components of aspirin and dipyridamole tablets.

Actions
Pharmacology: Antithrombotic action is the result of the additive antiplatelet effects of dipyridamole and aspirin.

Pharmacokinetics:

    Absorption –

        Dipyridamole: Peak plasma levels of dipyridamole are achieved ≈ 2 hours after administration of a daily dose of 400 mg dipyridamole and aspirin combination (given as 200 mg twice daily). The peak plasma concentration at steady-state is ≈ 1.98 mcg/mL and the steady-state trough concentration is ≈ 0.53 mcg/mL.

        Aspirin: Peak plasma levels of aspirin are achieved ≈ 0.63 hours after administration of a 50 mg/day aspirin dose from dipyridamole and aspirin combination (given as 25 mg twice/day). The peak plasma concentration at steady-state is ≈ 319 ng/mL. Aspirin undergoes moderate hydrolysis to salicylic acid in the liver and the GI wall, with 50% to 75% of an administered dose reaching the systemic circulation as intact aspirin.

    Distribution –

        Dipyridamole: Dipyridamole is highly lipophilic; however, it has been shown that the drug does not cross the blood-brain barrier to any significant extent in animals. The steady-state volume of distribution of dipyridamole is ≈ 92 L. Approximately 99% of dipyridamole is bound to plasma proteins, predominantly to α1-acid glycoprotein and albumin.

        Aspirin: Aspirin is poorly bound to plasma proteins and its apparent volume of distribution is low (10 L). Its metabolite, salicylic acid, is highly bound to plasma proteins, but its binding is concentration-dependent (nonlinear). At low concentrations (< 100 mcg/mL), ≈ 90% of salicylic acid is bound to albumin. Salicyclic acid is widely distributed to all tissues and fluids in the body, including the CNS, breast milk, and fetal tissues.

    Metabolism/Excretion –

        Dipyridamole: Dipyridamole is metabolized in the liver, primarily by conjugation with glucuronic acid, of which monoglucuronide, which has low pharmacodynamic activity, is the primary metabolite. In plasma, ≈ 80% of the total amount is present as parent compound and 20% as monoglucuronide. Most of the glucuronide metabolite (≈ 95%) is excreted via bile into the feces, with some evidence of enterohepatic circulation. Renal excretion of parent compound is negligible and urinary excretion of the glucuronide metabolite is low (≈ 5%).

        Aspirin: Aspirin is rapidly hydrolized in plasma to salicylic acid with a half-life of 20 minutes. Plasma levels of aspirin are essentially undetectable 2 to 2.5 hours after dosing, and peak salicylic acid concentration occurs 1 hour (range, 0.5 to 2 hours) after aspirin administration. Salicylic acid is primarily conjugated in the liver to form a number of minor metabolites. Salicylate metabolism is saturable and the total body clearance decreases at higher serum concentrations.

        The elimination of acetylsalicylic acid follows first-order kinetics with the dipyridamole and aspirin combination and has a half-life of 0.33 hours. The half-life of salicylic acid is 1.71 hours.

Contraindications

Hypersensitivity to dipyridamole, aspirin, or any of the other product components.

Allergy: Aspirin is contraindicated in patients with a known allergy to NSAIDs and in patients with asthma, rhinitis, and nasal polyps. Aspirin may cause severe urticaria, angioedema, or bronchospasms (asthma).

Reye's syndrome: Do not use in children or teenagers with viral infections with or without fever. There is a risk of Reye's syndrome with concomitant use of aspirin in certain viral illnesses.

Warnings

Alcohol: Counsel patients who consume ≥ 3 alcoholic drinks every day about the bleeding risks involved with chronic, heavy alcohol use while taking **aspirin**.

Coagulation abnormalities: Even low doses of **aspirin** can inhibit platelet function leading to an increase in bleeding time. This can adversely affect patients with inherited or acquired bleeding disorders (eg, liver disease, vitamin K deficiency).

Peptic ulcer disease: Avoid using **aspirin**, which can cause gastric mucosal irritation and bleeding in patients with a history of active peptic ulcer disease.

Renal function impairment: No changes were observed in the pharmacokinetics of **dipyridamole** or its glucuronide metabolite with creatinine clearances ranging from ≈ 15 mL/min to > 100 mL/min if data were corrected for differences in age. Avoid **aspirin** in patients with severe renal failure (glomerular filtration rate < 10 mL/min).

Hepatic function impairment: Elevations of hepatic enzymes and hepatic failure have been reported in association with **dipyridamole** administration. Dipyridamole can be dosed without restriction as long as there is no evidence of hepatic failure. Avoid **aspirin** in patients with severe hepatic insufficiency.

Mutagenesis: **Aspirin** induced chromosome aberrations in cultured human fibroblasts.

Fertility impairment: Aspirin inhibits ovulation in rats.

Elderly: Plasma concentrations (determined as AUC) of dipyridamole in healthy elderly subjects > 65 years of age were ≈ 40% higher than in subjects < 55 years of age receiving treatment with the dipyridamole and aspirin combination.

Pregnancy: Category B (dipyridamole); Category D (aspirin).

Lactation: Dipyridamole and aspirin are excreted in human breast milk in low concentrations.

Children: Safety and efficacy of dipyridamole and aspirin combination capsules in pediatric patients have not been studied. Because of the aspirin component, use of this product in the pediatric population is not recommended.

Precautions

Dipyridamole and aspirin combination is not interchangeable with the individual components of aspirin and dipyridamole tablets.

Coronary artery disease: Due to the vasodilatory effect of **dipyridamole**, use with caution in patients with severe coronary artery disease (eg, unstable angina, recently sustained MI). Chest pain may be aggravated in patients with underlying coronary artery disease who are receiving dipyridamole. For stroke or transient ischemic attack patients for whom **aspirin** is indicated to prevent recurrent MI or angina pectoris, the aspirin in this product may not provide adequate treatment for the cardiac indications.

Hypotension: **Dipyridamole** can produce peripheral vasodilation; use with caution in patients with hypotension.

Lab test abnormalities: **Aspirin** has been associated with elevated hepatic enzymes, blood urea nitrogen and serum creatinine, hyperkalemia, proteinuria, and prolonged bleeding time. **Dipyridamole** has been associated with elevated hepatic enzymes.

Drug Interactions

Drugs that may be affected by dipyridamole are adenosine and cholinesterase inhibitors.

Drugs that may be affected by aspirin include ACE inhibitors, acetazolamide, anticoagulants, anticonvulsants (hydantoins, valproic acid), beta blockers, diuretics, methotrexate, NSAIDs, oral hypoglycemics, and uricosuric agents (probenecid, sulfinpyrazone).

Drug/Lab test interactions: Over the course of 24 months, patients treated with dipyridamole and aspirin combination therapy showed a decline (mean change from baseline) in hemoglobin of 0.25 g/dL, hematocrit of 0.75%, and erythrocyte count of $0.13 \times 10^6/mm^3$.

Adverse Reactions

Adverse reactions that occurred in ≥ 3% of patients included the following: Headache; abdominal pain; dyspepsia; nausea; vomiting; diarrhea; hemorrhage; arthralgia; pain; fatigue; back pain.

TICLOPIDINE HCl

Tablets: 250 mg (*Rx*)   *Ticlid* (Syntex)

Warning:
Ticlopidine can cause life-threatening hematological adverse reactions, including neutropenia/agranulocytosis and thrombotic thrombocytopenic purpura (TTP).

Neutropenia/agranulocytosis: Neutropenia defined as an absolute neutrophil count (ANC) < 1200 neutrophils/mm³ occurred in 50 of 2048 (2.4%) stroke patients who received ticlopidine in clinical trials. Neutropenia is calculated as follows: ANC = WBC x % neutrophils. In 17 patients (0.8%) the neutrophil count was < 450/mm³.

Thrombotic thrombocytopenic purpura (TTP): TTP was not seen during clinical trials, but US physicians reported about 100 cases between 1992 and 1997. Based on an estimated patient exposure of 2 to 4 million, and assuming an event reporting rate of 10% (the true rate is not known), the incidence of ticlopidine-associated TTP may be as high as 1 case in every 2000 to 4000 patients exposed (see Warnings).

Monitoring clinical and hematologic status: Severe hematological adverse reactions may occur within a few days of initiating therapy. The incidence of TTP peaks after ≈ 3 to 4 weeks of therapy and neutropenia peaks at ≈ 4 to 6 weeks with both declining thereafter. Only a few cases have arisen after > 3 months of treatment. Hematological adverse reactions cannot be reliably predicted by any identified demographic or clinical characteristics. During the first 3 months of treatment, hematologically and clinically monitor patients receiving ticlopidine for evidence of neutropenia or TTP. Immediately discontinue ticlopidine if there is any evidence of neutropenia or TTP.

Indications

Thrombotic stroke: To reduce the risk of thrombotic stroke (fatal or nonfatal) in patients who have experienced stroke precursors, and in patients who have had a completed thrombotic stroke.

Because ticlopidine is associated with a risk of life-threatening blood dyscrasias including TTP and neutropenia/agranulocytosis (see Warnings), reserve for patients who are intolerant or allergic to aspirin therapy or who have failed aspirin therapy.

Administration and Dosage

Recommended dose: 250 mg twice daily taken with food.

Actions

Pharmacology: Ticlopidine is a platelet aggregation inhibitor. When taken orally, ticlopidine causes a time and dose-dependent inhibition of both platelet aggregation and release of platelet granule constituents, as well as a prolongation of bleeding time.

Ticlopidine interferes with platelet membrane function by inhibiting ADP-induced platelet-fibrinogen binding and subsequent platelet-platelet interactions. The effect on platelet function is irreversible for the life of the platelet.

After discontinuation of ticlopidine, bleeding time and other platelet function tests return to normal within 2 weeks in the majority of patients.

Pharmacokinetics: Ticlopidine is rapidly absorbed (> 80%), with peak plasma levels occurring at ≈ 2 hours after dosing, and is extensively metabolized. Administration after meals results in a 20% increase in the area under the plasma concentration-time curve (AUC). Ticlopidine displays non-linear pharmacokinetics and clearance decreases markedly on repeated dosing.

Ticlopidine binds reversibly (98%) to plasma proteins, mainly to serum albumin and lipoproteins. The binding to albumin and lipoproteins is nonsaturable over a wide concentration range. Ticlopidine also binds to alpha-1 acid glycoprotein; at concentrations attained with the recommended dose, ≤ 15% in plasma is bound to this protein.

Ticlopidine is metabolized extensively by the liver; only trace amounts of intact drug are detected in the urine. Following an oral dose, 60% is recovered in the urine and 23% in the feces. Approximately, 33% of the dose excreted in the feces is intact ticlopidine, possibly excreted in the bile. Approximately 40% to 50% of the metabolites circulating in plasma are covalently bound to plasma proteins, probably by acylation. Although analysis of urine and plasma indicates ≥ 20 metabolites, no metabolite that accounts for the activity of ticlopidine has been isolated.

Contraindications

Hypersensitivity to the drug; presence of hematopoietic disorders such as neutropenia and thrombocytopenia or a history of TTP; presence of a hemostatic disorder or active pathological bleeding; severe liver impairment.

Warnings

Neutropenia: Neutropenia may occur suddenly. Bone-marrow examination typically shows a reduction in myeloid precursors. After withdrawal of ticlopidine, the neutrophil count usually rises to > 1200/mm^3 within 1 to 3 weeks.

Thrombocytopenia: Rarely, thrombocytopenia may occur in isolation or together with neutropenia. If clinical evaluation and repeat laboratory testing confirm the presence of thrombocytopenia, discontinue the drug.

TTP: Clinically, fever might suggest neutropenia or TTP. Weakness, pallor, petechiae or purpura, dark urine (because of blood, bile pigments, or hemoglobin) or jaundice, or neurological changes might also suggest TTP. Have the patient discontinue ticlopidine and contact the physician immediately upon the occurrence of these findings.

Monitoring – Monitor patients for neutropenia, thrombocytopenia, and TTP prior to initiating ticlopidine and every 2 weeks through the third month of therapy. If therapy is stopped during this 3-month period, continue to monitor for 2 weeks after discontinuation. More frequent monitoring and monitoring after the first 3 months of therapy are necessary only in patients exhibiting clinical signs or hematological laboratory signs (eg, neutrophil count < 70% of baseline count, decrease in hematocrit or platelet count).

Laboratory monitoring includes complete blood count, especially the absolute neutrophil count, platelet count, and the appearance of the peripheral smear. Thrombocytopenia induced by ticlopidine is occasionally unrelated to TTP. Further investigate for a diagnosis of TTP with the occurrence of any acute, unexplained reduction in hemoglobin or platelet count. Discontinue ticlopidine if there are laboratory signs of TTP or the neutrophil count is < 1200/mm^3.

Cholesterol elevation: Ticlopidine therapy causes increased serum cholesterol and triglycerides. Serum total cholesterol levels are increased 8% to 10% within 1 month of therapy and persist at that level. The ratios of lipoprotein subfractions are unchanged.

Hematological effects: Rare cases of pancytopenia and TTP, some of which have been fatal, have occurred.

Anticoagulant drugs: If a patient is switched from an anticoagulant or fibrinolytic drug to ticlopidine, discontinue the former drug prior to ticlopidine administration.

Renal function impairment: There is limited experience in patients with renal impairment. No unexpected problems have been encountered in patients having mild renal impairment, and there is no experience with dosage adjustment in patients with greater degrees of renal impairment. Nevertheless, for renally impaired patients it may be necessary to reduce ticlopidine dosage or discontinue it altogether if hemorrhagic or hematopoietic problems are encountered.

Hepatic function impairment: The average plasma concentration in patients with advanced cirrhosis was slightly higher than that seen in older subjects. Because of limited experience in patients with severe hepatic disease, who may have bleeding diatheses, the use of ticlopidine is not recommended.

Elderly: Clearance of ticlopidine is somewhat lower in elderly patients and trough levels are increased. No overall differences in safety or efficacy were observed between elderly patients and younger patients, but greater sensitivity of some older individuals cannot be ruled out.

Pregnancy: Category B.

Lactation: It is not known whether this drug is excreted in human breast milk.

Children: Safety and efficacy in patients < 18 years of age have not been established.

Precautions

Increased bleeding risk: Use with caution in patients who may be at risk of increased bleeding from trauma, surgery, or pathological conditions. If it is desired to eliminate the antiplatelet effects of ticlopidine prior to elective surgery, discontinue the drug 10 to 14 days prior to surgery. Increased surgical blood loss has occurred in patients undergoing surgery during treatment with ticlopidine.

Prolonged bleeding time is normalized within 2 hours after administration of 20 mg methylprednisolone IV. Platelet transfusions also may be used to reverse the effect of ticlopidine on bleeding. If possible, avoid platelet transfusions because they may accelerate thrombosis in patients with TTP on ticlopidine.

GI bleeding: Ticlopidine prolongs template bleeding time. Use with caution in patients who have lesions with a propensity to bleed (such as ulcers). Use drugs that might induce such lesions with caution in patients on ticlopidine.

Drug Interactions

The dose of drugs metabolized by hepatic microsomal enzymes with low therapeutic ratios, or being given to patients with hepatic impairment, may require adjustment to maintain optimal therapeutic blood levels when starting or stopping concomitant therapy with ticlopidine.

Drugs that may interact include antacids, cimetidine, aspirin, digoxin, phenytoin, and theophylline.

Drug/Food interactions: The oral bioavailability of ticlopidine is increased by 20% when taken after a meal. Administration with food is recommended to maximize GI tolerance.

Adverse Reactions

Adverse reactions were relatively frequent, with > 50% of patients reporting at least one. Most involved the GI tract. Most adverse effects are mild, but 21% of patients discontinued therapy because of an adverse event, principally diarrhea, rash, nausea, vomiting, GI pain, and neutropenia. Most adverse effects occur early in the course of treatment, but a new onset of adverse effects can occur after several months. Ticlopidine has been associated with a number of bleeding complications such as ecchymosis, epistaxis, hematuria, conjunctival hemorrhage, GI bleeding, posttraumatic bleeding, and perioperative bleeding. The incidence of elevated alkaline phosphatase (> 2 times upper limit of normal) was 7.6% in ticlopidine patients. The incidence of elevated AST (> 2 times upper limit of normal) was 3.1% in ticlopidine patients.

CLOPIDOGREL

Tablets: 75 mg (*Rx*)   *Plavix* (Sanofi)

Indications
Atherosclerotic events: Reduction of atherosclerotic events (MI, stroke, and vascular death) in patients with atherosclerosis documented by recent stroke, recent MI, or established peripheral arterial disease.

Administration and Dosage
The recommended dose of clopidogrel is 75 mg once daily with or without food.

No dosage adjustment is necessary for elderly patients or patients with renal disease.

Actions
Pharmacology: Clopidogrel is a thienopyridine derivative, chemically related to ticlopidine, that inhibits platelet aggregation. It acts by irreversibly modifying the platelet ADP receptor. Consequently, platelets exposed to clopidogrel are affected for the remainder of their lifespan.

Dose-dependent inhibition of platelet aggregation can be seen 2 hours after single oral doses of clopidogrel. Platelet aggregation and bleeding time gradually return to baseline values after treatment is discontinued, generally in about 5 days.

Pharmacokinetics:
Absorption/Distribution – Clopidogrel absorption is ≥ 50% and is rapid after oral administration. Bioavailability is unaffected by food. Both the parent compound and the main metabolite bind reversibly in vitro to plasma protein (98% and 94%, resepectively).

Metabolism/Excretion – Clopidogrel is extensively metabolized by the liver. It undergoes rapid hydrolysis into its carboxylic acid derivative; glucuronidation also occurs.

The elimination half-life of the main circulating metabolite was 8 hours with ≈ 50% excreted in the urine and ≈ 46% in the feces 5 days after dosing.

Contraindications
Hypersensitivity to the drug or any component of the product; active pathological bleeding such as peptic ulcer or intracranial hemorrhage.

Warnings
Neutropenia/agranulocytosis: Ticlopidine, a drug chemically similar to clopidogrel, is associated with a 0.8% rate of neutropenia (< 450 neutrophils/mL).

Based on clinical trials, the risk of myelotoxicity with clopidogrel appears to be quite low. Consider this possibility when a patient receiving clopidogrel demonstrates fever or other signs of infection.

Hepatic function impairment: Experience is limited in patients with severe hepatic disease, who may have bleeding diatheses. Use with caution in this population.

Pregnancy: Category B.

Lactation: Studies in rats have shown that clopidogrel and its metabolites are excreted in milk. It is not known whether this drug is excreted in human breast milk.

Children: Safety and efficacy have not been established.

Precautions
Bleeding risk: As with other antiplatelet agents, use with caution in patients who may be at risk of increased bleeding from trauma, surgery, or other pathological conditions. If a patient is to undergo elective surgery and an antiplatelet effect is not desired, discontinue clopidogrel 7 days prior to surgery.

GI bleeding – Clopidogrel prolongs the bleeding time. Use with caution in patients who have lesions with a propensity to bleed (eg, ulcers). Cautiously use drugs that might increase such lesions (eg, aspirin, other NSAIDs) in patients taking clopidogrel.

Drug Interactions
At high concentrations in vitro, clopidogrel inhibits P450 2C9. Accordingly, clopidogrel may interfere with the metabolism of phenytoin, tamoxifen, tolbutamide, warfarin, torsemide, fluvastatin, and many nonsteroidal anti-inflammatory agents, but

there are no data with which to predict the magnitude of these interactions. Use caution when any of these drugs is coadministered with clopidogrel.

Adverse Reactions

Adverse reactions occurring in ≥ 3% of patients include flu-like symptoms, chest pain, edema, headache, dizziness, dyspepsia, abdominal pain, diarrhea, nausea, arthralgia, purpura, dyspnea, cough, rhinitis, rash, pruritus, depression, hypercholesteremia.

ANTICOAGULANTS

Blood coagulation resulting in the formation of a stable fibrin clot involves a cascade of proteolytic reactions involving the interaction of clotting factors, platelets, and tissue materials. Clotting factors (see table) exist in the blood in inactive form and must be converted to an enzymatic or activated form before the next step in the clotting mechanism can be stimulated. Each factor is stimulated in turn until an insoluble fibrin clot is formed.

Two separate pathways, intrinsic and extrinsic, lead to the formation of a fibrin clot. Both pathways must function for hemostasis.

Intrinsic pathway: All the protein factors necessary for coagulation are present in circulating blood. Clot formation may take several minutes and is initiated by activation of factor XII.

Extrinsic pathway: Coagulation is activated by release of tissue thromboplastin, a factor not found in circulating blood. Clotting occurs in seconds because factor III bypasses the early reactions.

Refer to the next page for the complete coagulation pathway.

Anticoagulants used therapeutically include heparin, warfarin (a coumarin derivative), and anisindione (an indandione derivative).

Blood Clotting Factors		
Factor	Synonym	Vitamin K-dependent
I	Fibrinogen	no
II	Prothrombin	yes
III	Tissue thromboplastin, tissue factor	no
IV	Calcium	no
V	Labile factor, proaccelerin	no
VII	Proconvertin	yes
VIII	Antihemophilic factor, AHF	no
IX	Christmas factor, plasma thromboplastin component, PTC	yes
X	Stuart factor, Stuart-Prower factor	yes
XI	Plasma thromboplastin antecedent, PTA	no
XII	Hageman factor	no
XIII	Fibrin stabilizing factor, FSF	no
HMW-K	High molecular weight Kininogen, Fitzgerald factor	no
PL	Platelets or phospholipids	no
PK	Prekallikrein, Fletcher factor	no
Protein C[1]		yes
Protein S[2]		yes

[1] Partially responsible for inhibition of the extrinsic pathway. Inactivates factors V and VIII and promotes fibrinolysis. Activity declines following warfarin administration.

[2] A cofactor to accelerate the anticoagulant activity of protein C. Decreased levels occur following warfarin administration.

COAGULATION PATHWAY

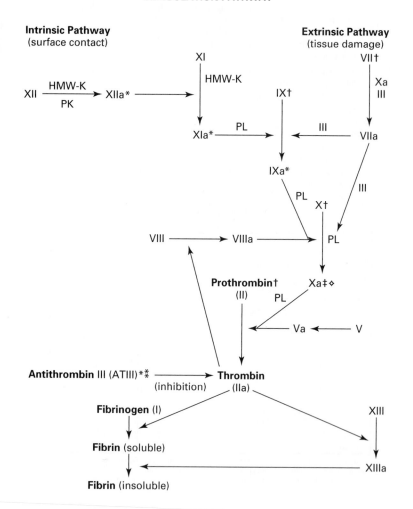

Intrinsic Pathway
(surface contact)

Extrinsic Pathway
(tissue damage)

* Major site of activity for unfractionated heparin
† Site of activity for warfarin and anisindione
‡ Major site of activity for fractionated heparin
※ Minor site of activity for fractionated heparin
◇ Minor site of activity for unfractionated heparin

LOW MOLECULAR WEIGHT HEPARINS

DALTEPARIN SODIUM

Solution: 16 mg/0.2 mL, 32 mg/0.2 mL, and 64 mg/mL (Rx)	*Fragmin* (Pharmacia & Upjohn)

ENOXAPARIN SODIUM

Injection:[1] 30 mg/0.3 mL, 40 mg/0.4 mL, 60 mg/0.6 mL, 80 mg/0.8 mL, 100 mg/mL, 90 mg/0.6 mL, 120 mg/0.8 mL, 150 mg/1 mL (Rx)	*Lovenox* (Aventis)

TINZAPARIN SODIUM

Injection: 40,000 IU/2 mL[2] (Rx)	*Innohep* (DuPont Pharma)

[1] Preservative free. Approximate anti-Factor Xa activity of 100 IU/1 mg (with standard reference to the WHO First International Low Molecular Weight Heparin Reference Standard).
[2] Anti-Factor Xa International Units.

Warning:

> When neuraxial anesthesia (epidural/spinal anesthesia) or spinal puncture is employed, patients who are anticoagulated or scheduled to be anticoagulated with low molecular weight heparins or heparinoids for prevention of thromboembolic complications are at risk of developing an epidural or spinal hematoma, which can result in long-term or permanent paralysis.
>
> The risk of these events is increased by the use of indwelling epidural catheters for administration of analgesia or by the concomitant use of drugs affecting hemostasis, such as nonsteroidal anti-inflammatory drugs (NSAIDs), platelet inhibitors, or other anticoagulants. The risk also appears to be increased by traumatic or repeated epidural or spinal puncture.
>
> Frequently monitor patients for signs and symptoms of neurological impairment. If neurological compromise is noted, urgent treatment is necessary.
>
> The physician should consider the potential benefit vs risk before neuraxial intervention in patients anticoagulated or scheduled to be anticoagulated for thromboprophylaxis.

Indications

Dalteparin: Prevention of deep-vein thrombosis (DVT), which may lead to pulmonary embolism (PE), following hip surgery or abdominal surgery who are at risk for thromboembolic complications; unstable angina/non-Q-wave MI.

Enoxaparin:

DVT prophylaxis – For prevention of DVT, which may lead to PE in patients undergoing hip replacement surgery (during and following hospitalization), knee replacement surgery, or abdominal surgery who are at risk for thromboembolic complications, or in medical patients at risk for thromboembolic complications due to severely restricted mobility during acute illness.

Abdominal surgery patients at risk include those who are > 40 years of age, obese, undergoing surgery under general anesthesia lasting > 30 minutes, or who have additional risk factors such as malignancy or a history of DVT or PE.

DVT/PE treatment – In conjunction with warfarin sodium for inpatient treatment of acute DVT with or without PE or for outpatient treatment of acute DVT without PE.

Unstable angina/Non-Q-wave MI – For the prevention of ischemic complications of unstable angina and non-Q-wave MI when coadministered with aspirin.

Tinzaparin: Treatment of acute symptomatic DVT with or without PE when administered in conjunction with warfarin sodium. The safety and effectiveness of tinzaparin were established in hospitalized patients.

Unlabeled uses: Systemic anticoagulation in venous and arterial thromboembolic complications (1 mg/kg **enoxaparin** SC twice/day); secondary prophylaxis for recurrent thromboembolic events (40 mg enoxaparin SC once daily).

Administration and Dosage
ENOXAPARIN:

Administration – Administer by SC injection only; do not administer IM. Screen patients prior to prophylactic administration of enoxaparin to rule out a bleeding disorder. There is usually no need for daily monitoring of the effect of enoxaparin in patients with normal presurgical coagulation parameters.

When using enoxaparin ampules, use a tuberculin syringe or equivalent to assure withdrawal of the appropriate volume of drug. Patients may self-inject only if their physician determines that it is appropriate and with medical follow-up as necessary.

DVT, prophylaxis –

Hip or knee replacement surgery: 30 mg every 12 hours by SC injection, with the initial dose given within 12 to 24 hours postoperatively provided hemostasis has been established. The average duration of administration is 7 to 10 days; up to 14 days has been well tolerated in controlled clinical trials.

For hip replacement surgery, consider a dose of 40 mg once daily SC, given initially 9 to 15 hours prior to surgery. Continue prophylaxis for 3 weeks.

Abdominal surgery: In adults at risk for thromboembolic complications, administer 40 mg once daily SC with the initial dose given 2 hours prior to surgery. The usual duration of administration is 7 to 10 days, up to 12 days.

Medical patients during acute illness: In medical patients at risk for thromboembolic complications due to severely restricted mobility during acute illness, the recommended dose is 40 mg once daily SC. The usual duration of administration is 6 to 11 days; up to 14 days has been well tolerated.

DVT/PE, treatment –

Outpatient treatment: For patients with acute DVT without PE who can be treated at home, the recommended dose is 1 mg/kg SC every 12 hours.

Inpatient treatment: For patients with acute DVT with PE or patients with acute DVT without PE (who are not candidates for outpatient treatment), the recommended dose is 1 mg/kg SC every 12 hours or 1.5 mg/kg SC once daily (same time each day).

Outpatient and inpatient treatment: Initiate warfarin therapy when appropriate (usually within 72 hours of enoxaparin). Continue enoxaparin for a minimum of 5 days and until a therapeutic anticoagulant effect has been achieved (INR 2-3). The average duration is 7 days; up to 17 days has been well tolerated.

Unstable angina/Non-Q-wave MI – In patients with unstable angina or non-Q-wave MI, the recommended dose is 1 mg/kg SC every 12 hours in conjunction with oral aspirin therapy (100 to 325 mg once daily). Treat with enoxaparin for ≥ 2 days and continue until clinical stabilization. The usual duration of treatment is 2 to 8 days; up to 12.5 days have been well tolerated. To minimize the risk of bleeding following vascular instrumentation during the treatment of unstable angina, adhere precisely to the intervals recommended between doses. Leave the vascular access sheath for instrumentation in place for 6 to 8 hours following a dose of enoxaparin. Give the next scheduled dose ≥ 6 to 8 hours after sheath removal. Observe site for signs of bleeding or hematoma formation.

SC injection technique – To avoid the loss of drug, do not expel the air bubble from the syringe before the injection. Administer by deep SC injection while patients are lying down. Alternate administration between the left and right anterolateral and left and right posterolateral abdominal wall. Introduce the whole length of the needle into a skin-fold held between the thumb and forefinger; hold the skin-fold throughout the injection. To minimize bruising, do not rub the injection site. An automatic injector, *Lovenox EasyInjector*, is available for patients to administer enoxaparin packaged in 30 and 40 mg prefilled syringes.

Renal function impairment – Consider dose adjustment for low weight (< 45 kg) patients and for those with severe renal impairment (Ccr < 30 mL/min).

Admixture incompatibility – Do not mix with other injections or infusions.

DALTEPARIN:

Administration – Administer by SC injection; do not administer IM. Dosage adjustment and routine monitoring of coagulation parameters are not required if the dosage and administration recommendations are followed.

Unstable angina/Non-Q-wave MI – The recommended dose of dalteparin injection is 120 IU/kg of body weight (but not more than 10,000 IU) SC every 12 hours with concurrent oral aspirin (75 to 165 mg/day) therapy. Continue treatment until the patient is clinically stabilized. In clinical trials, the usual duration of treatment was 5 to 8 days. Concurrent aspirin therapy is recommended except when contraindicated.

Volume of Dalteparin to be Administered by Patient Weight						
Patient weight (lb)	< 110	110 to 131	132 to 153	154 to 175	176 to 197	≥ 198
Patient weight (kg)	< 50	50 to 59	60 to 69	70 to 79	80 to 89	≥ 90
Volume of dalteparin (mL)[1]	0.55	0.65	0.75	0.9	1	1

[1] Calculated volume based on the 9.5 mL multiple-dose vial (10,000 anti-Factor Xa IU/mL).

DVT, prophylaxis –

Abdominal surgery: In patients undergoing abdominal surgery with a risk of thromboembolic complications, administer 2500 IU SC once daily, starting 1 to 2 hours prior to surgery and repeat once daily for 5 to 10 days postoperatively. Dosage adjustment and routine monitoring of coagulation parameters are not required if these dosage and administration recommendations are followed.

High-risk patients – In abdominal surgery in patients at high risk for thromboembolic complications (eg, malignancy), administer 5000 IU SC the evening before surgery and repeat once daily for 5 to 10 days postoperatively. Alternatively, in patients with malignancy, administer 2500 IU SC 1 to 2 hours prior to surgery with an additional 2500 IU SC dose 12 hours later and then 5000 IU once daily for 5 to 10 days.

Hip replacement surgery: The usual duration of administration is 5 to 10 days after surgery; up to 14 days was well tolerated in controlled clinical trials.

Dalteparin SC Dosing for Patients Undergoing Hip Replacement Surgery				
Timing of first dose of dalteparin	10 to 14 hours before surgery	≤ 2 hours before surgery	4 to 8 hours after surgery[1]	Postoperative period[2]
Postoperative start	—	—	2500 IU[3]	5000 IU qd
Preoperative start — day of surgery		2500 IU	2500 IU[3]	5000 IU qd
Preoperative start — evening before surgery[4]	5000 IU		5000 IU	5000 IU qd

[1] Or later, if hemostasis has not been achieved.
[2] Up to 14 days of treatment was well tolerated in controlled clinical trials, where the usual duration of treatment was 5 to 10 days postoperatively.
[3] Allow a minimum of 6 hours between this dose and the dose to be given on postoperative day 1. Adjust the timing of the dose on postoperative day 1 accordingly.
[4] Allow ≈ 24 hours between doses.

Coagulation parameters: Dosage adjustment and routine monitoring of coagulation parameters are not required if these dosage and administration recommendations are followed.

SC injection technique – Administer by deep SC injection while patient is sitting or lying down. Dalteparin may be injected in a U-shaped area around the navel, the upper outer side of the thigh, or the upper outer quadrangle of the buttock. Vary the injection site daily. When the area around the navel or the thigh is used, use the thumb and forefinger to lift up a fold of skin while giving the injection. Insert the entire length of the needle at a 45 to 90 degree angle.

TINZAPARIN: Evaluate all patients for bleeding disorders before administration of tinzaparin.

Adults: The recommended dose of tinzaparin for the treatment of DVT with or without PE is 175 anti-Xa IU/kg of body weight, adminstered SC once daily for ≥ 6 days and until the patient is adequately anticoagulated with warfarin (international normalizing ratio [INR] ≥ 2 for 2 consecutive days). Initiate warfarin sodium therapy when appropriate (usually within 1 to 3 days of tinzaparin initiation).

As tinzaparin may theoretically affect the prothrombin time (PT)/INR, draw blood for PT/INR determination just prior to the next scheduled dose of tinzaparin for patients receiving tinzaparin and warfarin.

The following table provides tinzaparin doses for the treatment of DVT with or without PE. It is necessary to calculate the appropriate tinzaparin dose for patient weights not displayed in the table.

Use an appropriately calibrated syringe to assure withdrawal of the correct volume of drug from tinzaparin vials.

Tinzaparin Weight-Based Dosing for Treatment of DVT With or Without Symptomatic PE			
	DVT Treatment		
	175 IU/kg SC once daily 20,000 IU/mL		
Body weight (lbs)	Dose (IU)	Amount (mL)	Patient body weight (kg)
68-80	6000	0.3	31-36
81-94	7000	0.35	37-42
95-107	8000	0.4	43-48
108-118	9000	0.45	49-53
119-131	10,000	0.5	54-59
132-144	11,000	0.55	60-65
145-155	12,000	0.6	66-70
156-168	13,000	0.65	71-76
169-182	14,000	0.7	77-82
183-195	15,000	0.75	83-88
196-206	16,000	0.8	89-93
207-219	17,000	0.85	94-99
220-232	18,000	0.9	100-105
233-243	19,000	0.95	106-110
244-256	20,000	1	111-116
257-270	21,000	1.05	117-122

Use the following equation to calculate the volume (mL) of tinzaparin 175 anti-Xa IU/kg SC dose for treatment of DVT:

Patient weight (kg) x 0.00875 mL/kg = volume to be given (mL) SC.

Administration: Inspect the solution visually for particulate matter and discoloration prior to administration. Administer tinzaparin by SC injection. Do not administer by IM or IV injection. Do not mix tinzaparin with other injections or infusions.

SC injection technique: Position patients either lying down (supine) or sitting, and administer tinzaparin by deep SC injection. Alternate administration between left and right anterolateral and left and right posterolateral abdominal wall. Vary the injection site daily. Introduce the whole length of the needle into a skin fold held between the thumb and forefinger; hold the skin fold throughout the injection. To minimize bruising, do not rub the injection site after completion of the injection.

Actions

Pharmacology: **Enoxaparin, tinzaparin,** and **dalteparin** are low molecular weight heparins (LMWHs) with antithrombotic properties. These agents enhance the inhibition of Factor Xa and thrombin by antithrombin III and potentiate preferentially the inhibition of coagulation factor Xa, while only slightly affecting thrombin and clotting time (eg, activated partial thromboplastin time [APTT] or prothrombin time [PT]).

Pharmacokinetics:

Approximate Pharmacokinetic Parameters of LMWHs Based on Anti-Xa Activity					
LMWH	Bioavailability (%)	T_{max} (hrs)	Vd (L)	Cl (mL/min)	Terminal $t_{1/2}$ (hrs)
Dalteparin	≈ 87	4	2.8 to 4.2[1]	28.7 and 18.2[1,2]	3 to 5
Enoxaparin	92	3 to 5	6	15	4.5
Tinzaparin	86.7	3.7[3]	3.1 to 5	28[4]	3 to 4[3]

[1] Based on a 70 kg patient.
[2] Following 30 and 120 IU/kg doses of anti-Factor Xa, respectively.
[3] Dosing based on 4500 IU; mean dose 64.3 IU/kg.
[4] Following 4500 IU IV.

Contraindications

Hypersensitivity to LMWHs, heparin, or pork products; hypersensitivity to sulfites or benzyl alcohol, history of heparin-induced thrombocytopenia (**tinzaparin**); active major bleeding; thrombocytopenia associated with positive in vitro tests for anti-platelet antibody in the presence of a LMWH.

Do not give **dalteparin** to patients undergoing regional anesthesia for unstable angina or non-Q-wave MI because of an increased risk of bleeding associated with the dosage of dalteparin recommended for unstable angina and non-Q-wave MI.

Warnings

Route of administration: For SC administration only; do not administer IM or IV.

Interchangeability with heparin: LMWHs cannot be used interchangeably (unit for unit) with unfractionated heparin or other low molecular weight heparins.

Spinal/Epidural anesthesia: As with other anticoagulants, there have been rare cases of neuraxial hematomas reported with the concurrent use of LMWHs and spinal/epidural anesthesia or spinal puncture resulting in long-term or permanent paralysis. The risk of these events may be higher with the use of postoperative indwelling epidural catheters or by the concomitant use of additional drugs affecting hemostasis such as NSAIDs (see Warning Box).

Hemorrhage: Use LMWHs, like other anticoagulants, with extreme caution in patients who have an increased risk of hemorrhage, such as those with severe uncontrolled hypertension, bleeding diathesis, diabetic retinopathy, bacterial endocarditis, congenital or acquired bleeding disorders (including hepatic failure and amyloidosis), active ulceration and angiodysplastic GI disease, hemorrhagic stroke or shortly after brain, spinal, or ophthalmological surgery, or in patients treated concomitantly with platelet inhibitors.

Thrombocytopenia: The incidence of thrombocytopenia with platelet counts between $50,000/mm^3$ and $100,000/mm^3$ was 1.3% in patients treated with **enoxaparin**, 1% with **tinzaparin**, and < 1% with **dalteparin**. Severe thrombocytopenia (platelet count < $50,000/mm^3$) occurred in 0.13% of tinzaparin-treated patients and 0.1% of enoxaparin-treated patients.

Heparin-induced thrombocytopenia: Use with extreme caution in patients with a history of this condition.

Priapism: Priapism has been reported from postmarketing surveillance of **tinzaparin** as a rare occurrence. In some cases, surgical intervention was required.

Renal/Hepatic function impairment: Delayed elimination of LMWHs may occur.

Elderly: Delayed elimination of **enoxaparin** and **tinzaparin** may occur.

Pregnancy: Category B.

Lactation: It is not known whether this drug is excreted in breast milk.

Children: Safety and efficacy in children have not been established.

Precautions

Monitoring: Periodic complete blood counts, including platelet count, urinalysis, and stool occult blood tests are recommended during the course of treatment. At recommended prophylaxis doses, routine coagulation tests such as PT and aPTT are relatively insensitive measures of activity and are, therefore, unsuitable for monitoring. Anti-Factor Xa may be used to monitor the anticoagulant effect in patients with significant renal impairment or if abnormal coagulation parameters or bleeding should occur.

General: Use with care in patients with a bleeding diathesis, uncontrolled arterial hypertension, or a history of recent GI ulceration, diabetic retinopathy, and hemorrhage.

Benzyl alcohol: The multiple-dose vials of **dalteparin** and **tinzaparin** contain benzyl alcohol as a preservative. Benzyl alcohol has been associated with a fatal "gasping syndrome" in premature infants. Because benzyl alcohol may cross the placenta, do not use dalteparin preserved with benzyl alcohol in pregnant women.

Thromboembolic events: If thromboembolic events occur despite LMWH prophylaxis, discontinue and initiate appropriate therapy.

Special risk: Use with care in patients with a bleeding diathesis, uncontrolled arterial hypertension, or a history of recent GI ulceration and hemorrhage, and diabetic retinopathy.

Sulfite sensitivity: **Tinzaparin** contains metabisulfite, a sulfite that may cause allergic-type reactions including anaphylactic symptoms and life-threatening or less severe asthmatic episodes.

Drug Interactions

Anticoagulants and platelet inhibitors: Use LMWHs with care in patients receiving oral anticoagulants or platelet inhibitors (eg, aspirin, salicylates, NSAIDs including ketorolac tromethamine, dipyridamole, sulfinpyrazone, dextran, ticlopidine) and thrombolytics because of increased risk of bleeding. If coadministration is essential, use close clinical and laboratory monitoring of these patients.

Drug/Lab test interactions: Asymptomatic reversible increases in aspartate (AST) and alanine (ALT) aminotransferase levels have occurred in patients treated with LMWHs and heparin. Because aminotransferase determinations are important in the differential diagnosis of MI, liver disease, and pulmonary emboli, interpret elevations that might be caused by LMWHs with caution.

Adverse Reactions

Adverse reactions associated with LMWHs include clinically significant bleeding, hemorrhage, injection site reactions, thrombocytopenia, local irritation following SC administration, fever, nausea, peripheral edema, wound hematoma, urinary tract infection, and hyochromic anemia.

Serious adverse events with **enoxaparin** in a clinical trial in patients with unstable angina or non-Q-wave MI include heart failure (0.95%); pneumonia (0.82%); atrial fibrillation and lung edema (0.7%). About 10% of pregnant women receiving **tinzaparin** experienced significant vaginal bleeding.

Lab test abnormalities: Asymptomatic increases in transaminase levels (AST and ALT) have been reported during treatment with LMWHs. Because transaminase determinations are important in the differential diagnosis of MI, liver disease, and pulmonary emboli, interpret elevations that might be caused by drugs like LMWHs with caution.

HEPARIN

HEPARIN SODIUM	
Injection: 1000, 5000, 10,000, and 20,000 units/mL (multiple dose vials) (*Rx*)	Various, *Liquaemin Sodium* (Organon)
1000, 5000, 10,000, and 20,000 units/mL (single dose amps and vials) (*Rx*)	Various, *Liquaemin Sodium Preservative Free* (Organon)
1000, 2500, 5000, 7500, 10,000, and 20,000 units/mL (unit dose vials) (*Rx*)	Various

HEPARIN SODIUM AND SODIUM CHLORIDE	
Injection: 1000 and 2000 units (*Rx*)	*Heparin Sodium and 0.9% Sodium Chloride* (Clintec)
12,500 and 25,000 units (*Rx*)	*Heparin Sodium and 0.45% Sodium Chloride* (Abbott)

HEPARIN SODIUM LOCK FLUSH	
Injection: 10 and 100 units/mL (*Rx*)	Various, *Hep-Lock* (Elkins-Sinn)

Indications

Prophylaxis and treatment: Prophylaxis and treatment of venous thrombosis and its extension; pulmonary embolism; peripheral arterial embolism; atrial fibrillation with embolization.

Diagnosis and treatment: Diagnosis and treatment of acute and chronic consumption coagulopathies (disseminated intravascular coagulation [DIC]).

Postoperative: Low dose regimen for prevention of postoperative deep venous thrombosis (DVT) and pulmonary embolism in patients undergoing major abdominothoracic surgery or patients who are at risk of developing thromboembolic disease.

According to National Institutes of Health Consensus Development Conference, low-dose heparin is treatment of choice as prophylaxis for DVT and pulmonary embolism in urology patients > 40 years of age; pregnant patients with prior thromboembolism; stroke patients; those with heart failure, acute MI or pulmonary infection; also recommended as suggested prophylaxis in high-risk surgery patients, moderate and high-risk gynecologic patients without malignancy, neurology patients with extracranial problems, and patients with severe musculoskeletal trauma.

Prevention: Prevention of clotting in arterial and heart surgery, blood transfusions, extracorporeal circulation, dialysis procedures, and blood samples for laboratory purposes.

Unlabeled uses: As an adjunct in treatment of coronary occlusion with acute MI. Although there is some controversy regarding the efficacy of heparin therapy with concurrent antiplatelet therapy (eg, aspirin) in the prevention of rethrombosis/reocclusion after primary thrombolysis with thrombolytics during acute MI, it is recommended by the American College of Cardiology and the American Heart Association. Generally, administer heparin IV immediately after thrombolytic therapy, usually within 2 to 8 hours (depending on the thrombolytic used), and maintain the infusion for at least 24 hours. Begin aspirin therapy immediately as soon as the patient is admitted, and continue its administration.

Administration and Dosage

Give by intermittent IV injection, continuous IV infusion or deep SC (ie, above the iliac crest of abdominal fat layer) injection. Continuous IV infusion is generally preferable due to the higher incidence of bleeding complications with other routes. Avoid IM injection because of the danger of hematoma formation.

Adjust dosage according to coagulation test results prior to each injection. Dosage is adequate when WBCT is ≈ 2.5 to 3 times control value, or when aPTT is 1.5 to 2 times normal.

When given by continuous IV infusion, perform coagulation tests every 4 hours in the early stages. When administered by intermittent IV infusion, perform coagulation tests before each dose during early stages and at appropriate intervals thereafter. After deep SC injection, perform tests 4 to 6 hours after the injections.

General heparin dosage guidelines: Although dosage must be individualized, the following may be used as guidelines:

Heparin Dosage Guidelines		
Method of administration	Frequency	Recommended dose[1]
Subcutaneous[2]	Initial dose	10,000 – 20,000 units[3]
	Every 8 hours	8000 – 10,000 units
	Every 12 hours	15,000 – 20,000 units
Intermittent IV	Initial dose	10,000 units[4]
	Every 4 to 6 hours	5000 – 10,000 units[4]
IV Infusion	Continuous	20,000 – 40,000 units/day[3]

[1] Based on a 68 kg (150 lb) patient.
[2] Use a concentrated solution.
[3] Immediately preceded by IV loading dose of 5000 units.
[4] Administer undiluted or in 50 to 100 mL 0.9% NaCl.

Children: In general, the following dosage schedule may be used as a guideline:
Initial dose – 50 units/kg IV bolus.
Maintenance dose – 100 units/kg/dose IV drip every 4 hours, or 20,000 units/m²/ 24 hours continuous IV infusion.

Low-dose prophylaxis of postoperative thromboembolism: Low-dose heparin prophylaxis, prior to and after surgery, will reduce the incidence of postoperative DVT in the legs and clinical pulmonary embolism. Give 5000 units SC 2 hours before surgery and 5000 units every 8 to 12 hours thereafter for 7 days or until the patient is fully ambulatory, whichever is longer. Administer by deep SC injection above the iliac crest or abdominal fat layer, arm, or thigh using a concentrated solution. Use a fine gauge needle (25 to 26 gauge) to minimize tissue trauma. Reserve such prophylaxis for patients > 40 years of age undergoing major surgery. Exclude patients on oral anticoagulants or drugs that affect platelet function or in patients with bleeding disorders, brain or spinal cord injuries, spinal anesthesia, eye surgery, or potentially sanguineous operations.

If bleeding occurs during or after surgery, discontinue heparin and neutralize with protamine sulfate. If clinical evidence of thromboembolism develops despite low-dose prophylaxis, give full therapeutic doses of anticoagulants until contraindicated. Prior to heparinization, rule out bleeding disorders; perform appropriate coagulation tests just prior to surgery. Coagulation test values should be normal or only slightly elevated at these times.

Surgery of the heart and blood vessels: Give an initial dose of not less than 150 units/kg to patients undergoing total body perfusion for open heart surgery. Often, 300 units/kg is used for procedures < 60 minutes and 400 units/kg is used for procedures > 60 minutes.

Extracorporeal dialysis: Follow equipment manufacturers' operating directions.

Laboratory samples: Add 70 to 150 units per 10 to 20 mL sample of whole blood to prevent coagulation of sample.

Clearing intermittent infusion (heparin lock) sets: To prevent clot formation in a heparin lock set, inject dilute heparin solution (Heparin Lock Flush Solution, USP; or a 10 to 100 units/mL heparin solution) via the injection hub in a quantity sufficient to fill the entire set to the needle tip. Replace this solution each time the heparin lock is used. If the administered drug is incompatible with heparin, flush the entire heparin lock set with sterile water or normal saline before and after the medication is administered; following the second flush, the dilute heparin solution may be reinstilled into the set. Consult the set manufacturer's instructions.

Converting to oral anticoagulant therapy: Perform baseline coagulation tests to determine prothrombin activity when heparin activity is too low to affect PT or INR. When the results of the initial prothrombin determinations are known, initiate the oral anticoagulant in the usual amount. Thereafter, perform coagulation tests and prothrombin activity at appropriate intervals. When the prothrombin activity reaches the desired therapeutic range, discontinue heparin and continue oral anticoagulants.

Actions

Pharmacology: Small amounts of heparin in combination with antithrombin III (heparin cofactor) inhibit thrombosis by inactivating factor Xa and inhibiting the conversion of prothrombin to thrombin. Once active thrombosis has developed, larger amounts of heparin can inhibit further coagulation by inactivating thrombin and preventing the conversion of fibrinogen to fibrin. In combination with antithrombin III, heparin inactivates factors IX, X, Xa, XI, XII, and thrombin, inhibiting conversion of fibrinogen to fibrin. The heparin-antithrombin III complex is 100 to 1000 times more potent as an anticoagulant than antithrombin III alone. Heparin also prevents the formation of a stable fibrin clot by inhibiting the activation of factor XIII (the fibrin stabilizing factor). Other effects include the inhibition of thrombin-induced activation of factors V and VIII.

Commercial products contain both low and high molecular weight heparin fractions. Low molecular weight heparin has a greater inhibitory effect on factor Xa, and less antithrombin activity than the high molecular weight fraction.

Heparin inhibits reactions that lead to clotting, but does not significantly alter the concentration of the normal clotting factors of blood. Although clotting time is prolonged by full therapeutic doses, in most cases it is not measurably affected by low doses of heparin. Bleeding time is usually unaffected.

Heparin also enhances lipoprotein lipase release (which clears plasma of circulating lipids), increases circulating free fatty acids, and reduces lipoprotein levels.

Pharmacokinetics:

Absorption/Distribution – Heparin is not adsorbed from the GI tract. An IV bolus results in immediate anticoagulant effects. The duration of action is dose-dependent. Peak plasma levels of heparin are achieved 2 to 4 hours following SC use. Once absorbed, heparin is distributed in plasma and is extensively protein bound.

Metabolism/Excretion – Following administration, heparin demonstrates a biphasic elimination curve. The lack of relationship between plasma and pharmacologic half-lives may reflect factors such as protein binding. Heparin is rapidly cleared from plasma with an average half-life of 30 to 180 minutes. Half-life is dose-dependent and may be significantly prolonged at higher doses. Heparin is partially metabolized by liver heparinase and the reticuloendothelial system. There may be a secondary site of metabolism in the kidneys. Apparent volume of distribution is 40 to 60 mL/kg. In patients with deep venous thrombosis, plasma clearance is more rapid and half-life is shorter than in patients with pulmonary embolism. Heparin is excreted in urine as unchanged drug (≤ 50%) particularly after large doses. Some urinary degradation products have anticoagulant activity.

Contraindications

Hypersensitivity to heparin; severe thrombocytopenia; uncontrolled bleeding (except when it is due to DIC); any patient for whom suitable blood coagulation tests cannot be performed at the appropriate intervals (there is usually no need to monitor coagulation parameters in patients receiving low-dose heparin).

Warnings

Hemorrhage: Hemorrhage can occur at virtually any site in patients receiving heparin. An unexplained fall in hematocrit, fall in blood pressure or any other unexplained symptom should lead to serious consideration of a hemorrhagic event. An overly prolonged coagulation test or bleeding can usually be controlled by withdrawing the drug. Signs and symptoms will vary according to the location and extent of bleeding and may present as paralysis, headache, chest, abdomen, joint or other pain, shortness of breath, difficulty breathing or swallowing, unexplained swelling, or unexplained shock. GI or urinary tract bleeding may indicate an underlying occult lesion. Certain hemorrhagic complications may be difficult to detect.

Use heparin with extreme caution in disease states in which there is increased danger of hemorrhage. These include:

Cardiovascular – Subacute bacterial endocarditis; arterial sclerosis; dissecting aneurysm; increased capillary permeability; severe hypertension.

CNS – During and immediately following spinal tap, spinal anesthesia, or major surgery, especially of the brain, spinal cord, or eye.

Hematologic – Hemophilia; some vascular purpuras; thrombocytopenia.

GI – Ulcerative lesions, diverticulitis or ulcerative colitis; continuous tube drainage of the stomach or small intestine.

Obstetric – Threatened abortion; menstruation.

Other – Liver disease with impaired hemostasis; severe renal disease.

Hyperlipidemia: Heparin may increase free fatty acid serum levels by induction of lipoprotein lipase. The catabolism of serum lipoproteins by this enzyme produces lipid fragments that are rapidly processed by the liver. Patients with dysbetalipoproteinemia (type III) are unable to catabolize the lipid fragments, resulting in hyperlipidemia.

Resistance: Increased resistance to the drug is frequently encountered in fever, thrombosis, thrombophlebitis, infections with thrombosing tendencies, MI, cancer, and postoperative states.

Thrombocytopenia: Thrombocytopenia has occurred in patients receiving heparin. The incidence of heparin-associated thrombocytopenia is higher with bovine than with porcine heparin. The severity also appears to be related to heparin dose.

Early thrombocytopenia – Early thrombocytopenia (Type I) develops 2 to 3 days after starting heparin, tends to be mild and is due to a direct action of heparin on platelets.

Delayed thrombocytopenia – Delayed thrombocytopenia (Type II) develops 7 to 12 days after either low-dose or full-dose heparin, can have serious consequences and may reflect the presence of an immunoglobulin that induces platelet aggregation.

Mild thrombocytopenia – Mild thrombocytopenia may remain stable or reverse even if heparin is continued. However, closely monitor thrombocytopenia of any degree. If a count falls below 100,000/mm^3 or if recurrent thrombosis develops, discontinue heparin. If continued heparin therapy is essential, administration of heparin from a different organ source can be reinstituted with caution.

White clot syndrome – Rarely, patients may develop new thrombus formation in association with thrombocytopenia resulting from irreversible aggregation of platelets induced by heparin, the so-called "white clot syndrome." The process may lead to severe thromboembolic complications. Monitor platelet counts before and during therapy. If significant thrombocytopenia occurs, immediately terminate heparin and institute other therapeutic measures.

Hypersensitivity reactions: Heparin is derived from animal tissue; use with caution in patients with a history of allergy. Before a therapeutic dose is given, a trial dose may be advisable. Have epinephrine 1:1000 immediately available.

Vasospastic reactions – Vasospastic reactions may develop 6 to 10 days after starting therapy and last 4 to 6 hours. The affected limb is painful, ischemic, and cyanotic. An artery to this limb may have been recently catheterized. After repeated injections, the reaction may gradually increase to generalized vasospasm with cyanosis, tachypnea, feeling of oppression, and headache. Itching and burning, especially on the plantar side of the feet, is possibly based on a similar allergic vasospastic reaction. Chest pain, elevated blood pressure, arthralgias, or headache also have been reported in the absence of definite peripheral vasospasm.

Hepatic function impairment: Heparin half-life may be prolonged in liver disease.

Elderly: A higher incidence of bleeding has occurred in women > 60 years of age.

Pregnancy: Category C.

Lactation: Heparin is not excreted in breast milk.

Children: Safety and efficacy have not been determined in newborns; germinal matrix intraventricular hemorrhage occurs more often in low-birth-weight infants receiving heparin.

Use heparin lock-flush solution with caution in infants with disease states in which there is an increased danger of hemorrhage. The use of the 100 unit/mL concentration is not advised because of bleeding risk, especially in low-birth-weight infants.

Precautions

Monitoring: The most common test used to monitor heparin's effect is aPTT. Other tests used include Activated Coagulation Time (ACT) and Lee White-Whole Blood Clotting Time (WBCT). If the coagulation test is unduly prolonged or if hemorrhage occurs, discontinue the drug promptly. Perform periodic platelet counts, hematocrit and tests for occult blood in stool during the entire course of therapy, regardless of route of administration.

Hyperkalemia: Hyperkalemia may develop, probably due to induced hypoaldosteronism. Use with caution in patients with diabetes or renal insufficiency. Monitor patient closely.

Drug Interactions

Drugs that may interact include cephalosporins, nitroglycerin, penicillins, and salicylates.

Drug/Lab test interactions: Significant elevations of aminotransferase (AST and ALT) levels have occurred in a high percentage of patients. Cautiously interpret aminotransferase increases that might be caused by heparin.

If heparin comprises ≥ 10% of the total volume of a sample for blood gas analysis, errors in measurements of carbon dioxide pressure, bicarbonate concentration, and base excess may occur.

Adverse Reactions

Adverse reactions associated with heparin include hemorrhage, chills, fever, urticaria, and thrombocytopenia.

COUMARIN AND INDANDIONE DERIVATIVES

WARFARIN SODIUM	
Tablets: 1, 2, 2.5, 4, 5, 7.5 and 10 mg (*Rx*)	*Coumadin* (DuPont)
ANISINDIONE	
Tablets: 50 mg (*Rx*)	*Miradon* (Schering)
DICUMAROL	
Tablets: 25 mg (*Rx*)	*Dicumarol* (Abbott)

Indications

Warfarin/Anisindione/Dicumarol: Prophylaxis and treatment of venous thrombosis and its extension; treatment of atrial fibrillation with embolization; prophylaxis and treatment of pulmonary embolism (PE).

Warfarin: Prophylaxis of atrial fibrillation with embolism. As an adjunct in the prophylaxis of systemic embolism after myocardial infarction (MI).

Anisindione/Dicumarol: As an adjunct in the treatment of coronary occlusion. Warfarin is generally the drug of choice.

Administration and Dosage

Dosage: Individualize dosage.

Available clinical evidence indicates that prolongation of the prothrombin time (PT) to 1.2 to 1.5 times control, when measuring with the less sensitive thromboplastin reagents, is sufficient for prophylaxis and treatment of venous thromboembolism and minimizes the risk of hemorrhage associated with more prolonged PT values. In cases where the risk of thromboembolism is great, such as in patients with recurrent systemic embolism, maintain a PT of 1.5 to 2 times control. A ratio of > 2 appears to provide no additional therapeutic benefit in most patients and is associated with a higher risk of bleeding.

For the 3 commercial rabbit brain thromboplastins currently used in North America, a PT ratio of 1.3 to 2 is equivalent to an INR of 2 to 4. For other thromboplastins, the INR can be calculated as:

$$INR = (observed\ PT\ ratio)^{ISI}$$

where the ISI (International Sensitivity Index) is the calibration factor and is available from the manufacturers of the thromboplastin reagent and observed PT ratio is:

$$\frac{PT\ observed}{PT\ control}$$

Following are the recommended therapeutic ranges for oral anticoagulant therapy from the American College of Chest Physicians (ACCP) and the National Heart, Lung, and Blood Institute (NHLBI):

ACCP/NHLBI Recommended Therapeutic Range for Oral Anticoagulant Therapy		
Condition	PT Ratio[1]	INR
Acute MI[2]	1.3 to 1.5	2 to 3
Atrial fibrillation[2]	1.3 to 1.5	2 to 3
Mechanical prosthetic valves	1.5 to 2	3 to 4.5
Pulmonary embolism, treatment	1.3 to 1.5	2 to 3
Systemic embolism		
Prevention	1.3 to 1.5	2 to 3
Recurrent	1.5 to 2	3 to 4.5
Tissue heart valves[2]	1.3 to 1.5	2 to 3
Valvular heart disease[2]	1.3 to 1.5	2 to 3
Venous thrombosis		
Prophylaxis (high-risk surgery)	1.3 to 1.5	2 to 3
Treatment	1.3 to 1.5	2 to 3

[1] ISI of 2.4
[2] To prevent systemic embolism

Transfer from heparin therapy: To provide continuous adequate anticoagulation in a patient on heparin, switch to oral anticoagulation. Because there is a delayed onset of oral anticoagulant effects, give heparin and warfarin simultaneously from the first day, or alternatively, start warfarin on the third to sixth day of heparin therapy. Use concurrent therapy until a therapeutic PT or INR is achieved.

Elderly: Lower dosages are recommended.

Duration of therapy: In the determination of the duration of long-term anticoagulant therapy, consider history of recurrent thromboembolism, underlying diseases, reason for anticoagulant therapy (eg, atrial fibrillation), and risks of adverse effects.

WARFARIN:

  Induction – Initiate with 10 mg/day for 2 to 4 days; adjust daily dosage according to PT or INR determinations. Use of a large loading dose (eg, 30 mg) may increase the incidence of hemorrhagic and other complications, does not offer more rapid protection against thrombi formation and is not recommended.

  Maintenance – 2 to 10 mg/day, based on PT or INR.

  Bioequivalence – Bioequivalence problems have been documented for warfarin sodium products marketed by different manufacturers. Brand interchange is not recommended.

  Treatment during dentistry and surgery – In patients who must be anticoagulated prior to, during or immediately following dental or surgical procedures, adjusting the dosage to maintain the PT at the low end of the therapeutic range (or maintain the corresponding INR value) may safely allow for continued anticoagulation. Limit the operative site to permit effective use of local measures for hemostasis. Under these conditions, dental and surgical procedures may be performed without undue risk of hemorrhage.

Minidose warfarin: Minidose warfarin may be beneficial as prophylaxis against venous thrombosis after major surgery. In 1 study, 1 mg/day given before surgery (mean 20 days) significantly lowered the incidence of DVT compared with controls; there was no difference between the 1 mg/day and the full-dose anticoagulation group. APTT and PT were not prolonged beyond normal on the day of surgery using the minidose therapy.

ANISINDIONE: 300 mg the first day, 200 mg the second day, 100 mg the third day, and 25 to 250 mg/day for maintenance.

DICUMAROL: 200 to 300 mg the first day, 25 to 200 mg on subsequent days.

Treatment during dentistry and surgery – If it is elected to administer anticoagulants prior to, during or immediately following dental or surgical procedures, it is recommended that the dosage of dicumarol be adjusted to maintain the prothrombin time at $\approx 1\frac{1}{2}$ to $2\frac{1}{2}$ times the control level.

Actions

Pharmacology: Coumarins (dicumarol and warfarin) and indandiones (anisindione) interfere with the hepatic synthesis of vitamin K-dependent clotting factors, which results in an in vivo depletion of clotting factors VII, IX, X, and II (prothrombin). Anticoagulant effects are dependent on the half-lives of these clotting factors, which are 6, 24, 36, and 50 hours, respectively. Hence, the reduction in the rate of synthesis of the clotting factors determines the clinical response. Although factor VII is quickly depleted and an initial prolongation of the PT is seen in 8 to 12 hours, maximum anticoagulation (thus, antithrombotic effects) is not approached for 3 to 5 days as the other factors are depleted and the drug achieves steady-state.

Warfarin is available as a racemic mixture containing the R(+) and S(–) enantiomers in equal proportions; however, the S-isomer is 3 to 6 times more potent as an anticoagulant than the R-isomer.

Pharmacokinetics:

Absorption – The oral anticoagulants are generally rapidly and completely absorbed.

Distribution – Oral anticoagulants are highly bound to plasma proteins (97% to > 99%), primarily albumin.

Metabolism/Excretion – These agents are metabolized by hepatic microsomal enzymes and are excreted primarily in the urine and feces as inactive metabolites.

Various Pharmacokinetic Parameters of Oral Anticoagulants			
Oral anticoagulant	Half-life (days)	Peak activity (days)	Duration[1] (days)
Coumarin derivatives			
Dicumarol	1-2	1.5-2	5-6
Warfarin	1-2.5[2]	1.5-3	2-5
Indandione derivative			
Anisindione	3-5	2-3	1-3

[1] Following drug discontinuation
[2] S-isomer $\approx$ 2 days; R-isomer $\approx$ 1.33 days

Contraindications

Pregnancy (see Warnings); hemorrhagic tendencies; hemophilia; thrombocytopenic purpura; leukemia; recent or contemplated surgery of the eye or CNS, major regional lumbar block anesthesia, or surgery resulting in large, open surfaces; patients bleeding from the GI, respiratory, or GU tract; threatened abortion; aneurysm (cerebral, dissecting aortic); ascorbic acid deficiency; history of bleeding diathesis; prostatectomy; continuous tube drainage of the small intestine; polyarthritis; diverticulitis; emaciation; malnutrition; cerebrovascular hemorrhage; eclampsia and preeclampsia; blood dyscrasias; severe uncontrolled or malignant hypertension; severe renal or hepatic disease; pericarditis and pericardial effusion; subacute bacterial endocarditis; visceral carcinoma; following spinal puncture and other diagnostic or therapeutic procedures (ie, IUD insertion) with potential for uncontrollable bleeding; unsupervised senility; alcoholism; psychosis; open wounds; history of warfarin-induced necrosis.

Warnings

Monitoring:

PT – Treatment is highly individualized. Control dosage by periodic determination of PT or other suitable coagulation tests (eg, INR). Monitor PT daily during the initiation of therapy and whenever any other drug is added to or discontinued from therapy that may alter the patient's response. Concurrent heparin therapy will elevate the PT 10% to 20%; if target PT levels are not increased by the same percentage during concurrent therapy, the patient could be inadequately anticoagulated when the heparin therapy is discontinued. Once stabilized, monitor PT every 4 to 6 weeks.

INR – INR is based on the determination of an International Normalized Ratio that provides a common basis for PT results and interpretations of therapeutic ranges. For a discussion of the relationship between PT and INR in clinical practice, refer to Administration and Dosage.

Hemorrhage/Necrosis: The most serious risks associated with anticoagulant therapy are hemorrhage in any tissue or organ and, less frequently, necrosis or gangrene of skin and other tissues; this has resulted in death or permanent disability. Discontinue therapy when anticoagulants are the suspected cause of developing necrosis; consider heparin therapy.

Hemorrhagic tendency may be manifested by hematuria, skin petechiae, hemorrhage into or from a wound or ulcerating lesion, or petechial and purpuric hemorrhages throughout the body.

Bleeding during anticoagulant therapy does not always correlate with prothrombin activity. Bleeding that occurs when the PT or INR is within the therapeutic range warrants investigation because it may unmask a previously unsuspected lesion (eg, tumor, ulcer).

Independent risk factors that may provide a basis for predicting major bleeding with anticoagulants include: ≥ 65 years of age; history of stroke; history of GI bleeding; serious comorbid condition (eg, recent MI, renal insufficiency, severe anemia); atrial fibrillation.

"Purple toe syndrome" – Anticoagulant therapy may enhance the release of atheromatous plaque emboli thereby increasing the risk of complications from systemic cholesterol microembolization including the "purple toe syndrome."

Excessive uterine bleeding may occur, but menstrual flow is usually normal. Women may be at risk of developing ovarian hemorrhage at the time of ovulation.

Oral anticoagulants should not be used in the treatment of acute completed strokes due to the risk of fatal cerebral hemorrhage.

Adrenal hemorrhage – Adrenal hemorrhage with resultant acute adrenal insufficiency has occurred.

Special risk patients: There is an increased risk with use of anticoagulants in the following conditions: Trauma; infection (concomitant antibiotic therapy may alter intestinal flora); renal insufficiency; prolonged dietary insufficiencies (eg, sprue, vitamin K deficiency); moderate to severe hypertension; polycythemia vera; vasculitis; severe allergic disorders; anaphylactic disorders; indwelling catheters; severe diabetes; surgery or trauma resulting in large exposed raw surfaces.

Use with caution in patients with active tuberculosis, severe diabetes, history of ulcerative disease of the GI tract, and during menstruation and the postpartum period.

Protein C deficiency: Known or suspected hereditary, familial, or clinical deficiency in protein C has been associated with necrosis following warfarin therapy.

Agranulocytosis and hepatitis: Agranulocytosis and hepatitis have been associated with anisindione use.

Rebound hypercoagulability: Rebound hypercoagulability was thought to occur upon sudden anticoagulant withdrawal, but has not been reproducible. Therefore, tapering the dose to discontinuation appears unnecessary, although tapering the dose gradually over 3 to 4 weeks is recommended if possible.

CHF: Patients with CHF may become more sensitive to dicumarol.

Hypersensitivity reactions: Delayed reactions are rare and occur within 1 to 3 months following the start of anisindione; 10% of cases are fatal. Discontinue the medication at the first sign of hypersensitivity reactions.

Renal/Hepatic function impairment: Use with caution.

Elderly: Older patients may be more sensitive to these agents.

Pregnancy: Category X.

If oral anticoagulants are used in pregnant women, do not administer during the first trimester, and discontinue prior to labor and delivery.

Some clinicians suggest the replacement of oral anticoagulants with heparin therapy before term. After 5 to 7 days, therapy with oral anticoagulants may be resumed if indicated.

Lactation: Warfarin appears in breast milk in an inactive form. Infants nursed by warfarin-treated mothers had no change in PT.

Anisindione and dicumarol or their metabolites may be excreted in breast milk in amounts sufficient to cause a prothrombopenic state and bleeding in the newborn.

Children: Safety and efficacy in children < 18 years of age have not been established. Oral anticoagulants may be beneficial in children with rare thromboembolic disorder secondary to other disease states such as the nephrotic syndrome or congenital heart lesions. Heparin is probably the initial anticoagulant of choice because of its immediate onset of action.

Precautions

Enhanced anticoagulant effects: Several endogenous factors that may result in an increased response to the oral anticoagulants or an increased PT or INR include: Carcinoma; hepatic disorders including hepatitis or obstructive jaundice; biliary fistula; febrile states; preparatory bowel sterilization; recent surgery; x-ray therapy; vitamin K deficiency; steatorrhea; CHF; diarrhea; poor nutritional state or collagen disease; renal insufficiency; hyperthyroidism; elevated temperature. Also, female and elderly patients are more sensitive to these agents.

Decreased anticoagulant effects: Endogenous factors that may reduce the response to the oral anticoagulants or decrease the PT or INR include: Edema; hyperlipidemia; diabetes mellitus; hypothyroidism; hereditary resistance to oral anticoagulants.

Drug Interactions

Oral anticoagulants have a great potential for clinically significant drug interactions. Warn all patients about potential hazards and instruct against taking **any** drug, including nonprescription products, without the advice of a physician or pharmacist.

Careful monitoring and appropriate dosage adjustments usually will permit safe administration of combined therapy. Critical times during therapy occur when an interacting drug is added to or discontinued from a patient stabilized on anticoagulants.

Coumarin and indandione derivatives are affected by many drugs. Those that may significantly affect coumarin and indandione derivatives include amiodarone, 17-alkyl androgens, barbiturates, clofibrate, dextrothyroxine, erythromycin, histamine H_2 antagonists, metronidazole, miconazole, phenylbutazones, quinine derivatives, salicylates, sulfinpyrazone, sulfonamides, thioamines, thyroid hormones, and vitamin E.

Drug/Lab test interactions: Oral anticoagulants may cause red-orange discoloration of alkaline urine; this may interfere with some lab tests.

Adverse Reactions

Hemorrhage – Hemorrhage is the principal adverse effect of oral anticoagulants. Other adverse reactions include nausea; diarrhea; pyrexia; dermatitis; exfoliative dermatitis; urticaria; alopecia; sore mouth; mouth ulcers; fever; abdominal cramping; leukopenia; red-orange urine; priapism (causal relationship not established); paralytic ileus and intestinal obstruction from submucosal or intramural hemorrhage.

LEPIRUDIN

Powder for injection: 50 mg (*Rx*)	*Refludan* (Hoechst-Marion Roussel)

Indications

Thrombocytopenia, heparin-induced: For anticoagulation in patients with heparin-induced thrombocytopenia (HIT) and associated thromboembolic disease in order to prevent further thromboembolic complications.

Administration and Dosage

Initial dosage: 0.4 mg/kg (≤ 110 kg) slowly IV (ie, over 15 to 20 seconds) as a bolus dose followed by 0.15 mg/kg (≤ 110 kg/hr) as a continuous IV infusion for 2 to 10 days or longer if clinically needed.

Normally the initial dosage depends on the patient's body weight; this is valid for patients ≤ 110 kg. In patients with a body weight > 110 kg, the initial dosage should not be increased beyond the 110 kg body weight dose (maximal initial bolus dose of 44 mg, maximal initial infusion dose of 16.5 mg/hr).

Determine patient baseline activated partial thromboplastin time (aPTT) prior to initiation of therapy with lepirudin, because lepirudin should not be started in patients presenting with a baseline aPTT ratio of ≥ 2.5 in order to avoid initial overdosing.

Monitoring: Adjust the dosage (infusion rate) according to the aPTT ratio.

The target range for the aPTT ratio during treatment (therapeutic window) should be 1.5 to 2.5. Data from clinical trials in HIT patients suggest that with aPTT ratios higher than this target range, the risk of bleeding increases, while there is no incremental increase in clinical efficacy. Do not start in patients with a baseline aPTT ratio of ≥ 2.5 in order to avoid initial overdosing.

The first aPTT determination for monitoring treatment should be done 4 hours after start of the lepirudin infusion. Follow-up aPTT determinations are recommended at least once daily, as long as treatment is ongoing.

More frequent aPTT monitoring is highly recommended in patients with renal impairment or serious liver injury or with an increased risk of bleeding.

Dose modifications: Any aPTT ratio out of the target range is to be confirmed at once before drawing conclusions with respect to dose modifications, unless there is a clinical need to react immediately.

If the confirmed aPTT ratio is above the target range, stop the infusion for 2 hours. At restart, decrease the infusion rate by 50% (no additional IV bolus should be administered). Determine the aPTT ratio again 4 hours later.

If the confirmed aPTT ratio is below the target range, increase the infusion rate in steps of 20%. Determine the aPTT ratio again 4 hours later.

Do not exceed an infusion rate of 0.21 mg/kg/hr without checking for coagulation abnormalities, which might be preventive of an appropriate aPTT response.

Renal function impairment: As lepirudin is almost exclusively excreted in the kidneys, consider individual renal function prior to administration. In case of renal impairment, relative overdose might occur even with the standard dosing regimen. Therefore, the bolus dose and infusion rate must be reduced in case of known or suspected renal insufficiency (Ccr < 60 mL/min or serum creatinine > 1.5 mg/dL).

There is only limited information on the therapeutic use of lepirudin in HIT patients with significant renal impairment. The following dosage recommendations are mainly based on single-dose studies in a small number of patients with renal impairment. Therefore, these recommendations are only tentative.

Base dose adjustments on Ccr values, whenever available, as obtained from a reliable method (24 hour urine sampling). If Ccr is not available, base the dose adjustments on the serum creatinine.

In all patients with renal insufficiency the bolus dose is to be reduced to 0.2 mg/kg.

The standard initial infusion rate must be reduced according to the recommendations given in the following table. Additional aPTT monitoring is highly recommended.

Reduction of Lepirudin Infusion Rate in Patients with Renal Impairment			
		Adjusted infusion rate	
Ccr (mL/min)	Serum creatinine (mg/dL)	% of standard initial infusion rate	mg/kg/hr
45 - 60	1.6 - 2	50%	0.075
30 - 44	2.1 - 3	30%	0.045
15 - 29	3.1 - 6	15%	0.0225
< 15[1]	> 6[1]	avoid or stop infusion[1]	

[1] In hemodialysis patients or in case of acute renal failure (Ccr < 15 mL/min or serum creatinine > 6 mg/dL), avoid or stop infusion of lepirudin. Consider additional IV bolus doses of 0.1 mg/kg every other day only if the aPTT ratio falls below the lower therapeutic limit of 1.5.

Concomitant use with thrombolytic therapy: Clinical trials in HIT patients have provided only limited information on the combined use of lepirudin and thrombolytic agents. The following dosage regimen of lepirudin was used in 9 HIT patients in the studies who presented with TECs at baseline and were started on both lepirudin and thrombolytic therapy (alteplase, urokinase, or streptokinase).

Pay special attention to the fact that thrombolytic agents per se may increase the aPTT ratio. Therefore, aPTT ratios with a given plasma level of lepirudin are usually higher in patients who receive concomitant thrombolysis than in those who do not.

Initial IV bolus – 0.2 mg/kg.

Continuous IV infusion – 0.1 mg/kg/hr.

Patients scheduled to switch to oral anticoagulation: If a patient is scheduled to receive coumarin derivatives (vitamin K antagonists) for oral anticoagulation after lepirudin therapy, the dose of lepirudin should first be gradually reduced in order to reach an aPTT ratio just above 1.5 before initiating oral anticoagulation. As soon as an international normalized ratio (INR) of 2 is reached, stop lepirudin therapy.

Preparation and dilution: Lepirudin should not be mixed with other drugs except Water for Injection, 0.9% Sodium Chloride Injection or 5% Dextrose Injection.
- For reconstitution, use Water for Injection or 0.9% Sodium Chloride Injection.
- For further dilution, 0.9% Sodium Chloride Injection or 5% Dextrose Injection are suitable.
- For rapid, complete reconstitution, inject 1 mL of diluent into the vial and shake it gently. After reconstitution a clear, colorless solution is usually obtained in a few seconds but definitely in < 3 minutes.
- Do not use solutions that are cloudy or contain particles.
- Immediately use the reconstitution solution. It remains stable for ≤ 24 hours at room temperature (eg, during infusion).
- Warm the preparation to room temperature before administration.
- Appropriately discard any unused solution.

Initial IV bolus: For IV bolus injection, use a solution with a concentration of 5 mg/mL. Preparation of lepirudin solution with a concentration of 5 mg/mL:
- Reconstitute one vial (50 mg) with 1 mL of Water for Injection or 0.9% Sodium Chloride Injection.
- The final concentration of 5 mg/mL is obtained by transferring the contents of the vial into a sterile, single-use syringe (of ≥ 10 mL capacity) and dilut-

ing the solution to a total volume of 10 mL using Water for Injection, 0.9% Sodium Chloride Injection, or 5% Dextrose Injection.

- The final solution is to be administered according to body weight (see following table).

IV injection of the bolus is to be carried out slowly (ie, over 15 to 20 seconds).

Standard Bolus Injection Volumes of Lepirudin According to Body Weight for a 5 mg/mL Concentration		
Body weight (kg)	Injection Volume	
	Dosage 0.4 mg/kg	Dosage 0.2 mg/kg[1]
50	4 mL	2 mL
60	4.8 mL	2.4 mL
70	5.6 mL	2.8 mL
80	6.4 mL	3.2 mL
90	7.2 mL	3.6 mL
100	8 mL	4 mL
≥ 110	8.8 mL	4.4 mL

[1] Dosage recommended for all patients with renal insufficiency.

IV infusion: For continuous IV infusion, solutions with concentration of 0.2 or 0.4 mg/mL may be used.

Preparation of a lepirudin solution with a concentration of 0.2 or 0.4 mg/mL:

- Reconstitute 2 vials (each containing 50 mg) with 1 mL each using either Water for Injection or 0.9% Sodium Chloride Injection.
- The final concentrations of 0.2 or 0.4 mg/mL are obtained by transferring the contents of both vials into an infusion bag containing 500 or 250 mL of 0.9% Sodium Chloride Injection or 5% Dextrose Injection.

The infusion rate (mL/hr) is to be set according to body weight (see following table).

Standard Infusion Rates of Lepirudin According to Body Weight		
	Infusion rate at 0.15 mg/kg/hr	
Body weight (kg)	500 mL infusion bag 0.2 mg/mL	250 mL infusion bag 0.4 mg/mL
50	38 mL/hr	19 mL/hr
60	45 mL/hr	23 mL/hr
70	53 mL/hr	26 mL/hr
80	60 mL/hr	30 mL/hr
90	68 mL/hr	34 mL/hr
100	75 mL/hr	38 mL/hr
≥ 110	83 mL/hr	41 mL/hr

Actions

Pharmacology: Lepirudin (rDNA), a recombinant hirudin derived from yeast cells, is a highly specific direct inhibitor of thrombin.

One molecule of lepirudin binds to one molecule of thrombin and thereby blocks the thrombogenic activity of thrombin. As a result, all thrombin-dependent coagulation assays are affected (eg, aPTT values increase in a dose-dependent fashion).

Pharmacokinetics:

Absorption/Distribution – Following IV administration, distribution is essentially confined to extracellular fluids and is characterized by an initial half-life of ≈ 10 minutes. Elimination follows a first-order process and is characterized by a terminal half-life of ≈ 1.3 hours in young healthy volunteers. As the IV dose is increased over the range of 0.1 to 0.4 mg/kg, the maximum plasma concentration and the AUC increase proportionally.

Metabolism/Excretion – Lepirudin is thought to be metabolized by release of amino acids via catabolic hydrolysis of the parent drug; however, conclusive data are not available. Approximately 48% of the administered dose is excreted in the urine, which consists of unchanged drug (35%) and other fragments of the parent drug.

The systemic clearance of lepirudin is proportional to the glomerular filtration rate or creatinine clearance. Dose adjustment based on creatinine clearance is recommended (see Administration and Dosage). In patients with marked renal insufficiency (creatinine clearance < 15 mL/min) and on hemodialysis, elimination half-lives are prolonged ≤ 2 days.

Special populations: The systemic clearance of lepirudin in women is ≈ 25% lower than in men. In elderly patients, the systemic clearance of lepirudin is 20% lower than in younger patients. This may be explained by the lower creatinine clearance in elderly patients compared with younger patients.

Contraindications
Hypersensitivity to hirudins.

Warnings
Intracranial bleeding: Following concomitant thrombolytic therapy with alteplase (tPA) or streptokinase may be life-threatening. Carefully assess the risk of lepirudin administration vs its anticipated benefit in patients with increased risk of bleeding. In particular, this includes the following conditions:
- Recent puncture of large vessels or organ biopsy
- Anomaly of vessels or organs
- Recent cerebrovascular accident, stroke, intracerebral surgery, or other neuraxial procedures
- Severe uncontrolled hypertension
- Bacterial endocarditis
- Advanced renal impairment (see Warnings)
- Hemorrhagic diathesis
- Recent major surgery
- Recent major bleeding (eg, intracranial, GI, intraocular, pulmonary)

Renal function impairment: With renal impairment, relative overdose might occur even with a standard dosage regimen. In patients with marked renal insufficiency (creatinine clearance < 15 mL/min) and on hemodialysis, elimination half-lives are prolonged ≤ 2 days. Reduce the bolus dose and rate of infusion in patients with known or suspected renal insufficiency (see Administration and Dosage).

Pregnancy: Category B. Use during pregnancy only if clearly needed.

Lactation: It is not known whether lepirudin is excreted in breast milk. Because of the potential for serious adverse reactions in nursing infants, decide whether to discontinue nursing or to discontinue the drug, taking into account the importance of the drug to the mother.

Children: Safety and efficacy have not been established.

Precautions
Antibodies: Formation of antihirudin antibodies was observed in ≈ 40% of HIT patients treated with lepirudin. This may increase the anticoagulant effect of lepirudin possibly because of delayed renal elimination of active lepirudin-antihirudin complexes. Therefore, strict monitoring of aPTT is necessary also during prolonged therapy. No evidence of neutralization of lepirudin or of allergic reactions associated with positive antibody test results was found.

Hepatic injury: Serious liver injury (eg, cirrhosis) may enhance the anticoagulant effect of lepirudin caused by coagulation defects secondary to reduced generation of vitamin K-dependent coagulation factors.

Reexposure: There is limited information to support any recommendations for reexposure to lepirudin. Of 13 patients reexposed in two studies, one experienced a mild allergic skin reaction during the second treatment cycle.

Allergic reactions: Approximately 53% of all allergic reactions or suspected allergic reactions occurred in patients who concomitantly received thrombolytic therapy (eg, streptokinase) for acute MI or contrast media for coronary angiography (see Adverse Reactions).

Lab test abnormalities: In general, adjust the dosage (infusion rate) according to the aPTT ratio (patient aPTT at a given time over an aPTT reference value, usually the median of the laboratory normal range for aPTT; see Administration and Dosage). Other thrombin- dependent coagulation assays are affected by lepirudin.

Drug Interactions
Drugs that may interact with lepirudin and increase the risk of bleeding include thrombolytics (eg, tPA, streptokinase) and coumarin derivatives (vitamin K antagonists).

Adverse Reactions
Adverse events occurring in ≥ 3% of patients include the following: Bleeding from puncture sites and wounds; anemia or isolated drop in hemoglobin; other hematoma and unclassified bleeding; hematuria; GI and rectal bleeding; epistaxis; fever; abnormal liver function; pneumonia; sepsis; allergic skin reactions; multiorgan failure.

ARGATROBAN

Injection: 100 mg/mL (*Rx*) | *Acova* (SmithKline Beecham)

Indications
Thrombosis, prophylaxis or treatment: As an anticoagulant for prophylaxis or treatment of thrombosis in heparin-induced thrombocytopenia.

Administration and Dosage
Preparation for IV administration: Dilute argatroban in 0.9% Sodium Chloride Injection, 5% Dextrose Injection, or Lactated Ringer's Injection to a final concentration of 1 mg/mL.

Initial dosage in heparin-induced thrombocytopenia: Before administering argatroban, discontinue heparin therpy and obtain a baseline activated partial thromboplastin time (aPTT). The recommended initial dose of argatroban for adults without hepatic impairment is 2 mcg/kg/min administered as a continuous infusion (see table).

| Standard Infusion Rates for 2 mcg/kg/min Dose of Argatroban (1 mg/mL Final Concentration) ||
Body weight (kg)	Infusion rate (mL/hr)
50	6
60	7
70	8
80	10
90	11
100	12
110	13
120	14
130	16
140	17

Monitoring and adjusting therapy:
Monitoring therapy – In general, therapy with argatroban is monitored using aPTT. Tests of anticoagulant effects (including aPTT) typically attain steady-state levels within 1 to 3 hours following initiation of argatroban. Dose adjustment may be required to attain the target aPTT. Check the aPTT 2 hours after initiation of therapy to confirm the aPTT is within the desired therapeutic range.

Dosage adjustment – After the initial dose of argatroban, the dose can be adjusted as clinically indicated (not to exeed 10 mcg/kg/min), until the steady-state aPTT is 1.5 to 3 times the initial baseline value (not to exceed 100 seconds).

Hepatically impaired patients – For patients with moderate hepatic impairment, an initial dose of 0.5 mcg/kg/min is recommended.

Conversion to oral anticoagulant therapy:

Initiating oral anticoagulant therapy – Recognize the potential for combined effects on International Normalized Ratio (INR) with coadministration of argatroban and warfarin. Do not use a loading dose of warfarin. Initiate therapy using the expected daily dose of warfarin.

Coadministration of warfarin and argatroban at doses ≤ 2 mcg/kg/min – Use of argatroban with warfarin results in prolongation of INR beyond that produced by warfarin alone. Measure INR daily while argatroban and warfarin are coadministered. In general, with doses of argatroban ≤ 2 mcg/kg/min, argatroban can be discontinued when the INR is > 4 on combined therapy. After argatroban is discontinued, repeat the INR measurement in 4 to 6 hours. If the repeat INR is below the desired therapeutic range, resume the infusion of argatroban and repeat the procedure daily until the desired therapeutic range on warfarin alone is reached.

Coadministration of warfarin and argatroban at doses > 2 mcg/kg/min – For doses > 2 mcg/kg/min, the relationship of INR on warfarin alone to the INR on warfarin plus argatroban is less predictable. In this case, in order to predict the INR on warfarin alone, temporarily reduce the dose of argatroban to a dose of 2 mcg/kg/min. Repeat the INR on argatroban and warfarin 4 to 6 hours after reduction of the argatroban dose and follow the process outlined above for administering argatroban at doses ≤ 2 mcg/kg/min.

Effect on INR: Because argatroban is a direct thrombin inhibitor, coadministration of argatroban and warfarin produces a combined effect on the laboratory measurement of the INR. However, concurrent therapy, compared with warfarin monotherapy, exerts no additional effect on vitamin K dependent factor Xa activity.

Actions

Pharmacology:

Mechanism of action – Argatroban, a synthetic, direct thrombin inhibitor derived from L-arginine, reversibly binds to the thrombin active site. It exerts its anticoagulant effects by inhibiting thrombin-catalyzed or induced reactions, including fibrin formation; activation of coagulation factors V, VIII, and XIII; protein C; and platelet aggregation.

Pharmacokinetics:

Distribution – Argatroban distributes mainly in the extracellular fluid; apparent steady-state volume of distribution is 174 mL/kg (12.18 L in a 70 kg adult). It is 54% bound to human serum proteins.

Metabolism – The main route of argatroban metabolism is hydroxylation and aromatization of the 3-methyltetrahydroquinoline ring in the liver by the human liver microsomal cytochrome P450 enzymes CYP3A4/5. Data suggest that CYP3A4/5 mediated metabolism is not an important elimination pathway in vivo.

Excretion – Total body clearance is ≈ 5.1 mL/min/kg (0.31 L/hr/kg) for infusion doses ≤ 40 mcg/kg/min. The terminal elimination half-life of argatroban ranges between 39 and 51 minutes. Argatroban is excreted primarily in the feces, presumably through biliary secretion.

Pharmacokinetic/Pharmacodynamic relationship – Steady-state levels of drug and anticoagulant effect are typically attained within 1 to 3 hours and are maintained until the infusion is discontinued or the dosage adjusted.

Contraindications

Overt major bleeding; hypersensitivity to this product or any of its components (see Warnings).

Warnings

Argatroban is intended for IV administration. Discontinue all parenteral anticoagulants before administration of argatroban.

Hemorrhage: Hemorrhage can occur at any site in the body in patients receiving argatroban. An unexplained fall in hematocrit or blood pressure, or any other unexplained symptom should lead to consideration of a hemorrhagic event. Use argatroban with extreme caution in disease states and other circumstances in which there is an increased danger of hemorrhage.

Hepatic function impairment: Exercise caution when administering argatroban to patients with hepatic disease by starting with a lower dose and carefully titrating until the desired level of anticoagulation is achieved. Also, upon cessation of argatroban infusion in the hepatically impaired patient, full reversal of anticoagulant effects may require > 4 hours because of decreased clearance and increased elimination half-life of argatroban (see Administration and Dosage).

Pregnancy: Category B.

Lactation: Discontinue nursing or discontinue the drug.

Children: The safety and effectiveness of argatroban in patients < 18 years of age have not been established.

Precautions

Lab test abnormalities: Anticoagulation effects associated with argatroban infusion at doses ≤ 40 mcg/kg/min are well correlated with the aPTT. Although other global clot-based tests including PT, the INR, ACT, and TT are affected by argatroban, the therapeutic ranges for these tests have not been identified for argatroban therapy. Plasma argatroban concentrations also correlate well with anticoagulant effects (see Pharmacology).

Drug Interactions

Concomitant use of argatroban with antiplatelet agents, thrombolytics, and other anticoagulants may increase the risk of bleeding (see Warnings).

Adverse Reactions

Adverse reactions occurring in ≥ 3% of patients include the following: Allergies, dyspnea, hypotension, fever, diarrhea, sepsis, cardiac arrest, nausea, ventricular tachycardia, pain, UTI, vomiting, infection, pneumonia, atrial fibrillation.

Major hemorrhagic events: GI (2.3%)

Minor hemorrhagic events: GI (14.4%); hematuria/GU (11.6%); decreased Hgb, HCT (10.4%); groin (5.4%); intracranial bleeding in post-MI patients receiving streptokinase (1%).

BIVALIRUDIN

Injection, lyophilized: 250 mg *(Rx)*   *Angiomax* (Medicines Co.)

Indications

Unstable angina: For use as an anticoagulant in patients with unstable angina undergoing percutaneous transluminal coronary angioplasty (PTCA). Bivalirudin is intended for use with aspirin and has been studied only in patients receiving concomitant aspirin.

Administration and Dosage

The recommended dosage of bivalirudin is an IV bolus of 1 mg/kg followed by a 4-hour IV infusion at a rate of 2.5 mg/kg/hr. After completion of the initial 4-hour infusion, an additional IV infusion of bivalirudin may be initiated at a rate of 0.2 mg/kg/hr for ≤ 20 hours, if needed. Bivalirudin is intended for use with aspirin (300 to 325 mg daily) and has been studied only in patients receiving concomitant aspirin. Initiate treatment with bivalirudin just prior to PTCA. The dose may need to be reduced, and anticoagulation status monitored, in patients with renal impairment.

Instructions for administration: Bivalirudin is intended for IV injection and infusion. To each 250 mg vial, add 5 mL of Sterile Water for Injection, USP. Gently swirl until all material is dissolved. Further dilute each reconstituted vial in 50 mL of 5% Dextrose in Water or 0.9% Sodium Chloride for Injection to yield a final concentration of 5 mg/mL (eg, 1 vial in 50 mL, 2 vials in 100 mL, 5 vials in 250 mL). Adjust the dose to be administered according to the patient's weight (see table below).

If the low-rate infusion is used after the initial infusion, prepare a lower concentration bag. In order to prepare this bag, reconstitute the 250 mg vial with 5 mL Sterile Water for Injection, USP. Gently swirl until all material is dissolved. Further dilute each reconstituted vial in 500 mL of 5% Dextrose in Water or 0.9% Sodium Chloride for Injection to yield a final concentration of 0.5 mg/mL. Select the infusion rate to be administered from the right-hand column of the table below.

Bivalirudin Dosing Table			
	Using 5 mg/mL concentration		Using 0.5 mg/mL concentration
Weight (kg)	Bolus (1 mg/kg) (mL)	Initial 4-hour infusion (2.5 mg/kg/hr) (mL/hr)	Subsequent low-rate infusion (0.2 mg/kg/hr) (mL/hr)
43 to 47	9	22.5	18
48 to 52	10	25	20
53 to 57	11	27.5	22
58 to 62	12	30	24
63 to 67	13	32.5	26
68 to 72	14	35	28
73 to 77	15	37.5	30
78 to 82	16	40	32
83 to 87	17	42.5	34
88 to 92	18	45	36
93 to 97	19	47.5	38
98 to 102	20	50	40
103 to 107	21	52.5	42
108 to 112	22	55	44
113 to 117	23	57.5	46
118 to 122	24	60	48
123 to 127	25	62.5	50
128 to 132	26	65	52
133 to 137	27	67.5	54
138 to 142	28	70	56
143 to 147	29	72.5	58
148 to 152	30	75	60

Administer bivalirudin via an IV line. Do not mix other medications with bivalirudin before or during administration. No incompatibilities have been observed with glass bottles or polyvinyl chloride bags and administration sets.

Inspect parenteral drug products visually for particulate matter and discoloration prior to administration. Do not use preparations of bivalirudin containing particulate matter.

Actions

Pharmacology: Bivalirudin directly inhibits thrombin by specifically binding to the catalytic site and to the anion-binding exosite of circulating and clot-bound thrombin. The binding of bivalirudin to thrombin is reversible.

Pharmacokinetics: Bivalirudin exhibits linear pharmacokinetics following IV administration to patients undergoing PTCA. In these patients, a mean steady-state bivalirudin concentration of ≈ 12.3 mcg/mL is achieved following an IV bolus of 1 mg/kg and a 4-hour 2.5 mg/kg/hr IV infusion. Bivalirudin is cleared from plasma by a combination of renal mechanisms and proteolytic cleavage, with a half-life in patients with normal renal function of 25 minutes. Drug elimination is related to glomular filtration rate (GFR). Total body clearance is similar for patients with normal renal function and with mild renal impairment (60 to 89 mL/min). Clearance is reduced ≈ 20% in patients with moderate and severe renal impairment and reduced ≈ 80% in dialysis-dependent patients. For patients with renal impairment, monitor the activated clotting time (ACT). Bivalirudin is hemodialyzable. Approximately 25% is cleared by hemodialysis.

Bivalirudin does not bind to plasma proteins (other than thrombin) or to red blood cells.

Special populations –

Bivalirudin Pharmacokinetic Parameters and Dose Adjustments in Renal Impairment			
Renal function (GFR, mL/min)	Clearance (mL/min/kg)	Half-life (minutes)	Percent reduction in infusion dose
Normal renal function (≥ 90 mL/min)	3.4	25	0
Mild renal impairment (60 to 90 mL/min)	3.4	22	0
Moderate renal impairment (30 to 59 mL/min)	2.7	34	20
Severe renal impairment (10 to 29 mL/min)	2.8	57	60
Dialysis-dependent patients (off dialysis)	1	3.5 hours	90

Contraindications
Active major bleeding; hypersensitivity to bivalirudin or any of its components.

Warnings
Immunogenicity/Reexposure: Among 494 subjects who received bivalirudin in clinical trials and were tested for antibodies, 2 subjects had treatment-emergent positive bivalirudin antibody tests. Neither subject demonstrated clinical evidence of allergic or anaphylactic reactions and repeat testing was not performed. Nine additional patients who had initial positive tests were negative on repeat testing.

Elderly: Of the total number of patients in clinical studies of bivalirudin undergoing PTCA, 41% were ≥ 65 years of age, while 11% were > 75 years of age. A difference of ≥ 5% between age groups was observed for heparin-treated but not bivalirudin-treated patients with regard to the percentage of patients with major bleeding events. There were no individual bleeding events that were observed with a difference of ≥ 5% between treatment groups, although puncture site hemorrhage and catheterization site hematoma were each observed in a higher percentage of patients ≥ 65 years of age than in patients < 65 years of age. This difference between age groups was more pronounced for heparin-treated than bivalirudin-treated patients.

Pregnancy: Category B.

Lactation: It is not known whether bivalirudin is excreted in breast milk. Exercise caution when bivalirudin is administered to a nursing woman.

Children: The safety and efficacy in pediatric patients have not been established.

Precautions
Monitoring: An unexplained fall in blood pressure or hematocrit, or any unexplained symptom, should lead to serious consideration of a hemorrhagic event and cessation of bivalirudin administration.

Drug Interactions
In clinical trials in patients undergoing PTCA, coadministration of bivalirudin with heparin, warfarin, or thrombolytics was associated with increased risks of major bleeding events compared with patients not receiving these concomitant medications. There is no experience with coadministration of bivalirudin and plasma expanders such as dextran. Use bivalirudin with caution in patients with disease states associated with an increased risk of bleeding.

Adverse Reactions
The most frequent adverse reactions reported were back pain, pain, nausea, headache, and hypotension. Percent of patients with major hemorrhage was 3.7%.

Adverse Events Other Than Bleeding Occurring in ≥ 5% of Patients in Either Treatment Group in Randomized Clinical Trials		
	Treatment group	
Adverse reaction	Bivalirudin (n = 2161)	Heparin (n = 2151)
Cardiovascular		
Hypotension	12	17
Hypertension	6	5
Bradycardia	5	8
CNS		
Headache	12	10
Insomnia	7	6
Anxiety	6	7
Nervousness	5	4
GI		
Nausea	15	16
Vomiting	6	8
Abdominal pain	5	5
Dyspepsia	5	5
Miscellaneous		
Back pain	42	44
Pain	15	17
Injection site pain	8	13
Pelvic pain	6	8
Fever	5	5
Urinary retention	4	5

Chapter 3

ENDOCRINE AND METABOLIC AGENTS

Estrogens, 91
   Vaginal Estrogens, 98
   Combined with Progestins, 99
Selective Estrogen Receptor Modulator, 100
   Raloxifene, 100
Progestins, 102
Contraceptive Products, 106
Levonorgestrel, 117
Medroxyprogesterone, 120
Androgens, 122
Androgen Hormone Inhibitor, 128
   Finasteride, 128
Danazol, 130
Adrenal Cortical Steroids, 132
   Glucocorticoids, 132
Antidiabetic Agents, 141
   Miglitol, 141
   Repaglinide, 142
   Nateglinide, 145
   Acarbose, 147
   Insulin, 148
   Insulin, Concentrated, 155
   Sulfonylureas, 156
   Metformin, 163
Thiazolidinediones, 167
Antidiabetic Combination Products, 171
   Glyburide/Metformin HCl, 171
Thyroid Hormones, 172
Antithyroid Agents, 177
Bisphosphonates, 179
Antidotes, 185
   Nalmefene, 186
   Naloxone, 189
   Naltrexone, 190
   Flumazenil, 192

ESTROGENS

ESTRONE AQUEOUS	
Injection: 5 mg/mL (*Rx*)	Various, *Kestrone 5* (Hyrex)
ESTRADIOL TRANSDERMAL SYSTEM	
Transdermal Patch: 0.025, 0.0375, 0.05, 0.075, and 0.1 mg per 24 hours (*Rx*)	*Estraderm* (Ciba), *Climara* (Berlex), *Vivelle* (Ciba-Geigy), *FemPatch* (Parke-Davis), *Esclim* (Serono), *Alora* (Procter & Gamble)
ESTRADIOL, ORAL	
Tablets: 0.5, 1, and 2 mg micronized estradiol (*Rx*)	Various, *Estrace* (Bristol-Myers Squibb)
ESTRADIOL VALERATE IN OIL	
Injection: 10, 20, and 40 mg per mL (*Rx*)	Various, *Delestrogen* (Bristol-Myers Squibb), *Estra-L 40* (Taylor), *Gynogen L.A. 20* (Forest), *Valergen 20* (Hyrex), *Valergen 40* (Hyrex)
CONJUGATED ESTROGENS, ORAL	
Tablets: 0.3, 0.625, 0.9, 1.25, and 2.5 mg (*Rx*)	*Premarin* (Wyeth-Ayerst)
CONJUGATED ESTROGENS, PARENTERAL	
Injection: 25 mg conjugated estrogens (*Rx*)	*Premarin Intravenous* (Wyeth-Ayerst)
ESTERIFIED ESTROGENS	
Tablets: 0.3, 0.625, 1.25, and 2.5 mg (*Rx*)	*Estratab* (Solvay Pharm.), *Menest* (SK-Beecham)
ESTROPIPATE	
Tablets: 0.75, 1.5, 3, and 6 mg estropipate (*Rx*)	Various, *Ogen* (Upjohn), *Ortho-Est* (Ortho)
ETHINYL ESTRADIOL	
Tablets: 0.02, 0.05, and 0.5 mg (*Rx*)	*Estinyl* (Schering)
SYNTHETIC CONJUGATED ESTROGENS, A	
Tablets: 0.625 and 0.9 mg (*Rx*)	*Cenestin* (Duramed)
ESTRADIOL HEMIHYDRATE	
Tablet, vaginal: 25 mcg (*Rx*)	*Vagifem* (Novo Nordisk)
ESTRADIOL CYPIONATE IN OIL	
Injection: 5 mg/mL (*Rx*)	Various, *depGynogen* (Forest), *Depo-Estradiol Cypionate* (Pharmacia & Upjohn), *DepoGen* (Hyrex)

Warning:

Estrogens have been reported to increase the risk of endometrial carcinoma.

When estrogens are used for the treatment of menopausal symptoms, use the lowest dose and discontinue medication as soon as possible. When prolonged treatment is indicated, reassess the patient at least semiannually to determine the need for continued therapy. Cyclic administration of low doses of estrogen may carry less risk than continuous administration.

Do not use estrogens during pregnancy.

The use of female sex hormones (both estrogens and progestins) during early pregnancy may seriously damage the offspring.

If estrogens are used during pregnancy, or if the patient becomes pregnant while taking estrogens, inform her of the potential risks to the fetus.

Indications

Estrogens are most commonly used as a component of combination contraceptives or as hormone replacement therapy in postmenopausal women. Benefits in postmenopausal women include relief of moderate to severe vasomotor symptoms, decreased risk of osteoporosis and cardiovascular disease. Hormone replacement therapy may also be used in female hypogonadism, castration, or primary ovarian failure. Less commonly, select breast or prostate cancer patients with advanced disease may receive estrogens as palliative therapy. **Estradiol hemihydrate** is used in the treatment of atrophic vaginitis.

Unlabeled uses: A 5 mcg ethinyl estradiol tablet is being investigated for use in the treatment of Turner's syndrome.

Administration and Dosage

Given cyclically for short-term use only: For treatment of moderate to severe vasomotor symptoms, atrophic vaginitis, or kraurosis vulvae associated with menopause. Administration should be cyclic (eg, 3 weeks on and 1 week off). Attempt to discontinue or taper medication at 3- to 6-month intervals.

Cyclical: Female hypogonadism or castration; primary ovarian failure; osteoporosis.

Chronic: Inoperable progressing prostatic cancer; inoperable progressing breast cancer.

Concomitant progestin therapy: Addition of a progestin for ≥ 10 to 13 days of a cycle of estrogen has lowered the incidence of endometrial hyperplasia. Morphological and biochemical studies of endometrium suggest that 10 to 14 days of progestin are needed to provide maximal maturation of the endometrium and to eliminate any hyperplastic changes. It is not established whether this will provide protection from endometrial carcinoma. There may be additional risks with the inclusion of progestin in estrogen replacement regimens, including adverse effects on carbohydrate and lipid metabolism (lowering HDL and raising LDL) which could diminish the purported cardioprotective effect of estrogen therapy; impairment of glucose tolerance; possible enhancement of mitotic activity in breast epithelial tissue, although few epidemiological data are available to address this point. Choice of progestin, cyclic or continuous mode, and dosage may be important in minimizing risks.

ESTRONE: Administer IM only. Shake vial and syringe well prior to withdrawal and injection (using a 21- to 23-gauge needle) to properly suspend medication.

> Cyclically –
>
> > *Replacement therapy of estrogen deficiency associated conditions (eg, hypogonadism, female castration, primary ovarian failure):* Initial relief of symptoms may be achieved through the administration of 0.1 to 1 mg of estrone weekly in single or divided doses. Some patients may require 0.5 to 2 mg/week.
> >
> > *Senile vaginitis and kraurosis vulvae:* Generally, 0.1 to 0.5 mg 2 or 3 times/week.
> >
> > *Abnormal uterine bleeding due to hormone imbalance:* May respond to brief courses of intensive therapy. Usual dose range is 2 to 5 mg/day for several days.
>
> Chronically –
>
> > *Inoperable progressing prostatic cancer:* For palliation in prostatic cancer, use estrone at 2 to 4 mg, 2 or 3 times/week. If a response to therapy is going to occur, it should be apparent within 3 months of beginning therapy. If a response does occur, continue the hormone until the disease is again progressive.
> >
> > *Inoperable progressing breast cancer in appropriately selected men and postmenopausal women:* 5 mg ≥ 3 times/week according to severity of pain.

ESTRADIOL TRANSDERMAL SYSTEM:

> Initiation of therapy –
>
> > *Treatment of menopausal symptoms:* Start with the 0.025 to 0.05 mg system applied to the skin twice weekly. Adjust dose as necessary to control symptoms. Use the lowest dosage necessary to control symptoms, especially in women with an intact uterus. Make attempts to taper or discontinue the drug at 3- to 6-month intervals.
> >
> > *Prophylaxis to prevent postmenopausal bone loss:* Initiate with 0.05 mg/day as soon as possible after menopause. Adjust dosage if necessary to control concurrent menopausal symptoms. Discontinuation may reestablish natural rate of bone loss.
> >
> > In women who are not taking oral estrogens, start treatment immediately. In women who are currently taking oral estrogens, start treatment 1 week after withdrawal of oral therapy or sooner if symptoms reappear in < 1 week.
> >
> > *Therapeutic regimen –* Therapy may be given continuously in patients who do not have an intact uterus. In patients with an intact uterus, therapy may be given on a cyclic schedule (eg, 3 weeks therapy followed by 1 week off).
> >
> > > *Estraderm, Alora, Esclim,* and *Vivelle* are applied twice a week; the *Climara* and *FemPatch* last for 7 days.
> > >
> > > *Application of system –* Place adhesive side of the system on a clean, dry area on the trunk of the body (including the buttocks and abdomen). Do not apply to breasts. Rotate application site with an interval of at least 1 week between applications to a particular site. The area should not be oily, damaged, or irritated. Avoid the

waistline, because tight clothing may rub the system off. Apply the system immediately after opening pouch and removing protective liner. Press firmly in place with the palm for ≈ 10 seconds. Make sure there is good contact, especially around the edges. In the unlikely event that a system should fall off, the same system may be reapplied. If necessary, apply a new system. In either case, continue the original treatment schedule.

ESTRADIOL, ORAL:

Moderate to severe vasomotor symptoms, vulva/vaginal atrophy associated with menopause, female hypogonadism, female castration, primary ovarian failure – Initiate treatment with 1 or 2 mg/day; adjust to control presenting symptoms. Titrate to determine the minimal effective dose for maintenance therapy.

Prostatic cancer (androgen-dependent, inoperable, progressing) – Administer 1 to 2 mg 3 times/day. Judge the effectiveness of therapy by phosphatase determinations and by symptomatic improvement of the patient.

Breast cancer (inoperable, progressing) – Given chronically in appropriately selected men and women, the usual dose is 10 mg 3 times/day for ≥ 3 months.

Osteoporosis prevention – Administer cyclically (eg, 23 days on, 5 days off) 0.5 mg/day as soon as possible after menopause. Adjust dosage if necessary to control concurrent menopause symptoms. Discontinuation may reestablish natural bone loss rate.

ESTRADIOL VALERATE IN OIL: Provides 2 to 3 weeks of estrogenic effect from a single IM injection.

For IM injection only.

Moderate to severe vasomotor symptoms, atrophic vaginitis or kraurosis vulvae associated with menopause, female hypogonadism, female castration, or primary ovarian failure – 10 to 20 mg every 4 weeks.

Prostatic carcinoma – ≥ 30 mg every 1 or 2 weeks.

CONJUGATED ESTROGENS, ORAL: Administer cyclically (3 weeks of daily estrogen and 1 week off) for all indications except selected cases of carcinoma.

Moderate to severe vasomotor symptoms associated with menopause – 1.25 mg/day. If the patient has not menstruated in ≥ 2 months, administration is started arbitrarily. If the patient is menstruating, begin administration on day 5 of bleeding.

Atrophic vaginitis and kraurosis vulvae associated with menopause – 0.3 to ≥ 1.25 mg/day, depending on tissue response of the patient.

Female hypogonadism – 2.5 to 7.5 mg/day, in divided doses for 20 days, followed by a rest period of 10 days. If bleeding does not occur by the end of this period, repeat dosage schedule. The number of courses of estrogen therapy necessary to produce bleeding may vary, depending on the responsiveness of the endometrium.

If bleeding occurs before the end of the 10-day period, begin a 20-day estrogen-progestin cyclic regimen with estrogen, 2.5 to 7.5 mg/day in divided doses. During the last 5 days of estrogen therapy, give an oral progestin. If bleeding occurs before this regimen is concluded, discontinue therapy and resume on the fifth day of bleeding.

Female castration and primary ovarian failure – 1.25 mg/day. Adjust according to severity of symptoms and patient response. For maintenance, adjust to lowest effective level.

Osteoporosis – 0.625 mg/day, cyclically.

Mammary carcinoma (for palliation) – 10 mg 3 times/day for ≥ 3 months.

Prostatic carcinoma (for palliation) – 1.25 to 2.5 mg 3 times/day. Effectiveness can be judged by phosphatase determinations as well as by symptomatic improvement.

CONJUGATED ESTROGENS, PARENTERAL: Treatment of abnormal uterine bleeding due to hormonal imbalance in the absence of organic pathology. Administration IV produces a more rapid response and is preferred. Usual dose is one 25 mg injection IV or IM. Repeat in 6 to 12 hours if necessary. Inject slowly to obviate the occurrence of flushes.

Compatibility – Infusion of conjugated estrogens with other agents is not recommended. However, in emergencies when an infusion has already been started, make the injection into the tubing just distal to the infusion needle. Solution is compatible with normal saline, dextrose, and invert sugar solutions. It is not compatible with protein hydrolysate, ascorbic acid, or any solution with an acid pH.

ESTERIFIED ESTROGENS:

Moderate to severe vasomotor symptoms, atrophic vaginitis or kraurosis vulvae associated with menopause – Cyclic therapy for short-term use. Average dose is 0.3 to ≥ 1.25 mg/day. Adjust dosage to the lowest effective level and discontinue as soon as possible.

Female hypogonadism – Administer 2.5 to 7.5 mg/day in divided doses for 20 days followed by a 10-day rest period. If bleeding does not occur by the end of this period, repeat the same dosage schedule. The number of courses of estrogen therapy necessary to produce bleeding varies, depending on endometrial responsiveness.

If bleeding occurs before the end of the 10-day period, begin a 20-day estrogen-progestin cyclic regimen of 2.5 to 7.5 mg/day in divided doses for 20 days. During the last 5 days of estrogen therapy, give an oral progestin. If bleeding occurs before this regimen is concluded, discontinue therapy; resume on the fifth day of bleeding.

Female castration and primary ovarian failure – Give 1.25 mg/day, cyclically.

Prostatic carcinoma (inoperable, progressing) – 1.25 to 2.5 mg 3 times/day. Judge the effectiveness of therapy by symptomatic response and phosphatase determinations.

Breast cancer (inoperable, progressing) – In appropriately selected men and postmenopausal women, give 10 mg 3 times/day for ≥ 3 months.

Osteoporosis prevention: Initiate therapy to prevent postmenopausal bone loss as soon as possible after menopause. Initiate at 0.3 mg/day and increase to a maximum daily dose of 1.25 mg/day if necessary to control concurrent menopausal symptoms.

ESTROPIPATE (Piperazine Estrone Sulfate):

Moderate to severe vasomotor symptoms, atrophic vaginitis or kraurosis vulvae associated with menopause – Give cyclically for short-term use. The lowest dose and regimen that will control symptoms should be chosen. Usual dosage range is 0.625 to 5 mg/day.

Female hypogonadism, female castration or primary ovarian failure – Administer cyclically, 1.5 to 9 mg estropipate (calculated as 1.25 to 7.5 mg estrone sulfate)/day for the first 3 weeks, followed by a rest period of 8 to 10 days. Repeat if bleeding does not occur by the end of the rest period. The duration of therapy necessary to produce withdrawal bleeding will vary according to the responsiveness of the endometrium. If satisfactory withdrawal bleeding does not occur, give an oral progestin in addition to estrogen during the third week of the cycle.

Osteoporosis prevention – 0.625 mg daily for 25 days of a 31 day cycle per month.

ETHINYL ESTRADIOL:

Moderate to severe vasomotor symptoms associated with menopause – Give cyclically for short-term use only. Choose the lowest dose that will control symptoms, and discontinue medication as promptly as possible. Administer cyclically (eg, 3 weeks on; 1 week off). Attempt to discontinue or taper medication at 3- to 6-month intervals. Usual dosage range is 0.02 to 0.5 mg/day. The effective dose may be as low as 0.02 mg every other day. Dosage schedule for early menopause, while spontaneous menstruation continues, is 0.05 mg once/day for 21 days followed by a 7-day rest period. May add a progestational agent during the latter part of the cycle.

For initial treatment of late menopause, the same regimen is indicated with 0.02 mg for the first few cycles, after which the 0.05 mg dosage may be substituted. In more severe cases, such as those due to surgical and roentgenologic castration, give 0.05 mg 3 times/day at the start of treatment. With adequate clinical improvement, usually obtainable in a few weeks, dosage may be reduced to 0.05 mg/day. A progestational agent may be added during the latter part of a planned cycle.

Female hypogonadism – 0.05 mg 1 to 3 times/day during the first 2 weeks of a theoretical menstrual cycle. Follow with a progestin during the last half of the arbitrary cycle. Continue for 3 to 6 months. The patient is then untreated for 2 months. Prescribe additional therapy if the cycle cannot be maintained without hormonal therapy.

Cancer of the female breast (inoperable, progressing) – In appropriately selected postmenopausal women, 1 mg 3 times/day given chronically for palliation.

Prostatic carcinoma (inoperable, progressing) – 0.15 to 2 mg/day given chronically for palliation.

SYNTHETIC CONJUGATED ESTROGENS, A:

Menopause – For treatment of moderate to severe vasomotor symptoms associated with menopause, choose the lowest dose and regimen that will control symptoms. Initial doses of 0.625 mg are recommended with titration up to 1.25 mg. Discontinue medication as promptly as possible. Attempt to discontinue or taper medication at 3- to 6-month intervals.

ESTRADIOL HEMIHYDRATE: Gently insert into the vagina as far as it can comfortably go without force, using the supplied applicator.

Initial dose – 1 tablet, inserted vaginally, once daily for 2 weeks. Have the patient administer treatment at the same time each day.

Maintenance dose – 1 tablet, inserted vaginally, twice weekly.

The physician should assess the need to continue therapy with the patient. Attempt to discontinue or taper medication at 3- to 6-month intervals.

ESTRADIOL CYPIONATE IN OIL: For IM use only.

Moderate to severe vasomotor symptoms associated with menopause – Usual dosage range is 1 to 5 mg IM, every 3 to 4 weeks. Attempt to discontinue or taper medication at 3- to 6-month intervals.

Female hypogonadism – 1.5 to 2 mg IM at monthly intervals.

Actions

Pharmacology: Although 6 different natural estrogens have been isolated from the human female, only 3 are present in significant quantities: Estradiol, estrone, and estriol. The most potent and major secretory product of the ovary, estradiol, is rapidly oxidized to estrone. Hydration of estrone produces the much weaker estriol. The estrogenic potency of estradiol is 12 times estrone's and 80 times estriol's.

Estrogens, important in developing and maintaining female reproductive system and secondary sex characteristics, promote growth and development of the vagina, uterus, fallopian tubes, and breasts. They affect release of pituitary gonadotropins; cause capillary dilatation, fluid retention, protein anabolism, and thin cervical mucus; inhibit or facilitate ovulation; prevent postpartum breast discomfort. Indirectly, they contribute to: Shaping the skeleton (conserving calcium and phosphorus and encouraging bone formation); maintenance of tone and elasticity of urogenital structures; changes in epiphyses of long bones that allow for pubertal growth spurt and its termination; growth of axillary and pubic hair; pigmentation of nipples and genitals.

Pharmacokinetics:

Absorption/Distribution – Absorption of most natural estrogens and their derivatives from the GI tract is complete. The limited oral effectiveness of natural estrogens and their esters is due to their metabolism. About 80% of estradiol is bound to sex hormone binding globulin; most of the rest is loosely bound to albumin and $\approx$ 2% is unbound. Estrone is highly bound to protein as it circulates in the blood, primarily as a conjugate with sulfate.

Transdermal system: In contrast to oral estradiol, the skin metabolizes estradiol via the transdermal system only to a small extent. Therefore, transdermal use produces therapeutic serum levels of estradiol with lower circulating levels of estrone and estrone conjugates, and requires smaller total doses. Transdermal use produces mean serum estradiol concentrations comparable with those produced by daily oral administration at $\approx$ 20 times the daily transdermal dose.

Metabolism/Excretion – Metabolism and inactivation occur primarily in the liver. During cyclic passage through the liver, estrogens are degraded to less active estrogenic compounds conjugated with sulfuric and glucuronic acids.

Contraindications

Breast cancer, except in appropriately selected patients being treated for metastatic disease; estrogen-dependent neoplasia; undiagnosed abnormal genital bleeding; active thrombophlebitis or thromboembolic disorders; history of thrombophlebitis, thrombosis or thromboembolic disorders associated with previous estrogen use (except when used in treatment of breast or prostatic malignancy); known or suspected pregnancy.

Warnings

Induction of malignant neoplasms: Estrogens may increase the risk of endometrial carcinoma.

Gallbladder disease: There is a 2- to 3-fold increase in risk of gallbladder disease in women receiving postmenopausal estrogens. This may be related to large doses.

Effects similar to those caused by estrogen-progestin oral contraceptives (OCs): Consider the following effects noted in OC users as potential risks of estrogen use:

Elevated blood pressure – Elevated blood pressure is common, but is less frequent with estrogen replacement therapy than with OC use.

Thromboembolic disease – OC users have an increased risk of thromboembolic and thrombotic vascular diseases, including thrombophlebitis, pulmonary embolism, stroke, and MI. Cases of retinal thrombosis, mesenteric thrombosis, and optic neuritis have been reported. The risk of several of these adverse reactions is dose-related. An increased risk of postsurgical thromboembolic complications has also been reported.

Some studies have shown that women taking estrogen replacement therapy have hypercoagulability, primarily related to decreased antithrombin activity. This effect appears dose- and duration-dependent and is less pronounced than that associated with oral contraceptive use. Also, postmenopausal women tend to have increased coagulation parameters at baseline compared with premenopausal women.

Do not use in people with active thrombophlebitis or thromboembolic disorders or in people with a history of such disorders associated with estrogen use (except in treatment of malignancy).

Large doses (conjugated estrogens 5 mg/day), comparable with those used to treat prostate and breast cancer, have increased risk of nonfatal MI, pulmonary embolism, and thrombophlebitis in men.

Familial hyperlipoproteinemia: Estrogen therapy may be associated with massive elevations of plasma triglycerides leading to pancreatitis and other complications in patients with familial defects of lipoprotein metabolism.

Hypercalcemia: Estrogens may lead to severe hypercalcemia in patients with breast cancer and bone metastases. If this occurs, discontinue the drug and take appropriate measures to reduce the serum calcium level.

Glucose tolerance: A worsening of glucose tolerance has been observed in a significant percentage of patients on estrogen-containing oral contraceptives. Carefully observe diabetic patients receiving estrogen.

Uterine leiomyomata: Preexisting uterine leiomyomata may increase in size during estrogen use.

Hepatic function impairment: Patients with a history of jaundice during pregnancy have an increased risk of recurrence while on estrogen-containing OCs. If jaundice develops in any patient on estrogen, discontinue medication and investigate the cause. Estrogens may be poorly metabolized in impaired liver function; use with caution.

Pregnancy: Category X (see Warning Box).

Lactation: Estrogens have been shown to decrease the quantity and quality of breast milk and may be excreted in breast milk. Administer only when clearly needed.

Children: Safety and efficacy are not established. Because of effects on epiphyseal closure, use judiciously in young patients in whom bone growth is incomplete.

Precautions

History/Physical exam: Before initiating estrogens, take complete medical and family history. Pretreatment and periodic history and physical exams every 12 months should include blood pressure, breasts, abdomen, pelvic organs, and a Papanicolaou smear.

Excessive estrogenic stimulation: Certain patients may develop undesirable manifestations of excessive estrogenic stimulation (eg, abnormal or excessive uterine bleeding, mastodynia). Advise the pathologist of estrogen therapy when relevant specimens are submitted.

Estropipate vaginal cream: Rule out gonorrhea or neoplasia before prescribing estropipate vaginal cream. Treat trichomonal, monilial, or bacterial infection with appropriate antimicrobial therapy.

Fluid retention: Estrogens may cause some degree of fluid retention; conditions which might be influenced by this factor (eg, asthma, epilepsy, migraine, cardiac or renal dysfunction) require careful observation.

Calcium and phosphorus metabolism: Calcium and phosphorus metabolism is influenced by estrogens; use caution in patients with metabolic bone diseases associated with hypercalcemia or in renal insufficiency.

Prolonged: Prolonged unopposed estrogen therapy may increase risk of endometrial hyperplasia.

Acute intermittent porphyria: Acute intermittent porphyria may be precipitated by estrogens.

Benzyl alcohol: Benzyl alcohol, contained in some of these products as a preservative, has been associated with a fatal "gasping syndrome" in premature infants.

Photosensitivity: Photosensitization may occur; therefore, caution patients to take protective measures (ie, sunscreens, protective clothing).

Tartrazine sensitivity: Some of these products contain tartrazine which may cause allergic-type reactions (including bronchial asthma) in susceptible individuals. Although the incidence of sensitivity is low, it is frequently seen in patients who also have aspirin hypersensitivity.

Drug Interactions
Drugs that may be affected by estrogens include oral anticoagulants, tricyclic antidepressants, hydantoins, and corticosteroids.

Drugs that may affect estrogens include barbiturates, rifampin, and hydantoins.

Drug/Lab test interactions: Certain endocrine and liver function tests may be affected by estrogen-containing OCs. Expect these similar changes with larger doses:

Increased sulfobromophthalein retention.

Increased prothrombin and factors VII, VIII, IX, and X; decreased antithrombin III; increased norepinephrine-induced platelet aggregability.

Increased thyroid binding globulin (TBG) leading to increased circulating total thyroid hormone, as measured by PBI, T_4 by column, or T_4 by radioimmunoassay. Free T_3 resin uptake is decreased, reflecting the elevated TBG; free T_4 concentration is unaltered.

Impaired glucose tolerance; decreased pregnanediol excretion; reduced response to metyrapone test; reduced serum folate concentration.

Increased plasma HDL and HDL-2 subfraction concentrations, reduced LDL cholesterol concentration levels, increased triglyceride levels.

Adverse Reactions
Significant adverse reactions include breakthrough bleeding; spotting; change in menstrual flow; dysmenorrhea; premenstrual-like syndrome; amenorrhea during and after treatment; nausea; vomiting; abdominal cramps; bloating; cholestatic jaundice; chloasma or melasma (may persist when drug is discontinued); erythema nodosum/multiforme; hemorrhagic eruption; urticaria; dermatitis; steepening of corneal curvature; intolerance to contact lenses; headache; migraine; dizziness; mental depression; convulsions; pain at injection site; sterile abscess; postinjection flare; redness and irritation at application site with the estradiol transdermal system (17%); aggravation of porphyria; edema; changes in libido; breast tenderness, enlargement, or secretion.

MISCELLANEOUS ESTROGENS, VAGINAL

Cream: 1.5 mg estropipate/g (*Rx*)	*Ogen* (Pharmacia & Upjohn)
0.1 mg estradiol/g (*Rx*)	*Estrace* (Bristol-Myers Squibb)
0.625 mg conjugated estrogens/g (*Rx*)	*Premarin* (Wyeth-Ayerst)
0.01% dienestrol (*Rx*)	*Ortho Dienestrol* (Ortho Pharm)
Ring: 2 mg estradiol (*Rx*)	*Estring* (Pharmacia & Upjohn)

Indications

Treatment of atrophic vaginitis (cream or ring) and kraurosis vulvae (cream) associated with menopause.

Administration and Dosage

Treatment of atrophic vaginitis, kraurosis vulvae associated with menopause: Choose the lower dose that will control symptoms and discontinue medication as promptly as possible. Make attempts to discontinue or taper medication at 3- to 6-month intervals.

Estropipate and conjugated estrogens – Administer cyclically; 3 weeks on and 1 week off. Give ½ to 2 g/day of conjugated estrogens and 2 to 4 g/day of estropipate intravaginally depending on severity of condition.

Estradiol –

Cream: 2 to 4 g/day for 1 or 2 weeks. Gradually reduce to 50% of the initial dosage for a similar period. A maintenance dose of 1 g 1 to 3 times/week may be used after restoration of the vaginal mucosa has been achieved.

Ring: Insert as deeply as possible into the upper one-third of the vaginal vault. The ring is to remain in place continuously for 3 months, after which it should be removed, and if appropriate, replaced by a new ring.

Should the ring be removed or fall out at any time during the 90-day treatment period, rinse the ring in lukewarm water and re-insert.

Dienestrol – Usual dosage is 1 applicatorful once or twice daily for 1 or 2 weeks, then reduce to initial dosage for a similar period. A maintenance dosage of 1 applicatorful 1 to 3 times/week may be used after restoration of vaginal mucosa has been achieved.

Actions

Pharmacology: The signs and symptoms of vulvovaginal epithelial atrophy (atrophic vaginitis) may be alleviated by the topical application of an estrogenic hormone.

Warnings

Vaginal bleeding: Uterine bleeding might be provoked by excessive administration in menopausal women. Evaluation may be required to differentiate this uterine bleeding from carcinoma. Breast tenderness and vaginal discharge may result from excessive estrogenic stimulation; endometrial withdrawal bleeding may occur if use is suddenly discontinued.

ESTROGENS AND PROGESTINS COMBINED

Tablets: 0.625 mg conjugated estrogens/5 mg medroxyprogesterone acetate, 0.625 mg conjugated estrogens/2.5 mg medroxyprogesterone acetate (*Rx*)

Prempro (Wyeth-Ayerst)

0.625 mg conjugated estrogens, 0.625 mg conjugated estrogens/5 mg medroxyprogesterone acetate (*Rx*)

Premphase (Wyeth-Ayerst)

5 mcg ethinyl estradiol/1 mg norethindrone acetate (*Rx*)

Femhrt (Parke-Davis)

1 mg estradiol/0.5 mg norethindrone acetate (*Rx*)

Activella (Pharmacia)

1 mg estradiol; 1 mg estradiol/0.09 mg norgestimate (*Rx*)

Ortho-Prefest (Ortho-McNeil)

Transdermal patch: 0.05 mg estradiol/0.14 mg norethindrone acetate; 0.05 mg estradiol/0.25 mg norethindrone acetate (*Rx*)

CombiPatch (Aventis)

Indications

In women with an intact uterus for the treatment of moderate to severe vasomotor symptoms associated with menopause; treatment of vulval and vaginal atrophy (*Femhrt* excluded); osteoporosis prevention (*CombiPatch* excluded); treatment of hypoestrogenism caused by hypogonadism, castration, or primary ovarian failure (*CombiPatch* only).

Unlabeled uses: May be an effective alternative to treat hypercholesterolemia in postmenopausal women (0.3 to 1.25 mg conjugated estrogens with 5 mg medroxyprogesterone).

Administration and Dosage

Prempro: One 0.625 mg/2.5 mg tablet once daily; can increase to 0.625 mg/5 mg once daily.

Premphase: One 0.625 mg conjugated estrogens tablet once daily on days 1 through 14 and one 0.625 mg conjugated estrogen/5 mg medroxyprogesterone tablet taken once daily on days 15 through 28.

Femhrt and Activella: One tablet/day.

Ortho-Prefest: One pink tablet/day for 3 days, followed by 1 white tablet/day for 3 days. This regimen is repeated continuously without interruption.

CombiPatch: Replace the patch system twice weekly. Advise women that monthly withdrawal bleeding often occurs.

Apply to a smooth (fold-free) clean, dry area of the skin on the lower abdomen. Do not apply to or near the breasts and avoid the waistline. The sites of application must be rotated; allow an interval of ≥ 1 week between applications to the same site.

Continuous combined regimen – Apply twice weekly during a 28-day cycle. Irregular bleeding may occur particularly in the first 6 months.

Continuous sequential regimen – It can be applied as a sequential regimen in combination with an estradiol-only transdermal delivery system.

Menopause and vulval/vaginal atrophy: Reevaluate patients at 3- to 6-month intervals to determine the need for continued treatment.

Osteoporosis: The mainstays of prevention and management of osteoporosis are estrogen and calcium; exercise and nutrition may be important adjuncts.

Monitoring: Monitor closely for signs of endometrial cancer; evaluate recurrent or persistent abnormal vaginal bleeding appropriately to rule out malignancy.

RALOXIFENE

Tablets: 60 mg (*Rx*)   *Evista* (Eli Lilly)

Indications

Osteoporosis, prevention and treatment: Prevention and treatment of osteoporosis in post-menopausal women.

Administration and Dosage

The recommended dosage is 60 mg/day, which may be administered any time of day without regard to meals.

Actions

Pharmacology: Raloxifene is a selective estrogen receptor modulator (SERM) that reduces resorption of bone and decreases overall bone turnover.

Pharmacokinetics:

Absorption – Raloxifene is absorbed rapidly after oral administration with ≈ 60% of an oral dose adsorbed. However, presystemic glucuronide conjugation is extensive and absolute bioavailability is only 2%.

Distribution – The apparent volume of distribution is 2348 L/kg and is not dose-dependent. Raloxifene and the monoglucuronide conjugates are highly bound to plasma proteins (95%).

Metabolism – Raloxifene undergoes extensive first-pass metabolism to the glucuronide conjugates. Raloxifene is not metabolized by cytochrome P450 pathways. Plasma elimination half-life to 27.7 hours after single dose oral dosing and 32.5 after multiple dose oral dosing.

Excretion – Raloxifene is primarily excreted in feces; < 6% of the raloxifene dose is eliminated in urine as glucuronide conjugates and < 0.2% is excreted unchanged in urine.

Contraindications

Women who are lactating or who are or may become pregnant (see Warnings); women with active or a history of venous thromboembolic events, including deep vein thrombosis, pulmonary embolism, and retinal vein thrombosis; hypersensitivity to raloxifene or other constituents of the drug.

Warnings

Venous thromboembolic events: An analysis of raloxifene-treated women showed an increased risk of venous thromboembolic events defined as DVT and pulmonary embolism. Other venous thromboembolic events could also occur. A less serious event, superficial thrombophlebitis, has been reported more frequently with raloxifene. The greatest risk for DVT and pulmonary embolism occurs during the first 4 months of treatment. Discontinue raloxifene ≥ 72 hours prior to and during prolonged immobilization (eg, postsurgical recovery, prolonged bed rest), and resume therapy only after the patient is fully ambulatory. Advise patients to avoid prolonged restrictions of movement during travel.

Premenopausal use: There is no indication for premenopausal use of raloxifene.

Carcinogenesis: In long term carcinogenicity studies in animals there was an increased incidence of ovarian tumors, testicular interstitial cell tumors, and prostatic adenocarcinomas.

Fertility impairment: Raloxifene delayed and disrupted embryo implantation resulting in prolonged gestation and reduced litter size.

Pregnancy: Category X.

Lactation: Raloxifene should not be used by lactating women.

Children: Raloxifene should not be used in pediatric patients.

Precautions

Concurrent estrogen therapy: The concurrent use of raloxifene and systemic estrogen or hormone replacement therapy (ERT or HRT) has not been studied in prospective clinical trials; therefore, concomitant use is not recommended.

Lipid metabolism: Raloxifene lowers serum total and LDL cholesterol by 6% to 11% but does not affect serum concentrations of total HDL cholesterol or triglycerides. Take these effects into account in therapeutic decisions for patients who may require therapy for hyperlipidemia.

Limited clinical data suggest that some women with a history of marked hypertriglyceridemia (> 5.6 mmol/L or > 500 mg/dL) in response to treatment with oral estrogen or estrogen plus progestin may develop increased levels of tryglycerides when treated with raloxifene. Women with this medical history should have serum triglycerides monitored when taking raloxifene.

Endometrium: Raloxifene has not been associated with endometrial proliferation. Investigate unexplained uterine bleeding as clinically indicated.

Supplemental calcium: Add supplemental calcium to the diet if daily intake is inadequate.

Drug Interactions

Highly protein-bound drugs: In vitro, raloxifene did not affect the binding of warfarin, phenytoin, or tamoxifen. However, use caution when raloxifene is coadministered with other highly protein-bound drugs, such as diazepam, diazoxide, and lidocaine.

Drugs that may interact with raloxifene include ampicillin and cholestyramine. Raloxifene may affect warfarin.

Adverse Reactions

Adverse reactions occurring in ≥ 3% of patients include hot flashes; depression; insomnia; vertigo; rash; sweating; nausea; diarrhea; dyspepsia; vomiting; flatulence; GI disorder; vaginits; UTI; cystitis; leukorrhea; uterine disorder; endometrial disorder; weight gain; peripheral edema; arthralgia; myalgia; leg cramps; arthritis; tendon disorder; sinusitis; rhinitis; bronchitis; pharyngitis; increased cough; infection; flu syndrome; headache; chest pain; fever.

Lab test abnormalities: Increased apolipoprotein A1; reduced serum total cholesterol, LDL cholesterol, fibrinogen, apolipoprotein B, and lipoprotein. Raloxifene modestly increases hormone-binding globulin concentrations, including sex steroid-binding globulin, thyroxine-binding globulin, and corticosteroid-binding globulin with corresponding increases in measured total hormone concentrations.

There were small decreases in serum total calcium, inorganic phosphate, total protein, and albumin which were generally of lesser magnitude than decreases observed during ERT/HRT. Platelet count was also decreased slightly and was not different from ERT.

Patient Information

Patient immobilization: Discontinue raloxifene ≥ 72 hours prior to and during prolonged immobilization (eg, post-surgical recovery, prolonged bed rest) and advise patients to avoid prolonged restrictions of movement during travel because of the increased risk of venous thromboembolic events.

PROGESTINS

HYDROXYPROGESTERONE IN OIL	
Injection: 125 and 250 mg/mL (*Rx*)	Various, *Hylutin* (Hyrex), *Hyprogest 250* (Keene)
MEDROXYPROGESTERONE	
Tablets: 2.5 mg and 5 mg (*Rx*)	*Cycrin* (ESI Pharma), *Provera* (Upjohn)
10 mg (*Rx*)	Various, *Amen* (Carnrick), *Curretab* (Solvay), *Provera* (Upjohn)
MEGESTROL ACETATE	
Tablets: 20 and 40 mg	Various, *Megace* (Bristol-Myers Oncology)
Suspension: 40 mg/mL (*Rx*)	*Megace* (Bristol-Myers Oncology)
NORETHINDRONE ACETATE	
Tablets: 5 mg (*Rx*)	*Aygestin* (Wyeth-Ayerst)
PROGESTERONE IN OIL	
Injection: 50 mg/mL (*Rx*)	Various
PROGESTERONE POWDER	
Powder (*Rx*)	Various
PROGESTERONE GEL	
Vaginal Gel: 8% (90 mg) (*Rx*)	*Crinone* (Wyeth Labs)

Warning:

Pregnancy: Progestins have been used beginning with the first trimester of pregnancy to prevent habitual abortion or treat threatened abortion; however, there is no adequate evidence that such use is effective. There is evidence of potential harm to the fetus when given during the first 4 months of pregnancy. Therefore, the use of such drugs during the first 4 months of pregnancy is not recommended.

The cause of abortion is generally a defective ovum, which progestational agents could not be expected to influence. In addition, progestational agents have uterine relaxant properties that may cause a delay in spontaneous abortion when given to patients with fertilized defective ova.

Indications

Amenorrhea; abnormal uterine bleeding; endometriosis (norethindrone only).

Megestrol: Treatment of anorexia, cachexia, or an unexplained significant weight loss in patients with a diagnosis of acquired immunodeficiency syndrome (AIDS).
Palliative treatment of advanced carcinoma of the breast or endometrium.

Progesterone gel: Progesterone supplementation or replacement as part of an Assisted Reproductive Technology (ART) treatment for infertile women with progesterone deficiency.

Unlabeled uses: Medroxyprogesterone acetate (10 mg/day) has been used in the treatment of menopausal symptoms and to stimulate respiration in obstructive sleep apnea and other forms of chronic hypoventilation.
Progesterone suppositories (rectal or vaginal, 200 to 400 mg twice daily) have been used in premenstrual syndrome (PMS).
Norethindrone (5 mg/day) appears to be effective in the treatment of hyperparathyroidism associated with mild hypercalcemia in postmenopausal women.

Administration and Dosage

HYDROXYPROGESTERONE IN OIL: For IM use.

Amenorrhea (primary and secondary); dysfunctional uterine bleeding; metrorrhagia – Usual adult dose: 375 mg.

Production of secretory endometrium and desquamation – Test for continuous endogenous estrogen production (Medical D and C). Usual adult dose 125 to 250 mg given on tenth day of cycle; repeat every 7 days until suppression is no longer desired.

MEDROXYPROGESTERONE ACETATE: For information on parenteral medroxyprogesterone acetate, refer to monograph in Antineoplastics chapter.

Secondary amenorrhea – 5 to 10 mg/day for 5 to 10 days. A dose for inducing an optimum secretory transformation of an endometrium that has been adequately primed with either endogenous or exogenous estrogen is 10 mg daily for 10 days. Start therapy any time. Withdrawal bleeding usually occurs 3 to 7 days after therapy ends.

Abnormal uterine bleeding due to hormonal imbalance in the absence of organic pathology – 5 to 10 mg/day for 5 to 10 days, beginning on the 16th or 21st day of the menstrual cycle. To produce an optimum secretory transformation of an endometrium that has been adequately primed with either endogenous or exogenous estrogen, give 10 mg/day for 10 days, beginning on the 16th day of the cycle. Withdrawal bleeding usually occurs 3 to 7 days after discontinuing therapy. Patients with recurrent episodes of abnormal uterine bleeding may benefit from planned menstrual cycling with medroxyprogesterone acetate.

MEGESTROL ACETATE: Initial dose is 800 mg/day (20 mL/day); daily doses of 400 and 800 mg/day were found to be clinically effective. Shake container well before using.

NORETHINDRONE ACETATE: Norethindrone acetate differs from norethindrone only in potency; the acetate is approximately twice as potent.

Secondary amenorrhea; abnormal uterine bleeding due to hormonal imbalance in the absence of organic pathology – 2.5 to 10 mg/day for 5 to 10 days during the second half of the theoretical menstrual cycle. Withdrawal bleeding usually occurs within 3 to 7 days.

Endometriosis –

Initial dose: 5 mg/day for 2 weeks; increase in increments of 2.5 mg/day every 2 weeks until 15 mg/day is reached. Therapy may be held at this level for 6 to 9 months or until breakthrough bleeding demands temporary termination.

PROGESTERONE: For IM use. The drug is irritating at the injection site.

Amenorrhea – Administer 5 to 10 mg/day for 6 to 8 consecutive days. If ovarian activity has produced a proliferative endometrium, expect withdrawal bleeding 48 to 72 hours after the last injection. Spontaneous normal cycles may follow.

Functional uterine bleeding – Administer 5 to 10 mg/day for 6 doses. Bleeding should cease within 6 days. When estrogen also is given, begin progesterone after 2 weeks of estrogen therapy. Discontinue injections when menstrual flow begins.

Progesterone is available as a micronized powder for prescription compounding.

PROGESTERONE GEL:

Infertility – For progesterone supplementation or replacement as part of an Assisted Reproductive Technology (ART) treatment for infertile women with progesterone deficiency. Administer 90 mg vaginally once daily in women who require progesterone supplementation. In women with partial or complete ovarian failure who require progesterone replacement, administer 90 mg vaginally twice daily. If pregnancy occurs, continue treatment until placental autonomy is achieved, ≤ 10 to 12 weeks.

Actions

Pharmacology: Progesterone, a principle of corpus luteum, is the primary endogenous progestational substance. Progestins (progesterone and derivatives) transform proliferative endometrium into secretory endometrium. They inhibit (at the usual dose range) the secretion of pituitary gonadotropins, which in turn prevents follicular maturation and ovulation. They also inhibit spontaneous uterine contraction. Progestins may demonstrate some estrogenic, anabolic, or androgenic activity. The precise mechanism by which megestrol produces effects in anorexia and cachexia is unknown.

Pharmacokinetics: Absorption of oral tablets and parenteral oily solutions of progestins is rapid; however, the hormone undergoes prompt hepatic transformation.

Contraindications

Hypersensitivity to progestins; thrombophlebitis, thromboembolic disorders, cerebral hemorrhage or patients with a history of these conditions; impaired liver function or disease; carcinoma of the breast; undiagnosed vaginal bleeding; missed abortion; as a diagnostic test for pregnancy; known or suspected pregnancy; prophylactic use to avoid weight loss (megestrol).

Warnings

Ophthalmologic effects: Discontinue medication pending examination if there is a sudden partial or complete loss of vision, or if there is sudden onset of proptosis, diplopia, or migraine. If papilledema or retinal vascular lesions are present, discontinue use.

Thrombotic disorders: Thrombotic disorders (thrombophlebitis, cerebrovascular disorders, retinal thrombosis, pulmonary embolism) occasionally occur in patients taking progestins.

HIV-infected women: Although megestrol has been used extensively in women for endometrial and breast cancers, its use in HIV-infected women has been limited. All the women in the clinical trials reported breakthrough bleeding.

Fertility impairment: Medroxyprogesterone acetate at high doses is an antifertility drug. High doses would be expected to impair fertility until the cessation of treatment.

Pregnancy: Category D (progesterone injection); *Category X* (norethindrone acetate). Use is not recommended. See Warning Box.

Lactation: Detectable amounts of progestins enter the milk of mothers receiving these agents. The effect on the nursing infant has not been determined.

Medroxyprogesterone does not adversely affect lactation and may increase milk production and duration of lactation if given in the puerperium.

Children: Safety and efficacy of megestrol acetate suspension in children have not been established.

Precautions

Causes of weight loss: Institute therapy with megestrol for weight loss only after treatable causes of weight loss are sought and addressed.

Respiratory infections: Long-term treatment may increase the risk of respiratory infections.

Pretreatment physical examination: Pretreatment physical examination should include breasts and pelvic organs, as well as Papanicolaou smear.

Fluid retention: Fluid retention may occur; therefore, conditions influenced by this factor (epilepsy, migraine, asthma, cardiac, or renal dysfunction) require careful observation.

Depression: Observe patients who have a history of psychic depression and discontinue the drug if the depression recurs to a serious degree.

Glucose tolerance: A decrease in glucose tolerance has been observed in a small percentage of patients on estrogen-progestin combination drugs. Carefully observe diabetic patients receiving progestin therapy.

Menopause: The age of the patient constitutes no absolute limiting factor, although treatment with progestins may mask the onset of the climacteric.

Photosensitivity: Photosensitization (photoallergy or phototoxicity) may occur.

Drug Interactions

Drugs that may interact with progestins include aminoglutethimide and rifampin.

Drug/Lab test interactions: Laboratory test results of hepatic function, coagulation tests (increase in prothrombin, Factors VII, VIII, IX, and X), thyroid, metyrapone test and endocrine functions, may be affected by progestins or estrogens. A decrease in glucose tolerance has been observed in a small percentage of patients on estrogen-progestin combination drugs. Pregnanediol determination may be altered by the use of progestins.

Adverse Reactions

Adverse reactions that may occur include breakthrough bleeding, spotting, change in menstrual flow, amenorrhea, changes in cervical erosion and cervical secretions; breast changes (tenderness); masculinization of the female fetus; edema; changes in weight (increase or decrease); cholestatic jaundice; rash (allergic) with and without pruritus; acne; melasma or chloasma; mental depression; alopecia; hirsutism; thromboembolic phenomena including thrombophlebitis and pulmonary embolism; sensitivity reactions ranging from pruritus and urticaria to generalized rash (medroxyprogesterone acetate).

For information concerning adverse reactions associated with combined estrogen-progestin therapy, refer to the Oral Contraceptives monograph.

Megestrol: Adverse reactions occuring in ≥ 3% of patients include diarrhea; impotence; rash; flatulence; hypertension; asthenia; insomnia; nausea; anemia; fever; libido decreased; hyperglycemia; headache.

CONTRACEPTIVE PRODUCTS

MONOPHASIC ORAL CONTRACEPTIVES

Tablets: Estrogens (ethinyl estradiol, mestranol), progestins (desogestrel, drospirenone, ethynodiol diacetate, levonorgestrel, norethindrone, norethindrone acetate, norgestimate, norgestrel) (*Rx*)

Alesse (Wyeth-Ayerst), *Apri, Aviane* (Duramed), *Brevicon* (Watson), *Demulen* (Searle), *Desogen* (Organon), *Levlen* (Berlex), *Levora* (Watson), *Levlite* (Berlex), *Loestrin* (Parke-Davis), *Lo/Ovral* (Wyeth Ayerst), *Low-Ogestrel* (Watson), *Microgestin Fe* (Watson), *Modicon* (Ortho-McNeil), *Necon* (Watson), *Nordette* (Monarch), *Norinyl* (Watson), *Nortrel* (Barr) *Ogestrel* (Watson), *Ortho-Cept, Ortho-Cyclen, Ortho-Novum* (Ortho-McNeil), *Ovcon* (Warner Chilcott), *Ovral* (Wyeth-Ayerst), *Yasmin* (Berlex), *Zovia* (Watson)

BIPHASIC ORAL CONTRACEPIVES

Tablets: Estrogen (ethinyl estradiol), progestin (norethindrone, desogestrel) (*Rx*)

Jenest-28, Mircette (Organon), *Necon 10/11* (Watson), *Ortho-Novum 10/11* (Ortho-McNeil)

TRIPHASIC ORAL CONTRACEPTIVES

Tablets: Estrogen (ethinyl estradiol), progestin (levonorgestrel, norethindrone, norgestimate) (*Rx*)

Estrostep 21, Estrostep Fe (Parke-Davis), *Ortho-Novum 777, Ortho Tri-Cyclen* (Ortho-McNeil), *Tri-Levlen* (Berlex), *Tri-Norinyl* (Watson), *Triphasil* (Wyeth-Ayerst) *Trivora-28* (Watson)

PROGESTIN-ONLY PRODUCTS

Tablets: Norethindrone 0.35 mg (*Rx*)

Micronor (Ortho-McNeil), *Nor-QD* (Watson)

Norgestrel 0.075 mg (*Rx*)

Ovrette (Wyeth-Ayerst)

EMERGENCY CONTRACEPTIVES

Tablets: 0.75 mg levonorgestrel (*Rx*)

Plan B (Women's Capital Corp.)

0.25 mg levonorgestrel, 0.05 mg ethinyl estradiol (*Rx*)

Preven (Gynètics)

NORELGESTROMIN/ETHINYL ESTRADIOL TRANSDERMAL SYSTEM

Patch: 6 mg norelgestromin, 0.75 mg ethinyl estradiol/total patch content

Ortho Evra (Ortho-McNeil)

Warning:

Cigarette smoking: Cigarette smoking increases the risk of cardiovascular side effects from hormonal contraceptive use. This risk increases with age and with heavy smoking ($\geq$ 15 cigarettes/day) and is quite marked in women > 35 years of age. Women who use hormonal contraceptives should not smoke.

Indications

Contraceptive: For the prevention of pregnancy. Start new patients on preparations containing $\leq$ 35 mcg estrogen.

Emergency contraception: For prevention of pregnancy following unprotected intercourse or a known or suspected contraceptive failure. To obtain efficacy, the first dose should be taken as soon as possible within 72 hours of intercourse. The second dose must be taken 12 hours later.

Acne vulgaris (Ortho Tri-Cyclen only): For the treatment of moderate acne vulgaris in females $\geq$ 15 years of age who have no known contraindications to oral contraceptive therapy, desire contraception, have achieved menarche, and are unresponsive to topical antiacne medications.

Administration and Dosage

Product choice: Only low-dose pills should be routinely used now; there is rarely a need for > 50 mcg estrogen component tablets.

Sunday-Start packaging: If the instructions recommend starting the regimen on Sunday, take the first tablet on the first Sunday after menstruation begins. If menstruation begins on Sunday, take the first tablet on that day.

21-Day regimen: Day 1 of the cycle is the first day of menstrual bleeding. Take 1 tablet daily for 21 days, beginning on day 5 of cycle. No tablets are taken for 7 days; whether bleeding has stopped or not, start a new course of 21 days.

28-Day regimen: To eliminate the need to count the days between cycles, some products contain 7 inert or iron-containing tablets to permit continuous daily dosage during the entire 28-day cycle. Take the 7 tablets on the last 7 days of the cycle.

Biphasic and triphasic OCs: Follow instructions on the dispensers or packs. As with the monophasic OCs, 1 tablet is taken each day; however, as the color of the tablet changes, the strength of the tablet also changes (ie, the estrogen/progestin ratio varies).

Missed dose:
    One tablet – Take it as soon as remembered, or take 2 tablets the next day; alternatively take 1 tablet, discard the other missed tablet, continue as scheduled and use another form of contraception for the 7 days after the pills missed, preferably for the remainder of the cycle.

    Two consecutive tablets – Take 2 tablets as soon as remembered with the next pill at the usual time, or take 2 tablets/day for the next 2 days, then resume the regular schedule. Use an additional form of contraception for the 7 days after pills are missed, preferably for the remainder of the cycle.

    Three consecutive tablets – Begin a new compact of tablets, starting on day 1 of the cycle after the last pill was taken or starting 7 days after the last tablet was taken.

Emergency contraception: If a positive pregnancy result is obtained, advise the patient not to take the pills in the kit.

    Take the initial 1 (*Plan B*) or 2 (*Preven*) pills as soon as possible but within 72 hours of unprotected intercourse. This is followed by the second dose of 1 (*Plan B*) or 2 (*Preven*) pills 12 hours later. Emergency contraception can be used at any time during the menstrual cycle. If the user vomits ≤ 1 hour of taking either dose of the medication, she should contact her health care professional to discuss whether or not to repeat that dose or take an antinausea medication.

Contraception:
    Progestin-only – One tablet every day at the same time. Administration is continuous, with no interruption between pill packs. Every time a pill is taken late, especially if a pill is missed, pregnancy is more likely.

       Missed dose: If the patient is > 3 hours late or misses ≥ 1 tablet, she should take a missed pill as soon as remembered, then go back to taking progestin-only pills (POPs) at the regular time, but be sure to use a backup method (such as a condom or spermicide) every time she has sexual intercourse for the next 48 hours.

Acne: The timing of dosing with *Ortho Tri-Cyclen* for acne should follow the guidelines for use of *Ortho Tri-Cyclen* as an OC. The dosage regimen for treatment of facial acne uses a 21-day active and a 7-day inert schedule. Take 1 active tablet daily for 21 days followed by 1 inert for 7 days. After 28 tablets have been taken, a new course is started the next day.

Postpartum administration: Postpartum administration in non-nursing mothers may begin at the first postpartum examination (4 to 6 weeks), regardless of whether spontaneous menstruation has occurred. Also, start no earlier than 4 to 6 weeks after a midtrimester pregnancy termination.

Switching pills: If switching from the combined pills to POPs, take the first POP the day after the last active combined pill is finished. Do not take any of the 7 inactive pills from the combined pill pack. Many women have irregular periods after switching to POPs; this is normal and to be expected. If switching from POPs to the combined pills, take the first active combined pill on the first day of menses, even if the POP pack is not finished. If switching to another brand of POPs, start the new brand any time. If breastfeeding, switch to another method of birth control at any time, except do not switch to the combined pills until breastfeeding is stopped or until ≥ 6 months after delivery.

Dosage adjustments:

Achieving Proper Hormonal Balance In An Oral Contraceptive			
Estrogen		Progestin	
Excess	Deficiency	Excess	Deficiency
Nausea, bloating Cervical mucorrhea, polyposis Melasma Hypertension Migraine headache Breast fullness or tenderness Edema	Early or midcycle breakthrough bleeding Increased spotting Hypomenorrhea	Increased appetite Weight gain Tiredness, fatigue Hypomenorrhea Acne, oily scalp[1] Hair loss, hirsutism[1] Depression Monilial vaginitis Breast regression	Late breakthrough bleeding Amenorrhea Hypermenorrhea

[1] Result of androgenic activity of progestins.

Pharmacological Effects of Progestins Used in Oral Contraceptives[1]	Progestin	Estrogen	Antiestrogen	Androgen
Norgestrel/levonorgestrel	+++	0	++	++++
Desogestrel	+++	0/+	0	0/+
Norgestimate	+++	0	0	0
Ethynodiol diacetate	++	+[2]	+[2]	+
Norethindrone acetate	+	+	+++	+
Norethindrone	+	+[2]	+[2]	+
Norethynodrel	+	+++	0	0

[1] Symbol Key: +++ *pronounced effect*   ++ *moderate effect*   + *slight effect*   0 *no effect*
[2] Has estrogenic effect at low doses; may have antiestrogenic effect at higher doses.

Progestin-only products: Administer daily, starting on the first day of menstruation. Take 1 tablet at the same time each day, every day of the year.

Postpartum administration – May be initiated no earlier than 4 weeks postpartum; however, consider the increased risk of thromboembolic disease associated with the postpartum period.

Missed dose –

One tablet: Take as soon as remembered, then take next tablet at regular time.

Two consecutive tablets: Do not take the missed tablets; discard and take the next tablet at the regular time (*Micronor* and *Nor-Q.D.*), or take 1 of the missed tablets, discard the other and take daily tablet at usual time (*Ovrette*).

Three consecutive tablets: Discontinue immediately.

Use an additional method of contraception if ≥ 2 tablets are missed until menses appears or pregnancy is ruled out. If menses does not occur within 45 days, regardless of circumstances, discontinue drug, use a nonhormonal method of contraception, and rule out pregnancy. Because of the slightly higher failure rate of the progestin-only products, a more conservative approach is to discontinue the regimen if only 1 tablet is missed and use other nonhormonal contraceptive methods until menses occurs or pregnancy is ruled out.

Patch:

Use – This system uses a 28-day (4-week) cycle. A new patch is applied each week for 3 weeks (21 days total). Week 4 is patch-free. Withdrawal bleeding is expected to begin during this time.

Apply every new patch on the same day of the week. This day is known as the "Patch Change Day."

On the day after week 4 ends, a new 4-week cycle is started by applying a new patch. Under no circumstances should there be more than a 7 day patch-free interval between dosing cycles. If there are > 7 patch-free days, the woman may not be protected from pregnancy and back-up contraception (eg, condoms, spermicide, diaphragm) must be used for 7 days. As with combined oral contraceptives, the risk of ovulation increases with each day beyond the recommended drug-free period. If intercourse has occurred during such an extended patch-free interval, consider the possibility of fertilization.

The patient must choose 1 option:

First day start – For first day start, the woman should apply her first patch during the first 24 hours of her menstrual period.

If therapy starts after day 1 of the menstrual cycle, a nonhormonal back-up contraceptive (eg, condoms, spermicide, diaphragm) should be used concurrently for the first 7 consecutive days of the first treatment cycle.

Sunday start – For Sunday start, the woman should apply her first patch on the first Sunday after her menstrual period starts. She must use back-up contraception for the first week of her first cycle.

If the menstrual period begins on a Sunday, the first patch should be applied on that day and no back-up contraception is needed.

Application – Apply the patch to clean, dry, intact, healthy skin on the buttock, abdomen, upper outer arm, or upper torso in a place where it will not be rubbed by tight clothing. The patch should not be placed on skin that is red, irritated, or cut, nor should it be placed on the breasts.

To prevent interference with the adhesive properties of the patch, no topical products should be applied to the skin area where the patch is or will be placed.

Patch changes may occur at any time on the change day. Apply each new patch to a new spot on the skin to help avoid irritation, although they may be kept within the same anatomic area.

If a patch is partially or completely detached –

For < 1 day (up to 24 hours): The woman should try to reapply it to the same place or replace it with a new patch immediately. No back-up contraception is needed. The woman's "patch change day" will remain the same.

For > 1 day (≥ 24 hours) or if the woman is not sure how long the patch has been detached: The woman may not be protected from pregnancy. She should stop the current contraceptive cycle and start a new cycle immediately by applying a new patch. There is now a new "day 1" and a new "patch change day." Back-up contraception (eg, condoms, spermicide, diaphragm) must be used for the first week of the new cycle.

Do not reapply a patch if it is no longer sticky, if it has become stuck to itself or another surface, if it has other material stuck to it, or if it has previously become loose or fallen off. If a patch cannot be reapplied, a new patch should be applied immediately. Do not use supplemental adhesives or wraps to hold the patch in place.

If the woman forgets to change her patch –

At the start of any patch cycle (week 1/day 1): She may not be protected from pregnancy. She should apply the first patch of her new cycle as soon as she remembers. There is now a new "patch change day" and a new "day 1." The woman must use back-up contraception (eg, condoms, spermicide, diaphragm) for the first week of the new cycle.

In the middle of the patch cycle (week 2/day 8 or week 3/day 15):

For 1 or 2 days (up to 48 hours) – She should apply a new patch immediately. The next patch should be applied on the usual "patch change day." No back-up contraception is needed.

For > 2 days (≥ 48 hours) – She may not be protected from pregnancy. She should stop the current contraceptive cycle and start a new 4-week cycle immediately by putting on a new patch. There is now a new "patch change day" and a new "day 1." The woman must use back-up contraception for 1 week.

At the end of the patch cycle (week 4/day 22): If the woman forgets to remove her patch, she should take it off as soon as she remembers. The next cycle should be started on the usual "patch change day," which is the day after day 28. No back-up contraception is needed.

Change day adjustment – If the woman wishes to change her patch change day, she should complete her current cycle, removing the third patch on the correct day. During the patch-free week, she may select an earlier patch change day by applying a new patch on the desired day. In no case should there be > 7 consecutive patch-free days.

Switching from an oral contraceptive – Treatment with the norelgestromin/ethinyl estradiol transdermal patch should begin on the first day of withdrawal bleeding. If there is no withdrawal bleeding within 5 days of the last active (hormone-containing) tablet, pregnancy must be ruled out. If therapy starts later than the first day of withdrawal bleeding, a nonhormonal contraceptive should be used concurrently for 7 days. If > 7 days elapse after taking the last active oral contraceptive tablet, consider the possibility of ovulation and conception.

Use after childbirth – Women who elect not to breastfeed should start contraceptive therapy with the norelgestromin/ethinyl estradiol transdermal patch no sooner than 4 weeks after childbirth. If a woman begins using the patch postpartum and has not yet had a period, consider the possibility of ovulation and conception occurring prior to use of the patch, and instruct her to use an additional method of contraception (eg, condoms, spermicide, diaphragm) for the first 7 days.

Use after abortion or miscarriage – After an abortion or miscarriage that occurs in the first trimester, the patch may be started immediately. An additional method of contraception is not needed if the patch is started immediately. If use of the patch is not started within 5 days following a first trimester abortion, the woman should follow the instructions for a woman starting the patch for the first time. In the meantime, advise her to use a nonhormonal contraceptive method. Ovulation may occur within 10 days after an abortion or miscarriage.

Do not start the patch any earlier than 4 weeks after a second trimester abortion or miscarriage. When the patch is used postpartum or postabortion, the increased risk of thromboembolic disease must be considered.

Breakthrough bleeding or spotting – In the event of breakthrough bleeding or spotting (bleeding that occurs on the days that the patch is worn), continue treatment. If breakthrough bleeding persists longer than a few cycles, consider a cause other than the patch.

In the event of no withdrawal bleeding (bleeding that should occur during the patch-free week), resume treatment on the next scheduled change day. If the patch has been used correctly, the absence of withdrawal bleeding is not necessarily an indication of pregnancy. Nevertheless, consider the possibility of pregnancy, especially if absence of withdrawal bleeding occurs in 2 consecutive cycles. Discontinue the patch if pregnancy is confirmed.

Skin irritation – If patch use results in uncomfortable irritation, the patch may be removed and a new patch may be applied to a different location until the next change day. Only 1 patch should be worn at a time.

Missed menstrual period – If the woman has not adhered to the prescribed schedule, consider the possibility of pregnancy at the time of the first missed period. Discontinue hormonal contraceptive use if pregnancy is confirmed.

If the woman has adhered to the prescribed regimen and misses 1 period, she should continue using her contraceptive patches.

If the woman has adhered to the prescribed regimen and misses 2 consecutive periods, rule out pregnancy. Discontinue use of the patch if pregnancy is confirmed.

Estimated Relative Oral Contraceptive Estrogen/Progestin Activity		
Product	Progestin activity	Estrogen activity
Monophasic		
Alesse, Levlite, Aviane	Low	Low
Brevicon, Modicon, Necon 0.5/35, Nortrel 0.5/35		
Ortho-Cyclen	Low	Low-Intermediate
Ovcon-35		
Levlen, Levora 0.15/30, Nordette	Intermediate	Low
Loestrin 1/20, Loestrin Fe 1/20, Microgestin Fe 1/20		
Lo/Ovral, Low-Ogestrel	Intermediate-High	Low
Loestrin 1.5/30, Loestrin Fe 1.5/30, Microgestin Fe 1.5/30		
Demulen 1/35, Zovia 1/35E	High	Intermediate
Desogen, Ortho-Cept, Apri		
Necon 1/50, Norinyl 1 + 50, Ortho-Novum 1/50	High	High
Necon 1/35, Norinyl 1 + 35, Ortho-Novum 1/35, Nortrel 1/35		
Ovcon 50		
Demulen 1/50, Zovia 1/50E		
Ovral-28, Ogestrel		
Yasmin	No data	Intermediate
Biphasic		
Jenest-28	Low	Low
Necon 10/11, Ortho-Novum 10/11		
Mircette	High	Intermediate
Triphasic		
Tri-Norinyl	Low	Low
Ortho-Novum 7/7/7		
Tri Levlen, Triphasil, Trivora	Low	Low-Intermediate
Ortho Tri-Cyclen		
Estrostep, Estrostep Fe, Cyclessa	Intermediate-High	Low

Actions

Pharmacology: Oral contraceptives (OCs) include estrogen-progestin combinations and progestin-only products.

Progestin-only – Progestin-only oral contraceptives prevent conception by suppressing ovulation in ≈ 50% of users, thickening the cervical mucus to inhibit sperm penetration, lowering the midcycle luteinizing hormone (LH) and follicle-stimulating hormone (FSH) peaks, slowing the movement of the ovum through the fallopian tubes, and altering the endometrium.

Combination OCs – Combination OCs inhibit ovulation by suppressing the gonadotropins, follicle-stimulating hormone (FSH) and luteinizing hormone (LH). Additionally, alterations in the genital tract, including cervical mucus (which inhibits sperm penetration) and the endometrium (which reduces the likelihood of implantation), may contribute to contraceptive effectiveness.

Contraceptive efficacy – If 100 women used emergency contraceptive pills (ECPs) correctly in 1 month, ≈ 2 women would become pregnant after a single act of intercourse. The use of ECPs results in a 75% reduction in the number of pregnancies expected if no ECPs were used after unprotected intercourse. Some clinical trials have shown that efficacy was greatest when ECPs were taken within 24 hours of unprotected intercourse, decreasing somewhat during each subsequent 24-hour period.

ECPs are not as effective as some other forms of contraception.

Pregnancy Rates for Various Means of Contraception (%)[1]		
Method of contraception	Lowest expected[2]	Typical[3]
Oral contraceptives		3
Combined	0.1	5
Progestin-only	0.5	5
Mechanical/Chemical		
Levonorgestrel implant	0.09	0.09
Medroxyprogesterone injection	0.3	0.3
IUD		
Progesterone	1.5	2
Copper T 380A	0.8	0.6
LNg 20	0.1	0.1
Cervical cap		
Parous	26	40
Nulliparous	9	20
Condom		
Without spermicide	3	14
With spermicide[4]	1.8	4 to 6
Spermicide alone	6	26
Diaphragm (with spermicidal cream or gel)	6	20
Female condom	5	21
Periodic abstinence (ie, rhythm; all methods)	1 to 9	25
Sterility		
Vasectomy	0.1	0.15
Tubal ligation	0.5	0.5
No contraception	85	85

[1] During first year of continuous use.
[2] Best guess of percentage expected to experience an accidental pregnancy among couples who initiate a method and use it consistently and correctly.
[3] A "typical" couple who initiate a method and experience an accidental pregnancy.
[4] Used as a separate product (not in condom package).

There are 3 types of combination OCs: Monophasic, biphasic, and triphasic. The biphasic and triphasic OCs are intended to deliver hormones in a fashion similar to physiologic processes.

Monophasic – Fixed dosage of estrogen to progestin throughout the cycle.

Biphasic – Amount of estrogen remains the same for the first 21 days of the cycle. Decreased progestin:estrogen ratio in first half of cycle allows endometrial proliferation. Increased ratio in second half provides adequate secretory development.

Triphasic – Estrogen amount remains the same or varies throughout cycle. Progestin amount varies.

Pharmacokinetics:

Estrogens – Ethinyl estradiol is rapidly absorbed with peak concentrations attained in 1 to 2 hours. It undergoes considerable first-pass elimination. Mestranol is demethylated to ethinyl estradiol. Ethinyl estradiol is ≈ 97% to 98% bound to plasma albumin. Half-life varies from 6 to 20 hours. It is excreted in bile and urine as conjugates, and undergoes some enterohepatic recirculation.

Progestins – Peak concentrations of norethindrone occur 0.5 to 4 hours after oral administration; it undergoes first-pass metabolism with an overall bioavailability around 65%. Levonorgestrel reaches peak concentrations between 0.5 to 2 hours, does not undergo a first-pass effect and is completely bioavailable. Desogestrel is rapidly and completely absorbed and converted into 3-keto-desogestrel, the biologically active metabolite. Relative bioavailability is ≈ 84%. Maximum concentrations of the metabolite are reached at 1.4 ± 0.8 hours. Norgestimate is well absorbed; peak serum concentrations are observed within 2 hours followed by a rapid decline to levels generally below assay within 5 hours. However, a major metabolite, 17-deacetyl norgestimate, appears rapidly in serum with concentrations greatly exceeding that of the parent. Both norethynodrel and ethynodiol diacetate are converted to norethindrone. Terminal half-life of the progestins are as follows: Norethindrone, 5 to 14 hours; levonorgestrel, 11 to 45 hours; desogestrel (metabolite), 38 ± 20 hours; norgestimate (metabolite), 12 to 30 hours. Progestin-only administration results in lower steady-state serum progestin levels and a shorter elimination half-life than concomitant administration with estrogens.

Patch – Norelgestromin is the active progestin largely responsible for the progestational activity that occurs in women following application of norelgestromin/ethinyl estradiol transdermal patch. Following application of the product, norelgestromin and ethinyl estradiol rapidly appear in the serum, reach a plateau by ≈ 48 hours, and are maintained at an approximate steady state throughout the wear period. Norelgestromin and norgestrel (a serum metabolite of norelgestromin) are highly bound (> 97%) to serum proteins. Because the patch is applied transdermally, first-pass metabolism (via the GI tract or liver) of norelgestromin and ethinyl estradiol that would be expected with oral administration is avoided. Following removal of patches, the elimination kinetics of norelgestromin and ethinyl estradiol were consistent for all studies with half-life values of ≈ 28 hours and 17 hours, respectively. The metabolites of norelgestromin and ethinyl estradiol are eliminated by renal and fecal pathways. For norelgestromin and ethinyl estradiol, increasing age, body weight, and body surface area each were associated with slight decreases in C_{ss} and AUC values.

Contraindications

Thrombophlebitis; thromboembolic disorders; history of deep-vein thrombophlebitis; cerebral vascular disease; myocardial infarction; coronary artery disease; valvular heart disease with complications; severe hypertension; diabetes with vascular involvement; headaches with focal neurological symptoms; major surgery with prolonged immobilization; known or suspected breast carcinoma or estrogen-dependent neoplasia; carcinoma of endometrium or other; acute or chronic hepatocellular disease with abnormal liver function; hepatic adenomas/carcinomas; undiagnosed abnormal genital bleeding; known or suspected pregnancy; cholestatic jaundice of pregnancy/jaundice with prior pill use; hypersensitivity to any component of the product; acute liver disease.

Warnings

Cigarette smoking: Cigarette smoking increases the risk of cardiovascular side effects from OCs. This risk increases with age and with heavy smoking (≥ 15 cigarettes/day) and is quite marked in women > 35 years of age. Women who use OCs should not smoke.

Hyperkalemia: Yasmin contains the progestin drospirenone that has antimineralocorticoid activity, including the potential for hyperkalemia in high-risk patients, comparable to a 25 mg dose of spironolactone. *Yasmin* should not be used in patients with conditions that predispose to hyperkalemia (eg, renal insufficiency, hepatic dysfunction, adrenal insufficiency). Women receiving daily, long-term treatment for chronic conditions or diseases with medications that may increase serum potassium should have their serum potassium level checked during the first treatment cycle. Drugs that may increase serum potassium include ACE inhibitors, angiotensin-II receptor antagonists, potassium-sparing diuretics, heparin, aldosterone antagonists, and NSAIDs.

Risks of OC use: The use of OCs is associated with increased risk of thromboembolism, stroke, MI, hypertension, hepatic neoplasia, and gallbladder disease, although risk of serious morbidity or mortality is very small in healthy women without underlying risk factors.

Mortality: Mortality associated with all methods of birth control is low and below that associated with childbirth, with the exception of OC use in women ≥ 35 who smoke and ≥ 40 who do not smoke. However, the Fertility and Maternal Health Drugs Advisory Committee recommended that the benefits of low-dose OC use by healthy non-smoking women > 40 years of age may outweigh the possible risks.

Thromboembolism: Be alert to the earliest symptoms of thromboembolic and thrombotic disorders. Should any of these occur or be suspected, discontinue the drug immediately.

MI – MI risk associated with OC use is increased. This risk is primarily in smokers or women with other underlying risk factors for coronary artery disease such as hypertension, hypercholesterolemia, morbid obesity, and diabetes.

Long-term use – Data suggest that the increased risk of MI persists after discontinuation of long-term OC use; the highest risk group includes women 40 to 49 years of age who used OCs for ≥ 5 years.

Smoking – Smoking in combination with OC use has been shown to contribute substantially to the incidence of MIs in women in their mid-30s or older, with smoking accounting for the majority of excess cases. Mortality rates associated with circulatory disease have been shown to increase substantially in smokers, especially in those ≥ 35 years of age who use OCs.

Cerebrovascular diseases – OCs increase the risks of cerebrovascular events (thrombotic and hemorrhagic strokes), although, in general, the risk is greatest in hypertensive women > 35 years of age who also smoke. The attributable risk is also greater in older women.

Vascular disease – A positive association is observed between the amount of estrogen and progestin in OCs and the risk of vascular disease. A decline in serum high density lipoproteins (HDL) has occurred with progestins. Because estrogens increase HDL cholesterol, the net effect depends on a balance achieved between doses of estrogen and progestin and the androgenic activity of the progestin.

Age – The risk of cerebrovascular and circulatory disease in OC users is substantially increased in women ≥ 35 years of age with other risk factors (eg, smoking, uncontrolled hypertension, hypercholesterolemia [LDL 190], obesity, diabetes).

Postsurgical thromboembolism – Risk is increased 2- to 4-fold. If possible, discontinue OCs ≥ 4 weeks before and 2 weeks after surgery and during and following prolonged immobilization because OCs are associated with an increased risk of thromboembolism.

Subarachnoid hemorrhage – Subarachnoid hemorrhage has been increased by OC use.

Dose-related risk – A positive association has been observed between the amount of estrogen and progestin in hormonal contraceptives and the risk of vascular disease.

Persistence of risk – There are 2 studies that have shown persistence of risk of vascular disease for ever-users of combination hormonal contraceptives.

Ocular lesions: Ocular lesions such as optic neuritis or retinal thrombosis have been associated with the use of OCs.

Risks of use before or during early pregnancy: Extensive epidemiological studies have revealed no increased risk of birth defects in women who have used oral contraceptives prior to pregnancy.

Gallbladder disease: Combination hormonal contraceptives such as norelgestromin/ethinyl estradiol transdermal patch may worsen existing gallbladder disease and may accelerate the development of this disease in previously asymptomatic women.

Carcinoma: While there are conflicting reports, the overall evidence in the literature suggests that use of OCs is not associated with an increase in the risk of developing any cancer, regardless of age and parity of first use.

Women with breast cancer should not use OCs because the role of female hormones in breast cancer has not been fully determined.

OC-users appear about half as likely to develop ovarian and endometrial cancer as women who have never used OCs. The protective effect from endometrial cancer lasts up to 15 years after the pills are stopped.

Hepatic lesions (adenomas, focal nodular hyperplasia, hepatocellular carcinoma, etc): Benign and malignant hepatic adenomas have been associated with the use of OCs. Severe abdominal pain, shock, or death may be due to rupture and hemorrhage of a liver tumor.

Pregnancy test: Do not administer progestin-only products or progestin-estrogen combinations to induce withdrawal bleeding as a test for pregnancy.

Carbohydrate metabolism: Glucose tolerance may decrease, which is directly related to estrogen dose.

Lipid profile: Triglycerides may increase. Some progestins decrease HDL, while some estrogens increase HDL.

Elevated blood pressure: Elevated blood pressure and hypertension may occur within a few months of beginning use. The prevalence increases with the duration of use and age. Incidence of hypertension may directly correlate with increasing dosages of progestin. Discontinue the OC if elevated blood pressure occurs.

Headaches: Onset or exacerbation of migraine or development of headache with focal neurological symptoms of a new pattern which is recurrent, persistent, or severe, requires OC discontinuation and evaluation.

Bleeding irregularities: Breakthrough bleeding (BTB), spotting, and amenorrhea are frequent reasons for discontinuing OCs. Progestin-only products are more likely to cause an alteration in menstrual patterns.

Progestin-only products – Episodes of irregular, unpredictable spotting, and BTB within the first year are the most frequently encountered side effects and are the major reasons why women discontinue OC use.

Menopause: Treatment with OCs may mask the onset of the climacteric.

Fertility impairment: Fertility impairment may occur in women discontinuing OCs; however, impairment diminishes with time.

Pregnancy: Category X. Rule out pregnancy before initiating or continuing the OCs, and always consider it if withdrawal bleeding does not occur.

Lactation: Oral contraceptives may interfere with lactation, decreasing both the quantity and the quality of breast milk. Furthermore, a small fraction of the hormones in OCs are excreted in breast milk. A few adverse effects on the nursing infant have been reported, including jaundice and breast enlargement.

If fully breastfeeding (not giving baby any food or formula), start pills 6 weeks after delivery. If partially breastfeeding (giving baby some food or formula), start taking pills by 3 weeks after delivery.

Children: Safety and efficacy are expected to be the same for postpubertal adolescents ≤ 16 years of age. Use of this product before menarche is not indicated.

Precautions

Monitoring: Pretreatment and annual exams should include blood pressure, breasts, abdomen and pelvic organs, including Papanicolaou smear.

Lipid disorders: HDL-C and total cholesterol may be increased, LDL-C may be increased or decreased, while LDL-C/HDL-C ratio may be decreased and triglycerides may be unchanged.

Uterine fibroids: Preexisting uterine leiomyomata (uterine fibroids) may increase in size. However, there is no evidence of this with low-dose OCs.

Pyridoxine deficiency: OC users may have relative pyridoxine deficiency.

Depression: The incidence of depression in OC users ranges from < 5% to 30%. Pyridoxine deficiency may be a factor in the depression.

Fluid retention: OCs may cause fluid retention.

Body weight ≥ 90 kg (198 lbs): Results of clinical trials suggest that the norelgestromin/ethinyl estradiol transdermal patch may be less effective in women with body weight ≥ 90 kg (198 lbs) than in women with lower body weights.

Hepatic function: Patients with a history of jaundice during pregnancy have an increased risk of recurrence of jaundice.

Contact lenses: Contact lens wearers who develop changes in vision or lens tolerance should be assessed by an ophthalmologist; consider temporary or permanent cessation of wear.

Serum folate levels: Serum folate levels may be depressed by therapy.

Acute intermittent porphyria: Estrogens have been reported to precipitate attacks of acute intermittent porphyria.

Vomiting/Diarrhea: Several cases of OC failure have been reported in association with vomiting or diarrhea. If significant GI disturbance occurs, a back-up method of contraception for the remainder of the cycle is recommended.

Sexually transmitted diseases (STDs): Advise patients that OCs do not protect against HIV infection and other STDs.

Photosensitivity: Photosensitization (photoallergy or phototoxicity) may occur.

Drug Interactions

Drugs that may affect oral contraceptives include acetaminophen, antibiotics, ascorbic acid, atorvastatin, barbiturates, carbamazepine, CYP3A4 inhibitors (eg, itraconazole, ketoconazole) felbamate, griseofulvin, hydantoins, oxcarbazepine, phenylbutazone, phenytoin, primidone, protease inhibitors, rifampin, St. John's wort, and topiramate. Drugs that may be affected by oral contraceptives include acetaminophen, anticoagulants, benzodiazepines, beta blockers, caffeine, clofibrate, corticosteroids, cyclosporine, morphine, prednisolone, salicylates, theophyllines, and tricyclic antidepressants.

Drug/Lab test interactions: Estrogen-containing OCs may cause the following alterations in serum, plasma or blood, unless specified otherwise.

   Increased – Factors I (prothrombin), VII, VIII, IX, X; fibrinogen; norepinephrine-induced platelet aggregation; thyroid binding globulin (TBG), leading to increased total thyroid hormone (as measured by protein bound iodine or T_4 by column or radioimmunoassay); corticosteroid levels; triglycerides and phospholipids; aldosterone; amylase; gamma-glutamyltranspeptidase; iron binding capacity; sex-hormone-binding globulins are increased and result in elevated levels of total circulating sex steroids (combination); corticoids; transferrin; prolactin; renin activity; vitamin A.

   Decreased – Antithrombin III; free T_3 resin uptake; response to metyrapone test; folate; glucose tolerance; albumin; cholinesterase; haptoglobin; zinc; vitamin B_{12}; sex-hormone-binding globulin, thyroxine due to decrease in thyroid-binding globulin (progestin-only).

Adverse Reactions

Serious adverse reactions that may occur include thrombophlebitis and venous thrombosis with or without embolism; pulmonary embolism; coronary thrombosis; MI; cerebral thrombosis; arterial thromboembolism; cerebral hemorrhage; hypertension; gallbladder disease; hepatic adenomas or benign liver tumors; mesenteric thrombosis. Other adverse reactions that may occur include nausea and vomiting (10% to 30% of patients during the first cycle, less common with low doses, and majority resolve in 3 months); abdominal cramps; bloating; breakthrough bleeding (majority,> 80%, resolve in 3 months); spotting; change in menstrual flow; amenorrhea during and after treatment; change in cervical erosion and cervical secretions; vaginal candidiasis; temporary infertility after discontinuation; breast changes; melasma (may persist); rash (allergic); migraine; mental depression; headache; dizziness; contact lens intolerance; edema; weight change (increase or decrease); changes in corneal curvature (steepening); neuro-ocular lesions (eg, retinal thrombosis, optic neuritis).

Emergency contraceptives: The most common adverse events in the clinical trial for women receiving emergency contraceptives include nausea; abdominal pain/cramps; fatigue; headache; menstrual irregularities; dizziness; breast tenderness; vomiting; diarrhea.

LEVONORGESTREL IMPLANTS

Kit: 6 capsules (each contains 36 mg levonorgestrel) (*Rx*)   *Norplant System* (Wyeth)

Indications

Prevention of pregnancy: The implant system is a long-term (≤ 5 years) reversible contraceptive system. Remove the capsules by the end of the 5th year; new capsules may be inserted at that time if continuing contraceptive protection is desired.

Administration and Dosage

Levonorgestrel implants consist of 6 *Silastic* capsules; each capsule is 2.4 mm in diameter and 34 mm in length and contains 36 mg levonorgestrel. Total administered (implanted) dose is 216 mg. Perform implantation of all 6 capsules during the first 7 days of menses onset. Insertion is subdermal in the mid-portion of the upper arm (see literature included with the product).

Actions

Pharmacology: Diffusion of levonorgestrel through the wall of each capsule provides a continuous low dose of the progestin. Because of the range of variability in blood levels and variation in individual response, blood levels alone are not predictive of the risk of pregnancy in an individual woman.

Pharmacokinetics: Levonorgestrel concentrations among women show considerable variation. They reach a maximum, or near maximum, within 24 hours after placement with mean values of 1600 pg/mL. Levels decline rapidly over the first month. Mean levels decline to values of around 400 pg/mL at 3 months to 258 pg/mL at 60 months.

Concentrations decrease with increasing body weight by a mean of 3.3 pg/mL/ kg. After capsule removal, mean concentrations drop to < 100 pg/mL by 96 hours and to below assay sensitivity (50 pg/mL) by 5 to 14 days.

Contraceptive efficacy –

	\multicolumn{6}{c}{Annual and 5-Year Cumulative Pregnancy Rates Per 100 Levonorgestrel Implant Users by Weight}

	\multicolumn{5}{c}{Year}	
Weight	1	2	3	4	5	Cumulative
< 50 kg (< 110 lbs)	0.2	0	0	0	0	0.2
50-59 kg (110-130 lbs)	0.2	0.5	0.4	2	0.4	3.4
60-69 kg (131-153 lbs)	0.4	0.5	1.6	1.7	0.8	5
≥ 70 kg (≥ 154 lbs)	0	1.1	5.1	2.5	0	8.5
All	0.2	0.5	1.2	1.6	0.4	3.9

Contraindications

Active thrombophlebitis or thromboembolic disorders; undiagnosed abnormal genital bleeding; known or suspected pregnancy; acute liver disease; benign or malignant liver tumors; known or suspected carcinoma of the breast; history of idiopathic intracranial hypertension; hypersensitivity to levonorgestrel or any component of the product.

Warnings

Insertion and removal complications: A surgical incision is required to insert the capsules. Complications related to insertion (eg, pain, edema, bruising, infection) may occur. There have been reports of arm pain, numbness, and tingling following the insertion and removal procedures. There also have been reports of nerve injury, most commonly associated with deep placement and removal. Expulsion of capsules has been reported more frequently when placement of the capsules was shallow or too close to the incision or when infection was present.

Bleeding irregularities: Most women can expect some variation in menstrual bleeding patterns. Irregular menstrual bleeding, intermenstrual spotting, prolonged episodes of bleeding and spotting, and amenorrhea occur in some women. Overall, these irregularities diminish with continuing use. After a pattern of regular menses, ≥ 6 weeks of amenorrhea may signal pregnancy. If pregnancy occurs, the capsules must be removed.

Delayed follicular atresia: If follicular development occurs, atresia of the follicle is sometimes delayed and the follicle may continue to grow beyond the size it would attain in a normal cycle.

Ectopic pregnancies: The risk of ectopic pregnancy may increase with the duration of use and, possibly, with increased weight of the user. Any patient who presents with lower abdominal pain must be evaluated to rule out ectopic pregnancy.

Foreign body carcinogenesis: Rarely, cancers have occurred at the site of foreign body intrusions or old scars.

Thromboembolic disorders: Patients who develop active thrombophlebitis or thromboembolic disease should have the levonorgestrel capsules removed. Also consider removal in women who will be immobilized for a prolonged period due to surgery or other illnesses.

Cerebrovascular disorders – Combination oral contraceptives have been shown to increase the relative and attributable risks of cerebrovascular events (thrombotic and hemorrhagic strokes), although, in general, the risk is greatest among older (> 35 years of age) hypertensive women who also smoke.

MI – An increased risk of MI has been attributed to combination oral contraceptive use.

Studies indicate a significant trend toward higher rates of MI and strokes with increasing doses of progestin in combination oral contraceptives. There have been postmarketing reports of MI coincident with levonorgestrel implant system use.

Idiopathic intracranial hypertension: There have been reports of idiopathic intracranial hypertension. A cardinal sign of idiopathic intracranial hypertension is papilledema; early symptoms may include headache (associated with a change in frequency, pattern, severity, or persistence; of particular importance are those headaches that are unremitting in nature) and visual disturbances.

Pregnancy: Category X.

Lactation: Levonorgestrel has been identified in breast milk. No significant effects were observed on growth or health of infants whose mothers used implants beginning 6 weeks after parturition.

Children: Safety and efficacy are expected to be similar for postpubertal adolescents < 16 years of age and users ≥ 16 years of age. Use of this product before menarche is not indicated.

Precautions

Physical examination and follow-up: Take a complete medical history and physical examination prior to the implantation or re-implantation of levonorgestrel implants and at least annually during its use. Carefully monitor women with a strong family history of breast cancer or who have breast nodules.

Carbohydrate and lipid metabolism: Effects of implants on carbohydrate metabolism appear to be minimal. Carefully observe diabetic and prediabetic patients.

Closely follow women who are being treated for hyperlipidemias.

Liver function: If jaundice develops consider removing the capsules.

Fluid retention: Prescribe with caution, and only with careful monitoring, in patients with conditions which might be aggravated by fluid retention.

Emotional disorders: Consider removing the capsules in women who become significantly depressed since the symptom may be drug-related. Carefully observe women with a history of depression and consider removal if depression recurs to a serious degree.

Contact lens: Contact lens wearers who develop changes in vision or in lens tolerance should be assessed by an ophthalmologist.

Autoimmune disease: There have been rare reports of various autoimmune diseases (eg, scleroderma, systemic lupus erythematosus, rheumatoid arthritis) in levonorgestrel implant users; however, the rate of reporting is significantly less than the expected incidence for these diseases.

Insertion and removal: To be sure that the woman is not pregnant at the time of capsule placement and to ensure contraceptive efficacy during the first cycle of use, insert capsules during the first 7 days of the cycle or immediately after an abortion. Insertion is not recommended before 6 weeks postpartum in breastfeeding women.

Infection: If infection occurs, institute suitable treatment. If infection persists, remove the capsules.

Expulsion: Expulsion of capsules occurs more frequently when placement of the capsules is extremely shallow, too close to the incision, or when infection is present. Replacement of an expelled capsule must be accomplished using a new sterile capsule. If infection is present, treat and cure before replacement. Contraceptive efficacy may be inadequate with < 6 capsules.

Provisions for removal: The removal should be done on such request or at the end of 5 years of usage by personnel instructed in the removal technique.

Drug Interactions

Carbamazepine and phenytoin: Reduced efficacy (pregnancy) has occurred. Warn users of the possibility of decreased efficacy with use of any related drugs.

Drug/Lab test interactions: Certain endocrine tests may be affected by levonorgestrel implants: Sex hormone binding globulin concentrations are decreased; thyroxine concentrations may be slightly decreased and triiodothyronine uptake increased.

Adverse Reactions

Adverse reactions occuring in ≥ 3% of patients include prolonged bleeding; spotting; amenorrhea; irregular bleeding; frequent bleeding onsets; removal difficulties affecting patients; scanty bleeding; breast discharge; cervicitis; musculoskeletal pain; abdominal discomfort; leukorrhea; vaginitis; pain or itching near implant site.

MEDROXYPROGESTERONE ACETATE

Injection: 150 mg/mL (Rx) *Depo-Provera* (Upjohn)

Indications

Prevention of pregnancy: It is a long-term injectable contraceptive in women when administered at 3-month intervals.

Administration and Dosage

Shake the vial vigorously just before use to ensure that the dose being administered represents a uniform suspension.

The recommended dose is 150 mg every 3 months administered by deep IM injection in the gluteal or deltoid muscle. To increase assurance that the patient is not pregnant at the time of the first administration, give this injection only during the first 5 days after the onset of a normal menstrual period; within 5 days postpartum if not breastfeeding; or, if breastfeeding, at 6 weeks postpartum. If the period between injections is > 14 weeks, determine that the patient is not pregnant before administering the drug.

Actions

Pharmacology: Medroxyprogesterone, when administered IM at the recommended dose to women every 3 months, inhibits the secretion of gonadotropins which, in turn, prevents follicular maturation and ovulation and results in endometrial thinning. These actions produce its contraceptive effect.

Pharmacokinetics: Following a single 150 mg IM dose, medroxyprogesterone concentrations increase for ≈ 3 weeks to reach peak plasma concentrations of 1 to 7 ng/mL. The levels then decrease exponentially until they become undetectable (< 100 pg/mL) between 120 to 200 days following injection. The apparent half-life following IM administration is ≈ 50 days.

Contraindications

Known or suspected pregnancy or as a diagnostic test for pregnancy; undiagnosed vaginal bleeding; known or suspected malignancy of breast; active thrombophlebitis, or current or past history of thromboembolic disorders, or cerebral vascular disease; liver dysfunction or disease; hypersensitivity to medroxyprogesterone or any of its other ingredients.

Warnings

Bleeding irregularities: Most women experience disruption of menstrual bleeding patterns. If abnormal bleeding persists or is severe, institute appropriate investigation to rule out the possibility of organic pathology, and institute appropriate treatment when necessary.

Bone mineral density changes: Use of medroxyprogesterone may be considered among the risk factors for development of osteoporosis. The rate of bone loss is greatest in the early years of use and then subsequently approaches the normal rate of age-related fall.

Thromboembolic disorders: Be alert to the earliest manifestations of thrombotic disorders. If any of these occur or are suspected, do not readminister the drug.

Ocular disorders: Do not readminister pending examination if there is a sudden partial or complete loss of vision or if there is a sudden onset of proptosis, diplopia, or migraine. If examination reveals papilledema or retinal vascular lesions, do not readminister.

Carcinogenesis: Long-term case-controlled surveillance of users found slight or no increased overall risk of breast cancer and no overall increased risk of ovarian, liver, or cervical cancer and a prolonged, protective effect of reducing the risk of endometrial cancer in the population of users.

Pregnancy: Category X.

Lactation: Detectable amounts of the drug have been identified in the milk of mothers receiving medroxyprogesterone. In nursing mothers treated with medroxyprogesterone, milk composition, quality, and amount are not adversely affected. Infants exposed to medroxyprogesterone via breast milk have been studied for developmental and behavioral effects through puberty; no adverse effects have been noted.

Precautions

Physical examination: The pretreatment and annual history and physical examination should include special reference to breast and pelvic organs, as well as a Papanicolaou smear.

Fluid retention: Because progestational drugs may cause some degree of fluid retention, conditions that might be influenced by this condition require careful observation.

Weight changes: There is a tendency for women to gain weight while on medroxyprogesterone therapy.

Return of fertility: Medroxyprogesterone has a prolonged contraceptive effect. It is expected that 68% of women who do become pregnant may conceive within 12 months, 83% may conceive within 15 months and 93% may conceive within 18 months from the last injection.

CNS disorders and convulsions: Carefully observe patients who have a history of psychic depression; do not readminister if the depression recurs.
There have been a few reported cases of convulsions. Association with drug use or preexisting conditions is not clear.

Carbohydrate metabolism: A decrease in glucose tolerance has been observed in some patients. Carefully observe diabetic patients during therapy.

Liver function: If jaundice develops, consider not readministering the drug.

Drug Interactions

Drugs that may interact with medroxyprogesterone include aminoglutethimide.

Drug/Lab test interactions: The following laboratory tests may be affected by medroxyprogesterone: Plasma and urinary steroid levels are decreased; gonadotropin levels are decreased; sex-hormone binding globulin concentrations are decreased; protein bound iodine and butanol extractable protein bound iodine may increase; T_3 uptake values may decrease; coagulation test values for prothrombin (Factor II), and Factors VII, VIII, IX, and X may increase. Sulfobromophthalein and other liver function test values may be increased; the effects of medroxyprogesterone acetate on lipid metabolism are inconsistent. Both increases and decreases in total cholesterol, triglycerides, low-density lipoprotein (LDL) cholesterol, and high-density lipoprotein (HDL) cholesterol have been observed.

Adverse Reactions

Common ($\geq$ 3%) adverse reactions include menstrual irregularities; weight changes; headache; nervousness; abdominal pain; discomfort; asthenia; dizziness.

ANDROGENS

FLUOXYMESTERONE	
Tablets: 2 mg, 5 mg (c-ɪɪɪ)	*Halotestin* (Pharmacia)
10 mg (c-ɪɪɪ)	Various, *Halotestin* (Pharmacia)
METHYLTESTOSTERONE	
Tablets: 10 mg (c-ɪɪɪ)	Various, *Methitest* (Global)
25 mg (c-ɪɪɪ)	Various, *Methitest* (Global)
Tablets (buccal): 10 mg (c-ɪɪɪ)	Various
Capsules: 10 mg (c-ɪɪɪ)	*Android* (ICN Pharm), *Testred* (ICN Pharm), *Virilon* (Star)
Injection: 200 mg/mL (c-ɪɪɪ)	*Virilon IM* (Star)
TESTOSTERONE, LONG-ACTING	
TESTOSTERONE ENANTHATE (IN OIL)	
Injection: 200 mg/mL (c-ɪɪɪ)	*Delatestryl* (BTG)
TESTOSTERONE CYPIONATE (IN OIL)	
Injection: 100 mg/mL, 200 mg/mL (c-ɪɪɪ)	*Depo-Testosterone* (Pharmacia)
TESTOSTERONE PELLETS	
Pellets: 75 mg (c-ɪɪɪ)	*Testopel* (Bartor Pharmacal)
TESTOSTERONE TRANSDERMAL SYSTEM	
Patch: 328 mg testosterone (c-ɪɪɪ)	*Testoderm TTS* (Alza)
24.3 mg testosterone (c-ɪɪɪ)	*Androderm* (Watson Pharma)
15 mg testosterone (c-ɪɪɪ)	*Testoderm, Testoderm with Adhesive* (Alza)
12.2 mg testosterone (c-ɪɪɪ)	*Androderm* (Watson Pharma)
10 mg testosterone (c-ɪɪɪ)	*Testoderm* (Alza)
TESTOSTERONE GEL	
Gel: 1% testosterone (c-ɪɪɪ)	*AndroGel 1%* (Unimed Pharm)

Anabolic steroids are classified as a *c-iii* controlled substance under the anabolic steroids act of 1990.

Indications

Males:

Replacement therapy – Replacement therapy in hypogonadism associated with a deficiency or absence of endogenous testosterone. Prior to puberty, androgen replacement therapy is needed for development of secondary sexual characteristics. Prolonged treatment is required to maintain sexual characteristics in these and other males who develop testosterone deficiency after puberty. Appropriate adrenal cortical and thyroid hormone replacement therapy are still necessary, however, and are of primary importance.

Primary hypogonadism (congenital or acquired): Testicular failure due to cryptorchidism, bilateral torsion, orchitis, vanishing testis syndrome, or orchidectomy; Klinefelter's syndrome, chemotherapy, or toxic damage from alcohol or heavy metals.

Hypogonadotropic hypogonadism (congenital or acquired): Idiopathic gonadotropin or luteinizing hormone releasing hormone (LHRH) deficiency or pituitary-hypothalamic injury from tumors, trauma, or radiation.

Delayed puberty: To stimulate puberty in carefully selected males with clearly delayed puberty. Brief treatment with conservative doses may be justified if these patients do not respond to psychological support.

Females:

Metastatic cancer – May be used secondarily in women with advancing inoperable metastatic (skeletal) breast cancer who are 1 to 5 years postmenopausal. Primary goals of therapy include ablation of the ovaries. This treatment has been used in premenopausal women with breast cancer who have benefited from oophorectomy and have a hormone-responsive tumor.

Administration and Dosage

FLUOXYMESTERONE:

Males –

Hypogonadism: 5 to 20 mg/day.

Delayed puberty: Carefully titrate dosage using a low dose, appropriate skeletal monitoring, and by limiting the duration of therapy to 4 to 6 months.

Females –

Inoperable breast carcinoma: 10 to 40 mg/day in divided doses. Continue for 1 month for a subjective response and 2 to 3 months for an objective response.

METHYLTESTOSTERONE:

Males –

Replacement therapy: Replacement therapy in androgen-deficient males is 10 to 50 mg of methyltestosterone daily.

Delayed puberty – Doses used in delayed puberty generally are in the lower range of that given above, and for a limited duration, for example, 4 to 6 months.

Females –

Inoperable breast cancer: 50 to 200 mg/day orally. Follow women closely because androgen therapy occasionally appears to accelerate the disease. Shorter acting androgen preparations may be preferred rather than those with prolonged activity for treating breast carcinoma, particularly during the early stages of androgen therapy.

TESTOSTERONE, LONG-ACTING: For IM use only. Individualize dosage. In general, > 400 mg/month is not required because of the prolonged action of the preparation.

Male hypogonadism –

Replacement therapy (eunuchism): 50 to 400 mg every 2 to 4 weeks.

Males with delayed puberty – 50 to 200 mg every 2 to 4 weeks for a limited duration.

Palliation of inoperable breast cancer in women – 200 to 400 mg every 2 to 4 weeks.

Androgen therapy occasionally appears to accelerate metastatic breast carcinoma.

TESTOSTERONE TRANSDERMAL SYSTEM:

Testoderm – Patients should start therapy with a 6 mg/day system applied daily; if scrotal area is inadequate, use a 4 mg/day system. Place the patch on clean, dry, scrotal skin. Dry-shave scrotal hair for optimal skin contact. Do not use chemical depilatories. The testosterone transdermal system should be worn 22 to 24 hours.

After 3 to 4 weeks of daily system use, blood should be drawn 2 to 4 hours after system application for determination of serum total testosterone. Because of variability in analytical values among diagnostic laboratories, this laboratory work and later analyses for assessing the effect of the transdermal testosterone therapy should be performed at the same laboratory.

If patients have not achieved desired results by the end of 6 to 8 weeks of use, consider another form of testosterone replacement therapy.

Testoderm TTS – One system is applied at about the same time each day. Place the adhesive side on a clean, dry area of skin on the arm, back, or upper buttocks immediately upon removal from the protective pouch. Do not apply to the scrotum. The area selected should not be oily, damaged, or irritated. Press the system firmly in place with the palm of the hand for ≈ 10 seconds, making sure there is good contact, especially around the edges. If the system falls off, the same system may be reapplied. If the system comes off after it has been worn for ≥ 12 hours and it cannot be reapplied, a new system may be applied at the next application time. In either case, continue the daily treatment schedule. Wear the system ≈ 24 hours and replace.

To ensure proper dosing, serum testosterone concentration may be measured 2 to 4 hours after an application of the system. If the concentrations are too low, the dosing regimen may be increased to 2 systems.

Androderm – The usual starting dose is one 5 mg system or two 2.5 mg systems applied nightly for 24 hours, providing a total dose of 5 mg/day.

Apply the adhesive side of the system to a clean, dry area of the skin on the back, abdomen, upper arms or thighs. Avoid bony prominences, such as the shoulder and hip areas. Do NOT apply to the scrotum. Rotate the sites of application, with an interval of 7 days between applications to the same site. The area selected should not be oily, damaged, or irritated.

To ensure proper dosing, the morning serum testosterone concentration may be measured following system application the previous evening. If the serum concentration is outside the normal range, repeat sampling with assurance of proper system adhesion as well as appropriate application time. Confirmed serum concentrations outside the normal range may require increasing the dosage regimen to 7.5 mg, or decreasing the regimen to 2.5 mg, maintaining nightly application. Because of variability in analytical values among diagnostic laboratories, this laboratory work and any later analysis for assessing the effect of therapy should be performed at the same laboratory so results can be more easily compared.

Non-virilized patient – Dosing may be initiated with 2.5 mg system nightly.

Storage/Stability – Do not store outside the pouch provided. Damaged systems should not be used. The drug reservoir may be burst by excessive pressure or heat. Discard systems in household trash in a manner that prevents accidental application or ingestion by children, pets, or others.

TESTOSTERONE PELLETS:

Replacement therapy – The dosage guideline for testosterone pellets for replacement therapy in androgen-deficient males is 150 to 450 mg SC every 3 to 6 months.

Delayed puberty – Dosages used in delayed puberty generally are in the lower range of that listed above, and for a limited time duration, for example 4 to 6 months.

Determination of dose – The number of pellets to be implanted depends upon the minimal daily requirement of testosterone propionate determined by a gradual reduction of the amount administered parenterally. The usual ratio is as follows: Implant two 75 mg pellets for each 25 mg testosterone propionate required weekly. It has been found that ≈ 33% of the material is absorbed in the first month, 25% in the second month, and 17% in the third month. Adequate effect of the pellets ordinarily continues for 3 to 4 months, sometimes as long as 6 months.

TESTOSTERONE GEL: The recommended starting dose of 1% testosterone gel is 5 g (to deliver 50 mg of testosterone) applied once daily (preferably in the morning) to clean, dry, intact skin of the shoulders and upper arms or abdomen. Upon opening the packet(s), squeeze the entire contents into the palm of the hand and immediately apply it to the application sites. Allow application sites to dry for a few minutes prior to dressing. Wash hands with soap and water after application. Cover the application sites with clothing after gel has dried.

Do not apply the gel to the genitals.

For optimal absorption of testosterone, it appears reasonable to wait ≥ 5 to 6 hours after application prior to showering or swimming. Showering or swimming after just 1 hour should have a minimal effect on the amount absorbed if done infrequently.

Measure serum testosterone levels 14 days after initiation of therapy to ensure proper dosing. If the serum testosterone concentration is below the normal range, or if the desired clinical response is not achieved, the dose may be increased from 5 to 7.5 g and from 7.5 to 10 g, as instructed by the physician.

The potential for dermal testosterone transfer following use exists. Washing the area of contact on the other person as soon as possible with soap and water will remove residual testosterone from the skin surface.

Storage/Stability: Store at controlled room temperature (20° to 25°C; 68° to 77°F).

Actions

Pharmacology: Testosterone, produced by the Leydig cells of the testis, is the primary natural androgen. In women, small amounts are synthesized by the ovary and adrenal cortex.

Endogenous androgens are responsible for the normal growth and development of the male sex organs and for maintenance of secondary sex characteristics. Androgens are responsible for the growth spurt of adolescence and for the termination of linear growth by fusion of the epiphyseal growth centers. During administration of exogenous androgens, endogenous testosterone release is inhibited through feedback inhibition of pituitary luteinizing hormone (LH). Large doses of exogenous androgens may suppress spermatogenesis through feedback inhibition of pituitary follicle stimulating hormone (FSH).

Pharmacokinetics:

Absorption –

Oral: Testosterone is metabolized by the gut and 44% is cleared by the liver in the first pass. The synthetic androgens are less extensively metabolized by the liver and have longer half-lives and are more suitable than testosterone for oral administration.

IM: Testosterone esters in oil injected IM are absorbed slowly from the lipid phase; thus, testosterone cypionate and enanthate can be given at intervals of 2 to 4 weeks.

Topical gel: Absorption of testosterone into the blood continues for the entire 24-hour dosing interval. Serum concentrations approximate the steady-state level by the end of the first 24 hours and are at steady state by the second or third day of dosing.

When the topical gel treatment is discontinued after achieving steady state, serum testosterone levels remain in the normal range for 24 to 48 hours but return to their pretreatment levels by the fifth day after the last application.

Transdermal:

Testoderm – Following placement of *Testoderm* on scrotal skin, the serum testosterone concentration rises to a maximum at 2 to 4 hours and returns toward baseline within $\approx$ 2 hours after system removal. Serum levels reach a plateau at 3 to 4 weeks.

Testoderm TTS – The 3 recommended skin sites (arm, back, and upper buttocks) are interchangeable based on equivalent testosterone $AUC_{(0-27)}$ values.

Androderm – Following application to non-scrotal skin, testosterone is continuously absorbed during the 24-hour dosing period. Daily application of 2 systems at $\approx$ 10:00 p.m. results in a serum testosterone concentration profile that mimics the normal circadian variation observed in healthy young men. Maximum concentrations occur in the early morning hours with minimum concentrations in the evening.

Distribution – Testosterone in plasma is $\approx$ 98% bound to a specific testosterone-estradiol binding globulin. There are considerable variations in the reported half-life of testosterone, ranging from 10 to 100 minutes. The half-life of testosterone cypionate IM is $\approx$ 8 days; for oral fluoxymesterone, it is $\approx$ 9.2 hours; and for methyltestosterone it is 2.5 to 3 hours.

Metabolism/Excretion – There are considerable variations in the reported half-life of testosterone, ranging from 10 to 100 minutes. The half-life of testosterone cypionate IM is $\approx$ 8 days; for oral fluoxymesterone, it is $\approx$ 9.2 hours; and for methyltestosterone it is 2.5 to 3 hours. Inactivation of testosterone occurs primarily in the liver. About 90% of a testosterone dose is excreted in the urine as conjugates of testosterone and its metabolites; about 6% of a dose is excreted in the feces.

Contraindications

Patients with serious cardiac, hepatic, or renal diseases; hypersensitivity to the drug; in men with carcinomas of the breast or prostate; pregnancy (see Warnings).

Pregnant women should avoid skin contact with *AndroGel* application sites in men. Testosterone may cause fetal harm. In the event that unwashed or unclothed skin to which *AndroGel* has been applied does come in direct contact with the skin of a pregnant woman, wash the general area of contact on the woman with soap and water as soon as possible. In vitro studies show that residual testosterone is removed from the skin surface by washing with soap and water.

Warnings

Athletic performance: Although the anabolic steroids are generally the agents that are abused for enhancement of athletic performance, these agents have also been used for such purposes. However, these drugs are not safe and effective for this use and have a potential risk of serious side effects.

Sleep apnea: The treatment of hypogonadal men with testosterone esters may potentiate sleep apnea in some patients, especially those with risk factors such as obesity or chronic lung diseases.

Product interchange: Do not use testosterone cypionate interchangeably with testosterone propionate because of differences in duration of action.

Breast cancer: Androgen therapy may cause hypercalcemia by stimulating osteolysis.

Hepatotoxicity: Prolonged use of high doses of androgens has been associated with the development of potentially life-threatening peliosis hepatis, hepatic neoplasms, and hepatocellular carcinoma. Cholestatic hepatitis and jaundice occur with fluoxymesterone and methyltestosterone at relatively low doses. Drug-induced jaundice is reversible when the medication is discontinued.

Oligospermia: Oligospermia and reduced ejaculatory volume may occur after prolonged administration or excessive dosage.

Edema: Edema, with or without CHF, may be a serious complication in patients with preexisting cardiac, renal, or hepatic disease.

Gynecomastia: Gynecomastia frequently develops and occasionally persists in patients being treated for hypogonadism.

Bone maturation: Use cautiously in healthy males with delayed puberty. Monitor bone maturation by assessing bone age of the wrist and hand every 6 months.

Carcinogenesis: There are rare reports of hepatocellular carcinoma in patients receiving long-term therapy with androgens in high doses.

Elderly: Elderly males, or men in general, treated with androgens may be at an increased risk of developing prostatic hypertrophy, prostatic carcinoma, and prostatic hyperplasia.

Pregnancy: Category X.

Lactation: It is not known whether androgens are excreted in breast milk.

Children: Use androgens very cautiously in children; the drugs should only be given by specialists who are aware of the adverse effects on bone maturation. Androgens may accelerate bone maturation without producing compensatory gain in linear growth. This adverse effect may result in compromised adult stature. The younger the child, the greater the risk of compromising final mature height.

Precautions

Monitoring: Frequently determine urine and serum calcium levels during the course of therapy in women with disseminated breast carcinoma. Periodically perform liver function tests, prostate specific antigen, cholesterol, and high-density lipoprotein. To ensure proper dosing, measure serum testosterone concentrations. Make periodic (every 6 months) x-ray examinations of bone age during treatment of prepubertal males to determine the rate of bone maturation and the effects of the androgen therapy on the epiphyseal centers. Check hemoglobin and hematocrit periodically for polycythemia in patients who are receiving high doses of androgens.

Virilization: Observe women for signs of virilization (deepening voice, hirsutism, acne, clitoromegaly, and menstrual irregularities). Discontinue therapy at the time of evidence of mild virilism to prevent irreversible virilization.

Benign prostatic hypertrophy: Patients with benign prostatic hypertrophy may develop acute urethral obstruction. Priapism or excessive sexual stimulation may develop. Oligospermia may occur after prolonged administration or excessive dosage.

Hypercholesterolemia: Serum cholesterol may be altered during therapy.

Drug Interactions

Androgens may affect anticoagulants, oxyphenbutazone, insulin, propranolol, corticosteroids/ACTH, and cyclosporine.

Drug/Lab test interactions:
   Thyroid function tests – Decreased levels of thyroxine-binding globulin, resulting in decreased total T_4 serum levels and increased resin uptake of T_3 and T_4. Free thyroid hormone levels remain unchanged, and there is no clinical evidence of thyroid dysfunction.

Adverse Reactions

Adverse reactions occurring in $\geq$ 3% of patients include headache, dizziness/vertigo, libido decreased, application site itching/erythema/discomfort, pruritus, burning sensation, acne, other application site reactions, burn-like blister under system, breast pain/tenderness, UTI/Prostatitis, prostate disorder, gynecomastia, abnormal lab tests (including abnormal hemoglobin, hematocrit, triglycerides, serum lipids, potassium glucose, creatinine, bilirubin, liver function tests).

Females: Amenorrhea and other menstrual irregularities; inhibition of gonadotropin secretion and virilization, including deepening voice and clitoral enlargement.

FINASTERIDE

Tablets: 1 mg (*Rx*)	*Propecia* (Merck)
5 mg (*Rx*)	*Proscar* (Merck)

Indications

Benign prostatic hyperplasia (BPH): Treatment of symptomatic BPH in men with an enlarged prostate to improve symptoms, reduce acute urinary retention risk, and reduce the risk of the need for surgery including transurethral resection of the prostate (TURP) and prostatectomy.

Androgenetic alopecia: Treatment of male pattern hair loss (vertex and anterior midscalp).

Administration and Dosage

Benign prostatic hyperplasia: Recommended dose is 5 mg once/day, with or without meals.
Prior to initiating therapy, perform appropriate evaluation to identify other conditions that might mimic BPH, such as infection, prostate cancer, stricture disease, hypotonic bladder, or other neurogenic disorders.

Although early improvement may be seen, at least 6 to 12 months of therapy may be necessary to assess whether a beneficial response has been achieved. Perform periodic follow-up evaluations to determine whether a clinical response has occurred.

Androgenetic alopecia: The recommended dosage is 1 mg once/day, with or without meals. In general, daily use ≥ 3 months is necessary before benefit is observed. Continued use is recommended to sustain benefit. Withdrawal of treatment leads to reversal of effect within 12 months.

Hepatic function impairment: Use caution in those patients with liver function abnormalities because finasteride is metabolized extensively in the liver.

Actions

Pharmacology: Finasteride, a synthetic 4-azasteroid compound, is a competitive and specific inhibitor of steroid 5α-reductase, an intracellular enzyme that converts testosterone into the potent androgen 5α-dihydrotestosterone (DHT).

Pharmacokinetics: Finasteride is well absorbed after oral administration, with a mean bioavailability of ≈ 64%, which is unaffected by food. The half-life of finasteride is 4.8 to 6 hours following 1 and 5 mg/day dosing, respectively.

Finasteride undergoes extensive hepatic metabolism through oxidative pathways to inactive compounds that are eliminated primarily through the bile; the mean urinary recovery of the parent drug within 24 hours of a dose was only 0.04%.

Approximately 90% is bound to plasma proteins. Finasteride crosses the blood-brain barrier.

Contraindications

Hypersensitivity to finasteride or any component of this product; use in women or children; pregnancy or use in women who may potentially be pregnant, including handling of crushed or broken tablets

Warnings

Hepatic function impairment: Use caution in those patients with liver function abnormalities since finasteride is metabolized extensively in the liver.

Pregnancy: Category X. Because of the potential risk to a male fetus, a woman who is pregnant or who may become pregnant should not handle crushed or broken finasteride tablets.

Lactation: Finasteride is not indicated for use in women. It is not known whether finasteride is excreted in breast milk.

Children: Finasteride is not indicated for use in children; safety and efficacy in children have not been established.

Precautions

Prostate cancer evaluation: Perform digital rectal examinations, as well as other evaluations for prostate cancer, on patients with BPH prior to initiating therapy and periodically thereafter.

Finasteride causes a decrease in serum prostate specific antigen (PSA) levels in patients with BPH even in the presence of prostate cancer. Consider this reduction of PSA levels when evaluating PSA laboratory data; it does not suggest a beneficial effect of finasteride on prostate cancer.

Carefully evaluate any sustained increases in PSA levels while on finasteride, including consideration of non-compliance to therapy.

Obstructive uropathy: Because not all patients demonstrate a response to finasteride, carefully monitor patients with a large residual urinary volume or severely diminished urinary flow for obstructive uropathy. These patients may not be candidates for this therapy.

Drug Interactions

Finasteride may affect theophylline.

Drug/Lab test interactions: When PSA laboratory determinations are evaluated, consider the fact that PSA levels are decreased in patients treated with finasteride.

Adverse Reactions

Adverse reactions occuring in ≥ 3% of patients include impotence and decreased libido. Breast tenderness and enlargement; hypersensitivity reactions, including lip swelling and skin rash have also been reported with finasteride 5 mg.

DANAZOL

Capsules: 50, 100, and 200 mg (*Rx*)   Various, *Danocrine* (Sanofi-Synthelabo)

Warning:

Use of danazol in pregnancy is contraindicated. A sensitive test (eg, beta subunit test if available) capable of determining early pregnancy is recommended immediately prior to start of therapy. Additionally, a nonhormonal method of contraception should be used during therapy. If a patient becomes pregnant while taking danazol, discontinue administration of the drug and apprise the patient of the potential risk to the fetus.

Thromboembolism, thrombotic and thrombophlebitic events, including sagittal sinus thrombosis and life-threatening or fatal strokes have been reported.

Experience with long-term therapy with danazol is limited. Peliosis hepatis and benign hepatic adenoma have been observed with long-term use. Peliosis hepatis and hepatic adenoma may be silent until complicated by acute, potentially life-threatening intra-abdominal hemorrhage. Therefore, alert the physician to this possibility. Attempts should be made to determine the lowest dose that will provide adequate protection (see Warnings).

Danazol has been associated with several cases of benign intracranial hypertension also known as pseudotumor cerebri. Early signs and symptoms of benign intracranial hypertension include papilledema, headache, nausea, and vomiting, and visual disturbances. Screen patients with these symptoms for papilledema and, if present, advise the patients to discontinue danazol immediately and refer them to a neurologist for further diagnosis and care.

Indications

Endometriosis: For the treatment of endometriosis amenable to hormonal management.

Fibrocystic breast disease: Danazol is usually effective in decreasing nodularity, pain, and tenderness, but it alters hormone levels; recurrence of symptoms is very common after cessation of therapy.

Hereditary angioedema: For the prevention of attacks of angioedema in males and females.

Administration and Dosage

Endometriosis: Begin therapy during menstruation or make sure the patient is not pregnant. Administer 800 mg/day in 2 divided doses to best achieve amenorrhea and rapid response to painful symptoms. Downward titration to a dose sufficient to maintain amenorrhea may be considered depending upon response. Initially, for mild cases, give 200 to 400 mg in 2 divided doses.

Fibrocystic breast disease: Begin therapy during menstruation or make sure patient is not pregnant. Dosage ranges from 100 to 400 mg/day in 2 divided doses.

Hereditary angioedema: Recommended starting dose is 200 mg 2 or 3 times/day. After a favorable initial response, determine continuing dosage by decreasing the dosage by ≤ 50% at intervals of ≥ 1 to 3 months if frequency of attacks prior to treatment dictates. If an attack occurs, increase dosage by ≤ 200 mg/day.

Actions

Pharmacology: A synthetic androgen derived from ethisterone, danazol suppresses the pituitary-ovarian axis by inhibiting the output of pituitary gonadotropins. Danazol depresses the output of both follicle-stimulating hormone (FSH) and luteinizing hormone (LH). Danazol acts by direct enzymatic inhibition of sex steroid synthesis and competitively inhibits binding of steroids to their cytoplasmic receptors in target tissues.

Endometriosis – In endometriosis, danazol alters the normal and ectopic endometrial tissue so that it becomes inactive and atrophic.

Hereditary angioedema – Danazol prevents attacks of the disease characterized by episodic edema of the abdominal viscera, extremities, face, and airway that may be disabling and, if the airway is involved, fatal. In addition, danazol partially or completely corrects the primary biochemical abnormality of hereditary angioedema. It increases the levels of the deficient C1 esterase inhibitor, thereby increasing the serum levels of the C4 component of the complement system.

Pharmacokinetics: Blood levels of danazol do not increase proportionately with increases in dose. When the dose is doubled, plasma levels increase only ≈ 35% to 40%.

Contraindications

Undiagnosed abnormal genital bleeding; markedly impaired hepatic, renal, or cardiac function; pregnancy and lactation; patients with porphyria.

Warnings

Thrombotic events: Thromboembolism, thrombotic and thrombophlebitic events including sagittal sinus thrombosis and life-threatening or fatal strokes have been reported.

Hepatic events: Experience with long-term therapy with danazol is limited. Peliosis hepatis and benign hepatic adenoma have been observed with long-term use (see Black Box Warning).

Intracranial hypertension: Danazol has been associated with several cases of benign intracranial hypertension (also known as pseudotumor cerebri) (see Black Box Warning).

Lipoprotein alterations: A temporary alteration of lipoproteins in the form of decreased high density lipoproteins (HDL) and possibly increased low density lipoproteins (LDL) has been reported during danazol therapy.

Carcinoma of the breast: Carcinoma of the breast should be excluded before initiating therapy for fibrocystic breast disease.

Long-term experience: Long-term experience with danazol is limited. Long-term therapy with other steroids alkylated at the 17 position has been associated with serious toxicity (cholestatic jaundice, peliosis hepatitis). Similar toxicity may develop after long-term danazol.

Androgenic effects: Androgenic effects may not be reversible even when the drug is discontinued. Watch patients closely for signs of virilization.

Pregnancy: Category X.

Lactation: Breastfeeding is contraindicated in patients taking danazol.

Children: Safety and efficacy in pediatric patients has not been established.

Precautions

Fluid retention: Conditions influenced by edema require careful observation.

Hepatic dysfunction: Hepatic dysfunction has been reported; perform periodic liver function tests.

Lipoproteins: Monitor HDL and LDL periodically.

Semen: Semen should be checked for volume, viscosity, sperm count, and motility every 3 to 4 months, especially in adolescents.

Porphyria: Danazol administration has been reported to cause exacerbation of the manifestations of acute intermittent porphyria.

Drug Interactions

Drugs that maybe affected by danazol are carbamazepine, cyclosporine, and warfarin.

Adverse Reactions

Significant adverse reactions include edema; vaginitis; nervousness; emotional lability; hepatic dysfunction; elevated blood pressure; pelvic pain; carpal tunnel syndrome; sleep disorders; fatigue; tremor; visual disturbances; anxiety; depression; gastroenteritis.

GLUCOCORTICOIDS

BETAMETHASONE

BETAMETHASONE, ORAL
Tablets: 0.6 mg (*Rx*)
Syrup: 0.6 mg/5 mL (*Rx*)

Celestone (Schering)

BETAMETHASONE SODIUM PHOSPHATE
Injection: 4 mg sodium phosphate/mL (*Rx*)

Celestone Phosphate (Schering)

BETAMETHASONE SODIUM PHOSPHATE AND ACETATE
Injection: 3 mg acetate and 3 mg sodium phosphate/mL (*Rx*) *Celestone Soluspan* (Schering)

BUDESONIDE
Capsules: 3 mg micronized budesonide

Entocort EC (AstraZeneca)

CORTISONE
Tablets: 5, 10, and 25 mg (*Rx*)
Injection: 50 mg/mL (*Rx*)

Various, *Cortisone Acetate* (Merck)
Cortone Acetate (Merck)

DEXAMETHASONE

DEXAMETHASONE, ORAL
Tablets: 0.25, 0.5, 0.75, 1, 1.5, 2, 4, and 6 mg (*Rx*)

Various, *Decadron* (Merck), *Dexone* (Solvay), *Hexadrol* (Organon)

Elixir: 0.5 mg/5 mL (*Rx*)

Various, *Decadron* (Merck), *Hexadrol* (Organon)

Oral Solution: 0.5 mg/5 mL (*Rx*)

Various

DEXAMETHASONE ACETATE
Injection: 8 and 16 mg/mL (*Rx*)

Various, *Dalalone L.A.* (Forest), *Dalalone D.P.* (Forest) *Decadron-LA* (Merck)

DEXAMETHASONE SODIUM PHOSPHATE
Injection: 4, 10, 20, and 24 mg/mL (*Rx*)

Various, *Dalalone* (Forest), *Decadron Phosphate* (Merck), *Hexadrol Phosphate* (Organon)

HYDROCORTISONE (CORTISOL)

HYDROCORTISONE
Tablets: 5, 10, and 20 mg (*Rx*)

Various, *Cortef* (Upjohn), *Hydrocortone* (Merck)

HYDROCORTISONE CYPIONATE
Oral Suspension: 10 mg/5 mL (*Rx*)

Cortef (Upjohn)

HYDROCORTISONE SODIUM PHOSPHATE
Injection: 50 mg/mL (*Rx*)

Hydrocortone Phosphate (Merck)

HYDROCORTISONE SODIUM SUCCINATE
Injection: 100, 250, 500, and 1000 mg per vial (*Rx*)

A-Hydrocort (Abbott), *Solu-Cortef* (Upjohn)

HYDROCORTISONE ACETATE
Injection: 25 and 50 mg/mL (*Rx*)

Various, *Hydrocortone Acetate* (Merck)

METHYLPREDNISOLONE

METHYLPREDNISOLONE, ORAL
Tablets: 2, 4, 8, 16, 24, and 32 mg (*Rx*)

Various, *Medrol* (Upjohn)

METHYLPREDNISOLONE SODIUM SUCCINATE
Powder for Injection: 40, 125, and 500 mg and 1 and 2 g per vial (*Rx*)

Various, *A-Methapred* (Abbott), *Solu-Medrol* (Upjohn)

METHYLPREDNISOLONE ACETATE
Injection: 20, 40, and 80 mg/mL (*Rx*)

Various, *Depo-Medrol* (Upjohn), *depMedalone* (Forest), *Adlone* (UAD)

PREDNISOLONE

PREDNISOLONE, ORAL
Tablets: 5 mg (*Rx*)
Syrup: 15 mg/5 mL (*Rx*)

Various, *Delta-Cortef* (Upjohn)
Prelone (Muro)

PREDNISOLONE ACETATE
Injection: 25 and 50 mg/mL (*Rx*)

Various, *Key-Pred 25* (Hyrex), *Key-Pred 50* (Hyrex)

PREDNISOLONE TEBUTATE
Injection: 20 mg/mL (*Rx*)

Various, *Hydeltra-T.B.A.*(Merck)

PREDNISOLONE SODIUM PHOSPHATE
Injection: 20 mg/mL (*Rx*)
Oral Liquid: 5 mg/5 mL (*Rx*)

Hydeltrasol (Merck)
Pediapred (Fisons)

PREDNISONE
Tablets: 1, 2.5, 5, 10, 20, and 50 mg (*Rx*) Various, *Meticorten* (Schering), *Orasone* (Solvay), *Deltasone* (Upjohn)

Oral Solution: 5 mg/5 mL (*Rx*) Various
Syrup: 5 mg/5 mL (*Rx*) *Liquid Pred* (Muro)

TRIAMCINOLONE

TRIAMCINOLONE, ORAL
Tablets: 1, 2, 4, and 8 mg (*Rx*) Various, *Aristocort* (Fujisawa)
TRIAMCINOLONE DIACETATE
Injection: 25 and 40 mg/mL (*Rx*) Various, *Aristocort Intralesional* (Fujisawa), *Aristocort Forte* (Fujisawa), *Triamolone 40* (Forest)

TRIAMCINOLONE HEXACETONIDE
Injection: 5 mg/mL (*Rx*) *Aristospan Intralesional* (Fujisawa)
20 mg/mL (*Rx*) *Aristospan Intra-articular* (Fujisawa)
TRIAMCINOLONE ACETONIDE
Injection: 3, 10, and 40 mg/mL (*Rx*) Various, *Tac-3* (Herbert), *Kenalog-10* (Westwood-Squibb), *Kenalog-40* (Westwood-Squibb), *Triamonide 40* (Forest)

Indications

Endocrine disorders: Primary or secondary adrenal cortical insufficiency (hydrocortisone or cortisone is the drug of choice; synthetic analogs may be used in conjunction with mineralocorticoids; in infancy, mineralocorticoid supplementation is important); congenital adrenal hyperplasia; nonsuppurative thyroiditis; hypercalcemia associated with cancer.

Parenteral – Acute adrenal cortical insufficiency (hydrocortisone or cortisone is drug of choice); preoperatively or in serious trauma or illness with known adrenal insufficiency or when adrenal cortical reserve is doubtful; shock unresponsive to conventional therapy if adrenal cortical insufficiency exists or is suspected.

Various rheumatic disorders.

Collagen diseases.

Dermatologic diseases.

Allergic states: Control of severe or incapacitating allergic conditions intractable to conventional treatment in serum sickness and drug hypersensitivity reactions. Parenteral therapy is indicated for urticarial transfusion reactions and acute noninfectious laryngeal edema (epinephrine is the drug of first choice).

Ophthalmic: Severe acute and chronic allergic and inflammatory processes involving the eye and its adnexa.

Respiratory diseases.

Hematologic disorders.

Neoplastic diseases.

Edematous states: To induce diuresis or remission of proteinuria in the nephrotic syndrome (without uremia) of the idiopathic type or that due to lupus erythematosus.

GI diseases: Crohn's disease and intractable sprue.

Multiple sclerosis.

Miscellaneous: Tuberculous meningitis with subarachnoid block or impending block when accompanied by appropriate antituberculous chemotherapy; in trichinosis with neurologic or myocardial involvement.

Intralesional administration: Keloids; localized hypertrophic, infiltrated, inflammatory lesions of lichen planus, psoriatic plaques, granuloma annulare, lichen simplex chronicus (neurodermatitis); discoid lupus erythematosus; necrobiosis lipoidica diabeticorum; alopecia areata. May be useful in cystic tumors of an aponeurosis or tendon (ganglia).

Triamcinolone: Treatment of pulmonary emphysema where bronchospasm or bronchial edema plays a significant role, and diffuse interstitial pulmonary fibrosis (Hamman-

Rich syndrome); in conjunction with diuretic agents to induce a diuresis in refractory CHF and in cirrhosis of the liver with refractory ascites; and for postoperative dental inflammatory reactions.

Unlabeled uses:

Glucocorticoid Unlabeled Uses	
Use	Drug/Comment
Acute mountain sickness	Dexamethasone 4 mg q 6 h; prevention or treatment
Antiemetic	Dexamethasone most common, 16 to 20 mg
Bacterial meningitis	Dexamethasone 0.15 mg/kg q 6 h; to decrease incidence of hearing loss
Bronchopulmonary dysplasia in preterm infants	Dexamethasone 0.5 mg/kg, then taper.
COPD	Prednisone 30 to 60 mg/day for 1 to 2 weeks, then taper
Depression, diagnosis of	Dexamethasone 1 mg
Duchenne's muscular dystrophy	Prednisone 0.75 to 1.5 mg/kg/day; to improve strength and function
Graves' ophthalmopathy	Prednisone 60 mg/day, taper to 20 mg/day
Hepatitis, severe alcoholic	Methylprednisolone 32 mg/day
Hirsutism	Dexamethasone 0.5 to 1 mg/day
Respiratory distress syndrome	Prevention in premature neonates (betamethasone most common); adults, methylprednisolone 30 mg/kg (controversial)
Septic shock	Methylprednisolone 30 mg/kg IV most common (very controversial)
Spinal cord injury, acute	Methylprednisolone IV within 8 hrs of injury; to improve neurologic function
Tuberculous pleurisy	Prednisolone 0.75 mg/kg/day, then taper; concurrently w/antituberculous therapy

Administration and Dosage

The maximal activity of the adrenal cortex is between 2 and 8 am, and it is minimal between 4 pm and midnight. Exogenous corticosteroids suppress adrenocortical activity the least when given at the time of maximal activity (am). Therefore, administer glucocorticoids in the morning prior to 9 am.

Initiation of therapy: The initial dosage depends on the specific disease entity being treated. Maintain or adjust the initial dosage until a satisfactory response is noted. If after a reasonable period of time there is a lack of satisfactory clinical response, discontinue the drug and transfer the patient to other appropriate therapy. For infants and children, the recommended dosage should be governed by the same considerations rather than by strict adherence to the ratio indicated by age or body weight. It should be emphasized that dosage requirements are variable and must be individualized.

Maintenance therapy: After a favorable response is observed, determine the maintenance dosage by decreasing the initial dosage in small amounts at intervals until the lowest dosage that will maintain an adequate clinical response is reached.

Withdrawal of therapy: If, after long-term therapy, the drug is to be stopped, it must be withdrawn gradually. If spontaneous remission occurs in a chronic condition, discontinue treatment gradually.

Alternate day therapy: Alternate day therapy is a dosing regimen in which twice the usual daily dose is administered every other morning. The purpose is to provide the patient requiring long-term treatment with the beneficial effects of corticosteroids while minimizing pituitary-adrenal suppression, the cushingoid state, withdrawal symptoms and growth suppression in children. The benefits of alternate day therapy are only achieved by using the intermediate-acting agents.

Intra-articular injection: Dose depends on the joint size and varies with the severity of the condition. In chronic cases, injections may be repeated at intervals of ≥ 1 to 5 weeks depending upon the degree of relief obtained from the initial injection. Injection must be made into the synovial space.

Miscellaneous (tendinitis, epicondylitis, ganglion): In the treatment of conditions such as tendinitis or tenosynovitis, inject into the tendon sheath rather than into the substance of the tendon. When treating conditions such as epicondylitis, outline the area of greatest tenderness and infiltrate the drug into the area.

Injections for local effect in dermatologic conditions: Avoid injection of sufficient material to cause blanching, since this may be followed by a small slough. One to four injections are usually employed.

BETAMETHASONE:
> *Betamethasone, oral –*
>> *Initial dosage:* 0.6 to 7.2 mg/day.
>
> *Betamethasone sodium phosphate –*
>> *Systemic and local:* The initial dosage may vary up to 9 mg/day.
>
> *Betamethasone sodium phosphate and acetate –* Betamethasone sodium phosphate provides prompt activity, while betamethasone acetate is only slightly soluble and affords sustained activity.
>> *Systemic:* Not for IV use.
>>> *Initial dose –* 0.5 to 9 mg/day. Dosage ranges are 33% to 50% of the oral dose given every 12 hours. In certain acute, life-threatening situations, dosages exceeding the usual may be justified and may be in multiples of oral dosages.
>>> *Bursitis, tenosynovitis, peritendinitis:* 1 mL given intrabursally.
>>> *Rheumatoid arthritis and osteoarthritis:* 0.5 to 2 mL given intra-articularly.
>>>> *Very large joints –* 1 to 2 mL.
>>>> *Large joints –* 1 mL.
>>>> *Medium joints –* 0.5 to 1 mL.
>>>> *Small joints –* 0.25 to 0.5 mL.
>>> *Dermatologic conditions:* 0.2 mL/cm^2 intradermally.
>>>> *Maximum dose –* 1 mL/week.
>> *Foot disorders –* The following doses are recommended at 3- to 7-day intervals:
>>> *Bursitis:*
>>>> *Under heloma durum or heloma molle –* 0.25 to 0.5 mL.
>>>> *Under calcaneal spur –* 0.5 mL.
>>>> *Over hallux rigidus or digiti quinti varus –* 0.5 mL.
>>> *Tenosynovitis, periostitis of cuboid:* 0.5 mL.
>>> *Acute gouty arthritis:* 0.5 to 1 mL.

BUDESONIDE:
> *Adults –* Take 9 mg once daily in the morning for up to 8 weeks. Swallow capsules whole; do not chew or break. Safety and efficacy of budesonide in the treatment of active Crohn's disease have not been established beyond 8 weeks. For recurring episodes of active Crohn's disease, a repeat 8-week course of budesonide can be given. Treatment with budesonide capsules can be tapered to 6 mg/day for 2 weeks prior to complete cessation.
>
> Patients with mild-to-moderately active Crohn's disease involving the ileum or ascending colon have been switched from oral prednisolone to budesonide with no reported episodes of adrenal insufficiency. Because prednisolone should not be stopped abruptly, tapering should begin concomitantly with initiating budesonide treatment.
>
>> *Hepatic insufficiency:* Consider reducing the dose of budesonide capsules in patients with hepatic insufficiency.

CORTISONE:
> *Initial dosage –* 25 to 300 mg/day. In less severe diseases, lower doses may suffice.

DEXAMETHASONE:
> *Dexamethasone, oral –*
>> *Initial dosage:* 0.75 to 9 mg/day.
>> *In acute, self-limited allergic disorders or acute exacerbations of chronic allergic disorders:* In acute, self-limited allergic disorders or acute exacerbations of chronic allergic disorders, the following dosage schedule combining parenteral (dexamethasone sodium phosphate injection, 4 mg/mL) and oral therapy (0.75 mg tablets) is suggested: First day, 1 or 2 mL IM; second day, 4 tablets in 2 divided doses; third day, 4 tablets in 2 divided doses; fourth day, 2 tablets in 2 divided doses; fifth day, 1 tablet; sixth day, 1 tablet; seventh day, no treatment; eighth day, follow-up visit.
>> *Suppression tests:* For Cushing's syndrome – Give 1 mg at 11 pm. Draw blood for plasma cortisol determination the following day at 8 am. For greater accuracy, give 0.5 mg every 6 hours for 48 hours. Collect 24 hour urine to determine 17-hydroxycorticosteroid excretion.
>> *Test to distinguish Cushing's syndrome due to pituitary ACTH excess from Cushing's syndrome due to other causes* – Give 2 mg every 6 hours for 48 hours. Collect 24 hour urine to determine 17-hydroxycorticosteroid excretion.
> *Dexamethasone acetate* – Not for IV use.
>> *Systemic:* 8 to 16 mg IM, may repeat in 1 to 3 weeks.
>> *Intralesional:* 0.8 to 1.6 mg.
>> *Intra-articular and soft tissue:* 4 to 16 mg; may repeat at 1 to 3 week intervals.
> *Dexamethasone sodium phosphate –*
>> *Systemic:*
>>> *Initial dosage* – 0.5 to 9 mg daily. Usual dose ranges are 33% to 50% of the oral dose given every 12 hours. However, in certain acute, life-threatening situations, dosages exceeding the usual may be justified and may be in multiples of the oral dosages.
>>> *Cerebral edema:* In adults, administer an initial IV dose of 10 mg, followed by 4 mg IM every 6 hours until maximum response has been noted. Response is usually noted within 12 to 24 hours. Dosage may be reduced after 2 to 4 days and gradually discontinued over 5 to 7 days. For palliative management of patients with recurrent or inoperable brain tumors, maintenance therapy with either the injection or tablets in a dosage of 2 mg 2 or 3 times daily may be effective.
>>> *Unresponsive shock* – Reported regimens range from 1 to 6 mg/kg as a single IV injection, to 40 mg initially followed by repeated IV injections every 2 to 6 hours while shock persists.

HYDROCORTISONE (Cortisol):
> *Hydrocortisone, oral –*
>> *Initial dosage:* 20 to 240 mg/day.
> *Hydrocortisone sodium phosphate* – Administer by IV, IM or SC injection. Initial dose is 15 to 240 mg/day. Usually, 33% to 50% of the oral dose every 12 hours. For acute diseases, doses> 240 mg may be required.
> *Hydrocortisone sodium succinate* – May be administered IV or IM. The initial dose is 100 to 500 mg, and may be repeated at 2, 4 or 6 hour intervals depending on patient response and clinical condition.
> *Hydrocortisone acetate* – For intralesional, intra-articular or soft tissue injection only. Not for IV use. Dosage range is 5 to 37.5 mg. If desired, a local anesthetic may be injected before hydrocortisone acetate or mixed in a syringe and given simultaneously.

METHYLPREDNISOLONE:
> *Methylprednisolone, oral –*
>> *Initial dose:* 4 to 48 mg/day; adjust until a satisfactory response is noted. Determine maintenance dose by decreasing initial dose in small decrements at appropriate intervals until reaching the lowest effective dose.
>> *Dosepak 21 therapy:* Follow manufacturer's directions.
> *Methylprednisolone sodium succinate –*
>> *Initial dose:* 10 to 40 mg IV, administered over 1 to several minutes. Give subsequent doses IV or IM.

Infants and children: Not less than 0.5 mg/kg/24 hours.

For high dose therapy, give 30 mg/kg IV, infused over 10 to 20 minutes. May repeat every 4 to 6 hours, not beyond 48 to 72 hours.

Methylprednisolone acetate – Not for IV use. As a temporary substitute for oral therapy, administer the total daily dose as a single IM injection. For prolonged effect, give a single weekly dose.

Adrenogenital syndrome: A single 40 mg injection IM every 2 weeks.

Rheumatoid arthritis: Weekly IM maintenance dose varies from 40 to 120 mg.

Dermatologic lesions: 40 to 120 mg IM weekly for 1 to 4 weeks. In severe dermatitis (eg, poison ivy), relief may result within 8 to 12 hours of a single dose of 80 to 120 mg IM. In chronic contact dermatitis, repeated injections every 5 to 10 days may be necessary. In seborrheic dermatitis, a weekly dose of 80 mg IM may be adequate.

Asthma and allergic rhinitis: 80 to 120 mg IM.

Intra-articular and soft tissue: 4 to 80 mg.

Intralesional: 20 to 60 mg.

PREDNISOLONE:
   Prednisolone –
      Initial dosage: 5 to 60 mg/day.
      Multiple sclerosis: In treatment of acute exacerbations of multiple sclerosis, 200 mg daily for a week followed by 80 mg every other day for 1 month.
   Prednisolone acetate – Not for IV use.
      Initial dosage: 4 to 60 mg/day, IM.
      Intralesional, intra-articular or soft tissue injection: 4 mg, up to 100 mg.
      Multiple sclerosis: 200 mg daily for a week, followed by 80 mg every other day or 4 to 8 mg dexamethasone every other day for 1 month.
   Prednisolone tebutate –
      Intra-articular, intralesional or soft tissue administration: 8 to 30 mg. Doses > 40 mg are not recommended.
   Prednisolone sodium phosphate –
      Parenteral: For IV or IM use.
         Initial dosage – 4 to 60 mg/day.
      Intra-articular, intralesional or soft tissue administration: 2 to 30 mg.
      Oral:
         Initial dosage – 5 to 60 mL (5 to 60 mg base) per day.
         Multiple sclerosis (acute exacerbations) – 200 mg daily for a week, followed by 80 mg every other day or 4 to 8 mg dexamethasone every other day for 1 month.

PREDNISONE: Initial dosage varies from 5 to 60 mg/day. Prednisone is inactive and must be metabolized to prednisolone. This may be impaired in patients with liver disease.

TRIAMCINOLONE:
   Triamcinolone, oral –
      Adrenocortical insufficiency: 4 to 12 mg, in addition to mineralocorticoid therapy.
      Rheumatic and dermatological disorders and bronchial asthma: 8 to 16 mg.
      Allergic states: 8 to 12 mg.
      Ophthalmological diseases: 12 to 40 mg.
      Respiratory diseases: 16 to 48 mg.
      Hematologic disorders: 16 to 60 mg.
      Tuberculous meningitis: 32 to 48 mg.
      Acute rheumatic carditis: 20 to 60 mg.
      Acute leukemia and lymphoma (adults): 16 to 40 mg. It may be necessary to give as much as 100 mg/day in leukemia.
      Acute leukemia (children): 1 to 2 mg/kg.
      Edematous states: 16 to 20 mg (up to 48 mg) until diuresis occurs.
      Systemic lupus erythematosus: 20 to 32 mg.
   Triamcinolone diacetate –
      Systemic: Not for IV use. May be administered IM for initial therapy; however, most clinicians prefer to adjust the dose orally until adequate control is attained.

The average dose is 40 mg IM per week. In general, a single parenteral dose 4 to 7 times the oral daily dose controls the patient from 4 to 7 days, up to 3 to 4 weeks.

Intra-articular and intrasynovial: 5 to 40 mg.

Intralesional or sublesional: 5 to 48 mg. Do not use > 12.5 mg/injection site. The usual average dose is 25 mg per lesion.

Triamcinolone hexacetonide – Not for IV use.

Intra-articular: 2 to 20 mg average.

Intralesional or sublesional: Up to 0.5 mg per square inch of affected area.

Triamcinolone acetonide –

Systemic:

Initial IM dose – 2.5 to 60 mg/day. Not for IV use.

Intra-articular or intrabursal administration and for injection into tendon sheaths:

Initial dose – 2.5 to 5 mg for smaller joints and 5 to 15 mg for larger joints. For adults, doses up to 10 mg for smaller areas and up to 40 mg for larger areas are usually sufficient.

Intradermal: Use only 3 or 10 mg/mL. Initial dose varies; limit to 1 mg per site.

Actions

Pharmacology: The naturally occurring adrenal cortical steroids have both anti-inflammatory (glucocorticoid) and salt-retaining (mineralocorticoid) properties. Glucocorticoids cause profound and varied metabolic effects. In addition, they modify the body's immune responses to diverse stimuli. These compounds are used as replacement therapy in adrenocortical deficiency states and may be used for their anti-inflammatory effects.

Pharmacokinetics: Hydrocortisone and most of its congeners are readily absorbed from the GI tract; greatly altered onsets and durations are usually achieved with injections of suspensions and esters. Hydrocortisone is metabolized by the liver, which is the rate-limiting step in its clearance. The metabolism and excretion of the synthetic glucocorticoids generally parallel hydrocortisone. Induction of hepatic enzymes will increase the metabolic clearance of hydrocortisone and the synthetic glucocorticoids.

The half-life values refer to the intrinsic activity of each agent; insoluble salts of these drugs are used as repository injections and have sustained effects due to delayed absorption from the injection site.

Glucocorticoid Equivalencies, Potencies and Half-Life					
Glucocorticoid	Approximate equivalent dose (mg)	Relative anti-inflammatory (glucocorticoid) potency	Relative mineralocorticoid potency	Plasma (min)	Biologic (hrs)
Short-acting					
Cortisone	25	0.8	2	30	8-12
Hydrocortisone	20	1	2	80-118	8-12
Intermediate-acting					
Prednisone	5	4	1	60	18-36
Prednisolone	5	4	1	115-212	18-36
Triamcinolone	4	5	0	200+	18-36
Methylprednisolone	4	5	0	78-188	18-36
Long-acting					
Dexamethasone	0.75	20-30	0	110-210	36-54
Betamethasone	0.6-0.75	20-30	0	300+	36-54

Contraindications

Systemic fungal infections; hypersensitivity to the drug; IM use in idiopathic thrombocytopenic purpura; administration of live virus vaccines (eg, smallpox) in patients receiving immunosuppressive corticosteroid doses (see Warnings).

Warnings

Infections: Corticosteroids may mask signs of infection, and new infections may appear during their use. There may be decreased resistance and inability of the host defense mechanisms to prevent dissemination of the infection. Restrict use in active tuberculosis to cases of fulminating or disseminated disease in which the corticosteroid is used for disease management with appropriate chemotherapy. Corticosteroids may exacerbate systemic fungal infections and may activate latent amebiasis.

Hepatitis: Corticosteroids may be harmful in chronic active hepatitis positive for hepatitis B surface antigen.

Ocular effects: Prolonged use may produce posterior subcapsular cataracts, glaucoma with possible damage to the optic nerves, and may enhance the establishment of secondary ocular infections due to fungi or viruses.

Fluid and electrolyte balance: Average and large doses of hydrocortisone or cortisone can cause elevation of blood pressure, salt and water retention and increased excretion of potassium. These effects are less likely to occur with the synthetic derivatives except when used in large doses.

Immunosuppression: During therapy, do not use live virus vaccines (eg, smallpox). Do not immunize patients who are receiving corticosteroids, especially high doses, because of possible hazards of neurological complications and a lack of antibody response. This does not apply to patients receiving corticosteroids as replacement therapy.

Adrenal suppression: Prolonged therapy of pharmacologic doses may lead to hypothalamic-pituitary-adrenal suppression. The degree of adrenal suppression varies with the dosage, relative glucocorticoid activity, biological half-life, and duration of glucocorticoid therapy within each individual. Adrenal suppression may be minimized by the use of intermediate-acting glucocorticoids (prednisone, prednisolone, methylprednisolone) on an alternate day schedule.

Stress: In patients receiving or recently withdrawn from corticosteroid therapy subjected to unusual stress, increased dosage of rapidly acting corticosteroids is indicated before, during, and after stressful situations, except in patients on high-dose therapy.

Cardiovascular: Reports suggest an apparent association between corticosteroid use and left ventricular free wall rupture after a recent MI.

Hypersensitivity reactions: Anaphylactoid reactions have occurred rarely with corticosteroid therapy.

Renal function impairment: Edema may occur in the presence of renal disease with a fixed or decreased glomerular filtration rate.

Elderly: Consider the risk/benefit factors of steroid use. Consider lower doses because of body changes caused by aging (ie, diminution of muscle mass and plasma volume).

Pregnancy: Corticosteroids cross the placenta (prednisone has the poorest transport). Chronic maternal ingestion during the first trimester has shown a 1% incidence of cleft palate in humans. Hypoadrenalism has occurred.

Lactation: Corticosteroids appear in breast milk and could suppress growth, interfere with endogenous corticosteroid production or cause other unwanted effects in the nursing infant. However, large doses for short periods may not harm the infant. Alternatives to consider include waiting 3 to 4 hours after the dose before breastfeeding and using prednisolone rather than prednisone.

Children: Carefully observe growth and development of infants and children on prolonged corticosteroid therapy.

Precautions

Monitoring: Observe patients for weight increase, edema, hypertension, and excessive potassium excretion, as well as for less obvious signs of adrenocortical steroid-induced untoward effects. Monitor for a negative nitrogen balance due to protein catabolism. Evaluate blood pressure and body weight, and do routine laboratory studies, including 2 hour postprandial blood glucose and serum potassium and a chest x-ray at regular intervals during prolonged therapy. Upper GI x-rays are desirable in patients with known or suspected peptic ulcer disease or significant dyspepsia or in patients complaining of gastric distress.

Use the lowest possible dose: Make a benefit/risk decision in each individual case as to the size of the dose, duration of treatment and the use of daily or intermittent therapy, since complications of treatment are dependent on these factors.

Steroid psychosis: Steroid psychosis is characterized by a delirious or toxic psychosis with clouded sensorium. Other symptoms may include euphoria, insomnia, mood swings, personality changes and severe depression. The onset of symptoms usually occurs within 15 to 30 days. Predisposing factors include doses > 40 mg prednisone equivalent, female predominance, and, possibly, a family history of psychiatric illness.

Multiple sclerosis: Although corticosteroids are effective in speeding the resolution of acute exacerbations of multiple sclerosis, they do not affect the ultimate outcome or natural history of the disease.

Repository injections: To minimize the likelihood and severity of atrophy, do not inject SC, avoid injection into the deltoid and avoid repeated IM injections into the same site, if possible. Repository injections are not recommended as initial therapy in acute situations.

Local injections: Intra-articular injection may produce systemic and local effects. A marked increase in pain accompanied by local swelling, further restriction of joint motion, fever and malaise is suggestive of septic arthritis. Frequent intra-articular injection may damage joint tissues.

Special risk: Use with caution in the following situations: Nonspecific ulcerative colitis if there is a probability of impending perforation, abscess or other pyogenic infection; diverticulitis; fresh intestinal anastomoses; hypertension; CHF; thromboembolitic tendencies; thrombophlebitis; osteoporosis; exanthema; Cushing's syndrome; antibiotic-resistant infections; convulsive disorders; metastatic carcinoma; myasthenia gravis; vaccinia; varicella; diabetes mellitus.; hypothyroidism, cirrhosis (enhanced effect of corticosteroids).

Drug Interactions

Drugs that may be affected by glucocorticoids include anticholinesterases, anticoagulants, cyclosporine, digitalis glycosides, isoniazid, nondepolarizing neuromuscular blockers, potassium-depleting agents (eg, diuretics), salicylates, somatrem and theophyllines. Drugs that may affect corticosteroids include aminoglutethimide, barbiturates, cholestyramine, oral contraceptives, ephedrine, estrogens, hydantoins, ketoconazole, macrolide antibiotics, and rifampin.

CYP3A4 inhibitors: If concomitant administration with a CYP3A4 inhibitor is indicated, closely monitor patients for increased signs or symptoms of hypercorticism. Consider reduction in **budesonide** dose.

Drug/Lab test interactions: Urine glucose and serum cholesterol levels may increase. Decreased serum levels of potassium, triiodothyronine (T_3), and a minimal decrease of thyroxine (T_4) may occur. Thyroid I^{131} uptake may be decreased. False-negative results with the nitroblue-tetrazolium test for bacterial infection. Dexamethasone, given for cerebral edema, may alter the results of a brain scan (decreased uptake of radioactive material).

Adverse Reactions

Adverse reactions that may occur include hypertension, myocardial rupture following recent MI, anaphylactoid/hypersensitivity reactions; sodium and fluid retention; hypokalemia; metabolic alkalosis; hypocalcemia; hypotension or shock-like reactions; muscle weakness; muscle mass loss; tendon rupture; osteoporosis; spontaneous fractures; thromboembolism or fat embolism; thrombophlebitis; cardiac arrhythmias or ECG changes due to potassium deficiency; syncopal episodes; pancreatitis; abdominal distension; ulcerative esophagitis; nausea; vomiting; increased appetite and weight gain; impaired wound healing; thin fragile skin; petechiae/ecchymoses; erythema; purpura; hirsutism; acneiform eruptions; allergic dermatitis; urticaria; convulsions; vertigo; headache; neuritis/paresthesias; aggravation of pre-existing psychiatric conditions; steroid psychoses; menstrual irregularities; development of Cushingoid state (eg, moonface, buffalo hump, supraclavicular fat pad enlargement, central obesity); suppression of growth in children; increased sweating; hyperglycemia; glycosuria; increased IOP; glaucoma; malaise; fatigue; insomnia.

MIGLITOL

Tablets: 25, 50, and 100 mg (Rx)	Glyset (Bayer)

Indications

Type 2 diabetes: Monotherapy adjunct to diet to improve glycemic control in patients with type 2 diabetes whose hyperglycemia cannot be managed by diet alone.

Combination therapy – In combination with a sulfonylurea when diet plus either miglitol or a sulfonylurea alone do not result in adequate glycemic control. The effect of miglitol to enhance glycemic control is additive to that of sulfonylureas when used in combination, presumably because the mechanism of action is different.

Administration and Dosage

The use of miglitol must be viewed as a treatment in addition to diet and not as a substitute for diet or as a convenient mechanism for avoiding dietary restraint.

Initial dosage: The recommended starting dosage is 25 mg, given orally 3 times/day at the start (with the first bite) of each main meal. However, some patients may benefit by starting at 25 mg once daily to minimize GI adverse effects and gradually increasing the frequency of administration to 3 times/day.

Maintenance dosage: The usual maintenance dose of miglitol is 50 mg 3 times/day although some patients may benefit from increasing the dose to 100 mg 3 times/day. In order to allow adaptation to potential adverse effects, initiate miglitol therapy at a dosage of 25 mg 3 times/day, the lowest effective dosage, and then gradually titrate upward. After 4 to 8 weeks of the 25 mg 3 times/day regimen, increase the dosage to 50 mg 3 times/day for ≈ 3 months. Measure glycosylated hemoglobin level is not satisfactory, the dosage may be further increased to 100 mg 3 times/day, the maximum recommended dosage. If no further reduction is postprandial glucose or glycosylated hemoglobin levels is observed with titration to 100 mg 3 times/day, consider lowering the dose.

Maximum dosage: The maximum recommended dosage is 100 mg 3 times/day.

Actions

Pharmacology: Miglitol is an alpha-glucoside inhibitor that delays the digestion of ingested carbohydrates resulting in a smaller rise in blood glucose concentration following meals. Miglitol reduces levels of glycosylated hemoglobin in patients with type 2 (non-insulin-dependent) diabetes mellitus.

In contrast to sulfonylureas and thiazolidinediones, miglitol does not enhance insulin secretion or increase insulin sensitivity.

Pharmacokinetics:

Absorption – Absorption of miglitol is saturable at high doses; a dose of 25 mg is completely absorbed, whereas a dose of 100 mg is only 50% to 70% absorbed. Peak concentrations are reached in 2 to 3 hours.

Distribution – The protein binding of miglitol is negligible (< 4%). Miglitol has a volume of distribution of 0.18 L/kg, consistent with distribution primarily into the extracellular fluid.

Metabolism – No metabolites have been detected in plasma, urine, or feces, indicating a lack of either systemic or presystemic metabolism.

Excretion – Miglitol is eliminated by renal excretion as unchanged drug. Following a 25 mg dose, > 95% of the dose is recovered in the urine within 24 hours. The elimination half-life from plasma is ≈ 2 hours.

Contraindications

Diabetic ketoacidoses; inflammatory bowel disease; colonic ulceration; partial intestinal obstruction; patients predisposed to intestinal obstruction; chronic intestinal diseases associated with marked disorders of digestion or absorption or with conditions that may deteriorate as a result of increased gas formation in the intestine; hypersensitivity to the drug or any of its components.

Warnings

Renal function impairment: Plasma concentrations of miglitol in renally impaired volunteers were proportionally increased relative to the degree of renal dysfunction. Patients with creatinine clearance < 25 mL/min taking 25 mg 3 times/day exhibited a > 2-fold increase in miglitol plasma levels as compared with subjects with creatinine clearance > 60 mL/min. Dosage adjustment to correct the increased plasma concentrations is not feasible because miglitol acts locally. Treatment of patients with creatinine clearance < 25 mL/min is not recommended.

Pregnancy: Category B.

Lactation: Althought the levels of miglitol reached in breast milk are exceedingly low, do not administer miglitol to a nursing woman.

Children: Safety and efficacy have not been established.

Precautions

Monitoring: Monitor therapeutic response to miglitol by periodic blood glucose tests. Measurement of glycosylated hemoglobin levels is recommended for the monitoring of long-term glycemic control.

Hypoglycemia: Because of its mechanism of action, miglitol, when administered alone, should not cause hypoglycemia. It may increase the hypoglycemic potential of the sulfonylurea. Use oral glucose (dextrose), whose absorption is not delayed by miglitol, instead of sucrose (cane sugar) in the treatment of mild to moderate hypoglycemia. Sucrose, whose hydrolysis to glucose and fructose is inhibited by miglitol, is unsuitable for the rapid correction of hypoglycemia. Severe hypoglycemia may require the use of either IV glucose infusion or glucagon injection.

Blood glucose control: When diabetic patients are exposed to stress such as fever, trauma, infection or surgery, a temporary loss of control of blood glucose may occur. At such times, temporary insulin therapy may be necessary.

Drug Interactions

Drugs that may affect miglitol include digestive enzymes and intestinal adsorbents. Drugs that may be affected by miglitol include digoxin, glyburide, metformin, propranolol, and ranitidine.

Adverse Reactions

Adverse reactions may include skin rash (4.3%, generally transient) and flatulence (41.5%). The incidence of diarrhea (28.7%) and abdominal pain (11.7%) diminish with continued treatment.

Lab test abnormalities: Low serum iron (9.2%) usually does not persist in the majority of cases and is not associated with reductions in hemoglobin or changes in other hematologic indices.

REPAGLINIDE

Tablets: 0.5, 1, and 2 mg *(Rx)*   *Prandin* (Novo Nordisk)

Indications

Type 2 diabetes mellitus: As an adjunct to diet and exercise to lower the blood glucose in patients with type 2 diabetes mellitus whose hyperglycemia cannot be controlled satisfactorily by diet and exercise alone.

In combination with metformin to lower blood glucose in patients whose hyperglycemia cannot be controlled by exercise, diet, and either agent alone.

Administration and Dosage

There is no fixed dosage regimen. Monitor the patient's blood glucose periodically to determine the minimum effective dose for the patient; to detect primary failure (ie, inadequate lowering of blood glucose at the maximum recommended dose of medication); and to detect secondary failure (ie, loss of adequate blood glucose-lowering response after an initial period of effectiveness). Glycosylated hemoglobin (HbA_{1c}) levels are of value in monitoring the patient's longer-term response to therapy.

Repaglinide doses are usually taken ≤ 15 minutes of the meal, but time may vary from immediately preceding the meal to as long as 30 minutes before the meal.

Starting dose: For patients not previously treated or whose glycosylated hemoglobin (HbA_{1c}) is < 8%, the starting dose is 0.5 mg. For patients previously treated with blood glucose-lowering agents and whose HbA_{1c} is ≥ 8%, the initial dose is 1 or 2 mg before each meal.

Dose adjustment: Determine dosing adjustments by blood glucose response, usually fasting blood glucose. Double the preprandial dose up to 4 mg until satisfactory blood glucose response is achieved. At least 1 week should elapse to assess response after each dose adjustment.

Dose range: Dose range is 0.5 to 4 mg taken with meals. Repaglinide may be dosed preprandially 2, 3, or 4 times/day in response to changes in the patient's meal pattern. Maximum recommended daily dose is 16 mg.

Patients receiving other oral hypoglycemic agents: When repaglinide is used to replace therapy with other oral hypoglycemic agents, it may be started the day after the final dose is given. Observe patients carefully for hypoglycemia because of potential overlapping of drug effects. When transferred from longer half-life sulfonylureas (eg, chlorpropamide), close monitoring may be indicated for up to ≥ 1 week.

Combination therapy: If repaglinide monotherapy does not result in adequate glycemic control, metformin may be added. Or, if metformin therapy does not provide adequate control, repaglinide may be added. The starting dose and dose adjustments for combination therapy are the same as repaglinide monotherapy. Carefully adjust the dose of each drug to determine the minimal dose required. Failure to do so could result in an increase in the incidence of hypoglycemic episodes. Use appropriate monitoring of fasting plasma glucose (FPG) and HbA_{1c}.

Actions

Pharmacology: Repaglinide is a non-sulfonylurea hypoglycemic agent of the meglitinide class (the non-sulfonylurea moiety of glyburide) used in the management of type 2 diabetes mellitus. It lowers blood glucose levels by stimulating the release of insulin from the pancreas. This action is dependent on functioning beta cells in the pancreatic islets. Insulin release is glucose-dependent and diminishes at low glucose concentrations.

Pharmacokinetics:

    Absorption – After oral administration, repaglinide is rapidly and completely absorbed from the GI tract. After single and multiple oral doses, peak plasma drug levels (C_{max}) occur within 1 hour (T_{max}). Repaglinide is rapidly eliminated from the blood stream with a half-life of ≈ 1 hour. The mean absolute bioavailability is 56%.

    Distribution – After IV dosing in healthy subjects, the volume of distribution at steady state was 31 L, and the total body clearance was 38 L/hr. Protein binding and binding to human serum albumin was > 98%.

    Metabolism – Repaglinide is completely metabolized by oxidative biotransformation and direct conjugation with glucuronic acid after either an IV or oral dose. The cytochrome P450 enzyme system, specifically 3A4, is involved in the N-dealkylation of repaglinide.

    Excretion – Within 96 hours after a single oral dose, ≈ 90% was recovered in the feces and ≈ 8% in the urine. Only 0.1% of the dose is cleared in the urine as parent compound. Less than 2% of the parent drug was recovered in feces.

Contraindications

Diabetic ketoacidosis, with or without coma (treat with insulin); type 1 diabetes; hypersensitivity to the drug or its inactive ingredients.

Warnings

Cardiovascular mortality: The administration of oral hypoglycemic drugs is associated with increased cardiovascular mortality as compared with treatment with diet alone or diet plus insulin.

Hepatic function impairment: Patients with impaired liver function may be exposed to higher concentrations of repaglinide and its associated metabolites than would patients with normal liver function receiving usual doses. Therefore, use repaglinide cautiously in patients with impaired liver function. Utilize longer intervals between dose adjustments to allow full assessment of response.

Pregnancy: Category C.

Lactation: It is not known whether repaglinide is excreted in breast milk.

Children: No studies have been performed in pediatric patients.

Precautions

Monitoring: Periodically monitor FPG and HbA_{1c} levels. During dose adjustment, fasting glucose can be used to determine response.

Hypoglycemia: Hepatic insufficiency may cause elevated repaglinide blood levels and may diminish gluconeogenic capacity, both of which increase the risk of serious hypoglycemia. Elderly, debilitated, or malnourished patients, and those with adrenal, pituitary, or hepatic insufficiency are particularly susceptible to the hypoglycemic action of glucose-lowering drugs.

Secondary failure: It may be necessary to discontinue repaglinide and administer insulin if the patient is exposed to stress (eg, fever, trauma, infection, surgery).

Drug Interactions

Repaglinide metabolism may be inhibited by antifungal agents like ketoconazole and miconazole, and antibacterial agents like erythromycin. Drugs that induce the cytochrome P450 enzyme system 3A4 may increase repaglinide metabolism (eg, troglitazone, rifampin, barbiturates, carbamazepine).

The actions of oral hypoglycemic agents may be potentiated by certain drugs including NSAIDs and other drugs that are highly protein bound, salicylates, sulfonamides, chloramphenicol, coumarins, probenecid, MAOIs, and beta blockers. Observe patient closely for loss of glycemic control when these agents are added to or withdrawn from repaglinide therapy.

Certain drugs tend to produce hyperglycemia and may lead to loss of glycemic control (eg, thiazides and other diuretics, corticosteroids, phenothiazines, thyroid products, estrogens, oral contraceptives, phenytoin, nicotinic acid, sympathomimetics, calcium channel blockers, isoniazid). Observe patient closely for loss of glycemic control when these agents are added to or withdrawn from repaglinide therapy.

Drug/Food interactions: When given with food, mean C_{max} and AUC of repaglinide were decreased 20% and 12.4%, respectively. Administer repaglinide before meals.

Adverse Reactions

The most common adverse events leading to discontinuation during trials were hyperglycemia, hypoglycemia, and related symptoms. Mild or moderate hypoglycemia occurred in 16% of repaglinide patients, 20% with glyburide, and 19% with glipizide. The adverse event profile of repaglinide was generally comparable with that for sulfonylurea drugs.

Adverse reactions occurring in ≥ 3% of patients include: URI, sinusitis, rhinitis, bronchitis, nausea, diarrhea, constipation, vomiting, dyspepsia, arthralgia, back pain, hypoglycemia, headache, paresthesia, chest pain, urinary tract infection.

NATEGLINIDE

Tablets: 60 and 120 mg (*Rx*)	*Starlix* (Novartis)

Indications
Type 2 diabetes mellitus:

   Monotherapy – To lower blood glucose in patients with type 2 diabetes whose hyperglycemia cannot be adequately controlled by diet and physical exercise and who have not been chronically treated with other antidiabetic agents.

   Combination therapy – In patients whose hyperglycemia is inadequately controlled with metformin, nateglinide may be added to, but not substituted for, metformin.

Do not switch patients whose hyperglycemia is not adequately controlled with glyburide or other insulin secretagogues to nateglinide; do not add nateglinide to their treatment regimen.

Administration and Dosage
Monotherapy and combination with metformin: The recommended starting and maintenance dose of nateglinide, alone or in combination with metformin, is 120 mg 3 times/day before meals.

   The 60 mg dose of nateglinide, alone or in combination with metformin, may be used in patients who are near goal HbA_{1c} when treatment is initiated.

Take 1 to 30 minutes prior to meals.

Actions
Pharmacology: Nateglinide is an amino-acid derivative that lowers blood glucose levels by stimulating insulin secretion from the pancreas. This action is dependent upon functioning beta-cells in the pancreatic islets. The extent of insulin release is glucose-dependent and diminishes at low glucose levels. Nateglinide is highly tissue selective with low affinity for heart and skeletal muscle.

   Nateglinide stimulates pancreatic insulin secretion within 20 minutes of oral administration. When nateglinide is dosed 3 times/day before meals there is a rapid rise in plasma insulin, with peak levels $\approx$ 1 hour after dosing and a fall to baseline by 4 hours after dosing.

Pharmacokinetics:

   Absorption – Following oral administration immediately prior to a meal, nateglinide is rapidly absorbed with mean peak plasma drug concentrations (C_{max}) generally occurring within 1 hour (T_{max}) after dosing. Absolute bioavailability is estimated to be $\approx$ 73%. When given with or after meals, the extent of nateglinide absorption remains unaffected. However, there is a delay in the rate of absorption characterized by a decrease in C_{max} and a delay in the time to peak plasma concentration T_{max}.

   Distribution – Based on data following IV administration of nateglinide, the steady-state volume of distribution is estimated to be $\approx$ 10 L in healthy subjects. Nateglinide is extensively bound (98%) to serum proteins, primarily serum albumin, and to a lesser extent α_1 acid glycoprotein.

   Metabolism – Nateglinide is metabolized by the mixed-function oxidase system prior to elimination. The major routes of metabolism are hydroxylation followed by glucuronide conjugation. The major metabolites are less potent antidiabetic agents than nateglinide.

   In vitro data demonstrate that nateglinide is predominantly metabolized by cytochrome P450 isoenzymes CYP2C9 (70%) and CYP3A4 (30%).

   Excretion – Nateglinide and its metabolites are rapidly and completely eliminated following oral administration. Nateglinide plasma concentrations decline rapidly with an average elimination half-life of $\approx$ 1.5 hours.

Contraindications
Known hypersensitivity to the drug or its inactive ingredients; type 1 diabetes; diabetic ketoacidosis (this condition should be treated with insulin).

Warnings

Diet/Exercise: In initiating treatment for patients with type 2 diabetes, emphasize diet and exercise as the primary form of treatment. In addition to regular physical activity, identify cardiovascular risk factors and take corrective measures.

Use of nateglinide must be viewed as a treatment in addition to diet and not as a substitute for diet or as a convenient mechanism for avoiding dietary restraint. Furthermore, loss of blood glucose control on diet alone may be transient, thus requiring only short-term administration of nateglinide.

Special populations: Patients with type 2 diabetes and renal failure on dialysis exhibited reduced overall drug exposure; however, hemodialysis patients also experienced reductions in plasma protein binding compared with the matched healthy volunteers.

Hepatic function impairment: Use nateglinide with caution in patients with chronic liver disease. Use with caution in patients with moderate to severe liver disease because such patients have not been studied.

Pregnancy: Category C.

Lactation: It is not known whether nateglinide is excreted in human milk. Because many drugs are excreted in human milk, do not administer nateglinide to a nursing woman.

Children: The safety and efficacy of nateglinide in pediatric patients have not been established.

Precautions

Monitoring: Periodically assess response to therapies with glucose values and HbA_{1c} levels.

Hypoglycemia: Geriatric patients, malnourished patients, and those with adrenal or pituitary insufficiency are more susceptible to the glucose-lowering effect of these treatments. Hypoglycemia may be difficult to recognize in patients with autonomic neuropathy or those who use beta-blockers. Administer nateglinide before meals to reduce the risk of hypoglycemia. Patients who skip meals should also skip their scheduled dose of nateglinide to reduce the risk of hypoglycemia.

Secondary failure: Transient loss of glycemic control may occur with fever, infection, trauma, or surgery. Insulin therapy may be needed instead of nateglinide therapy at such times. Secondary failure, or reduced effectiveness of nateglinide over a period of time, may occur.

Drug Interactions

Nateglinide is predominantly metabolized by the cytochrome P450 isozyme CYP2C9 (70%) and to a lesser extent CYP3A4 (30%). Nateglinide is a potential inhibitor of the CYP2C9 isoenzyme in vivo as indicated by its ability to inhibit the in vitro metabolism of tolbutamide. Inhibition of CYP3A4 metabolic reactions was not detected in in vitro experiments.

Drugs that may affect nateglinide include nonsteroidal anti-inflammatory agents (NSAIDs), salicylates, monoamine oxidase inhibitors, and non-selective beta-adrenergic blocking agents, thiazides, corticosteroids, thyroid products, and sympathomimetics.

Drug/Food interactions: Peak plasma levels were significantly reduced when nateglinide was administered 10 minutes prior to a liquid meal.

Adverse Reactions

Adverse reactions occurring in $\geq 3\%$ of patients include upper respiratory tract infection, back pain, flu symptoms, dizziness, arthropathy, diarrhea.

ACARBOSE

Tablets: 50 and 100 mg (*Rx*)   *Precose* (Bayer)

Indications

Hyperglycemia: As monotherapy as an adjunct to diet to lower blood glucose in patients with type 2 diabetes whose hyperglycemia cannot be managed on diet alone.

Acarbose also may be used with a sulfonylurea when diet plus either acarbose or a sulfonylurea do not result in adequate glycemic control.

Administration and Dosage

Dosage of acarbose must be individualized while not exceeding the maximum recommended dose of 100 mg 3 times/day.

Initial dosage: The recommended starting dosage is 25 mg (half of a 50 mg tablet) given 3 times/day at the start (with the first bite) of each main meal.

Maintenance dosage: Adjust dosage at 4- to 8-week intervals based on 1-hour postprandial glucose levels and on tolerance. After the initial dosage of 25 mg 3 times/day, the dosage can be increased to 50 mg 3 times/day. Some patients may benefit from further increasing the dosage to 100 mg 3 times/day. The maintenance dose ranges from 50 to 100 mg 3 times/day. However, because patients with low body weight may be at increased risk for elevated serum transaminases, consider only patients with body weight > 60 kg for dose titration above 50 mg 3 times/day. If no further reduction in postprandial glucose or glycosylated hemoglobin levels is observed with titration to 100 mg 3 times/day, consider lowering the dose. Once an effective and/tolerated dosage has been established, it should be maintained.

Actions

Pharmacology: Acarbose is a complex oligosaccharide that delays the digestion of ingested carbohydrates, thereby resulting in a smaller rise in blood glucose concentration following meals. As a consequence of plasma glucose reduction, acarbose reduces levels of glycosylated hemoglobin.

Because its mechanism of action is different, the effect of acarbose to enhance glycemic control is additive to that of sulfonylureas when used in combination.

Pharmacokinetics:

Absorption – Following oral dosing, peak plasma concentrations were attained 14 to 24 hours after dosing, while peak plasma concentrations of active drug were attained at ≈ 1 hour.

Metabolism – Acarbose is metabolized exclusively within the GI tract, principally by intestinal bacteria, but also by digestive enzymes. A fraction of these metabolites (≈ 34% of the dose) was absorbed and subsequently excreted in the urine.

Excretion – The fraction of acarbose that is absorbed as intact drug is almost completely excreted by the kidneys. When acarbose was given IV, 89% of the dose was recovered in the urine as active drug within 48 hours. In contrast, < 2% of an oral dose was recovered in the urine as active (ie, parent compound and active metabolite) drug. The plasma elimination half-life of acarbose activity is ≈ 2 hours in healthy volunteers.

Contraindications

Hypersensitivity to the drug; diabetic ketoacidosis or cirrhosis; inflammatory bowel disease; colonic ulceration; partial intestinal obstruction or predisposition to intestinal obstruction; chronic intestinal diseases associated with marked disorders of digestion or absorption; conditions that may deteriorate as a result of increased gas formation in the intestine.

Warnings

Renal function impairment: Patients with severe renal impairment (creatinine clearance [Ccr] < 25 mL/min/1.73 m^2) attained ≈ 5 times higher peak plasma concentrations of acarbose and 6 times larger AUCs than volunteers with normal renal function. Treatment of these patients with acarbose is not recommended.

Pregnancy: Category B.

Lactation: It is not known whether this drug is excreted in breast milk. Do not administer to a nursing woman.

Children: Safety and efficacy have not been established.

Precautions

Monitoring: Monitor therapeutic response to acarbose by periodic blood glucose tests. Measurement of glycosylated hemoglobin levels is recommended for the monitoring of long-term glycemic control. It is recommended that serum transaminase levels be checked every 3 months during the first year of the treatment with acarbose and periodically thereafter. If elevated transaminases are observed, a reduction in dosage or withdrawal of therapy may be indicated, particularly if the elevations persist.

Hypoglycemia: Because of its mechanism of action, acarbose alone should not cause hypoglycemia in the fasted or postprandial state. It may increase the hypoglycemic potential of the sulfonylurea. Use oral glucose (dextrose), whose absorption is not inhibited by acarbose, instead of sucrose (cane sugar) in the treatment of mild-to-moderate hypoglycemia. Severe hypoglycemia may require the use of either IV glucose infusion or glucagon injection.

Loss of blood glucose control: When diabetic patients are exposed to stress such as fever, trauma, infection or surgery, a temporary loss of control of blood glucose may occur. At such times, temporary insulin therapy may be necessary.

Drug Interactions

Drugs that may interact with acarbose include digestive enzymes, intestinal adsorbents (eg, charcoal) and digoxin.

Certain drugs tend to produce hyperglycemia and may lead to loss of blood glucose control. These drugs include the thiazides and other diuretics, corticosteroids, phenothiazines, thyroid products, estrogens, oral contraceptives, phenytoin, nicotinic acid, sympathomimetics, calcium channel blocking drugs, and isoniazid.

Adverse Reactions

GI symptoms are the most common reaction to acarbose. In trials, the incidences of abdominal pain, diarrhea, and flatulence were 21%, 33%, and 77%, respectively, with acarbose 50 to 300 mg 3 times/day.

INSULIN

INSULIN INJECTION

Injection: 100 units/mL (purified pork) (*otc*)	*Iletin* II *Regular* (Lilly)
100 units/mL (human insulin [rDNA]) (*otc*)	*Novolin R* (Novo Nordisk), *Velosulin BR* (Novo Nordisk)
Cartridges: 100 units/mL (human insulin [rDNA]). For use with *NovoPen* and *Novolin Pen.* (*otc*)	*Novolin R PenFill* (Novo Nordisk)
Injection: 100 units/mL (human insulin [rDNA]) (*otc*)	*Novolin R Prefilled* (Novo Nordisk)
100 units/mL (regular insulin [rDNA]) (*otc*)	*Humulin R* (Lilly)

ISOPHANE INSULIN SUSPENSION (NPH; insulin combined with protamine and zinc)

Injection: 100 units/mL (purified pork) (*otc*)	*NPH Iletin* II (Lilly)
100 units/mL (human insulin [rDNA]) (*otc*)	*Humulin N* (Lilly), *Novolin N* (Novo Nordisk), *Novolin N Prefilled* (Novo Nordisk)
Cartridges: 100 units/mL (human insulin [rDNA]). For use with *NovoPen* and *Novolin Pen.* (*otc*)	*Novolin N PenFill* (Novo Nordisk)

ISOPHANE INSULIN SUSPENSION (NPH) AND INSULIN INJECTION

70% isophane insulin and 30% insulin injection

Injection: 100 units/mL (human insulin [rDNA]) (*otc*)	*Humulin 70/30* (Lilly), *Novolin 70/30* (Novo Nordisk), *Novolin 70/30 Prefilled* (Novo Nordisk),
Cartridges: 100 units/mL (human insulin [rDNA]) (*otc*)	*Novolin 70/30 PenFill* (Novo Nordisk)

50% isophane insulin and 50% insulin injection

Injection: 100 units/mL (human insulin [rDNA]) (*otc*)	*Humulin 50/50* (Lilly)

INSULIN ZINC SUSPENSION (LENTE; 70% crystalline and 30% amorphous insulin suspension)	
Injection: 100 units/mL (purified pork) (*otc*)	*Lente Iletin II* (Lilly)
100 units/mL (human insulin [rDNA]) (*otc*)	*Humulin L* (Lilly), *Novolin L* (Novo Nordisk)
INSULIN ZINC SUSPENSION, EXTENDED (ULTRALENTE)	
Injection: 100 units/mL (human insulin [rDNA]) (*otc*)	*Humulin U Ultralente* (Lilly)
INSULIN ANALOG INJECTION	
Injection: 100 units/mL (human insulin lispro [rDNA]) (*Rx*)	*Humalog* (Lilly), *Humalog Mix 75/25*, *Humalog Mix 50/50*(Lilly), *Novolog* (Novo Nordisk)
HUMAN INSULIN LISPRO WITH PROTAMINE	
Injection: 100 units/mL (human insulin aspart [rDNA]) (Rx)	*Novolog* (Novo-Nordisk)
INSULIN GLARGINE	
Injection: 100 IU (3.6378 mg) insulin glargine (Rx)	*Lantus* (Aventis)

Indications

Type 1 diabetes mellitus (insulin-dependent).

Type 2 diabetes mellitus (non-insulin-dependent) that cannot be properly controlled by diet, exercise, and weight reduction.

In hyperkalemia, infusion of glucose and insulin produces a shift of potassium into cells and lowers serum potassium levels.

Severe ketoacidosis/diabetic coma: Severe ketoacidosis/diabetic coma insulin injection (regular insulin) may be given IV or IM for rapid effect in severe ketoacidosis or diabetic coma.

Highly purified (single component) and human insulins: Local insulin allergy, immunologic insulin resistance, injection site lipodystrophy; temporary insulin use (ie, surgery, acute stress type 2 diabetes, gestational diabetes); newly diagnosed diabetics.

Insulin aspart: Adults with diabetes mellitus for the control of hyperglycemia. Because insulin aspart has a more rapid onset and a shorter duration of action than human regular insulin, insulin aspart normally should be used in regimens together with an intermediate or long-acting insulin.

Insulin lispro: Treatment of patients with diabetes mellitus for the control of hyperglycemia. Insulin lispro has a more rapid onset and shorter duration of action than regular human insulin. Therefore, in patients with type 1 diabetes, use in regimens that include a longer-acting insulin. However, in patients with type 2 diabetes, insulin lispro may be used without a longer-acting insulin when used in combination therapy with sulfonylureas. It also may be used in combination with sulfonylureas in adults and children > 3 years of age.

> *Children (Humalog only)* – Safety and effectiveness in children < 18 years of age have not been determined for *Humalog Mix*. To improve accuracy of dosing in pediatric patients, a diluent may be used. If the diluent is added directly to the vial, the shelf life may be reduced.

Insulin glargine: Once-daily SC administration at bedtime in the treatment of adults and children with type 1 diabetes mellitus or adults with type 2 diabetes mellitus who require basal (long-acting) insulin for the control of hyperglycemia.

Administration and Dosage

INSULIN: Human regular insulin is best given 30 to 60 minutes before a meal.

The number and size of daily doses, time of administration and diet and exercise require continuous medical supervision. Dosage adjustment may be necessary when changing types of insulin, particularly when changing from single-peak to the more purified animal or human insulins.

Administer maintenance doses SC. Rotate administration sites to prevent lipodystrophy. A general rule is to not administer within 1 inch of the same site for 1 month. The rate of absorption is more rapid when the injection is in the abdomen (possibly > 50% faster), followed by the upper arm, thigh, and buttocks. Therefore, it may be best to rotate sites within an area rather than rotating areas.

Dosage guidelines –
  Children and adults: 0.5 to 1 U/kg/day.
  Adolescents (during growth spurt): 0.8 to 1.2 U/kg/day.
  Adjust doses to achieve premeal and bedtime blood glucose levels of 80 to
140 mg/dL (children < 5 years of age, 100 to 200 mg/dL).

INSULIN ASPART: Give immediately before a meal. Individualize dose. The total daily
  individual insulin requirement is usually between 0.5 and 1 unit/kg/day. In a meal-
  related treatment regimen, 50% to 70% of this requirement may be provided by
  insulin aspart and the remainder provided by an intermediate-acting or long-acting insulin. Patients may require more basal insulin in relation to bolus insulin
  and more total insulin when using insulin aspart compared with regular human insulin to prevent premeal hyperglycemia. Additional basal insulin injections may be
  necessary.
  Because of the fast onset of action of insulin aspart, administer close to a meal
  (start of meal within 5 to 10 minutes after injection). Regularly adjust dose according to blood glucose measurements.
  Administer by SC injection in the abdominal wall, the thigh, or the upper arm.
  Rotate injection sites within the same region. As with all insulins, the duration of
  action will vary according to the dose, injection site, blood flow, temperature, and
  level of physical activity.

INSULIN LISPRO: Insulin lispro is intended for SC administration. Pharmacokinetic
  and pharmacodynamic studies showed insulin lispro to be equipotent (1:1) to
  human regular insulin, but with more rapid activity. The quicker glucose-lowering
  effect of insulin lispro is related to the more rapid absorption rate from subcutaneous tissue. An adjustment of dose or schedule of basal insulin may be needed
  when a patient changes from other insulins to lispro, particularly to prevent premeal hyperglycemia.
  When used as a meal-time insulin, give insulin lispro within 15 minutes before
  or immediately after a meal. Human regular insulin is best given 30 to 60 minutes
  before a meal. To achieve optimal glucose control, the amount of longer-acting
  insulin being given may need to be adjusted when using insulin lispro.
  When not mixed in the same syringe with other insulins, lispro maintains its
  rapid onset of action and has less variability in its onset of action among injection
  sites compared with human regular insulin. After abdominal administration, insulin lispro concentrations are higher than those following deltoid or thigh injections.
  Also, the duration of action of insulin lispro is slightly shorter following abdominal injection, compared with deltoid and femoral injections. As with all insulin preparations, the time course of action of lispro may vary considerably in
  different individuals or within the same individual. Patients must be educated to
  use proper injection techniques.
  Compatibility – Insulin lispro may be diluted with sterile diluent for *Humalog,
  Humulin N, Humulin 50/50, Humulin 70/30,* and *NPH Iletin* to a concentration of
  1:10 (equivalent to U-10) or 1:2 (equivalent to U-50). Diluted insulin lispro may
  remain in patient use for 28 days when stored at 5°C (41°F) and for 14 days when
  stored at 30°C (86°F).

INSULIN GLARGINE: Insulin glargine is not intended for IV administration. The prolonged duration of activity of insulin glargine is dependent on injection into subcutaneous tissue.
  Insulin glargine must not be diluted or mixed with any other insulin or solution. If insulin glargine is diluted or mixed, the solution may become cloudy and
  the pharmacokinetic/pharmacodynamic profile (eg, onset of action, time to peak
  effect) of insulin glargine and/or the mixed insulin may be altered in an unpredictable manner.
  The potency of insulin glargine is approximately the same as human insulin. It
  exhibits a relatively constant glucose-lowering profile over 24 hours that permits
  once-daily dosing. Give insulin glargine SC once daily at bedtime. The desired

blood glucose levels as well as the doses and timing of antidiabetic medications must be determined individually. Blood glucose monitoring is recommended for all patients with diabetes.

As with all insulins, injection sites within an injection area (abdomen, thigh, or deltoid) must be rotated from one injection to the next.

In clinical studies, there was no relevant difference in insulin glargine absorption after abdominal, deltoid, or thigh SC administration. As for all insulins, the rate of absorption, and consequently the onset and duration of action, may be affected by exercise and other variables.

Insulin glargine is not the insulin of choice for the treatment of diabetic ketoacidosis. IV short-acting insulin is the preferred treatment.

Children – Insulin glargine can be safely administered to pediatric patients ≥ 6 years of age. Administration of pediatric patients < 6 years has not been studied. Based on the result of a study in pediatric patients, the dose recommendation for changeover to insulin glargine is the same as described for adults.

Initial dosing – In a clinical study with insulin-naive patients with type 2 diabetes already treated with oral antidiabetic drugs, insulin glargine was started at an average dose of 10 IU once daily, and subsequently adjusted according to the patient's need to a total daily dose ranging from 2 to 100 IU.

Changeover to insulin glargine – If changing from a treatment regimen with an intermediate- or long-acting insulin to a regimen with insulin glargine, the amount and timing of short-acting insulin or fast-acting insulin analog or the dose of any oral antidiabetic drug may need to be adjusted. In clinical studies, when patients were transferred from once-daily NPH human insulin or ultralente human insulin to once-daily insulin glargine, the initial dose was usually not changed. However, when patients were transferred from twice-daily NPH to insulin glargine once daily at bedtime, to reduce the risk of hypoglycemia, the initial dose (IU) was usually reduced by ≈ 20% (compared with total daily IU of NPH human insulin) within the first week of treatment and then adjusted based on patient response.

The dose may also have to be adjusted during intercurrent illness.

Preparation and handling – Use only if clear and colorless with no particles visible. The syringes must not contain any other medicinal product or residue.

Cartridge version only – If the *OptiPen One Insulin Delivery Device* malfunctions, insulin glargine may be drawn from the cartridge into a U 100 syringe and injected.

Actions

Pharmacology: Insulin and its analogs lower blood glucose levels by stimulating peripheral glucose uptake, especially by skeletal muscle and fat, and by inhibiting hepatic glucose production. Insulin, secreted by the beta cells of the pancreas, is the principal hormone required for proper glucose use in normal metabolic processes.

The bioavailability of the insulins is identical when given SC. The human insulins are slightly less antigenic than pork or beef insulins. Human insulin is the insulin of choice for patients with insulin allergy, insulin resistance, all pregnant patients with diabetes, and any patient who uses insulin intermittently.

Pharmacokinetics and Compatibility of Various Insulins						
	Insulin Preparations	Half-life (hrs)	Onset (hrs)	Peak (hrs)	Duration (hrs)	Compatible mixed with
Rapid-Acting	Insulin Injection (Regular)		0.5 to 1		8 to 12	All
	Prompt Insulin Zinc Suspension (Semilente)		1 to 1.5	5 to 10	12 to 16	Lente
	Lispro Insulin Solution	1	0.25	0.5 to 1.5	6 to 8	Ultralente, NPH
	Insulin Aspart Solution	1.5	0.25	1 to 3	3 to 5	[1]

Pharmacokinetics and Compatibility of Various Insulins					
Insulin Preparations	Half-life (hrs)	Onset (hrs)	Peak (hrs)	Duration (hrs)	Compatible mixed with
Intermediate-Acting Isophane Insulin Suspension (NPH)		1 to 1.5	4 to 12	24	Regular
Insulin Zinc Suspension (Lente)		1 to 2.5	7 to 15	24	Regular, semilente
Long-Acting Insulin Glargine Solution		1.1	5[2]	24[3]	None
Protamine Zinc Insulin Suspension (PZI)		4 to 8	14 to 24	36	Regular
Extended Insulin Zinc Suspension (Ultralente)		4 to 8	10 to 30	> 36	Regular, semilente

[1] See below.
[2] No pronounced peak; small amounts of insulin glargine are slowly released resulting in a relatively constant concentration/time profile over 24 hours.
[3] Studies only conducted up to 24 hours.

Mixing of insulins –

Insulin aspart: A clinical study in healthy male volunteers (n = 24) demonstrated that mixing insulin aspart with NPH human insulin immediately before injection produced some attenuation in the peak concentration of insulin aspart, but that the time to peak and the total bioavailability of insulin aspart were not significantly affected. If insulin aspart is mixed with NPH human insulin, draw insulin aspart into the syringe first. Inject immediately after mixing. Do not mix insulin aspart with crystalline zinc insulin preparations because of lack of compatability data.

The effects of mixing insulin aspart with insulins of animal source or insulin preparations produced by other manufacturers have not been studied (see Warnings).

Do not administer mixtures IV.

Insulin lispro: Mixing lispro with *Humulin N* or *Humulin U* does not decrease the absorption rate or the total bioavailability of insulin lispro. Given alone or mixed with *Humulin N*, insulin lispro results in a more rapid absorption and glucose-lowering effect compared with human regular insulin.

The effects of mixing lispro with insulins of animal source or insulin preparations produced by other manufacturers have not been studied.

If lispro is mixed with a longer-acting insulin such as *Humulin N* or *Humulin U*, draw lispro into the syringe first to prevent clouding of the lispro by the longer-acting insulin. Immediately make injection after mixing. Do not give mixtures IV.

Contraindications

During episodes of hypoglycemia and in patients sensitive to any ingredient of the product.

Warnings

Change insulins: Change insulins cautiously and under medical supervision. Changes in purity, strength, brand, type, or species source may require dosage adjustment.

Hypersensitivity reactions: May require discontinuation of insulin.

Local – Occasionally, redness, swelling, and itching at the injection site may develop. This reaction occurs if the injection is not properly made, if the skin is sensitive to the cleansing solution, or if the patient is allergic to insulin or insulin additives (eg, preservatives). The condition usually resolves in a few days to a few weeks. A change in the type or species source of insulin may be considered.

Systemic – Systemic reactions are less common and may present as a rash, short-ness of breath, fast pulse, sweating, a drop in blood pressure, bronchospasm, shock, anaphylaxis, or angioedema and may be life-threatening.

Insulin aspart – Localized reactions and generalized myalgias have been reported with the use of cresol as an injectable excipient.

Renal/Hepatic function impairment: Some studies with human insulin have shown increased circulating levels of insulin in patients with renal and hepatic failure. Careful glucose monitoring and dose adjustments of insulin may be necessary in these patients. Insulin requirements may be reduced in patients with renal function impairment.

Elderly: In elderly patients with diabetes, the initial dosing, dosing increments, and maintenance dosing should be conservative to avoid hypoglycemic reactions. Hypoglycemia may be difficult to recognize in the elderly.

Pregnancy: Category B; *Category* C (insulin glargine, insulin aspart).

Lactation: Lactating women may require adjustments in insulin dose and diet. It is unknown whether **insulin glargine** is excreted in significant amounts in breast milk. It is unknown whether **insulin aspart** is excreted in breast milk.

Children: Safety and efficacy in patients < 12 years of age have not been established.

Insulin glargine – Safety and effectiveness of insulin glargine have been established in children 6 to 15 years of age with type 1 diabetes.

Humalog – Humalog can be used in combination with sulfonylureas in children > 3 years of age.

Precautions

Symptoms of Hypoglycemia vs Ketoacidosis							
		Urine glucose/acetone	Symptoms				
Reaction	Onset		CNS	Respiration	Mouth/GI	Skin	Miscellaneous
Hypoglycemic reaction (insulin reaction)	sudden	0/0	fatigue, weakness, nervousness, confusion, headache, diplopia, convulsions, psychoses, dizziness, unconscious-ness	rapid, shallow	numb, tingling, hunger, nausea	pallor, moist, shallow, or dry	normal or non-characteristic pulse, eyeballs normal
Ketoacidosis (diabetic coma)	gradual (hours or days)	+/+	drowsiness, dim vision	air hunger	thirst, acetone breath, nausea, vomiting, abdominal pain, loss of appetite	dry, flushed	rapid pulse, soft eyeballs

Insulin resistance: Insulin resistance occurs rarely. Insulin-resistant patients require > 200 units of insulin/day for > 2 days in the absence of ketoacidosis or acute infection.

Hypoglycemia: Hypoglycemia may result from excessive insulin dose or may be due to: Increased work or exercise without eating; food not being absorbed in the usual manner because of postponement or omission of a meal or in illness with vomiting, fever or diarrhea; when insulin requirements decline.

Diabetic ketoacidosis: Diabetic ketoacidosis, a potentially life-threatening condition, requires prompt diagnosis and treatment. Hyperglucagonemia, hyperglycemia, and ketoacidosis may result. Diabetic ketoacidosis may result from stress, illness, or insulin omission, or may develop slowly after a long period of insulin control.

Lipodystrophy:

Lipoatrophy – Lipoatrophy is the breakdown of adipose tissue at the insulin injection site causing a depression in the skin.

Lipohypertrophy – Lipohypertrophy is the result of repeated insulin injection into the same site. This condition may be avoided by rotating the injection site.

Diet: Patients must follow a prescribed diet and exercise regularly. Determine the time, number and amount of individual doses and distribution of food among the meals of the day. Do not change this regimen unless prescribed otherwise.

Hyperthyroidism/Hypothyroidism: Hyperthyroidism may cause an increase in the renal clearance of insulin. Therefore, patients may need more insulin to control their diabetes. Hypothyroidism may delay insulin turnover, requiring less insulin to control diabetes.

Drug Interactions

Drugs That Decrease the Hypoglycemic Effect of Insulin	
Acetazolamide	Epinephrine
AIDS antivirals	Estrogens
Albuterol	Ethacrynic acid
Asparaginase	Isoniazid
Calcitonin	Lithium carbonate
Contraceptives, oral	Morphine sulfate
Corticosteroids	Niacin
Cyclophosphamide	Nicotine
Danazol	Phenothiazines
Dextrothyroxine	Phenytoin
Diazoxide	Somatropin
Diltiazem	Terbutaline
Diuretics	Thiazide diuretics
Dobutamine	Thyroid hormones

Drugs That Increase the Hypoglycemic Effect of Insulin	
ACE inhibitors	Lithium carbonate
Alcohol	MAO inhibitors
Anabolic steroids	Mebendazole
Antidiabetic products, oral	Pentamidine[2]
Beta blockers[1]	Phenylbutazone
Calcium	Propoxyphene
Chloroquine	Pyridoxine
Clofibrate	Salicylates
Clonidine	Somatostatin analog (eg, octreotide)
Disopyramide	Sulfinpyrazone
Fluoxetine	Sulfonamides
Guanethidine	Tetracyclines

[1] Nonselective beta blockers may delay recovery from hypoglycemic episodes and mask their signs/symptoms. Cardioselective agents may be alternatives.
[2] May sometimes be followed by hyperglycemia.

Adverse Reactions

Human insulin: Hypoglycemia and hypokalemia are among the potential clinical adverse events associated with the use of all insulins. Other adverse events commonly associated with human insulin therapy include the following:

Miscellaneous – Allergic reactions. Sodium retention and edema may occur, particularly if previously poor metabolic control is improved by intensified insulin therapy.

Dermatologic – Injection site reaction, lipodystrophy, pruritus, rash.

Lab test abnormalities – Hypoglycemia, hypokalemia.

INSULIN INJECTION CONCENTRATED

Injection: 500 units/mL (purified pork) (Rx)	Regular (Concentrated) Iletin II U-500 (Lilly)

Indications
Treatment of diabetic patients with marked insulin resistance (requirements > 200 units/day). A large dose may be administered SC in a reasonable volume.

Administration and Dosage
Administer SC. Do not inject IM or IV. It is inadvisable to inject concentrated insulin IV because of possible inadvertent overdosage.

Use a tuberculin-type or insulin syringe for dosage measurement. Dosage variations are frequent in the insulin-resistant patient, since the individual is unresponsive to the pharmacologic effect of the insulin. Nevertheless, encourage accuracy of measurement because of the potential danger of the preparations.

Actions
Pharmacology:
   Insulin resistance – Diabetes can usually be controlled with daily insulin doses ≤ 40 to 60 units; however, an occasional patient develops such resistance or becomes so unresponsive to the effect of insulin that daily doses of several hundred or even several thousand units are required. Patients who require doses in excess of 300 to 500 units daily usually have impaired insulin receptor function.

Pharmacokinetics: It frequently has a duration similar to repository insulin; a single dose demonstrates activity for 24 hours.

Contraindications
Hypoglycemia.

Warnings
General: This human insulin product differs from animal-source insulins because it is structurally identical to the insulin produced by the body's pancreas and because of its unique manufacturing process.
   Make any change of insulin cautiously and only under medical supervision. Changes in purity, strength, brand (manufacturer), type (eg, regular, NPH, lente), species (beef, pork, beef-pork, human), or method of manufacturer (rDNA vs animal-source insulin) may result in the need for a change in dosage.
   Some patients taking this product may require a change in dosage from that used with animal-source insulins. If an adjustment is needed, it may occur with the first dose or during the first several weeks or months.

Dosage adjustments: Closely observe every patient exhibiting insulin resistance who requires concentrated insulin for diabetic control until appropriate dosing is established. Response will vary among patients. Most patients will show a "tolerance" to insulin, so that minor dosage variations will not cause untoward symptoms of insulin shock. Some may require only 1 dose daily; others may require 2 or 3 injections per day.

Insulin shock: Observe extreme caution in the measurement of dosage; inadvertent overdose may result in irreversible insulin shock.

Hypoglycemic reactions: Hypoglycemia when using this concentrated insulin can be prolonged and severe. As with other human insulin preparations, hypoglycemia reactions may be associated with the administration of concentrated insulin. However, deep secondary hypoglycemic reactions may develop 18 to 24 hours after the original injection of concentrated insulin.

Lipodystrophy: Rarely, administration of insulin SC can result in lipoatrophy (depression in the skin) or lipohypertrophy (enlargement or thickening of tissue).

Hypersensitivity reactions: Less common than local allergic reactions, but potentially more serious, is systemic insulin allergy, which may cause generalized urticaria, dyspnea, or wheezing and may, on continued use, progress to anaphylaxis.

Pregnancy: Category B.

Lactation: It is not known whether insulin is excreted in significant amounts in breast milk. Exercise caution when administering to a nursing woman.

Precautions

Monitoring: Monitor blood and urine glucose, glycohemoglobin and urine ketones frequently. Monitor blood glucose closely and often until dosage is established.

Insulin resistance: Insulin resistance is frequently self-limited; after several weeks or months of high dosage, responsiveness may be regained and dosage reduced.

Drug Interactions

Oral hypoglycemic agents: Concurrent use of oral hypoglycemic agents is not recommended; there are no data to support such use.

Adverse Reactions

Hypoglycemic reactions (see Warnings); hypersensitivity (see Warnings).

SULFONYLUREAS

ACETOHEXAMIDE	
Tablets: 250 and 500 mg (*Rx*)	Various, *Dymelor* (Eli Lilly)
CHLORPROPAMIDE	
Tablets: 100 and 250 mg (*Rx*)	Various, *Diabinese* (Pfizer)
GLIMEPIRIDE	
Tablets: 1, 2, and 4 mg (*Rx*)	*Amaryl* (Hoechst Marion Roussel)
GLIPIZIDE	
Tablets: 5 and 10 mg (*Rx*)	Various, *Glucotrol* (Pfizer)
Tablets, extended-release: 5 and 10 mg (*Rx*)	*Glucotrol XL* (Pfizer)
GLYBURIDE	
Tablets: 1.25, 2.5, and 5 mg (*Rx*)	Various, *DiaBeta* (Hoechst Marion Roussel), *Micronase* (Upjohn)
Tablets, micronized: 1.5, 3, 4.5, and 6 mg (*Rx*)	*Glynase PresTab* (Pharmacia & Upjohn)
TOLAZAMIDE	
Tablets: 100, 250, and 500 mg (*Rx*)	Various, *Tolinase* (Pharmacia & Upjohn)
TOLBUTAMIDE	
Tablets: 500 mg (*Rx*)	Various, *Orinase* (Pharmacia & Upjohn)

Indications

As an adjunct to diet and exercise to lower the blood glucose in patients with type 2 (non-insulin-dependent) diabetes mellitus whose hyperglycemia cannot be controlled by diet and exercise alone.

Glimepiride:

Combination with insulin – Glimepiride is also indicated for use in combination with insulin to lower blood glucose in patients whose hyperglycemia cannot be controlled by diet and exercise in conjunction with an oral hypoglycemic agent. Combined use of glimepiride and insulin may increase the potential for hypoglycemia.

Glyburide:

Combination with metformin – Glyburide also may be used concomitantly with metformin when diet and glyburide or diet and metformin alone do not result in adequate glycemic control (see Metformin monograph).

Administration and Dosage

Short-term administration: Short-term administration of sulfonylureas may be sufficient during periods of transient loss of control in patients usually well controlled on diet.

Transfer from other hypoglycemic agents:

Sulfonylureas – When transferring patients from one oral hypoglycemic agent to another, no transitional period and no initial or priming dose is necessary. However, when transferring patients from chlorpropamide, exercise particular care during the first 2 weeks because the prolonged retention of chlorpropamide in the body and subsequent overlapping drug effects may provoke hypoglycemia.

Insulin – During insulin withdrawal period, test blood for glucose and urine for ketones 3 times/day and report results to physician daily.

Insulin Requirement When Instituting Sulfonylurea Therapy	
Insulin dose	Insulin requirement
< 20 units	Start directly on oral agent and discontinue insulin abruptly.
20-40 units	Initiate oral therapy with concurrent 25% to 50% reduction in insulin dose. Further reduce insulin as response is observed. With glyburide, insulin may be discontinued immediately.
> 40 units	Initiate oral therapy with concurrent 20% to 50% reduction in insulin dose. Further reduce insulin as response is observed.

Elderly patients: Elderly patients may be particularly sensitive to these agents; therefore, start with a lower initial dose before breakfast, and check blood and urine glucose during the first 24 hours of therapy.

Acute complications: During the course of intercurrent complications (eg, ketoacidosis, severe trauma, major surgery, infections, severe diarrhea, nausea, vomiting), supportive therapy with insulin may be necessary.

Combination insulin therapy: Concurrent administration of insulin and an oral sulfonylurea (generally glipizide or glyburide) has been used with some success in type 2 diabetic patients who are difficult to control with diet and sulfonylurea therapy alone.

ACETOHEXAMIDE:
   Initial dose – 250 mg to 1.5 g/day. Patients on ≤ 1 g/day can be controlled with once daily dosage. Those receiving 1.5 g/day usually benefit from twice daily dosage before morning and evening meals. Doses > 1.5 g/day are not recommended.

   Patients on other oral antidiabetic agents: When transfer is made, the initial dose of acetohexamide should be about half the tolbutamide dose and about double the chlorpropamide dose. A transition period usually is required because of the long half-life of chlorpropamide. Make subsequent dosage adjustments according to clinical response.

   Patients on insulin:

Transferral of Type 2 Diabetes Patients on Insulin to Acetohexamide Monotherapy		
Insulin dose	Initial acetohexamide dose	Insulin withdrawal
< 20	250 mg/day	Not necessary; may be discontinued abruptly.
> 20	250 mg/day	Reduce insulin dose by 25% to 30%; further reduce as response is observed. Consider hospitalization during the transition period.

CHLORPROPAMIDE:
   Initial dose – 250 mg/day in the mild to moderately severe, middle-aged, stable diabetic patient; use 100 to 125 mg/day in older, debilitated, or malnourished patients, and patients with impaired renal/hepatic function.

   Maintenance therapy – ≤ 100 to 250 mg/day. Severe diabetics may require 500 mg/day. Avoid doses > 750 mg/day.

   Patients on insulin –

Transferral of Type 2 Diabetes Patients on Insulin to Chlorpropamide Monotherapy		
Insulin dose	Initial chlorpropamide dose	Insulin withdrawal
≤ 40	250 mg/day	Not necessary; may be discontinued abruptly.
> 40	250 mg/day	Reduce insulin dose by 50%; further reduce as response is observed. Consider hospitalization during the transition period.

GLIMEPIRIDE:
   Initial dose – 1 to 2 mg once daily, given with breakfast or the first main meal. Patients sensitive to hypoglycemic drugs should begin at 1 mg once daily; titrate carefully.

Maximum starting dose is ≤ 2 mg.

Maintenance dose – 1 to 4 mg once daily. The maximum recommended dose is 8 mg once daily. After a dose of 2 mg is reached, increase dose at increments of ≤ 2 mg at 1 to 2 week intervals based on the patient's blood glucose response. Monitor long-term efficacy by measurement of HbA_{1c} levels, for example, every 3 to 6 months.

Combination insulin therapy – The recommended dose is 8 mg once daily with the first main meal with low-dose insulin.

Patients on other oral antidiabetic agents – When transferring patients to glimepiride, no transition period is necessary. No exact dosage relationship exists between glimepiride and the other oral hypoglycemic agents.

GLIPIZIDE:

Immediate release –

Initial dose: 5 mg, given ≈ 30 minutes before breakfast to achieve the greatest reduction in postprandial hyperglycemia. Geriatric patients or those with liver disease may be started on 2.5 mg of the immediate-release formulation.

Adjust dosage in 2.5 to 5 mg increments, as determined by blood glucose response. Several days should elapse between titration steps. If response to a single dose is not satisfactory, dividing that dose may prove effective. The maximum recommended once daily dose is 15 mg. The maximum recommended total daily dose is 40 mg.

Maintenance dose: Some patients may be controlled on a once-a-day regimen, while others show better response with divided dosing. Divide total daily doses > 15 mg and give before meals of adequate caloric content. Total daily doses > 30 mg have been safely given on a twice daily basis to long-term patients.

Extended release –

Initial dose: 5 mg/day, given with breakfast. The recommended dose for geriatric patients is also 5 mg/day. HbA_{1c} level measured at 3-month intervals is the preferred means of monitoring response to therapy. Measure HbA_{1c} as extended release therapy is initiated at the 5 mg dose and repeated ≈ 3 months later. If the first test result suggests that glycemic control over the preceding 3 months was inadequate, the dose may be increased to 10 mg. Make subsequent dosage adjustments at 3-month intervals. If no improvement is seen after 3 months of therapy with a higher dose, resume the previous dose. Base decisions that use fasting blood glucose to adjust therapy on ≥ 2 similar consecutive values obtained ≥ 7 days after the previous dose adjustment.

Maintenance dose: Most patients will be controlled with 5 or 10 mg taken once daily. However, some patients may require up to the maximum recommended daily dose of 20 mg. While the glycemic control of selected patients may improve with doses that exceed 10 mg, clinical studies conducted to date have not demonstrated an additional group average reduction of HbA_{1c} beyond what was achieved with the 10 mg dose.

Immediate vs extended release: Patients receiving immediate-release glipizide may be switched safely to the extended-release tablets once a day at the nearest equivalent total daily dose. Patients receiving immediate-release tablets also may be titrated to the appropriate dose of the extended-release tablets starting with 5 mg once daily.

Combination therapy: When used in combination with other oral blood glucose-lowering agents, add the second agent at the lowest recommended dose and observe patients carefully.

Patients on other oral antidiabetic agents – No transition period is necessary when transferring patients to the extended-release tablets. Observe patients carefully (1 to 2 weeks) when being transferred from longer half-life sulfonylureas (ie, chlorpropamide) to the extended release tablets due to potential overlapping of drug effect.

Patients on insulin –

Transferral of Type 2 Diabetes Patients on Insulin to Glipizide Monotherapy		
Insulin dose	Initial glipizide dose	Insulin withdrawal
< 20	5 mg/day	Not necessary; may be discontinued abruptly.
> 20	5 mg/day	Reduce insulin dose by 50%; further reduce as response is observed. Consider hospitalization during the transition period.

GLYBURIDE (Glibenclamide):
   Nonmicronized (DiaBeta/Micronase) –
      Initial dose: 2.5 to 5 mg/day, administered with breakfast or the first main meal. For patients who may be more sensitive to hypoglycemic drugs, start at 1.25 mg/day.
      Maintenance dose: 1.25 to 20 mg/day. Give as a single dose or in divided doses. Increase in increments of ≤ 2.5 mg at weekly intervals based on the patient's blood glucose response. Daily doses > 20 mg are not recommended.
   Micronized (Glynase) –
      Initial dose: 1.5 to 3 mg/day, administered with breakfast or the first main meal. For patients who may be more sensitive to hypoglycemic drugs, start at 0.75 mg/day.
      Maintenance dose: 0.75 to 12 mg/day. Give as a single dose or in divided doses; some patients, particularly those receiving > 6 mg/day, may have a more satisfactory response with twice-daily dosing. Increase in increments of ≤ 1.5 mg at weekly intervals based on the patient's blood glucose response. Daily doses > 12 mg are not recommended.
      Concomitant metformin: Add micronized glyburide gradually to the dosing regimen of patients who have not responded to the maximum dose of metformin monotherapy after 4 weeks. (Refer to the Metformin monograph.) The desired control of blood glucose may be obtained by adjusting the dose of each drug. With concomitant therapy, the risk of hypoglycemia associated with sulfonylurea therapy continues and may be increased.
      Patients on other oral antidiabetic agents: Transfer patients from other oral antidiabetic regimens to glyburide conservatively. When transferring patients from oral hypoglycemic agents other than chlorpropamide, no transition period and no initial priming dose is necessary. When transferring patients from chlorpropamide, exercise care during the first 2 weeks because the prolonged retention of chlorpropamide in the body and subsequent overlapping drug effects may provoke hypoglycemia.
      Patients on insulin:

Transferral of Type 2 Diabetes Patients on Insulin to Glyburide Monotherapy		
Insulin dose	Initial glyburide dose	Insulin withdrawal
< 20	1.5-3 mg/day micronized, 2.5-5 mg/day non-micronized	Not necessary; may be discontinued abruptly.
20-40	3 mg/day micronized, 5 mg/day non-micronized	Not necessary; may be discontinued abruptly.
> 40	3 mg/day micronized, 5 mg/day non-micronized	Reduce insulin dose by 50%; further reduce as response is observed. Consider hospitalization during the transition period.

TOLAZAMIDE:
   Initial dose – 100 to 250 mg/day with breakfast or the first main meal. If fasting blood sugar (FBS) is < 200 mg/dL, use 100 mg/day, or 250 mg/day if FBS is > 200 mg/dL. If patients are malnourished, underweight, elderly or not eating prop-

erly, use 100 mg once a day. Adjust dose to response. If > 500 mg/day is required, give in divided doses twice daily. Doses > 1 g/day are not likely to improve control.

Maintenance dose – The usual maintenance dose is 100 to 1000 mg/day with the average maintenance dose being 250 to 500 mg/day. Following initiation of therapy, dosage adjustment is made in increments of 100 to 250 mg at weekly intervals based on the patient's blood glucose response.

Patients on other oral antidiabetic agents – Transfer patients from other oral antidiabetes regimens to tolazamide conservatively. When transferring patients from oral hypoglycemic agents other than chlorpropamide to tolazamide, no transition period or initial priming dose is necessary. Consider 250 mg chlorpropamide to provide approximately the same degree of blood control as 250 mg tolazamide. Observe the patient carefully for hypoglycemia during the transition period from chlorpropamide to tolazamide (1 or 2 weeks) due to the prolonged retention of chlorpropamide in the body and the possibility of a subsequent overlapping drug effect. If patient is receiving < 1 g/day tolbutamide, begin at 100 mg/day of tolazamide. If patient is receiving ≥ 1 g/day, initiate 250 mg/day tolazamide as a single dose. Consider 100 mg tolazamide to provide approximately the same degree of blood glucose control as 250 mg acetohexamide.

Patients on insulin –

Transferral of Type 2 Diabetes Patients on Insulin to Tolazamide Monotherapy		
Insulin dose	Initial tolaza-mide dose	Insulin withdrawal
< 20	100 mg/day	Not necessary; may be discontinued abruptly.
20-40	250 mg/day	Not necessary; may be discontinued abruptly
> 40	250 mg/day	Reduce insulin by 50%; further reduce as response is observed. Consider hospitalization during the transition period.

TOLBUTAMIDE:

Initial dose – 1 to 2 g/day (range, 0.25 to 3 g). A maintenance dose > 2 g/day is seldom required. Daily doses > 3 g are not recommended. Total dose may be taken in the morning, but divided doses may allow increased GI tolerance.

Patients on other oral antidiabetic agents – Transfer patients from other oral antidiabetes regimens to tolbutamide conservatively. When transferring patients from oral hypoglycemic agents other than chlorpropamide to tolbutamide, no transition period and no initial or priming doses are necessary. However, when transferring patients from chlorpropamide, exercise particular care during the first 2 weeks because of the prolonged retention of chlorpropamide in the body and the possibility that subsequent overlapping drug effects might provoke hypoglycemia.

Patients on insulin –

Transferral of Type 2 Diabetes Patients on Insulin to Tolbutamide Monotherapy		
Insulin dose	Initial tolbu-tamide dose	Insulin withdrawal
< 20	1-2 g/day	Not necessary; may be discontinued abruptly.
20-40	1-2 g/day	Reduce insulin dose by 30% to 50%; further reduce as response is observed.
> 40	1-2 g/day	Reduce insulin dose by 20%; further reduce as response is observed. Consider hospitalization during the transition period.

Occasionally, conversion to tolbutamide in the hospital may be advisable in candidates who require > 40 units of insulin daily. During this conversion period when insulin and tolbutamide are being used, hypoglycemia rarely may occur. During insulin withdrawal, have patients test urine for glucose and acetone ≥ 3 times/day and report results to their physician. The appearance of persistent acetonuria with glycosuria indicates that the patient is a type 1 diabetes patient who requires insulin therapy.

Actions

Pharmacology: The sulfonylurea hypoglycemic agents appear to lower blood glucose by stimulating insulin release from beta cells in the pancreatic islets possibly due to increased intracellular cAMP. These agents are only effective in patients with some capacity for endogenous insulin production. They may improve the binding between insulin and insulin receptors or increase the number of insulin receptors.

General clinical characteristics that favor successful sulfonylurea monotherapy following insulin withdrawal include the following:

- Onset of diabetes at ≥ 35 years of age
- Obese or normal body weight
- Duration of diabetes < 10 years
- Absence of ketoacidosis
- Fasting serum glucose ≤ 200 mg/dL
- Postprandial blood glucose values < 250 mg/dL
- Insulin requirement < 40 units/day
- Absence of renal or hepatic dysfunction

Pharmacokinetics: All sulfonylureas are strongly bound to plasma proteins, primarily albumin.

Major Pharmacokinetic Parameters of the Sulfonylureas							
Sulfonylureas	Approximate equivalent doses (mg)	Doses/ day	Serum t½ (hrs)	Onset (hrs)	Duration (hrs)	Renal excretion (%)	Active metabolites
First generation							
Acetohexamide	500-750	1-2	≈ 6-8 (parent drug + metabolite)	1	12-24	100	Yes
Chlorpropamide	250-375	1	36	1	24-60	100	Yes
Tolazamide	250-375	1-2	7	4-6	12-24	100	Yes
Tolbutamide	1000-1500	2-3	4.5-6.5	1	6-12	100	No
Second generation							
Glipizide	10	1-2	2-4	1-3	10-24	80-85	No
Glyburide Nonmicronized	5	1-2	10	2-4	16-24	50	Yes[1]
Micronized	3	1-2	≈ 4	1	12-24	50	Yes[1]
Glimepiride	NA[2]	1	≈ 9	2-3	24	60	Yes

[1] Weakly active.
[2] Not applicable.

Contraindications

Hypersensitivity to sulfonylureas; diabetes complicated by ketoacidosis, with or without coma; sole therapy of type 1 (insulin-dependent) diabetes mellitus; diabetes when complicated by pregnancy.

Warnings

The administration of oral hypoglycemic drugs: The administration of oral hypoglycemic drugs has been associated with increased cardiovascular mortality as compared with treatment with diet alone or diet plus insulin.

Patients treated for 5 to 8 years with diet plus tolbutamide (1.5 g/day) had a rate of cardiovascular mortality ≈ 2.5 times that of patients treated with diet alone. A significant increase in total mortality was not observed.

Bioavailability: Micronized glyburide 3 mg tablets provide serum concentrations that are *not* bioequivalent to those from the conventional formulation (nonmicronized) 5 mg tablets.

Renal/Hepatic function impairment: Hepatic impairment may result in inadequate release of glucose in response to hypoglycemia. Renal impairment may cause decreased elimination of sulfonylureas leading to accumulation producing hypoglycemia.

Elderly: In elderly, debilitated, or malnourished patients, and patients with impaired renal or hepatic function, the initial and maintenance dosing should be conservative to avoid hypoglycemic reactions.

Pregnancy: Category C; Category B (glyburide).

Lactation: Chlorpropamide and tolbutamide are excreted in breast milk. It is not known if other sulfonylureas are excreted in breast milk.

Children: Safety and efficacy in children have not been established.

Precautions

Monitoring:

Treatment Goals for Type 2 Diabetes Mellitus		
Patient population	Average preprandial glucose (mg/dL)	HbA_{1c}^1 (%)
ADA general recommendations[2]	80-120	< 7
Healthy, relatively young	80-120	< 8
Elderly and patients with serious medical conditions	100-140	< 9

[1] Glycosylated hemoglobin.
[2] American Diabetes Association 1999 Clinical Practice Recommendations.

During the transitional period, test the urine for glucose and acetone at least 3 times/day and have the results reviewed by a physician frequently. Measurement of glycosylated hemoglobin also is useful. It is important that patients be taught to correctly and frequently self-monitor blood glucose.

Hypoglycemia: All sulfonylureas may produce severe hypoglycemia. Proper patient selection, dosage and instructions are important to avoid hypoglycemic episodes.

Asymptomatic patients: Controlling blood glucose in type 2 diabetes with sulfonylureas has not been definitely established to be effective in preventing the long-term cardiovascular or neural complications of diabetes.

Loss of blood glucose control: When a patient stabilized on any diabetic regimen is exposed to stress such as fever, trauma, infection, or surgery, a loss of control may occur. At such times, it may be necessary to discontinue the drug and give insulin.

Disulfiram-like syndrome: A sulfonylurea-induced facial flushing or breathlessness reaction may occur when some sulfonylureas are administered with alcohol.

Syndrome of inappropriate secretion of antidiuretic hormone (SIADH): Water retention and dilutional hyponatremia have occurred after administration of sulfonylureas to type 2 diabetes patients, especially those with CHF or hepatic cirrhosis.

Drug Interactions

Drugs that may affect sulfonylureas include androgens, anticoagulants, azole antifungals, barbiturates, beta blockers, calcium channel blockers, charcoal, chloramphenicol, cholestyramine, ciprofloxacin, clofibrate, corticosteroids, diazoxide, estrogens, ethanol, fluconazole, gemfibrozil, histamine H_2 antagonists, hydantoins, isoniazid, magnesium salts, methyldopa, MAO inhibitors, nicotinic acid, oral contraceptives, phenothiazines, probenecid, rifampin, salicylates, sulfinpyrazone, sulfonamides, sympathomimetics, thiazide diuretics, thyroid agents, tricyclic antidepressants, urinary acidifiers, and urinary alkalinizers. Drugs that may be affected by sulfonylureas include digitalis glycosides.

Drug/Lab test interactions: A metabolite of tolbutamide in the urine may give a false-positive reaction for albumin if measured by the acidification-after-boiling test, which causes the metabolite to precipitate. There is no interference with the sulfosalicylic acid test.

Drug/Food interactions: Absorption of glipizide is delayed by ≈ 40 minutes when taken with food; the drug is more effective when given ≈ 30 minutes before a meal. The other sulfonylureas may be taken with food.

Adverse Reactions

GI disturbances (eg, nausea, epigastric fullness, heartburn) are the most common reactions. Other adverse reactions may include hypoglycemia, disulfiram-like reactions; allergic skin reactions; eczema; pruritus; erythema; urticaria; photosensitivity reactions; leukopenia; thrombocytopenia; aplastic anemia; agranulocytosis; hemolytic anemia; pancytopenia; weakness; paresthesia; tinnitus; fatigue; dizziness; vertigo; malaise; elevated liver function tests.

METFORMIN HCl

Tablets: 500, 850, and 1000 mg (*Rx*)	*Glucophage* (Bristol-Myers Squibb)
Tablets, extended-release: 500 mg (*Rx*)	*Glucophage* XR (Bristol-Myers Squibb)

Warning:
> *Lactic acidosis:* Lactic acidosis is a rare, but serious, metabolic complication that can occur because of metformin accumulation during treatment; when it occurs, it is fatal in ≈ 50% of cases. See Warnings.

Indications

Type 2 diabetes: As monotherapy, as an adjunct to diet and exercise to improve glycemic control in patients with type 2 diabetes. Metformin is indicated in patients ≥ 10 years of age and metformin extended-release (ER) tablets are indicated in patients ≥ 17 years of age.

Metformin or metformin ER may be used concomitantly with a sulfonylurea or insulin to improve glycemic control in adults ≥ 17 years of age.

Administration and Dosage

Dosage must be individualized on the basis of effectiveness and tolerance, while not exceeding the maximum recommended daily dose of 2550 mg in adults and 2000 mg in pediatric patients (10 to 16 years of age); the maximum recommended daily dose of metformin ER in adults is 2000 mg. Give metformin in divided doses with meals while metformin ER generally should be given once daily with the evening meal. Start at a low dose, with gradual dose escalation as described below, to reduce GI side effects and to permit identification of the minimum dose required for adequate glycemic control of the patient.

During treatment initiation and dose titration, use fasting plasma glucose to determine therapeutic response to metformin and to identify minimum effective dose. Thereafter, measure glycosylated hemoglobin at intervals of ≈ 3 months.

Short-term administration may be sufficient during periods of transient loss of control in patients usually well controlled on diet alone.

Metformin ER must be swallowed whole and never crushed or chewed. Occasionally, the inactive ingredients will be eliminated in the feces as a soft, hydrated mass.

Adults:
Metformin – The usual starting dose is 500 mg twice/day or 850 mg once/day, given with meals. Make dosage increases in increments of 500 mg/week or 850 mg every 2 weeks, up to a total of 2000 mg/day given in divided doses. Patients can be titrated from 500 mg twice/day to 850 mg twice/day after 2 weeks. For those patients requiring additional glycemic control, it may be given to a maximum daily dose of 2550 mg/day. Doses > 2000 mg may be better tolerated given 3 times/day with meals.

Metformin ER – The usual starting dose is 500 mg once/day with the evening meal. Make dosage increases in increments of 500 mg/week, up to a maximum of 2000 mg once/day with the evening meal. If glycemic control is not achieved on 2000 mg once/day, consider a trial of 1000 mg twice/day. If higher doses of metformin are required, use metformin at total daily doses up to 2550 mg administered in divided daily doses, as described above.

Conversion from metformin to metformin ER – In a randomized trial, results suggest that patients receiving metformin treatment may be safely switched to metformin ER once daily at the same total daily dose, up to 2000 mg once/day. Following a switch from metformin to metformin ER, closely monitor glycemic control and make dosage adjustments accordingly.

Pediatrics: The usual starting dose of metformin is 500 mg twice/day, given with meals. Make dosage increases in increments of 500 mg/week up to a maximum of 2000 mg/day given in divided doses.

Transfer from other antidiabetic therapy: When transferring patients from standard oral hypoglycemic agents other than chlorpropamide to metformin, generally no transition period is necessary. When transferring patients from chlorpropamide, exercise care during the first 2 weeks because of the prolonged retention of chlorpropamide leading to overlapping drug effects and possible hypoglycemia.

Concomitant metformin and oral sulfonylurea therapy: If patients have not responded to 4 weeks of the maximum dose of metformin monotherapy, consider gradual addition of an oral sulfonylurea while continuing metformin at the maximum dose, even if prior primary or secondary failure to a sulfonylurea has occurred.

With concomitant metformin and sulfonylurea therapy, the desired control of blood glucose may be obtained by adjusting the dose of each drug. However, make attempts to identify the minimum effective dose of each drug. With concomitant metformin and sulfonylurea therapy, risk of hypoglycemia associated with sulfonylurea therapy continues and may be increased. Take appropriate precautions.

If patients have not satisfactorily responded to 1 to 3 months of concomitant therapy with the maximum doses of metformin and an oral sulfonylurea, consider institution of insulin therapy and discontinuation of these oral agents.

Concomitant metformin or metformin ER and insulin therapy in adults: Continue the current insulin dose upon initiation of metformin or metfomin ER therapy. Initiate metformin or metformin ER therapy at 500 mg once/day in patients on insulin therapy. For patients not responding adequately, increase the dose of metformin or metformin ER by 500 mg after $\approx$ 1 week and by 500 mg every week thereafter until adequate glycemic control is achieved. The maximum recommended daily dose is 2500 mg for metformin and 2000 mg for metformin ER. It is recommended that the insulin dose be decreased by 10% to 25% when fasting plasma glucose concentrations decrease to < 120 mg/dL in patients receiving concomitant insulin and metformin or metformin ER. Individualize further adjustment based on glucose-lowering response.

Special patient populations: Initial and maintenance dosing should be conservative in patients with advanced age due to the potential for decreased renal function in this population. Base any dosage adjustment on a careful assessment of renal function. Generally, elderly patients should not be titrated to the maximum dose.

In debilitated or malnourished patients, the dosing should also be conservative and based on a careful assessment of renal function.

Actions

Pharmacology: Metformin improves glucose tolerance in subjects with type 2 diabetes, lowering basal and postprandial plasma glucose. Metformin decreases hepatic glucose production, decreases intestinal absorption of glucose and improves insulin sensitivity (increases peripheral glucose uptake and utilization). Metformin does not produce hypoglycemia and does not cause hyperinsulinemia. With metfomin therapy, insulin secretion remains unchanged while fasting insulin levels and day-long plasma insulin response may actually decrease.

Pharmacokinetics:

Absorption/Distribution – The absolute bioavailability of 500 mg metformin given under fasting conditions is $\approx$ 50% to 60%. Food decreases the extent and slightly delays the absorption of metformin.

Metformin is negligibly bound to plasma proteins; steady-state plasma concentrations are reached within 24 to 48 hours and are generally < 1 mcg/mL.

The extent of metformin absorption (as measured by AUC) from metformin ER at 2000 mg once/day dose is similar to the same total daily dose administered as metformin tablets 1000 mg twice/day.

Metabolism/Excretion – Metformin is excreted unchanged in the urine and does not undergo hepatic metabolism nor biliary excretion. Renal clearance is $\approx$ 3.5 times greater than creatinine clearance (Ccr) which indicates that tubular secretion is the major route of elimination. The elimination half-life is $\approx$ 17.6 hours.

Contraindications

1.) Renal disease or dysfunction (eg, as suggested by serum creatinine levels ≥ 1.5 mg/dL [males], ≥ 1.4 mg/dL [females] or abnormal Ccr), which also may result from conditions such as cardiovascular collapse (shock), acute MI, and septicemia.

2.) CHF requiring pharmacologic treatment.

3.) Temporarily discontinue metformin in patients undergoing radiologic studies involving intravascular administration of iodinated contrast materials because use of such products may result in acute alteration of renal function (see Drug Interactions).

4.) Hypersensitivity to metformin.

5.) Acute or chronic metabolic acidosis, including diabetic ketoacidosis, with or without coma. Treat diabetic ketoacidosis with insulin.

Warnings

Lactic acidosis: Lactic acidosis is a rare, but serious, metabolic complication that can occur due to metformin accumulation during treatment; when it occurs, it is fatal in ≈ 50% of cases. When metformin is implicated as the cause of lactic acidosis, metformin plasma levels > 5 mcg/mL are generally found.

The reported incidence of lactic acidosis in patients receiving metformin is very low (≈ 0.03 cases/1000 patient-years, with ≈ 0.015 fatal cases/1000 patient-years). Reported cases have occurred primarily in diabetic patients with significant renal insufficiency, including intrinsic renal disease and renal hypoperfusion, often in the setting of multiple concomitant medical/surgical problems and multiple concomitant medications. Patients with CHF requiring pharmacologic management, in particular those with unstable or acute CHF who are at risk of hypoperfusion and hypoxemia, are at increased risk of lactic acidosis. The risk of lactic acidosis increases with the degree of renal dysfunction and the patient's age. The risk of lactic acidosis may be significantly decreased by regular monitoring of renal function in patients taking metformin and by use of the minimum effective dose. Treatment of the elderly should be accompanied by careful monitoring of renal function. Do not initiate metformin treatment in patients ≥ 80 years of age unless measurement of Ccr demonstrates that renal function is not reduced. Promptly withhold metformin in the presence of any condition associated with hypoxemia, dehydration, or sepsis. Generally avoid metformin in patients with evidence of hepatic disease. Caution patients against excessive alcohol intake (acute or chronic) because alcohol potentiates the effects of metformin on lactate metabolism. Temporarily discontinue metformin prior to any intravascular radiocontrast study and for any surgical procedure.

Instruct the patient to notify the physician immediately if symptoms occur. Withdraw metformin until the situation is clarified. Serum electrolytes, ketones, blood glucose and, if indicated, blood pH, lactate levels, and blood metformin levels may be useful. Once a patient is stabilized on any dose of metformin, GI symptoms, which are common during initiation of therapy, are unlikely to be drug related. Later occurrence of GI symptoms could be because of lactic acidosis or other serious disease.

Suspect lactic acidosis in any diabetic patient with metabolic acidosis lacking evidence of ketoacidosis (ketonuria and ketonemia).

In a patient with lactic acidosis who is taking metformin, discontinue the drug immediately and promptly institute general supportive measures. Because metformin is dialyzable (with a clearance of up to 170 mL/min under good hemodynamic conditions), prompt hemodialysis is recommended to correct the acidosis and remove the accumulated metformin. Such management often results in prompt reversal of symptoms and recovery.

Renal function impairment: Metformin is known to be excreted by the kidney, and the risk of metformin accumulation and lactic acidosis increases with the degree of impairment of renal function. Patients with serum creatinine levels above the upper limit of normal for their age should not receive metformin or metformin ER. In patients with decreased renal function, the plasma and blood half-life of metformin is prolonged, and the clearance is decreased in proportion to the decrease in Ccr.

Concomitant medication(s) that affect renal function, result in significant hemodynamic change, or interfere with the disposition of metformin (ie, cationic drugs that are eliminated by renal tubular secretion; see Drug Interactions) should be used with caution.

Hepatic function impairment: Because impaired hepatic function has been associated with cases of lactic acidosis, avoid metformin in patients with clinical or laboratory evidence of hepatic disease.

Pregnancy: Category B.

Lactation: Decide whether to discontinue nursing or to discontinue the drug, taking into account the importance of the drug to the mother.

Children: Safety and efficacy for metformin for the treatment of type 2 diabetes have been established in pediatric patients ages 10 to 16 years of age who demonstrated a similar response in glycemic control to that seen in adults. Adverse effects were similar to those described in adults. A maximum daily dose of 2000 mg is recommended.

Safety and efficacy in children for metformin ER have not been established.

Precautions

Monitoring: Before initiation of therapy and at least annually thereafter, assess renal function. In patients at risk of renal dysfunction, assess renal function more frequently and discontinue the drug if renal impairment is present.

Evaluate a patient previously well controlled on metformin who develops laboratory abnormalities or clinical illness for evidence of ketoacidosis or lactic acidosis. Evaluation should include serum electrolytes and ketones, blood glucose and, if indicated, blood pH, lactate, pyruvate, and metformin levels. If acidosis of either form occurs, metformin must be stopped immediately and other appropriate corrective measures initiated.

Monitor response to all diabetic therapies by periodic measurements of fasting blood glucose and glycosylated hemoglobin levels, with a goal of decreasing these levels toward the normal range. During initial dose titration, fasting glucose can be used to determine the therapeutic response. Thereafter, monitor both glucose and glycosylated hemoglobin.

Perform initial and periodic monitoring of hematologic parameters (eg, hemoglobin/hematocrit, red blood cell indices) and renal function (serum creatinine) at least on an annual basis. While megaloblastic anemia has rarely been seen with metformin therapy, if this is suspected, exclude vitamin B_{12} deficiency.

Hypoxic states: Cardiovascular collapse (shock), acute CHF, acute MI and other conditions characterized by hypoxemia have been associated with lactic acidosis and may also cause prerenal azotemia. If such events occur, discontinue metformin.

Surgical procedures: Temporarily suspend metformin for surgical procedures (unless minor and not associated with restricted intake of food and fluids). Do not restart until the patient's oral intake has resumed and renal function is normal.

Vitamin B_{12} levels: A decrease of previously normal serum vitamin B_{12} levels, without clinical manifestations, is observed in $\approx$ 7% of patients receiving metformin in controlled clinical trials of 29 weeks duration. Such decrease, possibly because of interference with B_{12} absorption from the B_{12}-intrinsic factor complex is very rarely associated with anemia and appears to be rapidly reversible with discontinuation of metform or vitamin B_{12} supplementation.

Certain individuals with inadequate vitamin B_{12} or calcium intake or absorption appear to be predisposed to developing subnormal vitamin B_{12} levels. In these patients, routine serum vitamin B_{12} measurements at 2 to 3 year intervals may be useful.

Hypoglycemia: Hypoglycemia does not occur in patients receiving metformin alone under usual circumstances, but could occur with deficient caloric intake, strenuous exercise not compensated by caloric supplementation, or during concomitant use with other glucose lowering agents (such as sulfonylureas) or ethanol.

Elderly, debilitated, or malnourished patients, and those with adrenal or pituitary insufficiency or alcohol intoxication are particularly susceptible to hypoglycemic effects. Hypoglycemia may be difficult to recognize in the elderly and in people who are taking beta-adrenergic blocking drugs.

Loss of control of blood glucose: When a patient stabilized on any diabetic regimen is exposed to stress such as fever, trauma, infection, or surgery, a temporary loss of glycemic control may occur. At such times, it may be necessary to withhold metformin and temporarily administer insulin. Metformin may be reinstituted after the acute episode is resolved.

Should secondary failure occur with metformin or sulfonylurea monotherapy, combined therapy with metformin and sulfonylurea may result in a response. Should secondary failure occur with combined therapy, it may be necessary to consider therapeutic alternatives including initiation of insulin therapy.

Drug Interactions

Drugs that may affect metformin include alcohol, cationic drugs, cimetidine, furosemide, iodinated contrast material, and nifedipine.

Drugs that may be affected by metformin include glyburide and furosemide.

Certain drugs tend to produce hyperglycemia and may lead to loss of glycemic control. These drugs include thiazide and other diuretics, corticosteroids, phenothiazines, thyroid products, estrogens, oral contraceptives, phenytoin, nicotinic acid, sympathomimetics, calcium channel blocking drugs, and isoniazid. When such drugs are administered to a patient receiving metformin, closely observe the patient to maintain adequate glycemic control.

Drug/Food interactions: Food decreases the extent and slightly delays the absorption of a single 850 mg dose of metformin as shown by an ≈ 40% lower peak concentration and 25% lower AUC in plasma and a 35 minute prolongation of time to peak plasma concentration compared with the same strength administered under fasting conditions. The clinical relevance of these decreases is unknown.

Adverse Reactions

Adverse reactions occurring in ≥ 3% of patients include the following:

Metformin – Diarrhea; nausea; vomiting; abdominal discomfort; flatulence; asthenia; ingestion; headache.

Metformin ER – Abdominal pain; constipation; abdominal distention; dyspepsia/heartburn; flatulence; dizziness; headache; upper respiratory tract infection; taste disturbance.

THIAZOLIDINEDIONES

ROSIGLITAZONE MALEATE
Tablets: 2, 4, and 8 mg (Rx)   *Avandia* (SmithKline Beecham)

PIOGLITAZONE HCl
Tablets: 15, 30, and 45 mg (Rx)   *Actos* (Takeda Pharm. America, Inc.)

Indications

Type 2 diabetes: Concomitantly with a sulfonylurea, insulin (**pioglitazone**), or metformin to improve glycemic control.

Monotherapy as an adjunct to diet and exercise to lower blood glucose.

Administration and Dosage

Rosiglitazone maleate:

Monotherapy – The usual starting dose is 4 mg as a single dose once daily or in divided doses twice daily. For patients who respond inadequately following 12 weeks of treatment as determined by reduction in fasting serum glucose (FSG), the dose may be increased to 8 mg administered as a single dose once daily or in divided doses twice daily.

Combination therapy –

Metformin: For patients inadequately controlled with a maximum dose of metformin, rosiglitazone should be added to, rather than substituted for, metformin. The usual starting dose in combination with metformin is 4 mg administered as either a single dose once daily or in divided doses twice daily. The rosiglitazone dose may be increased to 8 mg/day following 12 weeks of therapy if there is insufficient reduction in FSG. Rosiglitazone may be administered as a single daily dose in the morning or divided and administered in the morning and evening.

Renal impairment – Metformin is contraindicated in patients with renal impairment. Therefore, concomitant administration of rosiglitazone and metformin is contraindicated in these patients.

Hepatic impairment – Use with caution in patients with hepatic impairment. Do not initiate rosiglitazone therapy if the patient exhibits clinical evidence of active liver disease or increased serum transaminase levels (ALT > 2.5 times the ULN) at start of therapy. Liver enzyme monitoring is recommended in all patients prior to initiation of therapy with rosiglitazone and periodically thereafter.

Pioglitazone:

Monotherapy – Initiate monotherapy in patients not adequately controlled with diet and exercise at 15 or 30 mg once daily. For patients who respond inadequately to the initial dose of pioglitazone, the dose can be increased in increments up to 45 mg once daily. Consider combination therapy for patients not responding adequately to monotherapy.

Combination therapy –

Sulfonylureas: Initiate pioglitazone in combination with a sulfonylurea at 15 or 30 mg once daily. Continue the current sulfonylurea upon initiation of pioglitazone therapy. Decrease the dose of the sulfonlyurea if patients report hypoglycemia.

Metformin: Initiate pioglitazone in combination with metformin at 15 or 30 mg once daily. Continue the current metformin dose upon initiation of pioglitazone therapy. It is unlikely that the dose of metformin will require adjustment because of hypoglycemia during combination therapy with pioglitazone.

Insulin: Initiate pioglitazone in combination with insulin at 15 or 30 mg once daily. Continue the current insulin dose upon initiation of pioglitazone therapy. Decrease the insulin dose by 10% to 25% in patients receiving pioglitazone and insulin if the patient reports hypoglycemia or if plasma glucose concentrations decrease to < 100 mg/dL. Individualize further adjustments based on glucose-lowering response.

Maximum recommended dose – Do not exceed > 45 mg once daily of pioglitazone because doses > 45 mg once daily have not been studied in placebo-controlled clinical studies.

Hepatic disease – Do not initiate pioglitazone therapy if the patient exhibits clinical evidence of active liver disease or increased serum transaminase levels (ALT > 2.5 times the ULN) at the start of therapy. Liver enzyme monitoring is recommended in all patients prior to initiation of therapy with pioglitazone and periodically thereafter.

Children – The use of pioglitazone in pediatric patients < 18 years of age is not recommended.

Actions

Pharmacology: Thiazolidinediones are antidiabetic agents that increase insulin sensitivity through the modulation of several processes. These agents affect insulin receptor kinase activity, insulin receptor phosphorylation, insulin receptor numbers, and hepatic glucose metabolism. **Pioglitazone** and **rosiglitazone** decrease hepatic gluconeogenesis and increase insulin-dependent muscle glucose uptake.

Addition of thiazolidinediones to a sulfonylurea has a synergistic effect because both agents act to improve glucose tolerance by different but complementary mechanisms. Unlike sulfonylureas, thiazolidinediones are not insulin secretagogues.

Pharmacokinetics:

Pharmacokinetics of Thiazolidinediones		
Parameters	Pioglitazone	Rosiglitazone
Absorption	Food does not alter absorption extent	99% bioavailability
C_{max}[1]	—	Fasted 1, 2, 8 mg: 76, 156, 598 ng/mL Fed 8 mg: 432 ng/mL
T_{max}	Fasted: 2 hours Fed: 3 to 4 hr	Fasted 2 mg: 1.3 hr; Fed 2 mg: 3.5 hr
Distribution Vd Protein binding	≈ 0.63 L/kg[2] > 99%	17.6 L 99.8%
Metabolism	Hydroxylation and oxidation,[3] CYP450 3A4	N-demethylation, hydroxylation, and conjugation with sulfate and glucuronic acid
Excretion Site Elimination t½	Urine (15 to 30%) Pioglitazone: 3 to 7 hr Total pioglitazone: 16 to 24 hr	Urine (64%), feces (23%) 3 to 4 hr
Oral clearance[1]	83.3 to 116.7 mL/min	Fasted 1, 2, 8 mg: 50.5, 48.1, 47.5 mL/min Fed 8 mg: 49.5 mL/min

[1] C_{max} and oral clearance for **rosiglitazone** were calculated following single oral doses.
[2] Volume of distribution was calculated following a single-dose administration.
[3] Metabolites M-II and M-IV (hydroxy derivatives of **pioglitazone**) and M-III (keto derivatives) are pharmacologically active in animal models of type 2 diabetes.

Special populations –

Hepatic function impairment:

Rosiglitazone – Unbound oral clearance of rosiglitazone was significantly lower in moderate to severe liver disease patients (Child-Pugh class B/C) in comparison with healthy subjects. This resulted in an increased C_{max} by 2-fold and AUC by 3-fold, and a longer elimination half-life by 2 hours. Do not initiate rosiglitazone in patients exhibiting clinical evidence of active liver disease or increased serum transaminase levels (ALT > 2.5 times the ULN).

Pioglitazone – Compared with healthy controls, subjects with impaired hepatic function (Child-Pugh class B/C) have an $\approx 45\%$ reduction in pioglitazone and total pioglitazone mean peak concentrations but no change in the mean AUC values. Do not initiate pioglitazone if the patient exhibits clinical evidence of active liver disease or serum transaminase levels (ALT > 2.5 the ULN).

Contraindications

Hypersensitivity or allergy to **pioglitazone** or **rosiglitazone** or any of their components.

Warnings

Hepatotoxicity: Available clinical data show no evidence of **pioglitazone**- and **rosiglitazone**-induced hepatotoxicity or ALT elevations. It is recommended that patients undergo periodic monitoring of liver enzymes. Check liver enzymes prior to the initiation of therapy in all treated patients. Do not initiate therapy in patients with increased baseline liver enzyme levels (ALT > 2.5 times the ULN). In patients with normal baseline liver enzymes, it is recommended that liver enzymes be monitored every 2 months for the first 12 months and periodically thereafter. If at any time ALT levels increase to > 3 times the ULN in patients on therapy with rosiglitazone, recheck liver enzyme levels as soon as possible. If ALT levels remain > 3 times the ULN, discontinue therapy.

If any patient develops symptoms suggesting hepatic dysfunction (eg, unexplained nausea, vomiting, abdominal pain, fatigue, anorexia, dark urine), check liver enzymes. The decision whether to continue the patient on therapy with pioglitazone and rosiglitazone should be guided by clinical judgment pending laboratory evaluations. If jaundice is observed, discontinue therapy.

Ovulation: In premenopausal anovulatory patients with insulin resistance, thiazolidinedione treatment may result in resumption of ovulation. These patients may be at risk for pregnancy.

Pregnancy: Category C (**pioglitazone, rosiglitazone**).

Lactation: Do not administer to nursing women.

Children: Safety and efficacy have not been established in patients < 18 years of age.

Precautions

Monitoring: See Warnings. Perform periodic fasting blood glucose and HbA$_{1c}$ measurements to monitor therapeutic response. Liver enzyme monitoring is recommended prior to initiation of therapy in all patients and periodically thereafter.

Type 1 diabetes: **Pioglitazone** and **rosiglitazone** are active only in the presence of insulin. Therefore, do not use in type 1 diabetes patients or for the treatment of diabetic ketoacidosis.

Hypoglycemia: Patients receiving **pioglitazone** in combination with insulin or oral hypoglycemics (eg, sulfonylureas) may be at risk for hypoglycemia; reduction in the dose of insulin or sulfonylureas may be necessary.

Hematologic: **Rosiglitazone** and **pioglitazone** may cause decreases in hemoglobin and hematocrit. These changes primarily occurred within the first 4 to 12 weeks of therapy and remained relatively constant thereafter.

Edema: Use **pioglitazone** and **rosiglitazone** with caution in patients with edema. In controlled clinical trials of patients with type 2 diabetes, mild to moderate edema was reported in pioglitazone- and rosiglitazone-treated patients.

Cardiovascular effects: In preclinical studies, thiazolidinediones caused plasma volume expansion and pre-load-induced cardiac hypertrophy. **Rosiglitazone** is not indicated in patients with New York Heart Association (NYHA) Class 3 and 4 cardiac status unless the expected benefit is judged to outweigh the potential risk.

Drug Interactions

Drugs that may affect **pioglitazone** include ketoconazole. Drugs that may be affected by **pioglitazone** include oral contraceptives.

Adverse Reactions

Adverse reactions that were reported in ≥ 5% of patients include accidental injury (rosiglitazone), aggravated diabetes mellitus, myalgia, sinusitis, tooth disorder, pharyngitis (pioglitazone), upper respiratory tract infection (pioglitazone, rosiglitazone). Pioglitazone when used in combination with sulfonylureas, metformin, or insulin caused an increased incidence of edema.

Reports of anemia (7.1%) were greater in patients treated with a combination of rosiglitazone and metformin compared with rosiglitazone monotherapy.

Lab test abnormalities:

Lipids – Increases in HDL, LDL, and total cholesterol have been observed in thiazolidinedione-treated patients.

Serum transaminase levels – 0.2% of **rosiglitazone**-treated patients and 0.26% of **pioglitazone**-treated patients had reversible elevations in AST or ALT > 3 times the ULN, compared with 0.6%, 0.2%, and 0.25% respectively, of patients receiving placebo. Mean and median values for bilirubin, AST, ALT, alkaline phosphatase, and GGT were decreased at the final visit in pioglitazone-treated patients compared with baseline, while values for LDH were slightly increased.

GLYBURIDE/METFORMIN HCl

Tablets: 1.25/250, 2.5/500, and 5 mg/500 mg *(Rx)*   *Glucovance* (Bristol-Myers Squibb)

Indications
Type 2 diabetes: Initial and second-line therapy.

Administration and Dosage
Individualize dosage, not exceeding the maximum recommended daily dose of 20 mg glyburide/2000 mg metformin. Give with meals and initiate at a low dose with gradual dose escalation to avoid hypoglycemia, to reduce GI side effects, and to permit determination of the minimum effective dose for adequate control of blood glucose.

Use appropriate blood glucose monitoring to determine the therapeutic response and to identify the minimum effective dose for the patient. Thereafter, measure HbA$_{1c}$ at intervals of $\approx$ 3 months to assess the effectiveness of therapy.

Initial therapy:
Starting dose – 1.25 mg/250 mg once or twice daily with meals.

Previously treated patients (second-line therapy):
Starting dose – 2.5 mg/500 mg or 5 mg/500 mg twice daily with meals.
Patients previously treated with combination therapy of glyburide (or another sulfonylurea) plus metformin, if switched to glyburide/metformin HCl, the starting dose should not exceed the daily dose of glyburide (or equivalent dose of another sulfonylurea) and metformin already being taken.

Specific patient populations: Glyburide/metformin HCl is not recommended for use during pregnancy or in pediatric patients. Initial and maintenance dosing should be conservative in patients with advanced age because of the potential for decreased renal function in this population. Dosage adjustment requires a careful assessment of renal function. Do not titrate elderly, debilitated, or malnourished patients to the maximum dose to avoid the risk of hypoglycemia.

THYROID HORMONES

LEVOTHYROXINE SODIUM

Tablets: 0.025, 0.05, 0.075, 0.088, 0.1, 0.112, 0.125, 0.137, 0.15, 0.175, 0.2, and 3 mg (Rx)
Various, *Eltroxin* (Roberts), *Levo-T* (Lederle), *Levothroid* (Forest), *Levoxyl* (Daniels), *Synthroid* (Knoll)

Powder for injection, lyophilized: 200 and 500 mcg per vial (Rx)
Various, *Levothroid* (Forest), *Levoxine* (Daniels), *Synthroid* (Knoll)

LIOTHYRONINE SODIUM

Tablets: 5, 25, and 50 mcg (Rx)
Various, *Cytomel* (SK-Beecham)

Injection: 10 mcg/mL (Rx)
Triostat (SK-Beecham)

LIOTRIX (60 mg = 1 grain)

Tablets: ¼, ½, 1, 2, and 3 grains (T$_4$:T$_3$ content in a 4:1 ratio) (Rx)
Thyrolar (Forest)

THYROID DESSICATED (60 mg = 1 grain)

Tablets: 15, 30, 60, 90, 120, 180, 240, and 300 mg (Rx)
Thyroid USP (Various), *Armour Thyroid* (Rhone-Poulenc Rorer)

Indications

Hypothyroidism: As replacement or supplemental therapy in hypothyroidism of any etiology, except transient hypothyroidism during the recovery phase of subacute thyroiditis.

Pituitary TSH suppressants: In the treatment or prevention of various types of euthyroid goiters, including thyroid nodules, subacute, or chronic lymphocytic thyroiditis (Hashimoto's), multinodular goiter, and in the management of thyroid cancer.

Thyrotoxicosis: May be used with antithyroid drugs to treat thyrotoxicosis, to prevent goitrogenesis and hypothyroidism and thyrotoxicosis during pregnancy.

Diagnostic use: Diagnostic use in suppression tests to differentiate suspected hyperthyroidism from euthyroidism.

Administration and Dosage

Generally, institute thyroid therapy at relatively low doses and slowly increase in small increments until the desired response is obtained. Administer thyroid as a single daily dose, preferably before breakfast.

Treatment of choice: Treatment of choice for hypothyroidism is T$_4$ under most circumstances because of its consistent potency, restoration of normal constant serum levels of T$_4$ and T$_3$ and its prolonged duration of action. However, it has a slow onset of action and its effects are cumulative over several weeks.

Dosage equivalents of thyroid products: In changing from one thyroid product to another, the following dosage equivalents may be used. However, each patient may still require fine dosage adjustments because these dosage equivalents are only estimates.

Dosage Equivalents of Thyroid Products			
	Composition ratio		
Preparation	T$_4$	T$_3$	Dosage equivalents
Crude hormone			
Thyroid USP	2 to 5	1	60 mg (1 grain)
Thyroglobulin	2.5	1	60 mg
Thyroid Strong	3.1	1	45 mg
Synthetic hormone			
Levothyroxine	1	0	0.1 mg[1]
Liothyronine	0	1	25 mcg
Liotrix	4	1	1 grain

[1] Previously considered to be 0.1 mg.

LEVOTHYROXINE SODIUM (T$_4$; L-thyroxine):
    Hypothyroidism –
        Initial dosage: Usual starting dose is 0.05 mg, with increments of 0.025 mg every 2 to 3 weeks. Use ≤ 0.025 mg/day in patients with long-standing hypothyroidism, particularly if cardiovascular impairment is suspected.

Maintenance dosage: Most patients require no more than 0.2 mg/day; failure to respond to 0.3 mg doses suggests lack of compliance or malabsorption.

IV or IM injection can be substituted for the oral dosage form when oral ingestion is precluded for long periods of time. The initial parenteral dosage should be ≈ ½ of the previously established oral dosage.

Myxedema coma – Consider a medical emergency. Levothyroxine may be administered via nasogastric tube, but the IV route is preferred. A starting dose of 0.4 mg given rapidly is usually well tolerated, even in elderly.

The initial dose is followed by daily supplements of 0.1 to 0.2 mg IV. Normal T_4 levels are achieved in 24 hours followed in 3 days by threefold elevation of T_3. Maintain continued daily IV administration of lesser amounts until the patient is fully capable of accepting a daily oral dose.

A daily maintenance dose of 0.05 to 0.1 mg parenterally should suffice to maintain the euthyroid state, once established. Resume oral therapy as soon as the clinical situation has been stabilized and the patient is able to take oral medication.

TSH suppression in thyroid cancer, nodules and euthyroid goiters – Larger amounts of thyroid hormone than those used for replacement therapy are required. This therapy is also used in treating nontoxic solitary nodules and multi-nodular goiters, and to prevent thyroid enlargement in chronic (Hashimoto's) thyroiditis.

Thyroid suppression therapy – 2.6 mcg/kg/day for 7 to 10 days. These doses usually yield normal serum T_4 and T_3 levels and lack of response to TSH.

Children – Follow the recommendations in the following table. In infants with congenital hypothyroidism, institute therapy with full doses as soon as diagnosis is made.

Levothyroxine tablets may be given to infants and children who cannot swallow intact tablets. Crush the proper dose tablet and suspend in a small amount of formula or water. The suspension can be given by spoon or dropper. Do NOT store the suspension for any period of time. The crushed tablet may also be sprinkled over a small amount of food such as cooked cereal or applesauce.

Recommended Pediatric Dosage for Congenital Hypothyroidism		
Age	Dose/day (mcg)	Daily dose/kg (mcg)
0 to 6 months	25 to 50	8 to 10
6 to 12 months	50 to 75	6 to 8
1 to 5 years	75 to 100	5 to 6
6 to 12 years	100 to 150	4 to 5
> 12 years	> 150	2 to 3

Alternative suggested doses include: 0 to 1 year, 8 to 10 mcg/kg/day; 1 to 5 years, 4 to 6 mcg/kg/day; > 5 years to adolescence, 3 to 4 mcg/kg/day.

LIOTHYRONINE SODIUM (T_3):

Mild hypothyroidism – Starting dose is 25 mcg/day. Daily dosage may then be increased by 12.5 or 25 mcg every 1 or 2 weeks. Usual maintenance dose is 25 to 75 mcg/day. Smaller doses may be fully effective in some patients, while dosages of 100 mcg/day may be required in others.

Congenital hypothyroidism – Starting dose is 5 mcg/day, with a 5 mcg increment every 3 to 4 days until the desired response is achieved. Infants a few months old may require only 20 mcg/day for maintenance. At 1 year of age, 50 mcg/day may be required. Above 3 years, full adult dosage may be necessary.

Simple (nontoxic) goiter – Starting dose is 5 mcg/day. Dosage may be increased every 1 to 2 weeks by 5 or 10 mcg. When 25 mcg/day is reached, dosage may be increased every 1 to 2 weeks by 12.5 or 25 mcg. Usual maintenance dosage is 75 mcg/day.

T_3 *suppression test* – 75 to 100 mcg daily for 7 days, then repeat I^{131} Thyroid Uptake test.

Myxedema – Starting dose is 5 mcg/day. This may be increased by 5 to 10 mcg/day every 1 to 2 weeks. When 25 mcg/day is reached, dosage may be increased by 12.5 or 25 mcg every 1 or 2 weeks. Usual maintenance dose is 50 to 100 mcg/day.

Myxedema coma/precoma (injection only) – Liothyronine injection is for IV use only; do not give IM or SC. Proper administration of an adequate dose is important in determining clinical outcome. Give ≥ 4 hours, and ≤ 12 hours, apart. Giving ≥ 65 mcg/day initially is associated with lower mortality. There is limited experience with > 100 mg/day.

An initial IV dose ranging from 25 to 50 mcg is recommended in the emergency treatment of myxedema complications in adults. In patients with known or suspected cardiovascular disease, an initial dose of 10 to 20 mcg is suggested.

Switching to oral therapy: Resume oral therapy as soon as the clinical situation has been stabilized and the patient is able to take oral medication.

Elderly or children – Start therapy with 5 mcg/day; increase only by 5 mcg increments at the recommended intervals.

LIOTRIX:

Hypothyroidism –

Initial dosage: Usual starting dose is 30 mg with 15 mg increments every 2 to 3 weeks. Use 15 mg/day in patients with long-standing hypothyroidism, particularly if cardiovascular impairment is suspected.

Maintenance dosage: Most patients require 60 to 120 mg/day; failure to respond to 180 mg doses suggests lack of compliance or malabsorption.

Thyroid cancer: Larger amounts of thyroid hormone than those used for replacement therapy are required.

Children – In infants with congenital hypothyroidism, institute therapy with full doses as soon as diagnosis is made.

Recommended Pediatric Dosage for Congenital Hypothyroidism		
	Tetraiodothyronine (T$_4$, levothyroxine) sodium	
Age	Dose/day	Daily dose/kg of body weight
0-6 mos	25-50 mcg	8-10 mcg
6-12 mos	50-75 mcg	6-8 mcg
1-5 yrs	75-100 mcg	5-6 mcg
6-12 yrs	100-150 mcg	4-5 mcg
over 12 yrs	over 150 mcg	2-3 mcg

THYROID DESICCATED:

Hypothyroidism –

Initial dosage: Usual starting dose is 30 mg, with increments of 15 mg every 2 to 3 weeks. Use 15 mg/day in patients with long-standing myxedema, particularly if cardiovascular impairment is suspected.

Maintenance dosage: 60 to 120 mg/day; failure to respond to 180 mg doses suggests lack of compliance or malabsorption.

Thyroid cancer – Larger amounts of thyroid hormone than those used for replacement therapy are required.

Children – In infants with congenital hypothyroidism, institute therapy with full doses as soon as diagnosis is made.

Recommended Pediatric Dosage of Dessicated Thyroid for Congenital Hypothyroidism		
Age	Dose/day (mg)	Daily dose/kg (mg)
0 to 6 mos	15 to 30	4.8 to 6
6 to 12 mos	30 to 45	3.6 to 4.8
1 to 5 yrs	45 to 60	3 to 3.6
6 to 12 yrs	60 to 90	2.4 to 3
> 12 yrs	> 90	1.2 to 1.8

Actions

Pharmacology:

Preparations – Thyroid hormones include both natural and synthetic derivatives. The natural product, desiccated thyroid, is derived from beef or pork. Although this preparation is most economical, standardization by iodine content or bioassay is inexact; synthetic derivatives are generally preferred because of more uniform standardization of potency.

Physiological effects – The mechanisms by which thyroid hormones exert their physiologic action are not well understood. It is believed that most of their effects are exerted through control of DNA transcription and protein synthesis. Their principal effect is to increase metabolic rate of body tissues noted by increases in: Oxygen consumption; respiratory rate; body temperature; cardiac output; heart rate; blood volume; rate of fat, protein and carbohydrate metabolism; enzyme system activity; growth and maturation. Thyroid hormones exert a profound influence on every organ system and are particularly important in CNS development. Thyroid hormones are also concerned with growth and differentiation of tissues.

Regulation of thyroid secretion: Endogenous thyroid hormone secretion is suppressed when exogenous thyroid hormones are given to euthyroid individuals in excess of the normal gland's secretion. Thyroid administration increases basal metabolic rate. The primary effect of the thyroid hormones is the result of T_3 activity.

Pharmacokinetics:

Absorption – Absorption of T_4 from the GI tract varies from 48% to 79% of the dose administered. In 4 hours, T_3 is 95% absorbed.

Various Pharmacokinetic Parameters of Thyroid Hormones				
Hormone	Ratio released from thyroid gland	Biologic potency	Half-life (days)	Protein binding (%)[2]
Levothyroxine (T_4)	20	1	6-7[1]	99+
Liothyronine (T_3)	1	4	≤ 2	99+

[1] 3 to 4 days in hyperthyroidism, 9 to 10 days in myxedema.
[2] Includes TBg, TBPA and TBa.

Contraindications

Acute MI and thyrotoxicosis uncomplicated by hypothyroidism; where hypothyroidism and hypoadrenalism (Addison's disease) coexist, unless treatment of hypoadrenalism with adrenocortical steroids precedes the initiation of thyroid therapy; hypersensitivity to active or extraneous constituents.

Warnings

Obesity: Obesity has been treated with thyroid hormones. In euthyroid patients, hormonal replacement doses are ineffective for weight reduction. Larger doses may produce serious or even life-threatening toxicity, particularly when given with sympathomimetic amines such as anorexiants.

Cardiovascular disease: Use caution when the integrity of the cardiovascular system, particularly the coronary arteries, is suspect. This includes patients with angina or the elderly, in whom there is a greater likelihood of occult cardiac disease.

Observe patients with coronary artery disease during surgery, since the possibility of precipitating cardiac arrhythmias may be greater in those treated with thyroid hormones.

Endocrine disorders: Thyroid hormone therapy in patients with concomitant diabetes mellitus or insipidus or adrenal insufficiency (Addison's disease) exacerbates the intensity of their symptoms. Correct adrenal insufficiency with corticosteroids before administering thyroid hormones.

Morphologic hypogonadism and nephrosis – Rule out prior to initiating therapy.

Myxedema – Patients with myxedema are particularly sensitive to thyroid preparations. Begin treatment with small doses and gradual increments.

Hyperthyroid effects – In rare instances the administration of thyroid hormone may precipitate a hyperthyroid state or may aggravate existing hyperthyroidism.

Pregnancy: Category A.

Lactation: Minimal amounts of thyroid hormones are excreted in breast milk. Thyroid is not associated with serious adverse reactions.

Children: Congenital hypothyroidism – Pregnant women provide little or no thyroid hormone to the fetus. Routine determinations of serum T_4 or TSH are strongly advised in neonates in view of the deleterious effects of thyroid deficiency on growth and development. In infants, excessive doses of thyroid hormone preparations may produce craniosynostosis. In children, partial loss of hair may be experienced in the first few months of thyroid therapy; this is usually a transient phenomenon that results in later recovery.

Precautions

Monitoring: Treatment of patients with thyroid hormones requires the periodic assessment of thyroid status by means of appropriate laboratory tests. The TSH suppression test can be used to test the effectiveness of any thyroid preparation. Serum T_4 levels can be used to test the effectiveness of all thyroid medications except T_3. When the total serum T_4 is low but TSH is normal, a test specific to assess unbound (free) T_4 levels is warranted.

Decreased bone density: Long-term levothyroxine therapy has been associated with decreased bone density in the hip and spine in pre- and postmenopausal women.

Drug Interactions

Drugs that may affect thyroid hormones include cholestyramine, colestipol, and estrogens. Drugs that may be affected by thyroid hormones include anticoagulants, beta blockers, digitalis glycosides, and theophyllines.

Drug/Lab test interactions: Consider changes in TBg concentration when interpreting T_4 and T_3 values. In such cases, measure the unbound (free) hormone.

Effects of Drugs on Thyroid Function Tests

Blank space signifies no data ↑ Increased ⇑ Slightly increased ↓ Decreased ⇓ Slightly decreased 0 No effect	Free T_4	Serum T_4	T_3 uptake resin	Free thyroxine index (FTI)	Serum T_3	Serum TSH
p-aminosalicyclic acid		↓		↓		
Aminoglutethimide		↓				↑
Amiodarone	0/↑	↑		↑	↓	↑
Anabolic steroids/androgens	0	↓	↑	0	↓	0
Antithyroid (PTU, methimazole)	0	0	↓	0	↓	0
Asparaginase		↓	↑	0	↓	0
Barbiturates	0	↓	0/⇑	↓	0	0
Carbamazepine	0/↓	↓	0/↑	↓	0/↑	0/↑
Chloral hydrate		↓	0/⇑	0	⇓	0
Cholestiramine	0	↓		↓	0/↑	0
Clofibrate	0	↑	↓	0	↑	0
Colestipol	0	↓		↓	0/↑	0/↑
Contraceptives, oral	0	↑	↓	0	↓	0
Corticosteroids	0	↓	↑	0	↓	0/↓
Danazol	0	↓	↑	0	↓	0
Diazepam		↓		⇓		
Estrogens	0	↑	↓	0/⇑	↑	0
Ethionamide		↓				
Fluorouracil		↓	0/⇑	0	↓	0
Heparin (IV)		↓	0/↑	↑	0	
Insulin		↑				
Lithium carbonate		0/↓	0/↓	0/↓	0/↓	0/↑
Methadone		↑	↓	0	↑	0
Mitotane		↓	0/⇑	0	↓	0
Nitroprusside		↓				
Oxyphenbutazone/phenylbutazone		↓	0/⇑	0	↓	0

Effects of Drugs on Thyroid Function Tests						
Blank space signifies no data ↑ Increased ⇑ Slightly increased ↓ Decreased ⇓ Slightly decreased 0 No effect	Free T$_4$	Serum T$_4$	T$_3$ uptake resin	Free thyroxine index (FTI)	Serum T$_3$	Serum TSH
Perphenazine		↑	↓	↓	↑	
Phenytoin	0/↓	↓	0/⇑	↓	0/↑	0/↑
Propranolol	0	0/↓	0/↑	0/↓	0/↓	0
Resorcinol (excessive topical use)		↓	↓	↓	↓	↑
Salicylates (large doses)	0	↓	0/⇑	0	↓	0
Sulfonylureas		↓		0	0	
Thiazides		0			↑	

Drug/Food interactions: Fasting increases the absorption of T$_4$ from the GI tract.

Adverse Reactions

Adverse reactions other than those indicating hyperthyroidism due to therapeutic overdosage, either initially or during the maintenance period, are rare. Symptoms of overdosage include: Palpitations; tachycardia; arrhythmias; angina pectoris; cardiac arrest; tremors; headache; nervousness; insomnia; diarrhea; vomiting; weight loss; menstrual irregularities; sweating; heat intolerance; fever.

ANTITHYROID AGENTS

METHIMAZOLE
Tablets: 5 and 10 mg (*Rx*)　　　　　　　　　*Tapazole* (Lilly)
PROPYLTHIOURACIL
Tablets: 50 mg (*Rx*)　　　　　　　　　Various

Indications

Hyperthyroidism: Long-term therapy may lead to disease remission. Also used to ameliorate hyperthyroidism in preparation for subtotal thyroidectomy or radioactive iodine therapy.

PTU is also used when thyroidectomy is contraindicated or not advisable.

Administration and Dosage

METHIMAZOLE: Usually given in 3 equal doses at ≈ 8 hour intervals.

　Adults –
　　Initial: 15 mg daily for mild hyperthyroidism, 30 to 40 mg/day for moderately severe hyperthyroidism and 60 mg/day for severe hyperthyroidism.
　　Maintenance: 5 to 15 mg/day.
　Children –
　　Initial: 0.4 mg/kg/day.
　　Maintenance: ≈ ½ the initial dose.
　　Another suggested dosage for children is as follows:
　　Initial: 0.5 to 0.7 mg/kg/day or 15 to 20 mg/m^2/day in 3 divided doses.
　　Maintenance: ⅓ to ⅔ of intial dose beginning when the patient is euthyroid.
　　Maximum: 30 mg/24 hours.

PROPYLTHIOURACIL (PTU): Usually given in 3 equal doses at ≈ 8 hour intervals.

　Adults –
　　Initial: 300 mg/day. In patients with severe hyperthyroidism, very large goiters, or both, the initial dosage is usually 400 mg/day; an occasional patient will require 600 to 900 mg/day initially.
　　Maintenance: Usually, 100 to 150 mg/day.
　Children –
　　6 to 10 years of age: Initial dose is 50 to 150 mg/day.
　　≥ 10 years of age: Initial dose is 150 to 300 mg/day.

Maintenance: Determined by patient response.

Another suggested dosage for children is as follows:

Initial: 5 to 7 mg/kg/day or 150 to 200 mg/m^2/day in divided doses q8h.

Maintenance: $\frac{1}{3}$ to $\frac{2}{3}$ the intial dose beginning when the patient is euthyroid.

Actions

Pharmacology: Propylthiouracil (PTU) and methimazole inhibit the synthesis of thyroid hormones and, thus, are effective in the treatment of hyperthyroidism. They do not inactivate existing thyroxine (T$_4$) and triiodothyronine (T$_3$) nor do they interfere with the effectiveness of exogenous thyroid hormones. PTU partially inhibits the peripheral conversion of T$_4$ to T$_3$.

Pharmacokinetics:

Various Pharmacokinetic Parameters of Antithyroid Agents						
Antithyroid agent	Bioavailability (%)	Protein binding (%)	Transplacental passage	Breast milk levels (M:P)[1]	Half-life(hrs)	Excreted in urine (%)
Methimazole	80-95	0	High	High (1)	6-13	< 10
Propylthiouracil	80-95	75-80	Low	Low (0.1)	1-2	< 35

[1] Approximate milk:plasma ratio.

Contraindications

Hypersensitivity to antithyroid drugs; lactation.

Warnings

Agranulocytosis: Agranulocytosis is potentially the most serious side effect of therapy. Leukopenia, thrombocytopenia and aplastic anemia (pancytopenia) may also occur.

Pregnancy: Category D. These agents, used judiciously, are effective drugs in hyperthyroidism complicated by pregnancy. Because they readily cross the placenta and can induce goiter and even cretinism in the developing fetus, it is important that a sufficient, but not excessive, dose be given. If an antithyroid agent is needed, PTU is preferred because it is less likely than methimazole to cross the placenta and induce fetal/neonatal complications.

Lactation: Postpartum patients receiving antithyroid preparations should not nurse their babies. However, if necessary, the preferred drug is PTU.

Children: In several case reports, PTU hepatotoxicity has occurred in pediatric patients.

Precautions

Monitoring: Monitor thyroid function tests periodically during therapy.

Hemorrhagic effects: Because PTU may cause hypoprothrombinemia and bleeding, monitor prothrombin time during therapy, especially before surgical procedures.

Drug Interactions

Drugs that may interact with antithyroid agents include anticoagulants.

Adverse Reactions

Agranulocytosis is the most serious effect.

BISPHOSPHONATES

ALENDRONATE SODIUM		
Tablets: 5, 10, 35, 40, and 70 mg (*Rx*)	*Fosamax* (Merck)	
ETIDRONATE DISODIUM (ORAL)		
Tablets: 200 and 400 mg (*Rx*)	*Didronel* (Procter & Gamble)	
ETIDRONATE DISODIUM (PARENTERAL)		
Injection: 300 mg/amp (*Rx*)	*Didronel IV* (MGI Pharma)	
PAMIDRONATE DISODIUM		
Powder for injection, lyophilized: 30 and 90 mg (*Rx*)	*Aredia* (Novartis)	
RISEDRONATE SODIUM		
Tablets: 5 and 30 mg (*Rx*)	*Actonel* (Procter & Gamble)	
TILUDRONATE SODIUM		
Tablets: 240 mg (equiv. to 200 mg tiludronic acid) (*Rx*)	*Skelid* (Sanofi-Synthelabo)	
ZOLEDRONIC ACID		
Powder for injection: 4 mg zoledronic acid anhydrous (*Rx*)	*Zometa* (Novartis)	

Indications

Osteoporosis (alendronate, risedronate):

In postmenopausal women – For the treatment and prevention of osteoporosis in post-menopausal women.

Glucocorticoid-induced – Treatment (alendronate and risedronate) and prevention (risedronate) of glucocorticoid-induced osteoporosis in men and women receiving glucocorticoids in a daily dosage ≥ 7.5 mg of prednisone and who have low bone mineral density.

In men – To increase bone mass in men with osteoporosis (alendronate).

Paget's disease of bone: For treatment of patients with Paget's disease of bone having alkaline phosphatase at least two times the upper limit of normal, or those who are symptomatic or at risk for future complications from their disease (**alendronate, risedronate, tiludronate**); treatment of symptomatic Paget's disease (oral **etidronate**); treatment of moderate to severe Paget's disease (**pamidronate**).

Heterotopic ossification (oral etidronate): Prevention and treatment of heterotopic ossification following total hip replacement or caused by spinal injury.

Hypercalcemia of malignancy: In conjunction with adequate hydration for the treatment of moderate or severe hypercalcemia associated with malignancy, with or without bone metastases (**pamidronate**); when inadequately managed by dietary modification or oral hydration, concurrent therapy is recommended as soon as there is a restoration of urine output (parenteral **etidronate**); for hypercalcemia of malignancy which persists after adequate hydration has been restored (parenteral **etidronate, zoledronic acid**).

Breast cancer/Multiple myeloma (pamidronate): In conjunction with standard antineoplastic therapy for the treatment of osteolytic bone metastases of breast cancer and osteolytic lesions of multiple myeloma.

Unlabeled uses:

Etidronate – For the treatment of postmenopausal osteoporosis and prevention of bone loss in early postmenopausal women (intermittent cyclical therapy of 400 mg/day for 14 days followed by 76 days of elemental calcium, 500 mg/day); glucocorticoid-induced bone loss in postmenopausal women (400 mg/day × 1 month, then 400 mg/day for 2 weeks every third month plus calcium and ergocalciterol).

Risedronate – Prevention of bone loss in postmenopausal women (5 mg/day cyclically for 2 years on then 1 year off therapy).

Administration and Dosage

ALENDRONATE: Alendronate must be taken ≥ 30 minutes before the first food, beverage, or medication of the day with plain water only. Other beverages (including mineral water), food, and some medications are likely to reduce the absorption of alendronate. Waiting < 30 minutes or taking the drug with food, beverages (other than plain water), or other medications will lessen the effect of the drug by decreasing its absorption. To facilitate delivery to the stomach, and thus reduce the potential for esophageal irritation, swallow alendronate only upon arising for the day. Take with a full glass of water (6 to 8 ounces; 180 to 240 mL) and avoid lying down for ≥ 30 minutes and until after the first food of the day. Do not take alendronate at bedtime or before arising for the day. Failure to follow these instructions may increase the risk of esophageal adverse reactions (see Patient Information).

Patients with osteoporosis or Paget's disease should receive supplemental calcium and vitamin D if dietary intake is inadequate.

Osteoporosis in postmenopausal women –

Treatment: 70 mg once weekly or 10 mg once daily.

Prevention: 35 mg once weekly or 5 mg once daily.

The safety of treatment and prevention of osteoporosis with alendronate has been studied for ≤ 7 years.

Osteoporosis in men – 10 mg once daily.

Glucocorticoid-induced osteoporosis – 5 mg once daily. For postmenopausal women not receiving estrogen, the recommended dose is 10 mg once daily.

Patients also should receive adequate amounts of calcium and vitamin D.

Paget's disease of bone – 40 mg once a day for 6 months.

Retreatment: Relapses during the 12 months following therapy occurred in 9% of patients who responded to treatment. Retreatment with alendronate may be considered, following a 6-month post-treatment evaluation period, in patients who have relapsed based on increases in serum alkaline phosphatase.

ETIDRONATE DISODIUM (ORAL): Administer as a single dose. However, if GI discomfort occurs, divide the dose.

Paget's disease –

Initial treatment: 5 to 10 mg/kg/day (not to exceed 6 months) or 11 to 20 mg/kg/day (not to exceed 3 months). Reserve doses > 10 mg/kg/day for use when lower doses are ineffective, when there is an overriding requirement for suppression of increased bone turnover or when prompt reduction of elevated cardiac output is required. Doses > 20 mg/kg/day are not recommended.

Retreatment: Initiate only after an etidronate-free period of at least 90 days and if there is biochemical, symptomatic, or other evidence of active disease process. Retreatment regimens are the same as for initial treatment.

Heterotopic ossification –

Caused by spinal cord injury: 20 mg/kg/day for 2 weeks, followed by 10 mg/kg/day for 10 weeks; total treatment period is 12 weeks. Institute as soon as feasible following the injury, preferably prior to evidence of heterotopic ossification.

Complicating total hip replacement: 20 mg/kg/day for 1 month preoperatively, then 20 mg/kg/day for 3 months postoperatively; total treatment period is 4 months.

ETIDRONATE DISODIUM (PARENTERAL):

Recommended dose – Recommended dose is 7.5 mg/kg/day for 3 successive days.

Infusion time – Administer the diluted dose IV over a period of at least 2 hours. Slow infusion is important. The usual course of treatment is 1 infusion of 7.5 mg/kg/day on each of 3 consecutive days, but some patients have been treated for ≤ 7 days.

Retreatment – Retreatment may be appropriate if hypercalcemia recurs. There should be at least a 7-day interval between courses of treatment. With renal impairment, dose reduction may be advisable.

Oral etidronate – Oral etidronate may be started on the day after the last infusion. The recommended oral dose for patients who have had hypercalcemia is 20 mg/kg/day for 30 days. If serum calcium levels remain normal or clinically acceptable, treatment may be extended. Use for > 90 days is not adequately studied and is not recommended.

PAMIDRONATE DISODIUM:

Hypercalcemia of malignancy – Give consideration to the severity and the symptoms of hypercalcemia. Vigorous saline hydration alone may be sufficient for treating mild, asymptomatic hypercalcemia. Avoid overhydration in patients who have potential for cardiac failure. In hypercalcemia associated with hematologic malignancies, the use of glucocorticoid therapy may be helpful.

Moderate hypercalcemia: The recommended dose in moderate hypercalcemia (corrected serum calcium of ≈ 12 to 23.5 mg/dL) is 60 to 90 mg given as a *single-dose* IV infusion over ≥ 2 to 24 hours. Longer infusions (eg, > 2 hours) may reduce the risk for renal toxicity, particularly in patients with pre-existing renal insufficiency.

Severe hypercalcemia: Recommended dose (corrected serum calcium > 13.5 mg/dL) is 90 mg, which must be given by initial *single-dose*, IV infusion over 2 to 24 hrs. Longer infusions (eg, > 2 hours) may reduce the risk for renal toxicity, particularly in patients with pre-existing renal insufficiency.

Retreatment: Retreatment in patients who show complete or partial response initially may be carried out if serum calcium does not return to normal or remain normal after initial treatment. Allow a minimum of 7 days to elapse before retreatment to allow for full response to the initial dose. The dose and manner of retreatment are identical to that of the initial therapy.

Paget's disease – The recommended dose in patients with moderate to severe Paget's disease of bone is 30 mg daily, given as a 4 hour infusion on 3 consecutive days for a total dose of 90 mg.

Retreatment: When clinically indicated, retreat at the dose of initial therapy.

Osteolytic bone metastases of breast cancer – 90 mg administered over a 2-hour infusion every 3 to 4 weeks.

Osteolytic bone lesions of multiple myeloma – The recommended dose is 90 mg given as a 4-hour infusion on a monthly basis. Patients with marked Bence-Jones proteinuria and dehydration should receive adequate hydration prior to pamidronate infusion.

Preparation of solution – Reconstitute by adding 10 mL Sterile Water for Injection to each vial, resulting in a solution of 30 or 90 mg/10 mL. Allow drug to dissolve completely before withdrawing.

Hypercalcemia of malignancy: Administer the single dose as an IV infusion over ≥ 2 to 24 hours for the 60 and 90 mg doses. Dilute in 1 L Sterile 0.45% or 0.9% NaCl, or 5% Dextrose Injection. This infusion solution is stable for ≤ 24 hours at room temperature.

Paget's disease: Dilute the recommended daily dose of 30 mg in 500 mL Sterile 0.45% or 0.9% NaCl, or 5% Dextrose Injection and give over a 4-hour period for 3 consecutive days.

Osteolytic bone lesions of multiple myeloma: Dilute the recommended dose of 90 mg in 500 mL of Sterile 0.45% or 0.9% of NaCl, or 5% Dextrose Injection and give over 4 hours on a monthly basis.

Osteolytic bone metastases of breast cancer: Dilute the recommended dose of 90 mg in 250 mL of sterile 0.45% or 0.9% NaCl, or 5% Dextrose Injection and give over a 2-hour period every 3 to 4 weeks.

Admixture incompatibility – Do not mix with calcium-containing infusion solutions, such as Ringer's solution. Give in a single IV solution and line separate from all other drugs.

RISEDRONATE: Take once daily ≥ 30 minutes before the first food or drink of the day other than water.

Take while in an upright position with a full glass (6 to 8 ounces; 180 to 240 mL) of plain water and avoid lying down for 30 minutes to minimize the possibility of GI side effects.

Patients should receive supplemental calcium and vitamin D if dietary intake is inadequate. Take calcium supplements and calcium-, aluminum-, and magnesium-containing agents at a different time of the day to prevent interference with risedronate absorption.

Paget's disease – 30 mg once daily for 2 months. Retreatment may be considered (following post-treatment observation of ≥ 2 months) if relapse occurs or if treatment fails to normalize serum alkaline phosphatase. For retreatment, the dose and duration of therapy are the same as for initial treatment. No data are available on > 1 course of retreatment.

Treatment/Prevention of postmenopausal osteoporosis/glucocorticoid-induced osteoporosis – 5 mg orally daily.

Renal function impairment – Risedronate is not recommended for use in patients with severe renal impairment (Ccr < 30 mL/min). No dosage adjustment is necessary in patients with a Ccr ≥ 30 mL/min.

TILUDRONATE: Administer a single 400 mg/day oral dose, taken with 6 to 8 ounces of plain water only for a period of 3 months. Beverages other than plain water (including mineral water), food, and some medications are likely to reduce the absorption of tiludronate. Do not take within 2 hours of food. Take calcium or mineral supplements ≥ 2 hours before or after tiludronate. Take aluminum- or magnesium-containing antacids ≥ 2 hours after taking tiludronate. Do not take ≤ 2 hours of indomethacin.

Retreatment – Following therapy, allow an interval of 3 months to assess response.

ZOLEDRONIC ACID: Consider the severity of, as well as the symptoms of, tumor-induced hypercalcemia when considering use of zoledronic acid for injection. Vigorous saline hydration alone may be sufficient to treat mild, asymptomatic hypercalcemia.

Hydration – Initiate vigorous saline hydration, an integral part of hypercalcemia therapy, promptly and attempt to restore the urine output to ≈ 2 L/day throughout treatment. Mild or asymptomatic hypercalcemia may be treated with conservative measures (ie, saline hydration, with or without loop diuretics). Adequately hydrate patients throughout the treatment, but avoid overhydration, especially in those patients who have cardiac failure. Do not employ diuretic therapy prior to correction of hypovolemia.

Dose – The maximum recommended dose in hypercalcemia of malignancy (albumin-corrected serum calcium Albumin-corrected serum calcium (Cca, mg/dL) = Ca + 0.8 (mid-range albumin-measured albumin in mg/dL) ≥ 12 mg/dL [3 mmol/L]) is 4 mg. The 4 mg dose must be given as a single dose IV infusion over ≥ 15 minutes. Adequately rehydrate patients prior to administration of zoledronic acid.

Retreatment – Retreatment with 4 mg zoledronic acid may be considered if serum calcium does not return to normal or remain normal after initial treatment. It is recommended that a minimum of 7 days elapse before retreatment, to allow for a full response to the initial dose. Carefully monitor renal function in all patients receiving zoledronic acid and assess possible deterioration in renal function prior to retreatment with zoledronic acid.

Renal function deterioration – Because of the risk of clinically significant deterioration in renal function, which may progress to renal failure, single doses of zoledronic acid should not exceed 4 mg and the duration of infusion should be ≥ 15 minutes.

Actions

Pharmacology: Bisphosphonates act primarily on bone. Their major pharmacologic action is the inhibition of normal and abnormal bone resorption.

Pharmacokinetics:

Alendronate – There is no evidence that the bisphosphonates are metabolized. Mean steady-state volume of distribution (exclusive of bone) is ≥ 28 L. Protein binding in plasma is ≈ 78%.

Etidronate – Most absorbed drug is cleared from blood in 6 hours. Within 24 hours, about half the absorbed dose is excreted in urine. The remainder is chemically adsorbed to bone and is slowly eliminated. Unabsorbed drug is excreted intact in feces.

Pamidronate – A mean of 51% (32% to 80%) was excreted unchanged in urine within 72 hours. Urinary excretion rate profile after 60 mg over 4 hours exhibited biphasic disposition characteristics with an alpha half-life of 1.6 hours and a beta half-life of 27.2 hours.

Tiludronate – After administration of a single dose equivalent to 400 mg tiludronic acid to healthy male subjects, tiludronic acid was rapidly absorbed with peak plasma concentrations of ≈ 3 mg/L occurring within 2 hours.

Risedronate – Mean oral bioavailability is 0.63% and is decreased when administered with food.

Animal studies indicate that ≈ 60% of the dose is distributed to bone with the remainder excreted in the urine. The mean steady-state volume of distribution is 6.3 L/kg; plasma protein binding is ≈ 24%.

Contraindications

Hypersensitivity to bisphosphonates or any component of the products; hypocalcemia (**alendronate** and **risedronate**); Class Dc and higher renal impairment (serum creatinine > 5 mg/dL; **etidronate** only).

Warnings

Osteoporosis (alendronate): Consider causes other than estrogen deficiency and aging.

Paget's disease (etidronate): Response may be slow and may continue for months after treatment discontinuation. Do not increase dosage prematurely or resume treatment before there is evidence of reactivation of disease process.

Renal function impairment: It is likely that **alendronate** elimination via the kidney will be reduced in impaired renal function. Therefore, somewhat greater accumulation of alendronate in bone might be expected in impaired renal function. No dosage adjustment is necessary in mild to moderate renal insufficiency; alendronate use is not recommended in more severe renal insufficiency. Occasional mild-to-moderate renal function abnormalities (elevated BUN or serum creatinine) have occurred when **etidronate** was given to patients with hypercalcemia of malignancy. Reduction of the etidronate dose, if used at all, may be advisable in Class Cc renal functional impairment. In patients with Class Dc and higher renal functional impairment, withhold etidronate. Patients with hypercalcemia who receive an IV infusion of **pamidronate** should have periodic lab and clinical evaluations of renal function. **Tiludronate** and **risedronate** are not recommended for patients with severe renal failure (creatinine clearance < 30 mL/min). The plasma elimination half-life is longer with tiludronate. There must be strict adherence to the IV administration recommendations for **zoledronic acid** in order to decrease the risk of deterioration in renal function.

Pregnancy: Category B (oral etidronate); Category C (alendronate, parenteral etidronate, pamidronate, risedronate, and tiludronate).

Lactation: It is not known whether these drugs are excreted in breast milk. Do not give alendronate to a nursing mother.

Children: Safety and efficacy for use in children have not been established. Children have been treated with **etidronate** at doses recommended for adults, to prevent heterotopic ossifications or soft tissue calcifications.

Precautions

Monitoring: Carefully monitor standard hypercalcemia-related metabolic parameters, such as serum levels of calcium, phosphate, magnesium, and potassium following pamidronate initiation. Asymptomatic hypophosphatemia (16%), hypokalemia (7% to 9%), hypomagnesemia (11% to 12%), and hypocalcemia (5% to 12%) have occurred. Also, closely monitor electrolytes, creatinine as well as CBC, differential and hematocrit/hemoglobin. Carefully monitor patients who have preexisting anemia, leukopenia or thrombocytopenia in the first 2 weeks following treatment.

Nutrition: Patients should maintain adequate nutrition, particularly an adequate intake of calcium and vitamin D.

GI disorders: Use caution when using bisphosphonates in patients with active upper GI problems. **Etidronate** therapy has been withheld from patients with enterocolitis because diarrhea is seen in some patients, particularly at higher doses.

Osteoid: **Etidronate** suppresses bone turnover and may retard mineralization of osteoid laid down during the bone accretion process.

Fracture: In Paget's patients, treatment regimens of **etidronate** exceeding the recommended daily maximum dose of 20 mg/kg or continuous administration for periods > 6 months may be associated with an increased risk of fracture.

Hormone replacement therapy: Concomitant use with **alendronate** for osteoporosis in postmenopausal women is not recommended.

Hypocalcemia: Hypocalcemia has occurred with **etidronate** and **pamidronate**.

Hypocalcemia must be corrected before therapy initiation with **alendronate** and **risedronate**.

Drug Interactions

Drugs that may interact with **alendronate** include ranitidine and aspirin. Drugs that may interact with **tiludronate** include aspirin and indomethacin. Calcium supplements and antacids may interact with **alendronate**, **etidronate**, **risedronate**, or **tiludronate**. The patient should wait ≥ 30 minutes after taking alendronate before taking any other drug.

Drug/Food interactions: Absorption of **etidronate**, complete in 2 hours, may be reduced by foods or other preparations containing divalent cations. The bioavailability of **tiludronate** is reduced by food. Do not take within 2 hours of food. Mean oral bioavailability of **risedronate** is decreased when given with food. Take ≥ 30 minutes before the first food or drink of the day other than water.

Adverse Reactions

Adverse reactions occurring in ≥ 3% of patients include the following:

Alendronate: Abdominal pain, diarrhea, constipation, dyspepsia, nausea, back pain, accidental injury, influenza-like symptoms, and pain.

Etidronate: Convulsions, constipation, nausea, stomatitis, abnormal hepatic function, hypomagnesemia, hypophosphatemia, dyspnea, taste perversion, fever, fluid overload.

Pamidronate:

In patients receiving 90 mg over 24 hours: Atrial fibrillation, hypertension, syncope, somnolence, anorexia, constipation, GI hemorrhage, nausea, leukopenia, hypocalcemia, hypokalemia, hypomagnesemia, hypophosphatemia, rales/rhinitis, fatigue, fever, infusion site reaction, moniliasis, hypothyroidism.

In patients receiving 60 mg over 4 hours: Psychosis, anorexia, constipation, dyspepsia, nausea, vomiting, leukopenia, hypokalemia, hypomagnesemia, fever, uremia.

In patients receiving 60 mg over 24 hours: Hypokalemia, hypomagnesemia, hypophosphatemia, URI, fever, infusion site reaction.

Risedronate: Chest pain, dizziness, headache, abdominal pain, belching, colitis, constipation, dyspepsia, nausea, arthralgia, bone pain, leg cramps, myasthenia, bronchitis, sinusitis, amblyopia, dry eye, tinnitus, asthenia, edema/peripheral edema, influenza-like symptoms, rash, urticaria.

Tiludronate: Dizziness, headache, paresthesia, diarrhea, dyspepsia, nausea, vomiting, rales/rhinitis, sinusitis, URI.

ANTIDOTES

Drug	Trade Name (Distributor)	Toxic/Overdosed Substance
Dimercaprol (BAL)	BAL In Oil (H, W & D)	Arsenic, gold, mercury, lead
Deferoxamine Mesylate	Desferal Mesylate (Ciba)	Iron
Edetate Calcium Disodium	Calcium Disodium Versenate (Riker)	Lead
Sodium Thiosulfate		Arsenic, cyanide
Succimer	Chemet (Bock)	Lead
Narcotic Antagonists		Opioids
Naloxone	Narcan (DuPont)	
Physostigmine Salicylate	Antilirium (Forest Pharm.)	Anticholinergics (including tricyclic antidepressants) Diazepam, Morphine (CNS depression)
Fomepizole	Antizol (Orphan Medical)	Ethylene glycol or methanol
Pralidoxime Cl	Protopam (Ayerst)	Organophosphates; Anticholinesterases
Digoxin Immune Fab	Digibind (GlaxoSmithKline)	Digoxin
Methylene Blue	(Various)	Cyanide
Other agents used additionally as antidotes		
Leucovorin Calcium	Leucovorin Calcium (Lederle)	Folic acid antagonists (eg, methotrexate)
Hydroxocobalamin	(Various)	Cyanide poisoning from nitroprusside
Vitamin K	(Various)	Oral anticoagulants
Protamine Sulfate	(Various)	Heparin
Glucagon	(Lilly)	Insulin-induced hypoglycemia
Edetate Disodium	(Various)	Hypercalcemia Digitalis toxicity
Acetylcysteine	Mucomyst (Bristol-Myers) Mucosol (Dey Labs)	Acetaminophen
Atropine	(Various)	Cholinergic agents: Organophosphates, carbamates, pilocarpine, physostigmine or isofluorophate
Amyl nitrite, Na Nitrite, Na Thiosulfate	Cyanide antidote kit (Lilly)	Cyanide
Anticholinesterases		Anticholinergics, Nondepolarizing muscle relaxants
Pyridostigmine Br	Mestinon (Roche) Regonol (Organon)	
Neostigmine	Prostigmin (Roche)	
Edrophonium Cl	Tensilon (Roche)	

Drug	Trade Name (Distributor)	Toxic/Overdosed Substance
Nonspecific therapy of overdoses include:		
Osmotic diuretics		Nonspecific, supportive thera-pies of overdoses. See also General Management Guidelines.
Cathartics		
Peritoneal Dialysis Solutions		
Emetics		
Apomorphine Syrup of Ipecac	(Lilly) (Various)	
Activated Charcoal	(Various)	
Urinary Alkalinizers		
Urinary Acidifiers		

NALMEFENE HCl

Injection: 1 mg/mL (*Rx*)   *Revex* (Ohmeda)

Indications

Reversal of opioid effects: Complete or partial reversal of opioid drug effects, including respiratory depression, induced by either natural or synthetic opioids.

Opioid overdose: Management of known or suspected opioid overdose.

Administration and Dosage

Administration: Titrate nalmefene to reverse the undesired effects of opioids. Once adequate reversal has been established, additional administration is not required and actually may be harmful due to unwanted reversal of analgesia or precipitated withdrawal.

Duration of action: The duration of action of nalmefene is as long as most opioid analgesics. However, the apparent duration of action will vary depending on the half-life and plasma concentration of the narcotic being reversed, the presence or absence of other drugs affecting the brain or muscles of respiration and the dose of nalmefene administered. Partially reversing doses of nalmefene (1 mcg/kg) lose their effect as the drug is redistributed through the body, and the effects of these low doses may not last more than 30 to 60 minutes in the presence of persistent opioid effects. Fully reversing doses (1 mg/70 kg) last many hours, but may complicate the management of patients who are in pain, at high cardiovascular risk or who are physically dependent on opioids.

The recommended doses represent a compromise between a desirable controlled reversal and the need for prompt response and adequate duration of action. Using higher dosages or shorter intervals between incremental doses may increase the incidence and severity of symptoms related to acute withdrawal such as nausea, vomiting, elevated blood pressure, and anxiety.

Patients tolerant to or physically dependent on opioids: Nalmefene may cause acute withdrawal symptoms in individuals who have some degree of tolerance to and dependence on opioids. Closely observe these patients for symptoms of withdrawal. Administer subsequent doses with intervals of at least 2 to 5 minutes between doses to allow the full effect of each incremental dose of nalmefene to be reached.

Reversal of postoperative opioid depression: Use 100 mcg/mL dosage strength (blue label); refer to the following table for initial doses. The goal of treatment with nalmefene in the postoperative setting is to achieve reversal of excessive opioid effects without inducing a complete reversal and acute pain. This is best accomplished with an initial dose of 0.25 mcg/kg followed by 0.25 mcg/kg incremental doses at 2- to 5-minute intervals, stopping as soon as the desired degree of opioid reversal is obtained. A cumulative total dose > 1 mcg/kg does not provide additional therapeutic effect.

Nalmefene Dosage for Reversal of Postoperative Opioid Depression	
Body weight (kg)	Amount of nalmefene 100 mcg/mL solution (mL)
50	0.125
60	0.15
70	0.175
80	0.2
90	0.225
100	0.25

Cardiovascular risk patients: In cases where the patient is known to be at increased cardiovascular risk, it may be desirable to dilute nalmefene 1:1 with saline or sterile water and use smaller initial and incremental doses of 0.1 mcg/kg.

Management of known/suspected opioid overdose: Use 1 mg/mL dosage strength (green label). The recommended initial dose of nalmefene for nonopioid dependent patients is 0.5 mg/70 kg. If needed, this may be followed by a second dose of 1 mg/70 kg, 2 to 5 minutes later. If a total dose of 1.5 mg/70 kg has been administered without clinical response, additional nalmefene is unlikely to have an effect.

If there is a reasonable suspicion of opioid dependency, initially administer a challenge dose of 0.1 mg/70 kg. If there is no evidence of withdrawal in 2 minutes, follow the recommended dosing.

Repeated dosing: Nalmefene is the longest acting of the currently available parenteral opioid antagonists. If recurrence of respiratory depression does occur, titrate the dose again to clinical effect using incremental doses to avoid overreversal.

Hepatic and renal disease: Hepatic disease and renal failure substantially reduce the clearance of nalmefene. For single episodes of opioid antagonism, adjustment of nalmefene dosage is not required. However, in patients with renal failure, slowly administer the incremental doses (over 60 seconds).

Loss of IV access: Should IV access be lost or not readily obtainable, a single dose of nalmefene should be effective within 5 to 15 minutes after 1 mg IM or SC doses.

Actions

Pharmacology: Nalmefene, an opioid antagonist, is a 6-methylene analog of naltrexone. Nalmefene prevents or reverses the effects of opioids, including respiratory depression, sedation, and hypotension. Nalmefene has no opioid agonist activity; it does not produce respiratory depression, psychotomimetic effects or pupillary constriction, and no pharmacological activity was observed when it was administered in the absence of opioid agonists. Nalmefene can produce acute withdrawal symptoms in individuals who are opioid-dependent.

Pharmacokinetics:

  Absorption – Nalmefene is completely bioavailable following IM or SC administration. Nalmefene will be administered primarily as an IV bolus; however, it can be given IM or SC if venous access cannot be established. While the time to maximum plasma concentration was 2.3 hours following IM and 1.5 hours following SC administrations, therapeutic plasma concentrations are likely to be reached within 5 to 15 minutes after a 1 mg dose in an emergency.

  Distribution – Following a 1 mg parenteral dose, nalmefene was rapidly distributed. A 1 mg dose blocked > 80% of brain opioid receptors within 5 minutes after administration. The apparent volumes of distribution centrally and at steady state are 3.9 and 8.6 L/kg, respectively. Over a concentration range of 0.1 to 2 mcg/mL, 45% is bound to plasma proteins.

  Metabolism – Nalmefene is metabolized by the liver, primarily by glucuronide conjugation, and excreted in the urine; < 5% is excreted in the urine unchanged, and 17% is excreted in the feces.

  Excretion – After IV administration of 1 mg to healthy males, plasma concentrations declined biexponentially with a redistribution and a terminal elimination half-life of 41 ± 34 minutes and 10.8 ± 5.2 hours, respectively. The systemic clearance of nalmefene is 0.8 L/hr/kg and the renal clearance is 0.08 L/hr/kg.

Contraindications

Hypersensitivity to the product.

Warnings

Emergency use: Nalmefene is not the primary treatment for ventilatory failure. In most emergency settings, treatment with nalmefene should follow, not precede, the establishment of a patent airway, ventilatory assistance, administration of oxygen, and establishment of circulatory access.

Respiratory depression: Accidental overdose with long-acting opioids (eg, methadone, levomethadyl) may result in prolonged respiratory depression. Observe patients until there is no reasonable risk of recurrent respiratory depression. While nalmefene has a longer duration of action than naloxone in fully reversing doses, be aware that a recurrence of respiratory depression is possible.

Renal function impairment: There was a statistically significant 27% decrease in plasma clearance of nalmefene in the end-stage renal disease (ESRD) population during interdialysis (0.57 L/hr/kg) and a 25% decreased plasma clearance in the ESRD population during intradialysis (0.59 L/hr/kg) compared with controls (0.79 L/hr/kg). The elimination half-life was prolonged in ESRD patients from 10.2 (controls) to 26.1 hr.

Hepatic function impairment: Subjects with hepatic disease had a 28.3% decrease in plasma clearance of nalmefene compared with controls (0.56 vs 0.78 L/hr/kg, respectively). Elimination half-life increased from 10.2 to 11.9 hours in the hepatically impaired. No dosage adjustment is recommended because nalmefene will be administered as an acute course of therapy.

Elderly: Dose proportionality was observed in nalmefene AUC following 0.5 to 2 mg IV administration to elderly male subjects. There was an apparent age-related decrease in the central volume of distribution that resulted in a greater initial nalmefene concentration in the elderly group. While initial plasma concentrations were transiently higher in the elderly, it would not be anticipated that this population would require dosing adjustment.

Pregnancy: Category B.

Lactation: Exercise caution when nalmefene is administered to a nursing woman.

Children: Safety and efficacy have not been established. Only use nalmefene in the resuscitation of the newborn when the expected benefits outweigh the risks.

Precautions

Cardiovascular risks: Although nalmefene has been used safely in patients with preexisting cardiac disease, use all drugs of this class with caution in patients at high cardiovascular risk or who have received potentially cardiotoxic drugs.

Risk of precipitated withdrawal: Nalmefene is known to produce acute withdrawal symptoms and, therefore, should be used with extreme caution in patients with known physical dependence on opioids or following surgery involving high uses of opioids.

Incomplete reversal of buprenorphine: In animals, nalmefene doses up to 10 mg/kg (437 times the maximum recommended human dose) produced incomplete reversal of buprenorphine-induced analgesia. Hence, nalmefene may not completely reverse buprenorphine-induced respiratory depression.

Drug Interactions

Flumazenil: Flumazenil and nalmefene can induce seizures in animals. Remain aware of the potential risk of seizures from agents in these classes.

Adverse Reactions

Adverse reactions occurring in ≥ 3% of patients include nausea; vomiting; tachycardia; hypertension; postoperative pain; fever; dizziness.

NALOXONE HCl

Injection: 0.4 and 1 mg/mL (*Rx*)
Neonatal Injection: 0.02 mg/mL (*Rx*)

Various, *Narcan* (DuPont Pharm)

Indications

For the complete or partial reversal of narcotic depression, including respiratory depression, induced by opioids including natural and synthetic narcotics, propoxyphene, methadone, nalbuphine, butorphanol, and pentazocine. Also indicated for the diagnosis of suspected acute opioid overdosage.

Administration and Dosage

Give IV, IM, or SC. The most rapid onset of action is achieved with IV use, which is recommended in emergency situations.

Adults:
   Narcotic overdose (known or suspected) – Initial dose is 0.4 to 2 mg IV; may repeat IV at 2- to 3-minute intervals. If no response is observed after 10 mg has been administered, question the diagnosis of narcotic-induced or partial narcotic-induced toxicity.

   Postoperative narcotic depression (partial reversal) – Smaller doses are usually sufficient. Titrate dose according to the patient's response.

      Initial dose: Inject in increments of 0.1 to 0.2 mg IV at 2- to 3-minute intervals to the desired degree of reversal.

      Repeat doses: Repeat doses may be required within 1- or 2-hour intervals depending on the amount, type (ie, short- or long-acting) and time interval since last administration of narcotic. Supplemental IM doses have produced a longer lasting effect.

Children:
   Narcotic overdose (known or suspected) – Initial dose is 0.01 mg/kg IV; give a subsequent dose of 0.1 mg/kg if needed. If an IV route is not available, may be given IM or SC in divided doses.

   Postoperative narcotic depression – Follow the recommendations and cautions under adult administration guidelines. For initial reversal of respiratory depression, inject in increments of 0.005 to 0.01 mg IV at 2- to 3-minute intervals to desired degree of reversal.

Neonates:
   Narcotic-induced depression – Initial dose is 0.01 mg/kg IV, IM, or SC; may be repeated in accordance with adult administration guidelines.

Actions

Pharmacology: The mechanism of action is not fully understood; evidence suggests that it antagonizes the opioid effects by competing for the same receptor sites.

Pharmacokinetics:
   Distribution – After parenteral use, naloxone is rapidly distributed in the body. It is metabolized in the liver, primarily by glucuronide conjugation.

   Excretion – Naloxone is excreted in the urine. The serum half-life in adults ranged from 30 to 81 minutes; in neonates, 3.1 ± 0.5 hours.

   Onset, peak, and duration – Onset of action of IV naloxone is generally apparent within 2 minutes; it is only slightly less rapid when given SC or IM. Duration of action of 1 to 4 hours depends upon dose and route. IM use produces a more prolonged effect than IV use.

Contraindications

Hypersensitivity to these agents.

Warnings

Drug dependence: Administer cautiously to people who are known or suspected to be physically dependent on opioids, including newborns of mothers with narcotic dependence. Reversal of narcotic effect will precipitate acute abstinence syndrome.

Repeat administration: The patient who has satisfactorily responded should be kept under continued surveillance. Administer repeated doses as necessary, because the duration of action of some narcotics may exceed that of the narcotic antagonist.

Respiratory depression: Not effective against respiratory depression due to nonopioid drugs.

Pregnancy: Category B.

Lactation: It is not known whether the drug is excreted in breast milk.

Precautions

Other supportive therapy: Maintain a free airway and provide artificial ventilation, cardiac massage, and vasopressor agents; employ when necessary to counteract acute narcotic overdosage.

Cardiovascular effects: Several instances of hypotension, hypertension, pulmonary edema, and ventricular tachycardia and fibrillation have been reported in postoperative patients.

Adverse Reactions

Abrupt reversal of narcotic depression may result in nausea, vomiting, sweating, tachycardia, increased blood pressure, and tremulousness.

In postoperative patients, excessive dosage may result in excitement and significant reversal of analgesia, hypotension, hypertension, pulmonary edema, and ventricular tachycardia and fibrillation.

NALTREXONE HCl

Tablets: 50 mg (*Rx*)   *ReVia* (DuPont)

Indications

Narcotic addiction: Blockade of the effects of exogenously administered opioids.

Alcoholism: Treatment of alcohol dependence.

Administration and Dosage

If there is any question of occult opioid dependence, perform a naloxone challenge test. Do not attempt treatment until naloxone challenge is negative.

Alcoholism: A dose of 50 mg once daily is recommended for most patients. An initial 25 mg dose, splitting the daily dose and adjusting the time of dosing have met with limited success.

Narcotic dependence: Initiate treatment using the following guidelines:

1.) Do not attempt treatment until the patient has remained opioid-free for 7 to 10 days.

2.) Administer a naloxone challenge test (see below). If signs of opioid withdrawal are still observed following challenge, do not treat with naltrexone. The naloxone challenge can be repeated in 24 hours.

3.) Initiate treatment carefully, slowly increasing the dose. Administer 25 mg initially; observe patient for 1 hour. If no withdrawal signs occur, give the rest of the daily dose.

Maintenance treatment: Once the patient has been started on naltrexone, 50 mg every 24 hours will produce adequate clinical blockade of the actions of parenterally administered opioids. A flexible dosing regimen may be employed. Thus, patients may receive 50 mg every weekday with a 100 mg dose on Saturday, 100 mg every other day, or 150 mg every third day. Several studies have employed the following dosing regimen with success: 100 mg Monday, 100 mg Wednesday, and 150 mg Friday.

Actions

Pharmacology: Naltrexone blocks the effects of opioids by competitive binding at opioid receptors. This makes the blockade potentially surmountable.

Pharmacokinetics:

Absorption – Although well absorbed orally, naltrexone is subject to significant first-pass metabolism with oral bioavailability estimates ranging from 5% to 40%. Following oral administration, naltrexone undergoes rapid and nearly complete absorption with ≈ 96% of the dose absorbed from the GI tract. Peak plasma levels of naltrexone and 6-β-naltrexol occur ≤ 1 hour of dosing.

Distribution – The volume of distribution for naltrexone after IV administration is estimated to be 1350 L. In vitro, naltrexone is 21% bound to plasma proteins.

Metabolism/Excretion – The major metabolite of naltrexone is 6-β-naltrexol. The activity of naltrexone is believed to be due to both parent and the 6-β-naltrexol metabolite. The mean elimination half-life values for naltrexone and 6-β-naltrexol are 4 and 13 hours, respectively.

Renal elimination is primarily by glomerular filtration. Parent drug and metabolites are excreted primarily by the kidney; however, urinary excretion of unchanged naltrexone accounts for < 2% of an oral dose and fecal excretion is a minor elimination pathway. The urinary excretion of unchanged and conjugated 6-β-naltrexone accounts for 43% of an oral dose. Naltrexone and its metabolites may undergo enterohepatic recycling.

Contraindications

Patients receiving opioid analgesics; opioid-dependent patients; patients in acute opioid withdrawal; failed naloxone challenge; positive urine screen for opioids; history of sensitivity to naltrexone; acute hepatitis or liver failure.

Warnings

Hepatotoxicity: Naltrexone has the capacity to cause hepatocellular injury when given in excessive doses. It is contraindicated in acute hepatitis or liver failure, and its use in patients with active liver disease must be carefully considered in light of its hepatotoxic effects.

Warn patients of the risk of hepatic injury and advise them to stop naltrexone and seek medical attention if they experience symptoms of acute hepatitis.

Although no cases of hepatic failure have ever been reported, consider this as a possible risk of treatment.

Abstinence precipitation/syndrome: Unintended precipitation of abstinence or exacerbation of a preexisting subclinical abstinence syndrome may occur; therefore, patients should remain opioid-free for a minimum of 7 to 10 days before starting naltrexone.

Severe opioid withdrawal syndromes: Severe opioid withdrawal syndromes precipitated by accidental naltrexone ingestion have occurred in opioid-dependent individuals. Withdrawal symptoms usually appear ≤ 5 minutes of ingestion and may last up to 48 hours.

Surmountable blockade: While naltrexone is a potent antagonist with a prolonged pharmacologic effect (24 to 72 hours), the blockade produced by naltrexone is surmountable. This poses a potential risk to individuals who attempt to overcome the blockade by self-administering large amounts of opioids. Any attempt by a patient to overcome the antagonism by taking opioids is very dangerous and may lead to fatal overdose.

Use with narcotics: Patients taking naltrexone may not benefit from opioid-containing medicines. Use a nonopioid-containing alternative, if available.

Pregnancy: Category C.

Lactation: It is not known if naltrexone is excreted in breast milk.

Children: Safety for use in children < 18 years of age has not been established.

Precautions

Monitoring: A high index of suspicion for drug-related hepatic injury is critical if the occurrence of liver damage induced by naltrexone is to be detected at the earliest possible time.

Suicide: The risk of suicide is increased in patients with substance abuse with or without concomitant depression. This risk is not abated by treatment with naltrexone.

Drug Interactions

Drugs that may be affected by naltrexone include opioid-containing products and thioridazine.

Adverse Reactions

Adverse reactions associated with treatment of alcoholism include nausea, headache, dizziness, nervousness, fatigue, insomnia, and vomiting.

Reactions associated with treatment of narcotic addiction include difficulty sleeping, anxiety, nervousness, headache, low energy, irritability, increased energy, dizziness, abdominal cramps/pain, nausea, vomiting, loss of appetite, diarrhea, constipation, joint/muscle pain, delayed ejaculation, decreased potency, skin rash, chills, and increased thirst.

FLUMAZENIL

Injection: 0.1 mg/mL (*Rx*)   *Romazicon* (Hoffman-La Roche)

Indications

Reversal of benzodiazepine sedation: For the complete or partial reversal of the sedative effects of benzodiazepines in cases where general anesthesia has been induced or maintained with benzodiazepines, where sedation has been produced with benzodiazepines for diagnostic and therapeutic procedures, and for the management of benzodiazepine overdose.

Administration and Dosage

For IV use only. To minimize the likelihood of pain at the injection site, administer flumazenil through a freely running IV infusion into a large vein.

Individualization of dosage: In high-risk patients, it is important to administer the smallest amount of flumazenil that is effective. The 1-minute wait between individual doses in the dose-titration recommended for general clinical populations may be too short for high-risk patients because it takes 6 to 10 minutes for any single dose of flumazenil to reach full effects. Slow the rate of administration of flumazenil administered to high-risk patients.

Reversal of conscious sedation or in general anesthesia: The recommended initial dose is 0.2 mg (2 mL) administered IV over 15 seconds. If the desired level of consciousness is not obtained after waiting an additional 45 seconds, a further dose of 0.2 mg (2 mL) can be injected and repeated at 60 second intervals where necessary (up to a maximum of 4 additional times) to a maximum total dose of 1 mg (10 mL). Individualize the dose based on the patient's response, with most patients responding to doses of 0.6 to 1 mg.

In the event of resedation, repeated doses may be administered at 20-minute intervals as needed. For repeat treatment, administer no more than 1 mg (given as 0.2 mg/min) at any one time, and give no more than 3 mg in any 1 hour.

Suspected benzodiazepine overdose: The recommended initial dose is 0.2 mg (2 mL) administered IV over 30 seconds. If the desired level of consciousness is not obtained after waiting 30 seconds, a further dose of 0.3 mg (3 mL) can be administered over another 30 seconds. Further doses of 0.5 mg (5 mL) can be administered over 30 seconds at 1-minute intervals up to a cumulative dose of 3 mg.

Most patients with benzodiazepine overdose will respond to a cumulative dose of 1 to 3 mg, and doses beyond 3 mg do not reliably produce additional effects.

If a patient has not responded 5 minutes after receiving a cumulative dose of 5 mg, the major cause of sedation is likely not to be due to benzodiazepines, and additional flumazenil is likely to have no effect.

In the event of resedation, repeated doses may be given at 20-minute intervals if needed. For repeat treatment, give no more than 1 mg (given as 0.5 mg/min) at any one time and give no more than 3 mg in any 1 hour.

Actions

Pharmacology: Flumazenil antagonizes the actions of benzodiazepines on the CNS and competitively inhibits the activity at the benzodiazepine recognition site on the GABA/benzodiazepine receptor complex.

The duration and degree of reversal of benzodiazepine effects are related to the dose and plasma concentrations of flumazenil. The onset of reversal is usually evident within 1 to 2 minutes after the injection is completed. Within 3 minutes, 80% response will be reached, with the peak effect occurring at 6 to 10 minutes.

Pharmacokinetics: After IV administration, flumazenil has an initial distribution half-life of 7 to 15 minutes and a terminal half-life of 41 to 79 minutes. Peak concentrations of flumazenil are proportional to dose, with an apparent initial volume of distribution of 0.5 L/kg. After redistribution the apparent volume of distribution ranges from 0.77 to 1.6 L/kg. Protein binding is ≈ 50%.

Flumazenil is a highly extracted drug. Clearance of flumazenil occurs primarily by hepatic metabolism and is dependent on hepatic blood flow. In healthy volunteers, total clearance ranges from 0.7 to 1.3 L/hr/kg, with < 1% of the administered dose eliminated unchanged in urine. Elimination of drug is essentially complete within 72 hours, with 90% to 95% appearing in urine and 5% to 10% in feces.

Contraindications

Hypersensitivity to flumazenil or to benzodiazepines; benzodiazepine use for control of a potentially life-threatening condition; in patients who are showing signs of serious cyclic antidepressant overdose.

Warnings

Seizures: The use of flumazenil has been associated with the occurrence of seizures. These are most frequent in patients who have been on benzodiazepines for long-term sedation or in overdose cases where patients are showing signs of serious cyclic antidepressant overdose. Individualize the dosage of flumazenil and be prepared to manage seizures.

Seizure risk: The reversal of benzodiazepine effects may be associated with the onset of seizures in certain high-risk populations.

Most convulsions associated with flumazenil administration require treatment and have been successfully managed with benzodiazepines, phenytoin, or barbiturates.

Hypoventilation: Monitor patients who have received flumazenil for the reversal of benzodiazepine effects (after conscious sedation or general anesthesia) for resedation, respiratory depression or other residual benzodiazepine effects for an appropriate period (≤ 120 minutes) based on the dose and duration of effect of the benzodiazepine employed, because flumazenil has not been established as an effective treatment for hypoventilation due to benzodiazepine administration.

Flumazenil may not fully reverse postoperative airway problems or ventilatory insufficiency induced by benzodiazepines. In addition, even if flumazenil is initially effective, such problems may recur because the effects of flumazenil wear off before the effects of many benzodiazepines.

Hepatic function impairment: Mean total clearance is decreased to 40% to 60% of normal in patients with moderate liver dysfunction and to 25% of normal in patients with severe liver dysfunction compared with age-matched healthy subjects. This results in a prolongation of the half-life from 0.8 hours in healthy subjects to 1.3 hours in patients with moderate hepatic impairment and 2.4 hours in severely impaired patients.

Pregnancy: Category C.

Labor and delivery – The use of flumazenil to reverse the effects of benzodiazepines used during labor and delivery is not recommended because the effects of the drug in the newborn are unknown.

Lactation: It is not known whether flumazenil is excreted in breast milk.

Children: Flumazenil is not recommended for use in children.

Precautions

Monitoring: Monitor patients for resedation, respiratory depression, or other persistent or recurrent agonist effects for an adequate period of time after administration of flumazenil.

Return of sedation: Resedation is least likely in cases where flumazenil is adminstered to reverse a low dose of a short-acting benzodiazepine. It is most likely in cases where a large single or cumulative dose of a benzodiazepine has been given in the course of a long procedure along with neuromuscular blocking agents and multiple anesthetic agents.

Intensive Care Unit (ICU): Use with caution in the ICU because of the increased risk of unrecognized benzodiazepine dependence in such settings.

Overdose situations: Flumazenil is intended as an adjunct to, not as a substitute for, proper management of airway, assisted breathing, circulatory access and support, internal decontamination by lavage and charcoal, and adequate clinical evaluation.

Head injury: Use with caution in patients with head injury as flumazenil may be capable of precipitating convulsions or altering cerebral blood flow in patients receiving benzodiazepines.

Neuromuscular blocking agents: Do not use flumazenil until the effects of neuromuscular blockade have been fully reversed.

Psychiatric patients: Flumazenil may provoke panic attacks in patients with a history of panic disorder.

Drug and alcohol dependent patients: Use with caution in patients with alcoholism and other drug dependencies due to the increased frequency of benzodiazepine tolerance and dependence observed in these patient populations.

Tolerance to benzodiazepines: Flumazenil may cause benzodiazepine withdrawal symptoms in individuals who have been taking benzodiazepines long enough to have some degree of tolerance. Slower titration rates of 0.1 mg/min and lower total doses may help reduce the frequency of emergent confusion and agitation.

Physical dependence on benzodiazepines: Flumazenil is known to precipitate withdrawal seizures in patients who are physically dependent on benzodiazepines, even if such dependence was established in a relatively few days of high-dose sedation in ICU environments. The risk of either seizures or resedation in such cases is high and patients have experienced seizures before regaining consciousness. Use flumazenil in such settings with extreme caution, because use of flumazenil in this situation has not been studied and no information as to dose and rate of titration is available.

Pain on injection: To minimize the likelihood of pain or inflammation at the injection site, administer flumazenil through a freely flowing IV infusion into a large vein. Local irritation may occur following extravasation into perivascular tissues.

Respiratory disease: Appropriate ventilatory support is the primary treatment of patients with serious lung disease who experience serious respiratory depression due to benzodiazepines rather than the administration of flumazenil.

Ambulatory patients: Effects may wear off before a long-acting benzodiazepine is completely cleared from the body.

Mixed drug overdosage: Particular caution is necessary when using flumazenil in cases of mixed drug overdosage; toxic effects of other drugs taken in overdose (especially cyclic antidepressants) may emerge with reversal of the benzodiazepine effect by flumazenil.

Drug Interactions

Drug/Food interactions: Ingestion of food during an IV infusion of flumazenil results in a 50% increase in flumazenil clearance, most likely due to the increased hepatic blood flow that accompanies a meal.

Adverse Reactions

Adverse reactions may include death, convulsions, headache, injection site pain, increased sweating, fatigue, cutaneous vasodilation, nausea, vomiting, dizziness, agitation, dry mouth, tremors, palpitations, insomnia, dyspnea, hyperventilation, emotional lability, abnormal/blurred vision, and paresthesia.

Chapter 4

CARDIOVASCULAR AGENTS

Cardiac Glycosides, 197
Antianginal Agents, 205
    Nitrates, 205
Antiarrhythmic Agents, 209
    Quinidine, 212
    Procainamide, 215
    Disopyramide, 219
    Lidocaine, 222
    Tocainide, 225
    Propafenone, 226
    Flecainide, 228
    Bretylium, 231
    Amiodarone, 233
    Adenosine, 239
Calcium Channel Blockers, 241
Vasopressors for Shock, 253
Beta Blockers, 255
Alpha Beta Blockers, 269
    Labetalol, 269
    Carvedilol, 271

Antihypertensives, 274
    Methyldopa and Methyldopate, 278
    Clonidine, 280
    Alpha-1-Adrenergic Blockers, 283
    Hydralazine, 285
    Minoxidil, 287
    ACE Inhibitors, 289
    Angiotensin II Receptor Antagonists, 298
Antihyperlipidemics, 302
    Bile Acid Sequestrants, 304
    HMG-CoA Reductase Inhibitors, 306
    Gemfibrozil, 310
    Fenofibrate, 312

CARDIAC GLYCOSIDES

DIGOXIN

Capsules: 0.05, 0.1, and 0.2 mg (*Rx*)	*Lanoxicaps* (GlaxoSmithKline)
Tablets: 0.125 and 0.25 (*Rx*)	Various, *Lanoxin* (GlaxoSmithKline), *Digitek* (Vangard)
Elixir, pediatric: 0.05 mg/mL (*Rx*)	Various, *Lanoxin* (GlaxoSmithKline)
Injection: 0.25 mg/mL (*Rx*)	Various, *Lanoxin* (GlaxoSmithKline)
Injection, pediatric: 0.1 mg/mL (*Rx*)	Various, *Lanoxin* (GlaxoSmithKline)

Indications

Congestive heart failure (CHF) all degrees: Increased cardiac output results in diuresis and general amelioration of disturbances characteristic of right heart failure (venous congestion, edema) and left heart failure (dyspnea, orthopnea, cardiac asthma).

Atrial flutter: Digitalis slows the heart; normal sinus rhythm may appear. Often, flutter is converted to atrial fibrillation with a slow ventricular rate.

Administration and Dosage

Recommended dosages of digoxin may require considerable modification because of individual sensitivity of the patient to the drug, the presence of associated conditions, or the use of concurrent medications. In selecting a dose of digoxin, the following factors must be considered:

1.) The body weight of the patient. Calculate doses based upon lean (ie, ideal) body weight.
2.) The patient's renal function, preferably evaluated on the basis of estimated creatinine clearance.
3.) The patient's age. Infants and children require different doses of digoxin than adults.
4.) Concomitant disease states, concurrent medications, or other factors likely to alter the pharmacokinetic or pharmacodynamic profile of digoxin.

Serum digoxin concentrations: About 66% of adults considered adequately digitalized (without evidence of toxicity) have serum digoxin concentrations ranging from 0.8 to 2 ng/mL. Consequently, interpret the serum concentration of digoxin in the overall clinical context, and do not use an isolated measurement as the basis for increasing or decreasing the dose of the drug.

To allow adequate time for equilibration of digoxin between serum and tissue, perform sampling of serum concentrations just before the next scheduled dose of the drug. If this is not possible, perform sampling ≥ 6 to 8 hours after the last dose, regardless of the route of administration or the formulation used.

Heart failure:
    Adults – Digitalization may be accomplished by either of 2 general approaches that vary in dosage and frequency of administration but reach the same endpoint in terms of total amount of digoxin accumulated in the body.

1.) If rapid digitalization is considered medically appropriate, it may be achieved by administering a loading dose based upon projected peak digoxin body stores. Calculate maintenance dose as a percentage of the loading dose.
2.) Obtain more gradual digitalization beginning an appropriate maintenance dose, thus allowing digoxin body stores to accumulate slowly. Steady-state serum digoxin concentration will be achieved in ≈ 5 half-lives of the drug for the individual patient. Depending upon the patient's renal function, this will take between 1 and 3 weeks.

Atrial fibrillation: Peak digoxin body stores larger than the 8 to 12 mcg/kg required for most patients with heart failure and normal sinus rhythm have been used for control of ventricular rate in patients with atrial fibrillation. Titrate doses of digoxin used for the treatment of chronic atrial fibrillation to the minimum dose that achieves the desired ventricular rate control without causing undesirable side effects. Data are not available to establish the appropriate resting or exercise target rates that should be achieved.

Renal function impairment: In children with renal disease, digoxin must be carefully titrated based upon clinical response.

Rapid digitalization with a loading dose: Peak digoxin body stores of 8 to 12 mcg/kg should provide therapeutic effect with minimum risk of toxicity in most patients with heart failure and normal sinus rhythm. Because of altered digoxin distribution and elimination, projected peak body stores for patients with renal insufficiency should be conservative (ie, 6 to 10 mcg/kg; see Precautions).

Administer the loading dose in several portions, with roughly half the total given as the first dose. Additional fractions of this planned total dose may be given at 6- to 8-hour intervals, with careful assessment of clinical response before each additional dose.

If the patient's clinical reponse necessitates a change from the calculated loading dose of digoxin, then base calculation of the maintenance dose upon the amount actually given.

Digoxin injection is frequently used to achieve rapid digitalization, with conversion to digoxin tablets or capsules for maintenance therapy. If patients are switched from IV to oral digoxin formulations, make allowances for differences in bioavailability when calculating maintenance dosages (see Pharmacology).

Tablets – A single initial dose of 500 to 750 mcg (0.5 to 0.75 mg) of digoxin tablets usually produces a detectable effect in 0.5 to 2 hours that becomes maximal in 2 to 6 hours. Additional doses of 125 to 375 mcg (0.125 to 0.375 mg) may be given cautiously at 6- to 8-hour intervals until clinical evidence of an adequate effect is noted. The usual amount of digoxin tablets that a 70 kg patient requires to achieve 8 to 12 mcg/kg peak body stores is 750 to 1250 mcg (0.75 to 1.25 mg).

Capsules – A single initial dose of 400 to 600 mcg (0.4 to 0.6 mg) digoxin capsules usually produces a detectable effect in 0.5 to 2 hours that becomes maximal in 2 to 6 hours. Additional doses of 100 to 300 mcg (0.1 to 0.3 mg) may be given cautiously at 6- to 8-hour intervals until clinical evidence of an adequate effect is noted. The usual amount of the capsules that a 70 kg patient requires to achieve 8 to 12 mcg/kg peak body stores is 600 to 1000 mcg (0.6 to 1 mg).

Injection – A single initial IV dose of 400 to 600 mcg (0.4 to 0.6 mg) of injection usually produces a detectable effect in 5 to 30 minutes that becomes maximal in 1 to 4 hours. Additional doses of 100 to 300 mcg (0.1 to 0.3 mg) may be given cautiously at 6- to 8-hour intervals until clinical evidence of an adequate effect is noted. The usual amount of injection that a 70 kg patient requires to achieve 8 to 12 mcg/kg peak body stores is 600 to 1000 mcg (0.6 to 1 mg).

Dosage adjustment when changing preparations: The difference in bioavailability between digoxin injection or capsules and pediatric elixir or tablets must be considered when changing patients from 1 dosage form to another.

The absolute bioavailability of the capsule formulation is greater than that of the standard tablets and near that of the IV dosage form. As a result, the doses recommended for the capsules are the same as those for injection. Adjustments in dosage will seldom be necessary when converting a patient from the IV formulation to capsules.

Doses of 100 mcg (0.1 mg) and 200 mcg (0.2 mg) of digoxin capsules are approximately equivalent to 125 mcg (0.125 mg) and 250 mcg (0.25 mg) doses of tablets and pediatric elixir, respectively.

Maintenance dosing: The doses of digoxin used in controlled trials in patients with heart failure have ranged from 125 to 500 mcg (0.125 to 0.5 mg) once daily. In these studies, the digoxin dose has been generally titrated according to the patient's age, lean body weight, and renal function. Therapy is generally initiated at a dose of 250 mcg (0.25 mg) once daily in patients < 70 years of age with good renal function, at a dose of 125 mcg (0.125 mg) once daily in patients > 70 years of age or with impaired renal function, and at a dose of 62.5 mcg (0.0625 mg) in patients with marked renal impairment. Doses may be increased every 2 weeks according to clinical response.

In a subset of ≈ 1800 patients enrolled in a trial (wherein dosing was based on an algorithm similar to that in the table below) the mean (± SD) serum digoxin concentrations at 1 month and 12 months were ≈ 1.01 ng/mL and ≈ 0.97 ng/mL, respectively.

Base the maintenance dose upon the percentage of the peak body stores lost each day through elimination. The following formula has had wide clinical use:

Tablets:

Maintenance dosing –

Usual Digoxin Tablet Daily Maintenance Dose Requirements (mcg) for Estimated Peak Body Stores of 10 mcg/kg							Number of days before steady-state achieved[2]
Corrected Ccr (mL/min/70 kg)[1]	Lean Body Weight (kg/lbs)						
	50/110	60/132	70/154	80/176	90/198	100/220	
0	62.5	125	125	125	187.5	187.5	22
10	125	125	125	187.5	187.5	187.5	19
20	125	125	187.5	187.5	187.5	250	16
30	125	187.5	187.5	187.5	250	250	14
40	125	187.5	187.5	250	250	250	13
50	187.5	187.5	250	250	250	250	12
60	187.5	187.5	250	250	250	375	11
70	187.5	250	250	250	250	375	10
80	187.5	250	250	250	375	375	9
90	187.5	250	250	250	375	500	8
100	250	250	250	375	375	500	7

[1] Ccr is creatinine clearance, corrected to 70 kg body weight or 1.73 m^2 body surface area. For adults, if only serum creatinine concentrations (Scr) are available, a Ccr (corrected to 70 kg body weight) may be estimated in men as (140 – Age)/Scr. For women, multiply this result by 0.85. Note: This equation cannot be used for estimating Ccr in infants or children.
[2] If no loading dose is administered.

Infants and children – In general, divided daily dosing is recommended for infants and young children < 10 years of age. In the newborn period, renal clearance of digoxin is diminished and observe suitable dosage adjustments. This is especially pronounced in the premature infant. Beyond the immediate newborn period, children generally require proportionally larger doses than adults on the basis of body weight or body surface area. Children > 10 years of age require adult dosages in proportion to their body weight. Some researchers have suggested that infants and young children tolerate slightly higher serum concentrations than do adults.

Daily maintenance doses for each age group are given in the table below and should provide therapeutic effects with minimum risk of toxicity in most patients with heart failure and normal sinus rhythm. These recommendations assume the presence of normal renal function:

Daily Digoxin Maintenance Doses in Children with Normal Renal Function	
Age	Daily maintenance dose (mcg/kg)
2 to 5 years	10 to 15
5 to 10 years	7 to 10
> 10 years	3 to 5

Capsules: Because of the more complete absorption of digoxin from soft capsules, recommended oral doses are only 80% of those for tablets and elixir. Because the significance of the higher peak serum concentrations associated with once daily capsules is not established, divided daily dosing is presently recommended for the following:

1.) Infants and children < 10 years of age.
2.) Patients requiring a daily dose of ≥ 300 mcg (0.3 mg).
3.) Patients with a history of digitalis toxicity.

4.) Patients considered likely to become toxic.
5.) Patients in whom compliance is not a problem.

Usual Digoxin Solution-Filled Capsule Daily Maintenance Dose Requirements (mcg) for Estimated Peak Body Stores of 10 mcg/kg							
Corrected Ccr (mL/min/70 kg)[1]	Lean Body Weight (kg/lbs)						Number of days before steady-state achieved[2]
	50/110	60/132	70/154	80/176	90/198	100/220	
0	50	100	100	100	150	150	22
10	100	100	100	150	150	150	19
20	100	100	150	150	150	200	16
30	100	150	150	150	200	200	14
40	100	150	150	200	200	250	13
50	150	150	200	200	250	250	12
60	150	150	200	200	250	300	11
70	150	200	200	250	250	300	10
80	150	200	200	250	300	300	9
90	150	200	250	250	300	350	8
100	200	200	250	300	300	350	7

[1] Ccr is creatinine clearance, corrected to 70 kg body weight or 1.73 m^2 body surface area. For adults, if only serum creatinine concentrations (Scr) are available, a Ccr (corrected to 70 kg body weight) may be estimated in men as (140 − Age)/Scr. For women, multiply this result by 0.85. Note: This equation cannot be used for estimating Ccr in infants or children.
[2] If no loading dose is administered.

Infants and children – Individualize dosage. Divided daily dosing is recommended for infants and young children < 10 years of age. In these patients, where dosage adjustment is frequent and outside the fixed dosages available, digoxin capsules may not be the formulation of choice. In the newborn period, renal clearance of digoxin is diminished; observe suitable dosage adjustment. This is especially pronounced in the premature infant. Beyond the immediate newborn period, children generally require proportionally larger doses than adults on the basis of body weight or body surface area. Children > 10 years of age require adult dosages in proportion to body weight. Some researchers have suggested that infants and young children tolerate slightly higher serum concentrations than do adults.

Maintenance dosage – Daily maintenance doses for each age group are given below and should provide therapeutic effects with minimum risk of toxicity in most patients with heart failure and normal sinus rhythm. These recommendations assume the presence of normal renal function.

Usual Digitalizing and Maintenance Dosages for Digoxin Capsules in Children with Normal Renal Function Based on Lean Body Weight		
Age	Digitalizing[1] dose (mcg/kg)	Daily maintenance dose[2] (mcg/kg)
2 to 5 years	25 to 35	25% to 35% of the oral or IV digitalizing dose[3]
5 to 10 years	15 to 30	
> 10 years	8 to 12	

[1] IV digitalizing doses are the same as digitalizing doses of digoxin capsules.
[2] Divided daily dosing is recommended for children < 10 years of age.
[3] Projected or actual digitalizing dose providing desired clinical response.

Pediatric elixir:
Usual digitalizing and maintenance dosing –

Usual Digitalizing and Maintenance Dosages for Pediatric Elixir in Children with Normal Renal Function Based on Lean Body Weight		
Age	Oral digitalizing[1] dose (mcg/kg)	Daily maintenance dose[2] (mcg/kg)
Premature	20 to 30	20% to 30% of oral digitalizing dose[3]
Full-term	25 to 35	25% to 35% of oral digitalizing dose[3]
1 to 24 months	35 to 60	
2 to 5 years	30 to 40	
5 to 10 years	20 to 35	
> 10 years	10 to 15	

[1] IV digitalizing doses are 80% of oral digitalizing doses.
[2] Divided daily dosing is recommended for children < 10 years of age.
[3] Projected or actual digitalizing dose providing clinical response.

Gradual digitalization with a maintenance dose – More gradual digitalization also can be accomplished by beginning an appropriate maintenance dose. The range of percentages provided in the above table can be used in calculating this dose for patients with normal renal function.

Injection: Slow infusion of injection is preferable to bolus administration. Rapid infusion of digitalis glycosides has been shown to cause systemic and coronary arteriolar constriction, which may be clinically undesirable. Caution is thus advised and injection probably should be administered over a period of ≥ 5 minutes. Mixing injection with other drugs in the same container or simultaneous administration in the same intravenous line is not recommended.

Parenteral administration of digoxin should be used only when the need for rapid digitalization is urgent or when the drug cannot be taken orally. IM injection can lead to severe pain at the injection site, thus IV administration is preferred. If the drug must be administered by the IM route, inject it deep into the muscle followed by massage. Do not inject > 500 mcg (2 mL) into a single site.

If tuberculin syringes are used to measure very small doses, one must be aware of the problem of inadvertent overadministration of digoxin. Do not flush the syringe with the parenteral solution after its contents are expelled into an indwelling vascular catheter.

Admixture compatibility – Digoxin injection can be administered undiluted or diluted with a ≥ 4-fold volume of Sterile Water for Injection, 0.9% Sodium Chloride Injection, or 5% Dextrose Injection. The use of < 4-fold volume of diluent could lead to precipitation of the digoxin. Immediate use of the diluted product is recommended.

Maintenance Dose –

Usual Daily Maintenance Dose Requirements (mcg) of Digoxin Injection for Estimated Peak Body Stores of 10 mcg/kg[1]							
	Lean body weight (kg/lb)						
Corrected Ccr (mL/min/70 kg)[2]	50/110	60/132	70/154	80/176	90/198	100/220	Number of days before steady-state achieved[3]
0	75	75	100	100	125	150	22
10	75	100	100	125	150	150	19
20	100	100	125	150	150	175	16
30	10	125	150	150	175	200	14
40	100	125	150	175	200	225	13
50	125	150	175	200	225	250	12
60	125	150	175	200	225	250	11

Usual Daily Maintenance Dose Requirements (mcg) of Digoxin Injection for Estimated Peak Body Stores of 10 mcg/kg[1]	Lean body weight (kg/lb)						
Corrected Ccr (mL/min/70 kg)[2]	50/110	60/132	70/154	80/176	90/198	100/220	Number of days before steady-state achieved[3]
70	150	175	200	225	250	275	10
80	150	175	200	250	275	300	9
90	150	200	225	250	300	325	8
100	175	200	250	275	300	350	7

[1] Daily maintenance doses have been rounded to the nearest 25 mcg increment.
[2] Ccr is creatinine clearance, corrected to 70 kg body weight or 1.73 m^2 body surface area. For adults, if only serum creatinine concentrations (Scr) are available, a Ccr (corrected to 70 kg body weight) may be estimated in men as (140 − Age)/Scr. For women, this result should be multiplied by 0.85. Note: This equation cannot be used for estimating creatinine clearance in infants or children.
[3] If no loading dose is administered.

Pediatric injection:
  Digitalizing and maintenance dosages –

Usual Digitalizing and Maintenance Dosages for Digoxin Pediatric Injection in Children with Normal Renal Function Based on Lean Body Weight		
Age	IV digitalizing[1] dose (mcg/kg)	Daily IV maintenance dose[2] (mcg/kg)
Premature	15 to 25	20% to 30% of the IV digitalizing dose[3]
Full-term	20 to 30	25% to 35% of the IV digitalizing dose[3]
1 to 24 months	30 to 50	
2 to 5 years	25 to 35	
5 to 10 years	15 to 30	
≥ 10 years	8 to 12	

[1] IV digitalizing doses are 80% of oral digitalizing doses.
[2] Divided daily dosing is recommended for children < 10 years of age.
[3] Projected or actual digitalizing dose providing clinical response.

  Gradual digitalization with a maintenance dose – More gradual digitalization also can be accomplished by beginning an appropriate maintenance dose. The range of percentages provided in the table above can be used in calculating this dose for patients with normal renal function.

Actions

Pharmacology: Digoxin inhibits sodium-potassium ATPase, leading to an increase in the intracellular concentration of sodium and thus, (by stimulation of sodium-calcium exchange) an increase in the intracellular concentration of calcium. The pharmacologic consequences of these direct and indirect effects are the following: An increase in the force and velocity of myocardial systolic contraction (positive inotropic action); a decrease in the degree of activation of the sympathetic nervous system and renin-angiotensin system (neurohormonal deactivating effect); and slowing of the heart rate and decreased conduction velocity through the AV node (vagomimetic effect).

  Hemodynamic effects – Digoxin produces hemodynamic improvement in patients with heart failure. Short- and long-term therapy with the drug increases cardiac output and lowers pulmonary artery pressure, pulmonary capillary wedge pressure, and systemic vascular resistance.

Pharmacokinetics:
  Absorption – Following oral administration, peak serum concentrations of digoxin occur at 1 to 3 hours. Absorption of digoxin from the tablets has been demonstrated to be 60% to 80% complete compared with an identical IV dose of digoxin (absolute bioavailability) or capsules (relative bioavailability).

Distribution – Digoxin has a large apparent volume of distribution. Digoxin crosses the blood-brain barrier and the placenta. Approximately 25% of digoxin in the plasma is bound to protein. Serum digoxin concentrations correlate best with lean (ie, ideal) body weight, not total body weight.

Metabolism – Only a small percentage (16%) of a dose of digoxin is metabolized.

Excretion – Elimination of digoxin follows first-order kinetics. Following IV administration to healthy volunteers, 50% to 70% of a digoxin dose is excreted unchanged in the urine. Digoxin is not effectively removed from the body by dialysis, exchange transfusion, or during cardiopulmonary bypass because most of the drug is bound to tissue and does not circulate in the blood.

Contraindications

Ventricular fibrillation; hypersensitivity to digoxin or other digitalis preparations.

Warnings

Sinus node disease and AV block: The drug may cause severe sinus bradycardia or sino-atrial block in patients with pre-existing sinus node disease and may cause advanced or complete heart block in patients with pre-existing incomplete AV block. Consider inserting a pacemaker before treatment with digoxin.

Accessory AV pathway (Wolf-Parkinson-White syndrome): After IV digoxin therapy, some patients with paroxysmal atrial fibrillation or flutter and a coexisting accessory AV pathway have developed increased antegrade conduction across the accessory pathway bypassing the AV node, leading to a very rapid ventricular response or ventricular fibrillation. Unless conduction down the accessory pathway has been blocked (either pharmacologically or by surgery), do not use digoxin in such patients.

Use in patients with preserved left ventricular systolic function: Patients with certain disorders involving heart failure associated with preserved left ventricular ejection fraction may be particularly susceptible to toxicity of the drug.

Renal function impairment: Digoxin is primarily excreted by the kidneys; therefore, patients with impaired renal function require smaller than usual maintenance doses of digoxin (see Administration and Dosage).

Pregnancy: Category C.

Lactation: Exercise caution when digoxin is administered to a nursing woman.

Children: Newborn infants display considerable variability in tolerance. Premature and immature infants are particularly sensitive; reduce dosage and individualize digitalization according to infant's degree of maturity.

Precautions

Electrolyte disorders: In patients with hypokalemia or hypomagnesemia, toxicity may occur despite serum digoxin concentrations < 2 ng/mL, because potassium or magnesium depletion sensitizes the myocardium to digoxin. Therefore, it is desirable to maintain normal serum potassium and magnesium concentrations in patients being treated with digoxin.

Hypercalcemia from any cause predisposes the patient to digitalis toxicity. Calcium, particularly when administered rapidly by the IV route, may produce serious arrhythmias in digitalized patients. On the other hand, hypocalcemia can nullify the effects of digoxin in humans; thus, digoxin may be ineffective until serum calcium is restored to normal.

Thyroid disorders and hypermetabolic states: Hypothyroidism may reduce the requirements for digoxin. Heart failure or atrial arrhythmias resulting from hypermetabolic or hyperdynamic states (eg, hyperthyroidism, hypoxia, arteriovenous shunt) are best treated by addressing the underlying condition. Atrial arrhythmias associated with hypermetabolic states are particularly resistant to digoxin treatment. Care must be taken to avoid toxicity if digoxin is used.

Acute MI: Use digoxin with caution in patients with acute MI. The use of inotropic drugs in some patients in this setting may result in undesirable increases in myocardial oxygen demand and ischemia.

Electrical cardioversion: It may be desirable to reduce the dose of digoxin for 1 to 2 days prior to electrical cardioversion of atrial fibrillation to avoid the induction of ventricular arrhythmias, but physicians must consider the consequences of increasing the ventricular response if digoxin is withdrawn. If digitalis toxicity is suspected, delay elective cardioversion. If it is not prudent to delay cardioversion, select the lowest possible energy level to avoid provoking ventricular arrhythmias.

Lab test abnormalities: Periodically assess serum electrolytes and renal function (serum creatinine concentrations); the frequency of assessments will depend on the clinical setting.

Drug Interactions

Increased digoxin serum levels: The following agents may increase digoxin serum levels, possibly increasing its therapeutic and toxic effects: Alprazolam, amiodarone, anticholinergics, benzodiazepines, bepridil, captopril, cyclosporine, diltiazem, diphenoxylate, erythromycin, esmolol, felodipine, flecainide, hydroxychloroquine, ibuprofen, indomethacin, itraconazole, nifedipine, omeprazole, propafenone, propantheline, quinidine, quinine, tetracycline, tolbutamide, and verapamil.

Decreased GI absorption of digitalis glycosides: May be caused by the following agents, possibly decreasing the serum levels and therapeutic effects: Aminoglutethimide, aminoglycosides (oral), aminosalicylic acid, antacids (aluminum or magnesium salts), antihistamines, antineoplastics, barbiturates, cholestyramine, colestipol, hydantoins, hypoglycemic agents (oral), kaolin/pectin, metoclopramide, neomycin, penicillamine, rifampin, sucralfate, and sulfasalazine.

Other drugs that may interact with cardiac glycosides include the following: Albuterol, amphotericin B, beta blockers, calcium, disopyramide, loop diuretics, nondepolarizing muscle relaxants, potassium-sparing diuretics, succinylcholine, sympathomimetics, thiazide diuretics, thioamines, and thyroid hormones.

Drug/Lab test interactions: The use of therapeutic doses of digoxin may cause prolongation of the PR interval and depression of the ST segment on the electrocardiogram. Digoxin may produce false positive ST-T changes on the electrocardiogram during exercise testing.

Drug/Food interactions: When digoxin tablets are taken after meals, the rate of absorption is slowed but total amount absorbed is usually unchanged. However, when taken with meals high in bran fiber, the amount absorbed may be reduced.

Adverse Reactions

Digoxin adverse reactions are dose-dependent and occur at doses higher than those needed to achieve a therapeutic effect. Cardiac adverse reactions accounted for ≈ 50%, GI disturbances for ≈ 25%, and CNS and other toxicity for ≈ 25% of these adverse reactions. However, available evidence suggests that the incidence and severity of digoxin toxicity has decreased substantially in recent years.

Adverse reactions occurring in ≥ 3% of patients include the following: Headache, dizziness, mental disturbances, nausea, diarrhea, and death.

NITRATES

AMYL NITRITE	
Inhalant: 0.3 mL (*Rx*)	*Amyl Nitrite Vaporole* (GlaxoWellcome)
ISOSORBIDE DINITRATE (ORAL)	
Tablets: 5, 10, 20, 30, and 40 mg (*Rx*)	Various, *Isordil Titradose* (Wyeth-Ayerst)
Tablets, sustained-release: 40 mg (*Rx*)	Various, *Isordil Tembids* (Wyeth-Ayerst)
Capsules, sustained-release: 40 mg (*Rx*)	Various, *Isordil Tembids* (Wyeth-Ayerst), *Dilatrate-SR* (Schwarz Pharma)
ISOSORBIDE DINITRATE (SUBLINGUAL AND CHEWABLE)	
Tablets, sublingual: 2.5, 5, and 10 mg (*Rx*)	Various, *Isordil* (Wyeth-Ayerst)
Tablets, chewable: 5 and 10 mg (*Rx*)	*Sorbitrate* (ICI Pharma)
ISOSORBIDE MONONITRATE (ORAL)	
Tablets: 10 and 20 mg (*Rx*)	*Monoket* (Schwarz Pharma), *ISMO* (Wyeth-Ayerst)
Tablets, extended-release: 60 and 120 mg (*Rx*)	*Imdur* (Key)
NITROGLYCERIN (IV)	
Injection: 0.5 and 5 mg/mL (*Rx*)	Various, *Tridil* (Faulding)
Injection solution: 25, 50, 100, and 200 mg in 5% Dextrose (*Rx*)	Various
NITROGLYCERIN (SUBLINGUAL)	
Tablets, sublingual: 0.3, 0.4, and 0.6 mg (*Rx*)	*Nitrostat* (Parke-Davis), *NitroQuick* (Ethex)
NITROGLYCERIN (SUSTAINED RELEASE)	
Tablets, sustained-release: 2.6, 6.5, and 9 mg (*Rx*)	*Nitrong* (Rhone-Poulence Rorer)
Capsules, sustained-release: 2.5, 6.5, 9, and 13 mg (*Rx*)	Various, *Nitroglyn* (Kenwood), *Nitro-Time* (Time-Cap Labs)
NITROGLYCERIN (TOPICAL)	
Ointment: 2% in a lanolin-petroleum base (*Rx*)	Various, *Nitrol* (Adria)
NITROGLYCERIN TRANSDERMAL SYSTEMS	
Patch: 0.1, 0.2, 0.3, 0.4, 0.6, and 0.8 mg/hr (*Rx*)	*Nitro-Dur* (Key)
NITROGLYCERIN (TRANSLINGUAL)	
Spray: 0.4 mg/dose (*Rx*)	*Nitrolingual* (Rhone-Poulenc Rorer)
NITROGLYCERIN (TRANSMUCOSAL)	
Tablets, buccal, controlled-release: 1, 2, and 3 mg (*Rx*)	*Nitrogard* (Forest)

Indications

Acute angina (nitroglycerin sublingual, transmucosal or translingual spray; isosorbide dinitrate sublingual; amyl nitrite): For relief of acute anginal episodes; prophylaxis prior to events likely to provoke an attack.

Angina prophylaxis (nitroglycerin topical, transdermal, translingual spray, transmucosal and oral sustained release; isosorbide dinitrate; isosorbide mononitrate; erythrityl tetranitrate; pentaerythritol tetranitrate): Prophylaxis and long-term management of recurrent angina.

Nitroglycerin IV: Control of blood pressure in perioperative hypertension associated with surgical procedures, especially cardiovascular procedures, such as endotracheal intubation, anesthesia, skin incision, sternotomy, cardiac bypass, and in the immediate postsurgical period.

CHF associated with acute MI; treatment of angina pectoris unresponsive to organic nitrates or β-blockers; production of controlled hypotension during surgical procedures.

Administration and Dosage

AMYL NITRITE: Usual adult dose is 0.3 mL by inhalation, as required.

Crush the capsule and wave under the nose; 1 to 6 inhalations from one capsule are usually sufficient to produce the desired effect. May repeat in 3 to 5 minutes.

ISOSORBIDE DINITRATE, ORAL:
Tablets – Initial dose is 5 to 20 mg; maintenance dose is 10 to 40 mg every 6 hours.
Sustained release – The initial dose is 40 mg; maintenance controlled release dose is 40 to 80 mg every 8 to 12 hours. Do not crush or chew these preparations.

Tolerance – Tolerance to these agents may develop. Consider administering the short-acting preparations 2 or 3 times/day (last dose no later than 7 pm) and the sustained release preparations once daily or twice daily at 8 am and 2 pm.

ISOSORBIDE DINITRATE, SUBLINGUAL AND CHEWABLE:

Angina pectoris – Usual starting dose is 2.5 to 5 mg for sublingual tablets and 5 mg for chewable tablets.

Acute prophylaxis – 5 to 10 mg sublingual or chewable tablets every 2 to 3 hours. Limit use of sublingual or chewable isosorbide dinitrate for aborting an acute anginal attack in patients intolerant of or unresponsive to sublingual nitroglycerin.

Do not crush or chew sublingual tablets; do not crush chewable tablets before administering.

ISOSORBIDE MONONITRATE:

Tablets – 20 mg twice/day, with the 2 doses given 7 hours apart. A starting dose of 5 mg might be appropriate for people of particularly small stature, but should be increased to ≤ 10 mg by the second or third day of therapy. Suggested regimen is to give first dose on awakening and second dose 7 hours later.

Tablets, extended-release – Initially, 30 or 60 mg once daily. After several days, the dosage may be increased to 120 mg once daily. Rarely 240 mg may be required. Suggested regimen is to give in the morning on arising. Do not crush or chew extended release tablets, and swallow them with a half glassful of liquid.

NITROGLYCERIN, IV:

Dosage requirements – Initially, 5 mcg/min delivered through an infusion pump. Titrate to the clinical situation, initially in 5 mcg/min increments with increases every 3 to 5 minutes until some response is noted. If no response occurs at 20 mcg/min, use increments of 10 to 20 mcg/min. Once a partial blood pressure response is observed, reduce the dose and lengthen the interval between increments.

NITROGLYCERIN, SUBLINGUAL: Dissolve 1 tablet under tongue or in buccal pouch (between cheek and gum) at first sign of an acute anginal attack. Repeat approximately every 5 minutes until relief is obtained. Take no more than 3 tablets in 15 minutes. May be used prophylactically 5 to 10 minutes prior to activities which might precipitate an acute attack.

NITROGLYCERIN, SUSTAINED-RELEASE: The usual starting dose is 2.5 or 2.6 mg, 3 or 4 times/day. The dose generally may be increased by 2.5 or 2.6 mg increments 2 to 4 times/day over a period of days or weeks. Doses as high as 26 mg given 4 times/day have been reported effective.

Give the smallest effective dose 2 to 4 times/day.

Capsules must be swallowed; not for chewing or sublingual use.

NITROGLYCERIN, TOPICAL:

Usual therapeutic dose – 1 to 2 inches (25 to 50 mm) every 8 hours, up to 4 to 5 inches (100 to 125 mm) every 4 hours. Start with ½ inch (12.5 mm) every 8 hours; increase by ½ inch with each application to achieve desired effects.

One inch (25 mm) of ointment contains ≈ 15 mg nitroglycerin.

NITROGLYCERIN TRANSDERMAL SYSTEMS: Patient instructions for application are provided with products.

Apply once daily to a skin site free of hair and not subject to excessive movement. Do not apply to distal parts of extremities. Avoid areas with cuts/irritations.

Starting dose – 0.2 to 0.4 mg/hr. Doses between 0.4 and 0.8 mg/hr have shown continued effectiveness for 10 to 12 hours/day for ≥ 1 month of intermittent administration. Although the minimum nitrate-free interval has not been defined, data show that a nitrate-free interval of 10 to 12 hours is sufficient. Thus, an appropriate dosing schedule would include a daily "patch-on" period of 12 to 14 hours and a "patch-off" period of 10 to 12 hours. Tolerance is a major factor limiting efficacy when the system is used continuously for> 12 hours each day.

NITROGLYCERIN, TRANSLINGUAL: At the onset of attack, spray 1 or 2 metered doses onto or under the tongue. No more than 3 metered doses are recommended within 15 minutes. May use prophylactically 5 to 10 minutes prior to activities which might precipitate an acute attack. Do not inhale spray.

NITROGLYCERIN, TRANSMUCOSAL: 1 mg every 3 to 5 hours during waking hours. Place tablet between lip and gum above incisors, or between cheek and gum.

Actions

Pharmacology: Relaxation of vascular smooth muscle via stimulation of intracellular cyclic guanosine monophosphate production is the principal pharmacologic action of nitrates. Although venous effects predominate, nitroglycerin produces a dose-dependent dilation of both arterial and venous beds.

Pharmacokinetics:

Doseform, Onset, and Duration of Available Nitrates			
Nitrates	Dosage form	Onset (minutes)	Duration
Amyl nitrate	Inhalant	0.5	3 to 5 min
Nitroglycerin	IV	1 to 2	3 to 5 min
	Sublingual	1 to 3	30 to 60 min
	Translingual spray	2	30 to 60 min
	Transmucosal tablet	1 to 2	3 to 5 hours[1]
	Oral, sustained release	20 to 45	3 to 8 hours
	Topical ointment	30 to 60	2 to 12 hours[2]
	Transdermal	30 to 60	up to 24 hours[3]
Isosorbide dinitrate	Sublingual	2 to 5	1 to 3 hours
	Oral	20 to 40	4 to 6 hours
	Oral, sustained release	up to 4 hours	6 to 8 hours
Isosorbide mononitrate	Oral	30 to 60	nd[4]
Erythrityl tetranitrate	Sublingual and chewable	5	3 hours
	Oral	15 to 30	6 hours
Pentaerythritol tetranitrate	Oral	20 to 60	≈ 5 hours
	Oral, sustained release	30	up to 12 hours

[1] A significant antianginal effect can persist for 5 hours if the tablet has not completely dissolved.
[2] Depends on total amount used per unit of surface area.
[3] Tolerance may develop after 12 hours.
[4] nd = No data.

Contraindications

Hypersensitivity or idiosyncrasy to nitrates; severe anemia; closed-angle glaucoma; postural hypotension; early MI (sublingual nitroglycerin); head trauma or cerebral hemorrhage; allergy to adhesives (transdermal).

Amyl nitrate: Pregnancy.

Nitroglycerin IV: Hypotension or uncorrected hypovolemia; inadequate cerebral circulation; increased intracranial pressure; constrictive pericarditis; pericardial tamponade.

Warnings

MI: In acute MI, use nitrates only under close clinical observation and with hemodynamic monitoring. In general, do not use a long-acting form because its effects are difficult to terminate rapidly if excessive hypotension or tachycardia develop.

Arcing: A cardioverter/defibrillator should not be discharged through a paddle electrode that overlies a transdermal nitroglycerin system.

Postural hypotension: Postural hypotension may occur, even with small doses.

Angina: Nitrates may aggravate angina caused by hypertrophic cardiomyopathy.

Nitroglycerin IV:
    Hepatic or renal disease, severe – Use with caution.
    Hypotension – Avoid excessive prolonged hypotension, because of possible deleterious effects on the brain, heart, liver, and kidney from poor perfusion and the attendant risk of ischemia, thrombosis, and altered organ function. Paradoxical bradycardia and increased angina pectoris may accompany nitroglycerin-induced hypotension.
    Alcohol intoxication – Alcohol intoxication has developed in patients on high-dose IV nitroglycerin.

Sublingual nitroglycerin: Absorption is dependent on salivary secretion. Dry mough decreases absorption.

Transdermal nitroglycerin: Transdermal nitroglycerin is not for immediate relief of anginal attacks.

Pregnancy: Category C; Category X (amyl nitrite).

Lactation: It is not know whether nitrates are excreted in breast milk.

Children: Safety and efficacy for use in children have not been established.

Precautions

Tolerance: Tolerance to vascular and antianginal effects of nitrates may develop. The use of a low-nitrate or nitrate-free period should be part of the therapeutic strategy.

Glaucoma: Intraocular pressure may be increased; therefore, caution is required in administering to patients with glaucoma.

Excessive dosage: Excessive dosage may produce severe headache.

Volume depletion/hypotension: Severe hypotension (particularly with upright posture) may occur with even small doses of isosorbide mononitrate.

Withdrawal: In terminating treatment of angina, gradually reduce the dosage to prevent withdrawal reactions.

Drug Interactions

Drugs that may interact with nitrates include alcohol, aspirin, calcium channel blockers, dihydroergotamine, and heparin.

Drug/Lab test interactions: Nitrates may interfere with the *Zlatkis-Zak* color reaction causing a false report of decreased serum cholesterol.

Adverse Reactions

Cardiovascular: Tachycardia; palpitations; hypotension (sometimes with paradoxical bradycardia and increased angina pectoris); postural hypotension.

CNS: Headache that may be severe and persistent ($\leq$ 50%); apprehension; restlessness; weakness; vertigo; dizziness; agitation; anxiety; confusion; insomnia; nervousness.

Dermatologic: Drug rash or exfoliative dermatitis; cutaneous vasodilation with flushing; crusty skin lesions; pruritus; rash.

  Sublingual nitroglycerin – Sublingual nitroglycerin tablets may cause a local burning or tingling sensation in the oral cavity at the point of dissolution.

GI: Nausea; vomiting; diarrhea; dyspepsia; involuntary passing of urine and feces; abdominal pain.

GU: Dysuria; impotence; urinary frequency.

Miscellaneous: Arthralgia; bronchitis; muscle twitching; pallor; perspiration; cold sweat; asthenia; blurred vision; diplopia; edema; malaise; neck stiffness; increased appetite.

ANTIARRHYTHMIC AGENTS

Optimal therapy of cardiac arrhythmias requires documentation, accurate diagnosis, and modification of precipitating causes, and if indicated, proper selection and use of antiarrhythmic drugs. These drugs are classified according to their effects on the action potential of cardiac cells and their presumed mechanism of action.

Class I: Local anesthetics or membrane-stabilizing agents that depress phase 0.

IA *(quinidine, procainamide, disopyramide)* – Depress phase 0 and prolong the action potential duration.

IB *(tocainide, lidocaine, phenytoin, mexiletine)* – Depress phase 0 slightly and may shorten the action potential duration. Although arrhythmia is not a labeled indication for **phenytoin**, it is commonly used in treatment of digitalis-induced arrhythmias.

IC *(flecainide, encainide, propafenone)* – Marked depression of phase 0. Slight effect on repolarization. Profound slowing of conduction. **Encainide** was voluntarily withdrawn from the market, but is still available on a limited basis.

Moricizine – Moricizine is a Class I agent that shares some of the characteristics of the Class IA, B, and C agents.

Class II (propranolol, esmolol, acebutolol): Depress phase 4 depolarization.

Class III (bretylium, amiodarone): Produce a prolongation of phase 3 (repolarization).

Class IV (verapamil): Depress phase 4 depolarization and lengthen phases 1 and 2 of repolarization.

Sotalol: Sotalol has both Class II (beta blocking) and III properties; Class III effects are seen at doses > 160 mg.

Digitalis glycosides (digoxin): Digitalis glycosides (digoxin) cause a decrease in maximal diastolic potential and action potential duration and increase the slope of phase 4 depolarization.

Adenosine: Adenosine slows conduction time through the AV node and can interrupt the reentry pathways through the AV node.

Serum drug levels: Some antiarrhythmic drugs (eg, quinidine) can produce toxic effects that can be easily confused with the symptoms for which the drug has been prescribed. Drug serum levels are important in evaluating toxic or subtherapeutic dosage regimens of most of the antiarrhythmic drugs.

Proarrhythmic effects: Antiarrhythmic agents may cause new or worsened arrhythmias. It is essential that each patient be evaluated electrocardiographically and clinically prior to and during therapy to determine whether the response to the drug supports continued treatment.

Antiarrhythmic Electrophysiology/Electrocardiogram Effects

Group	Drug	Automaticity		Conduction velocity			Refractory period					ECG changes[1]				
		SA node	Ectopic pacemaker	Atrium	AV node	His-Purkinje	Atrium	AV node	His-Purkinje	Ventricle	Accessory pathways[2]	Heart rate	PR interval	QRS complex	QT_c interval	JT interval
I	Moricizine[3]	0	↓	0	↓	↓	±	0	0	0-↑	↑	0-↑	↑	↑	0	↓
	Quinidine	±	↓	↓	±	↓	↑↑	0-↑[4]	↑↑	↑	↑	±	±	↑	↑	↑
	Procainamide	±	↓	↓	±	↓	↑	0-↑[4]	↑↑	↑	↑↑	±	±	↑	↑	↑
	Disopyramide	±	↓	↓	±	↓	↑↑	0-↑[4]	↑↑	↑	↑	±	±	↑	↑	↑
	Lidocaine	0	↓	—	0	0	0	±	±	±	↑-↓	0	0	0	0-↓	0
	Phenytoin	↓-0	↓	-	0	0	0	±	±	±	-	±	0-↓	0	↓	0
	Tocainide	0-↓	↓	0	0	0	↓	↓	±	↓	↑	0	0	0	0-↓	0
	Mexiletine	↓	↓	0	0	0	0	±	↑	↑	↑	-	0	0	0	0
	Flecainide	↓	↓	↓↓	↓	↓↓	0	0	↑	↑	↑↑	0	↑[5]	↑↑[5]	0-↑[5]	0
	Encainide[6]	0-↓	↓	↓↓	↓	↓↓	0-↑	0-↑	↑	↑	↑↑	0	↑[5]	↑↑[5]	0-↑[5]	0
	Propafenone	0	↓	0	↓	↓	0	↑	↑	↑	↑	0	↑[5]	↑	0-↑[5]	0
II	Propranolol	↓	↓	±	↓	0-↓	±	↑	0	0	0-↑	↓	0-↑	0	0-↓	0
	Esmolol	↓	↓	±	↓	0-	±	↑	0	0	0-↑	↓	0-↑	0	0-↓	0
	Acebutolol	↓	↓	±	↓	0	±	↑	0	0	0-↑	↓	0-↑	0	0-↓	0
III	Bretylium	↑	↑	0	0	0-↑	0	↓-0-↑[7]	↑	0-↑	±	0	0	0	0	↑
	Amiodarone	↓	↓	↓	↓	↓	↑	↑	↑	↑	↑	↓	↑	↑	↑↑	↑↑
	Sotalol[8]	↓	↓	0	↓	0	↑↑	↑	↑↑	↑↑	↑	↓	↑	0	↑↑	↑↑
IV	Verapamil	↓	↓	0	↓	0	0	↑	0	0	0	↓	↑	0	0	0
—	Digoxin	0-↓	↑	±	↓	0-↑	±	↑	0	↓	↓-↑	↓	↑	0	↓	↓
—	Adenosine	↓	↓	0	↓	0	0	↑	0	0	0	↑	↑	0	0	—

[1] These values assume therapeutic levels.

[2] Accessory pathways occur in Wolff-Parkinson-White syndrome (preexcitation phenomena) and possibly other abnormal conditions.

[3] Does not belong to any of the 3 subclasses (A, B or C), but does have some properties of each.

[4] Retrograde AV node RP↑; antegrade RP not affected.

[5] Dose-related increases.

[6] Withdrawn from the market; however, available on a limited basis.

[7] Due to a complex balance of direct and indirect autonomic effects.

[8] Has both Class II (beta-blocking) and III properties; Class III effects are seen at doses > 160 mg.

Antiarrhythmic Pharmacokinetics

Group	Drug	Onset (hrs) (oral)[1]	Duration (hrs)	Half-life (hrs)	Protein binding (%)	Excreted unchanged (%)	Therapeutic serum level (mcg/mL)	Toxic serum levels (mcg/mL)
I A	Moricizine	2	10-24	1.5-3.5[2]	95	< 1	Not applicable	—
	Quinidine	0.5	6-8	6-7	80-90	10-50	2-6	> 8
	Procainamide	0.5	3+	2.5-4.7	14-23	40-70	4-8	> 16
	Disopyramide	0.5	6-7	4-10	20-60[3]	40-60	2-8	> 9
B	Lidocaine	—	0.25[4]	1-2	40-80	< 3	1.5-6	> 7
	Phenytoin	0.5-1	24+	22-36[5]	87-93	< 5	10-20	> 20
	Tocainide	—	—	11-15	10-20	28-55	4-10	> 10
	Mexiletine	—	—	10-12	50-60	10	0.5-2	> 2
C	Flecainide	—	—	12-27	40	30	0.2-1	> 1
	Encainide[6]	—	—	1-2[7]	75-85	< 5[8]	Not applicable	—
	MODE[9]			6-12	92		wide range	—
	ODE[9]			3-4	75-85		0.1-0.3	—
	Propafenone	—	—	2-10[10]	97	< 1	0.06-1	—
II	Propranolol	0.5	3-5	2-3	90-95	< 1	0.05-0.1	—
	Esmolol	< 5 min	very short	0.15	55	< 2	—	—
	Acebutolol	—	24-30	3-4	26	15-20	—	—
III	Bretylium	—	6-8	5-10	0-8	> 80	0.5-1.5	—
	Amiodarone	1-3 wks[11]	weeks to months	26-107 days	96	negligible	0.5-2.5	> 2.5
	Sotalol	—	—	12	0	100	—	—
IV	Verapamil	0.5	6	3-7	90	3-4	0.08-0.3	—
—	Digoxin	0.5-2	24+	30-40	20-25	60	0.5-2 ng/mL	> 2.5 ng/mL
—	Adenosine	(34 sec IV)	1-2 min	< 10 sec	—	0 (enters body pool)	Not applicable	—

[1] Within 1 to 5 minutes with IV use.
[2] Half-life may be prolonged in patients after multiple dosing.
[3] Protein binding is concentration-dependent.
[4] Very short after discontinuation of IV infusion.
[5] Half-life increases with increasing dosage.
[6] Withdrawn from the market; however, available on a limited basis.
[7] Half-life 6 to 11 hours in < 10% of patients (poor metabolizers).
[8] > 50% in poor metabolizers.
[9] MODE (3-methoxy-O-demethyl encainide) and ODE (O-demethyl encainide), metabolites more active than encainide on a per mg basis.
[10] Half-life 10 to 32 hours in < 10% of patients (slow metabolizers).
[11] Onset of action may occur in 2 to 3 days.

QUINIDINE

QUINIDINE SULFATE	
Tablets: 200 and 300 mg (*Rx*)	Various, *Quinora* (Key Pharm.)
Tablets, sustained-release: 300 mg (*Rx*)	Various, *Quinidex Extentabs* (Robins)
QUINIDINE GLUCONATE	
Tablets, sustained-release: 324 mg (*Rx*)	Various, *Quinaglute Dura-Tabs* (Berlex)
Injection: 80 mg/mL (*Rx*)	Various
QUINIDINE POLYGALACTURONATE	
Tablets: 275 mg (*Rx*)	*Cardioquin* (Purdue Frederick)

Indications

Oral: Premature atrial, AV junctional and ventricular contractions; paroxysmal atrial (supraventricular) tachycardia; paroxysmal AV junctional rhythm; atrial flutter; paroxysmal and chronic atrial fibrillation; established atrial fibrillation when therapy is appropriate; paroxysmal ventricular tachycardia not associated with complete heart block; maintenance therapy after electrical conversion of atrial fibrillation or flutter.

Parenteral: When oral therapy is not feasible or when rapid therapeutic effect is required.
Quinidine gluconate – Life-threatening *Plasmodium falciparum* malaria.

Administration and Dosage

Test dose: Administer a single 200 mg tablet of quinidine sulfate or 200 mg IM quinidine gluconate to determine whether the patient has an idiosyncratic reaction.

Adjust the dosage to maintain the plasma concentration between 2 to 6 mcg/mL.

Oral:

Premature atrial and ventricular contractions – 200 to 300 mg 3 or 4 times/day.

Paroxysmal supraventricular tachycardias – 400 to 600 mg every 2 or 3 hours until the paroxysm is terminated.

Atrial flutter – Administer quinidine after digitalization. Individualize dosage.

Conversion of atrial fibrillation – 200 mg every 2 or 3 hours for 5 to 8 doses, with subsequent daily increases until sinus rhythm is restored or toxic effects occur. Do not exceed a total daily dose of 3 to 4 g in any regimen.

Maintenance therapy – 200 to 300 mg 3 or 4 times/day. Other patients may require larger doses or more frequent administration than the usually recommended schedule.

Sustained release forms – 300 to 600 mg every 8 or 12 hours.

Parenteral:

IM – In the treatment of acute tachycardia, the initial dose is 600 mg quinidine gluconate. Subsequently, 400 mg quinidine gluconate can be repeated as often as every 2 hours.

IV – In ≈ 50% of patients who respond successfully to quinidine, the arrhythmia can be terminated by ≤ 330 mg quinidine gluconate (or its equivalent in other salts); as much as 500 to 750 mg may be required. Inject slowly.

QUINIDINE GLUCONATE – P. falciparum malaria – The following 2 regimens are effective empirically. As soon as practical, institute standard oral antiplasmodial therapy.

1) *Loading,* 15 mg/kg in 250 mL normal saline infused over 4 hours followed by: *Maintenance,* beginning 24 hours after the beginning of the loading dose, 7.5 mg/kg infused over 4 hours, every 8 hours for 7 days or until oral therapy can be instituted.

2) *Loading,* 10 mg/kg in 250 mL normal saline infused over 1 to 2 hours, followed immediately by: *Maintenance,* 0.02 mg/kg/min for up to 72 hours or until parasitemia decreases to < 1% or oral therapy can be instituted.

Children:

Oral (quinidine sulfate) – 30 mg/kg/day or 900 mg/m^2/day in 5 divided doses.

IV (quinidine gluconate) – 2 to 10 mg/kg/dose every 3 to 6 hours as needed; however, this route is not recommended.

Actions

Pharmacology: Quinidine, a class IA antiarrhythmic, depresses myocardial excitability, conduction velocity and contractility.

Pharmacokinetics:

Absorption/Distribution –

Anhydrous Quinidine Alkaloid Content in Various Salts			
	Quinidine content		
Quinidine salts	Active drug	Absorbed	Time to peak plasma levels (hours)
Quinidine sulfate	83%	73%	1 to 3[1]
Quinidine gluconate	62%	70%	3-5
Quinidine polygalacturonate	80%	—	6

[1] 3 to 5 hours for sustained release form.

Quinidine is rapidly absorbed from the GI tract. Maximum effects of quinidine gluconate occur 30 to 90 minutes after IM administration; onset is more rapid after IV administration. Activity persists for ≥ 6 to 8 hours. The average therapeutic serum levels are reported to be 2 to 7 mcg/mL. Toxic reactions may occur at levels from 5 to ≥ 8 mcg/mL. Quinidine is 80% to 90% bound to plasma proteins; the unbound fraction may be significantly increased in patients with hepatic insufficiency.

Metabolism/Excretion – From 60% to 80% of a dose is metabolized via the liver into several metabolites. Quinidine is excreted unchanged (10% to 50%) in the urine within 24 hours. The elimination half-life ranges from 4 to 10 hours in healthy patients, with a mean of 6 to 7 hours. Urinary acidification facilitates quinidine elimination, and alkalinization retards it. In patients with cirrhosis, the elimination half-life may be prolonged and the volume of distribution increased.

Contraindications

Hypersensitivity or idiosyncrasy to quinidine or other cinchona derivatives manifested by thrombocytopenia, skin eruption or febrile reactions; myasthenia gravis; history of thrombocytopenic purpura associated with quinidine administration; digitalis intoxication manifested by arrhythmias or AV conduction disorders; complete heart block; left bundle branch block or other severe intraventricular conduction defects exhibiting marked QRS widening or bizarre complexes; complete AV block with an AV nodal or idioventricular pacemaker; aberrant ectopic impulses and abnormal rhythms due to escape mechanisms; history of drug-induced torsade de pointes; history of long QT syndrome.

Warnings

Hepatotoxicity: Hepatotoxicity (including granulomatous hepatitis) due to quinidine hypersensitivity has occurred.

Atrial flutter or fibrillation: Reversion to sinus rhythm may be preceded by a progressive reduction in degree of AV block to a 1:1 ratio, which results in an extremely rapid ventricular rate. Prior to use in atrial flutter, pretreat with digitalis preparation.

Cardiotoxicity: Cardiotoxicity (eg, increased PR and QT intervals, 50% widening of QRS complex, ventricular tachyarrhythmias, frequent ventricular ectopic beats, or tachycardia) dictates immediate discontinuation of quinidine; closely monitor the ECG.

Large oral doses may reduce the arterial pressure by means of peripheral vasodilation. Serious hypotension is more likely with parenteral use.

Use quinidine with extreme caution in incomplete AV block, because complete block and asystole may result. The drug may cause unpredictable dysrhythmias in digitalized patients. Use cautiously in patients with partial bundle branch block, severe CHF, and hypotensive states due to the depressant effects of quinidine on myocardial contractility and arterial pressure.

Parenteral therapy: The dangers of parenteral use of quinidine are increased in the presence of AV block or absence of atrial activity. Administration is more hazardous in patients with extensive myocardial damage. Use of quinidine in digitalis-induced cardiac arrhythmia is extremely dangerous because the cardiac glycoside may already have caused serious impairment of intracardiac conduction system. Too rapid IV administration of as little as 200 mg may precipitate a fall of 40 to 50 mmHg in arterial pressure.

Syncope: Syncope occasionally occurs in patients on long-term quinidine therapy, usually resulting from ventricular tachycardia or fibrillation.

Renal, hepatic, or cardiac insufficiency: Use with caution in renal, cardiac, or hepatic insufficiency because of potential toxicity.

Hypersensitivity reactions: Asthma, muscle weakness, and infection with fever prior to quinidine administration may mask hypersensitivity reactions to the drug.

Pregnancy: Category C.

Lactation: Quinidine is excreted into breast milk with a milk:serum ratio of ≈ 0.71. The American Academy of Pediatrics considers quinidine to be compatible with breastfeeding.

Children: Safety and efficacy have not been established.

Precautions

Monitoring: Perform periodic blood counts and liver and kidney function tests. Discontinue use if blood dyscrasias or signs of hepatic or renal disorders occur. Frequently measure arterial blood pressure during IV use.

Potassium balance: The effect of quinidine is enhanced by potassium and reduced if hypokalemia is present. The risk of drug-induced torsade de pointes is increased by concomitant hypokalemia.

Drug Interactions

Drugs that may affect quinidine include amiodarone, antacids, barbiturates, cholinergic drugs, cimetidine, disopyramide, hydantoins, nifedipine, rifampin, sucralfate, urinary alkalinizers and verapamil. Drugs that may be affected by quinidine include anticholinergics, anticoagulants, beta blockers, cardiac glycosides, disopyramide, nondepolarizing neuromuscular blockers, procainamide, propafenone, succinylcholine, and tricyclic antidepressants.

Drug/Lab test interactions: Triamterene and quinidine have similar fluorescence spectra; thus, triamterene will interfere with the fluorescent measurement of quinidine serum levels.

Adverse Reactions

Adverse reactions may include nausea, vomiting, abdominal pain, diarrhea, anorexia; cinchonism (ringing in the ears, hearing loss, headache, nausea, dizziness, vertigo, lightheadedness, disturbed vision); headache; fever; vertigo; apprehension; excitement; confusion; delirium; dementia; depression; acute hemolytic anemia; hypoprothrombinemia; thrombocytopenic purpura; agranulocytosis; thrombocytopenia; leukocytosis; mydriasis; blurred vision; disturbed color perception; reduced vision field; night blindness, photophobia; rash; urticaria; cutaneous flushing with intense pruritus; photosensitivity; eczema; psoriasis; abnormalities of pigmentation; arthralgia; myalgia; disturbed hearing; lupus erythematosus; hepatitis; cardiac asystole; ventricular ectopy; idioventricular rhythms; paradoxical tachycardia; arterial embolism; hypotension; ventricular extrasystoles; complete AV block; ventricular flutter.

PROCAINAMIDE

Tablets: 250, 375, and 500 mg (*Rx*)	Various, *Pronestyl* (Princeton Pharm.)
Capsules: 250, 375, and 500 mg (*Rx*)	Various, *Pronestyl* (Princeton Pharm.)
Injection: 100 and 500 mg/mL (*Rx*)	Various, *Pronestyl* (Princeton Pharm.)
Tablets, sustained-release: 250, 500, 750, and 1000 mg (*Rx*)	Various, *Procan SR* (Parke-Davis), *Pronestyl-SR* (Princeton Pharm.)

Warning:
   The prolonged administration often leads to the development of a positive antinuclear antibody (ANA) test. If a positive ANA titer develops, assess the ben-
   efit/risk ratio related to continued therapy.

Indications
   Treatment of documented ventricular arrhythmias, such as sustained ventricular tachycardia, that are judged to be life-threatening.

Administration and Dosage
   Oral: Oral dosage forms are preferable for less urgent arrhythmias as well as for long-
   term maintenance after initial parenteral therapy. Individualize dosage based on
   clinical assessment of the degree of underlying myocardial disease, the patient's age
   and renal function.

   As a general guide, for younger adult patients with normal renal function, an initial total daily oral dose of $\leq$ 50 mg/kg may be used, given in divided doses every 3
   hours, to maintain therapeutic blood levels. For older patients, especially those >
   50 years of age, or for patients with renal, hepatic, or cardiac insufficiency, lesser
   amounts or longer intervals may produce adequate blood levels and decrease the
   probability of occurrence of dose-related adverse reactions. Administer the total
   daily dose in divided doses at 3-, 4-, or 6-hour intervals and adjust according to
   the patient's response.

Guidelines to Provide up to 50 mg/kg/day Procainamide			
Weight		Dose every 3 hours (standard formulation)	Dose every 6 hours (sustained release)
lb	kg		
88-110	40-50	250 mg	500 mg
132-154	60-70	375 mg	750 mg
176-198	80-90	500 mg	1 g
> 220	> 100	625 mg	1.25 g

[1] Initial dosage schedule guide only, to be adjusted for each patient individually, based on age, cardiorenal function, blood level (if available),
and clinical response.

   Sustained-release products are not recommended for initial therapy. Total dosage (50 mg/kg/day) may be given in divided doses every 6 hours.

   Parenteral: Useful for arrhythmias that require immediate suppression and for maintenance of arrhythmia control. IV therapy allows most rapid control of serious
arrhythmias, including those following MI; use in circumstances where close observation and monitoring of the patient are possible, such as in hospital or emergency facilities. IM administration is less apt to produce temporary high plasma
levels but therapeutic plasma levels are not obtained as rapidly as with IV administration.

   IM administration – IM administration may be used as an alternative to the oral
route for patients with less threatening arrhythmias but who are nauseated or vomiting, who are ordered to receive nothing by mouth preoperatively, or who may
have malabsorptive problems. An initial daily dose of 50 mg/kg may be estimated.
Divide this amount into fractional doses of $\frac{1}{8}$ to $\frac{1}{4}$ to be injected IM every 3 to
6 hours until oral therapy is possible. If > 3 injections are given, assess patient factors such as age and renal function, clinical response and, if available, blood levels of procainamide and NAPA in adjusting further doses for that individual. For

treatment of arrhythmias associated with anesthesia or surgery, the suggested dose is 100 to 500 mg by IM injection.

IV –

Dilutions and Rates for IV Infusions of Procainamide				
Infusion	Final concentration	Infusion volume[1]	Procainamide to be added	Infusion rate
Initial loading infusion	20 mg/mL	50 mL	1000 mg	1 mL/min (for up to 25 to 30 min)
Maintenance infusion[2]	2 mg/mL or	500 mL	1000 mg	1 to 3 mL/min
	4 mg/mL	250 mL	1000 mg	0.5 to 1.5 mL/min

[1] All infusions should be made up to final volume with 5% Dextrose Injection, USP.
[2] The maintenance infusion rates are calculated to deliver 2 to 6 mg/min depending on body weight, renal elimination rate and steady-state plasma level needed to maintain control of the arrhythmia. The 4 mg/mL maintenance concentration may be preferred if total infused volume must be limited.

Cautiously administer the IV injection to avoid a possible hypotensive response. Initial arrhythmia control, under blood pressure and ECG monitoring, may usually be accomplished safely within 30 minutes by either of the 2 methods that follow:

1) Slowly direct injection into a vein or into tubing of an established infusion line at a rate not to exceed 50 mg/min. It is advisable to dilute either the 100 or the 500 mg/mL concentrations prior to IV injection to facilitate control of dosage rate. Doses of 100 mg may be administered every 5 minutes at this rate until the arrhythmia is suppressed or until 500 mg has been administered, after which it is advisable to wait ≥ 10 minutes to allow for more distribution into tissues before resuming.

2) Alternatively, a loading infusion containing 20 mg/mL (1 g diluted to 50 mL with 5% Dextrose Injection, USP) may be administered at a constant rate of 1 mL/min for 25 to 30 minutes to deliver 500 to 600 mg. Some effects may be seen after infusion of the first 100 or 200 mg; it is unusual to require > 600 mg to achieve satisfactory antiarrhythmic effects.

The maximum advisable dosage to be given either by repeated bolus injections or such loading infusion is 1 g.

To maintain therapeutic levels, a more dilute IV infusion at a concentration of 2 mg/mL is convenient (1 g in 500 mL 5% Dextrose Injection, USP), and may be administered at 1 to 3 mL/min. If daily total fluid intake must be limited, a 4 mg/mL concentration (1 g in 250 mL of 5% Dextrose Injection, USP) administered at 0.5 to 1.5 mL/min will deliver an equivalent 2 to 6 mg/min. Assess the amount needed in a given patient to maintain the therapeutic level principally from the clinical response. Adjust for each patient based on close observation. A maintenance infusion rate of 50 mcg/kg/min to a person with a normal renal procainamide elimination half-life of 3 hours should produce a plasma level of ≈ 6.5 mcg/mL.

Terminate IV therapy if persistent conduction disturbances or hypotension develop. As soon as the patient's basic cardiac rhythm appears to be stabilized, oral antiarrhythmic maintenance therapy is preferable (if indicated and possible). A period of ≈ 3 to 4 hours (one half-life for renal elimination, ordinarily) should elapse after the last IV dose before administering the first dose of oral procainamide.

Children: The following doses have been suggested.

Oral – 15 to 50 mg/kg/day divided every 3 to 6 hours; maximum 4 g/day.

IM – 20 to 30 mg/kg/day divided every 4 to 6 hours; maximum 4 g/day.

IV – *Loading dose,* 3 to 6 mg/kg/dose over 5 minutes. *Maintenance,* 20 to 80 mcg/kg/min continuous infusion. Maximum 100 mg/dose or 2 g/day.

Actions

Pharmacology: Procainamide, a class IA antiarrhythmic, increases the effective refractory period of the atria, and to a lesser extent the bundle of His-Purkinje system and ventricles of the heart.

Electrophysiology – The ECG may show slight sinus tachycardia and widened QRS complexes and, less regularly, prolonged QT and PR intervals, as well as some decrease in QRS and T-wave amplitude.

Pharmacokinetics:

Absorption/Distribution – Oral procainamide is resistant to digestive hydrolysis, and the drug is well absorbed from the entire small intestinal surface, but individual patients vary in their completeness of absorption. Following oral use, plasma levels peak at ≈ 90 to 120 minutes. Following IM injection, plasma levels peak in 15 to 60 minutes. IV use can produce therapeutic plasma levels within minutes. About 15% to 20% is reversibly bound to plasma proteins. The apparent volume of distribution eventually reaches ≈ 2 L/kg with a half-life of ≈ 5 minutes.

Metabolism/Excretion – A significant fraction of the circulating procainamide may be metabolized in hepatocytes to N-acetylprocainamide (NAPA), ranging from 16% to 33% of an administered dose. NAPA also has significant antiarrhythmic activity and somewhat slower renal clearance than procainamide. The elimination half-life of procainamide is 3 to 4 hours in patients with normal renal function, but reduced creatinine clearance (Ccr) and advancing age each prolong the elimination half-life. Half-life and renal clearance are also reduced in infants. Thirty percent to 60% of the drug is excreted as unchanged procainamide, and 6% to 52% as the NAPA derivative. Both procainamide and NAPA are eliminated by active tubular secretion as well as by glomerular filtration.

Contraindications

Complete heart block; idiosyncratic hypersensitivity; lupus erythematosus; torsades de pointes.

Warnings

Blood dyscrasias: Agranulocytosis, bone marrow depression, neutropenia, hypoplastic anemia and thrombocytopenia in patients receiving procainamide have been reported at a rate of ≈ 0.5%. Fatalities have occurred (with ≈ 20% to 25% mortality in reported cases of agranulocytosis). Perform complete blood counts including white cell, differential, and platelet counts at weekly intervals for the first 3 months of therapy, and periodically thereafter. Perform complete blood counts promptly if the patient develops any signs of infection (eg, fever, chills, sore throat, stomatitis), bruising, or bleeding. If any of these hematologic disorders are identified, discontinue therapy. Blood counts usually return to normal within 1 month of discontinuation. Use caution in patients with preexisting marrow failure or cytopenia of any type.

Mortality: At present it is prudent to consider any antiarrhythmic agent to have a significant risk in patients with structural heart disease.

Complete heart block: Do not administer to patients with complete heart block because of its effects in suppressing nodal or ventricular pacemakers and the hazard of asystole. If significant slowing of ventricular rate occurs during treatment without evidence of AV conduction appearing, stop procainamide. In cases of second-degree AV block or various types of hemiblock, avoid or discontinue procainamide because of the possibility of increased severity of block, unless the ventricular rate is controlled by an electrical pacemaker.

Torsades de pointes: Procainamide may aggravate this special type of ventricular extrasystole or tachycardia instead of suppressing it.

Lupus erythematosus: If the lupus erythematosus-like syndrome develops in a patient with recurrent life-threatening arrhythmias not controlled by other agents, corticosteroid suppressive therapy may be used concomitantly with procainamide. Because the procainamide-induced lupoid syndrome rarely includes the dangerous pathologic renal changes, therapy may not necessarily have to be stopped unless the symptoms of serositis and the possibility of further lupoid effects are of greater risk than the benefit of procainamide in controlling arrhythmias. Patients with rapid acetylation capability are less likely to develop the lupoid syndrome after prolonged therapy.

Asymptomatic ventricular premature contractions: Avoid treatment of patients with this condition.

Digitalis intoxication: Exercise caution in the use of procainamide in arrhythmias associated with digitalis intoxication. Procainamide can suppress digitalis-induced arrhythmias; however, if there is concomitant marked disturbance of AV conduction, additional depression of conduction and ventricular asystole or fibrillation may result. Consider use of procainamide only if discontinuation of digitalis, and therapy with potassium, lidocaine, or phenytoin are ineffective.

First-degree heart block: Exercise caution if the patient exhibits or develops first-degree heart block while taking procainamide; dosage reduction is advised. If the block persists despite dosage reduction, evaluate the continuation of procainamide on the basis of current benefit vs risk of increased heart block.

Predigitalization for atrial flutter or fibrillation: Cardiovert or digitalize patients with atrial flutter or fibrillation prior to procainamide administration to avoid enhancement of AV conduction, which may result in ventricular rate acceleration beyond tolerable limits. Adequate digitalization reduces the possibility of sudden increase in ventricular rate.

CHF: Use with caution in patients with CHF and in those with acute ischemic heart disease or cardiomyopathy because even slight depression of myocardial contractility may further reduce cardiac output of the damaged heart.

Concurrent antiarrhythmic agents: Concurrent antiarrhythmic agents may produce enhanced prolongation of conduction or depression of contractility and hypotension, especially in patients with cardiac decompensation. Reserve concurrent use of procainamide with other Class IA antiarrhythmic agents (eg, quinidine, disopyramide) for patients with serious arrhythmias unresponsive to a single drug and use only if close observation is possible.

Myasthenia gravis: Procainamide administration in myasthenia gravis patients may be hazardous without optimal adjustment of anticholinesterase medications and other precautions. Immediately after initiation of therapy, closely observe patients for muscular weakness if myasthenia gravis is a possibility.

Renal insufficiency: Renal insufficiency may lead to accumulation of high plasma levels from conventional oral doses of procainamide, with effects similar to those of overdosage unless dosage is adjusted for the individual patient.

Hypersensitivity reactions: In patients sensitive to procaine or other ester-type local anesthetics, cross-sensitivity to procainamide is unlikely; however, consider the possibility. Do not use procainamide if it produces acute allergic dermatitis, asthma or anaphylactic symptoms.

Pregnancy: Category C.

Lactation: Discontinue nursing or the drug, taking into account the importance of the drug to the mother.

Children: Safety and efficacy have not been established.

Precautions

Monitoring: After achieving and maintaining therapeutic plasma concentrations and satisfactory ECG and clinical responses, continue frequent periodic monitoring of vital signs and ECG. If evidence of QRS widening of > 25% or marked prolongation of the QT interval occurs, concern for overdosage is appropriate; reduction in dosage is advisable if a 50% increase occurs. Elevated serum creatinine or urea nitrogen, reduced Ccr or history of renal insufficiency, as well as use in older patients (> 50 years of age), provide grounds to anticipate that less than the usual dosage and longer time intervals between doses may suffice. If facilities are available for measurement of plasma procainamide and NAPA levels or acetylation capability, individual dose adjustment for optimal therapeutic levels may be easier, but close observation of clinical effectiveness is the most important criterion.

Embolization: In conversion of atrial fibrillation to normal sinus rhythm by any means, dislodgement of mural thrombi may lead to embolization.

Tartrazine sensitivity: Some of these products contain tartrazine that may cause allergic-type reactions (including bronchial asthma). Although the overall incidence of tartrazine sensitivity in the general population is low, it is frequently seen in patients who also have aspirin hypersensitivity.

Sulfite sensitivity: Some of these products contain sulfites that may cause allergic-type reactions including anaphylactic symptoms and life-threatening or less severe asthmatic episodes. Sulfite sensitivity is seen more frequently in asthmatic or atopic nonasthmatic persons.

Drug Interactions

Drugs that may affect procainamide include beta blockers, ethanol, histamine H_2 antagonists, quinidine, and trimethoprim. Drugs that may be affected by procainamide include lidocaine and succinylcholine. Tests that depend on fluorescence measurement may also be affected.

Adverse Reactions

Significant adverse reactions include a lupus erythematosus-like syndrome of arthralgia, pleural or abdominal pain, and sometimes arthritis, pleural effusion, pericarditis, fever, chills, myalgia, and possibly related hematologic or skin lesions (after prolonged administration); neutropenia; thrombocytopenia; agranulocytosis (after repeated use; deaths have occurred); anorexia; nausea; vomiting; abdominal pain; bitter taste; diarrhea.

DISOPYRAMIDE

Capsules: 100 and 150 mg (*Rx*)	Various, *Norpace* (Searle)
Capsules, extended release: 100 and 150 mg (*Rx*)	Various, *Norpace* CR (Searle)

Indications

Treatment of documented ventricular arrhythmias (eg, sustained ventricular tachycardia) considered to be life-threatening.

Administration and Dosage

Individualize dosage. Initiate treatment in the hospital.

Adults: 400 to 800 mg/day. The recommended dosage for most adults is 600 mg/day. For patients < 50 kg (110 pounds), give 400 mg/day. Divide the total daily dose and administer every 6 hours in the immediate release form or every 12 hours in the controlled-release form.

Children: Divide daily dosage and administer equal doses every 6 hours or at intervals according to patient needs. Closely monitor plasma levels and therapeutic response. Hospitalize patients during initial treatment and start dose titration at the lower end of the ranges provided below:

Suggested Total Daily Disopyramide Dosage in Children[1]	
Age (years)	Disopyramide (mg/kg/day)
< 1	10 to 30
1 to 4	10 to 20
4 to 12	10 to 15
12 to 18	6 to 15

[1] Prepare a 1 to 10 mg/mL suspension by adding contents of the immediate release capsule to cherry syrup, NF. The resulting suspension, when refrigerated, is stable for 1 month; shake thoroughly before measuring dose. Dispense in an amber glass bottle. Do not use the controlled-release form to prepare the solution.

Initial loading dose: For rapid control of ventricular arrhythmia, give an initial loading dose of 300 mg immediate release (200 mg for patients < 50 kg [110 lbs]). Therapeutic effects are attained in 30 minutes to 3 hours. If there is no response or no evidence of toxicity within 6 hours of the loading dose, 200 mg every 6 hours may be administered instead of the usual 150 mg. If there is no response within 48 hours, discontinue the drug or carefully monitor subsequent doses of 250 or 300 mg every 6 hours.

Do not use the controlled-release form initially if rapid plasma levels are desired.

Severe refractory ventricular tachycardia: A limited number of patients have tolerated up to 1600 mg/day (400 mg every 6 hours), resulting in plasma levels up to 9 mcg/mL. Hospitalize patients for close evaluation and continuous monitoring.

Cardiomyopathy or possible cardiac decompensation: Do not administer a loading dose, and limit the initial dosage to 100 mg immediate release every 6 to 8 hours. Make subsequent dosage adjustments gradually.

Renal/Hepatic function impairment: For patients with moderate renal insufficiency (Ccr > 40 mL/min) or hepatic insufficiency, the recommended dosage is 400 mg/day given in divided doses (either 100 mg every 6 hours for immediate release or 200 mg every 12 hours for controlled release).

In severe renal insufficiency (Ccr ≤ 40 mL/min), the recommended dosage is 100 mg of the immediate release form given at the intervals shown in the table below, with or without an initial loading dose of 150 mg.

Disopyramide Dosage in Renal Impairment			
Creatinine clearance (mL/min)	Loading dose (mg)	Dose (mg)	Dosage interval (hours)
40-30	150	100	8
30-15	150	100	12
< 15	150	100	24

Transfer to disopyramide: Use the regular maintenance schedule, without a loading dose, 6 to 12 hours after the last dose of quinidine or 3 to 6 hours after the last dose of procainamide. Where withdrawal of quinidine or procainamide is likely to produce life-threatening arrhythmias, consider hospitalization.

When transferring from immediate to controlled release, start maintenance schedule of controlled release 6 hours after the last dose of immediate release.

Actions
Pharmacology:

Mechanism of action – Disopyramide is a class IA antiarrhythmic agent that decreases the rate of diastolic depolarization (phase 4), decreases the upstroke velocity (phase 0), increases the action potential duration of normal cardiac cells, and prolongs the refractory period (phases 2 and 3). It also decreases the disparity in refractoriness between infarcted and adjacent normally perfused myocardium.

Pharmacokinetics:

Absorption/Distribution – Following oral administration of immediate-release disopyramide, the drug is rapidly and almost completely absorbed. Peak plasma levels usually occur within 2 hours. Therapeutic plasma levels of disopyramide are 2 to 4 mcg/mL. Protein binding is concentration-dependent and varies from 50% to 65%; it is difficult to predict the concentration of the free drug when total drug is measured.

Metabolism/Excretion – About 50% is excreted in the urine as the unchanged drug and 30% as metabolites (20% mono-N-dealkyldisopyramide [MND]). The plasma concentration of MND is ≈ one-tenth that of disopyramide. The mean plasma half-life is 6.7 hours (range, 4 to 10 hours). In impaired renal function, half-life values ranged from 8 to 18 hours. Therefore, decrease the dose in renal failure to avoid drug accumulation.

Immediate-release vs controlled-release – Following multiple doses, steady-state plasma levels of between 2 and 4 mcg/mL were attained following either 150 mg every 6 hours (immediate release) or 300 mg every 12 hours (controlled release).

Contraindications
Cardiogenic shock; preexisting second- or third-degree AV block (if no pacemaker is present); congenital QT prolongation; sick sinus syndrome; hypersensitivity to disopyramide.

Warnings

Proarrhythmic effects: Because of the proarrhythmic effects, use with lesser arrhythmias is generally not recommended.

Asymptomatic ventricular premature contractions: Avoid treatment of patients with this condition.

Survival: Antiarrhythmic drugs have not been shown to enhance survival in patients with ventricular arrhythmias.

Negative inotropic properties:

    Heart failure/hypotension – May cause or aggravate CHF or produce severe hypotension, especially in patients with depressed systolic function. Do not use in patients with uncompensated or marginally compensated CHF or hypotension unless secondary to cardiac arrhythmia. Treat patients with a history of heart failure with careful attention to the maintenance of cardiac function, including optimal digitalization. If hypotension occurs or CHF worsens, discontinue use; restart at a lower dosage after adequate cardiac compensation has been established.

    Do not give a loading dose to patients with myocarditis or other cardiomyopathy; closely monitor initial dosage and subsequent adjustments.

    QRS widening – QRS widening (> 25%), although unusual, may occur; discontinue use in such cases.

    QT_c *prolongation* – QT_c prolongation and worsening of the arrhythmia, including ventricular tachycardia and fibrillation, may occur. Patients who have QT prolongation in response to quinidine may be at particular risk. Disopyramide has been associated with torsade de pointes. If QT prolongation > 25% is observed and if ectopy continues, monitor closely and consider discontinuing the drug.

Atrial tachyarrhythmias: Digitalize patients with atrial flutter or fibrillation prior to administration to ensure that enhancement of AV conduction does not increase ventricular rate beyond acceptable limits.

Conduction abnormalities: Use caution in patients with sick sinus syndrome, Wolff-Parkinson-White (WPW) syndrome or bundle branch block.

Heart block: If first-degree heart block develops, reduce dosage. If the block persists, drug continuation must depend upon the benefit compared with the risk of higher degrees of heart block. Development of second- or third-degree AV block or unifascicular, bifascicular, or trifascicular block requires discontinuation of therapy, unless ventricular rate is controlled by a ventricular pacemaker.

Concomitant antiarrhythmic therapy: Reserve concomitant use of disopyramide with other class IA antiarrhythmics or propranolol for life-threatening arrhythmias unresponsive to a single agent. Such use may produce serious negative inotropic effects or may excessively prolong conduction, particularly with cardiac decompensation.

Hypoglycemia: Hypoglycemia has been reported in rare instances. Monitor blood glucose levels in patients with CHF, chronic malnutrition, hepatic disease, and in those taking drugs which could compromise normal glucoregulatory mechanisms in the absence of food.

Anticholinergic activity: Do not use in patients with urinary retention, glaucoma, or myasthenia gravis unless adequate overriding measures are taken. Males with benign prostatic hypertrophy are at particular risk of having urinary retention. In patients with a family history of glaucoma, measure intraocular pressure before initiating therapy.

Renal function impairment: Reduce dosage in impaired renal function. Carefully monitor ECG for signs of overdosage. The controlled-release form is not recommended for patients with severe renal insufficiency.

Hepatic function impairment: Impairment increases plasma half-life; reduce dosage in such patients. Carefully monitor the ECG. Patients with cardiac dysfunction have a higher potential for hepatic impairment.

Pregnancy: Category C.

Lactation: Disopyramide has been detected in breast milk.

Precautions

Potassium imbalance: Disopyramide may be ineffective in *hypo*kalemia and its toxic effects may be enhanced in *hyper*kalemia. Correct any potassium deficit before instituting therapy.

Drug Interactions

Drugs that may affect disopyramide include beta blockers, erythromycin, hydantoins, quinidine, and rifampin. Drugs that may be affected by disopyramide include quinidine, anticoagulants, and digoxin.

Adverse Reactions

The most serious adverse reactions are hypotension and CHF. The most common reactions are anticholinergic and are dose-dependent. These may be transitory, but may be persistent or severe. Urinary retention is the most serious anticholinergic effect. Adverse reactions occurring in $\geq$ 3% of patients include urinary retention, frequency and urgency; dizziness; fatigue; headache; nausea; pain; bloating; gas; dry mouth; urinary hesitancy; constipation; blurred vision; dry nose; eyes and throat; muscle weakness; malaise; aches/pain.

LIDOCAINE HCl

Injection: (for IM administration) 300 mg/3 mL automatic injection device (*Rx*)	*LidoPen Auto-Injector* (Survival Technology)
(for direct IV administration) 1% (10 mg/mL), 2% (20 mg/mL) (*Rx*)	Various, *Xylocaine HCl IV for Cardiac Arrhythmias* (Astra)
(for IV admixtures) 10% (100 mg/mL) (*Rx*)	Various
(for IV admixtures) 4% (40 mg/mL), 20% (200 mg/mL) (*Rx*)	Various, *Xylocaine HCl IV for Cardiac Arrhythmias* (Astra)
(for IV infusion) 0.2% (2 mg/mL), 0.4% (4 mg/mL), 0.8% (8 mg/mL) (*Rx*)	Various

Indications

IV: Acute management of ventricular arrhythmias occurring during cardiac manipulation, such as cardiac surgery or in relation to acute myocardial infarction (MI).

IM: Single doses are justified in the following exceptional circumstances: When ECG equipment is not available to verify the diagnosis but the potential benefits outweigh the possible risks; when facilities for IV administration are not readily available; by the patient in the prehospital phase of suspected acute MI, directed by qualified medical personnel viewing the transmitted ECG.

Unlabeled uses: In pediatric patients with cardiac arrest, < 10% develop ventricular fibrillation, and others develop ventricular tachycardia; the hemodynamically compromised child may develop ventricular couplets or frequent premature ventricular beats. In these cases, administer 1 mg/kg lidocaine by the IV, intraosseous, or endotracheal route. A second 1 mg/kg dose may be given in 10 to 15 minutes. Start a lidocaine infusion if the second dose is required; a third bolus may be needed in 10 to 15 minutes to maintain therapeutic levels.

Administration and Dosage

IM: 300 mg. The deltoid muscle is preferred. Avoid intravascular injection. Use only the 10% solution for IM injection.

The *LidoPen Auto-Injector* unit is for self-administration into deltoid muscle or anterolateral aspect of thigh. Patient instructions are provided with product.

Replacement therapy – As soon as possible, change patient to IV lidocaine or to an oral antiarrhythmic preparation for maintenance therapy. However, if necessary, an additional IM injection may be administered after 60 to 90 minutes.

IV: Use only lidocaine injection without preservatives, clearly labeled for IV use. Monitor ECG constantly to avoid potential overdosage and toxicity.

IV bolus – IV bolus is used to establish rapid therapeutic blood levels. Continuous IV infusion is necessary to maintain antiarrhythmic effects. The usual dose is 50 to 100 mg, given at a rate of 25 to 50 mg/min. If the initial injection does not produce the desired clinical response, give a second bolus dose after 5 minutes. Give no more than 200 to 300 mg/hour.

Reduce loading (bolus) doses – Reduce loading (bolus) doses in patients with CHF or reduced cardiac output and in the elderly. However, some investigators recommend the usual loading dose be administered and only the maintenance dosage be reduced.

IV continuous infusion – IV continuous infusion is used to maintain therapeutic plasma levels following loading doses in patients in whom arrhythmias tend to recur and who cannot receive oral antiarrhythmic drugs. Administer at a rate of 1 to 4 mg/min (20 to 50 mcg/kg/min). Reduce maintenance doses in patients with heart failure or liver disease, or who are also receiving other drugs known to decrease clearance of lidocaine or decrease liver blood flow and in patients > 70 years of age. Reassess the rate of infusion as soon as the cardiac rhythm stabilizes or at the earliest signs of toxicity. Change patients to oral antiarrhythmic agents for maintenance therapy as soon as possible. It is rarely necessary to continue IV infusions for prolonged periods. Use a precision volume control IV set for continuous IV infusion.

Children – The American Heart Association's Standards and Guidelines recommend a bolus dose of 1 mg/kg, followed by an infusion of 30 mcg/kg/min. The following dosage has also been suggested:

Loading dose – Loading dose, 1 mg/kg/dose given IV or intratracheally every 5 to 10 min to desired effect, maximum total dose 5 mg/kg; *maintenance*, 20 to 50 mcg/kg/min.

Actions
Pharmacology: Therapeutic concentrations of lidocaine attenuate phase 4 diastolic depolarization, decrease automaticity and cause a decrease or no change in excitability and membrane responsiveness. Action potential duration and effective refractory period (ERP) of Purkinje fibers and ventricular muscle are decreased, while the ratio of ERP to action potential duration is increased. Lidocaine raises ventricular fibrillation threshold. AV nodal conduction time is unchanged or shortened. Lidocaine increases the electrical stimulation threshold of the ventricle during diastole.

Pharmacokinetics:
Absorption/Distribution – Lidocaine is ineffective orally; it is most commonly administered IV with an immediate onset (within minutes) and brief duration (10 to 20 minutes) of action following a bolus dose. Continuous IV infusion of lidocaine (1 to 4 mg/min) is necessary to maintain antiarrhythmic effects. Following IM administration, therapeutic serum levels are achieved in 5 to 15 minutes and may persist for up to 2 hours. Higher and more rapid serum levels are achieved by injection into the deltoid muscle. Therapeutic serum levels are 1.5 to 6 mcg/mL; serum levels > 6 to 10 mcg/mL are usually toxic. Lidocaine is ≈ 50% protein bound (concentration-dependent).

Metabolism/Excretion – Extensive biotransformation in the liver (≈ 90%) results in at least 2 active metabolites, monoethylglycinexylidide (MEGX) and glycinexylidide (GX). Lidocaine exhibits a biphasic half-life. The distribution phase is ≈ 10 minutes. The elimination half-life is 1.5 to 2 hours; half-life may be ≥ 3 hours following infusions of > 24 hours. Any condition that alters liver function, including changes in liver blood flow, which could result from severe congestive heart failure (CHF) or shock, may alter lidocaine kinetics. Less than 10% of the parent drug is excreted unchanged in the urine. Renal elimination plays an important role in the elimination of the metabolites.

Contraindications
Hypersensitivity to amide local anesthetics; Stokes-Adams syndrome; Wolff-Parkinson-White syndrome; severe degrees of sinoatrial, atrioventricular (AV), or intraventricular block in the absence of an artificial pacemaker.

Warnings

Survival: Prophylactic single dose lidocaine administered in a monitored environment does not appear to affect mortality in the earliest phase of acute MI, and may harm some patients who are later shown not to have suffered an acute MI.

Constant ECG monitoring: Constant ECG monitoring is essential for proper administration. Have emergency resuscitative equipment and drugs immediately available.

IV use: Signs of excessive depression of cardiac conductivity should be followed by dosage reduction and, if necessary, prompt cessation of IV infusion.

IM use: May increase creatine phosphokinase (CPK) levels. Use of the enzyme determination without isoenzyme separation, as a diagnostic test for acute MI, may be compromised.

Cardiac effects: Use with caution and in lower doses in patients with CHF, reduced cardiac output, digitalis toxicity accompanied by AV block and in the elderly.

In sinus bradycardia or incomplete heart block, lidocaine administration for the elimination of ventricular ectopy without prior acceleration in heart rate (eg, by atropine, isoproterenol or electric pacing) may promote more frequent and serious ventricular arrhythmias or complete heart block. Use with caution in patients with hypovolemia and shock, and all forms of heart block.

Acceleration of ventricular rate – Acceleration of ventricular rate may occur when administered to patients with atrial flutter or fibrillation.

Hypersensitivity: Hypersensitivity reactions may occur. Refer to Management of Acute Hypersensitivity Reactions.

Renal/Hepatic function impairment: Use caution with repeated or prolonged use in liver or renal disease; possible toxic accumulation may occur.

Pregnancy: Category B.

Lactation: Exercise caution when administering to a nursing woman.

Children: Safety and efficacy have not been established; reduce dosage. The IM auto-injector device is not recommended in children < 50 kg.

Precautions

Malignant hyperthermia: Amide local anesthetic administration has been associated with acute onset of fulminant hypermetabolism of skeletal muscle known as malignant hyperthermic crisis. Recognition of early unexplained signs of tachycardia, tachypnea, labile blood pressure, and metabolic acidosis may precede temperature elevation. Successful outcome depends on early diagnosis, prompt discontinuance of the triggering agent and institution of treatment, including oxygen, supportive measures, and IV dantrolene sodium.

Drug Interactions

Drugs that may affect lidocaine include beta blockers, cimetidine, procainamide, tocainide, and succinylcholine.

Adverse Reactions

Significant drug interactions include lightheadedness; nervousness; drowsiness; dizziness; apprehension; confusion; mood changes; hallucinations; tremors; convulsions; unconsciousness; hypotension; bradycardia; cardiovascular collapse, which may lead to cardiac arrest; febrile response; soreness/infection at the injection site; venous thrombosis or phlebitis extending from the site of injection; extravasation; vomiting; respiratory depression/arrest

TOCAINIDE HCl

| Tablets: 400 and 600 mg (Rx) | Tonocard (Astra Merck) |

Warning:

Blood dyscrasias: Agranulocytosis, bone marrow depression, leukopenia, neutropenia, aplastic/hypoplastic anemia, thrombocytopenia, and sequelae such as septicemia and septic shock have occurred in patients receiving tocainide. Fatalities have occurred (with ≈ 25% mortality in reported agranulocytosis cases). Because most of these events have been noted during the first 12 weeks of therapy, perform complete blood counts, including white cell, differential, and platelet counts, optimally, at weekly intervals for the first 3 months of therapy, and frequently thereafter. Perform complete blood counts promptly if the patient develops any signs of infection (eg, fever, chills, sore throat, stomatitis), bruising, or bleeding. If any of these hematologic disorders are identified, discontinue tocainide and institute appropriate treatment if necessary. Blood counts usually return to normal within 1 month of discontinuation. Use with caution in patients with preexisting bone marrow failure or cytopenia of any type.

Pulmonary fibrosis: Pulmonary fibrosis, interstitial pneumonitis, fibrosing alveolitis, pulmonary edema, and pneumonia have occurred in patients receiving tocainide. Many of these events occurred in patients who were seriously ill. Fatalities have occurred. The experiences are usually characterized by bilateral infiltrates on x-ray and are frequently associated with dyspnea and cough. Fever may be present. Instruct patients to promptly report any pulmonary symptoms (eg, exertional dyspnea, cough, wheezing). Chest x-rays are advisable at this time. If these pulmonary disorders develop, discontinue tocainide.

Indications

Treatment of life-threatening ventricular arrhythmias.

Unlabeled uses: Tocainide may be beneficial in the treatment of myotonic dystrophy (800 to 1200 mg/day) and trigeminal neuralgia (20 mg/kg/day in 3 divided doses).

Administration and Dosage

Individualize dosage. Guide dosage titration by clinical and ECG evaluation. Dose-related adverse effects tend to occur early in treatment, and they usually decrease in severity and frequency with time. These effects may be minimized by taking tocainide with food or by taking smaller, more frequent doses.

Initial dose: 400 mg every 8 hours. Range is 1200 to 1800 mg/day given in 3 divided doses. Doses > 2400 mg/day have been administered infrequently. Patients who tolerate the 3 times/day regimen may be tried on a twice-daily regimen with careful monitoring.

Some patients, particularly those with renal or hepatic impairment, may be adequately treated with < 1200 mg/day.

Actions

Pharmacology: Tocainide produces dose-dependent decreases in sodium and potassium conductance, decreasing the excitability of myocardial cells. Most patients who respond to lidocaine also respond to tocainide. Failure to respond to lidocaine usually predicts failure to respond to tocainide. Tocainide is a Class IB antiarrhythmic.

Pharmacokinetics:

Absorption/Distribution – Following oral administration the bioavailability of tocainide approaches 100%; peak serum concentrations are attained in 0.5 to 2 hours. Bioavailability is unaffected by food. Tocainide undergoes negligible first-pass hepatic degradation. Approximately 10% to 20% is plasma protein bound. The therapeutic range is 4 to 10 mcg/mL.

Metabolism/Excretion – Inactivated via conjugation in the liver. The average plasma half-life is ≈ 15 hours. About 40% is excreted unchanged in urine; alkalinization of urine reduces the percent of drug excreted unchanged, yet acidification causes no alterations. Half-life increased in severe renal dysfunction.

Contraindications

Hypersensitivity to tocainide or to amide-type local anesthetics; patients with second- or third-degree AV block in the absence of an artificial ventricular pacemaker.

Warnings

Proarrhythmia: Tocainide may increase arrhythmias in some patients.

Cardiac effects: Tocainide has not been shown to prevent sudden death in patients with serious ventricular ectopy. It has potentially serious adverse effects, including ability to worsen arrhythmias. Evaluate each patient by ECG and clinically prior to and during therapy to determine if response supports continued treatment.

In patients with known heart failure or minimal cardiac reserve, use with caution because of the potential for aggravating the degree of heart failure.

Use caution when instituting or continuing antiarrhythmic therapy in the presence of signs of increasing depression of cardiac conductivity.

Acceleration of ventricular rate – Acceleration of ventricular rate occurs infrequently when tocainide is administered to patients with atrial flutter or fibrillation.

Renal/Hepatic function impairment: In patients with severe liver or kidney disease, the rate of drug elimination may be significantly decreased.

Pregnancy: Category C.

Lactation: Decide whether to discontinue nursing or the drug, taking into account importance of the drug to the mother.

Children: Safety and efficacy for use in children have not been established.

Precautions

Hypokalemia: Because antiarrhythmic drugs may be ineffective in patients with hypokalemia, correct potassium deficits if present.

Drug Interactions

Drugs that may interact include cimetidine, metoprolol, and rifampin.

Adverse Reactions

Adverse reactions occurring in ≥ 3% of patients include dizziness/vertigo; nausea; vomiting; anorexia; diarrhea/loose stools; arthritis/arthralgia; paresthesia; tremor; confusion/disorientation/hallucinations; headache; nervousness; altered mood/awareness/ataxia; hypotension; tachycardia; worsening CHF (including arrhythmias); diaphoresis; rash/skin lesion; and blurred vision/visual disturbances. Adverse reactions leading to discontinuation of therapy occurred in 21% of patients and were usually related to the CNS or GI system.

PROPAFENONE HCl

Tablets: 150, 225, and 300 mg (Rx)	*Rythmol* (Knoll)

Indications

Treatment of documented life-threatening ventricular arrhythmias, such as sustained ventricular tachycardia.

Because of the proarrhythmic effects of propafenone, reserve its use for patients in whom the benefits of treatment outweigh the risks. The use of propafenone is not recommended in patients with less severe ventricular arrhythmias, even if the patients are symptomatic.

Administration and Dosage

Individually titrate on the basis of response and tolerance. Initiate with 150 mg every 8 hours (450 mg/day). Dosage may be increased at a minimum of 3 to 4 day intervals to 225 mg every 8 hours (675 mg/day) and, if necessary, to 300 mg every

8 hours (900 mg/day). The safety and efficacy of dosages exceeding 900 mg/day have not been established. In those patients in whom significant widening of the QRS complex or second- or third-degree AV block occurs, consider dose reduction.

As with other antiarrhythmics, in the elderly or patients with marked previous myocardial damage, increase dose more gradually during initial treatment phase.

Actions
Pharmacology: Propafenone is a Class IC antiarrhythmic with local anesthetic effects and direct stabilizing action on myocardial membranes.

Pharmacokinetics:

Absorption/Distribution – Propafenone is nearly completely absorbed after oral administration with peak plasma levels occurring ≈ 3.5 hours after administration. It exhibits extensive first-pass metabolism resulting in a dose-dependent and dosage-form-dependent absolute bioavailability. Propafenone follows a nonlinear pharmacokinetic disposition presumably due to saturation of first-pass hepatic metabolism as the liver is exposed to higher concentrations of propafenone and shows a very high degree of interindividual variability.

Metabolism/Excretion – There are 2 genetically determined patterns of propafenone metabolism. In > 90% of patients, the drug is rapidly and extensively metabolized with an elimination half-life of 2 to 10 hours. These patients metabolize propafenone into two active metabolites: 5-hydroxypropafenone and N-depropylpropafenone. They both are usually present in concentrations < 20% of propafenone. The saturable hydroxylation pathway is responsible for the nonlinear pharmacokinetic disposition.

Contraindications
Uncontrolled CHF; cardiogenic shock; sinoatrial, AV and intraventricular disorders of impulse generation or conduction (eg, sick sinus node syndrome, AV block) in the absence of an artificial pacemaker; bradycardia; marked hypotension; bronchospastic disorders; manifest electrolyte imbalance; hypersensitivity to the drug.

Warnings
Mortality: An excessive mortality or non-fatal cardiac arrest rate was seen in patients treated with encainide or flecainide compared with that seen in patients assigned to carefully matched placebo-treated groups.

Proarrhythmic effects: Propafenone may cause new or worsened arrhythmias. Such proarrhythmic effects range from an increase in frequency of PVCs to the development of more severe ventricular tachycardia, ventricular fibrillation or torsade de pointes, which may lead to fatal consequences. It is essential that each patient be evaluated electrocardiographically and clinically prior to, and during therapy to determine whether response to propafenone supports continued use.

Non-life-threatening arrhythmias: Use of propafenone is not recommended in patients with less severe ventricular arrhythmias, even if the patients are symptomatic.

Survival: There is no evidence from controlled trials that the use of propafenone favorably affects survival or the incidence of sudden death.

Nonallergic bronchospasm (eg, chronic bronchitis, emphysema): In general, these patients should not receive propafenone or other agents with beta-adrenergic blocking activity.

CHF: New or worsened CHF has occurred in 3.7% of patients.

As propafenone exerts both beta blockade and a (dose-related) negative inotropic effect on cardiac muscle, fully compensate patients with CHF before receiving propafenone. If CHF worsens, discontinue propafenone unless CHF is due to the cardiac arrhythmia and, if indicated, restart at a lower dosage only after adequate cardiac compensation has been established.

Conduction disturbances: Propafenone causes first-degree AV block. Average PR interval prolongation and increases in QRS duration are closely correlated with dosage increases and concomitant increases in propafenone plasma concentrations. Development of second- or third-degree AV block requires a reduction in dosage or discontinuation of propafenone. Bundle branch block and intraventricular conduction delay have occurred. Bradycardia has also occurred. Patients with sick sinus node syndrome should not be treated with propafenone.

Effects on pacemaker threshold: Pacing and sensing thresholds of artificial pacemakers may be altered. Monitor and program pacemakers accordingly during therapy.

Hematologic disturbances: Agranulocytosis with fever and sepsis has occurred. Unexplained fever or decrease in white cell count, particularly during the first 3 months of therapy, warrants consideration of possible agranulocytosis/granulocytopenia.

Renal function impairment: A considerable percentage of propafenone metabolites are excreted in the urine. Administer cautiously in impaired renal function.

Hepatic function impairment: Propafenone is highly metabolized by the liver; administer cautiously to patients with impaired hepatic function. The clearance of propafenone is reduced and the elimination half-life increased in patients with significant hepatic dysfunction. The dose of propafenone should be ≈ 20% to 30% of the dose given to patients with normal hepatic function.

Elderly: Because of the possible increased risk of impaired hepatic or renal function in this age group, use with caution. The effective dose may be lower in these patients.

Pregnancy: Category C.

Lactation: It is not known whether this drug is excreted in breast milk. Discontinue nursing or discontinue the drug.

Children: The safety and efficacy in children have not been established.

Precautions

Elevated ANA titers: Positive ANA titers have occurred. They have been reversible upon cessation of treatment and may disappear even with continued therapy. Carefully evaluate patients who develop an abnormal ANA test and, if persistent or worsening elevation of ANA titers is detected, consider discontinuing therapy.

Drug Interactions

Drugs that may affect propafenone include local anesthetics, cimetidine, quinidine, and rifampin. Drugs that may be affected by propafenone include anticoagulants, beta blockers, cyclosporine, and digoxin.

Adverse Reactions

Adverse reactions occurring in ≥ 3% of patients include angina; first-degree AV block; CHF; intraventricular conduction delay; palpitations; proarrhythmia; ventricular tachycardia; dizziness; fatigue; headache; constipation; dyspepsia; nausea/vomiting; unusual taste; blurred vision; dyspnea. About 20% of patients discontinued treatment due to adverse reactions.

FLECAINIDE ACETATE

Tablets: 50, 100, and 150 mg (*Rx*)   *Tambocor* (3M Pharm.)

Indications

Atrial fibrillation: For the prevention of paroxysmal atrial fibrillation/flutter (PAF) associated with disabling symptoms and paroxysmal supraventricular tachycardias (PSVT), including atrioventricular nodal reentrant tachycardia, atrioventricular reentrant tachycardia, and other supraventricular tachycardias of unspecified mechanism associated with disabling symptoms in patients without structural heart disease.

Ventricular arrhythmias: Prevention of documented life-threatening ventricular arrhythmias, such as sustained ventricular tachycardia.

Not recommended in patients with less severe ventricular arrhythmias even if the patients are symptomatic. Because of proarrhythmic effects of flecainide, reserve use for patients in whom benefits outweigh risks.

Administration and Dosage

For patients with sustained ventricular tachycardia, initiate therapy in the hospital and monitor rhythm.

Do not increase dosage more frequently than once every 4 days, because optimal effect may not be achieved during the first 2 to 3 days of therapy.

An occasional patient not adequately controlled by (or intolerant of) a dose given at 12-hour intervals may be dosed at 8-hour intervals.

Once the arrhythmia is controlled, it may be possible to reduce the dose, as necessary, to minimize side effects or effects on conduction.

PSVT and PAF: The recommended starting dose is 50 mg every 12 hours. Doses may be increased in increments of 50 mg twice daily every 4 days until efficacy is achieved. For PAF patients, a substantial increase in efficacy without a substantial increase in discontinuation for adverse experiences may be achieved by increasing the flecainide dose from 50 to 100 mg twice/day. The maximum recommended dose for patients with paroxysmal supraventricular arrhythmias is 300 mg/day.

Sustained ventricular tachycardia:
    Initial dose – 100 mg every 12 hours. Increase in 50 mg increments twice daily every 4 days until effective. Most patients do not require > 150 mg every 12 hours (300 mg/day). Maximum dose is 400 mg/day.

    Use of higher initial doses and more rapid dosage adjustments have resulted in an increased incidence of proarrhythmic events and CHF, particularly during the first few days of dosing. A loading dose is not recommended.

Renal function impairment: In severe renal impairment (Ccr ≤ 35 mL/min/1.73 m^2), the initial dosage is 100 mg once daily (or 50 mg twice/day). Frequent plasma level monitoring is required to guide dosage adjustments. In patients with less severe renal disease, initial dosage is 100 mg every 12 hours. Increase dosage cautiously at intervals > 4 days, observing the patient closely for signs of adverse cardiac effects or other toxicity. It may take > 4 days before a new steady-state plasma level is reached following a dosage change. Monitor plasma levels to guide dosage adjustments.

Transfer to flecainide: Theoretically, when transferring patients from another antiarrhythmic to flecainide, allow at least 2 to 4 plasma half-lives to elapse for the drug being discontinued before starting flecainide at the usual dosage. Consider hospitalization of patients in whom withdrawal of a previous antiarrhythmic is likely to produce life-threatening arrhythmias.

Plasma level monitoring: The majority of patients treated successfully had trough plasma levels between 0.2 and 1mcg/mL. The probability of adverse experiences, especially cardiac, may increase with higher trough plasma levels, especially levels > 1 mcg/mL. Monitor trough plasma levels periodically, especially in patients with severe or moderate chronic renal failure or severe hepatic disease and CHF, as drug elimination may be slower.

Actions

Pharmacology: Flecainide has local anesthetic activity and belongs to the membrane stabilizing (Class I) group of antiarrhythmic agents; it has electrophysiologic effects characteristic of the IC class of antiarrhythmics.

Pharmacokinetics:
    Absorption/Distribution – Oral absorption is nearly complete. Peak plasma levels are attained at ≈ 3 hours. The plasma half-life ranges from 12 to 27 hours after multiple oral doses. Steady-state levels are approached in 3 to 5 days; once at steady-state, no accumulation occurs during chronic therapy. Plasma levels are approximately proportional to dose. In patients with congestive heart failure (CHF; NYHA class III), the rate of flecainide elimination from plasma is moderately slower than for healthy subjects. Plasma protein binding is about 40% and is independent of plasma drug level over the range of 0.015 to about 3.4 mcg/mL.

    Metabolism/Excretion – About 30% of a single oral dose (range, 10% to 50%) is excreted in urine unchanged. The two major urinary metabolites are meta-O-dealkylated flecainide (active, but about as potent) and the meta-O-dealkylated lactam (inactive). These two metabolites (primarily conjugated) account for most of the remaining portion of the dose. With increasing renal impairment, the extent of unchanged drug in urine is reduced and the half-life is prolonged. Hemodialysis removes only about 1% of an oral dose as unchanged flecainide.

Contraindications

Preexisting second- or third-degree AV block, right bundle branch block when associated with a left hemiblock (bifascicular block), unless a pacemaker is present to sustain the cardiac rhythm if complete heart block occurs; recent myocardial infarction (MI); presence of cardiogenic shock; hypersensitivity to the drug.

Warnings

Mortality: An excessive mortality or non-fatal cardiac arrest rate was seen in patients treated with flecainide compared with that seen in a carefully matched placebo-treated group.

Ventricular pro-arrhythmic effects in patients with atrial fibrillation/flutter: Flecainide is not recommended for use in patients with chronic atrial fibrillation. Case reports of ventricular proarrhythmic effects in patients treated with flecainide for atrial fibrillation/flutter have included increased premature ventricular contractions (PVCs), ventricular tachycardia (VT), ventricular fibrillation (VF), and death.

Non-life-threatening ventricular arrhythmias: It is prudent to consider the risks of Class IC agents, coupled with the lack of any evidence of improved survival, generally unacceptable in patients whose ventricular arrhythmias are not life-threatening, even if the patients are experiencing unpleasant but not life-threatening symptoms or signs.

Proarrhythmic effects: Flecainide can cause new or worsened arrhythmias. Such proarrhythmic effects range from an increase in frequency of PVCs to the development of more severe ventricular tachycardia.

Sick sinus syndrome: Use only with extreme caution; the drug may cause sinus bradycardia, sinus pause, or sinus arrest. The frequency probably increases with higher trough plasma levels.

Heart failure: Flecainide has a negative inotropic effect and may cause or worsen CHF, particularly in patients with cardiomyopathy, preexisting severe heart failure (NYHA functional class III or IV), or low ejection fractions (< 30%). The initial dosage should be ≤ 100 mg twice/day; monitor patients carefully. Give close attention to maintenance of cardiac function, including optimal digitalis, diuretic or other therapy. Where CHF has developed or worsened during treatment, the time of onset has ranged from a few hours to several months after starting therapy. Some patients who develop reduced myocardial function while on flecainide can continue with adjustment of digitalis or diuretics; others may require dosage reduction or discontinuation of flecainide. When feasible, monitor plasma flecainide levels. Keep trough plasma levels < 1 mcg/mL.

Cardiac conduction: Flecainide slows cardiac conduction in most patients to produce dose-related increases in PR, QRS, and QT intervals. The degree of lengthening of PR and QRS intervals does not predict either efficacy or the development of cardiac adverse effects. Patients may develop new first-degree AV heart block. Use caution and consider dose reductions. The JT interval (QT minus QRS) only widens ≈ 4% on the average. Rare cases of torsade de pointes-type arrhythmias have occurred.

If second-or third-degree AV block, or right bundle branch block associated with a left hemiblock occurs, discontinue therapy unless a ventricular pacemaker is in place to ensure an adequate ventricular rate.

Electrolyte disturbance: Hypokalemia or hyperkalemia may alter the effects of Class I antiarrhythmic drugs. Correct preexisting hypokalemia or hyperkalemia before administration.

Effects on pacemaker thresholds: Flecainide increases endocardial pacing thresholds and may suppress ventricular escape rhythms. These effects are reversible. Use with caution in patients with permanent pacemakers or temporary pacing electrodes. Do not administer to patients with existing poor thresholds or nonprogrammable pacemakers unless suitable pacing rescue is available.

Hepatic function impairment: Because flecainide elimination from plasma can be markedly slower in patients with significant hepatic impairment, do not use in such patients unless the potential benefits outweigh the risks. If used, make dosage increases very cautiously when plasma levels have plateaued (after > 4 days).

Elderly: Patients ≤ 80 years of age and above have been safely treated with usual doses.

Pregnancy: Category C.

Lactation: Flecainide is excreted in breast milk; determine whether to discontinue nursing or discontinue the drug, taking into account the importance of the drug to the mother.

Children: Safety and efficacy for use in children < 18 years of age have not been established.

Based on several studies flecainide appears to be beneficial in treating supraventricular and ventricular arrhythmias in children. Elimination half-life is shorter and volume of distribution is smaller.

Drug Interactions
Drugs that may affect flecainide include amiodarone, cimetidine, disopyramide, propranolol, urinary acidifiers/alkalinizers, and verapamil. Smoking may also have an effect. Drugs that may be affected by flecainide include propranolol and digoxin.

Adverse Reactions
Adverse interactions occurring in ≥ 3% of patients include dizziness; dyspnea; headache; nausea; fatigue; palpitation; chest pain; asthenia; tremor; constipation; edema; abdominal pain; visual disturbances.

In post-MI patients with asymptomatic PVCs and non-sustained ventricular tachycardia, flecainide therapy was associated with a 5.1% rate of death and non-fatal cardiac arrest, compared with a 2.3% rate in a matched placebo group.

BRETYLIUM TOSYLATE

Injection: 50 mg/mL (*Rx*) 2 mg/mL (500 mg/vial) in 5% Dextrose, 4 mg/mL (1000 mg/vial) in 5% Dextrose (*Rx*)	Various, *Bretylol* (DuPont Critical Care) Various

Indications
For prophylaxis and therapy of ventricular fibrillation.

In the treatment of life-threatening ventricular arrhythmias (ie, ventricular tachycardia) which have failed to respond to first-line antiarrhythmic agents (eg, lidocaine).

Unlabeled uses: Bretylium is a second-line agent following lidocaine in the protocol for advanced cardiac life support during CPR. For resistant VF and VT (after lidocaine, defibrillation, and procainamide failures), give bretylium 5 to 10 mg/kg IV; repeat as needed up to 30 mg/kg; use a bolus every 15 to 30 minutes, infusion 1 to 2 mg/min. For life-threatening arrhythmia use an undiluted infusion of 1 g/250 mL.

Administration and Dosage
For short-term use only.

Keep patient supine during therapy or closely observe for postural hypotension. The optimal dose has not been determined. Dosages > 40 mg/kg/day have been used without apparent adverse effect. As soon as possible, and when indicated, change patient to an oral antiarrhythmic agent for maintenance therapy.

Immediate life-threatening ventricular arrhythmias (eg, ventricular fibrillation, hemo-dynamically unstable ventricular tachycardia): Administer undiluted, 5 mg/kg by rapid IV injection. If ventricular fibrillation persists, increase dosage to 10 mg/kg and repeat as necessary.

Maintenance: For continuous suppression, administer the diluted solution by continu-ous IV infusion at 1 to 2 mg/min. Alternatively, infuse the diluted solution at a dos-age of 5 to 10 mg/kg over > 8 minutes, every 6 hours. More rapid infusion may cause nausea and vomiting.

Other ventricular arrhythmias:

IV – Dilute before administration. Administer 5 to 10 mg/kg by IV infusion over > 8 minutes. More rapid infusion may cause nausea and vomiting. Give subsequent doses at 1 to 2 hour intervals if the arrhythmia persists. For maintenance therapy, the same dosage may be administered every 6 hours, or a constant infusion of 1 to 2 mg/min may be given.

IM – 5 to 10 mg/kg undiluted. Do not dilute prior to injection. Give subsequent doses at 1 to 2 hour intervals if the arrhythmia persists. Thereafter, maintain with same dosage every 6 to 8 hours.

Do not give > 5 mL in any one site. Do not inject into or near a major nerve; vary injection sites. Repeated injection into the same site may cause atrophy and necrosis of muscle tissue, fibrosis, vascular degeneration, and inflammatory changes.

Children: The following dosages have been suggested.

Acute ventricular fibrillation – 5 mg/kg/dose IV, followed by 10 mg/kg at 15- to 30-minute intervals, maximum total dose 30 mg/kg. *Maintenance,* 5 to 10 mg/kg/dose every 6 hours.

Other ventricular arrhythmias – 5 to 10 mg/kg/dose every 6 hours.

Actions

Pharmacology: Bretylium tosylate inhibits norepinephrine release by depressing adrener-gic nerve terminal excitability, inducing a chemical sympathectomy-like state. Bretylium blocks the release of norepinephrine in response to neuron stimulation. Peripheral adrenergic blockade causes orthostatic hypotension but has less effect on supine blood pressure. It has a positive inotropic effect on the myocardium.

Pharmacokinetics: Peak plasma concentration and peak hypotensive effects are seen within 1 hour of IM administration. However, suppression of premature ventricu-lar beats is not maximal until 6 to 9 hours after dosing, when mean plasma concen-tration declines to < 50% of peak level. Antifibrillatory effects occur within minutes of an IV injection. Suppression of ventricular tachycardia and other ven-tricular arrhythmias develops more slowly, usually 20 minutes to 2 hours after par-enteral administration.

The terminal half-life ranges from 6.9 to 8.1 hours. During dialysis, a 2-fold increase in clearance occurs. The drug is eliminated intact by the kidneys. Approxi-mately 70% to 80% of an IM dose is excreted in the urine during the first 24 hours, with an additional 10% excreted over the next 3 days.

Warnings

Hypotension: Hypotension (postural) occurs regularly in ≈ 50% of patients while they are supine, manifested by dizziness, lightheadedness, vertigo, or faintness. Toler-ance occurs unpredictably but may be present after several days. Hypotension with supine systolic pressure > 75 mmHg need not be treated unless symptomatic. If supine systolic pressure falls below 75 mmHg, infuse dopamine or norepinephrine to increase blood pressure; use dilute solution and monitor blood pressure closely because pressor effects are enhanced by bretylium. Perform volume expansion with blood or plasma and correct dehydration where appropriate.

Transient hypertension and increased frequency of arrhythmias: Transient hypertension and increased frequency of arrhythmias may occur due to initial release of norepin-ephrine from adrenergic postganglionic nerve terminals.

Fixed cardiac output: Avoid use with fixed cardiac output because severe hypotension may result from a fall in peripheral resistance without a compensatory increase in cardiac output. If survival is threatened by arrhythmia, the drug may be used, but give vasoconstrictive catecholamines promptly if severe hypotension occurs.

Renal function impairment: Because the drug is excreted principally via the kidney, increase the dosage interval in patients with impaired renal function.

Pregnancy: Category C. Reduced uterine blood flow with fetal hypoxia (bradycardia) is a potential risk. Give to a pregnant woman only if clearly needed.

Children: Safety and efficacy for use in children have not been established.

Drug Interactions
Drugs that may affect bretylium include catecholamines and digoxin.

Adverse Reactions
Adverse reactions occurring in ≥ 3% of patients include hypotension and postural hypotension; nausea and vomiting, primarily after rapid IV administration.

AMIODARONE HCl

Tablets: 200 and 400 mg (*Rx*)	Various, *Cordarone* (Wyeth-Ayerst), *Pacerone* (Upsher Smith)
Injection: 50 mg/mL (*Rx*)	*Cordarone* (Wyeth-Ayerst)

Indications
Ventricular arrhythmias:

Oral – Only for treatment of the following documented life-threatening recurrent ventricular arrhythmias that do not respond to documented adequate doses of other antiarrhythmics or when alternative agents are not tolerated:

1.) Recurrent ventricular fibrillation (VF).

2.) Recurrent hemodynamically unstable ventricular tachycardia (VT).

Parenteral – Initiation of treatment and prophylaxis of frequently recurring VF and hemodynamically unstable VT in patients refractory to other therapy. It can also be used to treat patients with VT/VF for whom oral amiodarone is indicated, but who are unable to take oral medication.

During or after treatment with IV amiodarone, patients may be transferred to oral amiodarone therapy. Use IV amiodarone for acute treatment until the patient's ventricular arrhythmias are stabilized. Most patients require this therapy for 48 to 96 hours, but IV amiodarone may be given safely for longer periods if needed.

Administration and Dosage
In order to ensure that an antiarrhythmic effect will be observed without waiting several months, loading doses are required. Individual patient titration is suggested.

Life-threatening ventricular arrhythmias (ventricular fibrillation or hemodynamically unstable ventricular tachycardia): Administer the loading dose in a hospital. Loading doses of 800 to 1600 mg/day are required for 1 to 3 weeks (occasionally longer) until initial therapeutic response occurs. Administer in divided doses with meals for total daily doses of ≥ 1000 mg, or when GI intolerance occurs. If side effects become excessive, reduce the dose. Elimination of recurrence of ventricular fibrillation and tachycardia usually occurs within 1 to 3 weeks, along with reduction in complex and total ventricular ectopic beats.

When starting amiodarone therapy, attempt to gradually discontinue prior antiarrhythmic drugs. When adequate arrhythmia control is achieved, or if side effects become prominent, reduce dose to 600 to 800 mg/day for 1 month and then to the maintenance dose, usually 400 mg/day. Some patients may require larger maintenance doses, up to 600 mg/day, and some can be controlled on lower doses.

Concurrent antiarrhythmic agents – In general, reserve the combination of amiodarone with other antiarrhythmic therapy for patients with life-threatening arrhythmias who are incompletely responsive to a single agent or incompletely responsive to amiodarone. During transfer to amiodarone, reduce the dose levels of previously administered agents by 30% to 50% several days after the addition of amiodarone when arrhythmia suppression should be beginning. Review the continued need for the other antiarrhythmic agent after the effects of amiodarone have been established, and attempt discontinuation. If the treatment is continued, carefully monitor these patients for adverse effects, especially conduction disturbances and exacerbation of tachyarrhythmias, as amiodarone is continued. In amiodarone-treated patients who require additional antiarrhythmic therapy, the initial dose of such agents should be ≈ 50% of the usual recommended dose.

Parenteral: Amiodarone shows considerable interindividual variation in response. Thus, although a starting dose adequate to suppress life-threatening arrhythmias is needed, close monitoring with adjustment of dose as needed is essential. The recommended starting dose of amiodarone IV is as follows.

Amiodarone IV Dose Recommendations During the First 24 Hours	
Loading infusions	
First rapid	150 mg over the *first* 10 minutes (15 mg/min). Add 3 mL amiodarone IV (150 mg) to 100 mL D5W (concentration, 1.5 mg/mL). Infuse 100 mL/10 min.
Followed by slow	360 mg over the *next* 6 hours (1 mg/min). Add 18 mL amiodarone IV (900 mg) to 500 mL D5W (concentration, 1.8 mg/mL).
Maintenance infusion	540 mg over the *remaining* 18 hours (0.5 mg/min). Decrease the rate of the slow loading infusion to 0.5 mg/min.

After the first 24 hours, continue the maintenance infusion rate of 0.5 mg/min (720 mg/24 hrs) utilizing a concentration of 1 to 6 mg/mL. In the event of breakthrough episodes of VF or hemodynamically unstable VT, 150 mg supplemental infusions of amiodarone IV mixed in 100 mL D5W may be given. Administer such infusions over 10 minutes to minimize the potential for hypotension. The rate of the maintenance infusion may be increased to achieve effective arrhythmia suppression.

The first 24-hour dose may be individualized for each patient; however, in controlled clinical trials, mean daily doses > 2100 mg were associated with an increased risk of hypotension. The initial infusion rate should not exceed 30 mg/min.

Based on the experience from clincial studies, a maintenance infusion of up to 0.5 mg/min can be cautiously continued for 2 to 3 weeks regardless of the patient's age, renal function, or left ventricular function. There has been limited experience in patients receiving amiodarone IV for > 3 weeks.

The surface properties of solutions containing injectable amiodarone are altered such that the drop size may be reduced. This reduction may lead to underdosage of the patient by up to 30%. If drop counter infusion sets are used, amiodarone must be delivered by a volumetric infusion pump.

Amiodarone IV concentrations > 3 mg/mL in D5W have been associated with a high incidence of peripheral vein phlebitis; however, concentrations of ≤ 2.5 mg/mL appear to be less irritating. Therefore, for infusions > 1 hour, amiodarone IV concentrations should not exceed 2 mg/mL unless a central venous catheter is used. Use an in-line filter during administration.

Amiodarone IV infusions exceeding 2 hours must be administered in glass or polyolefin bottles containing D5W.

Amiodarone adsorbs to polyvinyl chloride (PVC) tubing, and the clinical trial dose administration schedule was designed to account for this adsorption. Clinical trials were conducted using PVC tubing; therefore its use is recommended. The concentrations and rates of infusion provided in Administration and Dosage reflect doses identified in these studies. It is important that the recommended infusion regimen be followed closely.

Amiodarone IV has been found to leach out plasticizers, including DEHP (diphthalate) from IV tubing (including PVC tubing). The degree of leaching increases when infusing amiodarone IV at higher concentrations and lower flow rates than recommended.

Admixture incompatibility: Amiodarone IV in D5W, in a concentration of 4 mg/mL, forms a precipitate and is incompatible with the following drugs: Aminophylline, cefamandole, cefazolin, mezlocillin, heparin (no amiodarone concentration stated), and sodium bicarbonate (amiodarone concentration of 3 mg/mL).

IV to oral transition: During or after treatment with IV amiodarone, patients may be transferred to oral amiodarone therapy. Use IV amiodarone for acute treatment until the patient's ventricular arrhythmias are stabilized. Most patients require this therapy for 48 to 96 hours, but IV amiodarone may be given safely for longer periods if necessary. The optimal dose for changing from IV to oral administration will depend on the IV dose already administered, as well as the bioavailability of oral amiodarone.

The following table provides suggested doses of oral amiodarone to be initiated after varying durations of IV administration. These recommendations are made on the basis of a comparable total body amount of amiodarone delivered by the IV and oral routes, based on 50% bioavailability of oral amiodarone.

Recommendations for Oral Amiodarone Dosage After IV Infusion	
Duration of amiodarone IV infusions[1]	Initial daily dose of oral amiodarone
< 1 week	800 to 1600 mg
1 to 3 weeks	600 to 800 mg
> 3 weeks[2]	400 mg

[1] Assuming a 720 mg/day infusion (0.5 mg/min).
[2] Amiodarone IV is not intended for maintenance treatment.

Actions

Pharmacology: Amiodarone possesses electrophysiologic characteristics of all 4 Vaughan Williams Classes but has predominantly Class III antiarrhythmic effects. The antiarrhythmic effect may be due to ≥ 2 major properties: Prolongation of the myocardial cell-action potential duration and refractory period, and noncompetitive α- and β-adrenergic inhibition.

Pharmacokinetics:

Absorption – Following oral administration, amiodarone is slowly and variably absorbed; bioavailability is ≈ 50%. Maximum plasma concentrations are attained 3 to 7 hours after a single dose. Plasma concentrations with chronic dosing at 100 to 600 mg/day are approximately dose-proportional, with a mean 0.5 mg/L increase for each 100 mg/day.

Peak concentrations after 10-minute infusions of 150 mg in patients with VF or hemodynamically unstable VT range between 7 and 26 mg/L. Due to rapid distribution, serum concentrations decline to 10% of peak values within 30 to 45 minutes after the end of the infusion.

Distribution – Amiodarone has a very large but variable volume of distribution, averaging about 60 L/kg. One major metabolite, desethylamiodarone (DEA), accumulates to an even greater extent in almost all tissues. The drug is highly protein bound (≈ 96%).

Metabolism – Amiodarone is metabolized principally by CYP3A4 into DEA, the major active metabolite of amiodarone. DEA serum concentrations > 0.05 mg/L are not usually seen until after several days of continuous infusion but with prolonged therapy reach approximately the same concentration as amiodarone.

Excretion – Following discontinuation of chronic oral therapy, amiodarone has a biphasic elimination with an initial one-half reduction of plasma levels after 2.5 to 107 days. A much slower terminal plasma elimination phase shows a half-life of the parent compound of ≈ 53 days. For the metabolite, mean plasma elimination half-life was ≈ 61 days. Antiarrhythmic effects persist for weeks or months after the drug is discontinued.

The main route of elimination is via hepatic excretion into bile; some enterohepatic recirculation may occur. The drug has a very low plasma clearance with negligible renal excretion. Neither amiodarone nor its metabolite is dialyzable.

Contraindications

Hypersensitivity to the drug or any of its components.

Oral: Severe sinus-node dysfunction, causing marked sinus bradycardia; second- and third-degree AV block; when episodes of bradycardia have caused syncope (except when used in conjunction with a pacemaker).

Parenteral: Marked sinus bradycardia; second- and third-degree AV block unless a functioning pacemaker is available; cardiogenic shock.

Warnings

Potentially fatal toxicities: Potentially fatal toxicities with pulmonary toxicity have occurred with ventricular arrhythmias (at ≈ 400 mg/day), and symptomless abnormal diffusion capacity has occurred in much higher percentages. Pulmonary toxicity has been fatal ≈ 10% of the time. Hepatic injury is common, but usually mild, and evidenced by abnormal liver enzymes. Overt liver disease can occur and has been fatal. Amiodarone has made arrhythmia less well tolerated or more difficult to reverse. Significant heart block or sinus bradycardia has been seen. These events should be manageable in the proper clinical setting. Although such events do not appear more frequently with amiodarone than with other agents, effects are prolonged. In patients at high risk of arrhythmic death in whom amiodarone toxicity is an acceptable risk, amiodarone poses major management problems that could be life-threatening in a population at risk of sudden death so that every effort should be made to use alternative agents first.

Hospitalize patients while the loading dose is given. The time at which a life-threatening arrhythmia will recur after discontinuation or dose adjustment is unpredictable, ranging from weeks to months. The patient risk is greatest during this time. Substituting other antiarrhythmics when amiodarone must be stopped is made difficult by gradually, but unpredictably, changing amiodarone body stores. When amiodarone is ineffective, it still poses the risk of interacting with subsequent treatment.

Life-threatening arrhythmias: Use amiodarone only in patients with the indicated life-threatening arrhythmias because its use is accompanied by substantial toxicity.

Survival – There is no evidence that the use of amiodarone favorably affects survival.

Ophthalmologic effects: Optic neuropathy or neuritis may occur at any time following initiation of therapy, in some cases, visual impairment has progressed to permanent blindness. Corneal microdeposits appear in virtually all adults treated with amiodarone. They give rise to symptoms such as visual halos or blurred vision in as many as 10% of patients. Corneal microdeposits are reversible upon reduction of dose or drug discontinuation. Asymptomatic microdeposits are not a reason to reduce dose or stop treatment. Some patients develop photophobia and dry eyes. Vision is rarely affected and drug discontinuation is rarely needed.

Pulmonary toxicity:

Oral – Amiodarone may cause a clinical syndrome of cough and progressive dyspnea accompanied by functional, radiographic, gallium scan, and pathological data consistent with pulmonary toxicity. The frequency varies from 2% to 17%; fatalities occur in about 10% of cases. However, in patients with life-threatening arrhythmias, discontinuation of amiodarone therapy due to suspected drug-induced pulmonary toxicity should be undertaken with caution, as the most common cause of death in these patients is sudden cardiac death.

Any new respiratory symptom suggests pulmonary toxicity, therefore repeat and evaluate the history, physical exam, chest x-ray, gallium scan, and pulmonary function tests (with diffusion capacity). In some cases, rechallenge at a lower dose has not resulted in return of interstitial/alveolar pneumonitis.

Perform baseline chest x-rays and pulmonary function tests, including diffusion capacity before therapy initiation. A history and physicial exam and chest x-ray should be repeated every 3 to 6 months. Patients with preexisting pulmonary disease have a poorer prognosis if pulmonary toxicity does develop.

Hypersensitivity pneumonitis – Hypersensitivity pneumonitis usually appears earlier in the course of therapy, and rechallenging these patients results in a more rapid recurrence of greater severity.

Interstitial/alveolar pneumonitis – Interstitial/alveolar pneumonitis is characterized by findings of diffuse alveolar damage, interstitial pneumonitis or fibrosis in lung biopsy specimens. A diagnosis of amiodarone-induced interstitial/alveolar pneumonitis should lead to dose reduction or to withdrawal of amiodarone to establish reversibility. With these measures, a reduction in symptoms of amiodarone-induced pulmonary toxicity was usually noted within the first week. In some cases, rechallenge with amiodarone at a lower dose has not resulted in return of toxicity. Recent reports suggest that lower loading and maintenance doses of amiodarone are associated with a decrease incidence of amiodarone-induced pulmonary toxicity.

If a diagnosis of amiodarone-induced hypersensitivity pneumonitis is made, discontinue amiodarone and institute steroid treatment. If a diagnosis of amiodarone-induced interstitial/alveolar pneumonitis is made, institute steroid therapy and discontinue amiodarone or, at a minimum, reduce dosage.

Parenteral –

ARDS: 2% of patients were reported to have adult respiratory distress syndrome (ARDS) during clinical studies.

Pulmonary fibrosis: Only 1 of > 1000 patients treated with amiodarone IV in clincal studies developed pulmonary fibrosis.

Cardiac effects:

Proarrhythmias – Amiodarone can cause serious exacerbation of the presenting arrhythmia, a risk that may be enhanced by concomitant antiarrhythmics. In addition, amiodarone has caused symptomatic bradycardia, heart block, or sinus arrest with suppression of escape foci. Treat bradycardia by slowing the infusion rate or discontinuing amiodarone IV. In some patients, inserting a pacemaker is required. Cardiac conduction abnormalities are infrequent and reversible on discontinuation.

Hypotension – Hypotension is the most common adverse effect seen with amiodarone IV. Clinically significant hypotension during infusions was seen most often in the first several hours of treatment and appeared to be related to the rate of infusion. Hypotension necessitating alterations in therapy was reported in 3% of patients, with permanent discontinuation required in < 2% of patients. Treat hypotension initially by slowing the infusion; additional standard therapy may be needed.

Surgery:

Volatile anesthetic agents – Close perioperative monitoring is recommended in patients undergoing general anesthesia who are on amiodarone therapy as they may be more sensitive to the myocardial depressant and conduction effects of halogenated inhalational anesthetics.

Hypotension postbypass – Rare occasions of hypotension upon discontinuation of cardiopulmonary bypass during open-heart surgery in patients receiving amiodarone have been reported.

Hepatic effects:

Oral – Elevated hepatic enzyme levels (AST and ALT) are frequent, and in most cases are asymptomatic. If the increase exceeds 3 times normal, or doubles in a patient with an elevated baseline, consider discontinuation or dosage reduction.

Parenteral – Elevations of blood hepatic enzyme values, ALT, AST, and GGT, are seen commonly in patients with immediately life-threatening VT/VF.

In patients with life-threatening arrhythmias, weigh the potential risk of hepatic injury against the potential benefit of therapy. Monitor carefully for evidence of progressive hepatic injury. Give consideration to reducing the rate of administration or withdrawing amiodarone IV in such cases.

Elderly: Healthy subjects > 65 years of age show lower clearances of amiodarone than younger subjects and an increase in half-life.

Pregnancy: Category D.

Lactation: Amiodarone is excreted in breast milk. When amiodarone therapy is indicated, advise the mother to discontinue nursing.

Children: Safety and efficacy for use in children have not been established. Amiodarone is not recommended in children.

Precautions

Thyroid abnormalities: Amiodarone inhibits peripheral conversion of thyroxine (T_4) to triiodothyronine (T_3), prompting increased T_4 levels, increased levels of inactive reverse T_3 and decreased levels of T_3. It is also a potential source of large amounts of inorganic iodine. It can cause hypothyroidism or hyperthyroidism. High plasma iodide levels, altered thyroid function, and abnormal thyroid function tests may persist for several weeks or even months following amiodarone withdrawal.

Hypothyroidism – Hypothyroidism is best managed by dose reduction or thyroid hormone supplement.

Hyperthyroidism – Hyperthyroidism usually poses a greater hazard to the patient than hypothyroidism because of the possibility of arrhythmia breakthrough or aggravation. If any new signs of arrhythmia appear, consider the possibility of hyperthyroidism. Aggressive medical treatment is indicated, including, dose reduction or withdrawal of amiodarone.

Electrolyte disturbances: Correct potassium or magnesium deficiency before therapy begins as these disorders can exaggerate the degree of QTc prolongation and increase the potential for torsades de pointes.

Benzyl alcohol: Benzyl alcohol, contained in some of these products as a preservative, has been associated with a fatal "gasping syndrome" in premature infants.

Photosensitivity: Amiodarone has induced photosensitization in about 10% of patients. During long-term treatment, a blue-gray discoloration of the exposed skin may occur; some protection may be afforded by sun barrier creams or protective clothing. This is slowly and occasionally incompletely reversible on discontinuation of drug.

Drug Interactions

Drugs that may affect amiodarone include hydantoins, cholestyramine, fluoroquinolones, rifamycins, ritonavir, and cimetidine. Drugs that may be affected by amiodarone include anticoagulants, beta blockers, calcium channel blockers, cyclosporine, dextromethorphan, digoxin, disopyramide, fentanyl, flecainide, hydantoins, lidocaine, methotrexate, procainamide, quinidine, and theophylline.

Drug/Lab test interactions: Amiodarone alters the results of thyroid function tests, causing an increase in serum T_4 and serum reverse T_3 levels and a decline in serum T_3 levels. Despite these biochemical changes, most patients remain clinically euthyroid.

Drug/Food interactions: Food increases the rate and extent of absorption.

Adverse Reactions

Oral – Adverse reactions requiring discontinuation include: Pulmonary infiltrates or fibrosis; paroxysmal ventricular tachycardia; CHF; elevation of liver enzymes; visual disturbances; solar dermatitis; blue discoloration of skin; hyperthyroidism; hypothyroidism. Adverse reactions occurring in ≥ 3% of patients include CHF; GI complaints (nausea, vomiting, constipation, anorexia); dermatologic reactions (photosensitivity, solar dermatitis); neurologic problems (malaise, fatigue, tremor/abnormal involuntary movements, lack of coordination, abnormal gait/ataxia, dizziness, paresthesias); abnormal liver function tests.

Parenteral – The most important treatment-emergent adverse effects were hypotension, asystole/cardiac arrest/electromechanical dissociation (EMD), cardiogenic shock, CHF, bradycardia, liver function test abnormalities, VT, and AV block. The most common adverse effects leading to discontinuation of IV therapy were hypotension, asystole/cardiac arrest/EMD, VT, and cardiogenic shock. Adverse reactions occurring in ≥ 3% of patients include nausea.

ADENOSINE

Injection: 6 mg/2 mL (*Rx*)	*Adenocard* (Fujisawa)

Indications

Conversion to sinus rhythm of paroxysmal supraventricular tachycardia, including that associated with accessory bypass tracts (WPW syndrome). When clinically advisable, attempt appropriate vagal maneuvers (eg, Valsalva maneuver) prior to use.

Administration and Dosage

For rapid bolus IV use only. To be certain the solution reaches the systemic circulation, administer either directly into a vein or, if given into an IV line, as proximal as possible and follow with a rapid saline flush.

Initial dose: 6 mg as a rapid IV bolus (administered over a 1- to 2-second period).

Repeat administration: If first dose does not result in elimination of the supraventricular tachycardia within 1 to 2 minutes, give 12 mg as a rapid IV bolus. This 12 mg dose may be repeated a second time if required.

Children: The dosages used in neonates, infants, children, and adolescents were equivalent to those administered to adults on a weight basis.

> *< 50 kg –*
> *Initial dose:* 0.05 to 0.1 mg/kg as a rapid IV bolus given either centrally or peripherally. A saline flush should follow.
> *Repeat administration:* If conversion of PSVT does not occur within 1 to 2 minutes, additional bolus injections of adenosine can be administered at incrementally higher doses, increasing the amount given by 0.05 to 0.1 mg/kg. Follow each bolus with a saline flush. Continue this process until sinus rhythm is established or a maximum single dose of 0.3 mg/kg is used.
> *≥ 50 kg –* Administer the adult dose.

Doses > 12 mg are not recommended.

Actions

Pharmacology: Adenosine is an endogenous nucleoside occurring in all cells. It is not chemically related to other antiarrhythmic agents. Adenosine slows conduction time through the AV node, can interrupt the reentry pathways through the AV node and can restore normal sinus rhythm in patients with paroxysmal supraventricular tachycardia (PSVT), including PSVT associated with Wolff-Parkinson-White (WPW) syndrome.

Pharmacokinetics: Following an IV bolus, adenosine is taken up by erythrocytes and vascular endothelial cells. Half-life is estimated to be < 10 seconds. Adenosine enters the body pool and is primarily metabolized to inosine and adenosine monophosphate (AMP).

Contraindications

Second- or third-degree AV block or sick sinus syndrome (except in patients with a functioning artificial pacemaker); atrial flutter, atrial fibrillation and ventricular tachycardia (the drug is not effective in converting these arrhythmias to normal sinus rhythm); hypersensitivity to adenosine.

Warnings

Heart block: Adenosine may produce a short lasting first-, second- or third-degree heart block. In extreme cases, transient asystole may result. Institute appropriate therapy as needed. Patients who develop high-level block on 1 dose should not be given additional doses. These effects are generally self-limiting.

Arrhythmias: At the time of conversion to normal sinus rhythm, a variety of new rhythms may appear on the ECG. They generally last only a few seconds without intervention, and may take the form of premature ventricular contractions, atrial premature contractions, sinus bradycardia, sinus tachycardia, skipped beats, and varying degrees of AV nodal block. Such findings were seen in 55% of patients.

Treatment of other arrhythmias: Adenosine is not effective in converting rhythms other than PSVT, such as atrial flutter, atrial fibrillation, or ventricular tachycardia to normal sinus rhythm.

Ventricular response: In the presence of atrial flutter or atrial fibrillation, a transient modest slowing of ventricular response may occur immediately following use.

Hepatic and renal failure: Hepatic and renal failure should have no effect on the activity of a bolus adenosine injection.

Pregnancy: Category C.

Precautions

Asthma: A limited number of patients with asthma have received adenosine and have not experienced exacerbation of their asthma. However, inhaled adenosine induces bronchoconstriction in asthmatic patients but not in healthy individuals. Be alert to the possibility that adenosine could produce bronchoconstriction in patients with asthma.

Drug Interactions

Drugs that may interact with adenosine include carbamazepine, digoxin, dipyridamole, methylxanthines, and verapamil.

Adverse Reactions

Adverse reactions occurring in ≥ 3% of patients include facial flushing; shortness of breath/dyspnea; chest pressure; nausea.

CALCIUM CHANNEL BLOCKING AGENTS

AMLODIPINE
Tablets: 2.5, 5, and 10 mg (*Rx*) — *Norvasc* (Pfizer)

BEPRIDIL HCl
Tablets: 200, 300, and 400 mg (*Rx*) — *Vascor* (McNeil)

DILTIAZEM HCl
Tablets: 30, 60, 90, and 120 mg (*Rx*) — Various, *Cardizem* (Marion Merrell Dow)
Capsules, sustained-release: 60, 90, 120, 180, 240, 300, and 360 mg (*Rx*) — Various, *Cardizem SR* (Marion Merrell Dow), *Cardizem CD* (Marion Merrell Dow), *Dilacor XR* (Rhone-Poulenc Rorer), *Tiazac* (Forest)
Injection: 25 mg (5 mg/mL), 50 mg (5 mg/mL) (*Rx*) — *Cardizem* (Marion Merrell Dow)

FELODIPINE
Tablets, extended-release: 2.5, 5, and 10 mg (*Rx*) — *Plendil* (Merck)

ISRADIPINE
Capsules: 2.5 and 5 mg (*Rx*) — *DynaCirc* (Sandoz)

MIBEFRADIL
Tablets: 50 and 100 mg (*Rx*) — *Posicor* (Roche)

NICARDIPINE HCl
Capsules: 20 and 30 mg (*Rx*) — *Cardene* (Syntex)
Capsules, sustained-release: 30, 45, and 60 mg (*Rx*) — *Cardene SR* (Syntex)
Injection: 2.5 mg/mL (*Rx*) — *Cardene I.V.* (Wyeth)

NIFEDIPINE
Capsules: 10 and 20 mg (*Rx*) — Various, *Procardia* (Pfizer), *Adalat* (Bayer)
Tablets, sustained-release: 30, 60, and 90 mg (*Rx*) — *Procardia XL* (Pfizer), *Adalat CC* (Bayer)

NIMODIPINE
Capsules, liquid: 30 mg (*Rx*) — *Nimotop* (Bayer)

NISOLDIPINE
Tablets, extended-release: 10, 20, 30, and 40 mg (*Rx*) — *Sular* (Zeneca)

VERAPAMIL HCl
Tablets: 40, 80, and 120 mg (*Rx*) — Various, *Calan* (Searle), *Isoptin* (Knoll)
Tablets, sustained-release: 120, 180, and 240 mg (*Rx*) — Various, *Calan SR* (Searle), *Isoptin SR* (Knoll), *Covera-HS* (Searle)
Capsules, sustained-release: 120, 180, and 240 mg (*Rx*) — *Verelan* (Lederle)
Injection: 5 mg/2 mL (*Rx*) — Various, *Isoptin* (Knoll)

Indications

Calcium Channel Blocking Agents – Summary of Indications

Indications	Amlodipine	Bepridil	Diltiazem	Diltiazem SR	Diltiazem IV	Felodipine	Isradipine	Mibefradil	Nicardipine	Nicardipine SR	Nicardipine IV	Nifedipine	Nifedipine SR	Nimodipine	Nisoldipine	Verapamil	Verapamil SR	Verapamil IV
Angina pectoris																		
Vasospastic	✔			✔								✔	✔			✔		
Chronic stable	✔	✔	✔	✔				✔	✔							✔		
Unstable																✔		
Hypertension, essential	✔			✔		✔	✔	✔	✔	✔	✔		✔		✔	✔	✔	
Arrhythmias					✔											✔		
Supraventricular tachyarrhythmias																		✔
Subarachnoid hemorrhage														✔				

Administration and Dosage

Swallow extended-release tablets and sustained-release capsule forms whole; do not bite, open, chew, crush, or divide.

AMLODIPINE: May be taken without regard to meals.

Hypertension – Usual dose is 5 mg once daily. Maximum dose is 10 mg once daily. Small, fragile, or elderly patients or patients with hepatic insufficiency may be started on 2.5 mg once daily; this dose may also be used when adding amlodipine to other antihypertensive therapy. In general, titrate over 7 to 14 days; proceed more rapidly if clinically warranted with frequent assessment of the patient.

Angina (chronic stable or vasospastic) – 5 to 10 mg, using the lower dose for elderly and patients with hepatic insufficiency. Most patients require 10 mg.

BEPRIDIL HCl: Usual initial dose is 200 mg/day. After 10 days, dosage may be adjusted upward depending on response. Most patients are maintained at 300 mg. Maximum daily dose is 400 mg; minimum effective dose is 200 mg.

Elderly – Starting dose does not differ from that for younger patients; however, after therapeutic response is demonstrated, the elderly may require more frequent monitoring.

DILTIAZEM HCl:
Oral –

Tablets: Start with 30 mg 4 times/day before meals and at bedtime; gradually increase dosage to 180 to 360 mg (given in divided doses 3 or 4 times/day) at 1- to 2-day intervals until optimum response is obtained.

Sustained release:

Cardizem SR – Start with 60 to 120 mg twice daily. Adjust dosage when maximum antihypertensive effect is achieved (usually by 14 days chronic therapy). Optimum dosage range is 240 to 360 mg/day, but some patients may respond to lower doses.

Cardizem CD –

Hypertension: 180 to 240 mg once daily; some patients may respond to lower doses. Maximum antihypertensive effect is usually achieved by 14 days chronic therapy; therefore, adjust dosage accordingly. Usual range is 240 to 360 mg once daily; experience with doses > 360 mg is limited.

Angina: Start with 120 or 180 mg once daily. Some patients may respond to higher doses of up to 480 mg once daily. When necessary, titration may be carried out over a 7- to 14-day period.

Cardizem CD may be opened and administered, but do not crush.

Dilacor XR –

Hypertension: 180 to 240 mg once daily; adjust dose as needed. Individual patients, particularly those ≥ 60 years of age, may respond to a lower dose of 120 mg. Usual range is 180 to 480 mg once daily. Although current clinical experience with the 540 mg dose is limited, the dose may be increased to 540 mg with little or no increased risk of adverse reactions. Do not exceed 540 mg once daily.

Angina: Adjust dosage to each patient's needs, starting with a dose of 120 mg once daily, which may be titrated to doses of up to 480 mg once daily. when necessary, titration may be carried out over a 7- to 14-day period.

Hypertensive or anginal patients treated with other formulations of diltiazem can safely be switched to *Dilacor XR* at the nearest equivalent total daily dose. However, subsequent titration to higher or lower doses may be necessary and should be initiated as clinically indicated.

Administration in the morning on an empty stomach is recommended.

Parenteral –

Direct IV single injections (bolus): The initial dose is 0.25 mg/kg as a bolus administered over 2 minutes (20 mg is a reasonable dose for the average patient). If response is inadequate, a second dose may be administered after 15 minutes. The second bolus dose should be 0.35 mg/kg administered over 2 minutes (25 mg is a reasonable dose for the average patient). Individualize subsequent IV bolus doses. Dose patients with low body weights on a mg/kg basis. Some patients may respond to an initial dose of 0.15 mg/kg, although duration of action may be shorter.

Continuous IV infusion: For continued reduction of the heart rate (up to 24 hours) in patients with atrial fibrillation or atrial flutter, an IV infusion may be administered. Immediately following bolus administration of 20 mg (0.25 mg/kg) or 25 mg

(0.35 mg/kg) and reduction of heart rate, begin an IV infusion. The recommended initial infusion rate is 10 mg/hr. Some patients may maintain response to an initial rate of 5 mg/hr. The infusion rate may be increased in 5 mg/hr increments up to 15 mg/hr as needed, if further reduction in heart rate is required. The infusion may be maintained for up to 24 hours. Therefore, infusion duration > 24 hours and infusion rates > 15 mg/hr are not recommended.

Concomitant therapy: Concomitant therapy with β-blockers or digitalis is usually well tolerated, but the effects of coadministration cannot be predicted, especially in patients with left ventricular dysfunction or cardiac conduction abnormalities. Use caution in titrating dosages for impaired renal or hepatic function patients, since dosage requirements are not available.

FELODIPINE: The recommended starting dose is 5 mg once daily. Depending on the patient's response the dosage can be decreased to 2.5 mg or increased to 10 mg once daily. These adjustments should occur generally at intervals of not less than 2 weeks. The recommended dosage range is 2.5 to 10 mg once daily. Because they may develop higher plasma felodipine levels, closely monitor blood pressure in patients > 65 years old and in impaired hepatic function during dosage adjustment; generally, do not consider doses > 10 mg.

ISRADIPINE: Recommended initial dose is 2.5 mg twice daily. An antihypertensive response usually occurs within 2 to 3 hours; maximal response may require 2 to 4 weeks. If a satisfactory response does not occur after this period, the dose may be adjusted in increments of 5 mg/day at 2 to 4 week intervals up to a maximum of 20 mg/day. However, most patients show no additional response to doses > 10 mg/day, and adverse effects are increased in frequency above 10 mg/day.

MIBEFRADIL: The recommended dose is 50 or 100 mg once daily. Doses > 100 mg offer little or no additional benefit and induce a greater rate of adverse reactions. Exercise caution when administering to patients with severe hepatic impairment.

NICARDIPINE HCl:

Oral –

Angina and hypertension (immediate release only): Usual initial dose is 20 mg 3 times/day (range, 20 to 40 mg 3 times/day). The maximum blood pressure (BP) lowering effect occurs ≈ 1 to 2 hours after dosing. Allow at least 3 days before increasing dose to ensure achievement of steady-state plasma drug concentrations.

Hypertension (sustained release): Initial dose is 30 mg twice daily. Effective doses have ranged from 30 to 60 mg twice daily. The maximum BP lowering effect at steady-state is sustained from 2 to 6 hours after dosing.

The total daily dose of immediate-release nicardipine may not be a useful guide in judging the effective dose of the sustained-release form. Titrate patients currently receiving the immediate-release form with the sustained-release form starting at their current daily dose of immediate-release, then re-examine to assess adequacy of BP control.

Renal impairment: Use caution when titrating. Titrate dose beginning with 20 mg 3 times/day (immediate-release) or 30 mg twice/day (sustained-release).

Hepatic impairment: Use caution when titrating. Starting dose is 20 mg twice/day (immediate-release) with individual titration.

Parenteral –

Dosage:

Substitute for oral nicardipine – The IV infusion rate required to produce an average plasma concentration equivalent to a given oral dose at steady state is shown in the following table:

Equivalent Nicardipine Doses: Oral vs IV Infusion	
Oral dose	Equivalent IV infusion rate
20 mg q 8 hr	0.5 mg/hr
30 mg q 8 hr	1.2 mg/hr
40 mg q 8 hr	2.2 mg/hr

Initiation in a drug free patient – The time course of blood pressure decrease is dependent on the initial rate of infusion and the frequency of dosage adjustment. Administer by slow continuous infusion at a concentration of 0.1 mg/mL. With constant infusion, blood pressure begins to fall within minutes. It reaches about 50% of its ultimate decrease in about 45 minutes and does not reach final steady state for about 50 hours.

When treating acute hypertensive episodes in patients with chronic hypertension, discontinuation of infusion is followed by a 50% offset of action in 30 minutes but plasma levels of drug and gradually decreasing antihypertensive effects exist for ≈ 50 hours.

Titration – For gradual reduction in blood pressure, initiate therapy at 50 mL/hr (5 mg/hr). If desired reduction is not achieved at this dose, the infusion rate may be increased by 25 mL/hr (2.5 mg/hr) every 15 minutes up to a maximum of 150 mL/hr (15 mg/hr) until desired reduction of blood pressure is achieved. For more rapid reduction of blood pressure, initiate at 50 mL/hr. If desired reduction is not achieved at this dose, the infusion rate may be increased by 25 mL/hr every 5 minutes up to a maximum of 150 mL/hr until desired reduction of blood pressure is achieved. Following achievement of the blood pressure goal, decrease the infusion rate to 30 mL/hr.

Maintenance – Adjust the rate of infusion as needed to maintain desired response.

Conditions requiring infusion adjustment –

Hypotension or tachycardia: If there is concern of impending hypotension or tachycardia, discontinue the infusion. When blood pressure has stabilized, infusion may be restarted at low doses (eg, 30 to 50 mL/hr) and adjusted to maintain desired blood pressure.

Infusion site changes: Continue IV use as long as BP control is needed. Change the infusion site every 12 hours if administered via peripheral vein.

Transfer to oral antihypertensives – If treatment includes transfer to an oral antihypertensive other than nicardipine, generally initiate therapy upon discontinuation of the infusion. If oral nicardipine is to be used, administer the first dose of a 3-times-daily regimen 1 hour prior to discontinuation of the infusion.

NIFEDIPINE: Individualize dosage. Excessive doses can result in hypotension.

Initial dosage (capsule) – 10 mg 3 times/day. Usual range is 10 to 20 mg 3 times/day. Some patients, especially those with coronary artery spasm, respond only to higher doses, more frequent administration or both. In such patients, 20 to 30 mg 3 or 4 times/day may be effective. Doses > 120 mg/day are rarely necessary. More than 180 mg/day is not recommended.

Titrate throughout 7 to 14 days to assess response to each dose level; monitor blood pressure before proceeding to higher doses.

Sustained release –

Procardia XL: 30 or 60 mg once daily. Titrate over a 7- to 14-day period. Titration may proceed more rapidly if the patient is frequently assessed. Titration to doses > 120 mg is not recommended.

Angina patients maintained on the nifedipine capsule formulation may be switched to the sustained release tablet at the nearest equivalent total daily dose. Experience with doses > 90 mg in angina is limited; therefore, use with caution and only when clinically warranted.

Adalat CC: Adjust dosage according to the patient's needs. Administer once daily on an empty stomach. In general, titrate over a 7- to 14-day period starting with 30 mg once daily. Base upward titration on therapeutic efficacy and safety. Usual maintenance dose is 30 to 60 mg once daily. Titration to doses > 90 mg daily is not recommended.

Concomitant drug therapy – Concomitant drug therapy with β-blockers may be beneficial in chronic stable angina; however, the effects of concurrent treatment cannot be predicted, especially in patients with compromised left ventricular function or cardiac conduction abnormalities.

NIMODIPINE: Commence therapy within 96 hours of the subarachnoid hemorrhage (SAH), using 60 mg every 4 hours for 21 consecutive days.

If the capsule cannot be swallowed (eg, time of surgery, unconscious patient), make a hole in both ends of the capsule with an 18 gauge needle and extract the contents into a syringe. Empty the contents into the patient's in situ nasogastric tube and wash down the tube with 30 mg normal saline.

NISOLDIPINE: Administer nisoldipine orally once daily. Administration with a high fat meal can lead to excessive peak drug concentration and should be avoided. Avoid grapefruit products before and after dosing.

Initiate therapy with 20 mg orally once daily, then increase by 10 mg/week, or longer intervals, to attain adequate control of blood pressure. The usual maintenance dosage is 20 to 40 mg once daily. BP response increases over the 10 to 60 mg/day dose range, but adverse event rates also increase. Doses > 60 mg once daily are not recommended.

Elderly/Hepatic function impairment – Patients > 65 years of age or patients with impaired liver function are expected to develop higher plasma concentrations of nisoldipine. Monitor blood pressure closely during any dosage adjustment. A starting dose not exceeding 10 mg/day is recommended in these patient groups.

VERAPAMIL HCl: If heart failure is not severe or rate-related, use digitalis and diuretics, as appropriate, before verapamil. In moderately severe to severe cardiac dysfunction (pulmonary capillary wedge pressure [PCWP] > 20 mmHg, ejection fraction < 30%), acute worsening of heart failure may occur.

Do not exceed 480 mg/day; safety and efficacy are not established. Half-life increases during chronic use; maximum response may be delayed.

Oral –

Angina at rest and chronic stable angina: Usual initial dose is 80 to 120 mg 3 times/day. However, 40 mg 3 times/day may be warranted if patients may have increased response to verapamil (eg, decreased hepatic function, elderly). Base upward titration of safety and efficacy evaluated ≈ 8 hours after dosing. Increase dosage daily (eg, unstable angina) or weekly until optimum clinical response is obtained.

Arrhythmias: Dosage range in digitalized patients with chronic atrial fibrillation is 240 to 320 mg/day in divided doses 3 or 4 times/day. Dosage range for prophylaxis of paroxysmal supraventricular tachycardia (PSVT) (non-digitalized patients) is 240 to 480 mg/day in divided doses 3 or 4 times/day. In general, maximum effects will be apparent during the first 48 hours of therapy.

Essential hypertension: The usual initial monotherapy dose is 80 mg 3 times/day (240 mg/day). Daily dosages of 360 and 480 mg have been used, but there is no evidence that dosages > 360 mg provide added effect. Consider beginning titration at 40 mg 3 times/day in patients who might respond to lower doses, (eg, elderly or people of small stature). Antihypertensive effects are evident within the first week of therapy. Base upward titration on therapeutic efficacy, assessed at the end of the dosing interval.

Sustained-release (essential hypertension): Give with food. Usual daily dose is 240 mg/day in the morning. However, 120 mg/day may be warranted in patients who may have increased response (eg, elderly or people of small stature). Base upward titration on safety and efficacy evaluated ≈ 24 hours after dosing. If adequate response is not obtained, titrate upward to 240 mg/morning and 120 mg/evening, then 240 mg every 12 hours, if needed. When switching from immediate release tablets, total daily dose (in mg) may remain the same. Antihypertensive effects are evident within the first week.

Parenteral (supraventricular tachyarrhythmias): For IV use only. Give as slow IV injection over ≥ 2 minutes under continuous ECG and blood pressure monitoring. An IV infusion has been used (5 mg/hour); precede the infusion with an IV loading dose.

Initial dose – 5 to 10 mg (0.075 to 0.15 mg/kg) as IV bolus over 2 minutes.

Repeat dose – 10 mg (0.15 mg/kg) 30 minutes after the first dose if the initial response is not adequate.

Older patients – Give over ≥ 3 minutes to minimize risk of untoward drug effects.

Children –

≤ 1 year of age: 0.1 to 0.2 mg/kg (usual single dose range, 0.75 to 2 mg) as an IV bolus over 2 minutes (under continuous ECG monitoring).

1 to 15 years of age: 0.1 to 0.3 mg/kg (usual single dose range, 2 to 5 mg) IV over 2 minutes. Do not exceed 5 mg.

Repeat dose: Repeat above dose 30 minutes after the first dose if the initial response is not adequate (under continuous ECG monitoring). Do not exceed a single dose of 10 mg in patients 1 to 15 years of age.

Actions

Pharmacology: The calcium channel blockers share the ability to inhibit movement of calcium ions across the cell membrane. The effects on the cardiovascular system include depression of mechanical contraction of myocardial and smooth muscle and depression of both impulse formation (automaticity) and conduction velocity. **Bepridil** also inhibits fast sodium inward channels. Calcium channel blockers are classified by structure as follows: Diphenylalkylamines – verapamil; benzothiazepines – diltiazem; dihydropyridines – amlodipine, felodipine, isradipine, nicardipine, nifedipine, nimodipine, nisoldipine.

Pharmacokinetics:

Calcium Channel Blocking Agents: Pharmacology/Pharmacokinetics						
	Parameters	Diltiazem/SR	Nicardipine	Nifedipine/SR	Nisoldipine	Verapamil
Pharmacokinetics	Extent of absorption (%)[1]	80-90	≈ 100	90	nd	90
	Absolute bioavailability (%)[1]	40-67	35	45-70/86	5	20-35
	Onset of action - oral (min)	30-60	20	20	nd	30[2]
	Time of peak plasma levels (hrs)	2-3/6-11	0.5-2	0.5/6	6-12	1-2.2
	Protein binding (%)	70-80	> 95	92-98	> 99	83-92
	Therapeutic serum levels (ng/mL)	50-200	28-50	25-100	nd	80-300
	Metabolite	Desacetyl-diltiazem[5]	Glucuronide conjugates	Acid or lactone[3]	5 major urinary metabolites	Norverapamil[4]
	Excreted unchanged in urine (%)	2-4	< 1	1-2	trace	3-4
	Half-life, elimination (hrs)	3.5-6/5-7	2-4	2-5	7-12	3-7[7]
Electrophysiology	Effective refractory period (ERP)					
	Atrium	0	0	0	0	0
	AV node	↑*	↑↓*	±	0	↑↑*
	His-Purkinje	0	↓*	0	0	0
	Ventricle	0	0	0	0	0
	Accessory pathway	na	0	0	0	±
	SA node automaticity[8]	↓*	0	0	0	↓↓*
	AV node conduction[8]	↓↓*	0-↑*	±	0	↓↓↓*
	Sinus node recovery time	0[9]	0	0	0	0[9]

Calcium Channel Blocking Agents: Pharmacology/Pharmacokinetics

	Parameters	Diltiazem/SR	Nicardipine	Nifedipine/SR	Nisoldipine	Verapamil
ECG Changes	Heart rate	↓*-0	↑*	↑*	±	↑↓*
	QRS complex	0	0	0	0	0
	PR interval	↑*	nd	0	0	↑*
	QT interval	nd	↑*	nd	0	nd
Hemodynamics	Myocardial contractility[8]	↓*	0	↓*	0	↓↓*
	Cardiac output	0-↑*	↑↑*	↑↑*	0	↑↓*
	Peripheral vascular resistance	↓*	↓↓↓*	↓↓↓*	↓↓↓	↓↓*

* ↑↑↑ or ↓↓↓ = pronounced effect; ↑↑ or ↓↓ = moderate effect; ↑ or ↓ = slight effect; ± = negligible effect; nd = no data; na = not applicable
[1] Although these agents are well absorbed (80% to 90%) following oral administration, they are subject to extensive first-pass effects, resulting in an absolute bioavailability that is considerably less.
[2] Peak therapeutic effects occur within 3 to 5 minutes after IV administration.
[3] Inactive.
[4] Pharmacologic activity 20% of verapamil.
[5] Pharmacologic activity 25% to 50% of diltiazem; plasma levels 10% to 20% of parent drug.
[6] Of 6 metabolites identified, account for > 75%.
[7] 4.5 to 12 hours with multiple dosing; may be prolonged in elderly.
[8] Direct effects may be counteracted by reflex activity.
[9] Prolonged in sick sinus syndrome.
[10] Dose-related.

Calcium Channel Blocking Agents: Pharmacology/Pharmacokinetics

Amlodipine	Bepridil	Felodipine	Isradipine	Nimodipine	Parameters	
nd	≈ 100	≈ 100	90-95	nd	Extent of absorption (%)[1]	Pharmacokinetics
64-90	59	20	15-24	13	Absolute availability (%)[1]	
nd	60	120-300	120	nd	Onset of action - oral (min)	
6-12	2-3	2.5-5	1.5	≤ 1	Time of peak plasma levels (hrs)	
93	> 99	> 99	95	> 95	Protein binding (%)	
nd	1-2	nd	nd	nd	Therapeutic serum levels (ng/mL)	
90% converted to inactive	4-OH-N-phenylbepridil	Six inactive[2]	Monoacids and cyclic lactone[6]	Unknown[3]	Metabolite	
10	±	< 0.5	0	< 1	Excreted unchanged in urine (%)	
30-50	24	11-16	8	1-2	Half-life, elimination (hrs)	

Calcium Channel Blocking Agents: Pharmacology/Pharmacokinetics						
Amlodipine	Bepridil	Felodipine	Isradipine	Nimodipine	Parameters	
					Effective refractory period	Electrophysiology
0	↑*	0	0	na	Atrium	
0	↑*	0	0		AV node	
0	↑*	0	0		His-Purkinje	
0	↑*	0	0		Ventricle	
0	↑*	0	nd		Accessory pathway	
0	↓*	0	0		SA node automaticity[8]	
0	↓*	0	0		AV node conduction[8]	
0	nd	0	±		Sinus node recovery time	
±	↓*	±	±		Heart rate	ECG Changes
0	0	0	0		QRS complex	
0	↑*	0	0		PR interval	
0	↑↑[10]	0	↑*		QT interval	
↑*	↓*	↑*	0		Myocardial contractility[8]	Hemodynamics
↑*	0	↑*	↑*		Cardiac output	
↓↓↓*	↓*	↓↓↓*	↓↓↓*		Peripheral vascular resistance	

* ↑↑↑ or ↓↓↓ = pronounced effect; ↑↑ or ↓↓ = moderate effect; ↑ or ↓ = slight effect; ± = negligible effect; nd = no data; na = not applicable
[1] Although these agents are well absorbed (80% to 90%) following oral administration, they are subject to extensive first-pass effects, resulting in an absolute bioavailability that is considerably less.
[2] Peak therapeutic effects occur within 3 to 5 minutes after IV administration.
[3] Inactive.
[4] Pharmacologic activity 20% of verapamil.
[5] Pharmacologic activity 25% to 50% of diltiazem; plasma levels 10% to 20% of parent drug.
[6] Of 6 metabolites identified, account for > 75%.
[7] 4.5 to 12 hours with multiple dosing; may be prolonged in elderly.
[8] Direct effects may be counteracted by reflex activity.
[9] Prolonged in sick sinus syndrome.
[10] Dose-related.

Contraindications

Hypersensitivity to the drug; sick sinus syndrome or second- or third-degree AV block except with a functioning pacemaker, hypotension < 90 mm Hg systolic (bepridil, diltiazem, and verapamil).

Diltiazem: Acute MI and pulmonary congestion.

Verapamil: Severe left ventricular dysfunction; cardiogenic shock and severe CHF, unless secondary to a supraventricular tachycardia amenable to verapamil therapy and in patients with atrial flutter or atrial fibrillation and an accessory bypass tract.

Verapamil IV – Do not administer concomitantly with IV β-adrenergic blocking agents (within a few hours), because both may depress myocardial contractility and AV conduction; ventricular tachycardia (VT), because use in patients with wide-complex VT (QRS ≥ 0.12 sec) can result in marked hemodynamic deterioration and ventricular fibrillation.

Nicardipine: Advanced aortic stenosis.

Bepridil: History of serious ventricular arrhythmias; uncompensated cardiac insufficiency; congenital QT interval prolongation; use with other drugs that prolong QT interval.

Warnings

Induction of new serious arrhythmias (bepridil): Bepridil has Class I antiarrhythmic properties and, like other such drugs, can induce new arrhythmias, including VT/VF. In addition, because of its ability to prolong the QT interval, bepridil can cause torsades de pointes-type VT. Because of these properties, reserve for patients in whom other antianginal agents do not offer a satisfactory effect.

While the safe upper limit of QT is not defined, it is suggested that the interval not be permitted to exceed 0.52 seconds during treatment. If dose reduction does not eliminate the excessive prolongation, stop the drug. If concomitant diuretics are needed, consider low doses and the addition or primary use of a potassium-sparing diuretic and monitor serum potassium.

Hypotension: Hypotension, usually modest and well tolerated, may occasionally occur during initial therapy or with dosage increases, and may be more likely in patients taking concomitant β-blockers.

CHF: CHF has developed rarely, usually in patients receiving a β-blocker, after beginning **nifedipine.**

Oral verapamil, 1.8% developed CHF or pulmonary edema.

Use **diltiazem, nicardipine, isradipine, felodipine, amlodipine,** and **bepridil** with caution in CHF patients.

Cardiac conduction: **IV verapamil** slows AV nodal conduction and SA nodes; it rarely produces second- or third-degree AV block, bradycardia, and in extreme cases, asystole. This is more likely to occur in patients with sick sinus syndrome.

Oral verapamil – Oral verapamil may lead to first-degree AV block and transient bradycardia, sometimes accompanied by nodal escape rhythms.

Premature ventricular contractions (PVCs): During conversion or marked reduction in ventricular rate, benign complexes of unusual appearance (sometimes resembling PVCs) may occur after **IV verapamil.** Verapamil IV may produce potentially fatal ventricular fibrillation in patients with atrial fibrillation (AF) and WPW syndrome.

Hypertrophic cardiomyopathy (IHSS): Serious adverse effects were seen in 120 patients with IHSS (most refractory or intolerant to propranolol) who received oral **verapamil** at doses up to 720 mg/day. Sinus bradycardia occurred in 11%, second-degree AV block in 4% and sinus arrest in 2%.

β-blocker withdrawal/nifedipine: Patients recently withdrawn from β-blockers may develop a withdrawal syndrome with increased angina, probably related to increased sensitivity to catecholamines. Initiation of nifedipine will not prevent this occurrence and might exacerbate it by provoking reflex catecholamine release. Taper β-blockers rather than stopping them abruptly before beginning nifedipine.

Hepatic function impairment: The pharmacokinetics, bioavailability and patient response to **verapamil** and **nifedipine** may be significantly affected by hepatic cirrhosis.

Because **amlodipine, diltiazem, nicardipine, bepridil, felodipine,** and **nimodipine** are extensively metabolized by liver, use with caution in impaired hepatic function or reduced hepatic blood flow.

Renal function impairment: The pharmacokinetics of **diltiazem** and **verapamil** in patients with impaired renal function are similar to the pharmacokinetic profile of patients with normal renal function. However, caution is still advised. **Nifedipine's** plasma concentration is slightly increased in patients with renal impairment. **Nicardipine's** mean plasma concentrations, AUC and maximum concentration were ≈ 2-fold higher in patients with mild renal impairment. Use **bepridil** with caution in patients with serious renal disorders since the metabolites of bepridil are excreted primarily in the urine.

Increased angina: Occasional patients have increased frequency, duration or severity of angina on starting **nifedipine** or **nicardipine** or at the time of dosage increases.

Duchenne's muscular dystrophy: **Verapamil** may decrease neuromuscular transmission in patients with Duchenne's muscular dystrophy and prolong recovery from the neuromuscular blocking agent vecuronium.

Elderly: **Verapamil, nifedipine,** and **felodipine** may cause a greater hypotensive effect than that seen in younger patients, probably due to age-related changes in drug disposition.

Pregnancy: Category C.

Lactation: **Verapamil, diltiazem,** and **bepridil** are excreted in breast milk. One report suggests that diltiazem concentrations in breast milk may approximate serum levels. Bepridil is estimated to reach about one third the concentration in serum. Significant concentrations of **nicardipine** and **nimodipine** appear in maternal milk of rats. An insignificant amount of **nifedipine** is transferred into breast milk (over 24 hours, < 5% of a dose). It is not known if **isradipine, amlodipine,** or **felodipine** are excreted in breast milk.

Children: Safety and efficacy of **diltiazem, bepridil, felodipine, amlodipine,** and **isradipine** have not been established.

Controlled studies of **IV verapamil** have not been conducted in pediatric patients, but uncontrolled experience indicates that results of treatment are similar to those in adults. Patients < 6 months of age may not respond to IV verapamil; this resistance may be related to a developmental difference of AV node responsiveness.

Precautions

Acute hepatic injury: In rare instances, symptoms consistent with acute hepatic injury, as well as significant elevations in enzymes such as alkaline phosphatase, CPK, LDH, AST, and ALT have occurred with **diltiazem** and **nifedipine.**

Elevations of transaminases with and without concomitant elevations in alkaline phosphatase and bilirubin have occurred with **verapamil.**

Isolated cases of elevated LDH, alkaline phosphatase, and ALT levels have occurred rarely with **nimodipine.**

Clinically significant transaminase elevations have occurred in ≈ 1% of patients receiving **bepridil**; however, no patient became clinically symptomatic or jaundiced, and values returned to normal when the drug was stopped.

Edema: Edema, mild to moderate, typically associated with arterial vasodilation and not due to left ventricular dysfunction, occurs in 10% of patients receiving **nifedipine.** It occurs primarily in the lower extremities and usually responds to diuretics. In patients with CHF, differentiate this peripheral edema from the effects of decreasing left ventricular function.

Peripheral edema, generally mild and not associated with generalized fluid retention, may occur with **felodipine** within 2 to 3 weeks of therapy initiation. The incidence is both age- and dose-dependent, with frequency ranging from 10% in patients < 50 years of age taking 5 mg/day to 30% in patients > 60 years of age taking 20 mg/day.

Drug Interactions

Drugs that may affect calcium blockers include barbiturates, calcium salts, dantrolene, erythromycin, histamine H_2 antagonists, hydantoins, quinidine, rifampin, sulfinpyrazone, vitamin D and carbamazepine. Drugs that may be affected by calcium blockers include quinidine, anticoagulants, beta blockers, carbamazepine, cyclosporine, digitalis glycosides, encainide, etomidate, fentanyl, lithium, magnesium sulfate (parenteral), nondepolarizing muscle relaxants, prazosin, and theophyllines.

Drug/Food interactions: **Nifedipine, amlodipine,** and **verapamil** may be administered without regard to meals.

Bioavailability of **felodipine** is not affected by food, but increased > 2-fold when taken with doubly concentrated grapefruit juice vs water or orange juice.

High-fat meals and grapefruit juice with **nisolodipine** should be avoided.

Adverse Reactions
Generally not serious; rarely requires discontinuation or dosage adjustment.

Adverse Reactions of Calcium Channel Blockers (%)

	Adverse Reactions	Amlodipine	Bepridil	Diltiazem[1]	Felodipine	Isradipine	Nicardipine	Nifedipine[1]	Nimodipine	Nisoldipine	Verapamil (IV)
Central Nervous System	Dizziness/Light-headedness	1.1-3.4[2]	11.6-27	1.5-7	5.8	7.3	4-6.9	4.1-27	< 1	5	3.5 (1.2)
	Drowsiness		≥ 7			≤ 1					
	Nervousness	≤ 1	7.4-11.6	< 1	≤ 1.5	≤ 1	0.6	≤ 7			
	Headache	7.3	7-13.6	2.1-12	18.6	13.7	6.4-8.2	10-23	1.4-4.1	22	2.2 (1.2)
	Weakness/Shakiness/Jitteriness			1.2		1.2	0.6	≤ 12			< 1
	Asthenia	1-2	6.5-14	2.8-5	4.7			4.2-5.8	< 3		1.7
	Fatigue/Lethargy	4.5[2]				3.9					
	Tremor/Hand tremor	≤ 1	≤ 9.3	< 1						≤ 1	
Gastrointestinal	Nausea	2.9[2]	7-26	1.6-1.9	1.9	1.8	1.9-2.2	3.3-11	0.6-1.4	2	2.7 (0.9)
	Diarrhea	≤ 1	0-10.9	< 1	1.6	1.1		< 3	1.7-4.2	≤ 1	< 1
	Constipation	≤ 1	2.8	1.6	1.6	≤ 1	0.6	≤ 3.3			7.3
	Dry mouth/Thirst	≤ 1	3.4	< 1	≤ 1.5	≤ 1	0.4-1.4	< 3		≤ 1	< 1
	Flatulence	≤ 1	≤ 2		≤ 1.5			≤ 3		≤ 1	
Cardiovascular	Pharyngitis									5	
	Peripheral edema	1.8-14.6[2]	≤ 2	2.4-9	22.3	7.2	7.1-8	10-30	0.4-1.2	22	2.1
	Hypotension	≤ 1		1	≤ 1.5	≤ 1	< 0.4	≤ 5	1.2-8.1		2.5 (1.5)
	Palpitations	0.7-4.5[2]	≤ 6.5	< 1	1.8	42[2]	3.3-4.1	≤ 7	< 1	3	< 1
	AV block (1°, 2°, or 3°)			0.6-7.6	≤ 1.5		< 0.4				0.8-1.2
	Bradycardia	≤ 1	≤ 2	1.5-6					0.6-1		1.4 (1.2)
	Congestive heart failure			< 1		≤ 1			2-6.7	< 1	≤ 1	1.8
	Myocardial infarction				≤ 1.5	≤ 1	< 0.4	4-6.7		≤ 1	< 1
	Pulmonary edema							7			1.8
	Angina			< 1	≤ 1.5	2.4	5.6	≤ 1		2	
	Tachycardia	≤ 1	≤ 2	< 1	≤ 1.5	1.5	0.8-3.4	≤ 1	1		(1)
	Abnormal ECG			4.1			0.6		0.6-1.4		
	Vasodilation									4	
Dermatologic	Dermatitis/Rash	1-2	≤ 2	1-1.5	1.5	1.5	0.4-1.2	≤ 3	0.6-2.4	2	1.2
	Pruritus/Urticaria	1-2		< 1	≤ 1.5	≤ 1		≤ 3	< 1	≤ 1	< 1 (†)[3]

Adverse Reactions of Calcium Channel Blockers (%)										
Adverse Reactions	Amlodipine	Bepridil	Diltiazem[1]	Felodipine	Isradipine	Nicardipine	Nifedipine[1]	Nimodipine	Nisoldipine	Verapamil (IV)
Other Flushing	0.7-4.5[2]		1.7-3	6.4	2.6	5.6-9.7	< 3-25	1-2.1	4	< 1
Nasal or chest congestion/sinusitis/rhinitis	≤ 0.1	≤ 2	< 1	≤ 1.5		†	≤ 6		≤ 3	†
Sexual difficulties	1-2	≤ 2	< 1	≤ 1.5	≤ 1	†	≤ 3			< 1
Shortness of breath/dyspnea/wheezing	1-2	≤ 8.7	< 1	≤ 1.5	1.8	0.6	≤ 8	1.2		1.4
Muscle cramps/pain/inflammation	1-2			≤ 1.9			≤ 8	0.2-1.4		< 1
Joint stiffness/pain/arthritis	≤ 1		< 1			†	≤ 3			
Cough	≤ 0.1	≤ 2		2.9	≤ 1		6			
Anorexia	≤ 1	≤ 7	< 1							
Respiratory infection		2.8		≤ 5.5			≤ 1			

[1] Includes data for sustained release form.
[2] Appears to be dose-related.
[3] †Occurs, no incidence reported.

VASOPRESSORS USED IN SHOCK

Vasopressors: Sympathomimetic agents are used in shock to treat hypoperfusion in nor-movolemic patients and in patients unresponsive to whole blood or plasma volume expanders. These agents increase myocardial contractility, constrict capacitance vessels, and dilate resistance vessels. In cardiogenic shock or advanced shock from other causes associated with a low cardiac output, they may be combined with vasodilators (eg, nitroprusside, nitroglycerin) to maintain blood pressure while the vasodilator improves myocardial performance. Nitroprusside is used to reduce pre-load and afterload and improve cardiac output. Nitroglycerin directly relaxes the venous vasculature and decreases preload.

Pharmacology: Sympathomimetic agents produce α-adrenergic stimulation (vasoconstriction), β_1-adrenergic stimulation (increase myocardial contractility, heart rate, automaticity, and AV conduction), and β_2-adrenergic activity (peripheral vasodilation). Dopamine also causes vasodilation of the renal and mesenteric, cerebral, and coronary beds by dopaminergic receptor activation.

Monitoring: Monitoring shock patients and their response to drugs requires special vigilance. Monitor heart rate, blood pressure, and ECG continuously. Record urine output and fluid intake frequently. Due to rapid and life-threatening changes that can occur in the hemodynamically unstable patient, optimal drug selection, dose titration, and management is probably best achieved with the use of invasive hemodynamic monitoring.

Administration: Administration only should be via the IV route using a large-bore, free flowing IV in the antecubital vein, or a central vein due to unpredictable absorption. Small IVs in the extremities are both unreliable and unsafe for vasopressor administration. Frequent monitoring of the IV sites for extravasation injury is essential when vasopressor agents are being used.

Prolonged, high-dose therapy: Prolonged, high-dose therapy can produce cyanosis and tissue necrosis of distal extremities. The principle of using the lowest dose that produces an adequate response for the shortest period of time is very important when using these agents.

Plasma volume depletion: Prolonged use of vasopressors may result in plasma volume depletion; correct this by appropriate fluid and electrolyte replacement therapy. If plasma volumes are not corrected, hypotension may recur when these drugs are discontinued.

Acidosis: Acidosis lessens the response to vasopressors; therefore, correct acidosis if it exists or develops during the course of vasopressor therapy.

Avoid continuous IV therapy: Acute tolerance develops during continuous IV administration. High concentration/low volume (250 mL) vasopressor solutions administered with the aid of an infusion control device allows for maximum dosing flexibility because fluids and drugs can be regulated independently and the development of tolerance is minimized.

Effects of Vasopressors Used in Shock

| | | Sites of action | | | | Hemodynamic response | | | |
| | | Heart | | Blood vessels | | | | | |
+++ pronounced effect ++ moderate effect + slight effect 0 no effect ↑ increase ↓ decrease		Contractility (Inotropic) β₁	SA Node Rate (Chronotropic) β₁	Vasoconstriction α	Vasodilatation β₂	Renal Perfusion	Cardiac Output	Total Peripheral Resistance	Blood Pressure
Inotropic	Isoproterenol	+++	+++	0	+++	↑¹ or ↓²	↑	↓	↑³↓⁴
	Dobutamine	+++	0 to +⁵	0 to +⁵	+	0	↑	↓	↑
	Dopamine	+++	+ to ++⁵	+ to +++⁵	0 to +⁶	↑⁵	↓	↓⁵ or ↑	0 to ↑
Mixed	Epinephrine	+++	+++	+++⁵	++⁵	↓	↑	↓	↑³↓⁴
	Norepinephrine	++	++⁷	+++	0	↓	0 or ↓	↑	↑
	Ephedrine	++	++	+	0 to +	↓	↑	↑ or ↓	↑
	Mephentermine	+	+	+	++	↑ or ↓	↑	0 to ↑	↑
Pressors	Metaraminol	+	+	++	0	↓	↓	↑	↑
	Methoxamine	0	0⁷	+++	0	↓	0 or ↓	↑	↑
	Phenylephrine	0	0⁷	+++	0	↓	↓	↑	↑

[1] Cardiogenic or septicemic shock.
[2] Normotensive patient.
[3] Systolic effect.
[4] Diastolic effect.
[5] Effects are dose dependent.
[6] Dilates renal and splanchnic beds via dopaminergic effect at doses < 10 mcg/kg/min.
[7] Decreased heart rate may result from reflex mechanisms.

Common Dilutions and Infusion Rates for Selected Drugs Used in Shock

Drug	Usual Dilution for IV Infusion	Infusion Rate
Isoproterenol	2 mg (10 mL) in 500 mL D5W (4 mcg/mL) or 1 mg (5 mL) in 250 mL D5W	5 mcg/min
Dobutamine	250 mg in 250 to 500 mL NS or D5W (500 to 1000 mcg/mL)	2.5 to 15 mcg/kg/min
Dopamine	200 to 800 mg in 250 to 500 mL NS or D5W (400 to 3200 mcg/mL)	Low dose – 2.5 to 10 mcg/kg/min High dose – 20 to 50 mcg/kg/min
Norepinephrine	4 mg in 250 mL of D5W (16 mcg/mL)	Initial: 8 to 12 mcg/min Maintenance: 2 to 4 mcg/min

BETA-ADRENERGIC BLOCKING AGENTS

ACEBUTOLOL HCl
Capsules: 200 and 400 mg (*Rx*)   Various, *Sectral* (Wyeth-Ayerst)

ATENOLOL
Tablets: 25, 50, and 100 mg (*Rx*)   Various, *Tenormin* (AstraZeneca)
Injection: 5 mg/10 mL (*Rx*)   *Tenormin* (AstraZeneca)

BETAXOLOL HCl
Tablets: 10 and 20 mg (*Rx*)   *Kerlone* (Searle)

BISOPROLOL FUMARATE
Tablets: 5 and 10 mg (*Rx*)   *Zebeta* (Lederle)

CARTEOLOL HCl
Tablets: 2.5 and 5 mg (*Rx*)   *Cartrol* (Abbott)

ESMOLOL HCl
Injection: 10 or 250 mg/mL (*Rx*)   *Brevibloc* (Baxter)

METOPROLOL
Tablets: 50 and 100 mg (*Rx*)   *Lopressor* (Novartis)
Tablets, extended release: 25, 50, 100, and 200 mg (*Rx*)   *Toprol XL* (AstraZeneca)
Injection: 1 mg/mL (*Rx*)   Various, *Lopressor* (Novartis)

NADOLOL
Tablets: 20, 40, 80, 120, and 160 mg (*Rx*)   Various, *Corgard* (Bristol-Myers Squibb)

PENBUTOLOL SULFATE
Tablets: 20 mg (*Rx*)   *Levatol* (Schwarz Pharma)

PINDOLOL
Tablets: 5 and 10 mg (*Rx*)   Various, *Visken* (Novartis)

PROPRANOLOL
Tablets: 10, 20, 40, 60, 80, and 90 mg (*Rx*)   Various, *Inderal* (Wyeth-Ayerst)
Capsules, sustained release: 60, 80, 120, and 160 mg (*Rx*)   Various, *Inderal LA* (Wyeth-Ayerst)
Solution, oral: 4 and 8 mg/mL (*Rx*)   Various
Solution, concentrated oral: 80 mg/mL (*Rx*)   *Propranolol Intensol* (Roxane)
Injection: 1 mg/mL (*Rx*)   Various, *Inderal* (Wyeth-Ayerst)

SOTALOL HCl
Tablets: 80, 120, 160, and 240 mg (*Rx*)   Various, *Betapace* (Berlex)
80, 120, 160 mg (*Rx*)   *Betapace AF* (Berlex)

TIMOLOL MALEATE
Tablets: 5, 10, and 20 mg (*Rx*)   Various, *Blocadren* (Merck)

Warning:
To minimize the risk of induced arrhythmia, patients initiated or reinitiated on *Betapace* or *Betapace AF* should be placed for a minimum of 3 days (on their maintenance dose) in a facility that can provide cardiac resuscitation, continuous electrocardiographic monitoring, and calculations of creatinine clearance. For detailed instructions regarding dose selection and special cautions for people with renal impairment, see Administration and Dosage.

Do not substitute *Betapace* for *Betapace AF* because of significant differences in labeling (eg, patient package insert, dosing administration, safety information).

Indications

Indications ✔ = labeled x = unlabeled	Acebutolol	Atenolol	Betaxolol	Bisoprolol	Carteolol	Esmolol	Metoprolol[1]	Nadolol	Penbutolol	Pindolol	Propranolol[1]	Sotalol	Timolol
Hypertension	✔	✔	✔	✔	✔		✔	✔	✔	✔	✔		✔
Angina pectoris		✔					✔	✔			✔		
Cardiac arrhythmias													

Beta-Adrenergic Blocking Agents — Summary of Indications													
Indications ✔= labeled x = unlabeled	Acebutolol	Atenolol	Betaxolol	Bisoprolol	Carteolol	Esmolol	Metoprolol[1]	Nadolol	Penbutolol	Pindolol	Propranolol[1]	Sotalol	Timolol
Supraventricular arrhythmias/tachycardias						✔					✔		
Sinus tachycardia						✔							
Intraoperative and postoperative tachycardia and hypertension						✔							
Ventricular arrhythmias/tachycardias											✔	✔[2]	
Premature ventricular contractions (PVCs)	✔										✔		
Digitalis-induced tachyarrhythmias											✔		
Resistant tachyarrhythmias (during anesthesia)											✔		
Atrial ectopy						x							
Maintenance of normal sinus rhythm												✔	
MI		✔					✔				✔		✔
CHF (stable)[3]				x			✔[4]						
Pheochromocytoma											✔		
Migraine prophylaxis		x					x	x			✔		✔
Hypertrophic subaortic stenosis											✔		
Parkinsonian tremors								x			x[5]		
Akathisia, antipsychotic-induced							x				x		
Variceal bleeding in portal hypertension		x					x	x			x		x
Atrial fibrillation													
Rapid heart rate control						x							
Maintenance heart rate control						x							
Generalized anxiety disorder											x		
Angina													
Stable	x			x									
Unstable		x				x	x						

[1] Includes long-acting formulation.
[2] Not *Betapace AF*.
[3] See Precautions or Warnings.
[4] *Toprol-XL* 25 mg only.
[5] Sustained-release only.

Administration and Dosage

ACEBUTOLOL HCl:

Hypertension –

Initial dose: 400 mg in uncomplicated mild to moderate hypertension. May be given as a single daily dose, but 200 mg twice/day may be required for adequate control. Optimal response usually occurs with 400 to 800 mg/day (range, 200 to 1200 mg/day given twice daily).

Ventricular arrhythmia –

Initial dose: 400 mg (200 mg twice/day). Increase dosage gradually until optimal response is obtained, usually 600 to 1200 mg/day.

Elderly – Because bioavailability increases about 2-fold, older patients may require lower maintenance doses. Avoid doses > 800 mg/day.

Renal/Hepatic function impairment – Reduce the daily dose by 50% when creatinine clearance is < 50 mL/min/1.73^2. Reduce by 75% when it is < 25 mL/min/1.73^2. Use cautiously in impaired hepatic function.

ATENOLOL:

Hypertension (oral) –

Initial dosage: 50 mg once daily, used alone or in combination with other antihypertensive agents. If an optimal response is not achieved, increase to 100 mg/day. Dosage > 100 mg/day is unlikely to produce any further benefit.

Angina pectoris (oral) –

Initial dosage: 50 mg/day. If an optimal response is not achieved within 1 week, increase to 100 mg/day. Some patients may require 200 mg/day for optimal effect.

With once-daily dosing, 24-hour control is achieved by giving doses larger than necessary to achieve an immediate maximum effect. The maximum early effect on exercise tolerance occurs with doses of 50 to 100 mg, but the effect at 24 hours is attenuated, averaging ≈ 50% to 75% of that with once-daily doses of 200 mg.

Acute MI –

IV: Initiate treatment as soon as possible after the patient's arrival in the hospital and after eligibility is established. Begin treatment with 5 mg over 5 minutes followed by another 5 mg IV injection 10 minutes later. Dilutions in Dextrose Injection, Sodium Chloride Injection, or Sodium Chloride and Dextrose Injection may be used. These admixtures are stable for 48 hours if not used immediately.

Oral: In patients who tolerate the full 10 mg IV dose, initiate 50 mg tablets 10 minutes after the last IV dose followed by another 50 mg dose 12 hours later. Thereafter, administer 100 mg once daily or 50 mg twice/day for a further 6 to 9 days or until discharge from the hospital.

If there is any question concerning the use of IV atenolol, eliminate the IV administration and use the tablets at a dosage of 100 mg once daily or 50 mg twice/day for ≥ 7 days.

Renal function impairment –

Atenolol Dosage Adjustments in Severe Renal Impairment		
Creatinine clearance (mL/min/1.73 m^2)	Elimination half-life (hrs)	Maximum dosage
15 to 35	16 to 27	50 mg/day
< 15	> 27	50 mg every other day

Hemodialysis – Give 25 or 50 mg after each dialysis.

BETAXOLOL HCl:

Initial dose – 10 mg once daily, alone or added to diuretic therapy. If the desired response is not achieved the dose can be doubled. Increasing the dose > 20 mg has not produced a statistically significant additional hypertensive effect; however, the 40 mg dose is well tolerated.

Elderly – Cosider reducing the starting dose to 5 mg.

Renal function impairment – In patients with renal impairment, clearance of betaxolol declines with decreasing renal function.

In patients with severe renal impairment and those undergoing dialysis, the initial dose is 5 mg once daily. If the desired response is not achieved, dosage may be increased by 5 mg/day increments every 2 weeks to a maximum dose of 20 mg/day.

BISOPROLOL FUMARATE: May be given without regard to meals.

Initial dose – 5 mg once daily. In some patients, 2.5 mg may be appropriate. If the antihypertensive effect of 5 mg is inadequate, the dose may be increased to 10 mg and then, if necessary, to 20 mg once daily.

Renal/Hepatic function impairment – In patients with renal dysfunction (creatinine clearance < 40 mL/min) or hepatic impairment (hepatitis or cirrhosis), use an initial daily dose of 2.5 mg and use caution in dose titration.

Elderly – Dose adjustment is not necessary.

CARTEOLOL HCl:

Initial dose – 2.5 mg as a single daily dose, either alone or with a diuretic. If adequate response is not achieved, gradually increase to 5 and 10 mg as single daily doses. Doses > 10 mg/day are unlikely to produce further benefit, and may decrease response.

Maintenance – 2.5 to 5 mg once daily.

Renal function impairment –

Carteolol Dosage in Renal Impairment	
Creatinine clearance (mL/min/1.73 m²)	Dosage interval (hrs)
> 60	24
20 to 60	48
< 20	72

ESMOLOL HCl:

Supraventricular tachycardia – 50 to 200 mcg/kg/min; average dose is 100 mcg/kg/min although dosages as low as 25 mcg/kg/min have been adequate. Dosages as high as 300 mcg/kg/min provide little added effect and an increased rate of adverse effects, and are not recommended.

Dosage in Supraventricular Tachycardia				
Time	Loading dose (over 1 minute)		Maintenance dose (over 4 minutes)	
(minutes)	mcg/kg/min	mg/kg/min	mcg/kg/min	mg/kg/min
0 to 1	500	0.5		
1 to 5			50	0.05
5 to 6	500	0.5		
6 to 10			100	0.1
10 to 11	500	0.5		
11 to 15			150	0.15
15 to 16	—	—		
16 to 20			200[1]	0.2[1]
20 to (24 hours)			Maintenance dose titrated to heart rate or other clinical endpoint	

[1] As the desired heart rate or endpoint is approached, the loading infusion may be omitted and the maintenance infusion titrated to 300 mcg/kg/min (0.3 mg/kg/min) or downward as appropriate. Maintenance dosages > 200 mcg/kg/min (0.2 mg/kg/min) have not been shown to have significantly increased benefits. The interval between titration steps may be increased.

If adequate therapeutic effect is not observed within 5 minutes, repeat loading dose and follow with maintenance infusion increased to 100 mcg/kg/min. Continue titration procedure, repeating loading infusion, increasing maintenance infusion by increments of 50 mcg/kg/min (for 4 minutes). As desired heart rate or a safety end-point (eg, lowered blood pressure) is approached, omit loading infusion and titrate the maintenance dosage up or down to endpoint. Also, if desired, increase interval between titration steps from 5 to 10 minutes.

This specific dosage regimen has not been intraoperatively studied. Because of the time required for titration, it may not be optimal for intraoperative use.

The safety of dosages > 300 mcg/kg/min has not been studied.

In the event of an adverse reaction, reduce dosage or discontinue the drug. If a local infusion site reaction develops, use an alternative site. Avoid butterfly needles.

Transfer to alternative agents – After achieving adequate heart rate control and stable clinical status, transition to alternative antiarrhythmatic agents may be accomplished.

Reduce the dosage of esmolol as follows: 30 minutes after the first dose of the alternative agent, reduce esmolol infusion rate by 50%. Following the second dose of the alternative agent, monitor patient's response and, if satisfactory control is maintained for the first hour, discontinue esmolol infusion.

Intraoperative and postoperative tachycardia and hypertension – In the intraoperative and postoperative settings, it is not always advisable to slowly titrate the dose of esmolol to a therapeutic effect. Therefore, 2 dosing options are presented: Immediate control dosing and a gradual control when the physician has time to titrate.

Immediate control: For intraoperative treatment of tachycardia and hypertension, give an 80 mg ($\approx$ 1 mg/kg) bolus dose over 30 seconds followed by a 150 mcg/kg/min infusion, if necessary. Adjust the infusion rate as required up to 300 mcg/kg/min to maintain desired heart rate or blood pressure.

Gradual control: For postoperative tachycardia and hypertension, the dosing schedule is the same as that used in supraventricular tachycardia. To initiate treatment, administer a loading dosage infusion of 500 mcg/kg/min for 1 minute followed by a 4-minute maintenance infusion of 50 mcg/kg/min. If an adequate therapeutic effect is not observed within 5 minutes, repeat the same loading dosage and follow with a maintenance infusion increased to 100 mcg/kg/min (see Supraventricular tachycardia).

Withdrawal effects – The use of esmolol infusions $\leq$ 24 hours has been well documented. Limited data indicate that esmolol is well tolerated $\leq$ 48 hours.

Preparation of solution –

250 mg/mL amp: Aseptically prepare a 10 mg/mL infusion by adding two 2500 mg ampuls to a 500 mL container or one 2500 mg ampul to a 250 mL container of one of the IV fluids listed below (see Compatibility/Stability). This yields a final concentration of 10 mg/mL. The diluted solution is stable for $\geq$ 24 hours at room temperature. Esmolol has been well tolerated when administered via a central vein.

The 250 mg/mL strength is concentrated, and is not for direct IV injection; dilute prior to infusion. Do not mix with sodium bicarbonate. Do not mix with other drugs prior to dilution in a suitable IV fluid.

10 mg/mL: This dosage form is prediluted to provide a ready-to-use 10 mg/mL concentration. It may be used to administer an esmolol loading dose infusion by hand-held syringe while the maintenance infusion is being prepared.

Compatibility/Stability – Esmolol, at a final concentration of 10 mg/mL, is compatible with the following solutions and is stable for $\geq$ 24 hours at controlled room temperature or under refrigeration: 5% Dextrose Injection; 5% Dextrose in Lactated Ringer's Injection; 5% Dextrose in Ringer's Injection; 5% Dextrose and 0.9% or 0.45% Sodium Chloride Injection; Lactated Ringer's Injection; Potassium Chloride (40 mEq/L) in 5% Dextrose Injection; 0.9% or 0.45% Sodium Chloride Injection.

Esmolol is *not* compatible with 5% Sodium Bicarbonate Injection.

METOPROLOL:
Tablets (immediate-release) and injection –

Hypertension:

Initial dosage – 100 mg/day in single or divided doses, used alone or added to a diuretic taken with or immediately after meals. The dosage may be increased at weekly (or longer) intervals until optimum blood pressure reduction is achieved.

Maintenance dosage – 100 to 450 mg/day. Dosages > 450 mg/day have not been studied. While once daily dosing is effective and can maintain a reduction in blood pressure throughout the day, lower doses (especially 100 mg) may not maintain a full effect at the end of the 24-hour period; larger or more frequent daily doses may be required.

Angina pectoris:

Initial dosage – 100 mg/day in 2 divided doses. Dosage may be gradually increased at weekly intervals until optimum clinical response is obtained or a pronounced slowing of heart rate occurs. Effective dosage range is 100 to 400 mg/day. Dosages above 400 mg/day have not been studied.

MI:

Early treatment – During the early phase of definite or suspected acute MI, initiate treatment as soon as possible. Administer 3 IV bolus injections of 5 mg each at $\approx$ 2 minute intervals.

In patients who tolerate the full IV dose (15 mg), give 50 mg orally every 6 hours 15 minutes after the last IV dose and continue for 48 hours. Thereafter, administer a maintenance dosage of 100 mg twice daily.

In patients who do not tolerate the full IV dose, start with 25 or 50 mg orally every 6 hours (depending on the degree of intolerance) 15 minutes after the last IV dose or as soon as the clinical condition allows.

Late treatment – Patients with contraindications to early treatment, patients who do not tolerate the full early treatment, and patients in whom therapy is delayed for any other reason should be started at 100 mg orally, twice daily, as soon as their clinical condition allows. Continue for ≥ 3 months.

Tablets, extended release – The extended-release tablets are for once daily administration. When switching from immediate-release metoprolol tablets to extended-release, use the same daily dose.

Hypertension: The usual initial dosage is 50 to 100 mg/day in a single dose whether used alone or added to a diuretic. The dosage may be increased at weekly (or longer) intervals until optimum blood pressure reduction is achieved. Dosages > 400 mg/day have not been studied.

Angina pectoris: The usual initial dosage is 100 mg/day in a single dose. The dosage may be gradually increased at weekly intervals until optimum clinical response has been obtained or there is a pronounced slowing of the heart rate. Dosages > 400 mg/day have not been studied.

CHF: Dosage must be individualized and closely monitored during up-titration. Prior to initiation of therapy, stabilize the dosing of diuretics, ACE inhibitors, and digitalis (if used). The recommended starting dose is 25 mg once daily for 2 weeks in patients with NYHA Class II heart failure and 12.5 mg once daily in patients with more severe heart failure. Then double the dose every 2 weeks to the highest dosage level tolerated by the patient or up to 200 mg. If transient worsening of heart failure occurs, it may be treated with increased dose of diuretics, and it may be necessary to lower the dose of metoprolol or temporarily discontinue it. The dose should not be increased until symptoms of worsening heart failure have been stabilized; initial difficulty with titration should not preclude later attempts to introduce metoprolol. If heart failure patients experience symptomatic bradycardia, reduce the dose.

NADOLOL:

Angina pectoris –

Initial dose: 40 mg/day. Gradually increase dosage in 40 to 80 mg increments at 3- to 7-day intervals until optimum clinical response is obtained or there is pronounced slowing of the heart rate.

Maintenance dosage: Usual dose is 40 to 80 mg once daily. Up to 160 to 240 mg once daily may be needed. The safety and efficacy of dosages exceeding 240 mg/day have not been established.

Hypertension –

Initial dose: 40 mg once daily, alone or in addition to diuretic therapy. Gradually increase dosage in 40 to 80 mg increments until optimum blood pressure reduction is achieved.

Maintenance dose: Usual dose is 40 to 80 mg once daily. Up to 240 to 320 mg once daily may be needed.

Renal function impairment –

Nadolol Dosage Adjustments in Renal Failure	
Creatinine clearance (mL/min/1.73²)	Dosage interval (hours)
> 50	24
31 to 50	24 to 36
10 to 30	24 to 48
< 10	40 to 60

PENBUTOLOL SULFATE: Usual starting and maintenance dose is 20 mg once daily. Doses of 40 to 80 mg have been well tolerated but have not shown greater antihypertensive effect. A dose of 10 mg also lowers blood pressure, but the full effect is not seen for 4 to 6 weeks.

PINDOLOL:
Initial dose – 5 mg twice daily, alone or with other antihypertensive agents. If a satisfactory reduction in blood pressure does not occur within 3 to 4 weeks, adjust dose in increments of 10 mg/day at 3 to 4 week intervals, to a maximum of 60 mg/day.

PROPRANOLOL HCl:

Propranolol Dosage Based on Indication			
Indication	Initial dosage	Usual range	Maximum daily dosage
Arrhythmias		10 - 30 mg tid-qid (given ac-hs)	
Hypertension	40 mg bid or 80 mg once daily (SR)	120 - 240 mg/day (given bid-tid) or 120 - 160 mg once daily (SR)	640 mg
Angina	80 - 320 mg bid, tid, qid or 80 mg once daily (SR)	160 mg once daily (SR)	320 mg
MI		180 - 240 mg/day (given tid-qid)	240 mg
IHSS		20 - 40 mg tid-qid (given ac-hs) or 8 - 160 mg once daily (SR)	
Pheochromocytoma		60 mg/day x 3 days preoperatively (in divided doses)	
Inoperable tumor		30 mg/day (in divided doses)	
Migraine	80 mg/day once daily (SR) or in divided doses	160 - 240 mg/day (in divided doses)	
Essential tremor	40 mg bid	120 mg/day	320 mg

Parenteral –
Usual dose: 1 to 3 mg. Do not exceed 1 mg/min. If necessary, give a second dose after 2 minutes. Thereafter, do not give additional drug in < 4 hour. Transfer to oral therapy as soon as possible.

Pediatrics – IV use is not recommended; however, an unlabeled dose of 0.01 to 0.1 mg/kg/dose to a maximum of 1 mg/dose by slow infusion over 5 minutes has been used for arrhythmias.

Oral dosage for treating hypertension requires titration, beginning with a 1 mg/kg/day dosage regimen (eg, 0.5 mg/kg twice daily). May be increased at 3- to 5-day intervals to a maximum of 16 mg/kg/day.

The usual pediatric dosage range is 2 to 4 mg/kg/day in 2 equally divided doses (eg, 1 to 2 mg/kg twice daily). Dosage calculated by weight generally produces plasma levels in a therapeutic range similar to that in adults. Do not use doses > 16 mg/kg/day.

SOTALOL HCl:
Betapace – The recommended initial dose is 80 mg twice daily. This dose may be increased if necessary, after appropriate evaluation, to 240 or 320 mg/day (120 to 160 mg bid). In most patients, a therapeutic response is obtained at a total daily dose of 160 to 320 mg/day, given in 2 or 3 divided doses. Some patients with life-threatening refractory ventricular arrhythmias may require doses as high as 480 to 640 mg/day.

Adjust dosage gradually, allowing 3 days between dosing increments in order to attain steady-state plasma concentrations, and to allow monitoring of QT intervals.

Renal function impairment:

Sotalol Dosing Interval in Renal Impairment	
Creatinine clearance (mL/min)	Dosing interval (hours)[1]
≥ 60	12
30 to 59	24
10 to 29	36 to 48
< 10	Individualize dosage

[1] The initial dose of 80 mg and subsequent doses should be administered at these intervals. See following paragraph for dosage escalations.

Dose escalations in renal impairment should be done after administration of at least 5 to 6 doses at appropriate intervals (see above table).

Exercise extreme caution in the use of sotalol in patients with renal failure undergoing hemodialysis. The half-life of sotalol is prolonged ($\leq$ 69 hours) in anuric patients. However, sotalol can be partly removed by dialysis with subsequent partial rebound in concentrations when dialysis is completed. Safety (heart rate, QT interval) and efficacy (arrhythmia control) must be closely monitored.

Betapace AF – Therapy with *Betapace AF* must be initiated (and if necessary, titrated) in a setting that provides continuous ECG monitoring and in the presence of personnel trained in the management of serious ventricular arrhythmias. Continue to monitor patients in this way for a minimum of 3 days on the maintenance dose. In addition, do not discharge patients within 12 hours of electrical or pharmacological conversion to normal sinus rhythm.

The QT interval is used to determine patient eligibility for *Betapace AF* treatment and for monitoring safety during treatment. The baseline QT interval must be $\leq$ 450 msec in order for a patient to be started on *Betapace AF* therapy. During initiation and titration, monitor the QT interval 2 to 4 hours after each dose. If the QT interval prolongs to $\geq$ 500 msec, the dose must be reduced or the drug discontinued.

The dose of *Betapace AF* must be individualized according to creatinine clearance. Modify the dosing interval according to the following table.

Betapace AF Dosing Interval in Renal Impairment	
Creatinine clearance (mL/min)	Dosing interval (hours)
> 60	12
40 to 60	24
< 40	Contraindicated

The recommended initial dose of *Betapace AF* is 80 mg and is initiated as shown in the dosing algorithm described below. The 80 mg dose can be titrated upward to 120 mg during initial hospitalization or after discharge on 80 mg in the event of recurrence, by rehospitalization and repeating the same steps used during the initiation of therapy (see Upward Titration of Dose).

Anticoagulate patients with atrial fibrillation according to usual medical practice. Correct hypokalemia before initiation of *Betapace AF* therapy (see Warnings).

Patients to be discharged on *Betapace AF* therapy from an inpatient setting should have an adequate supply of *Betapace AF* to allow uninterrupted therapy until the patient can fill a *Betapace AF* prescription.

Initiation of therapy:
1.) Electrocardiographic assessment: Prior to administration of the first dose, the QT interval must be determined using an average of 5 beats. If the baseline QT is > 450 msec (JT $\geq$ 330 msec if QRS over 100 msec), *Betapace AF* is contraindicated.
2.) Starting dose: The starting dose of *Betapace AF* is 80 mg twice daily if the creatinine clearance is > 60 mL/min, and 80 mg once daily if the creatinine clearance is 40 to 60 mL/min. If the creatinine clearance is < 40 mL/min, *Betapace AF* is contraindicated.
3.) Administer the appropriate daily dose of *Betapace AF* and begin continuous ECG monitoring with QT interval measurements 2 to 4 hours after each dose.
4.) If the 80 mg dose level is tolerated and the QT interval remains < 500 msec after at least 3 days (after 5 or 6 doses if patient is receiving once daily dosing), the patient can be discharged. Alternatively, during hospitalization, the dose can be increased to 120 mg twice daily and the patient followed for 3 days on this dose (followed for 5 or 6 doses if the patient is receiving once daily doses).

Upward titration of dose: If the 80 mg dose level (given once or twice daily depending upon the creatinine clearance) does not reduce the frequency of relapses of

AFIB/AFL and is tolerated without excessive QT interval prolongation (ie, ≥ 520 msec), the dose level may be increased to 120 mg (once or twice daily depending on the creatinine clearance). As proarrhythmic events can occur not only at initiation of therapy, but also with each upward dosage adjustment, steps 2 through 5 used during initiation of *Betapace AF* therapy should be followed when increasing the dose level. In a US multicenter dose-response study, a 120 mg dose (once or twice daily) was found to be the most effective in prolonging the time to ECG documented symptomatic recurrence of AFIB/AFL. If the 120 mg dose does not reduce the frequency of early relapse of AFIB/AFL and is tolerated without excessive QT interval prolongation (≥ 520 msec), an increase to 160 mg (once or twice daily depending on the creatinine clearance) can be considered. Steps 2 through 5 used during the initiation of therapy should be used again to introduce such an increase.

Maintenance of Betapace AF therapy: Regularly re-evaluate renal function and QT if medically warranted. If QT is ≥ 520 msec (JT 430 msec or greater if QRS is > 100 msec), reduce the dose of *Betapace AF* therapy and carefully monitor patients until QT returns to < 520 msec. If the QT interval is ≥ 520 msec while on the lowest maintenance dose level (80 mg), discontinue the drug. If renal function deteriorates, reduce the daily dose in half by administering the drug once daily as described in Initiation of Therapy, step 3.

Special considerations: The maximum recommended dose in patients with a calculated creatinine clearance > 60 mL/min is 160 mg twice/day, doses > 160 mg twice/day have been associated with an increased incidence of torsades de pointes and are not recommended.

A patient who misses a dose should not double the next dose. The next dose should be taken at the usual time.

Transfer to sotalol from other antiarrhythmic therapy – Before starting sotalol, generally withdraw previous antiarrhythmic therapy under careful monitoring for a minimum of 2 to 3 plasma half-lives if the patient's clinical condition permits. Treatment has been initiated in some patients receiving IV lidocaine without ill effect. After discontinuation of amiodarone, do not initiate sotalol until the QT interval is normalized.

Transfer to Betapace AF from Betapace – Patients with a history of symptomatic atrial fibrillation/atrial flutter (AFIB/AFL) who are currently receiving *Betapace* for the maintenance of normal sinus rhythm should be transferred to *Betapace* AF because of the significant differences in labeling (ie, patient package insert for *Betapace* AF, dosing, administration, and safety information).

TIMOLOL MALEATE:

Hypertension –

Initial dosage: 10 mg twice/day used alone or added to a diuretic.

Maintenance dosage: 20 to 40 mg/day. Titrate, depending on blood pressure and heart rate. Increases to a maximum of 60 mg/day divided into 2 doses may be necessary. There should be an interval of at least 7 days between dosage increases.

MI (long-term prophylactic use in patients who have survived the acute phase of MI) – 10 mg twice/day.

Migraine – Initial dosage is 10 mg twice/day. During maintenance therapy the 20 mg/day dosage may be given as a single dose. Total daily dosage may be increased to a maximum of 30 mg in divided doses or decreased to 10 mg once daily depending on clinical response and tolerability. Discontinue if a satisfactory response is not obtained after 6 to 8 weeks of the maximum daily dosage.

Actions

Pharmacology:

Pharmacologic/Pharmacokinetic Properties of Beta-Adrenergic Blocking Agents									
0 – none + – low ++ – moderate +++ – high Drug	Adrenergic-receptor blocking activity	Membrane stabilizing activity	Intrinsic sympathomimetic activity	Lipid solubility	Extent of absorption (%)	Absolute oral bioavailability (%)	Half-life (hrs)	Protein binding (%)	Metabolism/Excretion
Acebutolol	β_1[1]	+[2]	+	Low	90	20-60	3-4	26	Hepatic; renal excretion 30% to 40%; nonrenal excretion 50% to 60% (bile; intestinal wall).
Atenolol	β_1[1]	0	0	Low	50	50-60	6-7	6-16	≈ 50% excreted unchanged in feces
Betaxolol	β_1[1]	+	0	Low	≈ 100	89	14-22	≈ 50	Hepatic; > 80% recovered in urine, 15% unchanged
Bisoprolol	β_1[1]	0	0	Low	≥ 90	80	9-12	≈ 30	≈ 50% excreted unchanged in urine, remainder as inactive metabolites; < 2% excreted in feces.
Esmolol	β_1[1]	0	0	Low	na[3]	na[3]	0.15	55	Rapid metabolism by esterases in cytosol of red blood cells
Metoprolol	β_1[1]	0[2]	0	Moderate	≈ 100	40-50	3-7	12	Hepatic; renal excretion, < 5% unchanged
Metoprolol, long-acting						77[4]			
Carteolol	β_1 β_2	0	++	Low	85	85	6	23-30	50% to 70% excreted unchanged in urine
Nadolol	β_1 β_2	0	0	Low	30	30-50	20-24	30	Urine, unchanged
Penbutolol	β_1 β_2	0	+	High	≈ 100	≈ 100	≈ 5	80-98	Hepatic (conjugation, oxidation); renal excretion of metabolites (17% as conjugate)
Pindolol	β_1 β_2	0	+++	Low	> 95	≈ 100	3-4[5]	40	Urinary excretion of metabolites (60% to 65%) and unchanged drug (35% to 40%)
Propranolol	β_1 β_2	++	0	High	< 90	30	3-5	90	Hepatic; < 1% excreted unchanged in urine
Propranolol, long-acting						9-18	8-11		
Sotalol	β_1 β_2	0	0	Low	nd[6]	90-100	12	0	Not metabolized; excreted unchanged in urine
Timolol	β_1 β_2	0	0	Low to moderate	90	75	4	< 10	Hepatic; urinary excretion of metabolites and unchanged drug

[1] Inhibits β_2 receptors (bronchial and vascular) at higher doses.
[2] Detectable only at doses much greater than required for beta blockade.
[3] Not applicable (available IV only).
[4] Average bioavailability; not absolute.
[5] In elderly hypertensive patients with normal renal function, t½ variable: 7 to 15 hours.
[6] No data.

Contraindications

Sinus bradycardia; greater than first degree heart block; cardiogenic shock; congestive heart failure (CHF) unless secondary to a tachyarrhythmia treatable with β-blockers; overt cardiac failure; hypersensitivity to β-blocking agents.

Acebutolol, carteolol: Persistently severe bradycardia.

Propranolol, nadolol, timolol, penbutolol, carteolol, sotalol, and pindolol: Bronchial asthma or bronchospasm, including severe chronic obstructive pulmonary disease.

Metoprolol: Treatment of MI in patients with a heart rate < 45 beats/min; significant heart block greater than first degree (PR interval ≥ 0.24 sec); systolic blood pressure < 100 mmHg; moderate to severe cardiac failure.

Sotalol: Congenital or acquired long QT syndromes.

Warnings

Proarrhythmia: Like other antiarrhythmic agents, **sotalol** can provoke new or worsened ventricular arrhythmias in some patients, including sustained ventricular tachycardia or ventricular fibrillation, with potentially fatal consequences. Because of its effect on cardiac repolarization, is the most common form of proarrhythmia associated with sotalol, occurring in ≈ 4% of high-risk patients.

Cardiac failure: Sympathetic stimulation is a vital component supporting circulatory function in CHF, and β-blockade carries the potential hazard of further depressing myocardial contractility and precipitating more severe failure.

Wolff-Parkinson-White syndrome: In several cases, the tachycardia was replaced by a severe bradycardia requiring a demand pacemaker after **propranolol** administration with as little as 5 mg.

Abrupt withdrawal: The occurrence of a β-blocker withdrawal syndrome is controversial. However, hypersensitivity to catecholamines has been observed in patients withdrawn from β-blocker therapy. Exacerbation of angina, MI, ventricular arrhythmias, and death have occurred after abrupt discontinuation of therapy. Reduce dosage gradually over 1 to 2 weeks and carefully monitor the patient.

Because coronary artery disease may be unrecognized, do not discontinue therapy abruptly, even in patients treated only for hypertension, as abrupt withdrawal may result in transient symptoms.

Peripheral vascular disease: Treatment with β-antagonists reduces cardiac output and can precipitate or aggravate the symptoms of arterial insufficiency in patients with peripheral or mesenteric vascular disease.

Nonallergic bronchospasm (eg, chronic bronchitis, emphysema): In general, do not administer β-blockers to patients with bronchospastic diseases. Administer **nadolol, timolol, penbutolol, propranolol, sotalol**, and **pindolol** with caution, because they may block bronchodilation produced by endogenous or exogenous catecholamine stimulation of $β_2$ receptors.

Because of their relative $β_1$ selectivity, low doses of **metoprolol, acebutolol, bisoprolol**, and **atenolol** may be used with caution in patients with bronchospastic disease who do not respond to, or cannot tolerate, other antihypertensive treatment.

Bradycardia: **Metoprolol** produces a decrease in sinus heart rate in most patients; this decrease is greatest among patients with high initial heart rates and least among patients with low initial heart rates.

Pheochromocytoma: It is hazardous to use **propranolol** or **atenolol** unless α-adrenergic blocking drugs are already in use, because this would predispose to serious blood pressure elevation.

Sinus bradycardia: Sinus bradycardia (heart rate < 50 bpm) occurred in 13% of patients receiving **sotalol** in clinical trials, and led to discontinuation in about 3%. Bradycardia itself increases risk of torsade de pointes.

Electrolyte disturbances: Do not use **sotalol** in patients with hypokalemia or hypomagnesemia prior to correction of imbalance.

Hypotension: If hypotension (systolic blood pressure ≤ 90 mmHg) occurs, discontinue drug and carefully assess patient's hemodynamic status and extent of myocardial damage.

Anaphylaxis: Anaphylaxis has occurred and may include symptoms such as profound hypotension, bradycardia with or without AV nodal block, severe sustained bronchospasm, hives, and angioedema. Deaths have occurred. Refer to Management of Acute Hypersensitivity Reactions.

Anesthesia and major surgery: Necessity, or desirability, of withdrawing β-blockers prior to major surgery is controversial. β-blockade impairs the heart's ability to respond to β-adrenergically mediated reflex stimuli. While this might help prevent arrhythmic response, risk of excessive myocardial depression during general anesthesia may be enhanced, and difficulty restarting and maintaining heart beat has occurred. If β-blockers are withdrawn, allow 48 hours between the last dose and anesthesia. Others may recommend withdrawal of β-blockers well before surgery takes place.

AV block: **Metoprolol** slows AV conduction and may produce significant first (PR interval ≥ 0.26 sec), second; or third-degree heart block. Acute MI also produces heart block.

Sick sinus syndrome: Use **sotalol** only with extreme caution in patients with sick sinus syndrome associated with symptomatic arrhythmias, because it may cause sinus bradycardia, sinus pauses, or sinus arrest.

Concomitant use of calcium channel blockers (atenolol): Bradycardia and heart block can occur and the left ventricular end diastolic pressure can rise when beta-blockers are administered with verapamil or diltiazem. Patients with preexisting conduction abnormalities or left ventricular dysfunction are particularly susceptible.

Recent acute MI (sotalol): Sotalol can be used safely and effectively in the long-term treatment of life-threatening ventricular arrhythmias following an MI. However, experience in the use of sotalol to treat cardiac arrhythmias in the early phase of recovery from acute MI is limited and at least at high initial doses is not reassuring. In the first 2 weeks post-MI, caution is advised and careful dose titration is especially important, particularly in patients with markedly impaired ventricular function.

Intraoperative and postoperative tachycardia and hypertension: Do not use esmolol as the treatment for hypertension in patients in whom the increased blood pressure is primarily caused by the vasoconstriction associated with hypothermia.

Renal/Hepatic function impairment: Use with caution.

Pregnancy: Category D (atenolol).

Category C (**betaxolol, esmolol, metoprolol, nadolol, timolol, propranolol, penbutolol, carteolol, bisoprolol**).

Category B (**acebutolol, pindolol, sotalol**).

Lactation: In general, nursing should not be undertaken by mothers receiving these drugs.

Children: Safety and efficacy for use in children have not been established.

IV administration of **propranolol** is not recommended in children; however, oral propranolol has been used.

Precautions

Diabetes/Hypoglycemia: β-adrenergic blockade may blunt premonitory signs and symptoms (eg, tachycardia, blood pressure changes) of acute hypoglycemia. Nonselective β-blockers may potentiate insulin-induced hypoglycemia.

Thyrotoxicosis: β-adrenergic blockers may mask clinical signs (eg, tachycardia) of developing or continuing hyperthyroidism. Abrupt withdrawal may exacerbate symptoms of hyperthyroidism, including thyroid storm.

In contrast, propranolol may be beneficial in reducing the symptoms of thyrotoxicosis.

Serum lipid concentrations: β-blockers may alter serum lipids including an increase in the concentration of total triglycerides, total cholesterol and LDL and VLDL cholesterol, and a decrease in the concentration of HDL cholesterol.

Muscle weakness: β-blockade has potentiated muscle weakness consistent with certain myasthenic symptoms (eg, diplopia, ptosis, generalized weakness).

Drug Interactions

Drugs that may affect beta blockers include aluminum salts, barbiturates, calcium salts, cholestyramine, cimetidine, colestipol, diphenhydramine, hydroxychloroquine, NSAIDs, penicillins (ampicillin), rifampin, salicylates, SSRIs, sulfinpyrazole, calcium blockers, oral contraceptives, flecainide, haloperidol, hydralazine, loop diuretics, MAO inhibitors, phenothiazines, propafenone, quinidine, quinolones (ciprofloxacin), thioamines, and thyroid hormones.

Drugs that may be affected by beta blockers include flecainide, gabapentin, haloperidol, hydralazine, phenothiazines, anticoagulants, benzodiazepines, clonidine, disopyramide, epinephrine, ergot alkaloids, lidocaine, nondepolarizing muscle relaxants, prazosin, sulfonylureas, and theophylline.

Drug/Lab test interactions: These agents may produce hypoglycemia and interfere with **glucose** or **insulin** tolerance tests. **Propranolol** and **betaxolol** may interfere with the glaucoma screening test due to a reduction in intraocular pressure.

Drug/Food interactions: Food enhances the bioavailability of **metoprolol** and **propranolol**; this effect is not noted with **nadolol**, **bisoprolol**, or **pindolol**. The rate of **carteolol** and **penbutolol** absorption is slowed by the presence of food; however, extent of absorption is not appreciably affected. **Sotalol** absorption is reduced ≈ 20% by a standard meal.

Adverse Reactions

Most adverse effects are mild and transient and rarely require withdrawal of therapy.

Cardiovascular: Bradycardia; torsade de pointes and other serious new ventricular arrhythmias; chest pain; hypertension; hypotension; peripheral ischemia; pallor; flushing; worsening of angina and arterial insufficiency; shortness of breath; peripheral vascular insufficiency; CHF; edema; pulmonary edema; vasodilation; presyncope and syncope; tachycardia; palpitations; first-, second-, and third-degree heart block; abnormal ECG; supraventricular tachycardia.

CNS: Dizziness; vertigo; tiredness/fatigue; headache; mental depression; peripheral neuropathy; paresthesias; lethargy; anxiety; nervousness; diminished concentration/memory; somnolence; restlessness; insomnia; sleep disturbances; sedation; change in behavior; mood change; incoordination; hallucinations; acute mental changes in the elderly; increase in signs and symptoms of myasthenia gravis.

It has been suggested that the more lipophilic the β-blocker, the higher the CNS penetration and subsequent incidence of adverse CNS effects.

Dermatologic: Rash; pruritus; skin irritation; increased pigmentation; sweating/hyperhidrosis; alopecia; dry skin; psoriasis; acne; eczema; flushing; purpura; erythematous rash.

Endocrine: Hyperglycemia; hypoglycemia; unstable diabetes.

GI: Gastric/epigastric pain; flatulence; gastritis; constipation; nausea; diarrhea; dry mouth; vomiting; heartburn; appetite disorder; anorexia; bloating; abdominal discomfort/pain; dyspepsia; taste distortion.

GU: Sexual dysfunction; impotence or decreased libido; dysuria; nocturia; urinary retention or frequency.

Hematologic: Agranulocytosis; nonthrombocytopenic or thrombocytopenic purpura; bleeding; thrombocytopenia; eosinophilia; leukopenia; hyperlipdemia.

Hypersensitivity: Pharyngitis; photosensitivity reaction; erythematous rash; fever combined with aching and sore throat; laryngospasm; respiratory distress; angioedema; anaphylaxis.

Musculoskeletal: Joint pain; arthralgia; muscle cramps/pain; back/neck pain; arthritis; twitching/tremor; localized pain; extremity pain; myalgia.

Ophthalmic: Eye irritation/discomfort; dry/burning eyes; blurred vision; conjunctivitis; ocular pain/pressure; abnormal lacrimation.

Respiratory: Bronchospasm; dyspnea; cough; bronchial obstruction; wheeziness; nasal stuffiness; pharyngitis; laryngospasm with respiratory distress; asthma; rhinitis; sinusitis.

Miscellaneous: Facial swelling; weight gain; weight loss; Raynaud's phenomenon; speech disorder; earache; asthenia; malaise; fever; death.

Lab test abnormalities: **Propranolol** may elevate blood urea levels in patients with severe heart disease. **Propranolol** and **metoprolol** may cause elevated serum transaminase, alkaline phosphatase and LDH.

Minor persistent elevations in AST and ALT have occurred in 7% of patients treated with **pindolol**. Elevations of AST and ALT of 1 to 2 times normal have occurred with **bisoprolol** (3.9% to 6.2%).

LABETALOL HCl

Tablets: 100, 200, and 300 mg (*Rx*)	*Normodyne* (Schering), *Trandate* (Glaxo-Wellcome)
Injection: 5 mg/ml (*Rx*)	*Normodyne* (Schering), *Trandate* (Glaxo-Wellcome)

Indications
Oral: Hypertension, alone or with other agents, especially thiazide and loop diuretics.

Parenteral: For control of blood pressure in severe hypertension.

Administration and Dosage
Oral:

Initial dose – 100 mg twice/day, alone or added to a diuretic. After 2 or 3 days, using standing BP as an indicator, titrate dosage in increments of 100 mg twice/day, every 2 or 3 days.

Maintenance dose – 200 to 400 mg twice/day. Patients with severe hypertension may require 1.2 to 2.4 g/day. Should side effects (principally nausea or dizziness) occur with twice daily dosing, the same total daily dose given 3 times/day may improve tolerability. Titration increments should not exceed 200 mg twice/day.

Parenteral:

Repeated IV injection – Initially, 20 mg (0.25 mg/kg for an 80 kg patient) slowly over 2 minutes. Additional injections of 40 or 80 mg can be given at 10 minute intervals until a desired supine BP is achieved or a total of 300 mg has been injected. The maximum effect usually occurs within 5 minutes of each injection.

Slow continuous infusion – Give at a rate of 3 ml/min (2 mg/min). Continue infusion until satisfactory response is obtained; then discontinue infusion and start oral labetalol. Effective IV dose range is 50 to 200 mg, up to 300 mg.

Transfer to oral dosing (hospitalized patients): Begin oral dosing when supine diastolic BP begins to rise. Recommended initial dose is 200 mg, then 200 or 400 mg, 6 to 12 hours later, depending on BP response. Thereafter, proceed as follows:

Inpatient Titration Instructions	
IV regimen	Oral daily dose[*]
200 mg bid	400 mg
400 mg bid	800 mg
800 mg bid	1600 mg
1200 mg bid	2400 mg

[*] Total daily dose may be given in 3 divided doses.

Actions
Pharmacology: Labetalol combines both selective, competitive postsynaptic α_1-adrenergic blocking, and nonselective, competitive β-adrenergic blocking activity. The α- and β-blocking actions decrease blood pressure (BP). Standing BP is lowered more than supine.

Pharmacokinetics:

Absorption/Distribution – Oral labetalol is completely absorbed; peak plasma levels occur in 1 to 2 hours. Steady-state plasma levels during repetitive dosing are reached by about the third day. Due to an extensive first-pass effect, absolute bioavailability is 25%. Protein binding is $\approx$ 50%.

Metabolism/Excretion – Metabolism is mainly through conjugation to glucuronide metabolites, which are excreted in urine and in feces (via bile). Elimination half-life is 5.5 to 8 hours. About 55% to 60% of a dose appears in urine as conjugates or unchanged drug in the first 24 hours.

Onset/Peak/Duration –

Oral: The peak effects of single oral doses occur within 2 to 4 hours and lasts 8 to 12 hours. The maximum, steady-state BP response upon oral, twice-a-day dosing occurs within 24 to 72 hours.

IV: The maximum effect of each IV injection of labetalol at each dose level occurs within 5 minutes. Following discontinuation of IV therapy, BP approaches pretreatment baseline values in 16 to 18 hours.

Contraindications

Bronchial asthma; overt cardiac failure; greater than first-degree heart block; cardiogenic shock; severe bradycardia.

Warnings

Cardiac failure: Avoid use in overt CHF; may be used with caution in patients with a history of heart failure who are well compensated. CHF has been observed in patients receiving labetalol.

Patients without history of cardiac failure (latent cardiac insufficiency): Continued depression of myocardium with β-blockers can lead to cardiac failure.

Withdrawal: Hypersensitivity to catecholamines has been seen in patients withdrawn from β-blockers. When discontinuing chronic labetalol, particularly in ischemic heart disease, gradually reduce dosage over 1 to 2 weeks and carefully monitor.

Nonallergic bronchospasm (eg, chronic bronchitis, emphysema): Patients with bronchospastic disease should, in general, not receive β-blockers.

Diabetes mellitus and hypoglycemia: β-blockade may prevent the appearance of premonitory signs and symptoms of acute hypoglycemia. β-blockade also reduces insulin release; it may be necessary to adjust antidiabetic drug dose.

Major surgery: Withdrawing β-blockers prior to major surgery is controversial. Protracted severe hypotension and difficulty restarting or maintaining heartbeat have been reported with beta blockers.

Rapid decreases of BP: Observe caution when reducing severely elevated BP. Achieve desired BP lowering over as long a time as possible.

Hepatic function impairment: Drug metabolism may be diminished.

   Jaundice or hepatic dysfunction – Jaundice or hepatic dysfunction has rarely been associated with labetalol.

Elderly: Bioavailability is increased in elderly patients.

Pregnancy: Category C.

Lactation: Small amounts are excreted in breast milk.

Children: Safety and efficacy for use in children have not been established.

Precautions

Hypotension: Symptomatic postural hypotension is most likely to occur 2 to 4 hours after a dose, especially following a large initial dose or upon large changes in dose. It is likely to occur if patients are tilted or allowed to assume the upright position ≤ 3 hours of receiving labetalol injection.

Drug Interactions

Drugs that may interact with labetalol include beta-adrenergic agonists, cimetidine, glutethimide, halothane, and nitroglycerin.

Drug/Lab test interactions: A labetalol metabolite may falsely increase urinary catecholamine levels when measured by a nonspecific trihydroxyindole reaction.

Drug/Food interactions: Food may increase bioavailability of the drug.

Adverse Reactions

Significant adverse reactions include fatigue; headache; drowsiness; paresthesias; difficulty in micturition; diarrhea; reversible increases in serum transaminases; dyspnea; bronchospasm; asthenia; muscle cramps; nausea; vomiting; fever with aching and sore throat; toxic myopathy; rashes; systemic lupus erythematosus; vision abnormality; hypoesthesia; ventricular arrhythmias; intensification of AV block; mental depression; scalp tingling.

CARVEDILOL

Tablets: 3.125, 6.25, 12.5, and 25 mg (Rx) Coreg (SmithKline Beecham)

Indications

Essential hypertension: Management of essential hypertension. It can be used alone or in combination with other antihypertensive agents, especially thiazide-type diuretics.

Congestive heart failure (CHF): For the treatment of mild or moderate NYHA class II or III heart failure of ischemic or cardiomyopathic origin, in conjunction with digitalis, diuretics, and ACE inhibitors, to reduce the progression of disease.

Unlabeled uses: Carvedilol appears to be beneficial in the treatment of the following conditions: Angina pectoris (25 to 50 mg twice daily); idiopathic cardiomyopathy (6.25 to 25 mg twice daily).

Administration and Dosage

Hypertension: The recommended starting dose is 6.25 mg twice daily. If this dose is tolerated, using standing systolic pressure measured about 1 hour after dosing as a guide, maintain the dose for 7 to 14 days, and then increase to 12.5 mg twice daily, if needed, based on trough blood pressure, again using standing systolic pressure 1 hour after dosing as a guide for tolerance. This dose also should be maintained for 7 to 14 days and can then be adjusted upward to 25 mg twice/day if tolerated and needed. The full antihypertensive effect of carvedilol is seen within 7 to 14 days. Total daily dose should not exceed 50 mg. Carvedilol should be taken with food to slow the rate of absorption and reduce the incidence of orthostatic effects.

CHF – Dosage must be indivualized and closely monitored during up-titration. Prior to initiation, stabilize the dosing of digitalis, diuretics, and ACE inhibitors.

The recommended starting dose is 3.125 mg twice/day for 2 weeks. If this dose is tolerated, it can then be increased to 6.25 mg twice/day. Dosing then should be doubled every 2 weeks to the highest level tolerated by the patient. The maximum recommended dose is 25 mg twice/day in patients weighing < 85 kg (187 lbs) and 50 mg twice/day in patients weighing > 85 kg.

Actions

Pharmacology: Carvedilol, an antihypertensive agent, is a racemic mixture in which non-selective β-adrenoreceptor blocking activity is present in the S(-) enantiomer and α-adrenergic blocking activity is present in both R(+) and S(-) enantiomers at equal potency. Carvedilol has no intrinsic sympathomimetic activity.

Carvedilol (1) reduces cardiac output, (2) reduces exercise- or isoproterenol-induced tachycardia, and (3) reduces reflex orthostatic tachycardia. Significant β-blocking effect is usually seen within 1 hour of drug administration.

Carvedilol also (1) attenuates the pressor effects of phenylephrine, (2) causes vasodilation, and (3) reduces peripheral vascular resistance. These effects contribute to the reduction of blood pressure and usually are seen within 30 minutes of drug administration.

Pharmacokinetics:

Absorption/Distribution – Carvedilol is rapidly and extensively absorbed following oral administration, with absolute bioavailability of ≈ 25% to 35% due to a significant degree of first-pass metabolism. Following oral administration, the apparent mean terminal elimination half-life generally ranges from 7 to 10 hours. Plasma concentrations achieved are proportional to the oral dose administered.

Carvedilol is > 98% bound to plasma proteins (primarily albumin). It has a steady-state volume of distribution of ≈ 115 L, indicating substantial distribution into extravascular tissues. Plasma clearance ranges from 500 to 700 mL/min.

Metabolism/Excretion – Carvedilol is extensively metabolized. Following oral administration in healthy volunteers, carvedilol accounted for only about 7% of the total in plasma as measured by area under the curve. Less than 2% of the dose was excreted unchanged in the urine. The metabolites of carvedilol are excreted primarily via the bile into the feces.

Contraindications

Patients with NYHA Class IV decompensated cardiac failure; bronchial asthma (2 cases of death from status asthmaticus have been reported in patients receiving single doses of carvedilol) or related bronchospastic conditions; second- or third-degree AV block; cardiogenic shock; severe bradycardia; hypersensitivity to the drug.

Warnings

Cardiac failure: Worsening cardiac failure or fluid retention may occur during up-titration of carvedilol. If such symptoms occur, increase diuretics and do not advance the carvedilol dose until clinical stability resumes. Occasionally, it is necessary to lower the carvedilol dose or temporarily discontinue it. Such episodes do not preclude subsequent successful titration of carvedilol.

Hepatic injury: Mild hepatocellular injury, confirmed by rechallenge, has occurred rarely with carvedilol therapy. At the first symptom/sign of liver dysfunction perform laboratory testing. If the patient has laboratory evidence of liver injury or jaundice, stop therapy and do not restart.

Peripheral vascular disease: β-blockers can precipitate or aggravate symptoms of arterial insufficiency in patients with peripheral vascular disease. Exercise caution.

Hypotension and postural hypotension: Hypotension and postural hypotension occurred in 9.7% and syncope in 3.4% of CHF patients receiving carvedilol, compared with 3.6% and 2.5% of placebo patients, respectively. The risk for these events was highest during the first 30 days of dosing.

Anesthesia and major surgery: If carvedilol treatment is to be continued perioperatively, take particular care with anesthetic agents which depress myocardial function.

Diabetes and hypoglycemia: β-blockers may mask some of the manifestations of hypoglycemia, particularly tachycardia. Nonselective β-blockers may potentiate insulin-induced hypoglycemia and delay recovery of serum glucose levels. Caution patients subject to spontaneous hypoglycemia, or diabetic patients receiving insulin or oral hypoglycemic agents about these possibilities and use carvedilol with caution.

Thyrotoxicosis: β-adrenergic blockade may mask clinical signs of hyperthyroidism, such as tachycardia. Abrupt withdrawal of β-blockade may be followed by an exacerbation of the symptoms of hyperthyroidism or may precipitate thyroid storm.

Pheochromocytoma: In patients with pheochromocytoma, an α-blocking agent should be initiated prior to use of any β-blocking agent. Although carvedilol has both α- and β-blocking pharmacologic activities, there has been no experience with its use in this condition. Therefore, use caution in administering carvedilol.

Prinzmetal's variant angina: Agents with non-selective β-blocking activity may provoke chest pain in patients with Prinzmetal's variant angina. Although the α-blocking activity of carvedilol may prevent such symptoms, take caution with patients suspected of having Prinzmetal's variant angina.

Congestive heart failure (CHF): Compared with healthy subjects, CHF patients had increased mean AUC and C_{max} values for carvedilol and its enantiomers.

Anaphylactic reaction: While taking β-blockers, patients with a history of severe anaphylactic reaction to a variety of allergens may be more reactive to repeated challenge, either accidental, diagnostic, or therapeutic. Such patients may be unresponsive to the usual doses of epinephrine used to treat allergic reaction.

Renal/Hepatic function impairment: Rarely, use of carvedilol in patients with CHF has resulted in deterioration of renal function. Patients at risk appear to be those with low blood pressure (systolic BP < 100 mmHg), ischemic heart disease, and diffuse vascular disease or underlying renal insufficiency. Renal function returned to baseline when carvedilol was stopped. Discontinue the drug or reduce dosage if worsening of renal function occurs.

Use of carvedilol in patients with clinically manifest hepatic impairment is not recommended.

Elderly: Plasma levels of carvedilol average about 50% higher in the elderly compared with young subjects. With the exception of dizziness (8.8% in the elderly vs 6%

in younger patients), there were no events for which the incidence in the elderly exceeded that in the younger population by > 2%.

Pregnancy: Category C.

Lactation: It is not known whether this drug is excreted in breast milk.

Children: Safety and efficacy in patients < 18 years of age have not been established.

Precautions

Cardiovascular effects: Because carvedilol has β-blocking activity, it should not be discontinued abruptly, particularly in patients with ischemic heart disease. Instead, discontinue over 1 to 2 weeks.

In clinical trials, carvedilol caused bradycardia in about 2% of patients. If pulse rate drops below 55 beats/min, reduce the dosage.

Bronchospasm, nonallergic (eg, chronic bronchitis, emphysema): In general, patients with bronchospastic disease should not receive β-blockers. Carvedilol may be used with caution, however, in patients who do not respond to, or cannot tolerate, other antihypertensive agents.

Drug Interactions

Drugs that may affect carvedilol include cimetidine, rifampin and strong inhibitors of CYP2D6 (eg, quinidine, fluoxetine, paroxetine, propafenone).

Drugs that may be affected by carvedilol include antidiabetic agents, calcium blockers, clonidine, catecholamine depleting agents (eg, reserpine), and digoxin.

Drug/Food interactions: When taken with food, rate of absorption is slowed but extent of bioavailability is not affected. Taking with food minimizes the risk of orthostatic hypotension.

Adverse Reactions

CHF patients: Reactions occurring in ≥ 3% of patients include dizziness; fatigue; upper respiratory tract infection; chest pain; diarrhea; hyperglycemia; pain; injury; generalized and dependent edema; abnormal vision; fever; bradycardia; hypotension; syncope; headache; nausea; abdominal pain; vomiting; weight increase; gout; BUN increase; NPN increase; hypercholesterolemia; back pain; arthralgia; myalgia; sinusitis; bronchitis; pharyngitis and urinary tract infection.

Hypertensive patients: Adverse reactions occurring in ≥ 3% of patients include dizziness and fatigue.

ANTIHYPERTENSIVES

Agents used in hypertension therapy are listed in the following tables:

Pharmacological Effects of Antihypertensive Agents													
↑ = increase ⇧ = slight increases 0 = no change ⇩ = slight decrease ↓ = decrease	Onset (min)	Peak effect[1] (hrs)	Duration of action[2] (hrs)	Plasma volume	Plasma renin activity	RBF/GFR[3]	Peripheral resistance	Cardiac output	Heart rate	LVH	Total cholesterol	HDL	LDL	Triglycerides
Antiadrenergic Agents – Centrally Acting													
Methyldopa	120	2-6	12-24	↑	⇩/0	⇩/0	↓	⇩/0	⇩/0	↓	0	0	0	0
Clonidine	30-60	2-5	12-24	↑	⇩	⇩/0	↓	⇩/0	↓	↓	0	0	0	0
Guanabenz	60	2-4	6-12	0	↓	0	↓	0	↓	↓	0	0	0	0
Guanfacine		1-4	24	⇩/0	↓		↓	0	⇩	↓	0	0	0	0
Antiadrenergic Agents – Peripherally Acting													
Reserpine	days	6-12	6-24	↑	⇩/0	⇩/0	↑	0/↓	↑					
Guanethidine		6-8	24-48	↑	⇩/0	⇩/0	↓	0/↓	↑					
Guanadrel	30-120	4-6	9-14	↑		0	↑	0	↓					
Doxazosin		2-3								↓	↓	↑	0/↓	↓
Prazosin	120-130	1-3	6-12	0/⇧	⇩/0	0	↓	0/⇧	0/⇧	↓	↓	↑	0/↑	↓
Terazosin	15	1-2	12-24	0	0	0	↓	⇧	⇧	↓	↓	↑	0/↓	↓
Antiadrenergic Agents – Beta-Adrenergic Blockers													
Acebutolol		3-8	24-30			⇩	↓	↓	0/↓	0/↑	↓	↑	0/↑	
Atenolol		2-4	24 +	⇩/0	↓	↓/0	0	↓	↓	↓	0/↑	↓	↑	0/↑
Betaxolol							↓	↓		0/↑	↓	↑	0/↑	
Bisoprolol							↓	↓		0			0	
Carteolol		1-3	24 +				↓	↓		0			0	
Metoprolol		1.5	13-19	⇩/0	↓	⇩/0	0/↓	↓	↓	↓	0/↑	↓	↑	0/↑
Nadolol		3-4	17-24	⇩/0	↓	0	0	↓	↓	↓	0/↑	↓	↑	0/↑
Penbutolol		1.5-3	20 +		↓	⇩	0	↓	↓		0	0/↑	0	↑/↓
Pindolol		1	24 +		0	0	↓	⇩	↓	0/↓	0	0/↑	0	↑/↓
Propranolol		2-4	8-12	⇩/0	↓	↓	⇩/0	↓	↓	↓	0	0/↑	0	↑/↓
Timolol		1-3	12	⇩/0	↓		0	↓	↓	↓	0	0/↑	0	↑/↓
Antiadrenergic Agents – Alpha/Beta-Adrenergic Blocker													
Labetalol		2-4	8-12	↑	↓	0/↑	↓	0	↓	↓				
Carvedilol	30						↓	↓	↓					
Angiotensin Converting Enzyme (ACE) Inhibitors													
Benazepril	60	0.5-1	24		↑	RBF ↑ GFR 0	↓	0/↑	0	↓	0	0	0	0
Captopril	15-30	0.5-1.5	6-12	⇧	↑	RBF ↑ GFR 0	↓	0/↑	0	↓	0	0	0	0
Enalapril	60	4-6	24	0/⇧	↑	RBF ↑ GFR 0	↓	↑	0	↓	0	0	0	0
Enalaprilat	15	3-4	≈ 6		↑	RBF ↑ GFR 0	↓	↑	0	↓	0	0	0	0
Fosinopril	60	≈ 3	24		↑	RBF ↑ GFR 0	↓	0/↑	0	↓	0	0	0	0
Lisinopril	60	≈ 7	24		↑	RBF ↑ GFR 0	↓	0	0	↓	0	0	0	0
Quinapril	60	1	24		↑	RBF ↑ GFR 0	↓	0/↑	0	↓	0	0	0	0
Ramipril	60-120	1	24		↑	RBF ↑ GFR 0	↓	0/↑	0	↓	0	0	0	0
Calcium Channel Blocking Agents													
Amlodipine	gradual	6-12	> 24	0	0	↑	↓↓↓	0	0	↓	0	0	0	0
Diltiazem SR	30-60	6-11					↓	0-↑	↓-0	↓	0	0	0	0

Pharmacological Effects of Antihypertensive Agents

Legend: ↑ = increase; ⇧ = slight increases; 0 = no change; ⇩ = slight decrease; ↓ = decrease

	Onset (min)	Peak effect[1] (hrs)	Duration of action[2] (hrs)	Plasma volume	Plasma renin activity	RBF[3] GFR[3]	Peripheral resistance	Cardiac output	Heart rate	LVH	Total cholesterol	HDL	LDL	Triglycerides
Felodipine	120-300	2.5-5					↓↓↓	↑	↑	↓	0	0	0	0
Isradipine	120	1.5					↓↓↓	↑	↑/↓	↓	0	0	0	0
Nicardipine	20	0.5-2			⇧/↑	⇧	↓	↑	↑	↓	0	0/⇧	0	0
Nifedipine SR	20	6					↓↓↓	↑↑	↑	↓	0	0	0	0
Verapamil	30	1-2.2			0/⇧	0	↓	↑/↓	↑/↓	↓	0	0/⇧	0	0
Diuretics														
Thiazides & deriv.	60-120	4-12	6-72	↓	↑	↓	↓	↓	0	0/??	↑	0	↑	↑
Loop diuretics	within 60	1-2	4-8	↓	↑	↓	↓	↓	0	0/??	↑	0	↑	↑
Amiloride	120	6-10	24	↓	↑	0	↓	↓	0					
Spironolactone	24-48 hr	48-72	48-72	↓	↑	0	↓	0	0					
Triamterene	2-4 hr	6-8	12-16											
Vasodilators														
Hydralazine	45	0.5-2	6-8	↑	↑	↑	↓	↑	↑	↑				
Minoxidil	30	2-3	24-72	↑	↑	0	↓	↑	↑	↑				
Agents For Hypertensive Emergencies/Urgencies														
Phentolamine	immed.		5-10 min	⇧	↑	↑	↓	0/↑	↑					
Phenoxybenzamine	gradual	2-3	24 +	⇧	↑	↑	↓	↑	↓					
Metyrosine		6 +	2-3 days				↓		↓					
Agents For Pheochromocytoma														
Nitroprusside	0.5-1		3-5 min	↑	↑	0	↓	⇩	⇧	NA				
Diazoxide	1-2	5 min	< 12	↑	↑	↑	↓	↑	↑					
Trimethaphan camsylate	1-2		10-15 min	↑	↓	0	↓	↓	↓					
Nitroglycerin (IV)	immed.		transient	0	0		↓	↑	↑					
Captopril[4]				⇧	↑	RBF ↑ GFR 0	↓	0/↑	0					
Enalaprilat[4]					↑	RBF ↑ GFR 0	↓	↑	0					
Hydralazine[4]	10-20		3-6											
Labetalol[4]	5-10		3-6	↑	↓	0/↑	↓	0	↓					
Nicardipine[4]	1-5		3-6		⇧/↑	⇧	↓	↑	↑					
Nifedipine[4]							↓↓↓	↑↑	↑					
Phentolamine[4]	1-2		3-10 min											
Miscellaneous Agents														
Mecamylamine	30-120		6-12+	↑	↓	↓	↓	↓	↑					
Pargyline		4-21 days	3 weeks		↓	↓	↓	0	0					
Tolazoline							↓							

[1] Peak clinical effect following a single oral dose, except where indicated.
[2] Duration of action is frequently dose-dependent.
[3] Renal blood flow and glomerular filtration rate.
[4] Unlabeled use.
[5] NA = Not applicable.

Stepped-Care Antihypertensive Regimen†:

Experience in treating essential hypertension (systolic blood pressure [BP] ≥ 140 mm Hg and/or diastolic BP ≥ 90 mm Hg) demonstrates the benefits of pharmacotherapy. Reducing BP decreases cardiovascular mortality and morbidity in patients with hypertension. Antihypertensive therapy protects against stroke, left ventricular hypertrophy, CHF, and progression to more severe hypertension. In addition to drug therapy, lifestyle modifications of adjunctive value include weight reduction, sodium and alcohol restriction, smoking cessation, regular exercise, and a diet low in saturated fat.

Hypertension Categories		
Range (mm Hg)		
Systolic	Diastolic	Category[1]
< 130	< 85	Normal BP
130-139	85-89	High normal BP
140-159	90-99	Stage 1 (mild) hypertension
160-179	100-109	Stage 2 (moderate) hypertension
180-209	110-119	Stage 3 (severe) hypertension
≥ 210	≥ 120	Stage 4 (very severe) hypertension

[1] When systolic and diastolic BP fall into different categories, select the higher category to classify the patient's BP (eg, classify 165/95 mm Hg as Stage 2, 170/115 mm Hg as Stage 3). Isolated systolic hypertension is systolic BP ≥ 140 mm Hg and diastolic BP < 90 mm Hg (stage appropriately).

For purposes of risk classification and management, specify presence or absence of target-organ disease and additional risk factors in addition to classifying hypertension stages. For example, classify a diabetic patient with Stage 3 hypertension and left ventricular hypertrophy as "Stage 3 hypertension with target-organ disease (left ventricular hypertrophy) and with one additional risk factor (diabetes)."

The *stepped-care approach* begins with lifestyle modifications. If BP remains ≥ 140/90 mm Hg for 3 to 6 months, start antihypertensive therapy, especially in patients with target-organ disease or other risk factors for cardiovascular disease. Initiate therapy with one agent, increase the dosage gradually, then add or substitute agents with gradual increases in doses until the therapeutic goal is achieved, side effects become intolerable or maximum dosages are reached. Try lifestyle modifications first.

Stepped-Care Approach		
I. Lifestyle modifications	Weight reduction Moderation of alcohol intake Regular physicial activity	Reduction of sodium intake Smoking cessation
II. Inadequate response	Continue lifestyle modifications Initial pharmacological selection[1] 1) Diuretics or beta blockers[2] 2) ACE inhibitors, calcium blockers, alpha$_1$ blockers, alpha-beta blocker[3]	
III. Inadequate response	1) Increase drug dose, or; 2) Substitute another drug, or; 3) Add a second agent from a different class.[4]	
IV. Inadequate response	Add a second or third agent or diuretic if not already prescribed.[4]	

[1] Initial drug therapy is monotherapy for Stage 1 and Stage 2 hypertension.

[2] Preferred because a reduction in morbidity and mortality has been demonstrated.

[3] Equally effective in reducing BP; however, these have not been tested in long-term controlled trials to demonstrate reduction of morbidity and mortality. Reserve for special indications or when preferred agents are unacceptable or ineffective.

[4] Supplemental antihypertensive agents, which include centrally acting alpha$_2$-agonists (clonidine, guanabenz, guanfacine, methyldopa), peripheral-acting adrenergic antagonists (guanadrel, guanethidine, rauwolfia alkaloids) and direct vasodilators (hydralazine, minoxidil), are not routinely well suited for initial monotherapy.

† The Fifth-Report of the Joint National Committee on Detection, Evaluation, and Treatment of High Blood Pressure. *Arch Intern Med* 1993;153:154-83.

Diuretics – Generally initiate therapy with a thiazide or other oral diuretic. Thiazide-type diuretics are drugs of choice; hydrochlorothiazide or chlorthalidone are generally preferred. Reserve loop diuretics for selected patients. This therapy alone may control many cases of mild hypertension. Consider treating diuretic-induced hypokalemia (< 3.5 mEq/L) with potassium supplementation or by adding a potassium-sparing diuretic to therapy.

Beta-adrenergic blocking agents – Beta-adrenergic blocking agents also may be used as initial drug monotherapy. Beta blockers are effective in older patients, but less effective in black people. Beta-adrenergic blocking agents decrease cardiac output without effects on vascular resistance. In addition, they inhibit renin release.

Calcium channel blockers, ACE inhibitors, labetalol, and alpha₁ blockers – Calcium channel blockers, ACE inhibitors, labetalol, and alpha$_1$ blockers may be used as initial monotherapy, although they are not routinely preferred over diuretics and beta blockers. Black people tend to respond better to calcium blockers than ACE inhibitors; labetalol may be more effective in black people than other beta blockers.

Antiadrenergic agents – Antiadrenergic agents (central and peripheral adrenergic inhibitors) are considered supplemental agents and are used when the initial drug therapy fails to achieve the desired effect. Diuretics are usually continued to provide synergistic effects and to prevent secondary fluid accumulation that may occur with use of antiadrenergic agents alone. Combination therapy also may minimize untoward reactions, which are more common at the higher doses necessary when a single drug is used alone.

Decreased adrenergic tone results in reduced cardiac output or decreased peripheral vascular resistance. Methyldopa, guanabenz, guanfacine, and clonidine act mainly in the CNS. Although reserpine has been used for years, other agents are preferred. Guanadrel is a peripheral antiadrenergic similar to guanethidine.

Vasodilators: Vasodilators also are considered supplemental agents and are not suited for initial monotherapy. A 3 drug regimen should include agents acting by different mechanisms. Hydralazine and minoxidil have direct vasodilating actions. In order to prevent reflex tachycardia caused by decreased peripheral resistance, these agents are most effective when used with a diuretic and a β-blocker. Minoxidil's undesirable side effects limit its use to severely hypertensive patients who do not respond to minimum doses of a diuretic and 2 other agents.

Antihypertensive drug withdrawal syndrome – Antihypertensive drug withdrawal syndrome may occur after discontinuation of antihypertensives.

To circumvent problems, encourage patient compliance, avoid excessive doses, avoid combining sympatholytics and β-blockers, and maintain antihypertensive medication in surgical patients. When discontinuing medication, taper the dose slowly, one drug at a time; use special caution in patients with coronary artery or cerebrovascular disease.

Treatment generally includes reinstitution of therapy, bed rest/sedation and, perhaps, therapy similar to treatment of malignant hypertension.

Step-down therapy – Attempt to decrease the dosage or the number of antihypertensive agents in patients; have them maintain lifestyle modifications. It may be possible to accomplish this in a deliberate, slow, progressive manner if the patient has been effectively controlled for 1 year and ≥ 4 visits.

METHYLDOPA AND METHYLDOPATE HCl

Tablets: 125 mg, 250 mg, and 500 mg methyldopa (*Rx*)	Various, *Aldomet* (Merck)
Oral Suspension: 250 mg methyldopa/5 mL (*Rx*)	Various, *Aldomet* (Merck)
Injection: 250 mg methyldopate HCl/5 mL (*Rx*)	Various, *Aldomet* (Merck)

Indications

Hypertension.

Methyldopate HCl may be used to initiate treatment of acute hypertensive crises; however, due to its slow onset of action, other agents may be preferred for rapid reduction of blood pressure.

Administration and Dosage

Impaired renal function: Methyldopa is largely excreted by the kidneys; patients with impaired renal function may respond to smaller doses.

Elderly: Syncope in older patients may be related to an increased sensitivity and advanced arteriosclerotic vascular disease. May be avoided by lower doses.

Adults: Initial therapy: 250 mg, 2 or 3 times a day in the first 48 hours. Adjust dosage at intervals of not less than 2 days until adequate response is achieved. To minimize sedation, increase dosage in the evening. By adjustment of dosage, morning hypotension may be prevented without sacrificing control of afternoon blood pressure.

Maintenance therapy – 500 mg to 3 g daily in 2 to 4 doses. Methyldopa is usually administered in 2 divided doses; some patients may be controlled with a single daily dose given at bedtime.

Concomitant drug therapy – When methyldopa is given with antihypertensives other than thiazides, limit the initial dosage to 500 mg/day in divided doses; when added to a thiazide, the dosage of thiazide need not be changed.

Children: Individualize dosage. Initial oral dosage is based on 10 mg/kg/day in 2 to 4 doses. The maximum daily dosage is 65 mg/kg or 3 g, whichever is less.

Tolerance: Tolerance may occur, usually between the second and third month of therapy. Adding a diuretic or increasing the dosage of methyldopa frequently restores blood pressure control. A thiazide is recommended if therapy was not started with a thiazide or if effective control of blood pressure cannot be maintained on 2 g methyldopa daily.

Discontinuation: Methyldopa has a relatively short duration of action; therefore, withdrawal is followed by return of hypertension, usually within 48 hours. This is not complicated by an overshoot of blood pressure above pretreatment levels.

IV: Add dose to 100 mL of 5% Dextrose or give in 5% Dextrose in Water in a concentration of 10 mg/mL. Administer over 30 to 60 minutes. When control has been obtained, substitute oral therapy starting with the same parenteral dosage schedule.

Adults – 250 to 500 mg every 6 hours as required (maximum 1 g every 6 hours).

Children – 20 to 40 mg/kg/day in divided doses every 6 hours. The maximum daily dosage is 65 mg/kg or 3 g, whichever is less.

Actions

Pharmacology: The mechanism of action of methyldopa has not been conclusively demonstrated, but is probably due to the drug's metabolism to alpha-methyl norepinephrine, which lowers arterial pressure by the stimulation of central inhibitory α-adrenergic receptors, false neurotransmission or reduction of plasma renin activity.

Pharmacokinetics:

Absorption/Distribution – Oral absorption of methyldopa is variable (range 8% to 62%); peak plasma levels are achieved in 2 to 4 hours. There is no correlation between plasma concentration and antihypertensive effect. Approximately 2 days are required to establish maximal antihypertensive effects and for hypertension to return after discontinuation of therapy. Effective IV doses cause a decline in blood pressure, which may begin in 4 to 6 hours and last 10 to 16 hours.

Metabolism – The elimination half-life is ≈ 2 hours; however, antihypertensive activity persists for up to 24 hours. The main metabolite, an inactive O-sulfate conjugate, is formed in intestinal cells. Approximately 70% of the absorbed drug is excreted in the urine as methyldopa and its mono-O-sulfate conjugate. The renal clearance is diminished in renal insufficiency. The plasma half-life of methyldopa is 105 minutes. After oral doses, excretion is essentially complete in 36 hours. Blood pressure reduction is pronounced and prolonged in renal failure. The drug is removed by dialysis.

Contraindications

Active hepatic disease, such as acute hepatitis or active cirrhosis; if previous methyldopa therapy has been associated with liver disorders; hypersensitivity to any component of these formulations.

Warnings

Positive Coombs' test/Hemolytic anemia: With prolonged therapy, 10% to 20% of patients develop a positive direct Coombs' test, usually between 6 and 12 months of therapy. This is associated rarely with hemolytic anemia, which could lead to potentially fatal complications and is difficult to predict. If a positive direct Coombs' test develops during therapy, determine whether hemolytic anemia exists and whether the positive Coombs' test may be a problem. Perform baseline and periodic blood counts to detect hemolytic anemia. A direct Coombs' test may be useful before therapy and at 6 and 12 months later. If Coombs'-positive hemolytic anemia occurs, discontinue methyldopa; anemia usually remits promptly. If not, give corticosteroids and consider other causes. If hemolytic anemia is related to methyldopa, do not reinstitute.

Liver disorders: Fever has occasionally occurred within the first 3 weeks of therapy, sometimes associated with eosinophilia or abnormalities in ≥ 1 liver function tests. Jaundice with or without fever may occur, usually within the first 2 to 3 months of therapy. In some patients, the findings are consistent with cholestasis. Fatal hepatic necrosis has been reported rarely. Incidence of elevated serum transaminase levels and impaired hepatic function ranges from 1% to 27%.

Perform periodic determinations of hepatic function, particularly during the first 6 to 12 weeks of therapy or when an unexplained fever occurs. If fever, abnormalities in liver function tests or jaundice appear, discontinue therapy; temperature and abnormalities in liver function revert to normal when the drug is discontinued. Do not reinstitute methyldopa therapy in such patients.

Hematologic disorders: Rarely, a reversible reduction of the white blood cell (WBC) count with a primary effect on granulocytes has been seen.

Renal function impairment: The active metabolites of methyldopa accumulate in uremia. Use with caution in renal failure. Prolonged hypotension has been reported.

Hypertension has recurred occasionally after dialysis in patients given methyldopa because the drug is removed by this procedure.

Hepatic function impairment: Use with caution in patients with previous liver disease or dysfunction.

Pregnancy: Category B.

Lactation: Methyldopa is excreted in breast milk.

Precautions

Paradoxical pressor response: Paradoxical pressor response has been reported with IV methyldopa.

Involuntary choreoathetotic movements: Involuntary choreoathetotic movements have been observed rarely in patients with severe bilateral cerebrovascular disease. Should these occur, discontinue methyldopa therapy.

Sedation: Sedation, usually transient, may occur during initial therapy or whenever the dose is increased; patients should observe caution while performing tasks requiring alertness during these periods.

Urine discoloration: Rarely, when urine is exposed to air, it may darken because of breakdown of methyldopa or its metabolites.

Sulfite sensitivity: These products contain sulfites that may cause allergic-type reactions in certain susceptible people. Sulfite sensitivity is seen more frequently in asthmatic or atopic nonasthmatic people.

Drug Interactions
Drugs that may affect methyldopa include haloperidol, levodopa, lithium, and propranolol.

Drugs that may be affected by methyldopa include haloperidol, levodopa, lithium, sympathomimetics, and tolbutamide.

Drug/Lab test interactions: Methyldopa may interfere with tests for: Urinary uric acid by phosphotungstate method; serum creatinine by alkaline picrate method; AST by colorimetric methods. Because methyldopa causes fluorescence in urine samples at the same wavelengths as catecholamines, falsely high levels of urinary catecholamines may occur and will interfere with the diagnosis of pheochromocytoma.

Adverse Reactions
Possible adverse reactions include fever; lupus-like syndrome; rise in BUN; myalgia; septic shock-like syndrome; headache; asthenia; weakness; dizziness; symptoms of cerebrovascular insufficiency; paresthesias; parkinsonism; Bell's palsy; decreased mental acuity; involuntary choreoathetotic movements; psychic disturbances; verbal memory impairment; bradycardia; prolonged carotid sinus hypersensitivity; aggravation of angina pectoris; pericarditis; myocarditis (fatal); orthostatic hypotension; edema/weight gain (usually relieved by a diuretic; discontinue methyldopa if edema progresses or signs of heart failure appear); nausea; vomiting; constipation; diarrhea; colitis; sore or "black" tongue; pancreatitis; liver disorders; positive Coombs' test, bone marrow depression; leukopenia; granulocytopenia; thrombocytopenia; positive tests for antinuclear antibody, LE cells and rheumatoid factor; rash; toxic epidermal necrolysis; gynecomastia; lactation; amenorrhea.

CLONIDINE HCl

Tablets: 0.1 mg, 0.2 mg, and 0.3 mg (*Rx*)	Various, *Catapres* (Boehringer-Ingelheim)
Transdermal system: 2.5 mg (release rate 0.1 mg/24 hrs) (*Rx*)	*Catapres-TTS-1* (Boehringer-Ingelheim)
5 mg (release rate 0.2 mg/24 hrs) (*Rx*)	*Catapres-TTS-2* (Boehringer-Ingelheim)
7.5 mg (release rate 0.2 mg/24 hrs) (*Rx*)	*Catapres-TTS-3* (Boehringer-Ingelheim)

Indications
Hypertension.

Unlabeled uses: Clonidine has been evaluated for use in the following conditions:

Clonidine Unlabeled Uses	
Use	Dosage[1]
Alcohol withdrawal	0.3 to 0.6 mg every 6 hours
Constitutional growth delay in children	0.0375 to 0.15 mg/m^2/day
Diabetic diarrhea	0.15 to 1.2 mg/day or 0.3 mg/24 hr patch (1 to 2 patches/week)
Gilles de la Tourette syndrome	0.15 to 0.2 mg/day
Hypertensive "urgencies" (diastolic> 120 mm Hg)	Initially 0.1 to 0.2 mg, followed by 0.05 to 0.1 mg every hour to a maximum of 0.8 mg
Menopausal flushing	0.1 to 0.4 mg/day or 0.1 mg/24 hr patch
Methadone/opiate detoxification	15 to 16 mcg/kg/day
Pheochromocytoma diagnosis (overnight clonidine suppression test)	0.3 mg

Clonidine Unlabeled Uses	
Use	Dosage[1]
Postherpetic neuralgia	0.2 mg/day
Reduction of allergen-induced inflammatory reactions in patients with extrinsic asthma	0.15 mg for 3 days
Smoking cessation facilitation	0.15 to 0.4 mg/day or 0.2 mg/24 hour patch
Ulcerative colitis	0.3 mg 3 times a day

[1] Dosage given as oral unless otherwise specified.

Administration and Dosage

Oral: Individualize dosage.

Initial dose – 0.1 mg twice daily. The elderly may benefit from a lower initial dose.

Maintenance dose – Increments of 0.1 or 0.2 mg/day may be made until desired response is achieved; most common range is 0.2 to 0.8 mg/day given in divided doses. The maximum dose is 2.4 mg/day. Minimize sedative effects by slowly increasing the daily dosage and giving the majority of the daily dose at bedtime.

Children – 5 to 25 mcg/kg/day in divided doses every 6 hours; increase at 5- to 7-day intervals.

Unlabeled route of administration – Sublingual clonidine, using a dosage of 0.2 to 0.4 mg/day, may be effective in hypertensive patients unable to take oral medication. The onset occurs within 30 to 60 minutes and blood pressure appears to be maintained on a twice daily regimen.

Renal Impairment – Adjust dosage according to degree of renal impairment and carefully monitor patients. Because only a minimal amount of clonidine is removed during hemodialysis, there is no need to give supplemental clonidine following dialysis.

Transdermal: Apply to a hairless area of intact skin on upper arm or torso, once every 7 days. Use a different skin site from the previous application. If the system loosens during the 7-day wearing, apply the adhesive overlay directly over the system to ensure good adhesion.

For initial therapy, start with the 0.1 mg system. If, after 1 or 2 weeks, desired blood pressure reduction is not achieved, add another 0.1 mg system or use a larger system. Dosage > two 0.3 mg systems usually does not improve efficacy. Note that the antihypertensive effect of the system may not commence until 2 to 3 days after application. Therefore, when substituting the transdermal system in patients on prior antihypertensive therapy, a gradual reduction of prior drug dosage is advised. Previous antihypertensive treatment may have to be continued, particularly in patients with severe hypertension.

Actions

Pharmacology: Initially, clonidine stimulates peripheral α-adrenergic receptors producing transient vasoconstriction. Stimulation of alpha-adrenergic in the brain stem results in reduced sympathetic outflow from the CNS and a decrease in peripheral resistance, renal vascular resistance, heart rate, and blood pressure.

Pharmacokinetics: Blood pressure declines within 30 to 60 minutes after an oral dose. The peak plasma level occurs in ≈ 3 to 5 hours with a plasma half-life of 12 to 16 hours. About 50% of the absorbed dose is metabolized in the liver. In patients with impaired renal function, half-life increases to 30 to 40 hours. Clonidine and its metabolites are excreted mainly in the urine. About 40% to 60% of the absorbed dose is recovered in the urine as unchanged drug in 24 hours.

Transdermal system – The system, a 0.2 mm thick film with 4 layers, contains a drug reservoir of clonidine, released at an approximately constant rate for 7 days.

Therapeutic plasma levels, achieved 2 to 3 days after initial application, are lower than during oral therapy with equipotent doses. When system is removed, therapeutic plasma clonidine levels persist for ≈ 8 hours and then decline slowly over several days; blood pressure returns gradually to pretreatment levels. Elimination half-life is ≈ 19 hours.

Contraindications

Hypersensitivity to clonidine or any component of adhesive layer of transdermal system.

Warnings

Use with caution in patients with severe coronary insufficiency, recent MI, cerebrovascular disease, or chronic renal failure.

Tolerance: Tolerance may develop, necessitating a reevaluation of therapy.

Pregnancy: Category C.

Lactation: Clonidine is excreted in breast milk.

Children: Safety and efficacy for use in children have not been established.

Precautions

Rebound hypertension: Do not discontinue therapy without consulting a physician. Discontinue therapy by reducing the dose gradually over 2 to 4 days to avoid a rapid rise in blood pressure.

If an excessive rise in blood pressure occurs, it can be reversed by resumption of therapy or by IV phentolamine, phenoxybenzamine, or prazosin. Direct vasodilators and captopril also have been used. If therapy is to be discontinued in patients receiving β-blockers and clonidine concurrently, discontinue β-blockers several days before the gradual withdrawal of clonidine.

Rebound hypertension also has occurred following discontinuation of the transdermal patch.

Ophthalmologic effects: Perform periodic eye examinations, because retinal degeneration has been noted in animal studies.

Perioperative use: Continue administration of clonidine to within 4 hours of surgery and resume as soon as possible thereafter. Carefully monitor blood pressure and institute appropriate measures to control it. If transdermal therapy is started during the perioperative period, note that therapeutic plasma levels are not achieved until 2 to 3 days after initial application.

Sensitization to transdermal clonidine: In patients who develop an allergic reaction to transdermal clonidine, oral clonidine HCl substitution may elicit a similar reaction.

Drug Interactions

Drugs that may interact with clonidine include beta-adrenergic blocking agents and tricyclic antidepressants.

Adverse Reactions

Oral – Adverse reactions may include dry mouth; drowsiness; dizziness; sedation; constipation; anorexia; malaise; nausea and vomiting; parotid pain; mild transient abnormalities in liver function tests; gynecomastia; CHF; orthostatic symptoms; palpitations, tachycardia and bradycardia; Raynaud's phenomenon; ECG abnormalities; conduction disturbances, arrhythmias, sinus bradycardia; dreams or nightmares; insomnia; hallucinations; delirium; nervousness; anxiety; depression; headache; rash, angioneurotic edema, hives, urticaria; hair thinning and alopecia; pruritus; impotence; decreased sexual activity; difficulty in micturition; weakness; muscle or joint pain; increased sensitivity to alcohol; dryness, itching or burning of the eyes; dryness of the nasal mucosa; pallor; fever; weakly positive Coombs' test.

Transdermal system – Adverse reactions may include dry mouth, drowsiness (the most frequent systemic reactions); constipation; nausea; change in taste; fatigue; headache; sedation; insomnia; nervousness; dizziness; impotence/sexual dysfunction; transient localized skin reactions; hyperpigmentation; edema; excoriation; burning; papules; throbbing; generalized macular rash.

ALPHA-1-ADRENERGIC BLOCKERS

DOXAZOSIN MESYLATE	
Tablets: 1, 2, 4, and 8 mg (*Rx*)	*Cardura* (Roerig)
PRAZOSIN	
Capsules: 1, 2, and 5 mg (*Rx*)	Various, *Minipress* (Pfizer)
TAMSULOSIN HCL	
Capsules: 0.4 mg (*Rx*)	*Flomax* (Boehringer-Ingelheim)
TERAZOSIN	
Capsules: 1, 2, 5, and 10 mg (*Rx*)	*Hytrin* (Abbott)

Indications

Hypertension: For the treatment of hypertension, alone or in combination with other antihypertensive agents (eg, diuretics, β-adrenergic blocking agents).

Terazosin and tamsulosin: Treatment of symptomatic benign prostatic hyperplasia.

Administration and Dosage

DOXAZOSIN MESYLATE:

    Hypertension –

      Initial dosage: 1 mg once daily. Postural effects are most likely to occur between 2 and 6 hours after a dose.

      Maintenance dose: Depending on the standing blood pressure response, dosage may be increased to 2 mg and thereafter, if necessary, to 4, 8 and 16 mg to achieve the desired reduction in blood pressure. Increases in dose beyond 4 mg increase the likelihood of excessive postural effects.

PRAZOSIN:

    Hypertension –

      Initial dose: 1 mg 2 or 3 times daily. When increasing dosages, give the first dose of each increment at bedtime to reduce syncopal episodes.

      Maintenance dose: 6 to 15 mg/day in divided doses. Doses > 20 mg usually do not increase efficacy; however, a few patients may benefit from up to 40 mg/day. After initial adjustment, some patients can be maintained on a twice-daily regimen.

      Children – A dose of 0.5 to 7 mg 3 times a day has been suggested.

      Concomitant therapy – When adding a diuretic or other antihypertensive agent, reduce dosage to 1 or 2 mg 3 times a day and then retitrate.

TAMSULOSIN:

    Benign prostatic hyperplasia – The recommended dose is 0.4 mg once daily, administered ≈ 30 minutes following the same meal each day.

      For those patients who fail to respond to the 0.4 mg dose after 2 to 4 weeks of dosing, the dose can be increased to 0.8 mg once daily. If administration is discontinued or interrupted for several days at either the 0.4 or 0.8 mg dose, start therapy again with the 0.4 mg once-daily dose.

TERAZOSIN:

    Hypertension – Adjust dose and the dose interval (12 or 24 hours) individually. The following is a guide:

      Initial dose: 1 mg at bedtime for all patients. Do not exceed this dose. Strictly observe this initial dosing regimen to avoid severe hypotensive effects.

      Subsequent doses: Slowly increase the dose to achieve the desired blood pressure response. The recommended dose range is 1 to 5 mg daily; however, some patients may benefit from doses as high as 20 mg/day. If response is substantially diminished at 24 hours, consider an increased dose or a twice-daily regimen.

    Benign prostatic hyperplasia –

      Initial dose: 1 mg at bedtime is the starting dose for all patients; do not exceed as an initial dose. Closely monitor patients to minimize the risk of severe hypotensive response.

      Subsequent doses: Increase the dose in a stepwise fashion to 2, 5 or 10 mg daily to achieve desired improvement of symptoms or flow rates. Doses of 10 mg once daily are generally required for clinical response; therefore, treatment with 10 mg for a minimum of 4 to 6 weeks may be required to assess whether a beneficial response has been achieved. There is insufficient data to support the use of doses > 20 mg in patients who do not respond.

Concomitant therapy – Observe caution when terazosin is administered concomitantly with other antihypertensive agents (eg, calcium antagonists) to avoid the possibility of significant hypotension. When adding a diuretic or other antihypertensive agent, dosage reduction and retitration may be necessary.

Actions

Pharmacology: **Prazosin, terazosin,** and **doxazosin** selectively block postsynaptic α-1-adrenergic receptors. These peripherally acting drugs dilate both resistance (arterioles) and capacitance (veins) vessels. Both supine and standing blood pressure are lowered. The effect is most pronounced on diastolic blood pressure.

In the treatment of benign prostatic hyperplasia (BPH), the reduction in symptoms and improvement in urine flow rates is related to relaxation of smooth muscle produced by blockade of alpha$_1$ adrenoceptors in the bladder neck and prostate.

Pharmacokinetics: **Prazosin** is extensively metabolized. The metabolites of prazosin are active. Duration of antihypertensive effect is 10 hours.

Terazosin undergoes minimal hepatic first-pass metabolism; nearly all of the circulating dose is in the form of parent drug.

Doxazosin is extensively metabolized in the liver.

Pharmacokinetics of Alpha-1-Adrenergic Blockers			
Parameters	Doxazosin	Prazosin	Terazosin
Oral bioavailability	65%	48% to 68%	90%
Affected by food	nd[1]	No	No
Peak plasma level, time	2 to 3 hrs	1 to 3 hrs	1 to 2 hrs
Protein binding	98%	92% to 97%	90% to 94%
Half-life	22 hrs	2 to 3 hrs	9 to 12 hrs
Excretion: Bile/feces	63%	< 90%	60%
Excretion: Urine	9%	< 10%	40%

[1] nd = no data

Contraindications

Hypersensitivity to quinazolines (eg, doxazosin, prazosin, terazosin).

Warnings

"First-dose" effect: **Prazosin, terazosin,** and **doxazosin,** like other α-adrenergic blocking agents, can cause marked hypotension (especially postural hypotension) and syncope with sudden loss of consciousness with the first few doses. Anticipate a similar effect if therapy is interrupted for more than a few doses, if dosage is increased rapidly, or if another antihypertensive drug is introduced.

The "first-dose" phenomenon may be minimized by limiting the initial dose to 1 mg of terazosin or prazosin (given at bedtime) or doxazosin.

Hepatic function impairment: Administer **doxazosin** with caution to patients with evidence of impaired hepatic function or to patients receiving drugs known to influence hepatic metabolism.

Pregnancy: Category C (**prazosin, terazosin**); Category B (**doxazosin**).

Lactation: Safety has not been established.

Children: Safety and efficacy for use in children have not been established.

Precautions

Weight gain: There was a tendency for patients to gain weight during **terazosin** therapy.

Cholesterol: During controlled clinical studies **prazosin, terazosin,** and **doxazosin** were associated with small decreases in LDL and cholesterol.

Drug Interactions

Drugs that interact may include beta blockers, indomethacin, verapamil, and clonidine.

Drug/Lab test interactions: False-positive results may occur in screening tests for pheochromocytoma in patients who are being treated with prazosin.

Adverse Reactions

	Hypertension			BPH
Adverse reaction	Doxazosin	Prazosin	Terazosin	Terazosin
Cardiovascular				
Palpitations	2%	5.3%	4.3%	0.9%
Postural hypotension/hypotension	0.3% to 1%	✔¹	1.3%	0.6% to 3.9%
CNS				
Dizziness	19%	10.3%	19.3%	9.1%
Somnolence	5%	no report	5.4%	3.6%
Asthenia	1% to 12%	≈ 7%	11.3%	7.4%
Drowsiness	✔¹	7.6%	✔¹	
GI				
Nausea	3%	4.9%	4.4%	1.7%
Musculoskeletal				
Shoulder/neck/back/extremity pain	< 0.5% to 2%	no report	1% to 3.5%	
Respiratory				
Dyspnea	1%	✔¹	3.1%	1.7%
Nasal congestion	no report	✔¹	5.9%	1.9%
Pharyngitis/rhinitis	3%	no report	1%	1.9%
Miscellaneous				
Headache	14%	7.8%	16.2%	4.9%
Edema	4%	✔¹	< 1%	
Peripheral edema	no report	no report	5.5%	0.9%

¹ Reactions associated with the drug; incidence unknown.

HYDRALAZINE HCl

Tablets: 10, 25, 50, and 100 mg (*Rx*)	Various, *Apresoline* (Ciba)
Injection: 20 mg/mL (*Rx*)	Various, *Apresoline* (Ciba)

Indications
Oral: Essential hypertension, alone or in combination with other agents.

Parenteral: Severe essential hypertension when the drug cannot be given orally or when the need to lower blood pressure is urgent.

Unlabeled uses: Hydralazine in doses up to 800 mg 3 times/day has been effective in reducing afterload in the treatment of congestive heart failure (CHF), severe aortic insufficiency, and after valve replacement.

Administration and Dosage
Bioavailability of hydralazine tablets is enhanced by the concurrent ingestion of food.

Initiate therapy: Initiate therapy in gradually increasing dosages; individualize dosage. Start with 10 mg 4 times daily for the first 2 to 4 days, increase to 25 mg 4 times daily for the balance of the first week.

Second and subsequent weeks: Increase dosage to 50 mg 4 times daily.

Maintenance: Adjust dosage to lowest effective level. Twice daily dosage may be adequate. In a few resistant patients, up to 300 mg/day may be required for a significant antihypertensive effect. In such cases, consider a lower dosage of hydralazine combined with a thiazide or reserpine or a beta blocker. However, when combining therapy, individual titration is essential to ensure the lowest possible therapeutic dose of each drug.

    Children –
      Initial: 0.75 mg/kg/day in 4 divided doses. Dosage may be increased gradually over the next 3 to 4 weeks to a maximum of 7.5 mg/kg or 200 mg daily.

Parenteral: Therapy in the hospitalized patient may be initiated IV or IM. Use parenterally only when the drug cannot be given orally. Usual dose is 20 to 40 mg, repeated as necessary. Certain patients (especially those with marked renal damage) may require a lower dose. Check blood pressure frequently; it may begin to fall within a few minutes after injection; average maximal decrease occurs in 10 to 80 minutes. Where there is a previously existing increased intracranial pressure, lowering the blood pressure may increase cerebral ischemia. Most patients can transfer to the oral form in 24 to 48 hours.

Children – 0.1 to 0.2 mg/kg/dose every 4 to 6 hours as needed.

Eclampsia – A dose of 5 to 10 mg every 20 minutes as an IV bolus has been recommended. If there is no effect after 20 mg, try another agent.

Stability: Use hydralazine injection as quickly as possible after drawing through a needle into a syringe. Hydralazine changes color after contact with a metal filter.

Actions

Pharmacology: Hydralazine exerts a peripheral vasodilating effect through a direct relaxation of vascular smooth muscle.

Pharmacokinetics: Hydralazine is rapidly absorbed after oral use. Half-life is 3 to 7 hours. Protein binding is 87%, and bioavailability is 30% to 50%. Plasma levels vary widely among individuals. Peak plasma concentrations occur 1 to 2 hours after ingestion; duration of action is 6 to 12 hours. Hypotensive effects are seen 10 to 20 minutes after parenteral use and last 2 to 4 hours. Slow acetylators generally have higher plasma levels of hydralazine and require lower doses to maintain control of blood pressure. Hydralazine undergoes extensive hepatic metabolism; it is excreted in the urine as active drug (12% to 14%) and metabolites.

Contraindications

Hypersensitivity to hydralazine; coronary artery disease; mitral valvular rheumatic heart disease.

Warnings

Lupus erythematosus: Hydralazine may produce a clinical picture simulating systemic lupus erythematosus including glomerulonephritis. Symptoms usually regress when the drug is discontinued, but residual effects have been detected years later. Long-term treatment with steroids may be necessary.

Perform complete blood counts and antinuclear antibody (ANA) titer determinations before and during prolonged therapy, even in the asymptomatic patient. These studies also are indicated if the patient develops arthralgia, fever, chest pain, continued malaise, or other unexplained signs or symptoms. If the ANA titer reaction is positive, carefully weigh benefits to be derived from hydralazine.

Renal function impairment: In hypertensive patients with normal kidneys who are treated with hydralazine, there is evidence of increased renal blood flow and a maintenance of glomerular filtration rate. Renal function may improve where control values were below normal prior to administration. Use with caution in patients with advanced renal damage.

Pregnancy: Category C.

Lactation: Hydralazine is excreted in breast milk.

Children: Safety and efficacy for use in children have not been established.

Precautions

Cardiovascular: The "hyperdynamic" circulation caused by hydralazine may accentuate specific cardiovascular inadequacies. It may reduce the pressor responses to epinephrine. Postural hypotension may result from hydralazine. Use with caution in patients with cerebral vascular accidents.

Coronary artery disease – Myocardial stimulation produced by hydralazine can cause anginal attacks and ECG changes of myocardial ischemia. The drug has been implicated in the production of MI. Use with caution in patients with suspected coronary artery disease.

Pulmonary hypertension – Use hydralazine with caution in patients with pulmonary hypertension. Severe hypotension may result. Monitor carefully.

Lipids – Hydralazine may cause some decrease in total cholesterol.

Peripheral neuritis: Peripheral neuritis evidenced by paresthesias, numbness, and tingling, has been observed. Add pyridoxine to the regimen if symptoms develop.

Hematologic effects: Blood dyscrasias consisting of reduction in hemoglobin and red cell count, leukopenia, agranulocytosis, and purpura have been reported. If such abnormalities develop, discontinue therapy. Periodic blood counts are advised.

Tartrazine sensitivity: Some of these products contain tartrazine, which may cause allergic-type reactions in susceptible individuals. Tartrazine sensitivity is frequently seen in patients who also have aspirin hypersensitivity.

Drug Interactions
Drugs that may interact with hydralazine include beta blockers (eg, metoprolol, propranolol) and indomethacin.

Drug/Food interactions: Taking with food results in higher plasma hydralazine levels.

Adverse Reactions
Possible adverse reactions include headache; anorexia; nausea; vomiting; diarrhea; palpitations; tachycardia; angina pectoris; toxic reactions (particularly the LE cell syndrome); lacrimation; conjunctivitis; dizziness; tremors; psychotic reactions; rash; urticaria; pruritus; fever; chills; arthralgia; eosinophilia; constipation; paralytic ileus; lymphadenopathy; splenomegaly; nasal congestion; flushing; edema; muscle cramps; hypotension; paradoxical pressor response; dyspnea; urination difficulty; adverse reactions with hydralazine are usually reversible when dosage is reduced. However, it may be necessary to discontinue the drug.

MINOXIDIL

Tablets: 2.5 and 10 mg (*Rx*)	Various, *Loniten* (Upjohn)

Warning:
Minoxidil may produce serious adverse effects. It can cause pericardial effusion, occasionally progressing to tamponade; it can exacerbate angina pectoris. Reserve for hypertensive patients who do not respond adequately to maximum therapeutic doses of a diuretic and 2 other antihypertensive agents.

Administer under close supervision, usually concomitantly with a beta-adrenergic blocking agent, to prevent tachycardia and increased myocardial workload. Usually, it must be given with a diuretic, frequently one acting in the ascending limb of the loop of Henle, to prevent serious fluid accumulation. When first administering minoxidil, hospitalize and monitor patients with malignant hypertension and those already receiving guanethidine to avoid too rapid or large orthostatic decreases in blood pressure.

Indications
Severe hypertension: Severe hypertension that is symptomatic or associated with target organ damage, and is not manageable with maximum therapeutic doses of a diuretic plus two other antihypertensives.

Topical minoxidil is used for the treatment of male pattern baldness (alopecia androgenetica) of the vertex of the scalp. Use of the tablets, in any formulation, to promote hair growth is not an approved use.

Administration and Dosage
Adults and children (≥ 12 years of age): Initial dosage is 5 mg/day as a single dose. Daily dosage can be increased to 10, 20, then 40 mg in single or divided doses if required. Effective range is usually 10 to 40 mg/day. Maximum dosage is 100 mg/day.

Children: Initial dosage is 0.2 mg/kg/day as a single dose. Dose may be increased in 50% to 100% increments until optimum BP control is achieved. Effective range is usually 0.25 to 1 mg/kg/day. Maximum dosage is 50 mg daily.

Dose frequency: If supine diastolic pressure has been reduced < 30 mm Hg, administer the drug only once a day; if reduced > 30 mm Hg, divide the daily dosage into 2 equal parts.

Dosage adjustment intervals: Dosage adjustment intervals, which must be carefully titrated, should be ≥ 3 days because the full response to a given dose is not obtained until then.

Actions

Pharmacology: Minoxidil is a direct-acting peripheral vasodilator. The exact mechanism of action on the vascular smooth muscle is unknown.

Pharmacokinetics:

Absorption/Distribution – Minoxidil is ≥ 90% absorbed from the GI tract. Plasma levels of the parent drug reach a maximum within the first hour and decline rapidly thereafter. Minoxidil is not protein bound; it concentrates in arteriolar smooth muscle.

Onset/Duration: The extent and time course of BP reduction by minoxidil do not correspond closely to its plasma concentration. When minoxidil is administered chronically, once or twice a day, the time required to achieve maximum effect on BP is inversely related to the size of the dose. Thus, maximum effect is achieved on 10 mg/day within 7 days, on 20 mg/day within 5 days and on 40 mg/day within 3 days.

Metabolism/Excretion – 90% is metabolized, predominantly by conjugation with glucuronic acid. Average plasma half-life is 4.2 hours.

Contraindications

Hypersensitivity to any component of the product; pheochromocytoma (because the drug may stimulate secretion of catecholamines from the tumor through its antihypertensive action); acute MI; dissecting aortic aneurysm.

Warnings

Mild hypertension: Because of the potential for serious adverse effects, use in milder degrees of hypertension is not recommended.

Cardiac lesions: Autopsies did not reveal right atrial or other hemorrhage pathology of the kind seen in animals.

ECG changes: Rarely, a large negative amplitude of the T wave may encroach upon the ST segment, but the ST segment is not independently altered. These changes usually disappear with continuance of treatment and revert to the pretreatment state if therapy is discontinued.

Fluid and electrolyte balance: Monitor fluid and electrolyte balance and body weight. Give with a diuretic to prevent fluid retention and possible CHF; a loop diuretic is usually required. If used without a diuretic, retention of several hundred mEq salt and corresponding volumes of water can occur in a few days, leading to increased plasma and interstitial fluid volume and local or generalized edema.

Refractory fluid retention rarely may require discontinuation of minoxidil. Under close medical supervision, it may be possible to resolve refractory salt retention by discontinuing the drug for 1 or 2 days, and then resuming treatment in conjunction with vigorous diuretic therapy.

Tachycardia: Minoxidil increases heart rate; this can be prevented by coadministration of a β-adrenergic blocking drug or other sympathetic nervous system suppressants. In addition, angina may worsen or appear for the first time during treatment, probably because of the increased oxygen demands associated with increased heart rate and cardiac output. This can usually be prevented by sympathetic blockade.

Pericardial effusion: Pericardial effusion, occasionally with tamponade, has occurred in ≈ 3% of treated patients not on dialysis, especially those with inadequate or compromised renal function. Many cases were associated with connective tissue disease, the uremic syndrome, CHF or fluid retention, but were instances in which these potential causes of effusion were not present. Observe patients closely for signs of pericardial disorder. Perform echocardiographic studies if suspicion arises. More vigorous diuretic therapy, dialysis, pericardiocentesis, or surgery may be required. If the effusion persists, consider drug withdrawal.

Hazard of rapid control of BP: In patients with very severe BP elevation, too rapid control of BP can precipitate syncope, cerebrovascular accidents, MI and ischemia of special sense organs with resulting decrease or loss of vision or hearing. Patients with compromised circulation or cryoglobulinemia also may suffer ischemic episodes of affected organs. Although such events have not been unequivocally associated with minoxidil use, experience is limited.

Hospitalize any patient with malignant hypertension during initial treatment to ensure that blood pressure is not falling more rapidly than intended.

Renal function impairment: Renal failure or dialysis patients may require smaller doses; closely supervise to prevent cardiac failure or exacerbation of renal failure.

Pregnancy: Category C.

Lactation: Minoxidil is excreted in breast milk; do not nurse while taking minoxidil.

Children: Use in children is limited, particularly in infants. The recommendations under Administration and Dosage are only a rough guide; careful titration is essential.

Precautions
Myocardial infarction: Minoxidil has not been used in patients who have had an MI within the preceding month. A reduction in arterial pressure with the drug might further limit blood flow to the myocardium, although this might be compensated by decreased oxygen demand because of lower BP.

Hypertrichosis: Elongation, thickening, and enhanced pigmentation of fine body hair develops within 3 to 6 weeks after starting therapy in ≈ 80% of patients. It is usually first noticed on the temples, between the eyebrows, between the hairline and the eyebrows, or in the sideburn area of the upper lateral cheek, later extending to the back, arms, legs, and scalp. After discontinuation, 1 to 6 months may be required for restoration to pretreatment appearance. No endocrine abnormalities have been found to explain the abnormal hair growth; thus, it is hypertrichosis without virilism.

Lab test abnormalities: Repeat tests that are abnormal at initiation of minoxidil therapy to ascertain whether improvement or deterioration is occurring under therapy. Initially, perform such tests frequently, at 1 to 3 month intervals, and as stabilization occurs, at 6 to 12 month intervals.

Drug Interactions
Drugs that may interact with minoxidil include guanethidine.

Adverse Reactions
Adverse reactions may include Stevens-Johnson syndrome; pericardial effusion; rebound hypertension (following gradual withdrawal in children); decreased initial hematocrit, hemoglobin and erythrocyte counts; nausea; vomiting; temporary edema; alkaline phosphatase/serum creatinine/BUN increase.

ACE INHIBITORS

BENAZEPRIL HCl	
Tablets: 5, 10, 20, and 40 mg (*Rx*)	*Lotensin* (Novartis)
CAPTOPRIL	
Tablets: 12.5, 25, 50, and 100 mg (*Rx*)	Various, *Capoten* (Bristol-Myers Squibb)
ENALAPRIL	
Tablets: 2.5, 5, 10, and 20 mg (*Rx*)	*Vasotec* (Merck)
Injection: 1.25 mg enalaprilat/mL (*Rx*)	*Vasotec I.V.* (Merck)
FOSINOPRIL SODIUM	
Tablets: 10, 20, and 40 mg (*Rx*)	*Monopril* (Bristol-Myers Squibb)
LISINOPRIL	
Tablets: 2.5, 5, 10, 20, and 40 mg (*Rx*)	*Prinivil* (Merck), *Zestril* (Zeneca)

MOEXIPRIL HCl	
Tablets: 7.5 and 15 mg (*Rx*)	*Univasc* (Schwarz Pharma)
PERINDOPRIL ERBUMINE	
Tablets: 2, 4, and 8 mg (*Rx*)	*Aceon* (Solvay Pharm.)
QUINAPRIL HCl	
Tablets: 5, 10, 20, and 40 mg (*Rx*)	*Accupril* (Parke-Davis)
RAMIPRIL	
Capsules: 1.25, 2.5, 5, and 10 mg (*Rx*)	*Altace* (Monarch)
TRANDOLAPRIL	
Tablets: 1, 2, and 4 mg (*Rx*)	*Mavik* (Knoll)

Warning:
>*Pregnancy:* When used in pregnancy during the second and third trimesters, ACEIs can cause injury and even death to the developing fetus. When pregnancy is detected, discontinue the ACEI as soon as possible.

Indications

Hypertension: The ACEIs are effective alone and in combination with other antihypertensive agents, especially thiazide-type diuretics. Blood pressure (BP)-lowering effects of ACEIs and thiazides are approximately additive.

Heart failure: Some ACEIs are effective in the management of CHF, usually as adjunctive therapy and in patients who demonstrate clinical signs of CHF or have evidence of left ventricular systolic dysfunction within the first few days after an AMI.

Myocardial infarction:
>*Lisinopril* – Treatment of hemodynamically stable patients within 24 hours of acute myocardial infarction (MI), to improve survival. Patients should receive, as appropriate, the standard recommended treatments such as thrombolytics, aspirin and beta blockers.

Left ventricular dysfunction (LVD): Various ACEIs have demonstrated improved survival and decreased rates of development of overt heart failure in patients with varying degrees of LVD (from modest, asymptomatic to severe with CHF).

Diabetic nephropathy:
>*Captopril* – Treatment of diabetic nephropathy (proteinuria > 500 mg/day) in patients with type 1 insulin-dependent diabetes mellitus and retinopathy.

Heart failure post-MI/left-ventricular dysfunction post-MI (Trandolapril, Ramipril): For stable patients who have evidence of left-ventricular systolic dysfunction (identified by wall motion abnormalities) or who are symptomatic from CHF within the first few days after sustaining acute MI. Administration to Caucasians decreases the risk of death (principally cardiovascular death) and decreases risk of heart failure-related hospitalization.

Perindopril:
>*Essential hypertension* – For the treatment of patients with essential hypertension. It may be used alone or given with other classes of antihypertensives, especially thiazide diuretics.

Ramipril:
>*Reduction in risk of MI, stroke, and death from cardiovascular causes* – In patients ≥ 55 years of age at high risk of developing a major cardiovascular event because of a history of coronary artery disease, stroke, peripheral vascular disease, or diabetes that is accompanied by ≥ 1 other cardiovascular risk factor (eg, hypertension, elevated total cholesterol levels, low HDL levels, cigarette smoking, documented microalbuminuria).

Unlabeled uses:
>*Captopril* – Management of hypertensive crises (25 mg initially, 100 mg 90 to 120 minutes later, 200 to 300 mg/day for 2 to 5 days, then adjusted). Sublingual captopril 25 mg has also been used effectively.

Severe childhood hypertension (0.3 mg/kg initial dose, titrated ≤ 6 mg/day given in 2 or 3 divided doses).

Rheumatoid arthritis (75 to 150 mg/day in divided doses).

Raynaud's syndrome (symptomatic relief) (37.5 mg/day).

Enalaprilat – May be used for hypertensive emergencies (1.25 to 5 mg every 6 hours), but the effects are often variable.

Administration and Dosage

BENAZEPRIL HCl:

Initial dose – 10 mg once daily for patients not receiving a diuretic.

Maintenance dosage – 20 to 40 mg/day as a single dose or 2 divided doses. A dose of 80 mg gives an increased response, but experience is limited.

Renal function impairment – 5 mg once daily in patients with Ccr of < 30 mL/min/ 1.73 m² (serum creatinine > 3 mg/dL). Dosage may be titrated upward until BP is controlled or to a maximum of 40 mg/day.

CAPTOPRIL: Administer 1 hour before meals.

Hypertension –

Initial: 25 mg 2 or 3 times/day. If satisfactory BP reduction is not achieved after 1 or 2 weeks, increase to 50 mg 2 or 3 times/day. If BP is not controlled after 1 or 2 weeks at this dose (and patient is not already on a diuretic), add a modest dose of a thiazide diuretic.

If further BP reduction is required, increase to 100 mg captopril 2 or 3 times/ day and then, if necessary, to 150 mg 2 or 3 times/day (while continuing diuretic). Usual dose is 25 to 150 mg 2 or 3 times/day. Do not exceed daily dose of 450 mg.

Accelerated or malignant hypertension: Promptly initiate captopril at 25 mg 2 or 3 times daily under close supervision. Increase dose every ≤ 24 hours until a satisfactory response is obtained or the maximum dose is reached.

Heart failure – Usual initial dosage is 25 mg 3 times daily. After 50 mg 3 times daily is reached, delay further dosage increases, where possible, for ≥ 2 weeks to determine if a satisfactory response occurs. Most patients have had a satisfactory clinical improvement at 50 or 100 mg 3 times daily. Do not exceed a daily dose of 450 mg. Captopril should generally be used in conjunction with a diuretic and digitalis.

LVD after MI – 50 mg 3 times daily is the target maintenance dose. Therapy may be initiated as early as 3 days following an MI. After a single 6.25 mg dose, initiate at 12.5 mg 3 times daily, then increase to 25 mg 3 times daily during the next several days and to a target of 50 mg 3 times daily over the next several weeks as tolerated.

Diabetic nephropathy – Recommended dose for long-term use is 25 mg 3 times daily.

Renal impairment – Reduce initial dosage and use smaller increments for titration, which should be quite slow (1- to 2-week intervals). After the desired therapeutic effect is achieved, slowly back-titrate to the minimal effective dose.

ENALAPRIL:

Oral –

Hypertension:

Patients taking diuretics – Discontinue the diuretic, if possible, for 2 to 3 days before beginning therapy with endapril to reduce the likelihood of hypotension. If the diuretic cannot be discontinued, use an initial dose of 2.5 mg under medical supervision for ≥ 2 hours and until BP has stabilized for at least an additional hour.

Patients not taking diuretics – Initial dose is 5 mg once a day. The usual dosage range is 10 to 40 mg/day as a single dose or in 2 divided doses.

Impaired renal function – Titrate the dosage upward until BP is controlled or until a maximum dose of 40 mg/day is reached. Use initial dose of 5 mg/day in normal renal function and mild impairment (Ccr 30 to 80 mL/min, serum creatinine ≤ 3 mg/dL); 2.5 mg/day in moderate-to-severe renal impairment (Ccr ≤ 30 mL/min, serum creatinine ≥ 3 mg/dL) and in dialysis patients on dialysis days.

Heart failure: As adjunctive therapy with diuretics and digitalis, the recommended starting dose is 2.5 mg twice daily. The usual therapeutic dosing range for the treatment of heart failure is 2.5 to 20 mg/day given in 2 divided doses. The maximum daily dose is 40 mg.

Renal impairment or hyponatremia –

Serum sodium < 130 mEq/L or with serum creatinine > 1.6 mg/dL: Initiate at 2.5 mg/day under close medical supervision. The dose may be increased to 2.5 mg twice daily, then 5 mg twice daily and higher as needed, usually at intervals of ≥ 4 days. The maximum daily dose is 40 mg.

Asymptomatic left ventricular dysfunction: 2.5 mg twice daily, titrated as tolerated to the targeted daily dose of 20 mg in divided doses.

Parenteral (enalaprilat) – For IV administration only.

Hypertension: 1.25 mg every 6 hours IV over 5 minutes.

The dose for patients being converted to IV from oral therapy is 1.25 mg every 6 hours. For conversion from IV to oral therapy, the recommended initial dose of tablets is 5 mg/day for patients with Ccr > 30 mL/min and 2.5 mg/day for patients with Ccr ≤ 30 mL/min. Adjust dosage according to BP response.

Patients taking diuretics: Starting dose for hypertension is 0.625 mg IV over 5 minutes. If there is inadequate clinical response after 1 hour, repeat the 0.625 dose. Give additional doses of 1.25 mg at 6-hour intervals.

For conversion from IV to oral therapy, the recommended initial dose of enalapril maleate tablets for patients who have responded to 0.625 mg enalaprilat every 6 hours is 2.5 mg once a day with subsequent dosage adjustment as needed.

High-risk patients: Hypertensive patients at risk of excessive hypotension include those with the following concurrent conditions or characteristics: Heart failure, hyponatremia, high-dose diuretic therapy, recent intensive diureses or increase in diuretic dose, renal dialysis, or severe volume or salt depletion of any etiology. Single doses of enalaprilat as low as 0.2 mg have produced excessive hypotension in normotensive patients with these diagnoses. Because of the potential for an extreme hypotensive response in these patients, initiate therapy under very close medical supervision. The starting dose should be ≤ 0.625 mg administered IV over a period of ≥ 5 minutes and preferably longer (up to 1 hour).

Renal function impairment: Administer 1.25 mg every 6 hours for patients with Ccr > 30 mL/min. For Ccr ≤ 30 mL/min, initial dose is 0.625 mg. If there is inadequate clinical response after 1 hour, the 0.625 mg dose may be repeated. May give additional 1.25 mg doses at 6-hour intervals. For dialysis patients, initial dose is ≤ 0.625 mg administered over ≥ 5 minutes preferably longer (≤ 1 hour).

For conversion from IV to oral therapy, the recommended initial dose is 5 mg once a day for patients with Ccr > 30 mL/min and 2.5 mg once daily for patients with Ccr ≤ 30 mL/min.

FOSINOPRIL SODIUM:

Initial dose – 10 mg once daily.

Maintenance dosage – Usual range needed to maintain a response is 20 to 40 mg/day but some patients appear to have a further response to 80 mg. If trough response is inadequate, consider dividing the daily dose.

LISINOPRIL:

Hypertension –

Initial therapy: 10 mg once/day in patients with uncomplicated essential hypertension not on diuretic therapy. The usual dosage range is 20 to 40 mg/day as a single daily dose.

Diuretic-treated patients: Discontinue the diuretic, if possible, for 2 to 3 days before beginning therapy with lisinopril to reduce the likelihood of hypotension. If the diuretic cannot be discontinued, use an initial dose of 5 mg under medical supervision for ≥ 2 hours and until BP has stabilized for at least an additional hour.

CHF –

Initial dose: 5 mg once daily with diuretics and digitalis. Usual effective dosage range is 5 to 20 mg/day as a single dose. In patients with hyponatremia (serum sodium < 130 mEq/L), initiate dose at 2.5 mg once daily. If used with diuretics, initial dose is 5 mg/day.

Elderly – Make dosage adjustments with particular caution.

Renal function impairment – For hypertension, titrate dosage upward until BP is controlled or to a maximum of 40 mg daily.

In acute MI, initiate lisinopril with caution in patients with evidence of renal dysfunction (serum creatinine concentration exceeding 2 mg/dL).

Lisinopril Dosage in Renal Impairment			
Renal status	Ccr (mL/min)	Serum creatinine (mg/dL)	Initial dose (mg/day)
Normal function to mild impairment	> 30	≤ 3	10
Moderate-to-severe impairment	≥ 10 to ≤ 30	≥ 3	5
Dialysis patients	< 10	—	2.5[1]

[1] Adjust dosage or dosing interval depending on the BP response.

Acute MI – In hemodynamically stable patients within 24 hours of the onset of symptoms of acute MI, the first dose is 5 mg, followed by 5 mg after 24 hours, 10 mg after 48 hours and then 10 mg once daily. Continue dosing for 6 weeks. Patients with a low systolic BP (≤ 120 mm Hg) when treatment is started or during the first 3 days after the infarct should be given a lower 2.5 mg dose. If hypotension occurs (systolic BP ≤ 100 mm Hg), a daily maintenance dose of 5 mg may be given with temporary reductions to 2.5 mg if needed. If prolonged hypotension occurs (systolic BP < 90 mm Hg for > 1 hour), withdraw lisinopril.

MOEXIPRIL HCl:

Initial dose – In patients not receiving diuretics, 7.5 mg 1 hour prior to meals once daily. If control is not adequate, increase the dose or divide the dosing.

Maintenance dose – 7.5 to 30 mg daily in 1 or 2 divided doses 1 hour before meals.

Renal function impairment – Cautiously use 3.75 mg once daily in patients with Ccr of ≤ 40 mL/min/1.73 m². Dosage may be titrated upward to a maximum of 15 mg/day.

PERINDOPRIL:

Use in uncomplicated hypertensive patients – In patients with essential hypertension, the recommended initial dose is 4 mg once a day. The dosage may be titrated upward until BP, when measured just before the next dose, is controlled or to a maximum of 16 mg/day. The usual maintenance dose range is 4 to 8 mg administered as a single daily dose. It also may be administered in 2 divided doses. When once-daily dosing was compared to twice-daily dosing in clinical studies, the twice-daily regimen was generally slightly superior, but not by more than ≈ 0.5 to 1 mmHg.

Use in elderly patients – As in younger patients, the recommended initial dosages for the elderly (> 65 years of age) is 4 mg daily in 1 or 2 divided doses. The daily dosage may be titrated upward until BP, when measured just before the next dose, is controlled, but experience with perindopril is limited in the elderly at doses > 8 mg. Administer dosages > 8 mg cautiously and under close medical supervision.

Use in concomitant diuretics – If BP is not adequately controlled with perindopril alone, a diuretic may be added. In patients currently being treated with a diuretic, symptomatic hypotension occasionally can occur following the initial dose of perindopril. To reduce likelihood of such reaction, the diuretic should, if possible, be discontinued 2 to 3 days prior to beginning perindopril therapy. Then, if BP is not controlled with perindopril alone, resume the diuretic.

If the diuretic cannot be discontinued, use an initial dose of 2 to 4 mg daily in 1 or 2 divided doses with careful medical supervision for several hours and until BP has stabilized. Titrate the dosage as described above.

Use in patients with impaired renal function – Perindoprilat elimination is decreased in renally impaired patients, with a marked increase in accumulation when Ccr drops < 30 mL/min. In patients with Ccr < 30 mL/min, safety and efficacy have not been established. For patients with lesser degrees of impairment (Ccr > 30 mL/min), the initial dosage should be 2 mg/day, and dosage should not exceed 8 mg/day because of limited clinical experience. During dialysis, perindopril is removed with the same clearance as in patients with normal renal function.

QUINAPRIL HCl:
> *Hypertension –*
>
>> *Initial dose:* 10 or 20 mg once daily for patients not on diuretics.
>>
>> *Elderly (≥ 65 years of age):* 10 mg once daily followed by titration to the optimal response.
>>
>> *Renal function impairment:* Initial dose is 10 mg with Ccr > 60 mL/min, 5 mg with Ccr 30 to 60 mL/min and 2.5 mg with Ccr 10 to 30 mL/min.
>
> CHF – The recommended starting dose is 5 mg twice/day. If the initial dose is well tolerated, titrate patients at weekly intervals until and effective dose, usually 20 to 40 mg/day given in 2 equally divided doses, is reached or undesirable hypotension, orthostasis, or azotemia prohibit reaching this dose.
>
>> *Renal impairment or hyponatremia:* In patients with heart failure and renal impairment, the recommended initial dose is 5 mg with Ccr > 30 mL/min and 2.5 mg with Ccr 10 to 30 mL/min. There is insufficient data for dosage recommendation in patients with Ccr < 10 mL/min.

RAMIPRIL:
> *Reduction in risk of MI, stroke, and death from cardiovascular causes –*
>
>> *Initial dose:* 2.5 mg once daily for 1 week, 5 mg once daily for the next 3 weeks, and then increased as tolerated to maintenance dose.
>>
>> *Maintenance dosage:* 10 mg once daily. If the patient is hypertensive or recently post-MI, it can also be given as a divided dose.
>>
>> *Renal function impairment:* In patients with Ccr of < 40 mL/min/1.73 m^2 (serum creatinine approximately > 2.5 mg/dL) doses only 25% of those normally used should be expected to induce full therapeutic levels of ramiprilat.
>>
>> *Hypertension –*
>>
>> *Initial dose:* 2.5 mg once daily in patients not receiving a diuretic.
>>
>> *Maintenance dosage:* 2.5 to 20 mg/day as a single dose or in two equally divided doses. If BP is not controlled with ramipril alone, a diuretic can be added.
>>
>> *Renal function impairment:* 1.25 mg once daily in patients with Ccr of < 40 mL/min/ 1.73 m^2 (serum creatinine approximately > 2.5 mg/dL). Dosage may be titrated upward until BP is controlled or to a maximum of 5 mg/day.
>
> Heart failure post-MI – Starting dose is 2.5 mg twice daily. A patient who becomes hypotensive at this dose may be switched to 1.25 mg twice daily, but all patients should then be titrated (as tolerated) toward a target dose of 5 mg twice daily, with dosage increases being ≈ 3 weeks apart. After the initial dose, observe for ≥ 2 hours and until BP has stabilized for at least an additional hour. If possible, reduce the dose of any concomitant diuretic.
>
>> *Renal function impairment:* 1.25 mg once daily in patients with Ccr of < 40 mL/min/ 1.73 m^2 (serum creatinine approximately > 2.5 mg/dL). Dosage may be increased to 1.25 mg twice daily up to a maximum dose of 2.5 mg twice daily depending on clinical response and tolerability.
>>
>> *Alternative route of administration* – Ramipril capsules are usually swallowed whole.
>
> However, the capsules may be opened and the contents sprinkled on a small amount of ≈ 4 oz applesauce or mixed in apple juice or water.

TRANDOLAPRIL:
> *Hypertension –*
>
>> *Initial dose:* The recommended initial dosage of trandolapril for patients not receiving a diuretic is 1 mg/day (2 mg in black patients). Adjust dosage according to the BP response. Make dosage adjustments at intervals of ≥ 1 week. Most patients have required dosages of 2 to 4 mg/day. There is little clinical experience with doses > 8 mg.
>>
>>> *Maintenance* – Patients inadequately treated with once daily dosing at 4 mg may be treated with twice-daily dosing. If BP is not adequately controlled with trandolapril monotherapy, a diuretic may be added.
>>>
>>> *Concomitant diuretic* – In patients being treated with a diuretic, symptomatic hypotension can occasionally occur following the initial dose of trandolapril. To reduce the likelihood of hypotension, if possible, discontinue the diuretic 2 to 3 days prior to beginning therapy with trandolapril. If BP is not controlled with

trandolapril alone, resume diuretic therapy. If the diuretic cannot be discontinued, give an initial dose of 0.5 mg trandolapril with careful medical supervision for several hours until BP has stabilized. Titrate dosage as described above to the optimal response.

Heart failure post-MI or LVD post-MI –

Initial dose: 1 mg/day

Maintenance dosage: Titrate to greatest tolerated dose.

Target dose: 4 mg/day.

Renal/Hepatic function impairment – For patients with a Ccr < 30 mL/min or with hepatic cirrhosis, the recommended starting dose, based on clinical and pharmacokinetic data, is 0.5 mg/day. Titrate as described above to the optimal response.

Actions

Pharmacology: The angiotensin-converting enzyme inhibitors (ACEIs) appear to act primarily through suppression of the renin-angiotensin-aldosterone system; however, no consistent correlation has been described between renin levels and drug response.

Synthesized by the kidneys, renin is released into the circulation where it acts on a plasma globulin substrate to produce angiotensin I. Angiotensin I is then converted by angiotensin converting enzyme (ACE) to angiotensin II. These agents prevent the conversion of angiotensin I to angiotensin II by inhibiting ACE. ACEIs may also inhibit local angiotensin II at vascular and renal sites and attenuate the release of catecholamines from adrenergic nerve endings.

Increased prostaglandin synthesis may also play a role in the antihypertensive action of captopril.

Some ACEIs have demonstrated a beneficial effect on the severity of heart failure and an improvement in maximal exercise tolerance in patients with heart failure. In these patients, ACEIs significantly decrease peripheral (systemic vascular) resistance, BP (afterload), pulmonary capillary wedge pressure (preload), pulmonary vascular resistance and heart size and increase cardiac output and exercise tolerance time.

Pharmacokinetics:

					Half-life		Elimination (24 hr)	
ACEI	Onset/ Duration (hrs)	Protein binding	Effect of food on absorption	Active metabolite	Normal renal function	Impaired renal function	Total	Un-changed
Benazepril	1/24	≈ 96.7% (≈ 95.3%)[1]	slightly reduced	benazeprilat	10-11 hr[1]	prolonged	11-12% bile[1]	trace
Captopril	nd[2]/ dose-related	≈ 25%-30%	reduced		< 2 hr	prolonged	> 95% urine	40%-50% in urine
Enalapril	1/24	nd[2]	none	enalaprilat	1.3 hr (11 hr)[1]	nd[2]	94% urine and feces	54% in urine (40%)[1]
Enalaprilat	0.25/≈6	na[3]	na[4]		11 hr	prolonged	nd[2]	> 90% in urine
Fosinopril	1/24	≈ 99.4%	slightly reduced	fosinoprilat	≈ 12 hr[1]	prolonged negligable clinical effect	50% urine, 50% feces	negligible
Lisinopril	1/24	na[3]	none	-	12 hr	prolonged	nd[2]	100% in urine
Moexipril	1.5/24	≈ 50%	markedly reduced	moexiprilat	2-9 hr[1]	prolonged	13% urine, 53% feces	1% in urine, 1% in feces
Quinapril	1/24	≈ 97%	reduced	quinaprilat	2 hr[1]	prolonged	≈60% urine, ≈37% feces	trace

Pharmacokinetics of the Active Moieties of ACEIs

Pharmacokinetics of the Active Moieties of ACEIs								
ACEI	Onset/ Duration (hrs)	Protein binding	Effect of food on absorption	Active metabolite	Half-life		Elimination (24 hr)	
					Normal renal function	Impaired renal function	Total	Un-changed
Ramipril	1-2/24	≈ 73% (≈ 56%)[1]	slightly reduced	ramiprilat	13-17 hr[1]	prolonged	≈ 60% urine, ≈ 40% feces	< 2%
Trandol-april	4/24	≈ 80%	reduced	trandolapri-lat	≈ 5 hr (≈ 10 hr)[1]	prolonged	33% urine, 56% feces	nd[2]

[1] Of active metabolite.
[2] nd – No data.
[3] na – Not applicable.
[4] na – Not applicable; available IV only.

Contraindications
Hypersensitivity to these products.

Warnings
Neutropenia/Agranulocytosis: Neutropenia (< 1000/mm^3) with myeloid hypoplasia resulted from **captopril** use. About half of the neutropenic patients developed systemic or oral cavity infections or other features of agranulocytosis. Neutropenia/agranulocytosis has occurred rarely with **enalapril** or **lisinopril** and in 1 patient on **quinapril**. Data are insufficient to show that **moexipril, ramipril, quinapril, benazepril, trandolapril,** or **fosinopril** do not cause agranulocytosis at similar rates. Periodically monitor WBC counts.

Angioedema: Angioedema has occurred. It may occur at any time during treatment, especially following the first dose of **enalapril** (0.2%), **captopril, lisinopril, trandolapril** (0.13%), **benazepril** (≈ 0.5%), **quinapril**(0.1%), or **moexipril** (< 0.5%). Angioedema associated with laryngeal edema may be fatal. Black patients receiving ACE inhibitor monotherapy have been reported to have a higher incidence of angioedema compared with non-blacks.

Proteinuria: Total urinary proteins > 1 g/day were seen in 0.7% of **captopril** patients. Nephrotic syndrome occurred in ≈ 20% of these cases.

Hypotension:
First-dose effect – ACE inhibitors may cause a profound fall in BP following the first dose.

Heart failure – In heart failure, where the BP was either normal or low, transient decreases in mean BP > 20% occurred in ≈ 50% of the patients.

Renal function impairment: Some hypertensive patients with renal disease, particularly those with severe renal artery stenosis, have developed increases in BUN and serum creatinine after reduction of BP.

In patients with severe CHF whose renal function may depend on the activity of the renin-angiotensin-aldosterone system, treatment with ACEIs may be associated with oliguria or progressive azotemia and, rarely, with acute renal failure or death.

Impaired renal function decreases **lisinopril** elimination. The elimination half-life of quinaprilat increases as Ccr decreases. Dosage adjustment may be necessary for **quinapril, benazepril, ramipril,** and **lisinopril**. Impaired renal function decreases total clearance of fosinoprilat and approximately doubles the AUC.

Hepatic function impairment: Patients with impaired liver function could develop markedly elevated plasma levels of unchanged **fosinopril** or **ramipril**. In patients with alcoholic or biliary cirrhosis, the rate, but not extent of fosinopril hydrolysis was reduced. Quinaprilat concentrations are reduced in alcoholic cirrhosis.

Elderly: Elderly patients may have higher blood levels and AUC of **lisinopril, ramiprilat, quinaprilat,** and **moexiprilat**. This may relate to decreased renal function rather than to age itself.

Pregnancy: Category C (first trimester); *Category* D (second and third trimesters). See Warning Box.

Lactation: Several ACEIs have been detected in breast milk. Do not administer **trandolapril** or **ramipril** to nursing mothers. It is not known whether **lisinopril**, **moexipril**, or **ramipril** is excreted in breast milk. Discontinue nursing or the drug.

Children: Safety and efficacy have not been established. Use **captopril** in children only when other measures for controlling BP have not been effective.

Precautions

Hyperkalemia: Elevated serum potassium (≥ 0.5 mEq/L greater than the upper limit of normal) was observed in 0.4% of hypertensive patients given **trandolapril**, $\approx 1\%$ of hypertensive patients given **benazepril**, **enalapril**, **ramipril**, or **moexipril**; $\approx 2\%$ of patients receiving **quinapril** or **lisinopril**, $\approx 2.6\%$ of hypertensive patients given **fosinopril**, and $\approx 4.8\%$ of CHF patients given lisinopril. Hyperkalemia also occurred with **captopril**.

Valvular stenosis: Theoretically, patients with aortic stenosis might be at risk of decreased coronary perfusion when treated with vasodilators, because they do not develop as much afterload reduction as others.

Surgery/Anesthesia: In patients undergoing major surgery or during anesthesia with agents that produce hypotension, ACEIs will block angiotensin II formation secondary to compensatory renin release.

Cough: Chronic cough has occurred with the use of all ACE inhibitors. Characteristically, the cough is nonproductive, persistent and resolves within 1 to 4 days after therapy discontinuation.

The incidence of cough, although still reported as 0.5% to 3% by some manufacturers, appears to range from 5% to 25% and has been reported to be as high as 39%, resulting in discontinuation rates as high as 15%.

Drug Interactions

Drugs that may affect ACE inhibitors may include antacids, capsaicin, indomethacin, phenothiazines, probenecid, and rifampin. Drugs that may be affected by ACE inhibitors include allopurinol, digoxin, lithium, potassium preparations/potassium-sparing diuretics, and tetracycline.

Drug/Lab test interactions: Captopril may cause a false-positive test for urine acetone.

Fosinopril may cause a false low measurement of serum digoxin levels with the *Digi-Tab RIA Kit for Digoxin* other kits such as the *Coat-A-Count RIA Kit*, may be used.

Drug/Food interactions: Food significantly reduces the bioavailability of **captopril** by 30% to 40%. Administer captopril 1 hour before meals. The rate and extent of **quinapril** absorption are diminished moderately (25% to 30%) when administered during a high-fat meal. The rate, but not extent, of **ramipril** and **fosinopril** absorption is reduced by food. Food does not reduce the GI absorption of **benazepril**, **enalapril**, and **lisinopril**.

Adverse Reactions

Adverse reactions may include chest pain, hypotension, headache, dizziness, fatigue, diarrhea, dysgeusia, cough, rash, dyspepsia, syncope, myalgia.

ANGIOTENSIN II RECEPTOR ANTAGONISTS

CANDESARTAN CILEXETIL	
Tablets: 4, 8, 16, and 32 mg (*Rx*)	*Atacand* (AstraZeneca)
EPROSARTAN MESYLATE	
Tablets: 400 and 600 mg (*Rx*)	*Teveten* (Unimed)
IRBESARTAN	
Tablets: 75, 150, and 300 mg (*Rx*)	*Avapro* (Bristol-Myers Squibb)
LOSARTAN POTASSIUM	
Tablets: 25, 50, and 100 mg (*Rx*)	*Cozaar* (Merck)
TELMISARTAN	
Tablets: 40 and 80 mg (*Rx*)	*Micardis* (Abbott)
VALSARTAN	
Capsules: 80 and 160 mg (*Rx*)	*Diovan* (Novartis)

Warning:

Pregnancy: When used in pregnancy during the second and third trimesters, drugs that act directly on the renin-angiotensin system can cause injury and even death to the developing fetus. When pregnancy is detected, discontinue angiotensin II receptor antagonists as soon as possible.

Indications

Hypertension: Treatment of hypertension alone or in combination with other antihypertensive agents.

Administration and Dosage

CANDESARTAN: Administer with or without food. The usual recommended starting dose is 16 mg once daily when used as monotherapy in patients who are not volume-depleted. Candesartan can be administered once or twice daily with total daily doses ranging from 8 to 32 mg. Larger doses do not appear to have a greater effect, and there is relatively little experience with such doses. If blood pressure is not controlled by candesartan alone, a diuretic may be added. Candesartan may be administered with other antihypertensive agents.

For patients with possible intravascular volume depletion (eg, patients treated with diuretics, particularly those with impaired renal function), initiate candesartan under close medical supervision and consider administering a lower dose.

EPROSARTAN: The usual recommended starting dosage is 600 mg once daily when used as monotherapy in patients who are not volume-depleted. Eprosartan can also be administered once or twice daily with total daily doses ranging from 400 to 800 mg. There is limited experience with doses > 800 mg/day.

If the antihypertensive effect measured at trough using once-daily dosing is inadequate, a twice-a-day regimen at the same total daily dose or an increase in dose may give a more satisfactory response. Achievement of maximum blood pressure (BP) reduction in most patients may take 2 to 3 weeks.

Eprosartan may be used in combination with other antihypertensive agents, such as thiazide diuretics or calcium channel blockers, if an additional BP-lowering effect is required. Discontinuation of treatment with eprosartan does not lead to a rapid rebound increase in blood pressure.

Elderly and Hepatic/Renal function impairment – No initial dosage adjustment is necessary for elderly, hepatically impaired patients, or those with renal impairment.

IRBESARTAN: The recommended initial dosage of irbesartan is 150 mg once daily with or without food. Patients may be titrated to 300 mg once daily.

Irbesartan may be administered with other antihypertensive agents. A low dose of a diuretic may be added if blood pressure is not controlled by irbesartan alone. Hydrochlorothiazide has been shown to have an additive effect. Patients not adequately treated by the maximum dose of 300 mg once daily are unlikely to derive additional benefit from a higher dose or twice-daily dosing.

LOSARTAN POTASSIUM: The usual starting dose is 50 mg once daily with 25 mg used in patients with possible depletion of intravascular volume (eg, patients treated with diuretics) and patients with a history of hepatic impairment. Losartan can be administered with or without food once or twice daily with total daily doses ranging from 25 to 100 mg.

If the antihypertensive effect measured at trough using once-daily dosing is inadequate, a twice-daily regimen at the same total daily dose or an increase in dose may give a more satisfactory response.

TELMISARTAN: The usual starting dose is 40 mg/day. BP response is dose-related over the range of 20 to 80 mg. May be administered with or without food. May be administered with other antihypertensive agents. When additional blood reduction beyond that achieved with 80 mg is required, a diuretic may be added.

Special risk patients – Patients on dialysis may develop orthostatic hypotension; monitor blood pressure closely. Initiate treatment under close medical supervision for patients with biliary obstructive disorders or hepatic insufficiency. Correct the condition of patients with depletion of intravascular volume before initiating therapy and monitor closely.

VALSARTAN: The recommended starting dose is 80 mg/day, with or without food, when used as monotherapy in patients who are not volume-depleted. Valsartan may be used over a dose range of 80 to 320 mg once daily.

If additional antihypertensive effect is required, the dosage may be increased to 160 or 320 mg or a diuretic may be added. Addition of a diuretic has a greater effect than dose increases beyond 80 mg. Valsartan may be administered with other antihypertensive agents.

Actions

Pharmacology: **Losartan**, **candesartan**, **irbesartan**, **telmisartan**, and **valsartan** are angiotensin II receptor (type AT_1) antagonists. Angiotensin II receptor antagonists (AIIRAs) block the vasoconstrictor and aldosterone-secreting effects of angiotensin II by selectively blocking the binding of angiotensin II to the AT_1 receptor found in many tissues.

AIIRAs do not inhibit ACE (kininase II, the enzyme that converts angiotensin I to angiotensin II and degrades bradykinin), nor do they bind to or block other hormone receptors or ion channels known to be important in cardiovascular regulation.

Pharmacokinetics:

Angiotensin II Antagonist Pharmacokinetics					
Parameters	Losartan (metabolite)[1]	Valsartan	Irbesartan	Candesartan	Telmisartan
Bioavailability	≈ 33%	≈ 25%	60% to 80%	≈ 15%	42%/58% (40 mg/160 mg)
Food effect (AUC/C_{max})	↓10%/↓	↓40%/↓50%	no effect	no effect	↓6%/↓20% (40 mg AUC/ 160 mg AUC)
Plasma bound	98.7% (99.8%)	95%	90%	> 99%	> 99.5%
C_{max}	1 hr (3 to 4 hrs)	2 to 4 hrs	1.5 to 2 hrs	3 to 4 hrs	0.5 to 1 hr
Volume of distribution	≈ 34 L (≈ 12 L)	17 L	53 to 93 L	0.13 L/kg	≈ 500 L
Converted to metabolites	(≈ 14%)	≈ 20%	< 20%	minor	≈ 11%
Metabolism enzymes, primary	CYP2C9; CYP3A4	unknown	CYP2C9	nd[3]	acylglucuronide
Terminal half-life	≈ 2 hrs (6 to 9 hrs)	≈ 6 hrs[2]	11 to 15 hrs	≈ 9 hrs	≈ 24 hrs
Total plasma clearance	≈ 600 mL/min (≈ 50 mL/min)	≈ 2 L/hr[2]	157 to 176 mL/min	0.37 mL/min/kg	> 800 mL/min
Renal clearance	≈ 75 mL/min (≈ 25 mL/min)	≈ 0.62 L/hr[2]	3 to 3.5 mL/min	0.19 mL/min/kg	nd[3]
Recovered in the urine	≈ 35%	13%	≈ 20%	≈ 33%	0.91%/ 0.49% (IV/oral)
Recovered in the feces	≈ 60%	83%	≈ 80%	≈ 67%	> 97%

[1] Active.
[2] IV dosing.
[3] nd = no data.

AIIRAs do not accumulate in plasma upon repeated once-daily dosing.

Losartan undergoes substantial first-pass metabolism and is converted to an active carboxylic acid metabolite (14% of dose) that is responsible for most of the angiotensin II receptor antagonism.

Valsartan is metabolized only to a small extent (< 10% of the systemically available dose), and the main metabolite is significantly less potent than valsartan in animal models.

In vitro studies of **irbesartan** oxidation by cytochrome P450 isoenzymes indicated irbesartan was oxidized primarily by 2C9; metabolism by 3A4 was negligible.

Telmisartan is metabolized by conjugation to form a pharmacologically inactive acylglucuronide.

Candesartan is rapidly and completely bioactivated by ester hydrolysis during absorption from the GI tract to candesartan, a selective AT_1 subtype angiotensin II receptor antagonist. Candesartan and its inactive metabolite do not accumulate in serum upon repeated once-daily dosing.

Contraindications

Hypersensitivity to any component of these products.

Warnings

Hypotension/Volume- or salt-depleted patients: In patients who are intravascularly volume-depleted (eg, those treated with diuretics), symptomatic hypotension may occur. Correct these conditions prior to administration.

Race: BP response with **telmisartan** in black patients (usually a low-renin population) is noticeably less than that in white patients. In controlled trials, **losartan** had an effect on blood pressure that was notably less in black patients than in non-blacks, a finding similar to ACE inhibitors. **Irbesartan** and **candesartan** were effective in reducing blood pressure regardless of race, although the effect was somewhat less in black.

Cough: In trials where **valsartan** was compared with an ACE inhibitor with or without placebo, the incidence of dry cough was significantly greater in the ACE inhibitor group (7.9%) than in the groups who received valsartan (2.6%) or placebo (1.5%). In patients who had dry cough when previously receiving ACE inhibitors, the incidences of cough in patients who received AIIRAs, HCTZ, or lisinopril were ≈ 22.5%, ≈ 18%, and 69%, respectively.

There was no significant difference in the incidence of cough between **losartan** or **irbesartan** and placebo.

Renal function impairment: In patients whose renal function may depend on the activity of the renin-angiotensin-aldosterone system (eg, patients with severe CHF), treatment with ACE inhibitors and angiotensin receptor antagonists has been associated with oliguria or progressive azotemia and with acute renal failure or death (rarely). No dosage adjustment is necessary for patients with renal impairment unless they are volume-depleted.

Hepatic function impairment:

Losartan – Compared with healthy subjects, the total plasma clearance in patients with hepatic insufficiency was ≈ 50% lower and the oral bioavailability was ≈ 2 times higher. A lower starting dose is recommended.

Valsartan – On average, patients with mild to moderate chronic liver disease have twice the exposure (measured by AUC values) to valsartan of healthy volunteers (matched by age, sex, and weight). In general, no dosage adjustment is needed in patients with mild to moderate liver disease. However, exercise care in this patient population.

Irbesartan – The pharmacokinetics of irbesartan following repeated oral administration were not significantly affected in patients with mild to moderate cirrhosis of the liver. No dosage adjustment is necessary in patients with hepatic insufficiency.

Candesartan – No differences in the pharmacokinetics were observed in patients with mild-to-moderate chronic liver disease. No initial dosage adjustment is necessary in patients with mild hepatic disease.

Telmisartan – As the majority of telmisartan is eliminated by biliary excretion, patients with biliary obstructive disorders or hepatic insufficiency can be expected to have reduced clearance. In patients with hepatic insufficiency, plasma concentrations of telmisartan are increased, and absolute bioavailability approaches 100%.

Elderly: No dosage adjustment is necessary when initiating AIIRAs in the elderly.

Pregnancy: Category C (first trimester); *Category D* (second and third trimesters).

Lactation: It is not known if AIIRAs are excreted in human breast milk.

Children: Safety and efficacy in patients < 18 years of age have not been established.

Precautions

Lab test abnormalities:

Liver function tests – Occasional elevations (> 150% in **valsartan**-treated patients) of liver enzymes or serum bilirubin have occurred.

Creatinine/Blood urea nitrogen (BUN) – Minor increases in BUN or serum creatinine were observed infrequently with **candesartan**, in < 0.1% of patients with essential hypertension treated with **losartan** alone, in 0.8% of patients taking **valsartan**, and < 0.7% with **irbesartan**. A ≥ 0.5 mg/dL rise in creatinine was observed in 0.4% **telmisartan** patients compared with 0.3% placebo patients.

Hemoglobin and hematocrit – A > 2 g/dL decrease in hemoglobin was observed in 0.8% **telmisartan** patients compared with 0.3% placebo patients. No patients discontinued therapy because of anemia.

Small decreases in hemoglobin and hematocrit occurred frequently in patients treated with **losartan** alone but were rarely of clinical importance. Decreases of > 20% in hemoglobin and hematocrit were observed in 0.4% and 0.8%, respectively, of **valsartan** patients, vs 0.1% and 0.1% with placebo.

Mean decreases in hemoglobin of 0.2 g/dL were observed in 0.2% of patients receiving **irbesartan**. Neutropenia (< 1000 cells/mm^3) occurred at similar frequencies (0.3%).

Small decreases in hemoglobin and hematocrit (mean decreases of ≈ 0.2 g/dL and 0.5 volume percent, respectively) were observed in patients treated with **candesartan** alone but were rarely of clinical importance.

Serum potassium – Increases of > 20% in serum potassium were observed in 4.4% of **valsartan**-treated patients vs 2.9% of placebo-treated patients.

A small increase (mean increase of 0.1 mEq/L) was observed in patients treated with **candesartan** alone but was rarely of clinical importance. One patient from a CHF trial was withdrawn for hyperkalemia (serum potassium, 7.5 mEq/L). This patient was also receiving spironolactone.

Hyperuricemia – Hyperuricemia was rarely found (0.6% with **candesartan** vs 0.5% with placebo.)

Drug Interactions

Drugs that may interact with losartan include cimetidine and phenobarbital.

Drugs that may interact with telmisartan include digoxin and warfarin.

In vitro studies show significant inhibition of the formation of oxidized **irbesartan** metabolites with the known cytochrome CYP2C9 substrates/inhibitors, tolbutamide, and nifedipine. However, clinical consequences were negligible.

Drug/Food interactions: A meal slows absorption of AIIRAs and decreases C_{max} but has only minor effects on **losartan** AUC or on the AUC of the metabolite (≈ 10% decrease). Food decreases **valsartan's** C_{max} by 50% and its AUC by 40%. Food slightly reduces the bioavailability of **telmisartan**, with an AUC reduction of ≈ 6% with the 40 mg tablet and ≈ 20% after a 160 mg dose. Food does not affect the bioavailability of **irbesartan** or **candesartan**.

Adverse Reactions

Adverse reactions occurring in ≥ 3% of patients include dizziness, upper respiratory tract infection, cough (**losartan**); viral infection (**valsartan**); fatigue, diarrhea, upper respiratory tract infection (**irbesartan**); dizziness, pain, and upper respiratory tract infection (**candesartan**); diarrhea, pain, upper respiratory tract infection, sinusitis (**telmisartan**).

ANTIHYPERLIPIDEMIC AGENTS

Lowering cholesterol levels can arrest or reverse atherosclerosis in all vascular beds and can significantly decrease the morbidity and mortality associated with atherosclerosis. Each 10% reduction in cholesterol levels is associated with an ≈ 20% to 30% reduction in the incidence of coronary heart disease. Hyperlipidemia, particularly elevated serum cholesterol and low density lipoprotein (LDL) levels, is a risk factor in the development of atherosclerotic cardiovascular disease.

Treatment of hyperlipidemia is based on the assumption that lowering serum lipids decreases morbidity and mortality of atherosclerotic cardiovascular disease.

The cornerstone of treatment in primary hyperlipidemia is diet restriction and weight reduction. Limit or eliminate alcohol intake. Use drug therapy in conjunction with diet, and after maximal efforts to control serum lipids by diet alone prove unsatisfactory, when tolerance to or compliance with diet is poor or when hyperlipidemia is severe and risk of complications is high. Treat contributory diseases such as hypothyroidism or diabetes mellitus.

Positive risk factors for CHD (other than high LDL) include: Age (men ≥ 45 years of age; women ≥ 55 years of age or women who go through premature menopause without estrogen replacement therapy); family history of premature CHD; smoking; hypertension (> 140/90 mmHg); low HDL cholesterol (< 35 mg/dL); obesity (> 30% overweight); and diabetes mellitus. Physical inactivity is not listed but should also be considered.

Negative risk factors include: High HDL cholesterol (≥ 60 mg/dL); subtract one risk factor if the patient's HDL is at this level.

All Americans (except children < 2 years of age) should adopt a diet that reduces total dietary fat, decreases intake of saturated fat, increases intake of polyunsaturated fat, and reduces daily cholesterol intake to ≤ 250 to 300 mg.

The following treatments guidelines are provided by the National Cholesterol Education Program Expert Panel on Detection, Evaluation and Treatment of High Blood Cholesterol in Adults ≥ 20 years of age.

Classification of Total and HDL Cholesterol Levels	
Level (mg/dL)	Classification
< 200 (5.2 mmol/L)	desirable
200-239 (5.2 - 6.2 mmol/L)	borderline-high
≥ 240 (6.2 mmol/L)	high
HDL < 35 (0.9 mmol/L)	low

1.) Total blood cholesterol < 200 mg/dL: HDL ≥ 35 mg/dL, repeat total cholesterol and HDL measurements within 5 years or with physical exam; provide education on general population eating pattern, physical activity, and risk factor education. HDL < 35 mg/dL, do lipoprotein analysis; base further action on LDL levels.

2.) Total blood cholesterol 200 to 239 mg/dL: HDL ≥ 35 mg/dL and < 2 risk factors, provide information on dietary modification, physical activity, and risk factor reduction; re-evaluate in 1 to 2 years, repeat total and HDL cholesterol measurements, and reinforce nutrition and physical activity education. HDL < 35 mg/dL or ≥ 2 risk factors, analyze lipoprotein; base further action on LDL levels.

3.) Total blood cholesterol ≥ 240 mg/dL: Analyze lipoprotein; base further action on LDL levels.

Classification of LDL- Cholesterol Levels	
Level (mg/dL)	Classification
< 130 (3.4 mmol/L)	desirable
130 -159 (3.4 - 4.1 mmol/L)	borderline-high
≥ 160 (4.1 mmol/L)	high

4.) LDL ≥ 160 mg/dL without CHD and with < 2 risk factors: Dietary treatment.
5.) LDL ≥ 130 mg/dL without CHD and with ≥ 2 risk factors: Dietary treatment.
6.) LDL ≥ 190 mg/dL without CHD and with < 2 other risk factors, or LDL ≥ 160 mg/dL without CHD and with ≥ 2 other risk factors: Drug treatment.

Elevations and treatment associated with each type of hyperlipidemia follow:

Hyperlipidemias and Their Treatment[1]						
	Hyperlipidemia type					
	I	IIa	IIb	III	IV	V
Lipids						
Cholesterol	N-⇑	↑	↑	N-↑	N-⇑	N-↑
Triglycerides	↑	N	↑	N-↑	↑	↑
Lipoproteins						
Chylomicrons	↑	N	N	N	N	↑
VLDL (pre-β)	N-⇑	N-↓	↑	N-⇑	↑	↑
ILDL (broad-β)[2]				↑		
LDL (β)	↓	↑	↑	↑	N-⇓	↓
HDL (α)	↓	N	N	N	N-⇓	↓
Treatment	Diet	Diet Bile acid sequestrants Dextrothyroxine Nicotinic acid Probucol HMG-CoA reductase inhibitors	Diet Bile acid sequestrants[3] Clofibrate[4] Gemfibrozil[5] Nicotinic acid HMG-CoA reductase inhibitors	Diet Clofibrate Gemfibrozil Nicotinic acid	Diet Clofibrate Gemfibrozil Nicotinic acid Fenofibrate	Diet Clofibrate Gemfibrozil Nicotinic acid Fenofibrate

[1] N = normal ↑ = increase ↓ = decrease ⇑ = slight increase ⇓ = slight decrease
[2] An abnormal lipoprotein.
[3] Particularly useful if hypercholesterolemia predominates.
[4] With high serum triglyceride levels and moderately elevated cholesterol.
[5] In patients with inadequate response to weight loss, bile acid sequestrants, and nicotinic acid.

Antihyperlipidemic Drug Effects[1]					
	Lipids		Lipoproteins		
Drug	Cholesterol	Triglycerides	VLDL (pre-β)	LDL (β)	HDL
Atorvastatin	↓	↓	↓	↓	↑
Cerivastatin	↓	↓	↓	↓	↑
Cholestyramine	↓	→↑	→↑	↓	→↑
Clofibrate[2]	↓	↓	↓	→↓	→↑
Colestipol	↓	→↑	↑	↓	→↑
Dextrothyroxine[2]	↓	→	→	↓	→
Fenofibrate	↓	↓	↓	↑	↑
Fluvastatin	↓	↓	↓	↓	↑
Gemfibrozil	↓	↓	↓	→↓	↑
Lovastatin	↓	↓	↓	↓	↑
Nicotinic Acid	↓	↓	↓	↓	↑
Pravastatin	↓	↓	↓	↓	↑
Simvastatin	↓	↓	↓	↓	↑

[1] ↓ = decrease ↑ = increase → = unchanged
[2] These agents are no longer commonly used as antihyperlipidemics.

BILE ACID SEQUESTRANTS

CHOLESTYRAMINE

Powder: 4 g anhydrous cholestyramine resin/9 g powder (*Rx*)	Various, *LoCHOLEST* (Warner Chilcott), *Questran* (Bristol-Myers Squibb)
4 g anhydrous cholestyramine resin/dose (*Rx*)	Various
4 g anhydrous cholestyramine resin/5.7 g powder (*Rx*)	*LoCHOLEST Light* (Warner Chilcott)
4 g anhydrous cholestyramine resin/5.5 g powder (*Rx*)	*Prevalite* (Upsher Smith)
4 g anhydrous cholestyramine resin/6.4 g powder (*Rx*)	*Questran Light* (Bristol-Myers Squibb)

COLESEVELAM HCl

Tablets: 625 mg (*Rx*)	*Welchol* (Sankyo Parke Davis)

COLESTIPOL HCl

Tablets: 1g (*Rx*)	*Colestid* (Pharmacia)
Granules: 5 g colestipol HCl/dose, 5 g colestipol HCl/7.5 g powder (*Rx*)	

Indications

Hyperlipoproteinemia: Adjunctive therapy for the reduction of elevated serum cholesterol in patients with primary hypercholesterolemia (elevated LDL) who do not respond adequately to diet.

Biliary obstruction (cholestyramine only): Relief of pruritus associated with partial biliary obstruction.

Administration and Dosage

Although generally given 3 to 4 times daily, there appears to be no advantage to dosing more frequently than twice daily.

CHOLESTYRAMINE:

Powder –

Adults: 4 g 1 to 2 times daily.

Maintenance dose: 8 to 16 g/day divided into 2 doses. Use gradual increases in dose with periodic assessment of lipid/lipoprotein levels at intervals of ≥ 4 weeks. Maximum recommended daily dose is 24 g.

Suggested time of administration is at mealtime but may be modified to avoid interference with absorption of other medications. Although the recommended dosing schedule is twice daily, it may be given in 1 to 6 per day.

COLESEVELAM: Take with liquid.

Monotherapy – The recommended starting dose is 3 tablets taken twice daily with meals or 6 tablets once daily with a meal. The dose can be increased to 7 tablets depending on desired therapeutic effect.

Combination therapy – For maximal therapeutic effect in combination with an HMG-CoA reductase inhibitor, the recommended dose of colesevalam is 3 tablets taken twice daily with meals or 6 tablets taken once daily with a meal. Doses of 4 to 6 tablets/day have been shown to be safe and effective when coadministered with an HMG-CoA reductase inhibitor or when the 2 drugs are dosed apart.

COLESTIPOL HCl:

Granules –

Adults: 5 to 30 g colestipol per day given once or in divided doses. The starting dose should be 5 g once or twice daily with a daily increment of 5 g at 1- or 2-month intervals.

Tablets – 2 to 16 g/day given once or in divided doses. The starting dose should be 2 g once or twice daily. Dosage increases of 2 g, once or twice daily, should occur at 1 or 2 month intervals.

Swallow tablets whole; do not cut, chew, or crush.

Actions

Pharmacology: Bile acid sequestering resins bind bile acids in the intestine to form an insoluble complex, which is excreted in the feces. This results in a partial removal of bile acids from the enterohepatic circulation, preventing their absorption. The lipid-lowering effect of 4 g cholestyramine equals 5 g colestipol.

Contraindications

Hypersensitivity to bile acid sequestering resins or any components of the products; complete biliary obstruction.

Warnings

Powder: To avoid accidental inhalation or esophageal distress, do not take powder or granules dry. Mix with fluids.

Pregnancy: These agents are not absorbed systemically and are not expected to cause fetal harm when given during pregnancy in recommended doses.

Lactation: Exercise caution when administering to a nursing woman. The possible lack of proper vitamin absorption may have an effect on nursing infants.

Children: Dosage schedules have not been established.

Precautions

Malabsorption: Because they sequester bile acids, these resins may interfere with normal fat absorption and digestion and may prevent absorption of fat-soluble vitamins such as A, D, E, and K.

Chronic use of resins may be associated with increased bleeding tendency due to hypoprothrombinemia associated with vitamin K deficiency.

Reduced folate: Reduction of serum or red cell folate has been reported over long-term administration of cholestyramine. Consider supplementation with folic acid.

Hyperchloremic acidosis: Prolonged use may cause hyperchloremic acidosis, especially in younger and smaller patients where relative dosage may be higher.

Constipation: These agents may produce or severely worsen preexisting constipation. Fecal impaction may occur and hemorrhoids may be aggravated.

Drug Interactions

These resins may delay or reduce the absorption of concomitant oral medication by binding the drugs in the gut. Take other drugs ≥ 1 hour before or 4 to 6 hours after these agents.

Drugs that may be affected by bile acid sequestrants include anticoagulants, aspirin, clindamycin, clofibrate, diclofenac, digitalis glycosides, furosemide, gemfibrozil, glipizide, hydrocortisone, imipramine, iopanoic acid, methyldopa, mycophenolate, nicotinic acid (niacin), penicillin G, phenytoin, phosphate supplements, piroxicam, propranolol, tetracyclines, thiazide diuretics, thyroid hormones, tolbutamide, ursodiol, and vitamins A, D, E, and K.

Adverse Reactions

GI:
> *Most common* – Constipation; infection; flatulence.
>
> *Less frequent* – Abdominal pain/distention/cramping; GI bleeding; belching; bloating; nausea; vomiting; diarrhea; loose stools; indigestion; dyspepsia; heartburn; anorexia; steatorrhea; rhinitis; pharyngitis.

Miscellaneous: Transient and modest elevations of AST, ALT, and alkaline phosphatase, (colestipol); liver function abnormalities (cholestyramine); pain, flu syndrome, accidental injury, asthenia (colesevelam); headache (including migraine and sinus); anxiety; vertigo; dizziness; lightheadedness; insomnia; fatigue; tinnitus; syncope; drowsiness; urticaria; dermatitis; asthma; wheezing; rash; backache; muscle/joint pains; hematuria; dysuria; burnt odor to urine; diuresis; uveitis; anorexia; weight loss/gain; increased libido; swollen glands; edema; weakness; shortness of breath; swelling of hands/feet.

HMG-CoA REDUCTASE INHIBITORS

ATORVASTATIN CALCIUM	
Tablets: 10, 20, 40, and 80 mg (*Rx*)	*Lipitor* (Parke-Davis)
FLUVASTATIN	
Capsules: 20 and 40 mg (*Rx*)	*Lescol* (Novartis)
Tablets, extended-release: 80 mg (*Rx*)	*Lescol XL* (Novartis)
LOVASTATIN	
Tablets: 10, 20, and 40 mg (*Rx*)	*Mevacor* (Merck)
PRAVASTATIN SODIUM	
Tablets: 10, 20, and 40 mg (*Rx*)	*Pravachol* (Bristol-Myers Squibb)
SIMVASTATIN	
Tablets: 5, 10, 20, 40, and 80 mg (*Rx*)	*Zocor* (Merck)

Indications

Antihyperlipidemics: Use HMG-CoA reductase inhibitors in addition to a diet restricted in saturated fat and cholesterol when diet and other nonpharmacological therapies alone have produced inadequate responses. Refer to individual product monographs.

HMG-CoA Reductase Inhibitor Indications					
Indication	Atorvastatin	Fluvastatin	Lovastatin	Pravastatin	Simvastatin
Primary hypercholesterolemia	✔[1]	✔[1]	✔[1]	✔[1]	✔[1]
Mixed dyslipidemia	✔[2]	✔[2]		✔[2]	✔[2]
Hypertriglyceridemia	✔[3]			✔[3]	✔[3]
Primary dysbetalipoproteinemia	✔[4]			✔[4]	✔[4]
Homozygous familial hyperlipidemia	✔				✔
Primary prevention coronary events			✔	✔	
Secondary prevention cardiovascular event(s)		✔	✔	✔	✔

[1] Includes heterozygous familial and nonfamilial hypercholesterolemia.
[2] Includes Fredrickson types IIa and IIb.
[3] Includes Fredrickson type IV.
[4] Includes Fredrickson type III.

Before initiating treatment with HMG-CoA reductase inhibitors, exclude secondary causes of hypercholesterolemia (eg, poorly controlled diabetes mellitus, hypothyroidism, nephrotic syndrome, dysproteinemias, obstructive liver disease, other drug therapy, alcoholism). Perform a lipid profile to measure total cholesterol (total-C), LDL cholesterol (LDL-C), HDL cholesterol (HDL-C), and triglycerides (TG). Estimate LDL-C in patients with TG < 100 mg/dL (< 4.5 mmol/L) using the following equation: LDL-C = total-C – ($\frac{1}{5}$TG + HDL-C). Determine LDL-C by ultracentrifugation for patients with TG > 400 mg/dL because this equation is less accurate.

Administration and Dosage

ATORVASTATIN CALCIUM:

Initial dose – 10 mg/day.

Dose range – 10 to 80 mg/day. Can be administered as a single dose at any time of the day, with or without food.

Concomitant therapy – Atorvastatin may be used in combination with a bile acid binding resin for additive effect. Avoid the combination of HMG-CoA reductase inhibitors and fibrates.

Renal function impairment – Dosage adjustment in renal dysfunction is not necessary.

FLUVASTATIN: May be taken without regard to meals.

Initial dose – 20 to 40 mg once daily at bedtime.

Dose range – 20 to 80 mg/day as a single dose in the evening. Administer the daily regimen of 80 mg in divided doses (eg, 40 mg twice a day) to those whose LDL-cholesterol response is inadequate at 40 mg/day. For patients requiring LDL cholesterol reduction to a goal of ≥ 25%, the recommended starting dose is 40 mg as 1 capsule, 80 mg as 1 tablet administered as a single dose in the evening, or 80 mg in divided doses of the 40 mg capsule given twice daily. For patients requiring LDL cholesterol reduction to a goal of < 25%, a starting dose of 20 mg may be used.

Concomitant therapy – Lipid-lowering effects on total cholesterol and LDL cholesterol are additive when fluvastatin is combined with a bile-acid binding resin or niacin. When administering a bile-acid resin (eg, cholestyramine) and fluvastatin, administer fluvastatin at bedtime, ≥ 2 hours following the resin, to avoid a significant interaction because of drug binding to resin.

Renal function impairment – Because fluvastatin is cleared hepatically with < 6% of the administered dose excreted in the urine, dose adjustments for mild to moderate renal impairment are not necessary. Exercise caution with severe impairment. Fluvastatin has not been studied at doses > 40 mg/day in patients with severe renal impairment; exercise caution when treating such patients at higher doses.

LOVASTATIN (MEVINOLIN): Place the patient on a standard cholesterol-lowering diet before starting lovastatin and continue on this diet during treatment. Give lovastatin with meals.

Initial dose is 20 mg/day with the evening meal in patients requiring reductions in LDL cholesterol of ≥ 20%; initiate at 10 mg/day in patients on immunosuppressants or in patients requiring smaller LDL reductions. Dosage range is 10 to 80 mg/day in single or 2 divided doses. Adjust at intervals of ≥ 4 weeks. Maximum dose is 80 mg/day, not to exceed 20 mg/day if given with immunosuppressants, fibrates, or niacin.

Renal function impairment – In patients with severe renal insufficiency (Ccr < 30 mL/min), use doses > 20 mg/day with caution.

PRAVASTATIN SODIUM: Place the patient on a standard cholesterol-lowering diet before starting pravastatin, and continue on this diet during treatment. May give without regard to meals. Initial dose is 10 to 40 mg once/day at bedtime; most patients on immunosuppressants start therapy with 10 mg/day pravastatin at bedtime and titrate to higher doses with caution. Most patients treated with this combination received a maximum of 20 mg/day pravastatin.

Concomitant lipid-lowering therapy – When administering a bile-acid binding resin (eg, cholestyramine, colestipol) and pravastatin, give pravastatin either ≥ 1 hour before or ≥ 4 hours following the resin.

Renal/Hepatic function impairment – Use a starting dose of 10 mg/day at bedtime.

Elderly – Initiate at 10 mg/day; LDL reductions may be achieved with ≤ 20 mg/day.

SIMVASTATIN: Place patient on a cholesterol-lowering diet before starting simvastatin; continue this diet during treatment. Give without regard to meals. Initial dose is 20 mg once daily in evening. Dosage may be started at 40 mg/night in patients requiring > 45% LDL reductions. For patients on immunosuppressants, use a starting dose of 5 mg/day (do not exceed 10 mg/day). Dosage range is 5 to 80 mg/day. Adjust dose at intervals of ≥ 4 weeks. Reduce dose if cholesterol falls below targeted range.

Renal function impairment – Initiate therapy with 5 mg/day and monitor closely.

Elderly – Use 5 mg/day starting dose; ≤ 20 mg/day may achieve maximum LDL reductions.

Actions

Pharmacology: These agents specifically competitively inhibit 3-hydroxy-3-methylglutaryl-coenzyme A (HMG-CoA) reductase, the enzyme which catalyzes the early rate-limiting step in cholesterol biosynthesis, conversion of HMG-CoA to mevalonate.

Pharmacokinetics:

Pharmacokinetics of HMG-CoA Reductase Inhibitors						
	Bioavailability	Excretion	t½ (hrs)	Major metabolites	Protein binding	Effects of renal/hepatic impairment
Atorva-statin	≈ 14% absolute bio-availability; first-pass metabolism (CYP3A4)	< 2% (urine)	≈ 14[1]	Metabolized to ortho- and parahydroxylated derivatives (active)	≥ 98%	Plasma levels not affected by renal disease; markedly increased with chronic alcoholic liver disease.
Fluva-statin	98% absorbed; absolute bioavailability 24%; extensive first-pass metabolism (CYP2C9)	< 6% (urine) ≈ 90% (feces)	< 1	Hydroxylated metabolites (active, do not circulate systemically)	98%	Potential drug accumulation with hepatic insufficiency.
Lova-statin	≈ 35% absorbed; extensive first-pass metabolism (CYP3A4); < 5% of oral dose reaches general circulation	10% (urine) 83% (feces)	3-4	Beta-hydroxyacid; 6'-hydroxyderivative; 2 additional metabolites	> 95%	Increased plasma concentration with severe renal disease.
Prava-statin	34% absorbed; absolute bioavailability 17%; extensive first-pass meta-bolism; plasma levels may not correlate with efficacy	≈ 20% (urine) 70% (feces)	1.8	Major degradation product: 3α-hydroxy isomeric metabolite	≈ 50%	Mean AUC varied 18-fold in cirrhotic patients and peak values varied 47-fold.
Simva-statin	60% to 80% absorbed; extensive first-pass metabolism (CYP3A4); < 5% of oral dose reaches general circulation	13% (urine) 60% (feces)	3	Beta-hydroxyacid; 6'-hydroxy, 6'-hydroxy-methyl, 6'-exomethylene derivatives	≈ 95%	Higher systemic exposure may occur in hepatic and severe renal insufficiency.

[1] For unmetabolized atorvastatin only. The t½ is 20 to 30 hours for the active metabolites.
[2] M1 and M23 metabolites; parent compound < 2%.

Contraindications

Hypersensitivity to any component of these products; active liver disease or unexplained persistent elevated liver function tests; pregnancy; lactation.

Warnings

Liver dysfunction: Use with caution in patients who consume substantial quantities of alcohol or who have a history of liver disease.

Pravastatin and **fluvastatin** plasma clearance is decreased but no dose adjustment is needed.

Skeletal muscle effects: Rhabdomyolysis with renal dysfunction secondary to myoglobinuria has occurred with some drugs in this class. Myalgia has occurred with **lovastatin**. Uncomplicated myalgia has been reported in **fluvastatin**-, and **atorvastatin**-treated patients.

Consider myopathy in any patient with diffuse myalgias, muscle tenderness or weakness, or marked elevation of CPK. Advise patients to report promptly muscle pain, tenderness or weakness, particularly with malaise or fever. Discontinue the drug if markedly elevated CPK levels occur or if myopathy is diagnosed.

Endocrine effects: Although cholesterol is the precursor of all steroid hormones, **lovastatin** has shown no effect on steroidogenesis. **Pravastatin** showed inconsistent results with regard to possible effects on basal steroid hormone levels; **fluvastatin** and **simvastatin** did not reduce basal plasma cortisol concentration or basal plasma testosterone concentration or impair adrenal reserve. Appropriately evaluate patients who display clinical evidence of endocrine dysfunction. Exercise caution when administering HMG-CoA reductase inhibitors with drugs that affect steroid levels or activity, such as ketoconazole, spironolactone, and cimetidine.

Hyperlipidemia, secondary causes: Prior to initiating therapy, exclude secondary causes of hyperlipidemia (eg, poorly controlled diabetes mellitus, hypothyroidism, nephrotic syndrome, dysproteinemias, obstructive liver disease, other drug therapy, alcoholism) and measure total-C, HDL-C, and triglycerides.

Hypersensitivity reactions: An apparent hypersensitivity syndrome has occurred. Refer to Management of Acute Hypersensitivity Reactions.

Renal function impairment: Closely monitor patients with renal impairment. Higher systemic exposure of **simvastatin** may occur in severe renal insufficiency.

Hepatic function impairment: Marked persistent increases (> 3 times ULN) in serum transaminases occurred in patients treated with all agents ranging in frequency from < 1% to 1.9%. When the drug was interrupted or discontinued or the dosage was reduced, transaminase levels usually fell slowly to pretreatment levels.

Elderly: In patients > 70 years of age, the AUC of **lovastatin** and **simvastatin** is increased. **Pravastatin** does not need dosage adjustment. The safety and efficacy of **atorvastatin** in patients ≥ 70 years of age were similar to those of patients < 70 years of age. Elderly patients (≥ 65 years of age) demonstrated a greater treatment response in respect to LDL-C, total-C and LDL/HDL ratio than patients < 65 years of age.

Pregnancy: Category X.

Lactation: **Lovastatin** and **atorvastatin** are excreted in the milk of rats; atorvastatin is likely to be excreted in breast milk; it is not known whether lovastatin and **simvastatin** are excreted in breast milk; a small amount of **pravastatin** is excreted in breast milk; **fluvastatin** is present in breast milk in a 2:1 ratio (milk:plasma).

Children: Safety and efficacy in individuals < 18 years of age have not been established; treatment in this age group is not recommended at this time.

Precautions

Monitoring: Perform liver function tests before initiating therapy, at 6 and 12 weeks after initiation of therapy, or after dose elevation and periodically thereafter (≈ 6-month intervals). Pay special attention to patients who develop elevated serum transaminase levels. If transaminase levels progress, particularly if they rise to 3 times the upper limit of normal and are persistent, discontinue the drug.

Because HMG-CoA reductase inhibitors may increase CPK and transaminase levels, consider this in the differential diagnosis of chest pain in patients treated with these agents.

Diet: Before instituting therapy, attempt to control hypercholesterolemia with diet, exercise, and weight reduction in obese patients.

Homozygous familial hypercholesterolemia: HMG-CoA reductase inhibitors are less effective in patients with the rare homozygous familial hypercholesterolemia, possibly because they have no functional LDL receptors.

Sleep disturbance: **Lovastatin** and **simvastatin** may interfere with sleep, causing insomnia, whereas **pravastatin** does not appear to disturb sleep.

Photosensitivity: Photosensitization (photoallergy or phototoxicity) may occur.

Drug Interactions

Drugs that may affect HMG-CoA reductase inhibitors include alcohol, antacids, azole antifungals, bile acid sequestrants, cimetidine, cyclosporine, erythromycin, gemfibrozil, isradipine, niacin, nicotinic acid, omeprazole, propranolol, ranitidine, and rifampin.

Drugs that may be affected by HMG-CoA reductase inhibitors include oral contraceptives, digoxin, and warfarin.

Atorvastatin, **lovastatin**, and **simvastatin** are primarily metabolized by CYP3A4; they may interact with CYP3A4 inhibitors.

Fluvastatin is primarily metabolized by CYP2C9; it may interact with CYP2C9 inhibitors.

Adverse Reactions

HMG-CoA Reductase Inhibitor Adverse Reactions (≥ 3%)[1]					
Adverse reaction	Atorvastatin	Fluvastatin (n = 2326)	Lovastatin	Pravastatin (n = 900)	Simvastatin (n = 1583)
CNS					
Headache	2.5 - 16.7	8.9	2.6 - 9.3	6.2	3.5
Dizziness	≥ 2	2.2	0.7 - 2	3.3	-
Asthenia	2.2 - 3.8	-	-	-	1.6
GI					
Nausea/Vomiting	≥ 2/< 2	3.2	1.9 - 4.7	7.3	1.3
Diarrhea	2.7 - 5.3	4.9	2.6 - 5.5	6.2	1.9
Abdominal pain/ cramps	2.1 - 3.8	4.9	2 - 5.7	5.4	3.2
Constipation	1.1 - 2.5	3.1	2 - 4.9	4	2.3
Flatulence	1.1 - 2.8	2.6	3.7 - 6.4	3.3	1.9
Dyspepsia	1.3 - 2.8	7.9	1.3 - 3.9	-	1.1
Musculoskeletal					
Localized pain	-	-	0.5 - 1	10	-
Myalgia	1.3 - 5.6	5	2.4 - 2.6	2.7	-
Back pain	1.1 - 3.8	5.7	-	-	-
Arthritis	≥ 2	2.1	-	-	-
Arthralgia	2 - 5.1	4	0.5 - 1	-	-
Respiratory					
Upper respiratory tract infection	-	16.2	-	-	2.1
Common cold	-	-	-	7	-
Rhinitis	≥ 2	4.7	-	4	-
Pharyngitis	1.3 - 2.5	3.8	-	-	-
Sinusitis	2.5 - 6.4	2.6	-	-	-
Bronchitis	≥ 2	-	-	-	-
Miscellaneous					
Chest pain	≥ 2	-	0.5 - 1	3.7	-
Rash/Pruritus	1.1 - 3.9/< 2	2.3	0.8 - 5.2	4	-
Cardiac chest pain	-	-	-	4	-
Fatigue	-	2.7	-	3.8	-
Influenza	2.2 - 3.2	5.1	-	2.4	-
Accidental trauma	1.3 - 4.2	5.2	-	-	-
Infection	2.8 - 10.3	-	-	-	-
Peripheral edema	≥ 2	-	-	-	-

[1] All events. Data are pooled from separate studies and are not necessarily comparable.

GEMFIBROZIL

Tablets: 600 mg (*Rx*)   *Gemcor* (Upsher-Smith), *Lopid* (Parke-Davis)
Capsules: 300 mg (*Rx*)   Various

Indications

Hypertriglyceridemia: Hypertriglyceridemia in adult patients (Types IV and V hyperlipidemia) who present a risk of pancreatitis and who do not respond to diet. Consider therapy for those with triglyceride elevations between 1000 and 2000 mg/dL, and who have a history of pancreatitis or of recurrent abdominal pain typical of pancreatitis.

Reducing coronary heart disease risk: Consider gemfibrozil therapy in those Type IIb patients who have low HDL-cholesterol levels in addition to elevated LDL-cholesterol and triglycerides and who have not responded to weight loss, dietary therapy, exercise, and other pharmacologic agents.

Gemfibrozil is not useful for the hypertriglyceridemia of Type I hyperlipidemia.

Administration and Dosage

Adults: 1200 mg/daily in 2 divided doses, 30 minutes before the morning and evening meals.

Actions

Pharmacology: Gemfibrozil is a lipid-regulating agent that decreases serum triglycerides and very low density lipoprotein (VLDL) cholesterol, and increases high density lipoprotein (HDL) cholesterol. While modest decreases in total and low density lipoprotein (LDL) cholesterol may be observed with gemfibrozil therapy, treatment of patients with elevated triglycerides due to Type IV hyperlipoproteinemia often results in a rise in LDL-cholesterol. Gemfibrozil usually raises HDL-cholesterol significantly in Type IIb patients with elevations of both serum LDL-cholesterol and triglycerides.

Pharmacokinetics:

Absorption/Distribution – Gemfibrozil is well absorbed from the GI tract. Peak plasma levels occur in 1 to 2 hours.

Metabolism/Excretion – Gemfibrozil mainly undergoes oxidation to form a hydroxymethyl and a carboxyl metabolite. It has a plasma half-life of 1.5 hours following multiple doses. Biological half-life is considerably longer, as some of the drug undergoes enterohepatic circulation and is reabsorbed in the GI tract. Approximately 70% is excreted in the urine, mostly as the glucuronide conjugate.

Contraindications

Hepatic or severe renal dysfunction, including primary biliary cirrhosis; pre-existing gallbladder disease; hypersensitivity to gemfibrozil.

Warnings

Cholelithiasis: If cholelithiasis is suspected, perform gallbladder studies. Discontinue therapy if gallstones are found.

Concomitant therapy: Concomitant therapy with gemfibrozil and lovastatin has been associated with rhabdomyolysis, markedly elevated creatine kinase (CK) levels and myoglobinuria, leading in a high proportion of cases to acute renal failure. In most subjects who have had an unsatisfactory lipid response to either drug alone, the possible benefit of combined therapy does not outweigh the risks. The use of gemfibrozil may occasionally be associated with myositis. If myositis is suspected or diagnosed, withdraw therapy.

Renal function impairment: There have been reports of worsening renal insufficiency upon the addition of gemfibrozil therapy in individuals with baseline plasma creatinine > 2 mg/dL. In such patients, consider the use of alternative therapy against the risks and benefits of a lower dose of gemfibrozil.

Pregnancy: Category C.

Lactation: Decide whether to discontinue nursing or discontinue the drug, taking into account the importance of the drug to the mother.

Children: Safety and efficacy in children have not been established.

Precautions

Estrogen therapy: Estrogen therapy is sometimes associated with massive rises in plasma triglycerides, especially in subjects with familial hypertriglyceridemia.

Contributory diseases: Contributory diseases such as hypothyroidism or diabetes mellitus should be adequately treated.

Monitoring therapy: Perform adequate pretreatment laboratory studies. Obtain periodic determinations of serum lipids during administration. Withdraw the drug after 3 months if response is inadequate.

Hematologic – Mild hemoglobin, hematocrit and white blood cell decreases have been observed. Perform periodic blood counts during the first 12 months of administration.

Liver function – Abnormal elevations of AST, ALT, LDH, bilirubin, and alkaline phosphatase have occurred, and are usually reversible on drug discontinuation. Perform periodic liver function studies and terminate therapy if abnormalities persist.

Blood glucose – Gemfibrozil has a moderate hyperglycemic effect; carefully monitor blood glucose levels during therapy.

Hazardous tasks: May produce drowsiness (dizziness or blurred vision); patients should observe caution while driving or performing other tasks requiring alertness, coordination and physical dexterity.

Drug Interactions
Drugs that may interact with gemfibrozil include oral anticoagulants and lovastatin.

Adverse Reactions
Adverse reactions occurring in $\geq 3\%$ of patients include dyspepsia; abdominal pain; diarrhea; fatigue.

FENOFIBRATE

Capsules: 67 mg (*Rx*)	*Tricor* (Abbott)

Indications
Hypertriglyceridemia: Adjunctive therapy to diet for treatment of adult patients with very high elevations of serum triglyceride levels (Types IV and V hyperlipidemia) who are at risk of pancreatitis and do not respond adequately to a determined dietary effort to control them.

Administration and Dosage
Patients should be placed on an appropriate triglyceride-lowering diet before receiving fenofibrate and should continue this diet during treatment.

Depending on the assessment of the patient's risk for pancreatitis, the initial dose is usually 67 mg/day given with meals to optimize bioavailability. Individualize dosage according to patient response, and increase sequentially, if necessary, following repeat serum triglyceride estimations at 4- to 8-week intervals. The maximum dose is 3 capsules/day (201 mg).

Withdraw therapy in patients who do not have an adequate response after 2 months of treatment with the maximum recommended dose of 3 capsules/day (201 mg).

Renal function impairment: Initiate treatment at 67 mg/day in patients having impaired renal function (Ccr < 50 mL/min), and increase only after evaluation of the effects on renal function and triglyceride levels at this dose.

Elderly: Limit the initial dose to 67 mg/day.

Actions
Pharmacology: Fenofibric acid, the active metabolite of fenofibrate, lowers plasma triglycerides apparently by inhibiting triglyceride synthesis, resulting in a reduction of very low density lipoprotein (VLDL) released into the circulation, and also by stimulating the catabolism of triglyceride-rich lipoprotein (eg, VLDL).

Pharmacokinetics:

Absorption/Distribution – Fenofibrate is well absorbed from the GI tract. Peak plasma levels of fenofibric acid occur within 6 to 8 hours after administration. Serum protein binding is $\approx 99\%$.

Metabolism – Fenofibrate is rapidly hydrolyzed by esterases to the active metabolite, fenofibric acid; no unchanged fenofibrate is detected in plasma. Fenofibric acid is primarily conjugated with glucuronic acid.

Excretion – Fenofibrate is eliminated with a half-life of 20 hours. It is mainly excreted in urine in the form of metabolites, primarily fenofibric acid and fenofibric acid glucuronide; $\approx 60\%$ of the dose appears in urine and 25% in feces.

Contraindications

Hepatic or severe renal dysfunction, including primary biliary cirrhosis, and patients with unexplained persistent liver function abnormality; preexisting gallbladder disease; hypersensitivity to fenofibrate.

Warnings

Mortality: Because of chemical, pharmacological, and clinical similarities between fenofibrate, clofibrate, and gemfibrozil, adverse events including excess total mortality determined in controlled clinical studies with these other fibrate drugs may also apply to fenofibrate.

Pancreatitis: Patients with a risk of pancreatitis typically have serum triglycerides > 2000 mg/dL and have elevations of VLDL-cholesterol as well as fasting chylomicrons (Type V hyperlipidemia).

Cholelithiasis: Fenofibrate, like clofibrate and gemfibrozil, may increase cholesterol excretion into the bile, leading to cholelithiasis. If cholelithiasis is suspected, gallbladder studies are indicated. Discontinue therapy if gallstones are found.

Myopathy/Myositis: The use of fibrates alone or in combination with HMG-CoA reductase inhibitors has been associated with rhabdomyolysis, markedly elevated creatine kinase (CK) levels and myoglobinuria, leading to a high proportion of acute renal failure cases. If myopathy/myositis is suspected or diagnosed, stop fenofibrate therapy.

Morbidity/Mortality: The effect of fenofibrate on coronary heart disease morbidity and mortality and non-cardiovascular mortality has not been established. Administer only to patients described under indications. If a significant reduction in fasting chylomicronemia does not occur, discontinue the drug.

Hypersensitivity reactions: Acute hypersensitivity reactions have occurred. Refer to Management of Acute Hypersensitivity Reactions.

Renal function impairment: Minimize the dosage in patients who have Ccr < 50 mL/min.

Hepatic function impairment: Fenofibrate is associated with significant increases in serum transaminases (AST or ALT). Increases to > 3 times the upper limit of normal (ULN) occurred. Hepatocellular, chronic active and cholestatic hepatitis associated with fenofibrate therapy have been reported after exposures of weeks to several years.

Pregnancy: Category C.

Lactation: Fenofibrate should not be used in nursing mothers.

Children: Safety and efficacy in children have not been established.

Precautions

Monitoring: Perform regular periodic monitoring of liver function, including serum ALT for the duration of therapy; discontinue therapy if enzyme levels persist > 3 times the normal limit. Rare spontaneous reports of thrombocytopenia and agranulocytosis have occurred. Thus, periodic blood counts are recommended during the first 12 months of fenofibrate administration.

Drug Interactions

Drugs that may affect fenofibrate include bile acid sequestrants.

Drugs that may be affected by fenofibrate include anticoagulants, cyclosporine, and HMG-CoA reductase inhibitors.

Drug/Food interactions: The absorption of fenofibrate is increased by ≈ 35% when administered with food.

Adverse Reactions

Adverse events occurring in ≥ 3% include rash, pruritis, dyspepsia, nausea/vomiting, diarrhea, abdominal pain, constipation, flatulence, rhinitis, infections, pain, headache, asthenia/fatigue, flu syndrome, and arthralgia.

Lab test abnormalities: Increases in creatinine and blood urea and decreases in hemoglobin and uric acid have occurred.

Anemia, leukopenia, eosinophilia, thrombocytopenia, and increased creatinine phosphokinase were reported.

Chapter 5

RENAL & GENITOURINARY AGENTS

Agents for Impotence, 317
  Alprostadil, 317
  Sildenafil Citrate, 319
Penicillamine, 322
Anticholinergics, 325
  Flavoxate, 325
  Oxybutynin, 325
  Tolterodine, 327
Thiazides and Related Diuretics, 330
  Loop Diuretics, 336
  Potassium-Sparing Diuretics, 341
    Amiloride HCl, 342
    Spironolactone, 343
    Triamterene, 345
  Carbonic Anhydrase Inhibitors, 347

ALPROSTADIL (Prostaglandin E$_1$; PGE$_1$)

Powder for injection, lyophilized: 6.15 mcg (5 mcg/mL), 11.9 mcg (10 mcg/mL) and 23.2 mcg (20 mcg/mL) (*Rx*)	*Caverject* (Pharmacia & Upjohn)
6.22 mcg (5 mcg/mL), 12.45 mcg (10 mcg/mL), 24.9 mcg (20 mcg/mL), 49.8 mcg (40 mcg/mL) (*Rx*)	*Edex* (Schwarz Pharma)
Pellet: 125, 250, 500, or 1000 mcg (*Rx*)	*Muse* (Vivus)

Indications

Erectile dysfunction: Treatment of erectile dysfunction caused by neurogenic, vasculogenic, psychogenic, or mixed etiology.

Intracavernosal alprostadil may be a useful adjunct to other diagnostic tests in the diagnosis of erectile dysfunction.

Unlabeled uses: Diagnostic peripheral arteriography (0.7 mcg/min for 10 minutes); treatment of atherosclerosis, gangrene, and pain caused by peripheral vascular disease.

Administration and Dosage

Initial titration:

Erectile dysfunction of vasculogenic, psychogenic, or mixed etiology – Initiate dosage titration at 2.5 mcg. If there is a partial response, the dose may be increased by 2.5 mcg to a dose of 5 mcg and then in increments of 5 to 10 mcg, depending on erectile response, until the dose that produces an erection suitable for intercourse and not exceeding a duration of 1 hour is reached. If there is no response to the initial 2.5 mcg dose, the second dose may be increased to 7.5 mcg, followed by increments of 5 to 10 mcg. If there is no response, then the next higher dose may be given within 1 hour. If there is a response, then there should be at least a 1-day interval before the next dose is given.

Erectile dysfunction of pure neurogenic etiology (spinal cord injury) – Initiate dosage titration at 1.25 mcg. The dose may be increased by 1.25 mcg to a dose of 2.5 mcg, followed by an increment of 2.5 mcg to a dose of 5 mcg, and then in 5 mcg increments until the dose that produces an erection suitable for intercourse and not exceeding a duration of 1 hour is reached. If there is no response, then the next higher dose may be given within 1 hour. If there is a response, then there should be at least a 1-day interval before the next dose is given.

Maintenance therapy: The first injections of alprostadil must be done at the physician's office by medically trained personnel. Self-injection therapy by the patient can be started only after the patient is properly instructed and well-trained in the self-injection technique. The recommended frequency of injection is ≤ 3 times/week, with at least 24 hours between each dose.

Intraurethral: Administer as needed to acheive an erection. The onset of effect is within 5 to 10 minutes after administration. The duration of effect is ≈ 30 to 60 minutes. A medical professional should instruct each patient on proper technique for administering alprostadil prior to self-administration. The maximum frequency of use is no more than 2 systems per 24-hour period.

Initiation of therapy – Titrate dose under the supervision of a physician to test a patient's response to alprostadil, to demonstrate proper administration technique and to monitor for evidence of hypotension. Individually titrate patients to the lowest dose that is sufficient for sexual intercourse. If necessary, increase the dose (or decrease) on separate occasions in a stepwise manner until the patient achieves an erection that is sufficient for sexual intercourse.

Actions

Pharmacology: Alprostadil induces erection by relaxation of trabecular smooth muscle and by dilation of cavernosal arteries.

Pharmacokinetics:

Distribution – Following intracavernosal injection, mean peripheral plasma concentrations at 30 and 60 minutes after injection were not significantly greater than baseline levels of endogenous alprostadil. Alprostadil is bound in plasma primarily to albumin (81% bound).

Intraurethral: Following intraurethral administration, alprostadil is absorbed from the urethral mucosa into the corpus spongosium. The half-life is short, varying between 30 seconds and 10 minutes.

Metabolism – Following IV administration, 60% to 90% of circulating alprostadil is metabolized in one pass through the lungs, primarily by beta- and omega-oxidation. The near-complete pulmonary first-pass metabolism of PGE_1 is the primary factor influencing the systemic pharmacokinetics of alprostadil and is a reason that peripheral venous plasma levels of PGE_1 are low or undetectable (< 2 pg/mL) following alprostadil administration. The enzyme catalyzing this process has been isolated from many tissues in the lower GU tract including the urethra, prostate, and corpus cavernosum.

Excretion – The metabolites of alprostadil are excreted primarily by the kidney, with almost 90% of an administered IV dose excreted in urine within 24 hours postdose. The remainder of the dose is excreted in the feces.

Contraindications

Hypersensitivity to the drug; conditions that might predispose patients to priapism (eg, sickle cell anemia or trait, multiple myeloma, leukemia); patients with anatomical deformation of the penis; patients with penile implants (intracavernosal); use in women, children, or newborns; use in men for whom sexual activity is inadvisable or contraindicated; for sexual intercourse with a pregnant woman unless the couple uses a condom barrier.

Warnings

Priapism: Priapism is known to occur following intracavernosal administration of vasoactive substances, including alprostadil. To minimize the chances of prolonged erection or priapism, titrate slowly to the lowest effective dose. Instruct the patient to seek immediate medical assistance for any erection that persists for > 6 hours. If priapism is not treated immediately, penile tissue damage, and permanent loss of potency may result.

Penile fibrosis: Regular follow-up of patients, with careful examination of the penis, is strongly recommended to detect signs of penile fibrosis. Discontinue treatment in patients who develop penile angulation, cavernosal fibrosis, or Peyronie's disease.

Penile pain: Penile pain after intracavernosal administration was reported. In the majority of the cases, penile pain was rated mild or moderate in intensity. Inject alprostadil slowly to decrease penile pain.

Hematoma/Ecchymosis: In most cases, hematoma/ecchymosis was judged to be a complication of a faulty injection technique.

Hemodynamic changes: Hemodynamic changes, manifested as decreases in blood pressure and increases in pulse rate, principally at doses > 20 mcg, were observed during clinical studies, and appeared to be dose-dependent.

Erectile dysfunction, causes: Diagnose and treat underlying treatable medical causes of erectile dysfunction prior to initiation of therapy.

Pulmonary disease: The pulmonary extraction of alprostadil following intravascular administration was reduced by 15% in patients with acute respiratory distress syndrome (ARDS).

Renal/Hepatic function impairment: Alterations in renal or hepatic function would not be expected to have a major influence on the pharmacokinetics of alprostadil.

Pregnancy: These products are not indicated for use in women. Do not use for sexual intercourse with a pregnant woman unless the couple uses a condom barrier.

Children: Caverject is not indicated for use in newborns or children. However, alprostadil (*Prostin VR Pediatric*) is used in newborns to maintain the patency of the ductus arteriosus in neonates with congenital heart defects.

Drug Interactions

Drugs that may interact with alprostadil include anticoagulants, cyclosporine, and vasoactive agents.

Adverse Reactions

Adverse reactions occurring in ≥ 3% of patients receiving alprostadil by intracaverno-sal administration include penile pain, prolonged erection, penile fibrosis, hema-toma, injection site hematoma, penis disorder, and upper respiratory infection.

Adverse reactions in ≥ 3% of patients receiving alprostadil by intraurethral adminis-tration include penile pain, urethral pain, urethral burning, urethral bleeding/spotting, testicular pain, headache, dizziness, URI, flu syndrome, hypotension, pain, and accidental injury.

SILDENAFIL CITRATE

Tablets: 25, 50, and 100 mg (*Rx*)   *Viagra* (Pfizer)

Indications

Erectile dysfunction: Treatment of erectile dysfunction.

Administration and Dosage

Sildenafil potentiated the hypotensive effects of nitrates; administration in patients who use nitric oxide donors (eg, sodium nitroprusside) or nitrates in any form is therefore contraindicated.

For most patients, the recommended dose is 50 mg taken as needed ≈ 1 hour before sexual activity. However, sildenafil may be taken anywhere from 4 hours to 30 min-utes before sexual activity. Based on effectiveness and tolerance, the dose may be increased to a maximum recommended dose of 100 mg or decreased to 25 mg. The maximum recommended dosing frequency is once per day.

Dosage adjustment: The following factors are associated with increased plasma levels of sildenafil: Age > 65 years (40% increase in AUC), hepatic impairment (eg, cirrho-sis, 80%), severe renal impairment (Ccr < 30 mL/min, 100%), and concomitant use of potent cytochrome P450 3A4 inhibitors (erythromycin, ketoconazole, itra-conazole, 200%). Because higher plasma levels may increase the efficacy and inci-dence of adverse events, consider a starting dose of 25 mg in these patients.

Actions

Pharmacology: Sildenafil, an oral therapy for erectile dysfunction, is a selective competi-tive inhibitor of cyclic guanosine monophosphate (cGMP)-specific phosphodiester-ase type 5 (PDE5). When sexual stimulation causes local release of nitric oxide (NO), inhibition of PDE5 by sildenafil causes increased levels of cGMP in the cor-pus cavernosum, resulting in smooth muscle relaxation and inflow of blood to the corpus cavernosum. Sildenafil at recommended doses has no effect in the absence of sexual stimulation.

Pharmacokinetics:

Absorption/Distribution – Sildenafil is rapidly absorbed, with absolute bioavailability of ≈ 40%. Its pharmacokinetics are dose-proportional over the recommended dose range. Maximum observed plasma concentrations are reached within 30 to 120 minutes (median, 60 minutes) of oral dosing in the fasted state. Sildenafil is distrib-uted into the tissues. Sildenafil and its major circulating N-desmethyl metabolite are ≈ 96% bound to plasma proteins.

Metabolism/Excretion – Sildenafil is cleared predominantly by the CYP3A4 (major route) and CYP2C9 (minor route) hepatic microsomal isoenzymes. It is converted into an active metabolite by N-desmethylation and is further metabolized. Silde-nafil and the metabolite have terminal half-lives of ≈ 4 hours.

Sildenafil is excreted as metabolites predominantly in the feces (≈ 80%) and to a lesser extent in the urine (≈ 13%).

Contraindications

Hypersensitivity to any component of the tablet; patients concurrently or intermit-tently using organic nitrates in any form (consistent with its known effects on the nitric oxide/cGMP pathway, sildenafil was shown to potentiate the hypotensive effects of nitrates).

Warnings

Renal function impairment: In volunteers with severe renal impairment (Ccr < 30 mL/min), sildenafil clearance was reduced. Consider an initial sildenafil dose of 25 mg in these patients.

Hepatic function impairment: In volunteers with hepatic cirrhosis, sildenafil clearance was reduced. Consider an initial sildenafil dose of 25 mg in these patients.

Elderly: Healthy elderly volunteers (≥ 65 years of age) had reduced sildenafil clearance with free plasma concentrations ≈ 40% greater than those in healthy younger volunteers. Consider an initial sildenafil dose of 25 mg in these patients.

Pregnancy: Category B.

Lactation: Sildenafil is not indicated for use in women.

Children: Sildenafil is not indicated for use in newborns and children.

Precautions

Erectile dysfunction: Undertake thorough medical history and physical examination to diagnose erectile dysfunction, determine potential underlying causes, and identify appropriate treatment.

The safety and efficacy of combinations of sildenafil with other treatments for erectile dysfunction have not been studied. Therefore, the use of such combinations is not recommended.

Cardiovascular status: Discuss with patients the potential cardiac risk of sexual activity in patients with preexisting cardiovascular disease. Treatments for erectile dysfunction, including sildenafil, generally should not be used in men for whom sexual activity is inadvisable because of their underlying cardiovascular status. Advise patients who experience symptoms (eg, angina pectoris, dizziness, nausea) upon initiation of sexual activity to refrain from further activity and discuss the episode with their physician.

There is no controlled clinical data on the safety or efficacy of sildenafil in patients who have suffered an MI, stroke, or life-threatening arrhythmia within the last 6 months; patients with resting hypotension (BP < 90/50 mmHg) or hypertension (BP > 170/110 mmHg); or patients with cardiac failure or coronary artery disease causing unstable angina. Use caution when prescribing sildenafil in these groups.

Deformation of penis/priapism: Use agents for the treatment of erectile dysfunction with caution in patients with anatomical deformation of the penis (such as angulation, cavernosal fibrosis, or Peyronie's disease) or in patients who have conditions that may predispose them to priapism (such as sickle cell anemia, multiple myeloma, or leukemia).

Warn patients that prolonged erections > 4 hours and priapism (painful erections > 6 hours in duration) have been reported infrequently since market approval of sildenafil. In the event of an erection that persists > 4 hours, advise the patient to seek immediate medical assistance.

Visual disturbances: Mild, transient, dose-related impairment of color discrimination (blue/green) was detected, with peak effects near the time of peak plasma levels.

Retinitis pigmentosa: A minority of patients with inherited retinitis pigmentosa have genetic disorders of retinal phosphodiesterases. Administer sildenafil with caution to these patients.

Drug Interactions

P450 system: Sildenafil metabolism is principally mediated by the cytochrome P450 (CYP) isoforms 3A4 (major route) and 2C9 (minor route). Therefore, inhibitors of these isoenzymes may reduce sildenafil clearance.

Strong CYP3A4 inhibitors such as ketoconazole, itraconazole, or mibefradil would be expected to increase sildenafil plasma levels, and population data from patients in clinical trials did indicate a reduction in sildenafil clearance when coadministered with CYP3A4 inhibitors (eg, ketoconazole, erythromycin, cimetidine). It can be expected that concomitant administration of CYP3A4 inducers, such as rifampin, will decrease plasma levels of sildenafil.

Sildenafil may affect nitrates and amlodipine. Sildenafil may be affected by amlodipine, beta-blockers, cimetidine, diuretics, and erythromycin.

Drug/Food interactions: When taken with a high-fat meal, the rate of sildenafil absorption is reduced, with a mean delay in T_{max} of 60 minutes and a mean reduction in C_{max} of 29%.

Adverse Reactions

Adverse reactions occurring in ≥ 3% of patients receiving sildenafil during clinical trials included headache, flushing, dyspepsia, nasal congestion, urinary tract infection, abnormal vision (mild and transient, predominantly color tinge to vision but also increased sensitivity to light or blurred vision), diarrhea.

PENICILLAMINE

Capsules: 125 and 250 mg (Rx)	*Cuprimine* (Merck)
Tablets, titratable: 250 mg (Rx)	*Depen* (Wallace)

Indications

Rheumatoid arthritis.

Wilson's disease (hepatolenticular degeneration).

Cystinuria.

Administration and Dosage

Give penicillamine on an empty stomach ≥ 1 hour before meals or 2 hours after meals and ≥ 1 hour apart from any other drug, food, or milk.

Wilson's disease: Initial dosage is 1 g/day for children or adults. This may be increased, as indicated by the urinary copper analyses, but it is seldom necessary to exceed 2 g/day. In patients who cannot tolerate 1 g/day initially, initiating dosage with 250 mg/day and increasing gradually allows closer control of the drug. Give on an empty stomach in 4 divided doses, 30 minutes to 1 hour before meals and at bedtime (≥ 2 hours after the evening meal).

Cystinuria:

Adult dosage – 2 g/day (range, 1 to 4 g/day) in 4 divided doses.

Pediatric dosage – 30 mg/kg/day in 4 divided doses. If 4 equal doses are not feasible, give the larger portion at bedtime. Initiating dosage with 250 mg/day, and increasing gradually, allows closer control of the drug and may reduce the incidence of adverse reactions.

Patients should drink about a pint of fluid at bedtime and another pint once during the night when urine is more concentrated and more acid than during the day. The greater the fluid intake, the lower the dosage of penicillamine required.

Rheumatoid arthritis: Administer on an empty stomach ≥ 1 hour before meals and ≥ 1 hour apart from any other drug, food, or milk.

Initial therapy: A single daily dose of 125 or 250 mg. Thereafter, increase dose at 1- to 3-month intervals by 125 or 250 mg/day as patient response and tolerance indicate. If satisfactory remission is achieved, continue the dose. If there is no improvement and if there are no signs of potentially serious toxicity after 2 to 3 months with doses of 500 to 750 mg/day, continue increases of 250 mg/day at 2- to 3-month intervals until satisfactory remission occurs or toxicity develops. If there is no discernible improvement after 3 to 4 months of treatment with 1 to 1.5 g/day, assume the patient will not respond and discontinue the drug.

Maintenance therapy: Many patients respond to ≤ 500 to 750 mg/day. In patients who respond but who evidence incomplete disease suppression after the first 6 to 9 months of treatment, increase daily dosage by 125 or 250 mg/day at 3-month intervals. Dosage > 1 g/day is unusual, but ≤ 1.5 g/day has been required.

Dosage frequency: Dosages ≤ 500 mg/day can be given as a single daily dose. Administer dosages > 500 mg/day in divided doses.

Actions

Pharmacology:

Rheumatoid arthritis – The mechanism of action of penicillamine in rheumatoid arthritis is unknown. The onset of therapeutic response may not be seen for 2 or 3 months in those patients who respond.

Wilson's disease: Penicillamine is a chelating agent that removes excess copper in patients with Wilson's disease. Noticeable improvement may not occur for 1 to 3 months.

Poisoning: Penicillamine also forms soluble complexes with iron, mercury, lead, and arsenic, which are readily excreted by the kidneys. The drug may be used to treat poisoning by these metals.

Cystinuria: Penicillamine reduces excess cystine excretion in cystinuria. Penicillamine with conventional therapy decreases crystalluria and stone formation and may decrease the size of or dissolve existing stones. This is done, at least in part, by disulfide interchange between penicillamine and cystine, resulting in a substance more soluble than cystine and readily excreted.

Pharmacokinetics: It is well absorbed from the GI tract after oral administration (40% to 70%); peak plasma levels occur in 1 to 3 hours. Most (80%) of the plasma penicillamine is protein bound, primarily to albumin. Penicillamine is rapidly excreted in the urine; 50% is excreted in the feces. Metabolites may be detected in the urine for up to 3 months after stopping the drug. Half-life ranges are 1.7 to 3.2 hours.

Contraindications

History of penicillamine-related aplastic anemia or agranulocytosis; rheumatoid arthritis patients with a history or other evidence of renal insufficiency; pregnancy; breastfeeding.

Warnings

Fatalities: Penicillamine has been associated with fatalities due to aplastic anemia, agranulocytosis, thrombocytopenia, Goodpasture's syndrome, and myasthenia gravis.

Hematologic: Leukopenia (2%) and thrombocytopenia (4%) have occurred. A reduction in WBC below 3500, neutrophils < 2000/mm^3, or monocytes > 500/mm^3 mandate permanent withdrawal of therapy.

Hepatotoxicity: Penicillamine has been associated with a mild elevation of hepatic enzymes that usually returns to normal even with continuation of the drug.

Autoimmune syndromes: Autoimmune syndromes that may be caused by penicillamine include polymyositis, diffuse alveolitis and dermatomyositis, Goodpasture's syndrome, myasthenic syndrome, pemphigus, and obliterative bronchiolitis.

    Pemphigoid-type – Pemphigoid-type reactions characterized by bullous lesions have required discontinuation of penicillamine and treatment with corticosteroids.

Lupus erythematosus: Certain patients will develop a positive antinuclear antibody (ANA) test and some may show a lupus erythematosus-like syndrome similar to other drug-induced lupus, but it is not associated with hypocomplementemia and may be present without nephropathy. A positive ANA test does not mandate drug discontinuance; however, a lupus erythematosus-like syndrome may develop later.

Sensitivity reactions: Once instituted for Wilson's disease or cystinuria, continue treatment with penicillamine on a daily basis. Interruptions for even a few days have been followed by sensitivity reactions after reinstitution of therapy.

Hypersensitivity reactions: Allergic reactions occur in ≈ 33% of patients. They are more common at the start of treatment, and occur as generalized rashes or drug fever. Discontinue treatment and reinstitute at a low dosage such as 250 mg/day, with gradual increases. Administering prednisolone 20 mg/day for the first few weeks of penicillamine therapy reduces the severity of these reactions. Antihistamines may control pruritus.

Renal function impairment: Proteinuria and hematuria may develop and may be a warning sign of membranous glomerulopathy, which can progress to a nephrotic syndrome.

Pregnancy: Category D.

Lactation: Safety has not been established.

Children: The efficacy of penicillamine in juvenile rheumatoid arthritis has not been established.

Precautions

Monitoring: When indicated, monitor drug toxicity or efficacy through urinalysis. In rheumatoid arthritis patients, discontinue the drug if unexplained gross hematuria or persistent microscopic hematuria develops. Perform liver function tests and an annual x–ray for renal stones.

    Monitor white and differential blood cell count, hemoglobin determination, and direct platelet count every 2 weeks for the first 6 months of penicillamine therapy and monthly thereafter.

Drug fever: Drug fever may appear in some patients, usually in the second to third week of therapy; it is sometimes accompanied by a macular cutaneous eruption.

Dermatologic – Skin rashes are the most frequent (44% to 50%) adverse reactions. Early rash occurs during the first few months of treatment and is more common.

A late rash – A late rash is less commonly seen, usually after 6 months or more of treatment, and requires drug discontinuation. It usually appears on the trunk, is accompanied by intense pruritus, and is usually unresponsive to topical corticosteroids.

Pemphigoid rash – Pemphigoid rash, the most serious dermatologic reaction occurs most often after 6 to 9 months of penicillamine.

Oral ulcerations: Oral ulcerations may develop that may have the appearance of aphthous stomatitis. Although rare, cheilosis, glossitis, and gingivostomatitis have been reported.

Hypogeusia: Hypogeusia occurs in 25% to 33% of patients, except for a lesser incidence in Wilson's disease (4%).

Dietary supplementation: Because of their dietary restriction, give patients with Wilson's disease, cystinuria, and rheumatoid arthritis whose nutrition is impaired 25 mg/day of pyridoxine during therapy, because penicillamine increases the requirement for this vitamin.

Iron deficiency may develop, especially in children and in menstruating women. This may be caused by diet. If necessary, give iron in short courses. A period of 2 hours should elapse between administration of penicillamine and iron, because orally administered iron reduces the effects of penicillamine.

Effects of penicillamine on collagen and elastin: Effects of penicillamine on collagen and elastin make it advisable to consider a reduction in dosage to 250 mg/day when surgery is contemplated.

Penicillamine may cause increased skin friability at sites subject to pressure or trauma, such as shoulders, elbows, knees, toes, and buttocks.

Drug Interactions

Drugs that may affect penicillamine include gold therapy, antimalarial or cytotoxic drugs, iron salts, antacids, and food.

Drugs that may be affected by penicillamine include digoxin.

Adverse Reactions

Penicillamine has a high incidence (> 50%) of untoward reactions, some of which are potentially fatal.

Adverse reactions that may occur in ≥ 3% of patients include anorexia; epigastric pain; nausea; vomiting; diarrhea; blunting/diminution/total loss of taste; taste perversion; thrombocytopenia; generalized pruritis; early and late rashes; proteinuria.

FLAVOXATE

Tablets: 100 mg (*Rx*)   *Urispas* (ALZA)

Indications
For the symptomatic relief of dysuria, urgency, nocturia, suprapubic pain, frequency, and incontinence as may occur in cystitis, prostatitis, urethritis, urethrocystitis/urethrotrigonitis.

Not indicated for definitive treatment but is compatible with drugs used to treat urinary tract infections.

Administration and Dosage
Adults and children > 12 years of age: 100 or 200 mg 3 or 4 times/day. Reduce the dose when symptoms improve.

Actions
Pharmacology: Counteracts smooth muscle spasm of the urinary tract and exerts its effect directly on the muscle.

Contraindications
Pyloric or duodenal obstruction; obstructive intestinal lesions or ileus; achalasia; GI hemorrhage; obstructive uropathies of the lower urinary tract.

Warnings
Glaucoma: Give cautiously in patients with suspected glaucoma.

Pregnancy: Category B.

Lactation: It is not known whether this drug is excreted in breast milk. Use caution when flavoxate is administered to a nursing woman.

Children: Safety and efficacy in children < 12 years of age have not been established.

Adverse Reactions
Nausea; vomiting; dry mouth; nervousness; vertigo; headache; drowsiness; mental confusion (especially in the elderly patient); hyperpyrexia; blurred vision; increased ocular tension; disturbance in eye accommodation; urticaria and other dermatoses; dysuria; tachycardia; palpitations; eosinophilia; leukopenia.

OXYBUTYNIN CHLORIDE

Tablets: 5 mg (*Rx*)   Various, *Ditropan* (ALZA)
Tablets, extended-release: 5, 10, 15 mg (*Rx*)   *Ditropan* XL (ALZA)
Syrup: 5 mg/5 mL (*Rx*)   Various, *Ditropan* (ALZA)

Indications
Bladder instability: For the relief of symptoms of bladder instability associated with voiding in patients with uninhibited and reflex neurogenic bladder (eg, urgency, frequency, urinary leakage, urge incontinence, dysuria).

For the treatment of overactive bladder with symptoms of urge urinary incontinence, urgency, and frequency (oxybutynin extended-release [ER] tablets).

Administration and Dosage
Oxybutynin immediate-release tablets:
Adults – 5 mg (tablets or syrup) 2 or 3 times/day. Maximum dose is 5 mg 4 times/day.
Children (> 5 years of age) – 5 mg (tablets or syrup) 2 times/day. Maximum dose is 5 mg 3 times/day.

Oxybutynin ER tablets: 5 mg once daily. Dosage may be adjusted in 5 mg increments to achieve a balance of efficacy and tolerability (up to a maximum of 30 mg/day). Dosage adjustments may proceed at approximately weekly intervals.

The ER tablets may be administered with or without food and must be swallowed whole with the aid of liquids, and not be chewed, divided, or crushed.

Actions

Pharmacology: Oxybutynin exerts direct antispasmodic effect on smooth muscle and inhibits the muscarinic action of acetylcholine on smooth muscle.

In patients with conditions characterized by involuntary bladder contractions, oxybutynin increases vesical capacity, diminishes frequency of uninhibited contractions of the detrusor muscle, and delays initial desire to void. Oxybutynin thus decreases urgency and the frequency of incontinent episodes and voluntary urination.

Oxybutynin is well tolerated in patients administered the drug from 30 days to 2 years.

Contraindications

Untreated angle-closure glaucoma; untreated narrow anterior chamber angles; GI obstruction; paralytic ileus; intestinal atony in the elderly or debilitated; megacolon; toxic megacolon complicating ulcerative colitis; severe colitis; myasthenia gravis; obstructive uropathy; unstable cardiovascular status in acute hemorrhage; hypersensitivity to the drug or any component of the product.

Warnings

Heat prostration: When administered in the presence of high environmental temperature, heat prostration (fever and heat stroke) may occur because of decreased sweating.

Diarrhea: Diarrhea may be an early symptom of incomplete intestinal obstruction, especially in patients with ileostomy or colostomy; discontinue treatment.

GI disorders: Doses administered to patients with ulcerative colitis may suppress GI motility and produce paralytic ileus and precipitate or aggravate toxic megacolon.

Administer ER tablets with caution to patients with GI obstructive disorders because of the risk of gastric retention.

The ER tablets, like other anticholinergic drugs, may decrease GI motility and should be used with caution in patients with conditions such as ulcerative colitis, intestinal atony, and myasthenia gravis.

Use the ER tablets with caution in patients who have gastroesophageal reflux or who are concurrently taking drugs (such as bisphosphonates) that can cause or exacerbate esophagitis.

As with other nondeformable material, use caution when administering the ER tablets to patients with preexisting severe GI narrowing (pathologic or iatrogenic). There have been rare reports of obstructive symptoms in patients with known strictures in association with the ingestion of other drugs in nondeformable controlled-release formulations.

Urinary retention: Administer ER tablets with caution to patients with clinically significant bladder outflow obstruction because of the risk of urinary retention.

Renal/Hepatic function impairment: Use ER tablets with caution in patients with hepatic or renal impairment.

Pregnancy: Category B.

Lactation: It is not known whether this drug is excreted in breast milk. Exercise caution when administering to a nursing woman.

Children: Safety and efficacy in children (< 5 years of age for immediate-release tablets) have not been established.

Precautions

Use with caution: Use with caution in the elderly and patients with autonomic neuropathy and hepatic or renal disease.

Cardiac and other effects: Symptoms of hyperthyroidism, coronary heart disease, CHF, cardiac arrhythmias, tachycardia, hypertension, hiatal hernia, and prostatic hypertrophy may be aggravated.

Hazardous tasks: Patients should use caution while driving or performing other tasks requiring alertness, coordination, or physical dexterity.

Drug Interactions

Drugs that interact with oxybutynin include atenolol, digoxin, haloperidol, phenothiazines, and amantadine.

Adverse Reactions

Adverse reactions occurring in ≥ 3% of patients – Palpitations; vasodilation; dizziness; insomnia; rash; constipation; dry mouth; nausea; urinary hesitance and retention.

Immediate-release tablets: Tachycardia; drowsiness; hallucinations; restlessness; decreased sweating; decreased GI motility; amblyopia; cycloplegia; decreased lacrimation; mydriasis; asthenia; impotence; suppression of lactation.

Extended-release tablets: Somnolence; headache; diarrhea; dyspepsia; blurred vision; dry eyes; asthenia; pain; rhinitis; urinary tract infection; hypertension; nervousness; confusion; dry skin; flatulence; gastroesophageal reflux; increased post-void residual volume; cystitis; upper respiratory tract infection; cough; sinusitis; bronchitis; dry nasal and sinus mucous membranes; pharyngitis; abdominal pain; accidental injury; back pain; flu syndrome; arthritis.

TOLTERODINE TARTRATE

Tablets: 1 and 2 mg *(Rx)*	*Detrol* (Pharmacia)
Capsules, extended-release: 2 and 4 mg *(Rx)*	*Detrol LA* (Pharmacia)

Indications

Overactive bladder: Treatment of patients with an overactive bladder with symptoms of urinary frequency, urgency, or urge incontinence.

Administration and Dosage

Immediate-release: The initial recommended dose is 2 mg twice/day. The dose may be lowered to 1 mg twice/day based on individual response and tolerability. For patients with significantly reduced hepatic function or who are currently taking drugs that are inhibitors of cytochrome P450 3A4, the recommended dose is 1 mg twice/day.

Extended-release (ER): The recommended dose is 4 mg once daily taken with liquids and swallowed whole. The dose may be lowered to 2 mg/day based on individual response and tolerability; however, limited efficacy data is available for the 2 mg capsules.

For patients with significantly reduced hepatic or renal function or who are currently taking drugs that are potent inhibitors of CYP3A4, the recommended dose of the ER capsules is 2 mg/day.

Actions

Pharmacology: Tolterodine is a competitive muscarinic receptor antagonist for overactive bladder. Urinary bladder contraction and salivation are mediated via cholinergic muscarinic receptors.

After oral administration, tolterodine is metabolized in the liver, resulting in the formation of the 5-hydroxymethyl derivative, a major active metabolite. The 5-hydroxymethyl metabolite, which exhibits antimuscarinic activity similar to that of tolterodine, contributes significantly to the therapeutic effect.

Tolterodine has a pronounced effect on bladder function in healthy volunteers. The main effects following a 6.4 mg single dose of tolterodine were an increase in residual urine, reflecting an incomplete emptying of the bladder, and a decrease in detrusor pressure.

Pharmacokinetics:

Absorption – Tolterodine is rapidly absorbed; ≥ 77% is absorbed, but absolute bioavailability is highly variable (10% to 74%). Maximum steady-state serum concentrations (C_{max}) typically occur within 1 to 2 hours. The pharmacokinetics of tolterodine are dose-proportional over the range of 1 to 4 mg.

Distribution – Tolterodine is highly bound to plasma proteins, primarily α_1-acid glycoprotein. The 5-hydroxymethyl metabolite is not extensively protein bound, with unbound fraction concentrations averaging ≈ 36%.

Metabolism – Tolterodine undergoes extensive and variable first-pass hepatic metabolism following oral dosing. The primary metabolic route involves the oxidation of the 5-methyl group mediated by the cytochrome P450 2D6 leading to the formation of an active 5-hydroxymethyl metabolite. Further metabolism leads to formation of the 5-carboxylic acid and N-dealkylated 5-carboxylic acid metabolites, which account for ≈ 51% and ≈ 29% of the metabolites recovered in the urine, respectively.

Variability in metabolism: A subset (≈ 7%) of the population is devoid of CYP2D6, the enzyme responsible for the formation of the 5-hydroxymethyl metabolite of tolterodine. The identified pathway of metabolism for these individuals ("poor metabolizers") is by dealkylation via cytochrome P450 3A4 (CYP3A4) to N-dealkylated tolterodine. The remainder of the population is referred to as "extensive metabolizers." Pharmacokinetic studies revealed that tolterodine is metabolized at a slower rate in poor metabolizers than in extensive metabolizers; this results in significantly higher serum concentrations of tolterodine and in negligible concentrations of the 5-hydroxymethyl metabolite.

Excretion – Following a 5 mg oral dose in healthy volunteers, 77% was recovered in urine and 17% was recovered in feces. Less than 1% (< 2.5% in poor metabolizers) of the dose was recovered as intact tolterodine, and 5% to 14% (< 1% in poor metabolizers) was recovered as the active 5-hydroxymethyl metabolite.

Special populations –

Renal insufficiency: Exposure levels of other metabolites of tolterodine were significantly higher (10- to 30-fold) in renally impaired patients.

Hepatic function impairment: The elimination half-life of tolterodine was longer in cirrhotic patients (mean, 8.7 hours) than in healthy, young, and elderly volunteers (mean, 2 to 4 hours). The clearance of oral tolterodine was substantially lower in cirrhotic patients (≈ 1.1 L/hr/kg) than in the healthy volunteers (≈ 5.7 L/hr/kg).

Contraindications

Urinary retention; gastric retention; uncontrolled narrow-angle glaucoma; hypersensitivity to the drug or its ingredients.

Warnings

Renal/Hepatic function impairment: Patients with significantly reduced hepatic function should not receive doses > 1 mg twice/day (> 2 mg/day for ER capsules). Treat patients with renal impairment with caution.

Pregnancy: Category C.

Lactation: It is not known whether tolterodine is excreted in human breast milk; therefore, discontinue administration during nursing.

Children: Safety and efficacy have not been established.

Precautions

Urinary/Gastric retention: Administer with caution to patients with clinically significant bladder outflow obstruction because of the risk of urinary retention and to patients with GI obstructive disorders, such as pyloric stenosis, because of the risk of gastric retention.

Controlled narrow-angle glaucoma: Use with caution in patients being treated for narrow-angle glaucoma.

Drug Interactions

Fluoxetine: Fluoxetine is a potent inhibitor of cytochrome P450 2D6 activity. No dose adjustment is required when tolterodine and fluoxetine are coadministered.

Cytochrome P450:

3A4 inhibitors – Patients receiving cytochrome P450 3A4 inhibitors, such as macrolide antibiotics (erythromycin and clarithromycin), antifungal agents (ketoconazole, itraconazole, and miconazole), or cyclosporine or vinblastine should not receive doses of tolterodine > 1 mg twice/day (> 2 mg/day for ER capsules).

2D6 – Tolterodine is not expected to influence the pharmacokinetics of drugs that are metabolized by cytochrome P450 2D6, such as flecainide, vinblastine, carbamazepine, and tricyclic antidepressants.

Drug/Food interactions: Food intake increases the bioavailability of tolterodine (average increase 53%). This change is not expected to be a safety concern and adjustment of dose is not needed.

Adverse Reactions

Adverse reactions occurring in ≥ 3% of patients include the following: Dry mouth, headache, dizziness, somnolence, abdominal pain, constipation, dyspepsia, xerophthalmia (extended- and immediate-release); diarrhea, fatigue, flu-like syndrome (immediate-release).

THIAZIDES AND RELATED DIURETICS

BENDROFLUMETHIAZIDE	
Tablets: 5 and 10 mg (*Rx*)	*Naturetin* (Princeton)
BENZTHIAZIDE	
Tablets: 50 mg (*Rx*)	*Exna* (Robins)
CHLOROTHIAZIDE	
Tablets: 250 and 500 mg (*Rx*)	Various, *Diuril* (Merck), *Diurigen* (Goldline)
Suspension: 250 mg/5 mL (*Rx*)	*Diuril* (Merck)
Powder for injection, lyophilized: 500 mg (as sodium) (*Rx*)	*Sodium Diuril* (Merck)
CHLORTHALIDONE	
Tablets: 15, 25, 50, and 100 mg (*Rx*)	Various, *Hygroton* (Rhone-Poulenc Rorer), *Thalitone* (Horus Therapeutics)
HYDROCHLOROTHIAZIDE	
Tablets: 25, 50, and 100 mg (*Rx*)	Various, *Esidrix* (Ciba), *Ezide* (Econo Med), *HydroDIURIL* (Merck), *Hydro-Par* (Parmed), *Oretic* (Abbott)
Solution: 50 mg/5 mL (*Rx*)	*Hydrochlorothiazide* (Roxane)
HYDROFLUMETHIAZIDE	
Tablets: 50 mg (*Rx*)	Various, *Diucardin* (Wyeth-Ayerst), *Saluron* (Apothecon)
INDAPAMIDE	
Tablets: 1.25 and 2.5 mg (*Rx*)	Various, *Lozol* (Rhone-Poulenc Rorer)
METHYCLOTHIAZIDE	
Tablets: 2.5 and 5 mg (*Rx*)	Various, *Aquatensen* (Wallace), *Enduron* (Abbott)
METOLAZONE	
Tablets: 2.5, 5 and 10 mg (*Rx*)	*Zaroxolyn* (Fisons)
0.5 mg (*Rx*)	*Mykrox* (Fisons)
POLYTHIAZIDE	
Tablets: 1, 2, and 3 mg (*Rx*)	*Renese* (Pfizer)
QUINETHAZONE	
Tablets: 50 mg (*Rx*)	*Hydromox* (Lederle)
TRICHLORMETHIAZIDE	
Tablets: 2 and 4 mg	Various, *Diurese* (American Urologicals), *Metahydrin* (Marion Merrell Dow), *Naqua* (Schering)

Indications

Edema: Adjunctive therapy in edema associated with congestive heart failure (CHF), hepatic cirrhosis, and corticosteroid and estrogen therapy. Useful in edema due to renal dysfunction (eg, nephrotic syndrome, acute glomerulonephritis, chronic renal failure).

> *Indapamide* – Indapamide alone is indicated for edema associated with CHF.

> *Metolazone* – Metolazone, rapidly acting (*Mykrox*), has not been evaluated for the treatment of CHF or fluid retention due to renal or hepatic disease, and the correct dosage for these conditions and other edematous states has not been established.

Hypertension: As the sole therapeutic agent or to enhance other antihypertensive drugs in more severe forms of hypertension.

Administration and Dosage

BENDROFLUMETHIAZIDE:

> *Edema* – 5 mg once daily, preferably in the morning.
>> *Initial:* Up to 20 mg once daily or divided into 2 doses.
>> *Maintenance:* 2.5 to 5 mg/day.
> *Hypertension* –
>> *Initial:* 5 to 20 mg/day.
>> *Maintenance:* 2.5 to 15 mg/day.

BENZTHIAZIDE:
> Edema –
>> Initial: 50 to 200 mg/day for several days, or until dry weight is attained. If dosages exceed 100 mg/day, give in 2 doses, following morning and evening meal.
>> Maintenance: 50 to 150 mg/day.
>
> Hypertension –
>> Initial: 50 to 100 mg/day. Give in 2 doses of 25 or 50 mg each, after breakfast and after lunch.
>> Maintenance: Maximal effective dose is 200 mg/day.

CHLOROTHIAZIDE:
> Adults –
>> Edema: 0.5 to 1 g once or twice/day, orally or IV. Reserve IV route for patients unable to take oral medication or for emergency situations.
>> Hypertension (oral forms only): Starting dose is 0.5 to 1 g/day as a single or divided dose. Rarely, some patients may require up to 2 g/day in divided doses.
>
> Infants and children –
>> Oral: 22 mg/kg/day (10 mg/lb/day) in 2 doses. Infants < 6 months of age may require up to 33 mg/kg/day (15 mg/lb/day) in 2 doses.
>> On this basis, infants up to 2 years of age may be given 125 to 375 mg/day in 2 doses. Children from 2 to 12 years of age may be given 375 mg to 1 g/day in 2 doses.
>> IV use is not generally recommended.

CHLORTHALIDONE: Give as a single dose with food in the morning. Maintenance doses may be lower than initial doses.
> Edema – Initiate therapy with 50 to 100 mg (Thalitone, 30 to 60 mg) daily, or 100 mg (Thalitone, 60 mg) on alternate days. Some patients may require 150 or 200 mg (Thalitone, 90 to 120 mg) at these intervals, or 120 mg Thalitone daily. However, dosages above this level do not usually create a greater response.
> Hypertension – Initiate therapy with a single dose of 25 mg/day (Thalitone, 15 mg). If response is insufficient after a suitable trial, increase to 50 mg (Thalitone, increase from 30 to 50 mg). For additional control, increase dosage to 100 mg once daily (except Thalitone), or add a second antihypertensive.
> Note: Doses > 25 mg/day are likely to potentiate potassium excretion but provide no further benefit in sodium excretion or blood pressure reduction.

HYDROCHLOROTHIAZIDE:
> Adults –
>> Edema:
>>> Initial – 25 to 200 mg/day for several days, or until dry weight is attained.
>>> Maintenance – 25 to 100 mg/day or intermittently. Refractory patients may require up to 200 mg/day.
>> Hypertension –
>>> Initial: 50 mg/day as a single or 2 divided doses. Doses > 50 mg are often associated with marked reductions in serum potassium. Patients usually do not require doses > 50 mg/day when combined with other antihypertensives.
>> Infants and children: Usual dosage is 2.2 mg/kg (1 mg/lb) daily in 2 doses. Pediatric patients with hypertension only rarely will benefit from doses > 50 mg/day.
>>> Infants (< 6 months of age) – Up to 3.3 mg/kg (1.5 mg/lb) daily in 2 doses.
>>> Infants (6 months to 2 years of age) – 12.5 to 37.5 mg/day in 2 doses. Base dosage on body weight.
>>> Children (2 to 12 years of age) – 37.5 to 100 mg/day in 2 doses. Base dosage on body weight.

HYDROFLUMETHIAZIDE:
> Edema –
>> Initial: 50 mg once or twice/day.
>> Maintenance: 25 mg to 200 mg/day. Administer in divided doses when dosage exceeds 100 mg/day.

Hypertension –
Initial: 50 mg twice/day.
Maintenance: 50 to 100 mg/day. Do not exceed 200 mg/day.

INDAPAMIDE:
Edema of congestive heart failure –
Adults: 2.5 mg as a single daily dose in the morning. If response is not satisfactory after 1 week, increase to 5 mg once daily.
Hypertension –
Adults: 1.25 mg as a single daily dose taken in the morning. If the response to 1.25 mg is not satisfactory after 4 weeks, increase the daily dose to 2.5 mg taken once daily. If the response to 2.5 mg is not satisfactory after 4 weeks, the daily dose may be increased to 5 mg taken once daily, but consider adding another antihypertensive.

METHYCLOTHIAZIDE:
Edema –
Adults: 2.5 to 10 mg once daily. Maximum effective single dose is 10 mg.
Hypertension –
Adults: 2.5 to 5 mg once daily. If blood pressure control is not satisfactory after 8 to 12 weeks with 5 mg once daily, add another antihypertensive.

METOLAZONE: Individualize dosage.
Zaroxolyn –
Mild to moderate essential hypertension: 2.5 to 5 mg once daily.
Edema of renal disease/cardiac failure: 5 to 20 mg once daily.
Mykrox –
Mild to moderate hypertension: 0.5 mg as a single daily dose taken in the morning. If response is inadequate, increase the dose to 1 mg daily. Do not increase dosage if blood pressure is not controlled with 1 mg. Rather, add another antihypertensive agent with a different mechanism of action.
Brand interchange – The metolazone formulations are not bioequivalent or therapeutically equivalent at the same doses. *Mykrox* is more rapidly and completely bioavailable. Do not interchange brands.

POLYTHIAZIDE:
Edema – 1 to 4 mg/day.
Hypertension – 2 to 4 mg/day.

QUINETHAZONE:
Adults – 50 to 100 mg once daily. Occasionally, 50 mg twice daily; 150 to 200 mg/day may be necessary infrequently.

TRICHLORMETHIAZIDE:
Edema – 2 to 4 mg once daily.
Hypertension – 2 to 4 mg once daily. In initiating therapy, doses may be given twice daily.

Actions

Pharmacology: Thiazide diuretics increase the urinary excretion of sodium and chloride in approximately equivalent amounts. They inhibit reabsorption of sodium and chloride in the cortical thick ascending limb of the loop of Henle and the early distal tubules. Other common actions include: Increased potassium and bicarbonate excretion, decreased calcium excretion and uric acid retention. At maximal therapeutic dosages all thiazides are approximately equal in diuretic efficacy.

The antihypertensive action requires several days to produce effects. Administration for ≤ 2 to 4 weeks is usually required for optimal therapeutic effect. The duration of the antihypertensive effect of the thiazides is sufficiently long to adequately control blood pressure with a single daily dose.

Pharmacokinetics:

Pharmacokinetics of Thiazides and Related Diuretics						
Diuretic	Onset (hours)	Peak (hours)	Duration (hours)	Equivalent dose (mg)	Percent absorbed	Half-life (hours)
Bendroflumethiazide	2	4	16 to 12	5	≈ 100	3 to 3.9
Benzthiazide	2	4 to 6	16 to 18	50	nd[1]	nd[1]
Chlorothiazide	2[2]	4[2]	16 to 12	500	10 to 21[3]	0.75 to 2
Chlorthalidone	2 to 3	2 to 6	24 to 72	50	64[3]	40
Hydrochlorothiazide	2	4 to 6	16 to 12	50	65 to 75	5.6 to 14.8
Hydroflumethiazide	2	4	16 to 12	50	50	≈ 17
Indapamide	1 to 2	≤ 2	up to 36	2.5	93	≈ 14
Methyclothiazide	2	6	24	5	nd[1]	nd[1]
Metolazone[4]	1	2	12 to 24	5	65	nd[1]
Polythiazide	2	6	24 to 48	2	nd[1]	25.7
Quinethazone	2	6	18 to 24	50	nd[1]	nd[1]
Trichlormethiazide	2	6	24	2	nd[1]	2.3 to 7.3

[1] nd = No data.
[2] Following IV use, onset of action is 15 minutes; peak occurs in 30 minutes.
[3] Bioavailability may be dose-dependent.
[4] *Mykrox* only: Peak plasma concentrations reached in 2 to 4 hrs, t½ $\approx$ 14 hrs.

Contraindications

Anuria; renal decompensation; hypersensitivity to thiazides or related diuretics or sulfonamide-derived drugs; hepatic coma or precoma (**metolazone**).

Warnings

Parenteral use: Use IV **chlorothiazide** only when patients are unable to take oral medication or in an emergency. In infants and children, IV use is not recommended.

Lupus erythematosus: Lupus erythematosus exacerbation or activation has occurred.

Hypersensitivity reactions: Hypersensitivity reactions may occur in patients with or without a history of allergy or bronchial asthma; cross-sensitivity with sulfonamides may also occur. Refer to Management of Acute Hypersensitivity Reactions.

Renal function impairment: Use with caution in severe renal disease because these agents may precipitate azotemia. Cumulative effects of the drug may develop in patients with impaired renal function. Monitor renal function periodically. **Metolazone** is the only thiazide-like diuretic that may produce diuresis in patients with GFR < 20 mL/min. Indapamide may also be useful in patients with impaired renal function.

Pregnancy: Category B (chlorothiazide, chlorthalidone, hydrochlorothiazide, indapamide, metolazone); Category C (bendroflumethiazide, benzthiazide, hydroflumethiazide, methyclothiazide, trichlormethiazide). Routine use during normal pregnancy is inappropriate.

Lactation: Thiazides may appear in breast milk. Discontinue nursing or the drug.

Children: Bendroflumethiazide, benzthiazide, chlorthalidone, hydrochlorothiazide, methyclothiazide, metolazone, hydroflumethiazide, trichlormethiazide – Safety and efficacy have not been established. Metolazone is not recommended for use in children. In infants and children, IV use of chlorothiazide has been limited and is generally not recommended.

Precautions

Fluid/Electrolyte balance: Perform initial and periodic determinations of serum electrolytes, BUN, uric acid and glucose. Observe patients for clinical signs of fluid or electrolyte imbalance (eg, hyponatremia, hypochloremic alkalosis, hypokalemia, changes in serum and urinary calcium).

Hypokalemia – Hypokalemia may develop during concomitant corticosteroids, ACTH, and especially with brisk diuresis, with severe liver disease or cirrhosis, vomiting or diarrhea, or after prolonged therapy.

Hyponatremia/Hypochloremia – A chloride deficit is generally mild and usually does not require specific treatment, except in extraordinary circumstances (as in liver or renal disease). Thiazide-induced hyponatremia has been associated with death and neurologic damage in elderly patients.

Hypomagnesemia – Thiazide diuretics have been shown to increase urinary excretion of magnesium, resulting in hypomagnesemia.

Hypercalcemia – Calcium excretion may be decreased by thiazide diuretics.

Hyperuricemia – Hyperuricemia may occur or acute gout may be precipitated in certain patients receiving thiazides, even in those patients without a history of gouty attacks.

Glucose tolerance – Hyperglycemia may occur with thiazide diuretics.

Lipids: Thiazides may cause increased concentrations of total serum cholesterol, total triglycerides and LDL (but not HDL) in some patients, although these appear to return to pretreatment levels with long-term therapy.

Photosensitivity: Photosensitization may occur.

Drug Interactions

Drugs that may be affected by thiazides include the following: Allopurinol; anesthetics; anticoagulants; antigout agents; antineoplastics; calcium salts; diazoxide; digitalis glycosides; insulin; lithium; loop diuretics; methyldopa; nondepolarizing muscle relaxants; sulfonylureas; vitamin D. Drugs that may affect thiazides include: Amphotericin B; anticholinergics; bile acid sequestrants; corticosteroids; methenamines; NSAIDs.

Drug/Lab test interactions: Thiazides may decrease serum PBI levels without signs of thyroid disturbance. Thiazides also may cause diagnostic interference of serum electrolyte, blood, and urine glucose levels (usually only in patients with a predisposition to glucose intolerance), serum bilirubin levels, and serum uric acid levels. In uremic patients, serum magnesium levels may be increased. **Bendroflumethiazide** and **trichlormethiazide** may interfere with the phenolsulfonphthalein test due to decreased excretion. In the phentolamine and tyramine tests, bendroflumethiazide may produce false-negative and trichlormethiazide may produce false-positive results.

Adverse Reactions

Adverse Reactions of Thiazides and Related Diuretics

Adverse reaction	Bendroflumethiazide	Benzthiazide	Chlorothiazide	Chlorthalidone	Hydrochlorothiazide	Hydroflumethiazide	Indapamide	Methyclothiazide	Metolazone	Polythiazide	Quinethazone	Trichlormethiazide
Cardiovascular												
Orthostatic hypotension	✔	✔	✔		✔	✔	<5%	✔	<2%[1]	✔	✔	✔
Palpitations							<5%		<2%[2]			✔
CNS												
Dizziness/Lightheadedness	✔	✔	✔	✔	✔	✔	≥5%	✔	10%[2]	✔	✔	✔
Vertigo	✔		✔	✔	✔	✔	<5%	✔	✔[3]	✔	✔	✔
Headache	✔	✔	✔	✔	✔	✔	≥5%	✔	9%[2]	✔	✔	✔
Paresthesias	✔	✔	✔	✔	✔	✔		✔	✔[3]	✔	✔	✔
Xanthopsia	✔	✔	✔	✔	✔	✔		✔		✔	✔	✔
Weakness	✔	✔	✔	✔	✔	✔	≥5%	✔	<2%[4]	✔	✔	✔
Restlessness/Insomnia	✔	✔	✔	✔	✔	✔	<5%	✔	✔[3]	✔	✔	✔
Drowsiness							<5%		✔[3]			✔

Adverse Reactions of Thiazides and Related Diuretics

Adverse reaction	Bendroflumethiazide	Benzthiazide	Chlorothiazide	Chlorthalidone	Hydrochlorothiazide	Hydroflumethiazide	Indapamide	Methyclothiazide	Metolazone	Polythiazide	Quinethazone	Trichlormethiazide
Fatigue/Lethargy/Malaise/Lassitude							≥5%		4%[2]			✔
Anxiety							≥5%		<2%[3]			
Depression							<5%		<2%[2]			✔
Nervousness							≥5%		<2%[3]			
Blurred vision (may be transient)	✔		✔		✔	✔	<5%		✔[3]			
GI												
Anorexia	✔	✔	✔	✔	✔	✔	<5%	✔	✔[3]	✔	✔	✔
Gastric irritation/epigastric distress	✔	✔	✔	✔	✔	✔	<5%	✔		✔	✔	✔
Nausea	✔	✔	✔	✔	✔	✔	<5%	✔	<2%[2]	✔	✔	✔
Vomiting	✔	✔	✔	✔	✔	✔	<5%	✔	<2%[4]	✔	✔	✔
Abdominal pain/cramping/bloating	✔	✔	✔	✔	✔	✔	<5%	✔	<2%[2]	✔	✔	✔
Diarrhea	✔	✔	✔	✔	✔	✔	<5%	✔	<2%[2]	✔	✔	✔
Constipation	✔	✔	✔	✔	✔	✔	<5%	✔	<2%[2]	✔	✔	✔
Jaundice (intrahepatic/cholestatic)	✔	✔	✔	✔	✔	✔		✔	✔[3]	✔	✔	✔
Pancreatitis	✔	✔	✔	✔	✔	✔		✔	✔[3]	✔	✔	✔
Dry mouth							<5%		<2%[1]			✔
GU												
Nocturia							<5%		<2%[1]			
Impotence/Reduced libido	✔	✔	✔	✔	✔	✔	<5%	✔	<2%[2]	✔	✔	✔
Hematologic												
Leukopenia	✔	✔	✔	✔	✔	✔		✔	✔[3]	✔	✔	✔
Thrombocytopenia	✔	✔	✔	✔	✔	✔		✔	✔	✔	✔	✔
Agranulocytosis	✔	✔	✔	✔	✔	✔		✔	✔[3]	✔	✔	✔
Aplastic/Hypoplastic anemia	✔	✔	✔	✔	✔	✔		✔	✔[3]	✔	✔	✔
Dermatologic												
Purpura	✔	✔	✔	✔	✔	✔		✔	✔[3]	✔	✔	✔
Photosensitivity/Photosensitivity dermatitis	✔	✔	✔	✔	✔	✔		✔	✔[3]	✔	✔	✔
Rash	✔	✔	✔	✔	✔	✔	<5%	✔	<2%[2]	✔	✔	✔
Urticaria	✔	✔	✔	✔	✔	✔		✔	✔[3]	✔	✔	✔
Necrotizing angiitis, vasculitis, cutaneous vasculitis	✔	✔	✔	✔	✔	✔	<5%	✔	✔[2]	✔	✔	✔
Pruritus	✔						<5%		<2%[1]			
Metabolic												
Hyperglycemia	✔	✔	✔	✔	✔	✔	<5%	✔	✔[3]	✔	✔	✔
Glycosuria	✔	✔	✔	✔	✔	✔	<5%	✔	✔[3]	✔	✔	✔
Hyperuricemia	✔	✔	✔	✔	✔	✔	<5%	✔		✔[3]		✔
Miscellaneous												
Muscle cramp/spasm	✔	✔	✔	✔	✔	✔	≥5%	✔	6%[2]	✔	✔	✔

[1] Percentage of occurrence refers to rapidly acting doseform; however this adverse reaction also occurred with the slow acting doseform.
[2] IV doseform.
[3] Possibly with life-threatening anaphylactic shock.
[4] Slow acting doseform only.
[5] Rapidly acting doseform only.

LOOP DIURETICS

BUMETANIDE	
Tablets: 0.5, 1, and 2 mg (*Rx*)	Various, *Bumex* (Roche)
Injection: 0.25 mg/mL (*Rx*)	
ETHACRYNIC ACID	
Tablets: 25 and 50 mg (*Rx*)	*Edecrin* (Merck)
Powder for Injection: 50 mg (as ethacrynate sodium) per vial (*Rx*)	*Edecrin Sodium* (Merck)
FUROSEMIDE	
Tablets: 20, 40, and 80 mg (*Rx*)	Various, *Lasix* (Hoechst-Roussel)
Oral Solution: 10 mg/mL (*Rx*)	
Injection: 10 mg/mL (*Rx*)	
TORSEMIDE	
Tablets: 5, 10, 20, and 100 mg (*Rx*)	*Demadex* (Boehringer Mannheim)
Injection: 10 mg/mL (*Rx*)	

> **Warning:**
> These agents are potent diuretics; excess amounts can lead to a profound diuresis with water and electrolyte depletion.

Indications

Edema: Edema associated with CHF, hepatic cirrhosis, and renal disease, including the nephrotic syndrome. Particularly useful when greater diuretic potential is desired.

Parenteral administration is indicated when a rapid onset of diuresis is desired (eg, acute pulmonary edema), when GI absorption is impaired or when oral use is not practical for any reason. As soon as it is practical, replace with oral therapy.

Hypertension (furosemide, oral; torsemide, oral): Alone or in combination with other antihypertensive drugs.

Ethacrynic acid:

Ascites – Short-term management of ascites due to malignancy, idiopathic edema, and lymphedema.

Congenital heart disease, nephrotic syndrome – Short-term management of hospitalized pediatric patients, other than infants.

Pulmonary edema, acute – Adjunctive therapy.

Administration and Dosage

BUMETANIDE:

Oral – 0.5 to 2 mg/day, given as a single dose. If diuretic response is not adequate, give a second or third dose at 4- to 5-hour intervals, up to a maximum daily dose of 10 mg. An intermittent dose schedule, given on alternate days or for 3 to 4 days with rest periods of 1 to 2 days in between, is the safest and most effective method for the continued control of edema. In patients with hepatic failure, keep the dose to a minimum, and if necessary, increase the dose carefully.

Parenteral – Initially, 0.5 to 1 mg IV or IM. Administer IV over a period of 1 to 2 minutes. If the initial response is insufficient, give a second or third dose at intervals of 2 to 3 hours; do not exceed a daily dosage of 10 mg. End parenteral treatment and start oral treatment as soon as possible.

Renal function impairment – In patients with severe chronic renal insufficiency, a continuous infusion of bumetanide (12 mg over 12 hours) may be more effective and less toxic than intermittent bolus therapy.

ETHACRYNIC ACID:

Oral –

Initial therapy: Give minimally effective dose (usually, 50 to 200 mg/day) on a continuous or intermittent dosage schedule to produce gradual weight loss of 2.2 to 4.4 kg/day (1 to 2 lb/day). Adjust dose in 25 to 50 mg increments. Higher doses, up to 200 mg twice daily, achieved gradually, are most often required in patients with severe, refractory edema.

Children: Initial dose is 25 mg. Make careful increments of 25 mg to achieve maintenance. Dosage for infants has not been established.

Maintenance therapy: Administer intermittently after an effective diuresis is obtained using an alternate daily schedule or more prolonged periods of diuretic therapy interspersed with rest periods.

Parenteral – Do not give SC or IM because of local pain and irritation. The usual IV dose for the average adult is 50 mg, or 0.5 to 1 mg/kg. Give slowly through the tubing of a running infusion or by direct IV injection over several minutes. Usually, only 1 dose is necessary; occasionally, a second dose may be required; use a new injection site to avoid thrombophlebitis. A single IV dose, not exceeding 100 mg, has been used. Insufficient pediatric experience precludes recommendation for this age group.

FUROSEMIDE:
    Oral –
    Edema: 20 to 80 mg/day as a single dose. Depending on response, administer a second dose 6 to 8 hours later. If response is not satisfactory, increase by increments of 20 or 40 mg, no sooner than 6 to 8 hours after previous dose, until desired diuresis occurs. This dose should then be given once or twice daily (eg, at 8 am and 2 pm). Dosage may be titrated up to 600 mg/day in patients with severe edema.

    Mobilization of edema may be most efficiently and safely accomplished with an intermittent dosage schedule; the drug is given 2 to 4 consecutive days each week. With doses > 80 mg/day, clinical and laboratory observations are advisable.

    Hypertension: 40 mg twice a day; adjust according to response. If the patient does not respond, add other antihypertensive agents. Reduce dosage of other agents by at least 50% as soon as furosemide is added to prevent excessive drop in blood pressure.

    Infants and children: 2 mg/kg. If diuresis is unsatisfactory, increase by 1 or 2 mg/kg, no sooner than 6 to 8 hours after previous dose. Doses > 6 mg/kg are not recommended. For maintenance therapy, adjust dose to the minimum effective level. A dose range of 0.5 to 2 mg/kg twice daily has also been recommended.

    CHF and chronic renal failure: It has been suggested that doses as high as 2 to 2.5 g/day or more are well tolerated and effective in these patients.

    Parenteral –
    Edema: Initial dose: 20 to 40 mg IM or IV. Give the IV injection slowly (1 to 2 minutes). If needed, another dose may be given in the same manner 2 hours later. The dose may be raised by 20 mg and given no sooner than 2 hours after previous dose, until desired diuretic effect is obtained. This dose should then be given once or twice daily. Administer high-dose parenteral therapy as a controlled infusion at a rate ≤ 4 mg/min.

    Acute pulmonary edema: The usual initial dose is 40 mg IV (over 1 to 2 minutes). If response is not satisfactory within 1 hour, increase to 80 mg IV (over 1 to 2 minutes).

    Infants and children: 1 mg/kg IV or IM given slowly under close supervision. If diuretic response after the initial dose is not satisfactory, increase the dosage by 1 mg/kg, no sooner than 2 hours after previous dose, until desired effect is obtained. Doses > 6 mg/kg are not recommended.

    CHF and chronic renal failure: It has been suggested that doses as high as 2 to 2.5 g/day or more are well tolerated and effective in these patients. For IV bolus injections, the maximum should not exceed 1 g/day given over 30 minutes.

TORSEMIDE: Torsemide may be given at any time in relation to a meal.

    Because of high bioavailability, oral and IV doses are therapeutically equivalent, so patients may be switched to and from the IV form with no change in dose. Administer the IV injection slowly over a period of 2 minutes.

    Congestive heart failure/chronic renal failure – The usual initial dose is 10 or 20 mg once daily oral or IV. If the diuretic response is inadequate, titrate the dose upward by approximately doubling until the desired diuretic response is obtained. Single doses > 200 mg have not been adequately studied.

Hepatic cirrhosis – The usual initial dose is 5 or 10 mg once daily oral or IV, administered together with an aldosterone antagonist or a potassium-sparing diuretic. If the diuretic response is inadequate, titrate the dose upward by approximately doubling until the desired diuretic response is obtained. Single doses > 40 mg have not been adequately studied.

Hypertension – The usual initial dose is 5 mg once daily. If the 5 mg dose does not provide adequate reduction in blood pressure within 4 to 6 weeks, the dose may be increased to 10 mg once daily.

Actions

Pharmacology: Furosemide and ethacrynic acid inhibit primarily reabsorption of sodium and chloride, not only in proximal and distal tubules, but also the loop of Henle. In contrast, bumetanide is more chloruretic than natriuretic and may have an additional action in the proximal tubule; it does not appear to act on the distal tubule. Torsemide acts from within the lumen of the thick ascending portion of the loop of Henle, where it inhibits the $Na^+/K^+/2Cl^-$-carrier system.

Pharmacokinetics: These agents are metabolized and excreted primarily through the urine. Protein binding of these agents exceeds 90%. Furosemide is metabolized $\approx$ 30% to 40%, and its urinary excretion is 60% to 70%. Oral administration of bumetanide revealed that 81% was excreted in urine, 45% of it as unchanged drug. Torsemide is cleared from the circulation by both hepatic metabolism ($\approx$ 80% of total clearance) and excretion into the urine ($\approx$ 20% of total clearance).

Pharmacokinetic Parameters of the Loop Diuretics								
Diuretic	Bioavail-ability (%)	Half-life (min)	Onset of action (min)	Peak (min)	Duration (hr)	Dosage (mg)	Relative potency	Doses/ day
Bumetanide								
Oral	72-96	60-90[5]	30-60	60-120	4-6	0.5-2	$\approx$ 40	1
IV			within minutes	15-30	0.5-1	0.5-1	$\approx$ 40	1-3
Ethacrynic acid								
Oral	$\approx$100	60	$\leq$ 30	120	6-8	50-100	0.6-0.8	1-2
IV			$\leq$ 5	15-30	2	50	0.6-0.8	1-2
Furosemide								
Oral	60-64[1]	$\approx$ 120[2]	$\leq$ 60	60-120[3]	6-8	20-80	1	1-2
IV or IM			$\leq$ 5[4]	30	2	20-40	1	
Torsemide								
Oral	$\approx$ 80	210	$\leq$ 60	60-120	6-8	5-20	2-4	1
IV			$\leq$ 10	$\leq$ 60	6-8	5-20	2-4	1

[1] Decreased in uremia and nephrosis.
[2] Prolonged in renal failure, uremia and in neonates.
[3] Decreased in CHF.
[4] Somewhat delayed after IM administration.
[5] Prolonged in renal disease.

Contraindications

Anuria; hypersensitivity to these compounds or to sulfonylureas; infants (ethacrynic acid); patients with hepatic coma or in states of severe electrolyte depletion until the condition is improved or corrected (bumetanide).

Warnings

Dehydration: Excessive diuresis may result in dehydration and reduction in blood volume with circulatory collapse and the possibility of vascular thrombosis and embolism, particularly in elderly patients.

Hepatic cirrhosis and ascites: In these patients, sudden alterations of electrolyte balance may precipitate hepatic encephalopathy and coma. Do not institute therapy until the basic condition is improved.

Ototoxicity: Tinnitus, reversible and irreversible hearing impairment, deafness, and vertigo with a sense of fullness in the ears have been reported. Deafness is usually reversible and of short duration (1 to 24 hours); however, irreversible hearing impairment has occurred. Usually, ototoxicity is associated with rapid injection, with severe renal impairment, with doses several times the usual dose, and with concurrent use with other ototoxic drugs.

Systemic lupus erythematosus: Systemic lupus erythematosus may be exacerbated or activated.

Thrombocytopenia: Because there have been rare spontaneous reports of thrombocytopenia with **bumetanide,** observe regularly for possible occurrence.

Hypersensitivity reactions: Patients with known sulfonamide sensitivity may show allergic reactions to **furosemide, torsemide,** or **bumetanide**. Bumetanide use following instances of allergic reactions to furosemide suggests a lack of cross-sensitivity. Refer to Management of Acute Hypersensitivity Reactions.

Renal function impairment: If increasing azotemia, oliguria, or reversible increases in BUN or creatinine occur during treatment of severe progressive renal disease, discontinue therapy.

Pregnancy: Category B (ethacrynic acid, torsemide); *Category C* (furosemide, bumetanide). Since furosemide may increase the incidence of patent ductus arteriosus in preterm infants with respiratory-distress syndrome, use caution when administering before delivery.

Lactation: **Furosemide** appears in breast milk.

Children: Safety and efficacy for use of **torsemide** in children, **bumetanide** in children < 18 years of age, and **ethacrynic acid** in infants (oral) and children (IV) have not been established.

    Furosemide – Furosemide stimulates renal synthesis of prostaglandin E_2 and may increase the incidence of patent ductus arteriosus when given in the first few weeks of life, to premature infants with respiratory-distress syndrome.

Precautions

Monitoring: Observe for blood dyscrasias, liver or kidney damage, or idiosyncratic reactions. Perform frequent serum electrolyte, calcium, glucose, uric acid, CO_2, creatinine, and BUN determinations during the first few months of therapy and periodically thereafter.

Cardiovascular effects: Too vigorous a diuresis, as evidenced by rapid and excessive weight loss, may induce an acute hypotensive episode. In elderly cardiac patients, avoid rapid contraction of plasma volume and the resultant hemoconcentration to prevent thromboembolic episodes, such as cerebral vascular thromboses and pulmonary emboli.

Electrolyte imbalance: Electrolyte imbalance may occur, especially in patients receiving high doses with restricted salt intake. Perform periodic determinations of serum electrolytes.

    Hypokalemia – Hypokalemia prevention requires particular attention to the following: Patients receiving digitalis and diuretics for CHF, hepatic cirrhosis, and ascites; in aldosterone excess with normal renal function; potassium-losing nephropathy; certain diarrheal states; or where hypokalemia is an added risk to the patient (eg, history of ventricular arrhythmias).

    Hypomagnesemia – Loop diuretics increase the urinary excretion of magnesium.

    Hypocalcemia – Serum calcium levels may be lowered (rare cases of tetany have occurred).

Hyperuricemia: Asymptomatic hyperuricemia can occur, and rarely, gout may be precipitated.

Glucose: Increases in blood glucose and alterations in glucose tolerance tests (fasting and 2 hour postprandial sugar) have been observed.

Lipids: Increases in LDL and total cholesterol and triglycerides with minor decreases in HDL cholesterol may occur.

Photosensitivity: Photosensitization (photoallergy or phototoxicity) may occur.

Drug Interactions

Loop diuretics may affect the following drugs: Aminoglycosides; anticoagulants; chloral hydrate; digitalis glycosides; lithium; nondepolarizing neuromuscular blockers; propranolol; sulfonylureas; theophyllines. Loop diuretics may be affected by the following drugs: Charcoal; cisplatin; clofibrate; hydantoins; NSAIDs; probenecid; salicylates; thiazide diuretics.

Drug/Food interactions: The bioavailability of **furosemide** is decreased and its degree of diuresis reduced when administered with food. Simultaneous food intake with **torsemide** delays the time to C_{max} by about 30 minutes, but overall bioavailability and diuretic activity are unchanged.

Adverse Reactions

Adverse reactions associated with loop diuretics include nausea; vomiting; diarrhea; gastric irritation; headache; fatigue; dizziness; thrombocytopenia; rash; orthostatic hypotension; hyperuricemia; hyperglycemia; electrolyte imbalance (decreased chloride, potassium and sodium); dehydration.

Bumetanide: Adverse reactions may include impaired hearing, ear discomfort, dry mouth, pain, renal failure, weakness, arthritic pain, muscle cramps, ECG changes, chest pain, hives, pruritus, itching, sweating, hyperventilation.

Ethacrynic acid: Adverse reactions may include anorexia, pain, GI bleeding, severe neutropenia, agranulocytosis, fever, chills, confusion, fatigue, malaise, sense of fullness in the ears, blurred vision, tinnitus, hearing loss (irreversible), rash.

Furosemide: Adverse reactions may include anorexia, cramping, constipation, blurred vision, hearing loss, restlessness, fever, anemia, purpura, thrombocytopenia, agranulocytosis, photosensitivity, urticaria, pruritus, thrombophlebitis, muscle spasm, weakness.

Torsemide: Adverse reactions may include excessive urination.

POTASSIUM-SPARING DIURETICS

Actions

Pharmacology: In the kidney, potassium is filtered at the glomerulus and then absorbed parallel to sodium throughout the proximal tubule and thick ascending limb of the loop of Henle, so that only minor amounts reach the distal convoluted tubule. As a result, potassium appearing in urine is secreted at the distal tubule and collecting duct. The potassium-sparing diuretics interfere with sodium reabsorption at the distal tubule, thus decreasing potassium secretion. They exert a weak diuretic and antihypertensive effect when used alone. Their major use is to enhance the action and counteract the kaliuretic effect of thiazide and loop diuretics.

Spironolactone – Spironolactone, a competitive inhibitor of aldosterone, binds to aldosterone receptors of the distal tubule and prevents the formation of a protein important in sodium transport. It is effective in primary and secondary hyperaldosteronism. Spironolactone is effective in lowering systolic and diastolic blood pressure in primary hyperaldosteronism and essential hypertension, although aldosterone secretion may be normal in benign essential hypertension.

Amiloride and triamterene – **Amiloride** and **triamterene** not only inhibit sodium reabsorption induced by aldosterone, but they also inhibit basal sodium reabsorption. They are not aldosterone antagonists, but act directly on the renal distal tubule, cortical collecting tubule and collecting duct. They induce a reversal of polarity of the transtubular electrical-potential difference and inhibit active transport of sodium and potassium. Amiloride may inhibit sodium, potassium-ATPase.

Potassium-Sparing Diuretics: Pharmacological and Pharmacokinetic Properties			
Parameters	Amiloride	Spironolactone	Triamterene
Pharmacology			
Tubular site of action	Proximal = distal	Distal	Distal
Mechanism of action	Na$^+$, K$^+$–ATPase inhibition; Na$^+$/H$^+$ exchange mechanism inhibition (proximal tubule)	Aldosterone antagonism	Membrane effect
Action:			
Onset (hours)	2	24 to 48	2 to 4
Peak (hours)	6 to 10	48 to 72	6 to 8
Duration (hours)	24	48 to 72	12 to 16
Pharmacokinetics			
Bioavailability	15% to 25%	> 90%	30% to 70%
Protein binding	23%	≥ 98%[1]	50% to 67%
Half-life (hours)	6 to 9	20[2]	3
Active metabolites	none	canrenone	hydroxytriamterene sulfate
Peak plasma levels (hours)	3 to 4	canrenone: 2 to 4	3
Excreted unchanged in urine	≈ 50%[3]	†[4]	≈ 21%
Dosage			
Daily dose (mg)	5 to 20	25 to 400	200 to 300

[1] Canrenone > 98%.
[2] 10 to 35 hours for canrenone.
[3] 40% excreted in stool within 72 hours.
[4] Metabolites primarily excreted in urine, but also in bile.

AMILORIDE HCl

Tablets: 5 mg (*Rx*) *Midamor* (Merck)

Indications

Adjunctive treatment with thiazide or loop diuretics in CHF or hypertension to: Help restore normal serum potassium in patients who develop hypokalemia on the kaliuretic diuretic; prevent hypokalemia in patients who would be at particular risk if hypokalemia were to develop (eg, digitalized patients or patients with significant cardiac arrhythmias).

Unlabeled uses: Amiloride (10 to 20 mg/day) may be useful in reducing lithium-induced polyuria without increasing lithium levels as is seen with thiazide diuretics.

Administration and Dosage

Administer with food.

Concomitant therapy: Add amiloride 5 mg/day to the usual antihypertensive or diuretic dosage of a kaliuretic diuretic. Increase dosage to 10 mg/day, if necessary; doses > 10 mg are usually not needed. If persistent hypokalemia is documented with 10 mg, increase the dose to 15 mg, then 20 mg, with careful titration of the dose and careful monitoring of electrolytes.

In patients with CHF, potassium loss may decrease after an initial diuresis; reevaluate the need or dosage for amiloride. Maintenance therapy may be intermittent.

Single drug therapy: The starting dose is 5 mg/day. Increase to 10 mg/day, if necessary; doses > 10 mg are usually not needed. If persistent hypokalemia is documented with 10 mg, increase the dose to 15 mg, then 20 mg, with careful monitoring of electrolytes.

Contraindications

Hypersensitivity to amiloride; serum potassium > 5.5 mEq/L; antikaliuretic therapy or potassium supplementation; renal function impairment patients receiving spironolactone or triamaterene.

Warnings

Hyperkalemia: Amiloride may cause hyperkalemia (serum potassium > 5.5 mEq/L) that, if uncorrected, is potentially fatal. Monitor serum potassium carefully. Symptoms of hyperkalemia include paresthesias, muscular weakness, fatigue, flaccid paralysis of the extremities, bradicardia, shock, and ECG abnormalities.

Diabetes mellitus: Avoid use of amiloride in diabetic patients. If it is used, monitor serum electrolytes and renal function frequently. Discontinue use ≥ 3 days before glucose tolerance testing.

Metabolic or respiratory acidosis: Cautiously institute amiloride in severely ill patients in whom respiratory or metabolic acidosis may occur, such as patients with cardiopulmonary disease or poorly controlled diabetes. Monitor acid-base balance frequently. Shifts in acid-base balance alter the ratio of extracellular/intracellular potassium; the development of acidosis may be associated with rapid increases in serum potassium.

Renal function impairment: Anuria, acute or chronic renal insufficiency and evidence of diabetic nephropathy are contraindications because potassium retention is accentuated and may result in the rapid development of hyperkalemia. Do not give to patients with evidence of renal impairment (BUN > 30 mg/dL or serum creatinine > 1.5 mg/dL) or diabetes mellitus without continuous monitoring of serum electrolytes, creatinine, and BUN levels.

Hepatic function impairment: In patients with preexisting severe liver disease, hepatic encephalopathy (manifested by tremors, confusion, and coma, and increased jaundice) may occur. Because amiloride is not metabolized by the liver, drug accumulation is not anticipated in patients with hepatic dysfunction, but accumulation can occur if hepatorenal syndrome develops.

Pregnancy: Category B.

Lactation: It is not known whether amiloride is excreted in breast milk.

Children: Safety and efficacy for use in children have not been established.

Precautions
Electrolyte imbalance and BUN increases: Hyponatremia and hypochloremia may occur when amiloride is used with other diuretics. Increases in BUN levels usually accompany vigorous fluid elimination, especially when diuretic therapy is used in seriously ill patients, such as those who have hepatic cirrhosis with ascites and metabolic alkalosis, or those with resistant edema.

Drug Interactions
Drugs that may interact include digoxin, potassium preparations, ACE inhibitors, and NSAIDs.

Adverse Reactions
Possible adverse reactions include headache, nausea, anorexia, diarrhea, vomiting.

SPIRONOLACTONE

Tablets: 25, 50, and 100 mg (Rx)	Various, *Aldactone* (Searle)

Indications
Primary hyperaldosteronism: Diagnosis of primary hyperaldosteronism.
> Short-term preoperative treatment of patients with primary hyperaldosteronism.
> Long-term maintenance therapy for patients with discrete aldosterone-producing adrenal adenomas who are poor operative risks, or who decline surgery.
> Long-term maintenance therapy for patients with bilateral micronodular or macronodular adrenal hyperplasia (idiopathic hyperaldosteronism).

Edematous conditions when other therapies are inappropriate or inadequate:
> CHF – Management of edema and sodium retention; also indicated with digitalis.
> *Cirrhosis of the liver accompanied by edema or ascites* – For maintenance therapy in conjunction with bed rest and the restriction of fluid and sodium.
> *Nephrotic syndrome.*

Essential hypertension: Usually in combination with other drugs.

Hypokalemia: Hypokalemia and the prophylaxis of hypokalemia in patients taking digitalis.

Unlabeled uses: Spironolactone has been used in the treatment of hirsutism (50 to 200 mg/day) due to its antiandrogenic properties. One study suggested that a lower dosage (50 mg twice/day on days 4 through 21 of the menstrual cycle) may help minimize the risk of metrorrhagia that occurs with higher doses.
> Symptoms of premenstrual syndrome (PMS) have been relieved at a dosage of 25 mg 4 times daily beginning on day 14 of the menstrual cycle.
> The combination of spironolactone (2 mg/kg/day) and testolactone (20 to 40 mg/kg/day) for ≥ 6 months may be effective for short-term treatment of familial male precocious puberty.
> Spironolactone 100 mg/day appears effective in short-term treatment of acne vulgaris.

Administration and Dosage
Spironolactone may be administered in single or divided doses.

Diagnosis of primary hyperaldosteronism: As initial diagnostic measure to provide presumptive evidence of primary hyperaldosteronism in patients on normal diets, as follows:
> *Long test* – 400 mg/day for 3 to 4 weeks. Correction of hypokalemia and hypertension provides presumptive evidence for diagnosis of primary hyperaldosteronism.

Short test – 400 mg/day for 4 days. If serum potassium increases but decreases when spironolactone is discontinued, consider a presumptive diagnosis of primary hyperaldosteronism.

Maintenance therapy for hyperaldosteronism: 100 to 400 mg/day in preparation for surgery. For patients unsuitable for surgery, employ the drug for long-term maintenance therapy at lowest possible dose.

Edema:

Adults (CHF, hepatic cirrhosis, nephrotic syndrome) – Initially, 100 mg/day (range, 25 to 200 mg/day). When given as the sole diuretic agent, continue for ≥ 5 days at the initial dosage level, then adjust to the optimal level. If after 5 days an adequate diuretic response has not occurred, add a second diuretic, which acts more proximally in the renal tubule. Because of the additive effect of spironolactone with such diuretics, an enhanced diuresis usually begins on the first day of combined treatment; combined therapy is indicated when more rapid diuresis is desired. Spironolactone dosage should remain unchanged when other diuretic therapy is added.

Children – 3.3 mg/kg/day (1.5 mg/lb/day) administered in single or divided doses.

Essential hypertension:

Adults – Initially, 50 to 100 mg/day in single or divided doses. May also be combined with diuretics, which act more proximally, and with other antihypertensive agents. Continue treatment for ≥ 2 weeks because the maximal response may not occur sooner. Individualize dosage.

Children – A dose of 1 to 2 mg/kg twice/day has been recommended.

Hypokalemia: 25 to 100 mg/day. Useful in treating diuretic-induced hypokalemia when oral potassium supplements or other potassium-sparing regimens are considered inappropriate.

Contraindications

Anuria; acute renal insufficiency; significant impairment of renal function; hyperkalemia; patients receiving amiloride or triamterene.

Warnings

Hyperkalemia: Carefully evaluate patients for possible fluid and electrolyte balance disturbances. Hyperkalemia may occur with impaired renal function or excessive potassium intake and can cause cardiac irregularities that may be fatal. Ordinarily, do not give potassium supplements with spironolactone.

Renal function impairment: Use of spironolactone may cause a transient elevation of BUN, especially in patients with preexisting renal impairment. The drug may cause mild acidosis.

Carcinogenesis: Spironolactone was a tumorigen in chronic toxicity studies in rats.

Pregnancy: Spironolactone or its metabolites may cross the placental barrier.

Lactation: Canrenone, a metabolite of spironolactone, appears in breast milk. The labeling suggests that an alternative method of infant feeding be instituted when using spironolactone; however, the American Academy of Pediatrics considers the drug to be compatible with breastfeeding.

Precautions

Hyponatremia: Hyponatremia may be caused or aggravated by spironolactone, especially in combination with other diuretics. Symptoms include dry mouth, thirst, lethargy, drowsiness.

Gynecomastia: Gynecomastia may develop and appears to be related to dosage and duration of therapy. It is normally reversible when therapy is discontinued.

Reversible hyperchloremic metabolic acidosis: Reversible hyperchloremic metabolic acidosis, usually in association with hyperkalemia, occurs in some patients with decompensated hepatic cirrhosis, even in the presence of normal renal function.

Drug Interactions

Drugs that may affect spironolactone include ACE inhibitors, salicylates, and food. Drugs that may be affected by spironolactone include anticoagulants, digitalis glycosides, mitotane, digoxin, and potassium preparations.

Adverse Reactions
Adverse reactions are usually reversible upon discontinuation of the drug.

Possible adverse reactions include cramping; diarrhea; gastric bleeding; ulceration; gastritis; vomiting; drowsiness; lethargy; headache; mental confusion; ataxia; irregular menses; carcinoma of the breast.

TRIAMTERENE

Capsules: 50 and 100 mg *(Rx)* | *Dyrenium* (Wellspring Pharmaceuticals)

Indications
Edema: Edema associated with CHF, hepatic cirrhosis, and the nephrotic syndrome; steroid-induced edema, idiopathic edema, and edema due to secondary hyperaldosteronism.

May be used alone or with other diuretics, either for additive diuretic effect or antikaliuretic (potassium-sparing) effect. It promotes increased diuresis in patients resistant or only partially responsive to other diuretics because of secondary hyperaldosteronism.

Administration and Dosage
Individualize dosage.

When used alone, the usual starting dose is 100 mg twice/daily after meals. When combined with other diuretics or antihypertensives, decrease the total daily dosage of each agent initially, and then adjust to the patient's needs. Do not exceed 300 mg/day.

Contraindications
Patients receiving spironolactone or amiloride; anuria; severe hepatic disease; hyperkalemia; hypersensitivity to triamterene; severe or progressive kidney disease or dysfunction, with the possible exception of nephrosis; preexisting elevated serum potassium (impaired renal function, azotemia) or patients who develop hyperkalemia while on triamterene.

Warnings
Hyperkalemia: Abnormal elevation of serum potassium levels (≥ 5.5 mEq/L) can occur. Hyperkalemia is more likely to occur in patients with renal impairment and diabetes (even without evidence of renal impairment), and in the elderly or severely ill. Because uncorrected hyperkalemia may be fatal, serum potassium levels must be monitored at frequent intervals, especially when dosages are changed or with any illness that may influence renal function.

When triamterene is added to other diuretic therapy, or when patients are switched to triamterene from other diuretics, discontinue potassium supplementation.

Hypersensitivity reactions: Monitor patients regularly for blood dyscrasias, liver damage, or other idiosyncratic reactions.

Renal function impairment: Perform periodic BUN and serum potassium determinations to check kidney function, especially in patients with suspected or confirmed renal insufficiency and in elderly or diabetic patients; diabetic patients with nephropathy are especially prone to develop hyperkalemia.

Hepatic function impairment: Triamterene is extensively metabolized in the liver. The overall diuretic response may not be affected.

Pregnancy: Category B.

Lactation: If the drug is essential, the patient should stop nursing.

Children: Safety and efficacy have not been established.

Precautions
Electrolyte imbalance: In CHF, renal disease, or cirrhosis, electrolyte imbalance may be aggravated or caused by diuretics. The use of full doses of a diuretic when salt intake is restricted can result in a low salt syndrome.

Renal stones: Triamterene has been found in renal stones with other usual calculus components. Use cautiously in patients with histories of stone formation.

Hematologic effects: Triamterene is a weak folic acid antagonist. Because cirrhotics with splenomegaly may have marked variations in hematological status, it may contribute to the appearance of megaloblastosis in cases where folic acid stores have been depleted. Perform periodic blood studies in these patients.

Metabolic acidosis: Triamterene may cause decreasing alkali reserve with a possibility of metabolic acidosis.

Diabetes mellitus: Triamterene may raise blood glucose levels for adult-onset diabetes; dosage adjustments of hypoglycemic agents may be necessary. Concurrent use with chlorpropamide may increase the risk of severe hyponatremia.

Photosensitivity: Photosensitization is likely to occur; avoid prolonged exposure to sunlight.

Drug Interactions

Drugs that may affect triamterene include ACE inhibitors, cimetidine, and indomethacin. Drugs that may be affected by triamterene include amantadine and potassium preparations. Triamterene will interfere with the fluorescent measurement of quinidine serum levels.

Adverse Reactions

Diarrhea; nausea; vomiting; jaundice; liver enzyme abnormalities. Azotemia; elevated BUN/creatinine; increased serum uric acid levels (in patients predisposed to gouty arthritis); thrombocytopenia; megaloblastic anemia; weakness; dizziness; hypokalemia; headache; dry mouth; anaphylaxis.

CARBONIC ANHYDRASE INHIBITORS

ACETAZOLAMIDE	
Tablets: 125 and 250 mg (*Rx*)	Various, *Diamox* (Lederle)
Capsules, sustained-release: 500 mg (*Rx*)	*Diamox Sequels* (Lederle)
DICHLORPHENAMIDE	
Tablets: 50 mg (*Rx*)	*Daranide* (Merck)
METHAZOLAMIDE	
Tablets: 25 and 50 mg (*Rx*)	Various, *GlaucTabs* (Akorn), *Neptazane* (Lederle)

Indications

Glaucoma: For adjunctive treatment of chronic simple (open-angle) glaucoma and secondary glaucoma; preoperatively in acute angle-closure glaucoma when delay of surgery is desired to lower intraocular pressure (IOP).

Acetazolamide:

Tablets, sustained-release capsules, and injection – For the prevention or amelioration of symptoms associated with acute mountain sickness in climbers attempting rapid ascent and in those who are susceptible to acute mountain sickness despite gradual ascent.

Tablets and injection only – For adjunctive treatment of edema due to CHF, drug-induced edema, and centrencephalic epilepsy (petit mal, unlocalized seizures).

Administration and Dosage

ACETAZOLAMIDE:

Chronic simple (open-angle) glaucoma –

Adults: 250 mg to 1 g/day, usually in divided doses for amounts > 250 mg. Dosage > 1 g/day does not usually increase the effect.

Secondary glaucoma and preoperative treatment of acute congestive (closed-angle) glaucoma –

Adults:

Short-term therapy – 250 mg every 4 hours or 250 mg twice/day.

Acute cases – 500 mg followed by 125 or 250 mg every 4 hours.

IV therapy may be used for rapid relief of increased intraocular pressure. A complementary effect occurs when used with miotics or mydriatics.

Children:

Parenteral – 5 to 10 mg/kg/dose, IM or IV, every 6 hours.

Oral – 10 to 15 mg/kg/day in divided doses, every 6 to 8 hours.

Diuresis in congestive heart failure –

Adults: Initially, 250 to 375 mg (5 mg/kg) once daily in the morning. If, after an initial response, the patient stops losing edema fluid, do not increase the dose; allow for kidney recovery by skipping medication for a day. Best diuretic results occur when given on alternate days, or for 2 days alternating with a day of rest. Failures in therapy may result from overdosage or from too frequent dosages.

Drug-induced edema – Most effective if given every other day or for 2 days alternating with a day of rest.

Adults: 250 to 375 mg once daily for 1 or 2 days.

Children: 5 mg/kg/dose, oral or IV, once daily in the morning.

Epilepsy –

Adults and children: 8 to 30 mg/kg/day in divided doses. The optimum range is 375 to 1000 mg/day. When given in combination with other anticonvulsants, the starting dose is 250 mg once daily.

Acute mountain sickness – 500 to 1000 mg/day, in divided doses of tablets or sustained release capsules. For rapid ascent (ie, in rescue or military operations), use the higher dose (1000 mg). If possible, initiate dosing 24 to 48 hours before ascent and continue for 48 hours while at high altitude, or longer as needed to control symptoms.

Sustained release – May be used twice daily, but is only indicated for use in glaucoma and acute mountain sickness.

Parenteral – Direct IV administration is preferred; IM administration is painful because of the alkaline pH of the solution.

DICHLORPHENAMIDE:

Glaucoma – Most effective when given with miotics. In acute angle-closure glaucoma, dichlorphenamide may be used with miotics and osmotic agents to rapidly reduce intraocular tension.

Adults:

Initial dose – 100 to 200 mg, followed by 100 mg every 12 hours, until the desired response is obtained.

Maintenance dosage – 25 to 50 mg 1 to 3 times/day.

METHAZOLAMIDE:

Glaucoma – 50 to 100 mg 2 or 3 times/day. May be used with miotic and osmotic agents.

Actions

Pharmacology: These agents are nonbacteriostatic sulfonamides that inhibit the enzyme carbonic anhydrase. This action reduces the rate of aqueous humor formation, resulting in decreased IOP.

Pharmacokinetics:

Pharmacokinetics of Carbonic Anhydrase Inhibitors				
Carbonic anhydrase inhibitor	IOP Lowering Effects			Relative inhibitor potency
	Onset (hours)	Peak effect (hours)	Duration (hours)	
Dichlorphenamide	within 1	2 to 4	6 to 12	30
Acetazolamide				
Tablets	1 to 1.5	1 to 4	8 to 12	1
Sustained release capsules	2	3 to 6	18 to 24	
Injection (IV)	2 min	15 min	4 to 5	
Methazolamide	2 to 4	6 to 8	10 to 18	†[1]

[1] † Quantitative data not available; reported to be more active than acetazolamide.

Contraindications

Hypersensitivity to these agents; depressed sodium or potassium serum levels; marked kidney and liver disease or dysfunction; suprarenal gland failure; hyperchloremic acidosis; adrenocortical insufficiency; severe pulmonary obstruction with inability to increase alveolar ventilation since acidosis may be increased (dichlorphenamide); cirrhosis (acetazolamide, methazolamide); long-term use in chronic noncongestive angle-closure glaucoma.

Warnings

Hepatic function impairment: Use of **methazolamide** in this condition could precipitate hepatic coma.

Pregnancy: Category C.

Lactation: Safety has not been established.

Children: Safety and efficacy for use in children have not been established.

Precautions

Monitoring: Monitor for hematologic reactions common to sulfonamides. Obtain baseline CBC and platelet counts before therapy and at regular intervals during therapy.

Hypokalemia – Hypokalemia may develop when severe cirrhosis is present, during concomitant use of steroids or ACTH, and with interference with adequate oral electrolyte intake.

Dose increases: Increasing the dose of **acetazolamide** does not increase diuresis and may increase drowsiness or paresthesia; it often results in decreased diuresis. However, very large doses have been given with other diuretics to promote diuresis in complete refractory failure.

Pulmonary conditions: Use **dichlorphenamide** with caution in patients with severe degrees of respiratory acidosis. These drugs may precipitate or aggravate acidosis. Use with caution in patients with pulmonary obstruction or emphysema when alveolar ventilation may be impaired.

Cross-sensitivity: Cross-sensitivity between antibacterial sulfonamides and sulfonamide derivative diuretics, including acetazolamide and various thiazides, has been reported.

Drug Interactions

Drugs that may interact with carbonic anhydrase inhibitors include cyclosporine, primidone, salicylates, and diflunisal.

Adverse Reactions

Sulfonamide-type adverse reactions may occur.

CNS: Convulsions; weakness; malaise; fatigue; nervousness; drowsiness; depression; dizziness; disorientation; confusion; ataxia; tremor; tinnitus; headache.

Dermatologic: Urticaria; pruritus; skin eruptions; rash (including erythema multiforme, Stevens-Johnson syndrome, toxic epidermal necrolysis); photosensitivity.

GI: Melena; anorexia; nausea; vomiting; constipation; taste alteration; diarrhea.

Hematologic: Bone marrow depression; thrombocytopenia; thrombocytopenic purpura; hemolytic anemia; leukopenia; pancytopenia; agranulocytosis.

Renal: Hematuria; glycosuria; urinary frequency.

Miscellaneous: Weight loss; fever; decreased/absent libido; impotence; electrolyte imbalance; hepatic insufficiency.

Chapter 6
RESPIRATORY AGENTS

Bronchodilators, 353
   Sympathomimetics, 353
   Xanthine Derivatives, 364
Respiratory Inhalant Products, 371
   Corticosteroids, 371
   Acetylcysteine, 378
   Ipratropium Bromide, 380
   Ipratropium Bromide and Albuterol Sulfate, 381
   Cromolyn Sodium, 382
   Nedocromil, 384
Nasal Decongestants, 386
Intranasal Steroids, 390
Antihistamines, 394
Narcotic Antitussives, 403
   Codeine, 403
Nonnarcotic Antitussives, 405
   Dextromethorphan, 405
   Diphenhydramine, 406
   Benzonatate, 406
   Dextromethorphan and Benzocaine, 407
Leukotriene Receptor Inhibitors, 408
   Zafirlukast, 408
   Zileuton, 409
   Montelukast Sodium, 410
Respiratory Inhalant Combinations, 412
   Fluticasone Propionate/Salmeterol, 412

SYMPATHOMIMETICS

ALBUTEROL

Tablets: 2 and 4 mg (as sulfate) (*Rx*)
Various, *Proventil* (Schering), *Ventolin* (GlaxoWellcome)

Tablets, extended-release: 4 mg (as sulfate) (*Rx*)
Proventil Repetabs (Schering), *Volmax* (Muro)

8 mg (as sulfate) (*Rx*)
Volmax (Muro)

Syrup: 2 mg (as sulfate)/5 mL (*Rx*)
Various, *Proventil* (Schering), *Ventolin* (GlaxoWellcome)

Aerosol: Each actuation delivers 90 mcg (*Rx*)
Various, *Proventil* (Schering), *Ventolin* (GlaxoWellcome)

Solution for Inhalation: 0.083% and 0.5% (as sulfate) (*Rx*)
Various, *Airet* (Medeva), *Proventil* (Schering), *Ventolin Nebules* (GlaxoWellcome)

0.63 mg (as sulfate)/3 mL, 1.25 mg/3 mL (*Rx*)
Proventil (Schering), *AccuNeb* (Dey)

BITOLTEROL

Solution for inhalation: 0.2% (*Rx*)
Tornalate (Dura)

EPHEDRINE SULFATE

Capsules: 25 mg (*otc*)
Various

Injection: 50 mg/mL (*Rx*)
Various

EPINEPHRINE

Solution for inhalation: 1:100 (10 mg/mL as HCl) (*Rx*)
Adrenalin Chloride Solution (Monarch)

2.25% racepinephrine HCl (1.125% epinephrine base) (*otc*)
microNefrin (Bird), *Nephron* (Nephron), *S2* (Nephron)

Topical solution: 1:1000 (1 mg/mL as HCl) (*Rx*)
Adrenalin Chloride Solution (Monarch)

Aerosol: 0.22 mg epinephrine/spray (*otc*)
Various, *Primatene Mist* (Whitehall Robins)

Injection: 1:1000 (1 mg as HCl/mL) solution (*Rx*)
Various, *Adrenalin Chloride Solution* (Monarch)

1:10,000 (0.1 mg/mL) solution (*Rx*)
Various

FORMOTEROL FUMARATE

Inhalation powder in capsules: 12 mcg
Foradil Aerolizer (Novartis)

ISOETHARINE HCl

Solution for inhalation: 1% (*Rx*)
Isoetharine HCl (Roxane)

ISOPROTERENOL

Injection: (1:5000 solution) 0.2 mg/mL (*Rx*)
Various, *Isuprel* (Abbott)

(1:50,000 solution) 0.02 mg/mL (*Rx*)
Isoproterenol HCl (Abbott)

LEVALBUTEROL HCl

Solution, inhalation: 0.63 mg levalbuterol/3 mL (as 0.73 mg levalbuterol HCl) and 1.25 mg levalbuterol/3 mL (as 1.44 mg levalbuterol HCl) (*Rx*)
Xopenex (Sepracor)

METAPROTERENOL SULFATE

Aerosol: Each dose delivers 0.65 mg (in 100 and 200 inhalation canisters) (*Rx*)
Alupent (Boehringer Ingelheim)

Solution for Inhalation: 0.4%, 0.6%, and 5% (*Rx*)
Various, *Alupent* (Boehringer Ingelheim)

PIRBUTEROL ACETATE

Aerosol: Delivers 0.2 mg (as acetate)/actuation (*Rx*)
Maxair Inhaler (3M Pharm), *Maxair Autohaler* (3M Pharm)

SALMETEROL

Aerosol: 25 mcg salmeterol base (as salmeterol xinafoate) per actuation (*Rx*)
Serevent (GlaxoSmithKline)

Inhalation powder: 50 mcg salmeterol (as salmeterol xinafoate salt) (*Rx*)
Serevent Diskus (GlaxoSmithKline)

TERBUTALINE SULFATE

Tablets: 2.5 and 5 mg (*Rx*)
Various, *Brethine* (Novartis)

Injection: 1 mg/mL (*Rx*)
Brethine (Novartis)

Indications

Sympathomimetics: According to the National Asthma Education and Prevention Program's Expert Panel Report II, long-acting β_2 agonists (eg, **salmeterol**) are used concomitantly with anti-inflammatory medications for long-term control of symptoms, especially nocturnal symptoms. They also prevent exercise-induced bronchospasm (EIB). Short-acting β_2 agonists (eg, **albuterol**, **bitolterol**, **pirbuterol**, **terbutaline**) are the therapy of choice for relief of acute symptoms and prevention of EIB.

Albuterol: Relief and prevention of bronchospasm in patients with reversible obstructive airway disease; prevention of exercise-induced bronchospasm.

Bitolterol: Prophylaxis and treatment of bronchial asthma and reversible bronchospasm. May be used with or without concurrent theophylline or steroid therapy.

Ephedrine sulfate:

Asthma – Ephedrine sulfate injection is indicated in the treatment of allergic disorders, such as bronchial asthma. Oral ephedrine is indicated for temporary relief of shortness of breath, tightness of chest, and wheezing due to bronchial asthma. Eases breathing for asthma patients by reducing spasms of bronchial muscles.

Epinephrine:

Inhalation – For temporary relief of acute paroxysms (eg, shortness of breath, tightness of chest, wheezing) of bronchial asthma; postintubation and infectious croup.

MicroNefrin: Chronic obstructive lung disease, chronic bronchitis, broncheolitis, bronchial asthma, and other peripheral airway diseases; croup (postintubation and infectious).

Injection – To relieve respiratory distress in bronchial asthma or during acute asthma attacks and for reversible bronchospasm in patients with chronic bronchitis, emphysema, and other obstructive pulmonary diseases; severe acute anaphylactic reactions, including anaphylactic shock and cardiac arrest, to restore cardiac rhythm.

Allergic reactions (eg, bronchospasm, urticaria, pruritus, angioneurotic edema, or swelling of the lips, eyelids, tongue, and nasal mucosa) due to anaphylactic shock caused by stinging insects (primarily of the order Hymenoptera, that includes bees, wasps, hornets, yellow jackets, bumble bees, and fire ants); severe allergic or anaphylactoid reactions caused by allergy injections; exposures to pollens, dusts, molds, foods, drugs, and exercise or unknown substances (so-called idiopathic anaphylaxis); severe, life-threatening asthma attacks characterized by wheezing, dyspnea, and inability to breathe.

Formoterol fumarate:

Asthma – For long-term, twice-daily (morning and evening) administration in the maintenance treatment of asthma and in the prevention of bronchospasm in adults and children ≥ 5 years of age with reversible obstructive airways disease, including patients with symptoms of nocturnal asthma, who require regular treatment with inhaled, short-acting, beta$_2$-agonists.

Exercise-induced bronchospasm (EIB) – For the acute prevention of EIB in adults and children ≥ 12 years of age when administered on an occasional, as-needed basis.

Concomitant therapy – Can be used concomitantly with short-acting beta$_2$-agonists, inhaled or systemic corticosteroids, and theophylline therapy. A satisfactory clinical response to formoterol does not eliminate the need for continued treatment with an anti-inflammatory.

Formoterol is not a substitute for inhaled or oral corticosteroids. Do not stop or reduce corticosteroids at the time formoterol is initiated.

Chronic obstructive pulmonary disease (COPD) – For long-term, twice daily (morning and evening) administration in the maintenance of bronchoconstriction in patients with COPD including chronic bronchitis and emphysema.

Isoetharine: For bronchial asthma and reversible bronchospasm that occurs with bronchitis and emphysema.

Isoproterenol:

Inhalation – Treatment of bronchospasm associated with acute and chronic bronchial asthma, pulmonary emphysema, bronchitis, and bronchiectasis.

Injection – Management of bronchospasm during anesthesia.

Sublingual – Management of patients with bronchopulmonary disease.

Isoproterenol and Phenylephrine Bitartrate: Treatment of bronchospasm associated with acute and chronic asthma; reversible bronchospasm which may be associated with emphysema or chronic bronchitis.

Levalbuterol: For the treatment or prevention of bronchospasm in adults and adolescents ≥ 12 years of age with reversible obstructive airway disease.

Metaproterenol: For bronchial asthma and reversible bronchospasm; treatment of acute asthmatic attacks in children ≥ 6 years of age (5% solution for inhalation *only*).

Pirbuterol: Prevention and reversal of bronchospasm in patients with reversible bronchospasm including asthma. Use with or without concurrent theophylline or steroid therapy.

Salmeterol:

Asthma/Bronchospasm – Long-term, twice-daily (morning and evening) administration in the maintenance treatment of asthma and in the prevention of bronchospasm in patients ≥ 12 years of age with reversible obstructive airway disease, including patients with symptoms of nocturnal asthma, who require regular treatment with inhaled, short-acting beta$_2$-agonists. It should not be used in patients whose asthma can be managed by occasional use of short-acting, inhaled beta$_2$-agonists. Salmeterol may be used with or without concurrent inhaled or systemic corticosteroid therapy.

Exercise-induced bronchospasm – Prevention of exercise-induced bronchospasm in patients ≥ 12 years of age.

COPD – Maintenance treatment of bronchospasm associated with COPD (including emphysema and chronic bronchitis).

Terbutaline: A bronchodilator for bronchial asthma and for reversible bronchospasm which may occur with bronchitis and emphysema.

Unlabeled uses: Oral and IV terbutaline have successfully inhibited premature labor. Initiate IV use at 10 mcg/min; titrate upward to a maximum of 80 mcg/min. Maintain IV dosage at the minimum effective dose for 4 hours. Oral doses of 2.5 mg every 4 to 6 hours have been used as maintenance therapy until term.

Administration and Dosage
ALBUTEROL:

Inhalation aerosol –

Adults and children ≥ 4 years of age (≥ 12 years of age for Proventil): 2 inhalations every 4 to 6 hours. In some patients, 1 inhalation every 4 hours may be sufficient. More frequent administration or a larger number of inhalations is not recommended. If previously effective dosage fails to provide relief, this may be a marker of destabilization of asthma and requires re-evaluation of the patient and treatment regimen.

Maintenance therapy (Proventil only): For maintenance therapy or to prevent exacerbation of bronchospasm, 2 inhalations 4 times/day should be sufficient.

Prevention of exercise-induced bronchospasm:

Adults and children ≥ 4 years of age (≥ 12 years of age for Proventil) – 2 inhalations 15 minutes prior to exercise.

Inhalation solution –

Adults and children ≥ 12 years of age : 2.5 mg 3 to 4 times/day by nebulization. Dilute 0.5 mL of the 0.5% solution with 2.5 mL sterile normal saline. Deliver over ≈ 5 to 15 minutes.

Children 2 to 12 years of age (≥ 15 kg): 2.5 mg (1 UD vial) 3 to 4 times/day by nebulization. Children weighing < 15 kg who require < 2.5 mg/dose (ie, less than a full UD vial) should use the 0.5% inhalation solution. Deliver over ≈ 5 to 15 minutes.

AccuNeb: The usual starting dosage for patients 2 to 12 years of age is 1.25 mg or 0.63 mg administered 3 or 4 times/day, as needed, by nebulization. More frequent administration is not recommended. Deliver over 5 to 15 minutes. *AccuNeb* has not been studied in the setting of acute attacks of bronchospasm.

Tablets –

Adults and children ≥ 12 years of age: Usual starting dosage is 2 or 4 mg 3 or 4 times/day. Do not exceed a total daily dose of 32 mg. Use doses > 4 mg 4 times/day only when the patient fails to respond. If a favorable response does not occur, cautiously increase stepwise, up to a max of 8 mg 4 times/day, as tolerated.

Children 6 to 12 years of age: Usual starting dosage is 2 mg 3 to 4 times/day. For those who fail to respond to the initial starting dosage, cautiously increase stepwise, but do not exceed 24 mg/day in divided doses.

Elderly patients and those sensitive to β-adrenergic stimulants: Start with 2 mg 3 or 4 times/day. If adequate bronchodilation is not obtained, increase dosage gradually to as much as 8 mg 3 or 4 times/day.

Tablets, extended release –

Volmax Extended Release:

Adults and children > 12 years of age – Usual recommended dose is 8 mg every 12 hours; in some patients, 4 mg every 12 hours may be sufficient. In unusual circumstances (eg, low adult body weight), initial doses may be 4 mg every 12 hours and progress to 8 mg every 12 hours according to response. The dose may be cautiously increased stepwise under physician supervision to a maximum of 32 mg/day in divided doses (eg, every 12 hours) if symptoms are not controlled.

Children 6 to 12 years of age – Usual recommended dose is 4 mg every 12 hours. The dose may be cautiously increased stepwise under physician supervision to a maximum of 24 mg/day in divided doses (eg, every 12 hours) if symptoms are not controlled.

Proventil Repetabs:

Adults and children > 12 years of age – The usual starting dose is 4 to 8 mg every 12 hours. Use doses > 8 mg twice/day when patients fail to respond to this dose. Increase the dose cautiously stepwise to a maximum of 16 mg twice/day as tolerated if a favorable response does not occur with the 8 mg twice/day dose.

Children 6 to 12 years of age – The usual starting dose is 4 mg every 12 hours. Use doses > 4 mg twice/day when patients fail to respond to this dose. Increase the dose cautiously stepwise to a maximum of 12 mg twice/day as tolerated if a favorable response does not occur with the 8 mg twice/day dose.

Switching to extended release tablets: Patients maintained on regular release albuterol can be switched to *Proventil Repetabs* or *Volmax Extended Release Tablets.* A 4 mg extended release tablet every 12 hours is equivalent to a regular 2 mg tablet every 6 hours. Multiples of this regimen up to the maximum recommended dose also apply.

Syrup –

Adults and children > 12 years of age: Usual dose is 2 or 4 mg 3 or 4 times/day. Give doses > 4 mg 4 times/day only when patient fails to respond. If a favorable response does not occur, cautiously increase, but do not exceed 8 mg 4 times/day.

Children (6 to 12 years of age): Usual starting dose is 2 mg 3 or 4 times/day. If patient does not respond to 2 mg 4 times/day, cautiously increase stepwise. Do not exceed 24 mg/day in divided doses.

Children (2 to 6 years of age): Initiate at 0.1 mg/kg 3 times/day. Do not exceed 2 mg 3 times/day. If the patient does not respond to the initial dose, increase stepwise to 0.2 mg/kg 3 times/day. Do not exceed 4 mg 3 times/day.

Elderly patients and those sensitive to β-adrenergic stimulation – Restrict initial dose to 2 mg 3 or 4 times/day. Individualize dosage thereafter.

BITOLTEROL:

Bronchospasm –

Adults and children > 12 years of age: 2 inhalations at an interval of at least 1 to 3 minutes, followed by a third inhalation if needed.

Solution for inhalation: Administer during a 10- to 15-minute period.

Dosing Regimens for Bitolterol Solution for Inhalation 0.2%				
	Continuous flow nebulization		Intermittent flow nebulization	
Doses	Volume (mL)	Bitolterol (mg)	Volume (mL)	Bitolterol (mg)
Usual dose	1.25	2.5	0.5	1
Decreased dose	0.75	1.5	0.25	0.5
Increased dose	1.75	3.5	0.75	1.5

Up to 1 mL solution for inhalation, 0.2% (2 mg) can be administered with the intermittent flow system to severely obstructed patients.

The usual frequency of treatments is 3 times/day. Treatments may be increased up to 4 times/day; however, the interval between treatments should be ≥ 4 hours. For some patients, 2 treatments a day may be adequate. Seek medical advice immediately if the previously effective dosage regimen fails to provide the usual relief as this is often a sign of seriously worsening asthma that would require reassessment of therapy.

Do not exceed the maximum daily dose of 8 mg with an intermittent flow nebulization system or 14 mg with a continuous flow nebulization system.

EPHEDRINE SULFATE: Ephedrine sulfate is a sympathomimetic alkaloid that stimulates alpha and beta receptors as well as the CNS. It is effective orally and parenterally. It is less potent than epinephrine.

Adults and children ≥ 12 years of age – Oral dosage is 12.5 to 25 mg every 4 hours, not to exceed 150 mg in 24 hours.

Adults – The usual parenteral dose is 25 to 50 mg administered SC or IM, or 5 to 25 mg administered slowly IV repeated every 5 to 10 minutes, if necessary.

Children –

Capsules: For use in children < 12 years of age, consult a physician.

Injection: The usual SC, IV, or IM dose is 0.5 to 0.75 mg/kg or 16.7 to 25 mg/m^2 every 4 to 6 hours.

EPINEPHRINE: Refer to specific product labeling for detailed administration and dosage information.

Inhalation aerosol – Start treatment at the first symptoms of bronchospasm. Individualize dosage.

Adults and children ≥ 4 years of age: Start with 1 inhalation, then wait ≥ 1 minute. If not relieved, use once more. Do not use again for ≥ 3 hours.

Nebulization –

Adults and children ≥ 4 years of age (AsthmaNefrin ≥ 12 years of age):

Hand pump nebulizer – Place 0.5 mL (10 drops) of epinephrine into the nebulizer reservoir. Place the nebulizer nozzle into the partially opened mouth. Squeeze the bulb 1 to 3 times. Inhale deeply. Do not administer more than every 3 hours. Supervise children during use.

Aerosol-nebulizer – Add 0.5 mL (≈ 10 drops) racemic epinephrine to 3 mL of diluent or 0.2 to 0.4 mL (≈ 4 to 8 drops) of MicroNefrin to 4.6 to 4.8 mL water. Administer for 15 minutes every 3 to 4 hours. Supervise children during use.

Children < 4 years of age: Consult a physician.

Topical solution – Apply locally as drops or spray, or with a sterile swab, as required. See product labeling for dilution instructions.

Injection –

Solution (1:1000):

Initial adult dose – 0.2 to 1 mL (0.2 to 1 mg) SC (preferred) or IM; repeat every 4 hours.

For infants and children – Give 0.01 mL/kg or 0.3 mL/m^2 (0.01 mg/kg or 0.3 mg/m^2) SC. Do not exceed 0.5 mL (0.5 mg) in a single pediatric dose. Repeat every 4 hours if necessary.

Solution (1:10,000): The adult IV dose for hypersensitivity reactions or to relieve bronchospasm usually ranges from 0.1 to 0.25 mg (1 to 2.5 mL of 1:10,000 solution) injected slowly. Neonates may be given a dose of 0.01 mg/kg; for the infant, 0.05 mg is an adequate initial dose and this may be repeated at 20- to 30-minute intervals in the management of asthma attacks.

Alternatively, if the patient has been intubated, epinephrine can be injected via the endotracheal tube directly into the bronchial tree at the same dosage for intravenous injection. It is rapidly absorbed through the lung capillary bed.

FORMOTEROL: Administer formoterol capsules only by the oral inhalation route and only using the *Aerolizer Inhaler*. Do not ingest formoterol (ie, swallowed) orally. Always store formoterol capsules in the blister, and only remove immediately before use.

When beginning treatment with formoterol, instruct patients who have been taking inhaled, short-acting beta$_2$-agonists on a regular basis (eg, 4 times/day) to discontinue the regular use of these drugs and use them only for symptomatic relief of acute asthma symptoms.

Asthma/Bronchospasm – For adults and children ≥ 5 years of age, the usual dosage is the inhalation of the contents of one 12-mcg formoterol capsule every 12 hours using the *Aerolizer Inhaler*. The patient must not exhale into the device. The total daily dose of formoterol should not exceed 1 capsule twice daily (24 mcg total daily dose). If symptoms arise between doses, take an inhaled short-acting beta$_2$ agonist for immediate relief.

Prevention of EIB – For adults and adolescents ≥ 12 years of age, the usual dosage is the inhalation of the contents of one 12-mcg formoterol capsule at least 15 minutes before exercise administered on an occasional as-needed basis.

Maintenance treatment of COPD – The usual dosage is the inhalation of the contents of one 12 mcg formoterol capsule every 12 hours using the *Aerolizer Inhaler*.

Prior to dispensing – Store in a refrigerator (2° to 8°C; 36° to 46°F).

After dispensing to patient – Store at 20° to 25°C (68° to 77°F). Protect from heat and moisture. Always store capsules in the blister and only remove from the blister immediately before use.

Always discard the capsules and *Aerolizer Inhaler* by the "Use by" date and always use the new *Aerolizer Inhaler* provided with each new prescription.

ISOETHARINE HCl:

Isoetharine Doses (Volume) Based on Strength of Solution		
Method of administration	Usual dose	Range of dose of 1:3 dilution[1]
Hand bulb nebulizer	4 inhalations	3 to 7 inhalations undiluted
Oxygen aerosolization[2]	0.5 mL	1 to 2 mL
IPPB[3]	0.5 mL	1 to 4 mL

[1] Dilution of 1 part isoetharine plus 3 parts of normal saline solution.
[2] Administered with oxygen flow adjusted to 4 to 6 L/min over 15 to 20 minutes.
[3] Usually an inspiratory flow rate of 15 L/min at a cycling pressure of 15 cm H_2O is recommended. It may be necessary, according to patient and type of IPPB apparatus, to adjust flow rate to 6 to 30 L/min, cycling pressure to 10 to 15 cm H_2O, and further dilution according to the needs of the patient.

ISOPROTERENOL:
Injection – For the management of bronchospasm during anesthesia, dilute 1 mL (0.2 mg) of a 1:5000 solution to 10 mL with Sodium Chloride Injection or 5% Dextrose Injection. Administer an initial dose of 0.01 to 0.02 mg (0.5 to 1 mL of diluted solution) IV; repeat when necessary; or use a 1:50,000 solutions undiluted and administer an initial dose of 0.01 to 0.02 mg (0.5 to 1 mL).

LEVALBUTEROL:
Adults and children ≥ 12 years of age – 0.63 mg administered 3 times/day, every 6 to 8 hours, by nebulization. May increase to 1.25 mg 3 times/day. Closely monitor patients receiving the higher dose for adverse systemic effect, and balance the risks of such effects against the potential for improved efficacy.

METAPROTERENOL:
Metered dose inhaler – 2 to 3 inhalations every 3 to 4 hours. Do not exceed 12 inhalations/day. Not recommended for children < 12 years of age.

Inhalant solutions – Usually, treatment need not be repeated more often than every 4 hours to relieve acute bronchospasm attacks. In chronic bronchospastic pulmonary diseases, give 3 to 4 times/day. A single dose of nebulized metaproterenol in the treatment of an acute attack of asthma may not completely abort an attack. Not recommended for children < 12 years of age.

Dosage and Dilution for Metaproterenol Inhalant Solutions			
Administration	Usual dose	Range	Dilution
Adults and children ≥ 12 years of age			
Hand bulb nebulizer	10 inhalations	5-15 inhalations	No dilution
IPPB[1]	0.3 mL	0.2-0.3 mL	In ≈ 2.5 mL saline or other diluent
Children 6 to 12 years of age			
Nebulizer	0.1 mL	0.1 to 0.2 mL	In saline to a total volume of 3 mL

[1] IPPB = intermittent positive pressure breathing

PIRBUTEROL:

Adults and children ≥ 12 years of age – 2 inhalations (0.4 mg) repeated every 4 to 6 hours. One inhalation (0.2 mg) may be sufficient for some patients.

Do not exceed a total daily dose of 12 inhalations.

If previously effective dosage regimen fails to provide the usual relief, seek medical advice immediately as this is often a sign of seriously worsening asthma that would require reassessment of therapy.

SALMETEROL:

Asthma/Bronchospasm – For maintenance of bronchodilatation and prevention of symptoms of asthma, including the symptoms of nocturnal asthma, the usual dosage for adults and children ≥ 12 years of age is 2 inhalations (42 mcg) twice daily (morning and evening, ≈ 12 hours apart). For asthma in children ≥ 4 years of age, use 1 inhalation/disk (50 mcg) twice daily (12 hours apart). Adverse effects are more likely to occur with higher doses of salmeterol, and more frequent administration or administration of a larger number of inhalations is not recommended.

To gain full therapeutic benefit, administer twice daily (morning and evening) in the treatment of reversible airway obstruction.

Prevention of exercise-induced bronchospasm – Two inhalations (1 inhalation ≥ 30 minutes for inhalation powder) ≥ 30 to 60 minutes before exercise protects against exercise-induced bronchospasm in many patients for ≤ 12 hours. Additional doses of salmeterol should not be used for 12 hours after the administration of this drug. Patients who are receiving salmeterol twice daily (morning and evening) should not use additional salmeterol for prevention of exercise-induced bronchospasm. When inhalation powder is used intermittently as needed for prevention of EIB, this protection may last ≤ 9 hours in adolescents and adults and ≤ 12 hours in patients 4 to 11 years of age.

COPD – For maintenance treatment of bronchospasm associated with COPD (including chronic bronchitis and emphysema), the usual dosage for adults is 2 inhalations (42 mcg) twice daily (morning and evening, ≈ 12 hours apart).

TERBUTALINE:

Oral –

Adults and children > 15 years of age: 5 mg, given at 6-hour intervals, 3 times/day during waking hours. If side effects are pronounced, dose may be reduced to 2.5 mg 3 times/day. Do not exceed 15 mg in 24 hours.

Children (12 to 15 years of age): 2.5 mg 3 times/day. Do not exceed 7.5 mg in 24 hours. Not recommended for children < 12 years of age.

Parenteral – Usual dose is 0.25 mg SC into the lateral deltoid area. If significant improvement does not occur in 15 to 30 minutes, administer a second 0.25 mg dose. Do not exceed a total dose of 0.5 mg in 4 hours. If a patient fails to respond to a second 0.25 mg dose within 15 to 30 minutes, consider other therapeutic measures.

Actions

Pharmacology: These agents are used to produce bronchodilation. They relieve reversible bronchospasm by relaxing the smooth muscles of the bronchioles in conditions associated with asthma, bronchitis, emphysema, or bronchiectasis. Bronchodilation may additionally facilitate expectoration.

The pharmacologic actions of these agents include: Alpha-adrenergic stimulation (vasoconstriction, nasal decongestion, pressor effects); β_1-adrenergic stimulation (increased myocardial contractility and conduction); and β_2-adrenergic stimulation (bronchial dilation and vasodilation, enhancement of mucociliary clearance, inhibition of cholinergic neurotransmission).

The relative selectivity of action of sympathomimetic agents is the primary determinant of clinical usefulness; it can predict the most likely side effects. The β_2 selective agents provide the greatest benefit with minimal side effects. Direct administration via inhalation provides prompt effects and minimizes systemic activity.

Sympathomimetic Bronchodilators: Pharmacologic Effects and Pharmacokinetic Properties					
Sympathomimetic	Adrenergic receptor activity	β_2 potency[1]	Route	Onset (minutes)	Duration (hrs)
Albuterol[2]	$\beta_1 < \beta_2$	2	PO	within 30	4-8
			Inh[3]	within 5	3-6
Bitolterol[2]	$\beta_1 < \beta_2$	5	Inh	2-4	5 ≥ 8
Ephedrine	$\alpha \quad \beta_1 \quad \beta_2$	—	PO	15-60	3-5
			SC	> 20	≤ 1
			IM	10-20	≤ 1
			IV	immediate	—
Epinephrine	$\alpha \quad \beta_1 \quad \beta_2$	—	SC	5-10	4-6
			IM	—	1-4
			Inh[3]	1-5	1-3
Isoetharine[2]	$\beta_1 < \beta_2$	6	Inh[3]	within 5	2-3
Isoproterenol	$\beta_1 \quad \beta_2$	1	IV	immediate	< 1
			Inh[3]	2-5	1-3
Metaproterenol[2]	$\beta_1 < \beta_2$	15	PO	≈ 30	4
			Inh[3]	5-30	1-6
Salmeterol[2]	$\beta_1 < \beta_2$	0.5	Inh	within 20	12
Pirbuterol[2]	$\beta_1 < \beta_2$	5	Inh	within 5	5
Terbutaline[2]	$\beta_1 < \beta_2$	4	PO	30	4-8
			SC	5-15	1.5-4
			Inh	5-30	3-6

[1] Relative molar potency: 1 = most potent.
[2] These agents all have minor β_1 activity.
[3] May be administered via aerosol or bulb nebulizer or IPPB administration.

Contraindications

Hypersensitivity to any component (allergic reactions are rare); cardiac arrhythmias associated with tachycardia; angina, preexisiting cardiac arrhythmias associated with tachycardia, known hypersensitivity to sympathomimetic amines, and ventricular arrhythmias requiring inotropic therapy, tachycardia or heart block caused by digitalis intoxication (**isoproterenol**); patients with organic brain damage, local anesthesia of certain areas (eg, fingers, toes) because of the risk of tissue sloughing, labor, cardiac dilitation, coronary insufficiency, cerebral arteriosclerosis, organic heart disease (**epinephrine**); in those cases where vasopressors may be contraindicated; narrow-angle glaucoma, nonanaphylactic shock during general anesthesia with halogenated hydrocarbons or cyclopropane (**epinephrine, ephedrine**).

Warnings

Special risk patients: Administer with caution to patients with diabetes mellitus, hyperthyroidism, prostatic hypertrophy (ephedrine) or history of seizures; elderly; psychoneurotic individuals, patients with long-standing bronchial asthma and emphysema who have developed degenerative heart disease (epinephrine).

In patients with status asthmaticus and abnormal blood gas tensions, improvement in vital capacity and blood gas tensions may not accompany apparent relief of bronchospasm following isoproterenol.

Diabetes – Large doses of IV **albuterol** and IV **terbutaline** may aggravate preexisting diabetes mellitus and ketoacidosis. Relevance to the use of oral or inhaled albuterol and oral terbutaline is unknown. Diabetic patients receiving any of these agents may require an increase in dosage of insulin or oral hypoglycemic agents.

Cardiovascular effects: Use with caution in patients with cardiovascular disorders including coronary insufficiency, ischemic heart disease, history of stroke, coronary artery disease, cardiac arrhythmias, CHF, and hypertension.

Closely monitor patients receiving **epinephrine**. Inadvertently induced high arterial blood pressure may result in angina pectoris, aortic rupture, or cerebral hemorrhage. Cardiac arrhythmias develop in some individuals even after therapeutic doses.

Beta-adrenergic agonists can produce significant cardiovascular effects measured by pulse rate, blood pressure, symptoms, or ECG changes (eg, flattening of T-waves, prolongation of the QTc interval, and ST-segment depression).

Isoproterenol doses sufficient to increase the heart rate > 130 bpm may increase the likelihood of inducing ventricular arrhythmias.

Ephedrine may cause hypertension resulting in intracranial hemorrhage. It may induce anginal pain in patients with coronary insufficiency or ischemic heart disease.

Large doses of inhaled or oral **salmeterol** (12 to 20 times the recommended dose) have been associated with clinically significant prolongation of the QTc interval, which has the potential for producing ventricular arrhythmias.

Paradoxical bronchospasm: Occasionally patients have developed severe paradoxical airway resistance with repeated, excessive use of inhalation preparations; the cause is unknown. Discontinue the drug immediately and institute alternative therapy.

Usual dose response: Advise patients to contact a physician if they do not respond to their usual dose of a sympathomimetic amine.

Further therapy with the bronchodilator **isoproterenol** aerosol alone is inadvisable when 3 to 5 treatments within 6 to 12 hours produce minimal or no relief.

Reduce **epinephrine** dose if bronchial irritation, nervousness, restlessness, or sleeplessness occurs. Do not continue to use epinephrine, but seek medical assistance immediately if symptoms are not relieved within 20 minutes or become worse.

CNS effects: Sympathomimetics may produce CNS stimulation.

Long-term use: Prolonged use of **ephedrine** may produce a syndrome resembling an anxiety state; many patients develop nervousness; a sedative may be needed.

Acute symptoms: Do not use **salmeterol** to relieve acute asthma symptoms. If the patient's short-acting, inhaled β_2-agonist becomes less effective (eg, the patient needs more inhalations than usual), medical evaluation must be obtained immediately.

Excessive use of inhalants – Deaths have been reported; the exact cause is unknown, but cardiac arrest following an unexpected severe acute asthmatic crisis and subsequent hypoxia is suspected.

Morbidity/Mortality – Regularly scheduled, daily use of beta agonists is not recommended.

Use with short-acting β_2-agonists – When patients begin treatment with salmeterol, advise those who have been taking short-acting, inhaled β_2-agonists on a regular daily basis to discontinue their regular daily-dosing regimen and clearly instruct them to use short-acting, inhaled β_2-agonists only for symptomatic relief if they develop asthma symptoms while taking salmeterol.

Overdosage or inadvertent IV injection: Overdosage or inadvertent IV injection of conventional SC **epinephrine** doses may cause severe or fatal hypertension or cerebrovascular hemorrhage resulting from the sharp rise in blood pressure. Fatalities may also occur from pulmonary edema resulting from peripheral constriction and cardiac stimulation.

Hypersensitivity: Hypersensitivity (allergic) reactions can occur after administration of **bitolterol, albuterol, metaproterenol, terbutaline, ephedrine, salmeterol**, and possibly other bronchodilators.

Elderly: Lower doses may be required due to increased sympathomimetic sensitivity.

Pregnancy: Category B (terbutaline). *Category* C (albuterol, bitolterol, ephedrine, epinephrine, isoetharine, isoproterenol, metaproterenol, salmeterol, pirbuterol).

Labor and delivery – Use of β_2 active sympathomimetics inhibits uterine contractions. Other reactions include increased heart rate, transient hyperglycemia, hypokalemia, cardiac arrhythmias, pulmonary edema, cerebral and myocardial ischemia, and increased fetal heart rate and hypoglycemia in the neonate. Although these effects are unlikely with aerosol use, consider the potential for untoward effects.

Do not use parenteral **ephedrine** in obstetrics when maternal blood pressure exceeds 130/80.

Lactation: **Terbutaline, ephedrine**, and **epinephrine** are excreted in breast milk. It is not known whether other agents are excreted in breast milk.

Children:

Inhalation – Safety and efficacy for use of **bitolterol, pirbuterol, isoetharine, salmeterol**, and **terbutaline** in children ≤ 12 years of age have not been established. **Albuterol** aerosol and inhalation powder in children < 4 years of age and **albuterol** solution for inhalation in children < 2 years of age have not been established. **Metaproterenol** may be used in children ≥ 6 years of age.

Injection – Parenteral **terbutaline** is not recommended for use in children < 12 years of age. Administer **epinephrine** with caution to infants and children. Syncope has occurred following administration to asthmatic children.

Oral – **Metaproterenol** is not recommended for use in children < 6 years of age. **Terbutaline** is not recommended for use in children < 12 years of age. Safety and efficacy of **albuterol** have not been established for children < 2 years (syrup), < 6 years (tablets) and < 12 years (tablets, timed-release) of age.

In children, **ephedrine** is effective in the oral therapy of asthma. Because of its CNS-stimulating effect, it is rarely used alone. This effect is usually countered by an appropriate sedative; however, its rationale has been questioned.

Precautions

Tolerance: Tolerance may occur with prolonged use of sympathomimetic agents, but temporary cessation of the drug restores its original effectiveness.

Hypokalemia: Decreases in serum potassium levels have occurred, possibly through intracellular shunting, which can produce adverse cardiovascular effects.

Hyperglycemia: **Isoproterenol** causes less hyperglycemia than does **epinephrine**.

Parkinson's disease: Epinephrine may temporarily increase rigidity and tremor.

Parenteral use: Administer **epinephrine** with great caution and in carefully circumscribed quantities in areas of the body served by end arteries or with otherwise limited blood supply (eg, fingers, toes, nose, ears, genitals) or if peripheral vascular disease is present to avoid vasoconstriction-induced tissue sloughing.

Combined therapy: Concomitant use with other sympathomimetic agents is not recommended, as it may lead to deleterious cardiovascular effects. This does not preclude the judicious use of an adrenergic stimulant aerosol bronchodilator in patients receiving tablets. Do not give on a routine basis. If regular coadministration is required, consider alternative therapy.

Do not use ≥ 2 beta-adrenergic aerosol bronchodilators simultaneously because of the potential of additive effects.

Patients must be warned not to stop or reduce corticosteroid therapy without medical advice, even if they feel better when they are being treated with β_2 agonists. These agents are not to be used as a substitute for oral or inhaled corticosteroids.

Sulfites: Some of these products contain sulfites that may cause allergic-type reactions (including anaphylactic symptoms and life-threatening or less severe asthmatic episodes) in certain susceptible people. The overall prevalence of sulfite sensitivity in the general population is unknown and probably low. It is seen more frequently in asthmatic or atopic nonasthmatic people. Specific products containing sulfites are identified in the product listings.

Drug abuse and dependence: Prolonged abuse of **ephedrine** can lead to symptoms of paranoid schizophrenia. Patients exhibit such signs as tachycardia, poor nutrition and hygiene, fever, cold sweat, and dilated pupils. Some measure of tolerance develops, but addiction does not occur.

Drug Interactions
Most interactions listed apply to sympathomimetics when used as vasopressors; however, consider the interaction when using the bronchodilator sympathomimetics. Drugs that may interact include antihistamines, alpha-adrenergic blockers, beta blockers, cardiac glycosides, diuretics, ergot alkaloids, furazolidine, general anesthetics, guanethidine, levothyroxine, methyldopa, MAO inhibitors, nitrates, oxytocic drugs, phenothiazines, rauwolfia alkaloids, tricyclic antidepressants, digoxin, theophylline, insulin, or oral hypoglycemic agents.

Drug/Lab test interactions: Isoproterenol causes false elevations of bilirubin as measured in vitro by a sequential multiple analyzer. Isoproterenol inhalation may result in enough absorption of the drug to produce elevated urinary epinephrine values. Although small with standard doses, the effect is likely to increase with larger doses.

Adverse Reactions

Sympathomimetic Bronchodilator Adverse Reactions (≥ 3%)[1]										
Adverse reaction	Albuterol	Bitolterol	Ephedrine	Epinephrine	Isoetharine	Isoproterenol	Metaproterenol	Pirbuterol	Salmeterol	Terbutaline
Cardiovascular										
Palpitations	< 1-10	1.5-3	✔	7.8-30	✔[2]	< 5-22	0.3-4	1.3-1.7	1-3	≤ 23
Tachycardia	1-10	< 3.7	✔	≤ 2.6	✔	2-12	< 17	1.2-1.3	1-3	1.3-3
Blood pressure changes/hypertension	1-5	< 1		✔	✔	2-5	0.3			< 1
Chest tightness/pain/discomfort, angina	< 3	≤ 1.5		≤ 2.6		✔	0.2	< 1.3		1.3-1.5
PVCs, arrhythmias, skipped beats		0.5	✔	✔		< 1-3		< 1		≈ 4
CNS										
Tremor	< 1-24.2	9-26.6		16-18	✔	< 15	1-33	1.3-6	4	< 5-38
Dizziness/vertigo	< 1-7	1-4	✔	3.3-7.8	✔	1.5-5	1-4	0.6-1.2	≥ 3	1.3-10
Shakiness/nervousness/tension	1-20	1.5-11.1	✔	8.5-31	✔	< 15	2.6-14	4.5-7	1-3	< 5-31
Drowsiness	< 1			8.2-14		< 5	0.7			< 5-11.7
Hyperactivity/Hyperkinesia, excitement	1-20	< 1			✔	✔		< 1		
Headache	2-22	≤ 8.4	✔	3.3-10	✔	1.5-10	≤ 4	1.3-2	28	7.8-10
Insomnia	1-11	< 1	✔	✔	✔	1.5	1.8	< 1		✔
GI										
Nausea/Vomiting	2-15	≤ 3	✔	1-11.5	✔	< 15	< 14	≤ 1.7	1-3	1.3-10
Heartburn/GI distress/disorder	≤ 5					≤ 5-10	≤ 4		1-3	< 10
Diarrhea	1						0.7	< 1.3	1-3	

	Sympathomimetic Bronchodilator Adverse Reactions (≥ 3%)[1]									
Adverse reaction	Albuterol	Bitolterol	Ephedrine	Epinephrine	Isoetharine	Isoproterenol	Metaproterenol	Pirbuterol	Salmeterol	Terbutaline
Respiratory — Cough	< 1-5	≤ 4.1				1-5	≤ 4	1.2	7	
Respiratory — Bronchospasm	1-15.4	≤ 1.5				≤ 18				
Respiratory — Throat dryness/irritation, pharyngitis	≤ 6	2.5-5				3.1	≤ 4	< 1	≥ 3	✔

[1] Data pooled for all routes of administration, all age groups, from separate studies, and are not necessarily comparable.
[2] ✔ = Reported; no incidence given.

Adverse reactions are generally transient, and no cumulative effects have been reported. It is usually not necessary to discontinue treatment; however, in selected cases temporarily reduce dosage.

Albuterol:
> *Respiratory* – Bronchitis (1.5% to 4%); epistaxis (1% to 3%).
> *Miscellaneous* – Increased appetite, stomachache (3%); muscle cramps (1% to 3%).

Bitolterol: Lightheadedness (6.8%). The overall incidence of cardiovascular effects was ≈ 5%.

Isoproterenol: Bronchitis (5%).

Metaproterenol: Asthma exacerbation (1% to 4%).

Salmeterol:
> *Respiratory* – Upper respiratory tract infection, nasopharyngitis (14%); nasal cavity/sinus disease (6%); sinus headache, lower respiratory tract infection (4%); allergic rhinitis (> 3%); rhinitis, laryngitis, tracheitis/bronchitis (1% to 3%).
> *Musculoskeletal* – Joint/back pain, muscle cramp/contraction, myalgia/myositis, muscular soreness (1% to 3%).
> *Miscellaneous* – Giddiness, influenza (> 3%); viral gastroenteritis, urticaria, dental pain, malaise/fatigue, rash/skin eruption, dysmenorrhea (1% to 3%).

XANTHINE DERIVATIVES

AMINOPHYLLINE

Tablets: 100 mg (equiv. to 79 mg theophylline), 200 mg (equiv. to 158 mg theophylline) (*Rx*) — Various

Tablets, controlled-release (12 hours): 225 mg (equiv. to 178 mg theophylline) (*Rx*) — *Phyllocontin* (Purdue Frederick)

Oral liquid: 105 mg (equiv. to 90 mg theophylline) per 5 mL (*Rx*) — Various

Injection: 250 mg (equiv. to 197 mg theophylline) per 10 mL (*Rx*) For IV use. — Various

Suppositories: 250 mg (equiv. to 197.5 mg theophylline) and 500 mg (equiv. to 395 mg theophylline) (*Rx*) — Various, *Truphylline* (G & W)

DYPHYLLINE

Tablets: 200 or 400 mg (*Rx*) — Various, *Dilor* (Savage)

Elixir: 100 or 160 mg/15 mL (33.3 or mg/5 mL) (*Rx*) — *Lufyllin* (Wallace), *Dilor* (Savage)

Injection: 250 mg/mL (*Rx*) — *Lufyllin* (Wallace)

OXTRIPHYLLINE

Tablets: 100 mg (equiv. to 64 mg theophylline) and 200 mg (equiv. to 127 mg theophylline) (*Rx*) — Various, *Choledyl* (Parke-Davis)

Tablets, sustained-action: 400 mg (equiv. to 254 mg theophylline) and 600 mg (equiv. to 382 mg theophylline) (*Rx*) — *Choledyl SA* (Parke-Davis)

Syrup, pediatric: 50 mg (equiv. to 32 mg theophylline) per 5 mL (*Rx*) — Various, *Choledyl* (Parke-Davis)

Elixir: 100 mg (equiv. to 64 mg theophylline) per 5 mL (*Rx*) — Various, *Choledyl* (Parke-Davis)

THEOPHYLLINE

Tablets: 100, 125, 200, 250, and 300 mg (*Rx*)	Various, *Slo-Phyllin* (Rhone-Poulenc Rorer), *Theolair* (3M Pharm), *Quibron-T Dividose* (Bristol Labs)
Capsules: 100 and 200 mg (*Rx*)	*Bronkodyl* (Winthrop),
Syrup: 80 mg and 150 mg/15 mL (26.7 or 50 mg/5 mL) (*Rx*)	*Aquaphyllin* (Ferndale), *Accurbron* (Marion Merrell Dow)
Elixir: 80 mg/15 mL (26.7 mg/5 mL) (*Rx*)	Various, *Asmalix* (Century), *Elixomin* (Cenci), *Elixophyllin* (Forest), *Theolair* (3M Pharmaceuticals), *Lanophyllin* (Lannett)
Solution: 80 mg/15 mL (26.7 mg/5 mL) (*Rx*)	Various, *Theolair* (3M Pharm)
Capsules, timed-release (8 to 12 hours): 50, 60, 65, 75, 100, 125, 130, 200, 250, 260, and 300 mg (sustained-release) (*Rx*)	*Aerolate* (Fleming), *Slo-bid Gyrocaps* (Rhone-Poulenc Rorer), *Slo-Phyllin Gyrocaps* (Rhone-Poulenc Rorer)
Capsules, timed-release (24 hours): 100, 200, and 300 mg (*Rx*)	*Theo-24* (Whitby)
Capsules, timed-release (12 hours): 125, 130, 250, and 260 mg (*Rx*)	*Theovent* (Schering), *Theoclear L.A.* (Central), *Theospan SR* (Laser)
Capsules, extended-release: 100, 125, 200, and 300 mg (*Rx*)	Various
Tablets, timed-release (12 to 24 hours): 100, 200, 300, and 450 mg (*Rx*)	Various
Tablets, extended-release: 450 mg (*Rx*)	Various
Tablets, extended-release (12 to 24 hours): 100, 200, and 300 mg (*Rx*)	*Theochron* (Various)
Tablets, extended-release (24 hours): 400 and 600 mg (*Rx*)	*Uni-Dur* (Key)
Tablets, timed-release (8 to 12 hours): 200, 250, 300, and 500 mg (*Rx*)	*Theolair-SR* (3M Pharm), *T-Phyl* (Purdue Frederick), *Quibron-T/SR* (Roberts), *Respbid* (Boehringer Ingelheim)
Tablets, sustained-release (8 to 12 hours): 100 and 300 mg (*Rx*)	*Sustaire* (Pfizer Labs)
Tablets, timed-release (8 to 24 hours): 100, 200, 300, and 450 mg (*Rx*)	*Theo-Dur* (Key)
Tablets, controlled-release (12 to 24 hours): 100, 200, and 300 mg (*Rx*)	*Theo-X* (Carnrick)
Tablets, timed-release (24 hours): 400 mg (*Rx*)	*Uniphyl* (Purdue Frederick)

THEOPHYLLINE AND DEXTROSE

Injection: 200, 400, and 800 mg/container (*Rx*)	Various

Indications

Symptomatic relief or prevention of bronchial asthma and reversible bronchospasm associated with chronic bronchitis and emphysema.

Unlabeled uses: Theophylline 10 mg/kg/day may significantly improve pulmonary function and dyspnea in patients with chronic obstructive pulmonary disease.

Administration and Dosage

AMINOPHYLLINE:

IV – The loading dose may be infused into 100 to 200 mL of 5% Dextrose Injection or 0.9% Sodium Chloride Injection. Do not exceed 25 mg/min infusion rate.

Parenteral administration – Inject aminophylline slowly, ≤ 25 mg/min, when given IV. Substitute oral therapy for IV aminophylline as soon as adequate improvement is achieved.

Loading dose:

In patients currently not receiving theophylline products – 6 mg/kg.

In patients currently receiving theophylline products – Each 0.5 mg/kg theophylline (0.6 mg/kg aminophylline) will increase the serum theophylline concentration by ≈ 1 mcg/mL. When respiratory distress warrants a small risk, 2.5 mg/kg theophylline (3.1 mg aminophylline IV) increases serum concentration by ≈ 5 mcg/mL. If the patient is not experiencing theophylline toxicity, this is unlikely to result in dangerous side effects.

Maintenance infusions – Administer by a large volume infusion to deliver the desired amount of drug each hour.

Aminophylline Maintenance Infusion Rates (mg/kg/hr)		
Patient group	First 12 hours	> 12 hours
Neonates to infants < 6 months of age	Not recommended	
Children 6 months to 9 years of age	1.2	1
Children 9 to 16 years of age and young adult smokers	1	0.8
Otherwise healthy nonsmoking adults	0.7	0.5
Older patients and those with cor pulmonale	0.6	0.3
Patients with CHF, liver disease	0.5	0.1-0.2

DYPHYLLINE: Dyphylline is a derivative of theophylline; it is not a theophylline salt, and is not metabolized to theophylline in vivo. Although dyphylline is 70% theophylline by molecular weight ratio, the amount of dyphylline equivalent to a given amount of theophylline is not known. Specific dyphylline serum levels may be used to monitor therapy; serum theophylline levels will not measure dyphylline. The minimal effective therapeutic concentration is 12 mcg/mL.

Oral –

Adults: Up to 15 mg/kg every 6 hours.

IM – (Not for IV administration.)

Adults: 250 to 500 mg injected slowly every 6 hours. Do not exceed 15 mg/kg every 6 hours.

Children: Safety and efficacy have not been established.

OXTRIPHYLLINE:

Adults – 4.7 mg/kg every 8 hours.

Children (9 to 16 years of age) and adult smokers – 4.7 mg/kg every 6 hours.

Children (1 to 9 years of age) – 6.2 mg/kg every 6 hours.

Sustained action – If total daily maintenance dosage is established at ≈ 800 or 1200 mg, 1 sustained-action tablet every 12 hours may be substituted.

THEOPHYLLINE: Individualize dosage. Base dosage adjustments on clinical response and improvement in pulmonary function with careful monitoring of serum levels. If possible, monitor serum levels to maintain levels in the therapeutic range of 10 to 20 mcg/mL. Levels > 20 mcg/mL may produce toxicity, and it may even occur with levels between 15 to 20 mcg/mL, particularly when factors known to reduce theophylline clearance are present. Once stabilized on a dosage, serum levels tend to remain constant.

Calculate dosages on the basis of lean body weight, because theophylline does not distribute into fatty tissue. Regardless of salt used, dosages should be equivalent based on anhydrous theophylline content.

Individualize frequency of dosing – Individualize frequency of dosing. With immediate release products, dosing every 6 hours is generally required, especially in children; intervals ≤ 8 hours may be satisfactory in adults. Some children and adults requiring higher than average doses (those having rapid rates of clearance; eg, half-lives < 6 hours) may be more effectively controlled during chronic therapy with sustained-release products. Determine dosage intervals to produce minimal fluctuations between peak and trough serum theophylline concentrations. Consider the absorption profile and the elimination rate. When converting from an immediate-release to a sustained-release product, the total daily dose should remain the same, and only the dosing interval adjusted.

Acute symptoms requiring rapid theophyllinization in patients not receiving theophylline – To achieve a rapid effect, an initial loading dose is required. Dosage recommendations are for theophylline anhydrous.

Dosage Guidelines for Rapid Theophyllinization		
Patient Group	Oral loading	Maintenance
Children 1 to 9 years of age	5 mg/kg	4 mg/kg q 6 h
Children 9 to 16 years of age and young adult smokers	5 mg/kg	3 mg/kg q 6 h
Otherwise healthy non-smoking adults	5 mg/kg	3 mg/kg q 8 h
Older patients, patients with cor pulmonale	5 mg/kg	2 mg/kg q 8 h
Patients with CHF	5 mg/kg	1-2 mg/kg q 12 h

Infants (preterm to < 1 year) –

Theophylline Dosage Guidelines for Infants	
Age	Initial maintenance dose
Premature infants	
≤ 24 days postnatal	1 mg/kg q 12 h
> 24 days postnatal	1.5 mg/kg q 12 h
Infants (6 to 52 weeks)	[(0.2 x age in weeks) = 5] x kg = 24 hr dose in mg
Up to 26 weeks	Divide into q 8 h dosing
26 to 52 weeks	Divide into q 6 h dosing

Acute symptoms requiring rapid theophyllinization in patients receiving theophylline – Each 0.5 mg/kg theophylline administered as a loading dose will increase the serum theophylline concentration by ≈ 1 mcg/mL. Ideally, defer the loading dose if a serum theophylline concentration can be obtained rapidly.

If this is not possible, exercise clinical judgment. When there is sufficient respiratory distress to warrant a small risk, then 2.5 mg/kg of theophylline administered in rapidly absorbed form is likely to increase serum concentration by ≈ 5 mcg/mL. If the patient is not experiencing theophylline toxicity, this is unlikely to result in dangerous adverse effects.

Chronic therapy – Slow clinical titration is generally preferred.

Initial dose: 16 mg/kg/24 hours or 400 mg/24 hours, whichever is less, of anhydrous theophylline in divided doses at 6- or 8-hour intervals.

Increasing dose: The above dosage may be increased in ≈ 25% increments at 3-day intervals so long as the drug is tolerated or until the maximum dose (indicated below) is reached.

Maximum dose (where the serum concentration is not measured) – Do not attempt to maintain any dose that is not tolerated.

Maximum Daily Theophylline Dose Based on Age	
Age	Maximum daily dose[1]
1 to 9 years	24 mg/kg/day
9 to 12 years	20 mg/kg/day
12 to 16 years	18 mg/kg/day
> 16 years	13 mg/kg/day

[1] Not to exceed listed dose or 900 mg, whichever is less.

Exercise caution in younger children who cannot complain of minor side effects. Older adults and those with cor pulmonale, CHF, or liver disease may have unusually low dosage requirements; they may experience toxicity at the maximal dosages recommended.

Measurement of serum theophylline concentrations during chronic therapy – The table below provides guidance to dosage adjustments based on serum theophylline level determinations:

Dosage Adjustment After Serum Theophylline Measurement		
If serum theophylline is:		Directions
Too low	5 to 10 mcg/mL	Increase dose by about 25% at 3-day intervals until either the desired clinical response or serum concentration is achieved.[1]
Within desired range	10 to 20 mcg/mL	Maintain dosage if tolerated. Recheck serum theophylline concentration at 6- to 12-month intervals.[2]
Too high	20 to 25 mcg/mL	Decrease doses by ≈ 10%. Recheck serum theophylline concentration after 3 days.[2]
	25 to 30 mcg/mL	Skip next dose and decrease subsequent doses by 25%. Recheck serum theophylline after 3 days.
	> 30 mcg/mL	Skip next 2 doses and decrease subsequent doses by 50%. Recheck serum theophylline after 3 days.

[1] The total daily dose may need to be administered at more frequent intervals if asthma symptoms occur repeatedly at the end of a dosing interval.
[2] Finer adjustments in dosage may be needed for some patients.

Timed-release capsules – These dosage forms gradually release the active medication so that the total daily dosage may be administered in 1 to 3 doses divided by 8 to 24 hours, depending on the patient's pharmacokinetic profile, thus reducing the number of daily doses required. These products are not necessarily interchangeable. If patients are switched from one brand to another, closely monitor their theophylline serum levels; serum concentrations may vary greatly following brand interchange.

THEOPHYLLINE and DEXTROSE: Substitute oral therapy for IV theophylline as soon as adequate improvement is achieved.

Children (< 6 months of age) – Due to marked variation in theophylline metabolism, use this drug only if clearly needed in infants.

Actions

Pharmacology: The methylxanthines (theophylline, its soluble salts and derivatives) directly relax the smooth muscle of the bronchi and pulmonary blood vessels, stimulate the CNS, induce diuresis, increase gastric acid secretion, reduce lower esophageal sphincter pressure, and inhibit uterine contractions. Theophylline is also a central respiratory stimulant. Aminophylline has a potent effect on diaphragmatic contractility in healthy people and may then be capable of reducing fatigability and thereby improve contractility in patients with chronic obstructive airways disease.

Pharmacokinetics:

Absorption – Theophylline is well absorbed from oral liquids and uncoated plain tablets; maximal plasma concentrations are reached in 2 hours. Rectal absorption from suppositories is slow and erratic, the oral route is generally preferred. Enteric-coated tablets and some sustained-release dosage forms may be unreliably absorbed.

Distribution – Average volume of distribution is 0.45 L/kg (range, 0.3 to 0.7 L/kg). Theophylline does not distribute into fatty tissue. Approximately 40% is bound to plasma protein. Therapeutic serum levels generally range from 10 to 20 mcg/mL. Although some bronchodilatory effect occurs at lower concentrations, stabilization of hyperreactive airways is most evident at levels > 10 mcg/mL, and adverse effects are uncommon at levels < 20 mcg/mL.

Metabolism/Excretion – Xanthines are biotransformed in the liver (85% to 90%) to 1, 3-dimethyluric acid, 3-methylxanthine and 1-methyluric acid; 3-methylxanthine accumulates in concentrations ≈ 25% of those of theophylline.

Excretion is by the kidneys; < 15% of the drug is excreted unchanged. Elimination kinetics vary greatly. Plasma elimination half-life averages about 3 to 15 hours in adult nonsmokers, 4 to 5 hours in adult smokers (1 to 2 packs per day), 1 to 9 hours in children, and 20 to 30 hours for premature neonates. In the neonate, theophylline is metabolized partially to caffeine. The premature neonate excretes ≈ 50% unchanged theophylline and may accumulate the caffeine metabolite.

Equivalent dose – Because of differing theophylline content, the various salts and derivatives are not equivalent on a weight basis.

Theophylline Content and Equivalent Dose of Various Theophylline Salts		
Theophylline salts	Theophylline %	Equivalent dose
Theophylline anhydrous	100	100 mg
Theophylline monohydrate	91	110 mg
Aminophylline anhydrous	86	116 mg
Aminophylline dihydrate	79	127 mg
Oxtriphylline	64	156 mg

Dyphylline – Dyphylline, a chemical derivative of theophylline, is not a theophylline salt as are the other agents. It is about one-tenth as potent as theophylline. Following oral administration, dyphylline is 68% to 82% bioavailable. Peak plasma concentrations are reached within 1 hour, and its half-life is 2 hours. The minimal effective therapeutic concentration is 12 mcg/mL. It is not metabolized to theophylline and 83% ± 5% is excreted unchanged in the urine.

Contraindications

Hypersensitivity to any xanthine; peptic ulcer; underlying seizure disorders (unless receiving appropriate anticonvulsant medication).

Aminophylline: Hypersensitivity to ethylenediamine.

Aminophylline rectal suppositories: Irritation or infection of rectum or lower colon.

Warnings

Status asthmaticus: Status asthmaticus is a medical emergency and is not rapidly responsive to usual doses of conventional bronchodilators. Oral theophylline products alone are not appropriate for status asthmaticus.

Toxicity: Excessive doses may cause severe toxicity; monitor serum levels to ensure maximum benefit with minimum risk.

Serious side effects such as ventricular arrhythmias, convulsions, or even death may appear as the first sign of toxicity without any previous warning. Less serious signs of toxicity (eg, nausea, restlessness) may occur frequently when initiating therapy, but are usually transient; when such signs are persistent during maintenance therapy, they are often associated with serum concentrations > 20 mcg/mL. Serious toxicity is not reliably preceded by less severe side effects.

Cardiac effects: Theophylline may cause dysrhythmias or worsen pre-existing arrhythmias.

Pregnancy: Category C.

Lactation: Theophylline distributes readily into breast milk.

Children: Sufficient numbers of infants < 1 year of age have not been studied in clinical trials to support use in this age group; however, there is evidence that the use of dosage recommendations for older infants and young children may result in the development of toxic serum levels.

Precautions

Use with caution: Cardiac disease; hypoxemia; hepatic disease; hypertension; CHF; alcoholism; elderly (particularly males); and neonates.

GI effects: Use cautiously in peptic ulcer. Local irritation may occur.

Drug Interactions

Agents that may decrease theophylline levels include aminoglutethimide, barbiturates, charcoal, hydantoins, ketoconazole, rifampin, smoking (cigarettes and marijuana), sulfinpyrazone, sympathomimetics (β-agonists), thioamines, carbamazepine, isoniazid, and loop diuretics.

Agents that may increase theophylline levels include allopurinol, beta blockers (nonselective), calcium channel blockers, cimetidine, oral contraceptives, corticosteroids, disulfiram, ephedrine, influenza virus vaccine, interferon, macrolides, mexiletine, quinolones, thiabendazole, thyroid hormones, carbamazepine, isoniazid, and loop diuretics.

The following agents may be affected by theophylline: Benzodiazepines, halothane, ketamine, lithium, nondepolarizing muscle relaxants, and propofol. Probenecid may increase the effects of dyphylline.

Drug/Food interactions: Theophylline elimination is increased (half-life shortened) by a low carbohydrate, high protein diet, and charcoal broiled beef (due to a high polycyclic carbon content). Conversely, elimination is decreased (prolonged half-life) by a high carbohydrate low protein diet. Food may alter the bioavailability and absorption pattern of certain sustained-release preparations. Some sustained-release preparations may be subject to rapid release of their contents when taken with food, resulting in toxicity. It appears that consistent administration in the fasting state allows predictability of effects.

Adverse Reactions

Adverse reactions/toxicity are uncommon at serum theophylline levels < 20 mcg/mL.

Levels > 20 mcg/mL – 75% of patients experience adverse reactions (eg, nausea, vomiting, diarrhea, headache, insomnia, irritability).

Levels > 35 mcg/mL – Hyperglycemia; hypotension; cardiac arrhythmias; tachycardia (> 10 mcg/mL in premature newborns); seizures; brain damage; death.

Other – Fever; flushing; hyperglycemia; inappropriate antidiuretic hormone syndrome; rash; alopecia. Ethylenediamine in aminophylline can cause sensitivity reactions, including exfoliative dermatitis and urticaria.

Cardiovascular: Palpitations; tachycardia; extrasystoles; hypotension; circulatory failure; life-threatening ventricular arrhythmias.

CNS: Irritability; restlessness; headache; insomnia; reflex hyperexcitability; muscle twitching; convulsions.

GI: Nausea; vomiting; epigastric pain; hematemesis; diarrhea; rectal irritation or bleeding (aminophylline suppositories). Therapeutic doses of theophylline may induce gastroesophageal reflux during sleep or while recumbent, increasing the potential for aspiration, which can aggravate bronchospasm.

Renal: Proteinuria; potentiation of diuresis.

Respiratory: Tachypnea; respiratory arrest.

CORTICOSTEROIDS

BECLOMETHASONE

Aerosol: 40 mcg/actuation (*Rx*)	*QVAR* (McNeil Consumer Healthcare)
42 mcg/actuation (*Rx*)	*Vanceril* (Schering)
80 mcg/actuation (*Rx*)	*QVAR* (McNeil Consumer Healthcare)
84 mcg/actuation (*Rx*)	*Vanceril Double Strength* (Schering/Key)

BUDESONIDE

Powder: Each actuation delivers ≈ 160 mcg *(Rx)*	*Pulmicort Turbuhaler* (AstraZeneca)
Inhalation suspension: 0.25 mg/2 mL, 0.5 mg/2 mL *(Rx)*	*Pulmicort Respules* (AstraZeneca)

FLUNISOLIDE

Aerosol: Each actuation delivers ≈ 250 mcg *(Rx)*	*AeroBid* (Forest), *AeroBid-M* (Forest)

FLUTICASONE

Aerosol: 44, 110, and 220 mcg *(Rx)*	*Flovent* (GlaxoWellcome)
Powder: 50, 100, and 250 mcg *(Rx)*	*Flovent Rotadisk* (GlaxoWellcome)

TRIAMCINOLONE

Aerosol: Each actuation delivers ≈ 100 mcg. Contains 60 mg triamcinolone acetonide *(Rx)*	*Azmacort* (Aventis)

Warning:

Adrenal insufficiency: Deaths caused by adrenal insufficiency have occurred in asthmatic patients during and after transfer from systemic corticosteroids to aerosol steroids. After withdrawal from systemic corticosteroids, several months are required for recovery of hypothalamic-pituitary-adrenal (HPA) function. During this period of HPA suppression, patients may exhibit symptoms of adrenal insufficiency when exposed to trauma, surgery, or infections, particularly gastroenteritis. Although aerosolized glucocorticoids may control asthmatic symptoms during these episodes, they do not provide the systemic steroid necessary for the treatment of these emergencies. Patients previously maintained on ≥ 20 mg of prednisone (or equivalent) may be most susceptible, especially when their systemic corticosteroids have been almost completely withdrawn.

Stress/Severe asthma attack: During periods of stress or a severe asthmatic attack, patients withdrawn from systemic corticosteroids should resume them (in large doses) immediately and contact physician. Patients should carry a warning card indicating they may need supplementary systemic steroids during such periods. To assess the risk of adrenal insufficiency in emergency situations, routine tests of adrenal cortical function, including measurement of early morning resting cortisol levels, should be performed periodically in all patients. An early morning resting cortisol level may be accepted as normal only if it falls at or near the normal mean level.

Indications

Asthma, chronic: Maintenance and prophylactic treatment of asthma; includes patients who require systemic corticosteroids and those who may benefit from systemic dose reduction/elimination; for the maintenance treatment of asthma and as prophylactic therapy in children 12 months to 8 years of age (budesonide respules).

Not indicated for relief of asthma that can be controlled by bronchodilators and other nonsteroid medications, in patients who require systemic corticosteroid treatment infrequently, or in the treatment of nonasthmatic bronchitis.

Administration and Dosage

Estimated Comparative Daily Dosages for Inhaled Corticosteroids (Adults)[1]			
Drug	Low dose	Medium dose	High dose
Beclomethasone dipropionate 42 mcg/puff 84 mcg/puff	168 to 504 mcg 4 to 12 puffs 2 to 6 puffs	504 to 840 mcg 12 to 20 puffs 6 to 10 puffs	> 840 mcg > 20 puffs > 10 puffs

Estimated Comparative Daily Dosages for Inhaled Corticosteroids (Adults)[1]			
Drug	Low dose	Medium dose	High dose
Budesonide *Turbuhaler* 200 mcg/dose	200 to 400 mcg 1 to 2 inhalations	400 to 600 mcg 2 to 3 inhalations	> 600 mcg > 3 inhalations
Flunisolide 250 mcg/puff	500 to 1000 mcg 2 to 4 puffs	1000 to 2000 mcg 4 to 8 puffs	> 2000 mcg > 8 puffs
Fluticasone MDI:[2] 44, 110, 220 mcg/puff	88 to 264 mcg 2 to 6 puffs (44 mcg) or 2 puffs (110 mcg)	264 to 660 mcg 2 to 6 puffs (110 mcg)	> 660 mcg > 6 puffs (110 mcg) or> 3 puffs (220 mcg)
DPI:[3] 50, 100, 250 mcg/puff	2 to 6 inhalations (50 mcg)	3 to 6 inhalations (100 mcg)	> 6 inhalations (100 mcg) or > 2 inhalations (250 mcg)
Triamcinolone acetonide 100 mcg/puff	400 to 1000 mcg 4 to 10 puffs	1000 to 2000 mcg 10 to 20 puffs	> 2000 mcg > 20 puffs

[1] *Guidelines for the Diagnosis and Management of Asthma.* Expert Panel Report 2. National Institutes of Health. National Heart, Lung, and Blood Institute. February 1997. http://www.lungusa.org/asthma/astnhlbi.html
[2] MDI = Metered dose inhaler.
[3] DPI = Dry powder inhaler.

Estimated Comparative Daily Dosages for Inhaled Corticosteroids (Children)[1]			
Drug	Low dose	Medium dose	High dose
Beclomethasone dipropionate (6 to 12 years of age) 42 mcg/puff 84 mcg/puff	84 to 336 mcg 2 to 8 puffs 1 to 4 puffs	336 to 672 mcg 8 to 16 puffs 4 to 8 puffs	> 672 mcg > 16 puffs > 8 puffs
Budesonide *Turbuhaler* (≥ 6 years of age) 200 mcg/dose	100 to 200 mcg	200 to 400 mcg 1 to 2 inhalations	> 400 mcg > 2 inhalations
Flunisolide (6 to 15 years of age) 250 mcg/puff	500 to 750 mcg 2 to 3 puffs	1000 to 1250 mcg 4 to 5 puffs	> 1250 mcg > 5 puffs
Fluticasone (≥ 12 years of age) MDI:[2] 44, 110 mcg/puff	88 to 176 mcg 2 to 4 puffs (44 mcg)	176 to 440 mcg 4 to 10 puffs (44 mcg) or 2 to 4 puffs (110 mcg)	> 440 mcg > 4 puffs (110 mcg)
DPI:[3] 50, 100, 250 mcg/dose	2 to 4 inhalations (50 mcg)	2 to 4 inhalations (100 mcg)	> 4 inhalations (100 mcg) or > 2 inhalations (250 mcg)
Triamcinolone acetonide (6 to 12 years of age) 100 mcg/puff	400 to 800 mcg 4 to 8 puffs	800 to 1200 mcg 8 to 12 puffs	> 1200 mcg > 12 puffs

[1] *Guidelines for the Diagnosis and Management of Asthma.* Expert Panel Report 2. National Institutes of Health. National Heart, Lung, and Blood Institute. February 1997. http://www.lungusa.org/asthma/astnhlbi.html
[2] MDI = Metered dose inhaler.
[3] DPI = Dry powder inhaler.

Patients receiving concomitant systemic steroids: Slowly wean patients from systemic corticosteroids after transferring to steroid inhalers. Monitor lung function (FEV_1 or AM PEFR), beta-agonist use, and asthma symptoms during withdrawal of oral corticosteroids. Transfer to steroid inhalant and subsequent management may be more difficult because of slow HPA function recovery that may last up to 12 months. These agents may be effective and may permit replacement or significant reduction in corticosteroid dosage.

Stabilize the patient's asthma before treatment is started. Initially, use aerosol concurrently with usual maintenance dose of systemic steroid. After ≈ 1 week, start gradual withdrawal of the systemic steroid by reducing the daily or alternate daily dose. Make the next reduction after 1 to 2 weeks, depending on response. Generally, these decrements should not exceed 25% of the prednisone dose or its equivalent. A slow rate of withdrawal cannot be overemphasized.

During withdrawal, some patients may experience symptoms of steroid withdrawal (eg, joint or muscular pain, lassitude, depression) despite maintenance or even improvement of respiratory function. Encourage continuance with the inhaler, but observe for objective signs of adrenal insufficiency (eg, fatigue, lassitude, weakness, nausea and vomiting, hypotension). If adrenal insufficiency occurs, increase the systemic steroid dose temporarily and continue further withdrawal more slowly.

During periods of stress or severe asthma attack, transfer patients will require supplementary systemic steroids.

BECLOMETHASONE: 50 mcg released at the valve delivers ≈ 42 mcg to the patient.

Beclovent –

Adults and children ≥ 12 years of age: 2 inhalations (84 mcg) 3 or 4 times/day. Alternatively, 4 inhalations (168 mcg) given twice daily has been effective in some patients. In patients with severe asthma, start with 12 to 16 inhalations (504 to 672 mcg) a day and adjust dosage downward according to response. Do not exceed 20 inhalations (840 mcg) daily.

Children 6 to 12 years of age: 1 or 2 inhalations (42 to 84 mcg) 3 or 4 times/day according to response. Alternatively, 4 inhalations (168 mcg) twice daily have been effective in some patients. Do not exceed 10 inhalations (420 mcg) daily. Clinical data are insufficient with respect to administration in children < 6 years of age.

Vanceril –

Adults: The usual recommended dosage is 2 inhalations (84 mcg) given 3 or 4 times/day. In some patients, 4 inhalations (168 mcg) given twice daily has been effective. In patients with severe asthma, it is advisable to start with 12 to 16 inhalations per day and adjust the dosage downward according to patient response. The maximal daily intake should not exceed 20 inhalations (840 mcg) in adults.

Children 6 to 12 years of age: The usual recommended dosage is 1 or 2 inhalations (42 to 84 mcg) given 3 or 4 times/day. The maximal daily intake should not exceed 10 inhalations (420 mcg) in children. Insufficient information is available to warrant use in children < 6 years of age.

Vanceril Double Strength –

Adults: 2 inhalations (168 mcg) twice daily. In patients with severe asthma, it is advisable to start with 6 to 8 inhalations a day and adjust the dosage downward according to the response of the patient. The maximal daily intake should not exceed 10 inhalations (840 mcg) in adults.

Children 6 to 12 years of age: 2 inhalations (168 mcg) twice daily. The maximal daily intake should not exceed 5 inhalations (420 mcg) in children. Insufficient data exist with respect to the administration to children < 6 years of age.

Patients not receiving systemic steroids – Follow above directions. In responsive patients, pulmonary function usually improves within 1 to 4 weeks.

Test aerosol by spraying 2 times into the air before first use and in cases where the product has not been used for > 7 days (≥ 10 days for *QVAR*). Rinse mouth after inhalation.

QVAR – The safety and efficacy in children < 12 years of age have not been established.

Solution aerosol does not require shaking. Two actuations of the 40 mcg strength should provide a dose comparable to 1 actuation of the 80 mcg strength. The recommended dosage relative to CFC-based beclomethasone dipropionate (CFC-BDP) inhalation aerosols is lower caused by differences in delivery characteristics between the products.

Recommended Doses in Patients ≥ 12 Years of Age for *QVAR*		
Previous therapy	Recommended starting dose	Highest recommended dose
Bronchodilators alone	40 to 80 mcg twice/day	320 mcg twice/day
Inhaled corticosteroids	40 to 160 mcg twice/day	320 mcg twice/day

BUDESONIDE:

Budesonide Recommended Starting Dose and Highest Recommended Dose		
Previous therapy	Recommended starting dose[1]	Highest recommended dose
Turbuhaler		
Adults		
Bronchodilators alone	200-400 mcg twice/day	400 mcg twice/day
Inhaled corticosteroids[2]	200-400 mcg twice/day	800 mcg twice/day
Oral corticosteroids	400-800 mcg twice/day	800 mcg twice/day
Children ≥ 6 years of age[3]		
Bronchodilators alone	200 mcg twice/day	400 mcg twice/day
Inhaled corticosteroids[2]	200 mcg twice/day	400 mcg twice/day
Oral corticosteroids	The highest recommended dose in children is 400 mcg twice/day.	
Respules		
Children 12 months to 8 years of age		
Bronchodilators alone	0.5 mg total daily dose administered either once or twice daily in divided doses	0.5 mg total daily dose
Inhaled corticosteroids	0.5 mg total daily dose administered either once or twice daily in divided doses	1 mg total daily dose
Oral corticosteroids	1 mg total daily dose administered either as 0.5 mg twice/day or 1 mg once daily	1 mg total daily dose

[1] 200 mcg released with each actuation delivers ≈ 160 mcg to the patient (*Turbuhaler*).
[2] In patients with mild to moderate asthma who are well controlled on inhaled corticosteroids, dosing budesonide 200 mcg or 400 mcg once daily may be considered. Administer budesonide once daily either in the morning or evening.
[3] Insufficient information is available to warrant use in children < 6 years of age.

Budesonide turbuhaler – In all patients, it is desirable to titrate to the lowest effective dose once asthma stability is achieved.

Each actuation delivers ≈ 160 mcg budesonide.

Improvement in asthma control following inhaled administration of budesonide can occur within 24 hours of treatment initiation, although maximum benefit may not be achieved for ≥ 1 to 2 weeks.

Budesonide respules – Administer by the inhaled route via jet nebulizer connected to an air compressor in asthmatic patients 12 months to 8 years of age. Improvement in asthma control following inhaled administration of budesonide can occur within 2 to 8 days of initiation of treatment, although maximum benefit may not be achieved for 4 to 6 weeks. It is desirable to downward-titrate to the lowest effective dose once asthma stability is achieved. In symptomatic children not responding to nonsteroidal therapy and in patients who require maintenance therapy of their asthma, a starting dose of 0.25 mg once daily may also be considered.

If once-daily treatment with budesonide does not provide adequate control of asthma symptoms, increase the total daily dose or administer as a divided dose.

Ultrasonic nebulizers are not suitable for the adequate administration of budesonide respules and therefore, are not recommended. The effects of mixing budesonide respules with other nebulizable medications has not been adequately assessed; administer separately in the nebulizer.

Patients maintained on chronic oral corticosteroids – Initially use concurrently with the patient's usual maintenance dose of systemic corticosteroid. Initiate at 1 mg/day.

FLUNISOLIDE: Each actuation delivers ≈ 250 mcg flunisolide.

Adults – 2 inhalations (500 mcg) twice daily, morning and evening (total daily dose 1000 mcg). Do not exceed 4 inhalations twice daily (2000 mcg).

Children 6 to 15 years of age – 2 inhalations twice daily, morning and evening (total daily dose 1000 mcg). Higher doses have not been studied. Safety and efficacy for use in children < 6 years of age have not been established. With chronic use, monitor children for growth as well as for effects on the HPA axis. Insufficient information is available to warrant use in children < 6 years of age.

Patients not receiving systemic steroids – In responsive patients, pulmonary function usually improves within 1 to 4 weeks.

FLUTICASONE:
Fluticasone aerosol (≥ 12 years of age) –

Recommended Doses for Fluticasone Aerosol		
Previous therapy	Recommended starting dose	Highest recommended dose
Bronchodilators alone	88 mcg twice/day	440 mcg twice/day
Inhaled corticosteroids	88-220 mcg twice/day[1]	440 mcg twice/day
Oral corticosteroids	880 mcg twice/day	880 mcg twice/day

[1] Starting doses > 88 mcg twice/day may be considered for patients with poorer asthma control or those who have previously required doses of inhaled corticosteroids that are in the higher range for that specific agent.

Fluticasone powder (≥ 4 years of age) –

Recommended Doses for Fluticasone Powder		
Previous therapy	Recommended starting dose	Highest recommended dose
Adults and adolescents		
Bronchodilators alone	100 mcg twice/day	500 mcg twice/day
Inhaled corticosteroids	100-250 mcg twice/day[1]	500 mcg twice/day
Oral corticosteroids	1000 mcg twice/day	1000 mcg twice/day
Children 4 to 11 years of age		
Bronchodilators alone	50 mcg twice/day	100 mcg twice/day
Inhaled corticosteroids	50 mcg twice/day	100 mcg twice/day

[1] Starting doses > 100 mcg twice/day for adults and adolescents and 50 mcg twice daily for children 4 to 11 years of age may be considered for patients with poorer asthma control or those who have previously required doses of inhaled corticosteroids that are in the higher range for that specific agent.

TRIAMCINOLONE: 200 mcg released with each actuation delivers ≈ 100 mcg.

Adults – The usual dosage is 2 inhalations (≈ 200 mcg) 3 to 4 times/day or 4 inhalations (400 mcg) twice daily. Do not exceed a maximum daily intake of 16 inhalations (1600 mcg). Higher initial doses (12 to 16 inhalations/day) may be advisable in patients with more severe asthma.

Children 6 to 12 years of age – The usual dosage is 1 or 2 inhalations (100 to 200 mcg) 3 to 4 times/day or 2 to 4 inhalations (200 to 400 mcg) twice daily. Do not exceed a maximum daily intake of 12 inhalations (1200 mcg). Clinical data are insufficient with respect to use in children < 6 years of age. Maximum benefit may not be achieved for ≥ 2 weeks.

Patients not receiving systemic steroids – Follow above directions. In responsive patients, an improvement in pulmonary function is usually apparent within 1 to 2 weeks but maximum benefit may not be achieved for ≥ 2 weeks.

Actions

Pharmacology: These agents are synthetic adrenocortical steroids with basic glucocorticoid actions and effects. Glucocorticoids may decrease number and activity of inflammatory cells, enhance effect of beta-adrenergic drugs on cyclic AMP production, inhibit bronchoconstrictor mechanisms, or produce direct smooth muscle relaxation. Inhaler use provides effective local steroid activity with minimal systemic effect.

Pharmacokinetics:

	Pharmacokinetics of Inhaled Corticosteroids				
Parameters	Corticosteroids				
	Beclomethasone	Budesonide	Flunisolide	Fluticasone	Triamcinolone
Absorption					
Systemic bioavailability from lungs	≈ 20%	25%	40%	20	21.5%
Distribution					
Vd (L/kg)	NA	4.3	1.8	3.5	1.4
Protein binding	87%	85% to 90%	NA	91%	≈ 68%
Metabolism					
Site	liver (CYP3A)	liver (CYP3A)	liver	liver (CYP3A4)	mostly from liver, less extensively from the kidneys
Metabolites (Activity)	beclomethasone 17-mono-propionate (active), free beclomethasone (very weak anti-inflammatory effects)	16α-hydroxy-prednisolone and 6β-hydroxy-budesonide (< 1% of parent)	6β-OH (low corticosteroid potency)	17β-carboxylic acid (negligible in animal studies)	6β-hydroxy-triamcinolone acetonide, 21-carboxy-triamcinolone acetonide, and 21-carboxy-6β-hydroxytriamcinolone acetonide (less active than parent)
Excretion					
Site	feces, urine (< 10%)	urine (≈ 60%), feces	renal (50%), feces (40%)	feces, urine (< 0.02%)	urine (≈ 40%), feces (≈ 60%)
T½	2.8 hr	2.8 hr	≈ 1.8 hr	3.1 hr	1.5 hr

Contraindications

Relief of acute bronchospasm; primary treatment of status asthmaticus or other acute episodes of asthma when intensive measures are required; hypersensitivity to any ingredient; systemic fungal infections; persistently positive sputum cultures for *Candida albicans*.

Vanceril: Relief of asthma that can be controlled by bronchodilators and other nonsteroid medications; in patients who require systemic corticosteroid treatment infrequently; treatment of nonasthmatic bronchitis.

Warnings

Infections: Localized fungal infections with *Candida albicans* or *Aspergillus niger* have occurred in the mouth, pharynx, and occasionally in the larynx. The incidence of clinically apparent infection is low, and may require treatment with appropriate antifungal therapy or discontinuance of aerosol steroid treatment. Use inhaled corticosteroids with caution, if at all, in patients with active or quiescent tuberculous infection of the respiratory tract, untreated systemic fungal, bacterial, parasitic or viral infection, or ocular herpes simplex.

Acute asthma: These products are not bronchodilators and are not for rapid relief of bronchospasm. See Black Box Warning.

Bronchospasm: Bronchospasm may occur with an immediate increase in wheezing following dosing; treat immediately with a fast-acting inhaled bronchodilator. See Black Box Warning.

Combination with prednisone: Combination therapy of inhaled corticosteroids with systemic corticosteroids may increase the risk of HPA suppression compared with a therapeutic dose of either one alone. Use inhaled corticosteroids with caution in patients already receiving prednisone.

Replacement therapy: Transfer from systemic steroid therapy may unmask allergic conditions previously suppressed. During withdrawal from oral steroids, some patients may experience withdrawal symptoms despite maintenance or improvement of respiratory function.

Pregnancy: Category C.

Lactation: Glucocorticoids are excreted in breast milk. It is not known whether inhaled corticosteroids are excreted in breast milk, but it is likely.

Children: Insufficient information is available to warrant use in children < 6 years of age or < 12 years of age with **fluticasone** and **beclomethasone**. Monitor growth in children and adolescents because there is evidence that oral corticosteroids may suppress growth in a dose-related fashion, particularly in higher doses for extended periods.

Precautions

Steroid withdrawal: During withdrawal from oral steroids, some patients may experience symptoms of systemically active steroid withdrawal (eg, joint or muscular pain, lassitude, depression), despite maintenance or even improvement of respiratory function. Although steroid withdrawal effects are usually transient and not severe, severe and even fatal exacerbation of asthma can occur if the previous daily oral corticosteroid requirement had significantly exceeded 10 mg/day of prednisone or equivalent.

HPA suppression: In responsive patients, inhaled corticosteroids may permit control of asthmatic symptoms with less HPA suppression. Because these agents are absorbed and can be systemically active, the beneficial effects in minimizing or preventing HPA dysfunction may be expected only when recommended dosages are not exceeded. Take particular care in observing patients postoperatively or during periods of stress for evidence of a decrease in adrenal function.

Flunisolide – Because of the possibility of higher systemic absorption, monitor patients using **flunisolide** for any evidence of systemic corticosteroid effect. If such changes occur, discontinue slowly, consistent with accepted procedures for discontinuing oral corticosteroids. When flunisolide is used chronically at 2 mg/day, monitor patients periodically for effects on the HPA axis.

Glaucoma: Rare instances of glaucoma, increased intraocular pressure, and cataracts have been reported following the inhaled administration of corticosteroids.

Long-term effects: The effects of long-term glucocorticoid inhalation are unknown. Although there is no clinical evidence of adverse effects, the local and systemic effects on developmental or immunologic processes in the mouth, pharynx, trachea, and lung are unknown.

There is no information about effects on acute, recurrent, or chronic pulmonary infection (including active or quiescent tuberculosis) or effects of long-term use on lung or other tissues. Use with caution (see Warnings).

Pulmonary infiltrates: Pulmonary infiltrates with eosinophilia may occur with beclomethasone or flunisolide.

Reduction in growth velocity: Closely follow the growth of adolescents taking corticosteroids, and weigh the benefits of corticosteroid therapy and asthma control against the possibility of growth suppression.

Drug Interactions

Ketoconazole: A potent inhibitor of cytochrome P450 3A4 may increase plasma levels of **budesonide** and **fluticasone** during concomitant dosing. The clinical significance is unknown. Use caution.

Adverse Reactions

Local: Throat irritation; hoarseness/dysphonia, coughing; dry mouth; rash; wheezing; facial edema; flu syndrome.

Systemic: Suppression of HPA function has occurred. Deaths caused by adrenal insufficiency have occurred during and after transfer from systemic to aerosol corticosteroids.

Beclomethasone – Adverse reactions occurring in ≥ 3% of patients include headache; nasal congestion; dysmenorrhea; dyspepsia; rhinitis; pharyngitis; coughing; upper respiratory tract infection; viral infections; sinusitis.

Budesonide – Adverse reactions occurring in ≥ 3% of patients include pain; fever; back pain; upper respiratory tract infection; sinusitis; pharyngitis; coughing; conjunctivitis; headache; rhinitis; epistaxis; otitis media; ear infection; viral infections; flu syndrome; voice alteration.

Flunisolide – Adverse reactions occurring in ≥ 3% of patients include palpitations; chest pain; dizziness; irritability; nervousness; shakiness; nausea; vomiting; abdominal pain; anorexia; heartburn; upper respiratory tract infection; nasal and sinus congestion; unpleasant taste; loss of smell or taste; edema; fever; menstrual disturbance; eczema; itching/pruritus; rash; sore throat; diarrhea; upset stomach; general flu; oral candidiasis; headache; rhinitis; sinusitis; cold symptoms; runny nose; sinus drainage/infection; hoarseness; sputum; wheezing; chest congestion; coughing; sneezing; ear infection.

Fluticasone – Adverse reactions occurring in ≥ 3% of patients include headache; pharyngitis; nasal congestion; sinusitis; rhinitis; upper respiratory tract infection; influenza; oral candidiasis; diarrhea; dysphonia; menstrual disturbance; nasal discharge; allergic rhinitis; fever.

Triamcinolone – Adverse reactions occurring in ≥ 3% of patients include pharyngitis; sinusitis; flu syndrome; headache; back pain.

ACETYLCYSTEINE (N-Acetylcysteine)

Solution: 10% and 20% (*Rx*)   Various, *Mucomyst* (Apothecon), *Mucosil-10* (Dey Labs)

Indications

Mucolytic: Adjuvant therapy for abnormal, viscid, or inspissated mucus secretions in chronic bronchopulmonary disease (chronic emphysema, emphysema with bronchitis, chronic asthmatic bronchitis, tuberculosis, bronchiectasis, primary amyloidosis of lung).

> Acute bronchopulmonary disease (pneumonia, bronchitis, tracheobronchitis).
> Pulmonary complications of cystic fibrosis.
> Tracheostomy care.
> Pulmonary complications associated with surgery.
> Use during anesthesia.
> Posttraumatic chest conditions.
> Atelectasis due to mucus obstruction.
> Diagnostic bronchial studies (bronchograms, bronchospirometry, bronchial wedge catheterization).

Antidote: To prevent or lessen hepatic injury that may occur following ingestion of a potentially hepatotoxic quantity of acetaminophen.

Administration and Dosage

Nebulization (face mask, mouth piece, tracheostomy): 1 to 10 mL of the 20% solution or 2 to 20 mL of the 10% solution every 2 to 6 hours; the dose for most patients is 3 to 5 mL of the 20% solution or 6 to 10 mL of the 10% solution 3 to 4 times/day.

Nebulization (tent, croupette): Very large volumes are required, occasionally up to 300 mL during a treatment period. The dose is the volume of solution that will maintain a very heavy mist in the tent or croupette for the desired period. Administration for intermittent or continuous prolonged periods, including overnight, may be desirable.

Instillation:

>*Direct* – 1 to 2 mL of a 10% to 20% solution as often as every hour.

>*Tracheostomy* – 1 to 2 mL of a 10% to 20% solution every 1 to 4 hours by instillation into the tracheostomy.

May be introduced directly into a particular segment of the bronchopulmonary tree by inserting (under local anesthesia and direct vision) a plastic catheter into the trachea. Instill 2 to 5 mL of the 20% solution by a syringe connected to the catheter.

Percutaneous intratracheal catheter – 1 to 2 mL of the 20% solution or 2 to 4 mL of the 10% solution every 1 to 4 hours by a syringe attached to the catheter.

Diagnostic bronchograms: 2 or 3 administrations of 1 to 2 mL of the 20% solution or 2 to 4 mL of the 10% solution by nebulization or by instillation intratracheally, prior to the procedure.

Equipment compatibility: Certain materials in nebulization equipment react with acetylcysteine, especially certain metals (notably iron and copper) and rubber. Where materials may come into contact with acetylcysteine solution, use parts made of the following materials: Glass, plastic, aluminum, anodized aluminum, chromed metal, tantalum, sterling silver, or stainless steel. Silver may become tarnished after exposure, but this is not harmful to the drug action or to the patient.

Admixture incompatibility: Tetracycline, chlortetracycline, oxytetracycline, erythromycin lactobionate, amphotericin B, and sodium ampicillin are incompatible when mixed in the same solution with acetylcysteine. Administer from separate solutions. Iodized oil, chymotrypsin, trypsin, and hydrogen peroxide are also incompatible.

Actions

Pharmacology: The mucolytic action of acetylcysteine is related to the sulfhydryl group in the molecule, which acts directly to split disulfide linkages between mucoprotein molecular complexes, resulting in depolymerization and a decrease in mucus viscosity. The mucolytic activity of acetylcysteine increases with increasing pH.

Acetylcysteine also reduces the extent of liver injury following acetaminophen overdose. It is thought that acetylcysteine protects the liver by maintaining or restoring glutathione levels, or by acting as an alternate substrate for conjugation with, and thus, detoxification of, the reactive metabolite of acetaminophen.

Pharmacokinetics: Following a 200 to 400 mg oral dose, peak plasma concentrations of 0.35 to 4 mg/L are achieved within 1 to 2 hours. Protein binding is $\approx$ 50% 4 hours post-dose. Volume of distribution is 0.33 to 0.47 L/kg. The terminal half-life of reduced acetylcysteine is 6.25 hours. Approximately 70% of total body clearance is nonrenal.

Contraindications

Hypersensitivity to acetylcysteine. As an antidote, there are no contraindications.

Warnings

Bronchial secretions: An increased volume of liquefied bronchial secretions may occur; when cough is inadequate, maintain an open airway by mechanical suction if necessary. When there is a large mechanical block due to a foreign body or local accumulation, clear the airway by endotracheal aspiration, with or without bronchoscopy.

Asthmatics: Carefully observe asthmatics under treatment with acetylcysteine. If bronchospasm progresses, discontinue medication immediately.

Antidotal use:

Allergic effects – Generalized urticaria has been observed rarely. If this or other allergic symptoms appear, discontinue treatment unless it is deemed essential and the allergic symptoms can be otherwise controlled.

Hepatic effects – If encephalopathy due to hepatic failure occurs, discontinue treatment to avoid further administration of nitrogenous substances.

Vomiting – Vomiting, occasionally severe and persistent, occurs as a symptom of acute acetaminophen overdose. Treatment with oral acetylcysteine may aggravate vomiting. Evaluate patients at risk of gastric hemorrhage concerning the risk of upper GI hemorrhage vs the risk of developing hepatic toxicity. Diluting acetylcysteine minimizes its propensity to aggravate vomiting.

Pregnancy: Category B.

Lactation: It is not known whether this drug is excreted in breast milk.

Precautions

Disagreeable odor: Administration may initially produce a slight disagreeable odor which soon disappears.

Face mask use: A face mask may cause stickiness on the face after nebulization; remove with water.

Solution color: Solution color may change in the opened bottle, but does not significantly impair the drug's safety or efficacy.

Continued nebulization: Continued nebulization of acetylcysteine with a dry gas results in concentration of drug in the nebulizer due to evaporation. Extreme concentration may impede nebulization and drug delivery. Dilute with Sterile Water for Injection as concentration occurs.

Adverse Reactions

Adverse reactions may include stomatitis; nausea; vomiting; fever; rhinorrhea; drowsiness; clamminess; chest tightness; bronchoconstriction; bronchospasm; irritation to the tracheal and bronchial tracts.

Antidotal use – Large doses of oral acetylcysteine may result in nausea, vomiting, and other GI symptoms. Rash (with or without mild fever), pruritus, angioedema, bronchospasm, tachycardia, hypotension, and hypertension have occurred.

IPRATROPIUM BROMIDE

Aerosol: Each actuation delivers 18 mcg (*Rx*)
Solution for Inhalation: 0.02% (500 mcg/vial) (*Rx*)
Nasal spray: 0.03% (21 mcg/spray) and
0.06% (42 mcg/spray) (Rx)

Atrovent (Boehringer Ingelheim)
Various, *Atrovent* (Boehringer Ingelheim)
Atrovent (Boehringer Ingelheim)

Indications

Bronchospasm (solution and aerosol): Used alone or in combination with other bronchodilators (especially beta-adrenergics) as a bronchodilator for maintenance treatment of bronchospasm associated with chronic obstructive pulmonary disease (COPD), including chronic bronchitis and emphysema. Ipratropium is not indicated for the initial treatment of acute episodes of bronchospasms.

Rhinorrhea:

Perennial rhinitis (0.03% nasal spray) – Symptomatic relief of rhinorrhea associated with allergic and nonallergic perennial rhinitis in patients ≥ 6 years of age.

Common cold (0.06% nasal spray) – Symptomatic relief of rhinorrhea associated with the common cold in patients ≥ 5 years of age.

Administration and Dosage

Aerosol: The usual dose is 2 inhalations (36 mcg) 4 times/day. Patients may take additional inhalations as required; however, do not exceed 12 inhalations in 24 hours.

Solution: The usual dose is 500 mcg (1 unit dose vial) administered 3 to 4 times/day by oral nebulization, with doses 6 to 8 hours apart. The solution can be mixed in the nebulizer with albuterol if used within 1 hour.

Nasal spray:

0.03% (patients ≥ 6 years of age) – The usual dose is 2 sprays (42 mcg) per nostril 2 or 3 times/day (total dose, 168 to 252 mcg/day). Optimum dosage varies.

0.06% (patients ≥ 5 years of age) – Recommended dose is 2 sprays (84 mcg) per nostril 3 or 4 times/day (total dose, 504 to 672 mcg/day). Optimum dosage varies.

Children 5 to 11 years of age: Recommended dose is 2 sprays (84 mcg) per nostril 3 times/day (total dose, 504 mcg/day).

The safety and efficacy of use > 4 days in patients with the common cold have not been established.

Actions

Pharmacology: Ipratropium for oral inhalation is a synthetic quaternary anticholinergic (parasympatholytic) ammonium compound chemically related to atropine. It appears to inhibit vagally mediated reflexes by antagonizing the action of acetylcholine. The bronchodilation following inhalation is primarily a local, site-specific effect, not a systemic one.

Pharmacokinetics: Much of an inhaled dose is swallowed as shown by fecal excretion studies. Ipratropium is not readily absorbed into the systemic circulation either from the surface of the lung or from the GI tract as confirmed by blood levels and renal excretion studies. The elimination half-life is $\approx$ 1.6 hours.

Contraindications

Hypersensitivity to ipratropium, atropine, or its derivatives; a history of hypersensitivity to soya lecithin or related food products such as soy bean or peanut (inhalation aerosol).

Warnings

Acute bronchospasm: Ipratropium is not indicated as a single agent for relief of bronchospasm in acute COPD exacerbation.

Special risk patients: Use with caution in patients with narrow-angle glaucoma, prostatic hypertrophy, or bladder neck obstruction.

Pregnancy: Category B.

Lactation: It is not known whether this drug is excreted in breast milk.

Children: Safety and efficacy in children < 12 years of age (aerosol and solution), < 6 years of age (0.03% nasal spray), and < 5 years of age (0.06% nasal spray) have not been established.

Drug Interactions

Ipratropium has been used concomitantly with other drugs, including sympathomimetic bronchodilators, methylxanthines, steroids, and cromolyn sodium, commonly used in the treatment of chronic obstructive pulmonary disease, without adverse drug reactions.

Adverse Reactions

Adverse reactions from **inhalational products** may include nervousness, cough, dryness of the oropharynx, irritation from aerosol, exacerbation of symptoms, dizziness, headache, GI distress, dry mouth, influenza-like symptoms, back or chest pain, nausea, dyspnea, bronchitis, upper respiratory tract infection, epistaxis, pharyngitis, nasal dryness, and miscellaneous nasal symptoms.

Adverse reactions from **nasal spray** may include epistaxis, nasal dryness, headache, and upper respiratory tract infection.

IPRATROPIUM BROMIDE AND ALBUTEROL SULFATE

Aerosol: Each actuation delivers 18 mcg ipratropium bromide and 103 mcg albuterol sulfate (*Rx*)   *Combivent* (Boehringer Ingelheim)

Indications

Bronchospasm: Use in patients with chronic obstructive pulmonary disease (COPD) on a regular aerosol bronchodilator who continue to have evidence of bronchospasm and require a second bronchodilator.

Administration and Dosage

Shake well before using.

The recommended dose is 2 inhalations 4 times/day. Patients may take additional inhalations as required; however, advise the patient not to exceed 12 in 24 hours. It is recommended to "test spray" 3 times before using the first time and in cases where the aerosol has not be used for > 24 hours.

CROMOLYN SODIUM (Disodium Cromoglycate)

Inhalation (for nebulization): 20 mg/2 mL (Rx)   Various
Solution (for nebulizer only): 20 mg/amp (Rx)   Intal (Rhone-Poulenc Rorer)
Aerosol spray: Each actuation delivers 800 mcg (Rx)
Nasal Solution: 40 mg/mL.   Nasalcrom (McNeil)
Each actuation delivers 5.2 mg (otc)
Oral concentrate: 5 mL/100 mg (Rx)   Gastrocrom (Medeva)

Indications

Severe bronchial asthma (nebulization solution, inhalation capsules, aerosol): Prophylactic management of severe bronchial asthma where the frequency, intensity, and predictability of episodes indicate the continued use of symptomatic medication. Such patients must have a significant bronchodilator-reversible component to their airway obstruction as demonstrated by pulmonary function tests.

Prevention of exercise-induced bronchospasm (nebulization solution, capsules, aerosol): Prevention of acute bronchospasm induced by toluene diisocyanate, environmental pollutants, and known antigens (aerosol).

Allergic rhinitis (nasal solution): Prevention and treatment of allergic rhinitis.

Mastocytosis (oral): Improves diarrhea, flushing, headaches, vomiting, urticaria, abdominal pain, nausea and itching in some patients.

Administration and Dosage

Nebulizer solution:

 Adults and children ≥ 2 years of age – Initially, 20 mg inhaled 4 times/day at regular intervals. Carefully instruct patients in the use of the inhaler. The effectiveness of therapy depends upon administration at regular intervals.

 Administer solution from a power operated nebulizer having an adequate flow rate and equipped with a suitable face mask or mouthpiece. *Hand operated nebulizers are not suitable.*

 Introduce cromolyn into the patient's therapeutic regimen when the acute episode has been controlled, the airway has been cleared, and the patient is able to inhale adequately.

Prevention of exercise-induced bronchospasm: Inhale 20 mg of the nebulizer solution no more than 1 hour before anticipated exercise (ie, within 10 to 15 minutes). The drug's protective effect will be stronger the shorter the interval between inhalation and exercise. Repeat inhalation as required for protection during prolonged exercise.

Concomitant corticosteroid treatment: Continue concomitant corticosteroid treatment and bronchodilators following the introduction of cromolyn. If the patient improves, attempt to decrease corticosteroid dosage. Even if the steroid-dependent patient fails to improve following cromolyn use, attempt gradual tapering of steroid dosage while maintaining close patient supervision. Consider reinstituting steroid therapy for a patient subjected to significant stress while being treated or within 1 year (occasionally up to 2 years) after steroid treatment has been terminated, in case of adrenocortical insufficiency. When the inhalation of cromolyn is impaired, a temporary increase in the amount of steroids or other agents may be required.

 Cautiously withdraw cromolyn in cases where its use has permitted a reduction in the maintenance dose of steroids as there may be a sudden reappearance of asthma that will require immediate therapy and possible reintroduction of corticosteroids.

Aerosol: For management of bronchial asthma in adults and children ≥ 5 years of age, the usual starting dose is two metered sprays inhaled 4 times/day at regular intervals. Do not exceed this dose. Not all patients will respond to the recommended dose, and a lower dose may provide efficacy in younger patients.

 Advise patients with chronic asthma that the effect of therapy is dependent upon its administration at regular intervals, as directed. Introduce therapy into the patient's therapeutic regimen when the acute episode has been controlled, the airway has been cleared and the patient is able to inhale adequately.

For the prevention of acute bronchospasm that follows exercise, exposure to cold dry air, or environmental agents – The usual dose is inhalation of 2 metered dose sprays shortly (ie, 10 to 15 minutes but not more than 60 minutes) before exposure to the precipitating factor.

Nasal solution:

Adults and children ≥ 6 years of age – One spray in each nostril 3 to 6 times/day at regular intervals every 4 to 6 hours. Maximum effects may not be seen for 1 to 2 weeks. Clear the nasal passages before administering the spray and inhale through the nose during administration.

Seasonal (pollenotic) rhinitis – Seasonal (pollenotic) rhinitis, and for prevention of rhinitis caused by exposure to other types of specific inhalant allergens – Treatment will be more effective if started prior to contact with the allergen. Continue treatment throughout exposure period.

Perennial allergic rhinitis – Effects of treatment may require 2 to 4 weeks of treatment. Concomitant use of antihistamines or nasal decongestants may be necessary during the initial phase of treatment, but the need for this medication should diminish and may be eliminated when the full benefit of therapy is achieved.

Oral:

Adults – Two ampules 4 times/day, 30 minutes before meals and at bedtime.

Children < 2 years of age – Not recommended.

2 to 12 years of age: One ampule 4 times/day 30 minutes before meals and bedtime.

If satisfactory control of symptoms is not achieved within 2 to 3 weeks, the dosage may be increased but should not exceed 40 mg/kg/day.

The effect of therapy is dependent upon its administration at regular intervals as directed. Not for inhalation or injection.

Maintenance – Once a therapeutic response has been achieved the dose may be reduced to the minimum required to maintain the patient with a lower degree of symptomatology. To prevent relapses, maintain the dosage.

Administer as a solution in water ≥ 30 minutes before meals after preparation according to the following directions.

1.) Break open and squeeze liquid contents of ampule(s) into a glass of water.

2.) Stir solution.

3.) Drink all of the liquid.

Compatibility: Cromolyn **nebulizer solution** is compatible with metaproterenol sulfate, isoproterenol HCl, 0.25% isoetharine HCl, epinephrine HCl, terbutaline sulfate, and 20% acetylcysteine solution for ≥ 1 hour after their admixture.

Actions

Pharmacology: Cromolyn is an anti-inflammatory agent. It has no intrinsic bronchodilator, antihistaminic, anticholinergic, vasoconstrictor, or glucocorticoid activity. The drug inhibits the release of mediators, histamine, and SRS-A (the slow-reacting substance of anaphylaxis, a leukotriene) from the mast cell. Cromolyn acts locally on the lung to which it is directly applied.

Bronchial asthma – Improvement ordinarily occurs within the first 4 weeks of administration, although some patients may demonstrate an immediate response.

Pharmacokinetics: After inhalation, ≈ 8% is absorbed from the lung and is rapidly excreted unchanged in bile and urine. The remainder is either exhaled, or deposited in the oropharynx, swallowed and excreted via the alimentary tract.

Cromolyn is poorly absorbed from the GI tract. No more than 1% of an administered dose is absorbed after oral administration, the remainder excreted in the feces.

Contraindications

Hypersensitivity to cromolyn or to any ingredient contained in these products.

Warnings

Acute asthma: Cromolyn has no role in the treatment of acute asthma, especially status asthmaticus; it is a prophylactic drug with no benefit for acute situations.

Hypersensitivity reactions: Severe anaphylactic reactions may occur rarely.

Renal/Hepatic function impairment: Decrease the dose or discontinue the drug in these patients.

Pregnancy: Category B.

Lactation: Safety for use in the nursing mother has not been established.

Children:

> *Aerosol* – Safety and efficacy in children < 5 years of age are not established.
> *Nebulizer solution* – Safety and efficacy in children < 2 years of age not established.
> *Nasal solution* – Safety and efficacy in children < 6 years of age are not established.

> *Oral* – Reserve use in children < 2 years of age for patients with severe disease in which potential benefits clearly outweigh risks.

Precautions

Bronchospasm: Occasionally, patients experience cough or bronchospasm following inhalation.

Asthma: Asthma may recur if drug is reduced below recommended dosage or discontinued.

Eosinophilic pneumonia: Pulmonary infiltrates with eosinophilia — If this occurs during the course of therapy, discontinue the drug.

Nasal stinging or sneezing: Nasal stinging or sneezing may be experienced by some patients immediately following instillation of the nasal solution.

Aerosol: Because of the propellants in this preparation, use with caution in patients with coronary artery disease or cardiac arrhythmias.

Adverse Reactions

Adverse reactions associated with **aerosol** may include lacrimation, swollen parotid gland, dysuria, urinary frequency, dizziness, headache, rash, urticaria, angioedema, joint swelling and pain, and nausea.

Reactions from the **nebulizer solution** may include cough, nasal congestion, wheezing, sneezing, nasal itching, epistaxis, nose burning, and abdominal pain.

Adverse events associated with the **nasal solution** may include sneezing, nasal stinging, nasal burning, nasal irritation, headache, and bad taste in mouth.

Adverse reactions from oral concentrate may include headache and diarrhea.

NEDOCROMIL SODIUM

Aerosol: 1.75 mg/actuation (*Rx*)   *Tilade* (Fisons)

Indications

Bronchial asthma: Maintenance therapy in the management of patients with mild to moderate bronchial asthma.

Administration and Dosage

The recommended dosage for symptomatic adults and children (≥ 12 years of age) is 2 inhalations 4 times/day at regular intervals to provide 14 mg/day. Initiate maintenance therapy at the same dose. In patients under good control on 4 times/day dosing (ie, patients whose only medication need is occasional [not more than twice a week] inhaled or oral beta-agonists, and who have no serious exacerbations with respiratory infections), a lower dose can be tried. If use of lower doses is attempted, first reduce to a 3 times/day regimen (10.5 mg/day) then, after several weeks on continued good control, to twice a day (7 mg/day).

Add nedocromil to the patient's existing treatment regimen (eg, bronchodilators). When a clinical response to nedocromil is evident and if the asthma is under good control, an attempt may be made to decrease concomitant medication usage gradually.

Proper inhalational technique is essential.

Advise patients that the optimal effect of nedocromil therapy depends on its administration at regular intervals, even during symptom-free periods.

Actions

Pharmacology: Nedocromil is an inhaled anti-inflammatory agent for the preventive management of asthma. It inhibits the in vitro activation of, and mediator release from, a variety of inflammatory cell types associated with asthma, including eosinophils, neutrophils, macrophages, mast cells, monocytes and platelets. Nedocromil inhibits the development of early and late bronchoconstriction responses to inhaled antigen.

Pharmacokinetics: Systemic bioavailability is low.

The mean 24 hour urinary excretion after either single- or multiple-dose administration represented ≈ 5% of the administered dose.

Nedocromil is ≈ 89% bound to plasma protein over a concentration range of 0.5 to 50 mcg/mL. This binding is reversible. It is not metabolized after IV administration and is excreted unchanged.

Contraindications

Hypersensitivity to nedocromil or other ingredients in the preparation.

Warnings

Acute bronchospasm: Nedocromil is not a bronchodilator and, therefore, should not be used for the reversal of acute bronchospasm, particularly status asthmaticus.

Pregnancy: Category B.

Lactation: It is not known whether this drug is excreted in breast milk.

Children: Safety and efficacy in children < 12 years of age have not been established.

Precautions

Coughing/Bronchospasm: Inhaled medications can cause coughing and bronchospasm in some patients.

Corticosteroids: If systemic or inhaled steroid therapy is at all reduced, monitor patients carefully.

Adverse Reactions

Adverse reactions associated with nedocromil may include coughing, pharyngitis, rhinitis, upper respiratory tract infection, bronchospasm, nausea, headache, chest pain, and unpleasant taste.

NASAL DECONGESTANTS

EPHEDRINE

Spray: 0.25% ephedrine sulfate (*otc*)
Pretz-D (Parnell)

Drops: 0.5% ephedrine sulfate (*otc*)
Vicks Vatronol (Richardson-Vicks)

EPINEPHRINE

Solution: 0.1% (*otc*)
Adrenalin Chloride (Parke-Davis)

NAPHAZOLINE

Drops: 0.05% solution (*otc*)
Privine (Ciba Consumer)

Spray: 0.05% solution (*otc*)

OXYMETAZOLINE

Solution: 0.025% (*otc*)
Afrin Children's Nose Drops (Schering-Plough)

0.05% (*otc*)
Various, *Afrin* (Schering-Plough), *Afrin Sinus* (Schering-Plough), *Allerest 12 Hour Nasal* (Ciba Cons.), *Cheracol Nasal* (Roberts), *Chlorphed-LA* (Roberts-Hauck), *Dristan 12 Hr Nasal* (Whitehall), *Duramist Plus* (Pfeiffer), *Duration* (Schering-Plough), *4-Way Long Lasting Nasal* (Bristol-Myers), *Nostrilla* (Ciba Consumer), *NTZ Long Acting Nasal* (Sterling Health), *Sinarest 12 Hour* (Ciba Cons.), *Vicks Sinex 12-Hour* (Richardson-Vicks)

PHENYLEPHRINE

Solution: 0.125% (*otc*)
Neo-Synephrine (Sterling Health)

0.16% (*otc*)
Alconefrin 12 (PolyMedica)

0.25% (*otc*)
Various, *Alconefrin 25* (PolyMedica), *Neo-Synephrine* (Sterling Health), *Children's Nostril* (Ciba), *Rhinall* (Scherer)

0.5% (*otc*)
Alconefrin (PolyMedica), *Neo-Synephrine* (Sterling Health), *Nostril* (Ciba), *Sinex* (Richardson-Vicks)

1% (*otc*)
Various, *Neo-Synephrine* (Sterling Health)

PSEUDOEPHEDRINE HCl

Tablets: 30 mg (*otc*)
Various, *Halofed* (Halsey), *Sudafed* (Warner Lambert Consumer), *Sudex* (Roberts)

60 mg (*otc*)
Various, *Cenafed* (Century Pharm.), *Halofed* (Halsey), *Sudafed* (Warner Lambert Consumer)

240 mg (*otc*)
Efidac/24 (Ciba)

Tablets, extended-release: 120 mg (*otc*)
Sudafed 12 Hour Caplets (Warner Lambert Consumer)

Capsules: 60 mg (*otc*)
Allermed (Murdock), *Sinustop Pro* (Murdock)

Capsules, timed-release: 120 mg (*Rx*)
Novafed (Marion Merrell Dow)

Liquid: 15 mg/5 mL (*otc*)
Dorcol Children's Decongestant (Sandoz), *Triaminic AM Decongestant Formula* (Sandoz)

30 mg/5 mL (*otc*)
Various, *Cenafed Syrup* (Century Pharm.), *Children's Sudafed* (Warner Lambert Consumer)

Drops: 7.5 mg/0.8 mL (*otc*)
PediaCare Infants' Decongestant (McNeil)

PSEUDOEPHEDRINE SULFATE

Tablets, extended-release: 120 mg (60 mg immediate-release/60 mg delayed-release) (*otc*)
Afrin (Schering-Plough), *Drixoral Non-Drowsy Formula* (Schering-Plough)

TETRAHYDROZOLINE

Solution: 0.05% (*Rx*)
Tyzine Pediatric Drops (Kenwood/Bradley)

0.1% (*Rx*)
Tyzine (Kenwood/Bradley)

XYLOMETAZOLINE

Solution: 0.05% (*otc*)
Otrivin Pediatric Nasal Drops (Ciba Consumer)

0.1% (*otc*)
Otrivin (Ciba Consumer)

MISCELLANEOUS NASAL DECONGESTANTS

Capsules: 5 mg phenylephrine HCl, 40 mg phenylpropanolamine HCl, 40 mg pseudoephedrine HCl (*Rx*)
No-Hist (Dunhall)

MISCELLANEOUS NASAL DECONGESTANT INHALERS

Inhaler: 250 mg propylhexedrine (*otc*)
Benzedrex (Menley & James)

50 mg l-desoxyephedrine (*otc*)
Vicks Inhaler (Richardson-Vicks)

MISCELLANEOUS NASAL DECONGESTANT COMBINATIONS

Solution: 0.25% phenylphrine HCl, 0.15% pyrilamine maleate *Myci-Spray* (Misemer) (*otc*)

0.5% phenylephrine HCl and 0.2% pheniramine maleate (*otc*)   *Dristan Nasal* (Whitehall)
0.5% phenylephrine HCl, 0.05% naphazoline HCl and 0.2%   *4-Way Fast Acting Original* (Bristol-Myers)
pyrilamine maleate (*otc*)

Indications

Oral: For temporary relief of nasal congestion due to the common cold, hay fever, or other upper respiratory allergies, and nasal congestion associated with sinusitis; to promote nasal or sinus drainage; relief of eustachian tube congestion.

Topical: Symptomatic relief of nasal and nasopharyngeal mucosal congestion due to the common cold, sinusitis, hay fever, or other upper respiratory allergies.

Adjunctive therapy of middle ear infections by decreasing congestion around the eustachian ostia. Nasal inhalers may relieve ear block and pressure pain in air travel.

Administration and Dosage

Systemic effects are less likely from topical use, but use caution in the conditions listed for oral agents. Adverse reactions are more likely with excessive use, in the elderly and in children.

EPHEDRINE: Dosage is product-specific; see labeling.

EPINEPHRINE:
    Adults and children (≥ 6 years of age) – Apply locally as drops or spray, or with a sterile swab, as required. Do not use in children < 6 years of age, except on physician's advice.

NAPHAZOLINE:
    Adults and children (≥ 12 years of age) – 1 or 2 drops or sprays in each nostril as needed, no more than every 6 hours (spray). Do not use in children < 12 years of age, unless directed by physician.

OXYMETAZOLINE:
    Adults and children (≥ 6 years of age) – 2 or 3 sprays or 2 or 3 drops of 0.05% solution in each nostril twice daily, morning and evening or every 10 to 12 hours (*Allerest*).
    Children (2 to 5 years of age) – 2 or 3 drops of 0.025% solution in each nostril twice daily, morning and evening.

PHENYLEPHRINE HCl:
    Adults (≥ 12 years of age) – 2 to 3 sprays or drops in each nostril. Repeat every 3 to 4 hours (0.25% and 0.5%). Do not repeat the 1% solution any more often than every 4 hours. The 0.25% solution is adequate in most cases. However, in resistant cases or if more powerful decongestion is desired, use the 0.5% or 1% solution.
    Children (6 to 12 years of age) – 0.25% – 2 to 3 sprays or drops in each nostril every 3 to 4 hours.
    Infants (> 6 months of age) – 0.16% – 1 or 2 drops in each nostril every 3 hours.

PSEUDOEPHEDRINE HCl:
    Adults – 60 mg every 4 to 6 hours (120 mg sustained release every 12 hours). Do not exceed 240 mg in 24 hours.
    Children – 30 mg every 4 to 6 hours. Do not exceed 120 mg in 24 hours.
      (2 to 5 years of age): 15 mg every 4 to 6 hours. Do not exceed 60 mg in 24 hours.
      (1 to 2 years of age): 7 drops (0.2 mL)/kg every 4 to 6 hours up to 4 doses/day.
      (3 to 12 months of age): 3 drops/kg every 4 to 6 hours up to 4 doses/day.

PSEUDOEPHEDRINE SULFATE:
    Adults and children ≥ 12 years of age – 120 mg every 12 hours.
    Do not crush or chew sustained-release preparations.

TETRAHYDROZOLINE:
    Adults and children (≥ 6 years of age) – 2 to 4 drops of 0.1% solution in each nostril every 3 to 4 hours as needed, or 3 to 4 sprays in each nostril every 4 hours as needed.

Children (2 to 6 years of age) – 2 to 3 drops of 0.05% solution in each nostril every 4 to 6 hours, as necessary. Do not use the 0.1% solution in children < 6 years of age.

XYLOMETAZOLINE:

Adults (≥ 12 years of age) – 2 to 3 drops or 2 to 3 sprays (0.1%) in each nostril every 8 to 10 hours.

Children (2 to 12 years of age) – 2 to 3 drops (0.05%) in each nostril every 8 to 10 hours.

MISCELLANEOUS NASAL DECONGESTANT INHALER:

Adults and children (≥ 6 years of age) – 1 to 2 inhalations in each nostril (while blocking the other nostril) not more than every 2 hours. Do not exceed recommended dosage. Do not use propylhexedrine for > 3 days or l-desoxyephedrine for > 7 days. If symptoms persist beyond this time, consult physician.

Actions

Pharmacology: Decongestants stimulate α-adrenergic receptors of vascular smooth muscle (vasoconstriction, pressor effects, nasal decongestion), although some retain β-adrenergic properties (eg, ephedrine, pseudoephedrine). The α-adrenergic effects cause intense vasoconstriction when applied directly to mucous membranes; systemically, the products have similar muted effects and decongestion occurs without drastic changes in blood pressure, vascular redistribution, or cardiac stimulation. Constriction in the mucous membranes results in their shrinkage; this promotes drainage, thus improving ventilation and the stuffy feeling.

Oral agents are not as effective as topical products, especially on an immediate basis, but generally have a longer duration of action, cause less local irritation and are not associated with rebound congestion (rhinitis medicamentosa).

Contraindications

Monoamine oxidase inhibitor (MAOI) therapy; hypersensitivity or idiosyncrasy to sympathomimetic amines manifested by insomnia, dizziness, weakness, tremor, or arrhythmias.

Oral: Severe hypertension and coronary artery disease.

Sustained release pseudoephedrine and naphazoline – Children < 12 years of age.

Topical:

Tetrahydrozoline – 0.1% solution in children < 6 years of age; 0.05% solution in infants < 2 years of age.

Naphazoline – Glaucoma.

Warnings

Special risk patients: Administer with caution to patients with hyperthyroidism, diabetes mellitus, cardiovascular disease, coronary artery disease, ischemic heart disease, increased intraocular pressure, or prostatic hypertrophy. Sympathomimetics may cause CNS stimulation and convulsions or cardiovascular collapse with hypotension.

Hypertension: Hypertensive patients should use these products only with medical advice, as they may experience a change in blood pressure because of the added vasoconstriction.

Excessive use: Excessive use of decongestants may cause systemic effects (eg, nervousness, dizziness, sleeplessness), which are more likely in infants and in the elderly. Habituation and toxic psychosis have followed long-term high-dose therapy.

Rebound congestion (rhinitis medicamentosa): May occur following topical application after the vasoconstriction subsides. Patients may increase the amount of drug and frequency of use, producing toxicity and perpetuating the rebound congestion.

Treatment – A simple but uncomfortable solution is to completely withdraw the topical medication. A more acceptable method is to gradually withdraw therapy by initially discontinuing the medication in one nostril, followed by total withdrawal. Substituting an oral decongestant for a topical one may also be useful.

Elderly: Patients ≥ 60 years of age are more likely to experience adverse reactions to sympathomimetics. Overdosage may cause hallucinations, convulsions, CNS depression, and death. Demonstrate safe use of a short-acting sympathomimetic before use of a sustained action formulation in elderly patients.

Pregnancy: Category C.

Lactation: Oral pseudoephedrine is contraindicated in the nursing mother because of the higher than usual risks to infants from sympathomimetic agents.

Other oral preparations – Consult a physician before using.

Topical – It is not known if these agents are excreted in breast milk.

Children: Use in children is product specific.

Precautions

Acute use: Use topical decongestants only in acute states and not longer than 3 to 5 days. Use sparingly (especially the imidazolines) in all patients, particularly infants, children and patients with cardiovascular disease.

Stinging sensation: Some individuals may experience a mild, transient stinging sensation after topical application. This often disappears after a few applications.

Drug Interactions

Most interactions listed apply to sympathomimetics when used as vasopressors; however, consider the interaction when using the nasal decongestants.

Drugs that may affect nasal decongestants include beta blockers, furazolidone, guanethidine, indomethacin, methyldopa, MAO inhibitors, rauwolfia alkaloids, tricyclic antidepressants, urinary acidifiers, and urinary alkalinizers.

Drugs that may be affected by nasal decongestants include bromocriptine, caffeine, guanethidine, insulin or oral hypoglycemic agents, and theophylline.

Adverse Reactions

Adverse reactions may include fear, anxiety, tenseness, restlessness, headache, lightheadedness, dizziness, drowsiness, tremor, insomnia, hallucinations, psychological disturbances, prolonged psychosis, convulsions, CNS depression, weakness, arrhythmias and cardiovascular collapse with hypotension, palpitations, nausea, vomiting, pallor, respiratory difficulty, orofacial dystonia, sweating, dysuria, and blepharospasm.

Reactions associated with topical use include burning, stinging, sneezing, dryness, local irritation, and rebound congestion.

INTRANASAL STEROIDS

BECLOMETHASONE DIPROPIONATE
Aerosol: 42 mcg (*Rx*)

Beconase (GlaxoWellcome), *Vancenase* (Schering), *Vancenase Pockethaler* (Schering)

Spray: 0.042% (*Rx*)
0.084% (*Rx*)

Beconase AQ (GlaxoWellcome)
Vancenase AQ (Schering)

BUDESONIDE
Inhaler: ≈ 32 mcg budesonide/actuation (*Rx*)
Spray: 32 mcg budesonide/spray (*Rx*)

Rhinocort (AstraZeneca)
Rhinocort Aqua (AstraZeneca)

FLUNISOLIDE
Spray: ≈ 25 mcg flunisolide (*Rx*)

Nasalide (Dura), *Nasarel* (Dura)

FLUTICASONE
Spray: 0.05% (each actuation delivers 50 mcg) (*Rx*)

Flonase (GlaxoSmithKline)

MOMETASONE FUROATE MONOHYDRATE
Spray: each actuation delivers 50 mcg mometasone furoate

Naxonex (Schering)

TRIAMCINOLONE
Inhaler: 55 mcg triamcinolone acetonide/actuation (*Rx*)
Spray: 55 mcg triamcinolone acetonide/actuation (*Rx*)
50 mcg trimacinolone acetonide/spray (*Rx*)

Nasacort (Aventis)
Nasacort AQ (Aventis)
Tri-Nasal (Muro)

Indications

Beclomethasone Dipropionate: Relief of the symptoms of seasonal or perennial rhinitis in cases poorly responsive to conventional treatment.

Prevention of recurrence of nasal polyps following surgical removal.

Spray formulations – For nonallergic (vasomotor) and perennial allergic rhinitis.

Budesonide: Management of symptoms of seasonal or perennial allergic rhinitis in adults and children ≥ 6 years of age and nonallergic perennial rhinitis in adults (*Rhinocort only*).

Flunisolide: Relief of the symptoms of seasonal or perennial rhinitis when effectiveness of or tolerance to conventional treatment is unsatisfactory.

Fluticasone: Management of nasal symptoms of seasonal and perennial allergic and non-allergic rhinitis in adults and children ≥ 4 years of age.

Mometasone furoate monohydrate: Treatment of the nasal symptoms of seasonal allergic and perennial allergic rhinitis in adults and children ≥ 3 years of age; prophylaxis of the nasal symptoms of seasonal allergic rhinitis and the treatment of the nasal symptoms of perennial allergic rhinitis in adults and adolescents ≥ 12 years of age.

Triamcinolone: Treatment of seasonal and perennial allergic rhinitis symptoms in adults and children ≥ 6 years of age (*Nasacort* and *Nasacort AQ*) or ≥ 12 years of age (*Tri-Nasal*).

Administration and Dosage

Improvement in symptoms usually becomes apparent within a few days. However, relief may not occur in some patients for as long as 2 weeks. Do not continue beyond 3 weeks in absence of significant symptomatic improvement.

BECLOMETHASONE DIPROPIONATE:

Adults and children ≥ 12 years of age –

Beconase, Vancenase: 1 inhalation (42 mcg) in each nostril 2 to 4 times/day (total dose 168 to 336 mcg/day). Patients can often be maintained on a maximum dose of 1 inhalation in each nostril 3 times/day (252 mcg/day).

Beconase AQ: Usual dosage is 1 or 2 inhalations (42 to 84 mcg) in each nostril twice a day (168 to 336 mcg/day).

Vancenase Pockethaler: Usual dosage is 1 inhalation (42 mcg) in each nostril 2 to 4 times/day (total dose 168 to 336 mcg/day). Maintenance dosage is 1 inhalation in each nostril 3 times/day (252 mcg/day).

Children 6 to 12 years of age –

Beconase, Vancenase: 1 inhalation in each nostril 3 times/day (252 mcg/day). Not recommended for children < 6 years of age because safety and efficacy studies have not been conducted in this age group.

Beconase AQ: Start with 1 inhalation in each nostril twice daily; patients not adequately responding to 168 mcg or those with more severe symptoms may use 336 mcg (2 inhalations in each nostril). Not recommended for children < 6 years of age.

Vancenase Pockethaler: Usual dosage is 1 inhalation in each nostril 3 times/day (252 mcg/day). Not recommended for children < 6 years of age.

Adults and children ≥ 6 years of age –

Vancenase AQ: The usual dosage is 1 or 2 inhalations in each nostril once daily (total dose 168 to 336 mcg/day). Use once daily at a regular interval. Not recommended in children < 6 years of age. Before initial use, prime the pump by actuating 6 times or until a fine spray appears. If pump is unused for > 4 days, reprime once or until fine spray appears.

Nasal polyps – Treatment may have to be continued for several weeks or more before a therapeutic result can be fully assessed. Recurrence of symptoms caused by polyps can occur after stopping treatment, depending on the severity of the disease.

BUDESONIDE:
Rhinocort –

Adults and children ≥ 6 years of age: Recommended starting dose is 256 mcg/day, given as either 2 sprays in each nostril in the morning and evening or as 4 sprays in each nostril in the morning. Doses exceeding 256 mcg/day (4 sprays/nostril) are not recommended. After the desired clinical effect has been obtained, reduce the maintenance dose to the smallest amount necessary for control of symptoms; gradually decrease the dose every 2 to 4 weeks as long as desired effect is maintained. If symptoms return, increase dose briefly to starting dose.

Rhinocort Aqua –

Adults and children ≥ 6 years of age: Recommended starting dose is 64 mcg/day administered as 1 spray/nostril once daily. Some patients who do not achieve symptom control at the recommended starting dose may benefit from an increased dose. It is always desirable to titrate an individual patient to the minimum effective dose to reduce the possibility of side effects.

Maximum recommended doses:

Adults ≥ 12 years of age – 256 mcg/day administered as 4 sprays/nostril once daily.

Children 6 through 11 years of age – 128 mcg/day administered as 2 sprays/ nostril once daily.

FLUNISOLIDE:
Adults – Starting dose is 2 sprays (50 mcg) in each nostril 2 times/day (total dose 200 mcg/day). May increase to 2 sprays in each nostril 3 times/day (total dose 300 mcg/day). Maximum daily dose is 8 sprays in each nostril (400 mcg/day).

Children (6 to 14 years of age) – Starting dose is 1 spray (25 mcg) in each nostril 3 times/day or 2 sprays (50 mcg) in each nostril 2 times/day (total dose 150 to 200 mcg/day). Maximum daily dose is 4 sprays in each nostril (200 mcg/day).

Maintenance dose – After desired clinical effect is obtained, reduce maintenance dose to smallest amount necessary to control symptoms. Approximately 15% of patients with perennial rhinitis may be maintained on 1 spray in each nostril/day.

FLUTICASONE:
Adults – Recommended starting dose is 2 sprays (50 mcg each) per nostril once daily (total daily dose, 200 mcg). The same dosage divided into 100 mcg given twice daily (eg, 8:00 am and 8:00 pm) is also effective. After the first few days, dosage may be reduced to 100 mcg (1 spray per nostril) once daily for maintenance therapy. Maximum total daily dosage should not exceed 200 mcg/day.

Adolescents ≥ 4 years of age – Start most adolescents with 100 mcg (1 spray/nostril/ day). Patients not adequately responding to 100 mcg may use 200 mcg (2 sprays/ nostril). Depending on response, dosage may be decreased to 100 mcg daily. Total daily dosage should not exceed 200 mcg/day.

Children < 4 years of age – Use not recommended.

MOMETASONE FUROATE MONOHYDRATE:

Adults and children ≥ 12 years of age – The usual recommended dose for prophylaxis and treatment of the nasal symptoms of seasonal allergic rhinitis and treatment of the nasal symptoms of perennial allergic rhinitis is 2 sprays (50 mcg/spray) in each nostril once daily (total daily dose, 200 mcg).

In patients with a known seasonal allergen that precipitates nasal symptoms of seasonal allergic rhinitis, prophylaxis with mometasone (200 mcg/day) is recommended 2 to 4 weeks prior to the anticipated start of the pollen season.

Children 3 to 11 years of age – The usual recommended dose for treatment of the nasal symptoms of seasonal allergic and perennnial allergic rhinitis is 1 spray (50 mcg) in each nostril once daily (total daily dose, 100 mcg).

TRIAMCINOLONE:

Adults and children ≥ 12 years of age –

Nasacort: The recommended starting dose is 220 mcg/day given as 2 sprays (55 mcg/spray) in each nostril once a day. The dose may be increased to 440 mcg/day (55 mcg/spray) either as once-a-day dosage or divided up to 4 times/day (ie, twice a day [2 sprays/nostril] or 4 times/day [1 spray/nostril]). After desired effect is obtained, some patients (≈ 50%) may be maintained on as little as 1 spray in each nostril once a day. The degree of relief does not seem to be significantly different when comparing 2 or 4 times/day dosing with once-a-day dosing.

A dose response between 110 and 440 mcg/day is not clearly discernible. In general, the highest dose tends to provide relief sooner. This suggests an alternative approach to starting therapy: Start treatment with 440 mcg (4 sprays/nostril/day), and then, depending on response, decrease the dose by 1 spray/day every 4 to 7 days.

Nasacort AQ: The recommended starting and maximum dose is 220 mcg/day as 2 sprays in each nostril once daily. When the maximum benefit has been achieved and symptoms have been controlled in patients initially controlled at 220 mcg/day, decreasing the dose to 110 mcg/day (1 spray in each nostril/day) has been demonstrated to be effective in allergic rhinitis symptoms.

Tri-Nasal: The recommended starting dose for most patients is 200 mcg (2 sprays/nostril) once daily. The dose may be increased to a maximum of 400 mcg (4 sprays/nostril) once daily. An alternative 400 mcg/day dosing regimen may be given as 200 mcg twice daily (two 50 mcg sprays in each nostril twice daily). Do not exceed the maximum daily dose of 400 mcg. After symptoms have been brought under control, the patient should be titrated to the minimum effective dose.

Children 6 to 12 years of age –

Nasacort: The recommended starting dose is 220 mcg/day given as 2 sprays (55 mcg/spray) in each nostril once a day. Once the maximal effect has been achieved, titrate the patient to the minimum effective dose.

Nasacort AQ: The recommended starting dose is 110 mcg/day given as 1 spray in each nostril once daily. The maximum recommended dose is 220 mcg/day as 2 sprays/nostril once daily. Once symptoms are controlled, pediatric patients may be maintained on 110 mcg/day (1 spray in each nostril per day).

Nasacort and *Nasacort AQ* are not recommended for children < 6 years of age.

Actions

Pharmacology: These drugs have potent glucocorticoid and weak mineralocorticoid activity. The mechanisms responsible for the anti-inflammatory action of corticosteroids on the nasal mucosa are unknown. However, glucocorticoids have a wide range of inhibitory activities against multiple cell types and mediators involved in allergic and nonallergic/irritant-mediated inflammation. These agents, when administered topically in recommended doses, exert direct local anti-inflammatory effects with minimal systemic effects.

Pharmacokinetics: The amount of an intranasal dose that reaches systemic circulation is generally low, and metabolism is rapid.

Contraindications

Untreated localized infections involving the nasal mucosa; hypersensitivity to the drug or any component of the product.

Warnings

Systemic corticosteroids: The combined administration of alternate day systemic prednisone with these products may increase the likelihood of HPA suppression.

Excessive doses/sensitivity: If recommended doses of intranasal beclomethasone are exceeded or if individuals are particularly sensitive or predisposed by virtue of recent systemic steroid therapy, symptoms of hypercorticism may occur, including, very rarely, menstrual irregularities, acneiform lesions, and cushingoid features.

Hypersensitivity reactions: Rare cases of immediate and delayed hypersensitivity reactions, including angioedema, urticaria, rash, and bronchospasm, have occurred.

Pregnancy: Category C.

Carefully observe infants born of mothers who have received substantial doses of corticosteroids during pregnancy for signs of adrenal insufficiency.

Lactation: Advise mothers taking pharmacologic doses not to nurse.

Beclomethasone, budesonide, flunisolide, triamcinolone – It is not known whether these drugs are excreted in breast milk.

Children: Safety and efficacy for use in children < 6 years of age (< 12 years of age for **triamcinolone**, ≤ 4 years of age for **fluticasone**) have not been established. Use in children < 6 years of age is not recommended; carefully follow growth and development if prolonged therapy is used.

Precautions

Infections: Localized infections of the nose and pharynx with *Candida albicans* have developed only rarely.

Use with caution in patients with active or quiescent tuberculosis infections of the respiratory tract, or in untreated fungal, bacterial or systemic viral infections, or ocular herpes simplex.

Individuals receiving immunosuppressant agents are more susceptible to infections than healthy individuals. Avoid exposure to chicken pox or measles.

Wound healing: Because of the inhibitory effect of corticosteroids on wound healing in patients who have experienced recent nasal septal ulcers, recurrent epistaxis, nasal surgery or trauma, use nasal steroids with caution until healing has occurred.

Vasoconstrictors: In the presence of excessive nasal mucosa secretion or edema of the nasal mucosa, the drug may fail to reach the site of intended action. In such cases, use a nasal vasoconstrictor during the first 2 to 3 days of therapy.

Systemic effects: Although systemic absorption is low when used in recommended dosage, HPA suppression and other systemic effects may occur, especially with excessive doses.

Long-term treatment: Examine patients periodically over several months or longer for possible changes in the nasal mucosa.

Drug Interactions

Use caution when coadministering **fluticasone** with ketoconazole and other known cytochrome P450 inhibitors.

Adverse Reactions

Adverse reactions associated with intranasal steroids include mild nasopharyngeal irritation, nasal irritation, burning, stinging, dryness, and headache.

Those associated with budesonide in particular include epistaxis, pharyngitis, and increased cough.

ANTIHISTAMINES

AZATADINE MALEATE
Tablets: 1 mg (*Rx*) *Optimine* (Key)

AZELASTINE HCl
Nasal spray: 137 mcg (as HCl)/spray (*Rx*) *Astelin* (Wallace Laboratories)

CETIRIZINE HCl
Tablets: 5 and 10 mg (*Rx*) *Zyrtec* (Pfizer)
Syrup: 5 mg/5 mL (*Rx*) *Zyrtec* (Pfizer)

CHLORPHENIRAMINE MALEATE
Tablets, chewable: 2 mg (*otc*) *Chlo-Amine* (Hollister-Stier)
Tablets: 4 mg (*otc*) Various, *Aller-Chlor* (Rugby), *Allergy* (Major), *Chlor-Trimeton Allergy 4 hour* (Schering-Plough Healthcare)
Tablets, timed-release: 8 and 12 mg (*otc*) *Chlor-Trimeton Allergy 8 Hour, Chlor-Trimeton Allergy 12 Hour* (Schering-Plough Healthcare)
Capsules, sustained-release: 8 and 12 mg (*Rx*) Various
Syrup: 2 mg/5 mL (*otc*) *Aller-Chlor* (Rugby)

CLEMASTINE FUMARATE
Tablets: 1.34 mg (*otc*[1]) Various, *Antihist-1* (Various, eg, Goldline)
2.68 mg (*Rx*) Various, *Tavist* (Novartis)
Syrup: 0.67 mg/5 mL (*Rx*) *Tavist* (Novartis)

CYPROHEPTADINE HCl
Tablets: 4 mg (*Rx*) Various, *Periactin* (Merck)
Syrup: 2 mg/5 mL (*Rx*) Various

DESLORATADINE
Tablets: 5 mg *Clarinex* (Schering)

DIPHENHYDRAMINE HCl
Capsules, soft gels: 25 mg (*otc/Rx*) Various, *Benadryl Allergy Kapseals* (Warner Lambert Consumer), *Benadryl Dye-Free Allergy Liqui-Gels* (Warner Lambert Consumer)
Capsules: 25 mg (*otc*) Various, *Banophen* (Major)
50 mg (*otc/Rx*) Various
Tablets: 25 mg (*otc*) *Banophen Caplets* (Major), *Benadryl Allergy* (Warner Lambert Consumer), *Benadryl Allergy Ultratabs* (Warner Lambert Consumer), *Diphenhist Captabs* (Rugby)
50 mg (*otc*) *AllerMax Caplets* (Pfeiffer), *Nighttime Sleep Aid* (Rugby)
Tablets, chewable: 12.5 mg (*otc*) *Benadryl Allergy* (Warner Lambert Consumer)
Liquid: 6.25 mg/5 mL (*otc*) *AllerMax Allergy & Cough Formula* (Pfeiffer), *Diphen AF* (Morton Grove)
12.5 mg/5 mL (*otc/Rx*) *Genahist* (Goldline), *Benadryl Allergy* (Warner Lambert Consumer), *Benadryl Dye-Free Allergy* (Warner Lambert Consumer), *Scot-Tussin Allergy DM* (Scot-Tussin Pharmacal
Solution: 12.5 mg/5 mL (*otc*) *Diphenhist* (Rugby)
Elixir: 12.5 mg/5 mL (*otc*) *Siladryl* (Silarx)
Syrup: 12.5 mg/5 mL (*otc/Rx*) Various, *Diphen Cough* (Morton Grove), *Tusstat* (Century Pharm)
Injection: 10 mg/mL and 50 mg/mL (*Rx*) Various, *Benadryl* (Parke-Davis), *Hyrexin-50* (Hyrex)

DEXCHLORPHENIRAMINE MALEATE
Tablets: 2 mg (*Rx*) *Polaramine* (Schering-Plough)
Tablets, timed-release: 4 and 6 mg (*Rx*) Various, *Polaramine Repetabs* (Schering-Plough)
Syrup: 2 mg/5 mL (*Rx*) *Polaramine* (Schering-Plough)

FEXOFENADINE HCl
Tablets: 30, 60, and 180 mg (*Rx*) *Allegra* (Aventis)
Capsules: 60 mg (*Rx*)

HYDROXYZINE

Tablets (as HCl): 10, 25, 50 mg (*Rx*)	Various, *Atarax* (Roerig)
100 mg (*Rx*)	*Atarax 100* (Roerig)
Capsules (as pamoate equiv. to HCl): 25, 50, and 100 mg (*Rx*)	Various, *Vistaril* (Pfizer)
Syrup (as HCl): 10 mg/5mL (*Rx*)	Various, *Atarax* (Roerig)
Oral suspension (as pamoate equiv. to HCl): 25 mg/5 mL (*Rx*)	*Vistaril* (Pfizer)
Injection (as HCl): 25 mg/mL and 50 mg/mL (*Rx*)	Various, *Vistaril* (Pfizer)

LORATADINE

Tablets: 10 mg (*Rx*)	*Claritin* (Schering)
Tablets, rapidly-disintegrating: 10 mg (*Rx*)	*Claritin Reditabs* (Schering)
Syrup: 1 mg/mL (*Rx*)	*Claritin* (Schering)

PHENINDAMINE TARTRATE

Tablets: 25 mg (*Rx*)	*Nolahist* (Amarin)

PROMETHAZINE HCl

Tablets: 12.5, 25, and 50 mg (*Rx*)	Various, *Phenergan* (Wyeth-Ayerst)
Syrup: 6.25 mg/5 mL, 25 mg/5 mL (*Rx*)	Various, *Phenergan Plain, Phenergan Fortis* (Wyeth-Ayerst)
Suppositories: 12.5, 25, and 50 mg (*Rx*)	Various, *Phenergan* (Wyeth-Ayerst)
Injection: 25 mg/mL, 50 mg/mL (*Rx*)	Various, *Phenergan* (Wyeth-Ayerst), *Anergan 50* (Forest)

TRIPELENNAMINE HCl

Tablets: 25 and 50 mg (*Rx*)	*PBZ* (Novartis)
Tablets, extended-release: 100 mg (*Rx*)	*PBZ-SR* (Novartis)

Indications

Oral: Relief of symptoms associated with: Perennial and seasonal allergic rhinitis; vasomotor rhinitis; allergic conjunctivitis; temporary relief of runny nose and sneezing caused by the common cold; allergic and non-allergic pruritic symptoms; mild, uncomplicated urticaria and angioedema; amelioration of allergic reactions to blood or plasma; dermatographism; adjunctive therapy in anaphylactic reactions; idiopathic chronic urticaria; lacrimation.

Parenteral: Amelioration of allergic reactions to blood or plasma; in anaphylaxis as an adjunct to epinephrine and other measures; for other uncomplicated allergic conditions of the immediate type when oral therapy is not possible.

Cyproheptadine: In addition to the general uses discussed in the antihistamine monograph, cyproheptadine is also indicated for hypersensitivity reactions, Type I.

Diphenhydramine: In addition to the general uses, diphenhydramine is indicated for active and prophylactic treatment of motion sickness; as a nighttime sleep aid (oral only); for parkinsonism (including drug-induced) in the elderly intolerant of more potent agents, for mild cases in other age groups and in combination with centrally acting anticholinergics; as a nonnarcotic cough suppressant (syrup only).

Hydroxyzine: In addition to uses discussed in the general monograph, hydroxyzine is indicated for: Sedation (oral only); analgesia, adjunctive therapy (parenteral only); antiemetic (parenteral only); used for management of anxiety, tension and psychomotor agitation in conditions of emotional stress.

Promethazine: In addition to uses discussed in the general monograph, promethazine is indicated for: Active and prophylactic treatment of motion sickness; preoperative, postoperative, or obstetric sedation; prevention and control of nausea and vomiting associated with anesthesia and surgery; an adjunct to analgesics for control of postoperative pain; sedation and relief of apprehension, and to produce light sleep; antiemetic effect in postoperative patients.

IV – Special surgical situations such as repeated bronchoscopy, ophthalmic surgery, poor risk patients, and with reduced amounts of meperidine or other narcotic analgesics as an adjunct to anesthesia and analgesia.

Administration and Dosage
AZATADINE MALEATE:
> *Adults and children > 12 years of age* – 1 or 2 mg twice/day.

AZELASTINE: Before initial use, replace the screw cap on the bottle with the pump unit and prime the delivery system with 4 sprays or until a fine mist appears. When ≥ 3 days have elapsed since last use, reprime the pump with 2 sprays or until a fine mist appears.
> *Seasonal allergic rhinitis –*
>> *Adults and children ≥ 12 years of age:* 2 sprays per nostril twice daily.
>> *Children 5 to 11 years of age:* 1 spray per nostril twice daily.
>
> *Vasomotor rhinitis –*
>> *Adults and children ≥ 12 years of age:* 2 sprays per nostril twice daily.
>
> *Caution* – Avoid spraying in the eyes.

CETIRIZINE HCl:
> *Adults and children ≥ 12 years of age* – 5 or 10 mg once daily depending on symptom severity. May be given with or without food.
>
> *Children 6 to 11 years of age* – 5 or 10 mg once daily depending on symptom severity.
>
> *Children 2 to 5 years of age* – 2.5 mg once daily. The dosage in this age group can be increased to a maximum dose of 5 mg/day as 5 mg once daily or as 2.5 mg given every 12 hours, depending on symptom severity and patient response.
>
> *Renal/Hepatic function impairment* – In patients ≥ 12 years of age with decreased renal function (creatinine clearance 11 to 31 mL/min), hemodialysis patients (creatinine clearance < 7 mL/min), and in hepatically impaired patients, 5 mg once daily is recommended. Similarly, pediatric patients 6 to 11 years of age with impaired renal or hepatic function should use the lower recommended dose. Because of the difficulty in reliably administering doses of < 2.5 mg of syrup and in the absence of pharmacokinetic and safety information in children < 6 years of age with impaired renal or hepatic function, its use in this impaired patient population is not recommended.

CHLORPHENIRAMINE MALEATE: Individualize dosage.
> *Tablets or syrup* – Administration with food delays absorption but does not affect bioavailability.
>> *Adults and children ≥ 12 years of age:* 4 mg every 4 to 6 hours. Do not exceed 24 mg in 24 hours.
>> *Children:*
>>> 6 to 12 years of age – 2 mg (break 4 mg tablets in half) every 4 to 6 hours. Do not exceed 12 mg in 24 hours.
>>> 2 to 6 years of age – 1 mg (¼ of a 4 mg tablet) every 4 to 6 hours.
>
> *Timed-release tablets –*
>> *Adults and children ≥ 12 years of age:* 8 mg every 8 to 12 hours; 12 mg every 12 hours. Do not exceed 24 mg in 24 hours.
>
> *Sustained-release capsules –*
>> *Adults and children ≥ 12 years of age:* 8 or 12 mg every 12 hours, up to 16 to 24 mg/day.
>> *Children 6 to 12 years of age:* 8 mg at bedtime or during the day as indicated.

CLEMASTINE FUMARATE:
> *Allergic rhinitis –*
>> *Adults:* 1.34 mg twice/day. Do not exceed 8.04 mg/day.
>> *Children 6 to 12 years of age (syrup only):* 0.67 mg twice/day. Do not exceed 4.02 mg/day.
>
> *Urticaria/angioedema –*
>> *Adults:* 2.68 mg 1 to 3 times/day. Do not exceed 8.04 mg/day.
>> *Children 6 to 12 years of age (syrup only):* 1.34 mg twice/day. Do not exceed 4.02 mg/day.

CYPROHEPTADINE HCl:

Adults – 4 to 20 mg/day. Initiate therapy with 4 mg 3 times/day. A majority of patients require 12 to 16 mg/day and occasionally as much as 32 mg/day. Do not exceed 0.5 mg/kg/day (0.23 mg/lb/day).

Children – Calculate total daily dosage as ≈ 0.25 mg/kg (0.11 mg/lb) or 8 mg/m^2.

Children 7 to 14 years of age: 4 mg 2 or 3 times/day. Do not exceed 16 mg/day.

Children 2 to 6 years of age: 2 mg 2 or 3 times/day. Do not exceed 12 mg/day.

DESLORATADINE:

Adults and children ≥ 12 years of age – The recommended dose is 5 mg once daily. In patients with liver or renal impairment, a starting dose of one 5 mg tablet every other day is recommended based on pharmacokinetic data.

DEXCHLORPHENIRAMINE MALEATE:

Adults ≥ 12 years of age – 2 mg every 4 to 6 hours, or 4 to 6 mg timed-release tablets at bedtime, or every 8 to 10 hours during the day.

Children –

6 to 11 years of age: 1 mg every 4 to 6 hours or a 4 mg timed-release tablet once daily at bedtime.

2 to 5 years of age: 0.5 mg every 4 to 6 hours. Do not use timed-release form.

DIPHENHYDRAMINE HCl:

Oral –

Adults: 25 to 50 mg every 4 to 8 hours.

Children (over 10 kg): 12.5 to 25 mg 3 or 4 times/day or 5 mg/kg/day or 150 mg/m^2/day. Maximum daily dosage is 300 mg.

In motion sickness – In motion sickness, give full dosage for prophylactic use; give the first dose 30 minutes before exposure to motion and similar doses before meals and at bedtime for the duration of exposure.

Parenteral – Administer IV or deeply IM.

Adults: 10 to 50 mg; 100 mg if required; maximum daily dosage is 400 mg.

Children: 5 mg/kg/day or 150 mg/m^2/day. Maximum daily dosage is 300 mg divided into 4 doses.

Nighttime sleep aid –

Adults and children ≥ 12 years of age: 50 mg at bedtime.

Antitussive (syrup only) –

Adults: 25 mg (10 mL) every 4 hours, not to exceed 100 mg (40 mL) in 24 hours.

Children:

6 to 12 years of age – 12.5 mg (5 mL) every 4 hours, not to exceed 50 mg (20 mL) in 24 hours.

2 to 6 years of age – 6.25 mg (2.5 mL) every 4 hours, not to exceed 25 mg (10 mL) in 24 hours.

FEXOFENADINE:

Seasonal allergic rhinitis –

Adults and children ≥ 12 years of age: 60 mg twice/day or 180 mg once daily.

Children 6 to 11 years of age: 30 mg twice/day.

Chronic idiopathic urticaria –

Adults and children ≥ 12 years of age: 60 mg twice/day.

Children 6 to 11 years of age: 30 mg twice/day.

Renal function impairment –

Adults and children ≥ 12 years of age: 60 mg once daily as a starting dose.

Children 6 to 11 years of age: 30 mg once daily as a starting dose.

HYDROXYZINE:

Pruritus –

Oral:

Adults – 25 mg 3 or 4 times/day.

Children –

> 6 years: 50 to 100 mg/day in divided doses.

< 6 years: 50 mg/day in divided doses.

Parenteral:

Adults – 25 mg 3 to 4 times/day.

Sedation (oral only) –

Adults: 50 to 100 mg as premedication or following general anesthesia. Hydroxyzine may potentiate concomitant narcotics and barbiturates; reduce dosages accordingly. Atropine and other belladonna alkaloids may be give as appropriate.

Children: 0.6 mg/kg.

Antiemetic/Analgesia, adjunctive therapy (parenteral only) –

Adults: 25 to 100 mg IM as pre- and postoperative and pre- and post-partum adjunctive medication to permit reduction of narcotic dosage and control emesis.

Children: 0.5 mg/lb IM as pre- and postoperative adjunctive therapy to permit reduction of narcotic dosage and control emesis.

Oral suspension – Shake vigorously until product is completely resuspended.

LORATADINE:

Adults and children ≥ 6 years of age – 10 mg once daily.

Children 2 to 5 years of age – 5 mg (5 mL) syrup once daily.

Hepatic/Renal function impairment (GFR < 30 mL/min) –

Adults and children ≥ 6 years of age: 10 mg every other day as starting dose.

Children 2 to 5 years of age: 5 mg every other day as starting dose.

Rapidly disintegrating tablets – Place rapidly disintegrating tablets on the tongue. Tablet disintegration occurs rapidly. Administer with or without water.

Use within 6 months of opening laminated foil pouch and immediately upon opening individual tablet blister.

PHENINDAMINE TARTRATE:

Adults and children > 12 years of age – 25 mg every 4 to 6 hours. Do not exceed 150 mg in 24 hours.

Children 6 to < 11 years of age – 12.5 mg every 4 to 6 hours. Do not exceed 75 mg in 24 hours.

PROMETHAZINE HCl: The preferred parenteral route of administration is deep IM injection; properly administered IV doses are well tolerated, but this method is associated with increased hazard. IV administration should be ≤ 25 mg/mL at a rate ≤ 25 mg/min. Avoid SC and intra-arterial injection because tissue necrosis and gangrene can result.

Individualize dosage; after initiation, adjust to smallest effective dose.

Hypersensitivity reactions, Type I –

Oral/Rectal: May be administered rectally or parenterally if the oral route is not feasible; however, resume oral administration as soon as possible if continued therapy is warranted.

Adults – Usual dose is 25 mg at bedtime; 12.5 mg before meals and at bedtime may be given, if necessary.

Children > 2 years of age – Single 25 mg dose at bedtime or 6.25 to 12.5 mg 3 times daily.

Parenteral:

Adults – 25 mg; may repeat dose within 2 hours if needed. Resume oral therapy as soon as patient's circumstances permit.

Children 2 to 12 years of age – ≤ 12.5 mg; dose should not exceed half the adult dose.

Sedation –

Oral/Rectal: If used for preoperative sedation, administer the night before surgery to relieve apprehension and produce quiet sleep.

Adults – 25 to 50 mg at bedtime.

Children > 2 years of age – 12.5 to 25 mg at bedtime.

Parenteral:

Adults – 25 to 50 mg at bedtime for nighttime sedation. May be combined with hypnotic agents for pre- and postoperative sedation; reduce concomitant hypnotic, analgesic and barbiturate dosage accordingly. Doses of 50 mg provide sedation and relieve apprehension during early stages of labor. Do not exceed 100 mg/24 hours for patients in labor.

Children 2 to 12 years of age – Do not exceed half the adult dose.

Antiemetic –

  Oral/Rectal:

    Adults – Usual dose is 25 mg; doses of 12.5 to 25 mg may be repeated every 4 to 6 hours as needed for prophylaxis or treatment of active nausea/vomiting.

    Children > 2 years of age – Usual dose is 25 mg or 0.5 mg/lb; doses of 12.5 to 25 mg may be repeated every 4 to 6 hours as needed for prophylaxis or treatment of active nausea/vomiting. Adjust dose to the age, weight, and severity of condition for the patient being treated.

  Parenteral:

    Adults – Usual dose is 12.5 to 25 mg, may repeat every 4 hours as needed. If used postoperatively, reduce doses of concomitant hypnotics, analgesics, or barbiturates accordingly.

    Children 2 to 12 years of age – Do not exceed half the adult dose. Do not use when etiology of vomiting is unknown.

  Motion sickness (oral and rectal only) –

    Adults: Usual dose is 25 mg twice/day; take first dose 30 to 60 minutes before anticipated travel; repeat 8 to 12 hours later if needed. On successive travel days, take on rising and again before the evening meal.

    Children > 2 years of age: 12.5 to 25 mg twice/day.

  Analgesia – As an adjunct to pre- and postoperative medications.

  Oral/Rectal:

    Adults – 50 mg administered with an equal amount of meperidine and an appropriate dose of belladonna alkaloid.

    Children > 2 years of age – 0.5 mg/lb in combination with an equal dose of meperdine and an atropine-like agent as appropriate.

  Parenteral:

    Adults – 25 to 50 mg in combination with appropriately reduced doses of analgesics and hypnotics; administer atropine-like drugs as appropriate.

    Children 2 to 12 years of age – 0.5 mg/lb in combination with an equal dose of analgesic or barbiturate and an appropriate dose of an atropine-like agent.

TRIPELENNAMINE HCl:

  Tablets and elixir –

    Adults: 25 to 50 mg every 4 to 6 hours. As little as 25 mg may control symptoms; as much as 600 mg/day may be given in divided doses.

    Children and infants: 5 mg/kg/day or 150 mg/m^2/day divided into 4 to 6 doses. Maximum total dose is 300 mg/day.

  Extended-release tablets –

    Adults: 100 mg in the morning and evening. In difficult cases, 100 mg every 8 hours may be required. Do not crush or chew extended release tablets.

    Children: Do not use in children.

Actions

Pharmacology:

Antihistamines: Dosage and Effects						
Antihistamine	Dose^1 (mg)	Dosing interval^2 (hrs)	Sedative effects	Antihistaminic activity	Anticholinergic activity	Antiemetic effects
First-Generation (non-selective)						
Alkylamines						
Brompheniramine	4	4 to 6	+	+++	++	—
Chlorpheniramine	4	4 to 6	+	++	++	—
Dexchlorpheniramine	2	4 to 6	+	+++	++	—
Ethanolamines						
Clemastine	1	12	++	+ to ++	+++	++ to +++
Diphenhydramine	25 to 50	6 to 8	+++	+ to ++	+++	++ to +++
Phenothiazines						
Promethazine	12.5 to 25	6 to 24	+++	+++	+++	++++

Antihistamines: Dosage and Effects						
Antihistamine	Dose[1] (mg)	Dosing interval[2] (hrs)	Sedative effects	Antihistaminic activity	Anticholinergic activity	Antiemetic effects
Piperazines						
Hydroxyzine	25 to 100	4 to 8	+++	++ to +++	++	+++
Piperidines						
Azatadine	1 to 2	12	++	++	++	—
Cyproheptadine	4	8	+	++	++	—
Phenindamine	25	4 to 6	±	++	++	—
Second-Generation (peripherally selective)						
Phthalazinone						
Azelastine[3]	0.5	12	±	++ to +++	±	—
Piperazine						
Cetirizine	5 to 10	24	±	++ to +++	±	—
Piperidines						
Fexofenadine	60	12	±	—	±	—
Loratadine	10	24	±	++ to +++	±	—

* ++++ = very high, +++ = high, ++ = moderate, + = low, ± = low to none. — = No data.
[1] Usual single adult dose.
[2] For conventional dosage forms.
[3] Some effects may be enhanced or reduced as a result of administration via the nasal route.

Pharmacokinetics:
Pharmacokinetics – Pharmacokinetics of first-generation agents have not been extensively studied. With a few exceptions, these agents are well absorbed following oral administration, have an onset of action within 15 to 30 minutes, are maximal within 1 to 2 hours and have a duration of ≈ 4 to 6 hours, although some are much longer acting. Most are metabolized by liver. Antihistamine metabolites and small amounts of unchanged drug are excreted in urine.
Second-generation agents –

Pharmacokinetics of Peripherally Selective H₁ Antagonists						
	Onset of action	T_{max} (hours)	Elimination t½ (hours)	Protein binding (%)	P450 metabolism	Food effect on absorption
Cetirizine	rapid	1	8.3	93	↓; 50% excreted unchanged	delayed 1.7 hours
Fexofenadine	rapid	2.6	14.4	60-70	↓↓; 95% excreted unchanged	—
Loratadine	rapid	1.3-2.5[1]	8.4-28[2]	97 (75)[2]	↑; 3A4, 2D6	delayed 1 hour

↑ = High ↓ = Low ↓↓ = Very low
[1] All active constituents (parent drug and active metabolites)
[2] Active metabolite
— = No data

Contraindications

First-generation antihistamines: Hypersensitivity to specific or structurally related antihistamines; newborn or premature infants (see Warnings); nursing mothers (see Warnings); narrow-angle glaucoma; stenosing peptic ulcer; symptomatic prostatic hypertrophy; bladder neck obstruction; pyloroduodenal obstruction; monoamine oxidase inhibitor (MAOI) use (see Drug Interactions); elderly, debilitated patients (**cyproheptadine**).

Second-generation antihistamines: Hypersensitivity to specific or structurally related antihistamines.

Warnings

Respiratory disease: In general, antihistamines are not recommended to treat *lower* respiratory tract symptoms including asthma, as their anticholinergic (drying) effects may cause thickening of secretions and impair expectoration.

Pre- and postoperative adjunctive therapy: Nonselective antihistamines may potentiate CNS depressants, such as narcotics, nonnarcotic analgesics, and barbiturates. Narcotic requirements may be reduced by as much as 50%. Reduce dosage appropriately.

Seizure threshold: **Promethazine** may lower the seizure threshold; consider this when giving to people with known seizure disorders or when giving in combination with narcotics or local anesthetics that may also affect seizure threshold.

Sleep apnea: Avoid sedatives and CNS depressants in patients with a history of sleep apnea.

Drug abuse: Nonmedical parenteral use of concurrent **butorphanol** and **diphenhydramine** has also been reported.

Hypersensitivity reactions: Hypersensitivity reactions may occur, and any of the usual manifestations of drug allergy may develop.

Renal/Hepatic function impairment: Use a lower initial dose of **loratadine** (10 mg every other day) in patients with renal or hepatic impairment.

Elderly: Antihistamines are more likely to cause dizziness, excessive sedation, syncope, toxic confusional states, and hypotension in elderly patients. Dosage reduction may be required. Phenothiazine side effects are more prone to develop in the elderly.

Pregnancy: (*Category B* – chlorpheniramine, dexchlorpheniramine, brompheniramine, cetirizine, diphenhydramine, cyproheptadine, clemastine, azatadine, loratadine. *Category C* – azelastine, promethazine, fexofenadine, hydroxyzine). Do not use during the third trimester; newborn and premature infants may have severe reactions (eg, convulsions).

Lactation: Due to the higher risk of adverse effects for infants generally, and for newborns and prematures in particular, antihistamine therapy is contraindicated in nursing mothers.

Children: Antihistamines may diminish mental alertness; conversely, they may occasionally produce excitation, particularly in the young child.

Avoid using **phenothiazines** in children with hepatic diseases, Reye's syndrome, a history of sleep apnea, or a family history of sudden infant death syndrome (SIDS).

Precautions

Hematologic: Use **promethazine** with caution in bone marrow depression. Leukopenia and agranulocytosis have been reported, usually when used with other toxic agents.

Anticholinergic effects: Antihistamines have varying degrees of atropine-like actions; use with caution in patients with a predisposition to urinary retention, history of bronchial asthma, increased intraocular pressure, hyperthyroidism, cardiovascular disease, or hypertension.

Phenothiazines: Use phenothiazines with caution in patients with cardiovascular disease, liver dysfunction, or ulcer disease. Promethazine has been associated with cholestatic jaundice.

Use cautiously in people with acute or chronic respiratory impairment, particularly children, because phenothiazines may suppress the cough reflex. If hypotension occurs, epinephrine is not recommended because phenothiazines may reverse its usual pressor effect and cause a paradoxical further lowering of blood pressure. Because these drugs have an antiemetic action, they may obscure signs of intestinal obstruction, brain tumor, or overdosage of toxic drugs.

Photosensitivity: Photosensitization may occur.

Hazardous tasks: May cause drowsiness and reduce mental alertness; patients should not drive or perform other tasks requiring alertness, coordination, or physical dexterity. Astemizole, loratadine, and fexofenadine appear to cause less sedation.

Drug Interactions

Drugs that may affect antihistamines include MAO inhibitors. Drugs that may affect antihistamines, specifically loratadine, include ketoconazole, cimetidine, and erythromycin. Drugs that may be affected by antihistamines include MAO inhibitors, alcohol, and CNS depressants.

See the Antipsychotic Agents monograph for drug interactions that relate to the 3 phenothiazine antihistamines: Promethazine, trimeprazine, and methdilazine.

Drug/Lab test interactions: Diagnostic pregnancy tests based on immunological reactions between HCG and anti-HCG may result in false-negative or false-positive interpretations in patients on promethazine. Increased blood glucose has occurred in promethazine patients.

Phenothiazines may increase **serum cholesterol, spinal fluid protein**, and **urinary urobilinogen levels**; decrease **protein bound iodine (PBI)**; yield false-positive **urine bilirubin tests**; interfere with **urinary ketone** and **steroid determinations**.

Discontinue antihistamines ≈ 4 days prior to skin testing procedures; these drugs may prevent or diminish otherwise positive reactions to dermal reactivity indicators.

Adverse Reactions

Adverse reactions may include: Peripheral, angioneurotic, and laryngeal edema; anaphylactic shock; photosensitivity; reflex tachycardia; extrasystoles; venous thrombosis at injection site (**IV promethazine**); cardiac arrest; ECG changes, including blunting of T-waves and prolongation of the QT interval; disturbed coordination; dermatitis; asthma; lupus erythematosus-like syndrome; urticaria; drug rash; postural hypotension; palpitations; bradycardia; tachycardia; faintness; increases and decreases in blood pressure; drowsiness (often transient); sedation; dizziness; headache (loratadine); epigastric distress, especially ethylenediamines; urinary frequency; dysuria; urinary retention; anemias; thrombocytopenia; leukopenia; agranulocytosis; pancytopenia; thickening of bronchial secretions; tingling, heaviness and weakness of the hands; bitter taste, eye pain/tearing, sneezing (nasal spray).

CODEINE

Tablets: 15, 30, and 60 mg (c-II)   Various

Indications

Cough: For suppression of cough induced by chemical or mechanical respiratory tract irritation.

Pain: Relief of mild to moderate pain.

Administration and Dosage

Adults: 10 to 20 mg every 4 to 6 hours. Maximum 120 mg/day.

Children:

6 to 12 years – 5 to 10 mg every 4 to 6 hours. Maximum 60 mg/day.

2 to 6 years – 2.5 to 5 mg every 4 to 6 hours. Maximum 30 mg/day.

Codeine is also available in many multi-ingredient respiratory preparations as an antitussive.

Actions

Pharmacology: Codeine has good antitussive activity. The dose required to suppress coughing is lower than the dose required for analgesia.

Pharmacokinetics: Codeine and its salts are well absorbed. Codeine is metabolized primarily in the liver and is excreted primarily in the urine within 24 hours, 5% to 15% as unchanged codeine and the remainder as the products of glucuronide conjugation and metabolites. The plasma half-life of codeine is ≈ 2.9 hours.

Contraindications

Hypersensitivity to the drug; premature infants or during labor when delivery of a premature infant is anticipated.

Warnings

Head injury and increased intracranial pressure: The respiratory depressant effects of the opiates and their capacity to elevate cerebrospinal fluid pressure may be markedly exaggerated in the presence of head injury, intracranial lesions or a preexisting increase in intracranial pressure. Usual oral doses of codeine produce little respiratory depression; however, exercise caution, particularly with larger doses.

Asthma and other respiratory conditions: Use with extreme caution in patients having an acute asthmatic attack, patients with chronic obstructive pulmonary disease or cor pulmonale, patients having a substantially decreased respiratory reserve, and patients with preexisting respiratory depression, hypoxia, or hypercapnia.

Acute abdominal conditions: Administration of codeine or other opiates may obscure the diagnosis or clinical course in patients with acute abdominal conditions.

Pregnancy: Category C.

Labor and delivery – Opiates cross the placental barrier. The closer to delivery and the larger the dose used, the greater the possibility of respiratory depression in the newborn. Avoid use during labor if a premature infant is anticipated.

Lactation: Some studies have reported detectable amounts of codeine in breast milk.

Children: Do not use opiates, including codeine, in premature infants. Give opiates to infants and small children only with great caution and carefully monitor dosage. Safety and efficacy of codeine in newborn infants have not been established.

Precautions

Administer with caution: Administer with caution, and reduce the initial dose in patients with acute abdominal conditions, convulsive disorders, significant hepatic or renal impairment, fever, hypothyroidism, Addison's disease, ulcerative colitis, prostatic hypertrophy, urethral stricture, patients with recent GI or urinary tract surgery, and in very young, elderly, or debilitated patients.

Drug abuse and dependence: The abuse potential of codeine is less than that of heroin or morphine. Psychological dependence, physical dependence, and tolerance may occur.

Drug Interactions

CNS depressants and alcohol. Use codeine cautiously and in reduced dosage to avoid additive effects when given concomitantly.

Drug/Lab test interactions: Because opiates may increase biliary tract pressure, with resultant increases in plasma amylase or lipase levels, determination of these enzyme levels may be unreliable for 24 hours after an opiate has been given.

Adverse Reactions

Adverse reactions associated with codeine may include nausea, vomiting, sedation, dizziness, constipation, lightheadedness, euphoria, dysphoria, weakness, headache, hallucinations, disorientation, visual disturbances, convulsions, pruritus, giant urticaria, and laryngeal edema.

DEXTROMETHORPHAN HBr

Capsules: 30 mg (otc)	*Drixoral Cough Liquid Caps* (Schering-Plough)
Lozenges: 2.5, 5, 7.5, and 15 mg (otc)	*Scot-Tussin DM Cough Chasers* (Scot-Tussin), *Children's Hold* (Menley & James), *Hold DM* (Menley & James), *Robitussin Cough Calmers* (Robins), *Sucrets Cough Control* (SK-Beecham), *Suppress* (Ferndale), *Trocal* (Hauck), *Sucrets 4-Hour Cough* (SK-Beecham)
Liquid: 10 mg/15 mL (3.33 mg/5 mL) (otc)	*Creo-Terpin* (Lee)
3.5, 7.5, and 15 mg/5 mL (otc)	*Pertussin CS* (Pertussin), *Robitussin Pediatric* (Robins), *Benylin Pediatric* (Warner Wellcome), *St. Joseph Cough Suppressant* (Schering–Plough), *Benylin Adult* (Warner Wellcome), *Pertussin ES* (Pertussin), *Vicks Dry Hacking Cough* (Richardson-Vicks)
10 mg/5 mL (otc)	*Various, Benylin DM* (Parke-Davis), *Silphen DM* (Silarx)
Liquid, sustained action: Dextromethorphan polistirex equivalent to 30 mg dextromethorphan HBr/5 mL (otc)	*Delsym* (Fisons)

Indications

To control nonproductive cough.

Administration and Dosage

Liquid, lozenges, and syrup: Adults and children (> 12 years of age) - 10 to 30 mg every 4 to 8 hours. Do not exceed 120 mg in 24 hours.

Children (6 to 12 years of age) – 5 to 10 mg every 4 hours or 15 mg every 6 to 8 hours. Do not exceed 60 mg in 24 hours.

Children (2 to 6 years of age) – 2.5 to 7.5 mg every 4 to 8 hours. Do not exceed 30 mg/day.

Children (< 2 years of age) – Use only as directed by a physician.

Sustained action liquid:
Adults – 60 mg every 12 hours.
Children (6 to 12 years of age) – 30 mg every 12 hours.
Children (2 to 5 years of age) – 15 mg every 12 hours.

Actions

Pharmacology: Dextromethorphan is the d-isomer of the codeine analog of levorphanol; it lacks analgesic and addictive properties. Its cough suppressant action is due to a central action on the cough center in the medulla. Dextromethorphan 15 to 30 mg equals 8 to 15 mg codeine as an antitussive.

Contraindications

Hypersensitivity to any component.

Warnings

Do not use: Do not use for persistent or chronic cough or cough accompanied by excessive secretions.

Drug abuse and dependence: Anecdotal reports of abuse of dextromethorphan-containing cough/cold products has increased, especially among teenagers.

Drug Interactions

Drugs that may interact with dextromethorphan include MAO inhibitors.

DIPHENHYDRAMINE HCl

Syrup: 12.5 mg/5 mL (*otc*)[1]   Various, *Silphen Cough* (Silarx), *Tusstat* (Century)

[1] Products available *otc* or *Rx* depending on product labeling.

Indications
For the control of cough due to colds or allergy.

Administration and Dosage
Adults: 25 mg every 4 hours, not to exceed 150 mg in 24 hours.

Children (6 to 12 years of age): 12.5 mg every 4 hours, not to exceed 75 mg in 24 hours.

Children (2 to 6 years of age): 6.25 mg every 4 hours, not to exceed 25 mg in 24 hours.

BENZONATATE

Capsules: 100 mg (*Rx*)   Various, *Tessalon Perles* (Forest)

Indications
Symptomatic relief of cough.

Administration and Dosage
Adults and children (> 10 years of age): 100 mg 3 times/day, up to 600 mg/day.

Actions
Pharmacology: Benzonatate is related to tetracaine. It anesthetizes stretch receptors in respiratory passages, lungs, and pleura, dampening their activity, and reducing the cough reflex at its source. It has no inhibitory effect on the respiratory center in recommended dosage. Onset of action is 15 to 20 minutes; effects last 3 to 8 hours.

Contraindications
Hypersensitivity to benzonatate or related compounds (eg, tetracaine).

Warnings
Pregnancy: Category C.

Lactation: It is not known whether this drug is excreted in breast milk.

Precautions
Local anesthesia: Release of benzonatate in the mouth can produce a temporary local anesthesia of the oral mucosa. Swallow the capsules without chewing.

Adverse Reactions
Sedation; headache; mild dizziness; constipation; nausea; GI upset; pruritus; skin eruptions; nasal congestion; sensation of burning in the eyes; a vague "chilly" sensation; chest numbness; hypersensitivity.

DEXTROMETHORPHAN HBr and BENZOCAINE

Lozenges: 10 mg dextromethorphan HBr and 10 mg benzocaine (*otc*)	*Spec-T* (Apothecon)
5 mg dextromethorphan and 2 mg benzocaine (*otc*)	*Cough-X* (Ascher)
5 mg dextromethorphan HBr and 1.25 mg benzocaine (*otc*)	*Vicks Formula 44 Cough Control Discs* (Richardson-Vicks)
2.5 mg dextromethorphan HBr and 1 mg benzocaine (*otc*)	*Vicks Cough Silencers* (Richardson-Vicks)

Administration and Dosage

Vicks Formula 44:

Adults and children ≥ 12 years of age – 2 lozenges dissolved in mouth, one at a time, every 4 hours. Do not exceed 12 lozenges in 24 hours.

Children 3 to 12 years of age – 1 lozenge every 4 hours. Do not exceed 6 in 24 hours.

Children < 3 years of age – Use only as directed by physician.

Vicks Cough Silencers:

Adults and children ≥ 12 years of age – 4 lozenges dissolved in mouth, one at a time, every 4 hours. Do not exceed 48 lozenges in 24 hours.

Children 6 to < 12 years of age – 2 to 4 lozenges every 4 hours. Do not exceed 24 in 24 hours.

Children 2 to < 6 years of age – 1 to 2 lozenges every 4 hours. Do not exceed 12 in 24 hours.

Children < 2 years of age – Use only as directed by physician.

Spec-T:

Adults and children ≥ 6 years of age – 1 every 3 hours. Do not exceed 6 in 24 hours.

Children < 6 years of age – Use only as directed.

Cough-X:

Adults and children ≥ 6 years of age – 1 every 2 hours, up to 12/day.

Children 2 to 6 years of age – 1 every 4 hours, up to 6/day.

Children < 2 of age – Use only as directed by physician.

ZAFIRLUKAST

Tablets: 20 mg (*Rx*)   *Accolate* (Zeneca)

Indications

Asthma: Prophylaxis and chronic treatment of asthma in adults and children ≥ 12 years of age.

Administration and Dosage

The recommended dose of zafirlukast is 20 mg twice/day in adults and children ≥ 12 years of age. Because food reduces bioavailability of zafirlukast, take ≥ 1 hour before or 2 hours after meals.

Actions

Pharmacology: Zafirlukast is a selective and competitive leukotreine receptor antagonist (LTRA) of leukotreine D_4 and E_4 (LTD_4 and LTE_4), components of slow-reacting substance of anaphylaxis (SRSA).

Pharmacokinetics: Oral zafirlukast is rapidly absorbed. Peak plasma concentrations are achieved 3 hours after dosing. The mean terminal elimination half-life of zafirlukast is ≈ 10 hours in both healthy subjects and patients with asthma. Zafirlukast is > 99% bound to plasma proteins, predominantly albumin.

Zafirlukast is extensively metabolized. Urinary excretion accounts for ≈ 10% of the dose and the remainder is excreted in the feces. Liver microsomes that hydroxylate metabolites of zafirlukast are formed through the cytochrome P450 2C9 (CYP2C9) enzyme pathway.

Contraindications

Hypersensitivity to zafirlukast or any of its inactive ingredients.

Warnings

Acute asthma attacks: Zafirlukast is not indicated for use in the reversal of bronchospasm in acute asthma attacks, including status asthmaticus.

Infection: An increased proportion of zafirlukast patients > 55 years of age reported infections as compared to placebo-treated patients.

Hepatic function impairment: The clearance of zafirlukast is reduced in patients with stable alcoholic cirrhosis.

Elderly: The clearance of zafirlukast is reduced in elderly patients (≥ 65 years of age), such that C_{max} and AUC are approximately twice those of younger adults.

Pregnancy: Category B.

Lactation: Zafirlukast is excreted in breast milk.

Children: The safety and effectiveness of zafirlukast in patients < 12 years of age have not been established.

Drug Interactions

Due to zafirlukast's inhibition of cytochrome P450 2C9 and 3A4 isoenzymes, use caution with coadministration of drugs known to be metabolized by these isoenzymes.

Drugs that may affect zafirlukast include aspirin, erythromycin, and theophylline.

Drugs that may be affected by zafirlukast include warfarin.

Drug/Food interactions: The bioavailability of zafirlukast may be decreased when taken with food. Take zafirlukast at least 1 hour before or 2 hours after meals.

Adverse Reactions

Adverse reactions occurring in ≥ 3% of patients include headache, nausea, infection.

ZILEUTON

Tablets: 600 mg (*Rx*)   *Zyflo* (Abbott)

Indications

Asthma: The prophylaxis and chronic treatment of asthma in adults and children ≥ 12 years of age.

Administration and Dosage

The recommended dosage of zileuton for the symptomatic treatment of patients with asthma is 600 mg 4 times/day for a total daily dose of 2400 mg. For ease of administration, zileuton may be taken with meals and at bedtime.

Actions

Pharmacology: Zileuton is a specific inhibitor of 5-lipoxygenase and thus inhibits leukotriene (LTB_1, LTC_1, LTD_1, LTe_1) formation.

Zileuton inhibits leukotriene-dependent smooth muscle contractions. Pretreatment with zileuton attenuated bronchoconstriction caused by cold air challenge in patients with asthma.

Pharmacokinetics:

Absorption – Zileuton is rapidly absorbed upon oral administration with a mean time to peak plasma concentration (T_{max}) of 1.7 hours and a mean peak level (C_{max}) of 4.98 mcg/mL. Plasma concentrations of zileuton are proportional to dose.

Distribution – The apparent volume of distribution of zileuton is ≈ 1.2 L/kg. Zileuton is 93% bound to plasma proteins, primarily to albumin, with minor binding to alpha-acid glycoprotein.

Metabolism – Several zileuton metabolites have been identified in plasma and urine. These include two diastereomeric O-glucuronide conjugates (major metabolites) and an N-dehydroxylated metabolite and unchanged zileuton each accounted for < 0.5% of the dose. Liver microsomes have shown that zileuton and its N-dehydroxylated metabolite can be oxidatively metabolized by the cytochrome P450 isoenzymes 1A2, 2C9, and 3A4 (CYP1A2, CYP2C9, and CYP3A4).

Excretion – Elimination of zileuton is predominantly via metabolism with a mean terminal half-life of 2.5 hours. Zileuton activity is primarily because of the parent drug. Orally administered zileuton is well absorbed into the systemic circulation with 94.5% and 2.2% of the dose recovered in urine and feces, respectively.

Contraindications

Active liver disease or transaminase elevations ≥ 3 times the upper limit of normal, hypersensitivity to zileuton or any of its inactive ingredients.

Warnings

Hepatotoxicity: Elevations of ≥ 1 liver function tests may occur during zileuton therapy. These laboratory abnormalities may progress, remain unchanged or resolve with continued therapy.

Acute asthma attacks: Zileuton is not indicated for use in the reversal of bronchospasm in acute asthma attacks, including status asthmaticus.

Hematologic: Occurrences of low white blood cell count (≤ 2.8×10^9/L) were observed in 1% of 1678 patients taking zileuton and 0.6% of 1056 patients taking placebo.

Hepatic function impairment: Use with caution in patients who consume substantial quantities of alcohol or have a history of liver disease.

Pregnancy: Category C.

Lactation: Zileuton and its metabolites are excreted in rat milk. It is not known if zileuton is excreted in breast milk.

Children: The safety and effectiveness of zileuton in pediatric patients < 12 years of age have not been established.

Precautions

Monitoring: Evaluate hepatic transaminases at initiation of and during therapy with zileuton. Monitor serum ALT before treatment begins, once-a-month for the first 3 months, every 2 to 3 months for the remainder of the first year and periodically thereafter for patients receiving long-term zileuton therapy. If symptoms of liver dysfunction develop or transaminase elevations > 5 time the ULN occur, discontinue therapy and follow transaminase levels until normal.

Drug Interactions

Liver microsomes have shown that zileuton and its N-dehydroxylated metabolite can be oxidatively metabolized by the cytochrome P450 isoenzymes 1A2, 2C9, and 3A4. Use caution when prescribing a medication that inhibits any of these enzymes.

Drugs that may be affected by zileuton include propranolol, terfenadine, theophylline, and warfarin.

Drugs that may affect zileuton include digoxin, oral contraceptives, phenytoin, and prednisone.

Adverse Reactions

Adverse reactions occurring ≥ 3% of patients include headache; pain; abdominal pain; asthenia; accidental injury; dyspepsia; nausea; ALT elevation; myalgia.

MONTELUKAST SODIUM

| **Tablets**: 10 mg (*Rx*) | *Singulair* (Merck & Co.) |
| **Tablets, chewable**: 4 and 5 mg (*Rx*) | *Singulair* (Merck & Co.) |

Indications

Asthma: Prophylaxis and chronic treatment of asthma in adults and pediatric patients ≥ 2 years of age.

Administration and Dosage

Adults and adolescents ≥ 15 years of age: One 10 mg tablet daily, taken in the evening. No additional clinical benefit to doses > 10 mg/day.

Pediatric patients 6 to 14 years of age: One 5 mg chewable tablet daily, taken in the evening.

Pediatric patients 2 to 5 years of age: One 4 mg chewable tablet daily, taken in the evening. Safety and effectiveness in pediatric patients < 2 years of age have not been established.

Actions

Pharmacology: Montelukast is a selective and orally active leukotriene receptor antagonist that inhibits the cysteinyl leukotrine ($CysLT_1$) receptor.

Montelukast causes inhibition of airway CysLT receptors as demonstrated by the ability to inhibit bronchoconstriction caused by inhaled LTD_4 in asthmatics.

Pharmacokinetics:

Absorption – Montelukast is rapidly absorbed following oral administration. After administration of the 10 mg film-coated tablet to fasted adults, the mean peak plasma concentration (C_{max}) is achieved in 3 to 4 hours (T_{max}). The mean oral bioavailability is 64%. The oral bioavailability and C_{max} are not influenced by a standard meal in the morning.

Distribution – Montelukast is > 99% bound to plasma proteins.

Metabolism – Montelukast is extensively metabolized.

Excretion – The plasma clearance of montelukast averages 45 mL/min in healthy adults. Montelukast and its metabolites are excreted almost exclusively via the bile.

The mean plasma half-life ranged from 2.7 to 5.5 hours in healthy young adults.

Contraindications

Hypersensitivity to any component of this product.

Warnings

Pregnancy: Category B.

Lactation: It is not known if montelukast is excreted in human breast milk.

Children: Safety and efficacy in children < 6 years of age have not been established.

Precautions

Bronchospasm: Montelukast is not indicated for use in the reversal of bronchospasm in acute asthma attacks, including status asthmaticus.

Do not use montelukast as monotherapy for the treatment and management of exercise-induced bronchospasm.

Rescue medication: Advise patients to have appropriate rescue medication available. Therapy with montelukast can be continued during acute exacerbations of asthma.

Concurrent corticosteroids: While the dose of inhaled corticosteroid may be reduced gradually under medical supervision, montelukast should not be abruptly substituted for inhaled or oral corticosteroids.

Aspirin sensitivity: Patients with known aspirin sensitivity should continue avoidance of aspirin or nonsteroidal anti-inflammatory agents while taking montelukast.

Drug Interactions

Drugs that may interact with montelukast include phenobarbital and rifampin.

Adverse Reactions

Adverse reactions occurring in ≥ 3% of patients include headache; respiratory influenza. Pediatric patients 6 to 14 years of age demonstrated a ≥ 2% frequency of diarrhea; laryngitis; pharyngitis; nausea; otitis; sinusitis; viral infection.

Pediatric patients 2 to 5 years of age: In patients 2 to 5 years of age receiving montelukast, the following events occurred with a frequency of ≥ 2%: Rhinorrhea; otitis; ear pain; bronchitis; leg pain; thirst; sneezing; rash; urticaria.

FLUTICASONE PROPIONATE/SALMETEROL

Powder for inhalation: 100 mg fluticasone propionate/50   *Advair Diskus* (GlaxoWellcome)
mcg salmeterol, 250 mcg fluticasone propionate/50 mcg salme-
terol, 500 mcg fluticasone propionate/50 mcg salmeterol (*Rx*)

Indications

Asthma, chronic: For the long-term, twice-daily maintenance treatment of asthma in
patients ≥ 12 years of age.

Not indicated for the relief of acute bronchospasm.

Administration and Dosage

Administer by the orally inhaled route only. The maximum recommended dose of fluticasone propionate/salmeterol is 500 mcg/50 mcg twice/day.

Adults and children ≥ 12 years of age: 1 inhalation twice/day (morning and evening,
≈ 12 hours apart).

More frequent administration or a higher number of inhalations of the prescribed
strength is not recommended, as some patients are more likely to experience
adverse effects with higher doses of salmeterol. The safety and efficacy of fluticasone propionate/salmeterol when administered in excess of recommended doses have
not been established.

Patients not currently on an inhaled corticosteroid: A starting dose of fluticasone propionate/
salmeterol 100 mcg/50 mcg twice/day is recommended for patients who are not
currently on an inhaled corticosteroid and whose disease severity warrants treatment with 2 maintenance therapies, including patients on noncorticosteroid maintenance therapy.

Patients currently on an inhaled corticosteroid: The following table provides the recommended
starting dose for patients currently on an inhaled corticosteroid.

Recommended Starting Doses of Fluticasone Propionate/Salmeterol for Patients Taking Inhaled Corticosteroids		
Current daily dose of inhaled corticosteroid		Recommended strength and dosing schedule of fluticasone propionate/salmeterol diskus
Beclomethasone dipropionate	≤ 420 mcg	100 mcg/50 mcg twice/day
	462-840 mcg	250 mcg/50 mcg twice/day
Budesonide	≤ 400 mcg	100 mcg/50 mcg twice/day
	800-1200 mcg	250 mcg/50 mcg twice/day
	1600 mcg[1]	500 mcg/50 mcg twice/day
Flunisolide	≤ 1000 mcg	100 mcg/50 mcg twice/day
	1250-2000 mcg	250 mcg/50 mcg twice/day
Fluticasone propionate inhalation aerosol	≤ 176 mcg	100 mcg/50 mcg twice/day
	440 mcg	250 mcg/50 mcg twice/day
	660-880 mcg[1]	500 mcg/50 mcg twice/day
Fluticasone propionate inhalation powder	≤ 200 mcg	100 mcg/50 mcg twice/day
	500 mcg	250 mcg/50 mcg twice/day
	1000 mcg[1]	500 mcg/50 mcg twice/day
Triamcinolone acetonide	≤ 1000 mcg	100 mcg/50 mcg twice/day
	1100-1600 mcg	250 mcg/50 mcg twice/day

[1] Do not use fluticasone propionate/salmeterol for transferring patients from systemic
corticosteroid therapy.

For all patients, titrate to the lowest effective strength after adequate asthma stability is achieved.

If symptoms arise in the period between doses, administer an inhaled, short-acting
beta$_2$-agonist for immediate relief.

Patients who are receiving fluticasone propionate/salmeterol twice daily should not
use salmeterol for prevention of exercise-induced bronchospasm, or for any other
reason.

Improvement in asthma control following inhaled administration of fluticasone pro-
pionate/salmeterol can occur within 30 minutes of beginning treatment, although

maximum benefit may not be achieved for ≥ 1 week. Individual patients will experience a variable time to onset and degree of symptom relief.

Replacing the current strength of fluticasone propionate/salmeterol with a higher strength may provide additional asthma control for patients who do not respond adequately to the starting dose after 2 weeks of therapy.

If a previously effective dosage regimen fails to provide adequate asthma control, reevaluate the therapeutic regimen and consider additional therapeutic options, such as replacing the current strength of fluticasone propionate/salmeterol with a higher strength, adding additional inhaled corticosteroid, or initiating oral corticosteroids.

Advise patients to rinse mouth after inhalation.

Elderly: No dosage adjustment is recommended based on available data for fluticasone propionate/salmeterol and its active components.

Chapter 7

CENTRAL NERVOUS SYSTEM AGENTS

Amphetamines, 417
Anorexiants, 420
Narcotic Agonist Analgesics, 423
Narcotic Agonist-Antagonist Analgesics, 445
    Pentazocine, 445
    Pentazocine Combinations, 447
    Nalbuphine, 447
    Buprenorphine, 449
Central Analgesics, 451
    Tramadol, 451
Acetaminophen, 453
Salicylates, 455
    Diflunisal, 459
Nonnarcotic Analgesic Combinations, 461
    Diclofenac Sodium and Misoprostol, 461
NSAIDs, 463
Sulfasalazine, 477
Agents for Gout, 478
    Probenecid, 478
    Allopurinol, 480
    Colchicine, 483
Agents for Migraine, 485
    Serotonin 5-HT$_1$ Receptor Agonists, 485
    Methysergide Maleate, 490
    Ergotamine Derivatives, 491
Isometheptene Mucate/Dichloralphenazone/Acetaminophen, 493
Antiemetic/Antivertigo Agents, 494
    Cyclizine and Meclizine, 498
    Buclizine, 499
    Diphenhydramine, 499
    Dimenhydrinate, 500
    Trimethobenzamide, 501
    Dronabinol, 502
    5-HT$_3$ Receptor Antagonists, 503

Antianxiety Agents, 508
    Meprobamate, 508
    Benzodiazepines, 509
    Miscellaneous,
        Buspirone, 514
        Hydroxyzine, 515
        Doxepin, 517
Antidepressants, 518
    Tricyclic Compounds, 519
    Tetracyclic Compounds, 525
    Trazodone, 528
    Bupropion, 529
    Venlafaxine, 532
    Nefazodone, 535
    SSRIs, 537
    MAO Inhibitors, 545
Antipsychotic Agents, 548
    Phenothiazine and Thioxanthene Derivatives, 553
    Phenylbutylpiperadine Derivatives, 559
    Molindone, 561
    Dibenzapine Derivatives, 562
    Benzisoxazole Derivatives, 565
    Risperidone, 565
    Lithium, 566
Miscellaneous Psychotherapeutics, 569
    Dexmethylphenidate HCl, 569
    Methylphenidate, 571
    Pemoline, 574
    Tacrine, 576
    Rivastigmine, 578
    Galantamine HBr, 580
    Donepezil, 582
    Amphetamines, 583
    Ergoloid Mesylates, 583
Sedatives/Hypnotics, Nonbarbiturate, 585
    Zolpidem Tartrate, 585
    Zaleplon, 587
    Benzodiazepines, 589
Sedatives/Hypnotics, Barbiturate, 592

Anticonvulsants, 597
   Hydantoins, 598
   Zonisamide, 603
   Clonazepam, 605
   Clorazepate Dipotassium, 605
   Diazepam, 606
   Lamotrigine, 607
   Levetiracetam, 611
   Primidone, 613
   Valproic Acid, 615
   Carbamazepine, 621
   Gabapentin, 624
   Tiagabine, 625
   Topiramate, 627
   Magnesium Sulfate, 630
   Oxcarbazepine, 631
Skeletal Muscle Relaxants, 635
   Cyclobenzaprine, 635
   Diazepam, 636
   Baclofen, 637
   Dantrolene Sodium, 639

Parkinson's Disease, 642
   Anticholinergics, 642
   Levodopa/Carbidopa, 645
   Entacapone, 646
   Amantadine, 649
   Bromocriptine, 650
   Selegiline, 650
   Pergolide, 651
   Dopamine Receptor Agonists,
    Non-Ergot, 652
Antialcoholic Agents, 655
   Disulfiram, 655
Smoking Deterrents, 657
    Nicotine, 657
    Bupropion HCl, 660

AMPHETAMINES

AMPHETAMINE SULFATE (Racemic Amphetamine Sulfate)
Tablets: 5 and 10 mg (*c-ii*)	Various

DEXTROAMPHETAMINE SULFATE
Tablets: 5 mg (*c-ii*)	Various, *Dexedrine* (GlaxoSmithKline)
Tablets: 10 mg (*c-ii*)	Various
Capsules, sustained-release: 5 and 10 mg (*c-ii*)	*Dexedrine Spansules* (GlaxoSmithKline)
Capsules, sustained-release: 15 mg (*c-ii*)	Various, *Dexedrine Spansules* (GlaxoSmithKline)

METHAMPHETAMINE HCl (Desoxyephedrine HCl)
Tablets: 5 mg (*c-ii*)	*Desoxyn* (Abbott)
Tablets, long-acting: 5, 10, and 15 mg (*c-ii*)	*Desoxyn Gradumet* (Abbott)

AMPHETAMINE MIXTURES
Tablets: 10 and 20 mg mixed salts of a single entity amphetamine product (*c-ii*)	*Adderall* (Richwood)

Warning:
> *Drug dependence:* Amphetamines have a high potential for abuse. Abrupt cessation following prolonged high dosage results in extreme fatigue, mental depression, and changes on the sleep EEG. Use in weight reduction programs only when alternative therapy has been ineffective. Administration for prolonged periods may lead to drug dependence. Prescribe or dispense sparingly.

Indications
Narcolepsy: Treatment of narcolepsy.

Attention deficit disorder (ADD) with hyperactivity: Indicated as an integral part of a total treatment program that includes other remedial measures (psychological, educational, social) for a stabilizing effect in children with a behavioral syndrome characterized by moderate to severe distractibility, short attention span, hyperactivity, emotional lability, and impulsivity.

Exogenous obesity: As a short-term adjunct in a regimen of weight reduction based on caloric restriction for patients refractory to alternative therapy.

Administration and Dosage
Administer at the lowest effective dosage and adjust individually. Avoid late evening doses, particularly with the long-acting form, because of the resulting insomnia.

ADD: When treating the attention deficit disorder in children, occasionally interrupt drug administration to determine if there is a recurrence of behavioral symptoms sufficient to require continued therapy.

Obesity: When used for obesity, intermittent or interrupted courses of therapy may be useful. A 3- to 6-week course of therapy followed by a discontinuation period of half the original treatment length has been suggested.

AMPHETAMINE SULFATE:
Narcolepsy – 5 to 60 mg/day in divided doses.

Children (6 to 12 years of age): Narcolepsy seldom occurs in children < 12 years of age. When it does, initial dose is 5 mg/day; increase in increments of 5 mg at weekly intervals until optimal response is obtained (maximum 60 mg/day).

Adults (≥ 12 years of age): Start with 10 mg/day; raise in increments of 10 mg/day at weekly intervals. If adverse reactions appear (eg, insomnia, anorexia), reduce dose. Long-acting forms may be used for once-a-day dosage. With tablets or elixir, give first dose on awakening; additional doses (1 or 2) at intervals of 4 to 6 hours.

ADD – Not recommended for children < 3 years of age.

Children (3 to 5 years of age): 2.5 mg/day; increase in increments of 2.5 mg/day at weekly intervals until optimal response is obtained. Usual range is 0.1 to 0.5 mg/kg/dose every morning.

Children (≥ 6 years of age): 5 mg once or twice/day; increase in increments of 5 mg/day at weekly intervals until optimal response is obtained. Dosage will rarely exceed 40 mg/day. Usual range is 0.1 to 0.5 mg/kg/dose every morning.

Long-acting forms may be used for once-a-day dosage. With tablets or elixir, give first dose on awakening; additional doses (1 or 2) may be given at intervals of 4 to 6 hours.

Exogenous obesity – 5 to 30 mg/day in divided doses of 5 to 10 mg, 30 to 60 minutes before meals. Long-acting form: 10 or 15 mg in the morning. Not recommended for children < 12 years of age.

DEXTROAMPHETAMINE SULFATE: Refer to Administration and Dosage for Amphetamine Sulfate.

METHAMPHETAMINE HCl:

ADD – Initially, 5 mg once or twice/day; increase in increments of 5 mg/day at weekly intervals until an optimum response is achieved. Usual effective dose is 20 to 25 mg/day.

Total daily dose may be given as conventional tablets in 2 divided doses, or once/day using the long-acting form. Do not use the long-acting form for initiation of dosage or until the titrated daily dose is equal to or greater than the dosage provided in a long-acting tablet.

Obesity – 5 mg, 30 minutes before each meal.

Long-acting form: 10 to 15 mg in the morning.

Treatment duration should not exceed a few weeks. Do not use in children < 12 years of age.

AMPHETAMINE MIXTURES: These mixtures contain various salts of amphetamine and dextroamphetamine. Refer to Administration and Dosage for Amphetamine Sulfate.

Actions

Pharmacology: Amphetamines are sympathomimetic amines with CNS stimulant activity. CNS effects are mediated by release of norepinephrine from central noradrenergic neurons. Peripheral alpha and beta activity includes elevation of systolic and diastolic blood pressures and weak bronchodilator and respiratory stimulant action.

Pharmacokinetics:

Absorption/Distribution – Following oral use, amphetamines are completely absorbed within 3 hours. They are widely distributed in the body, with high concentrations in the brain.

Metabolism/Excretion – Amphetamine is metabolized in the liver. Accumulated hydroxylated metabolites have been implicated in the development of amphetamine psychosis. Urinary excretion of the unchanged drug is pH dependent.

Contraindications

Advanced arteriosclerosis; symptomatic cardiovascular disease; moderate to severe hypertension; hyperthyroidism; hypersensitivity or idiosyncrasy to the sympathomimetic amines; glaucoma; agitated states; history of drug abuse; during or within 14 days following administration of MAO inhibitors (hypertensive crises may result).

Warnings

Tolerance: When tolerance to the anorectic effect develops, do not exceed recommended dose in an attempt to increase the effect; rather, discontinue the drug.

Pregnancy: Category C.

Lactation: Amphetamines are excreted in breast milk.

Children: Do not use as anorectic agents in children < 12 years of age. Amphetamine and dextroamphetamine are not recommended in children < 3 years of age for ADD.

Precautions

Hypertension: Use cautiously.

ADD: Drug treatment is not indicated in all cases.

Hazardous tasks: May cause dizziness. Observe caution while driving or performing other tasks requiring alertness.

Drug Interactions

Drugs that may interact with amphetamines include guanethidine, monoamine oxidase (MAO) inhibitors, tricyclic antidepressants, urinary acidifiers, and urinary alkalinizers.

Drug/Lab test interactions: Plasma **corticosteroid** levels may be increased. **Urinary steroid** determinations may be altered by amphetamines.

Adverse Reactions

Adverse reactions may include palpitations; tachycardia; elevation of blood pressure; reflex decrease in heart rate; arrhythmias (at larger doses); overstimulation; restlessness; dizziness; insomnia; euphoria; dysphoria; tremor; headache; changes in libido; dry mouth; unpleasant taste; diarrhea; constipation; urticaria; impotence.

ANOREXIANTS

BENZPHETAMINE HCL	
Tablets: 50 mg *(c-III)*	*Didrex* (Pharmacia)
DIETHYLPROPION HCl	
Tablets: 25 mg *(c-IV)*	Various, *Tenuate* (Aventis)
Tablets, sustained-release: 75 mg *(c-IV)*	Various, *Tenuate Dospan* (Aventis)
PHENDIMETRAZINE TARTRATE	
Tablets: 35 mg *(c-III)*	Various, *Bontril PDM* (Amerin)
Capsules, sustained-release: 105 mg *(c-III)*	*Prelu-2* (Roxane), *Melfiat-105 Unicelles* (Numark), *Bontril Slow-Release* (Amerin)
PHENTERMINE HCl	
Tablets: 8 and 37.5 mg *(c-IV)*	Various, *Zantryl* (Ion), *Adipex-P* (Gate), *Pro-Fast SA* (American Pharm.)
Capsules: 15, 18.75, 30, and 37.5 mg *(c-IV)*	Various, *Adipex-P* (Gate), *Ionamin* (Celltech), *Pro-Fast HS* (American Pharm.), *Pro-Fast SR* (American Pharm.)
SIBUTRAMINE	
Capsules: 5, 10, and 15 mg *(c-IV)*	*Meridia* (Knoll)

Indications

Exogenous obesity: As a short-term (8 to 12 weeks) adjunct in a regimen of weight reduction based on caloric restriction. Measure the limited usefulness of these agents against their inherent risks.

Sibutramine:

Obesity treatment – Management of obesity, including weight loss and maintenance of weight loss, in conjunction with a reduced calorie diet.

Administration and Dosage

Intermittent or interrupted courses of therapy may be useful in the treatment of obesity. A 3- to 6-week course of therapy followed by a discontinuation period of half the original treatment length has been suggested.

BENZPHETAMINE HCl: Initiate dosage with 25 to 50 mg once/day; increase according to response. Dosage ranges from 25 to 50 mg, 1 to 3 times/day.

DIETHYLPROPION HCl:

Tablets – 25 mg 3 times/day, 1 hour before meals and in mid-evening if needed to overcome night hunger.

Sustained release tablets – 75 mg once/day, in mid-morning.

PHENDIMETRAZINE TARTRATE:

Tablets and capsules – 35 mg 2 or 3 times/day, 1 hour before meals.

Sustained-release capsules – 105 mg once/day in the morning 30 to 60 minutes before breakfast.

PHENTERMINE HCl: Take 8 mg 3 times/day, 30 minutes before meals, or 15 to 37.5 mg as a single daily dose before breakfast or 10 to 14 hours before retiring.

Take *Pro-Fast HS* and *Pro-Fast SR* capsules ≈ 2 hours after breakfast for appetite control. Take *Adipex-P* capsules and tablets before breakfast or 1 to 2 hours after breakfast; the tablet dosage may be adjusted to the patient's need (ie, ½ tablet [18.75 mg] daily or 18.75 mg 2 times/day may be adequate).

Swallow *Ionamin* capsules whole.

Avoid late-evening medication because of the possibility of resulting insomnia.

SIBUTRAMINE: The recommended starting dose is 10 mg administered once/day with or without food. If there is inadequate weight loss, the dose may be titrated after 4 weeks to a total of 15 mg once/day. Reserve the 5 mg dose for patients who do not tolerate the 10 mg dose. Blood pressure and heart rate changes should be taken into account when making decisions regarding dose titration.

Doses > 15 mg/day are not recommended. In most of the clinical trials, sibutramine was given in the morning.

The safety and efficacy of sibutramine have not been determined > 2 years at this time.

Actions

Pharmacology: Adrenergic agents (eg, **diethylpropion, benzphetamine, phendimetrazine, phentermine**) act by modulating central norepinephrine and dopamine receptors through the promotion of catecholamine release. Aside from phentermine, other adrenergic agents are infrequently used, perhaps because of the lack of long-term, well-controlled data or the fear of their potential abuse. Older adrenergic weight-loss drugs (eg, amphetamine, methamphetamine, phenmetrazine), which strongly engage in dopamine pathways, are no longer recommended because of the risk of their abuse.

Pharmacokinetics:

Absorption – **Diethylpropion** is rapidly absorbed from the GI tract after oral administration and is extensively metabolized through a complex pathway of biotransformation involving N-dealkylation and reduction. Many of these metabolites are biologically active and may participate in the therapeutic action of diethylpropion.

Sibutramine is rapidly absorbed from the GI tract (T_{max} 1.2 hours) following oral administration.

Metabolism – Sibutramine is metabolized in the liver principally by the cytochrome P450 ($3A_4$) isoenzyme.

Excretion – Most of the drug and metabolites are excreted via the kidneys.

Contraindications

Advanced arteriosclerosis; symptomatic cardiovascular disease; moderate to severe hypertension; hyperthyroidism; known hypersensitivity or idiosyncrasy to sympathomimetic amines; glaucoma; agitated states; history of drug abuse; during or ≤ 14 days following the administration of MAO inhibitors (hypertensive crises may result); coadministration with other CNS stimulants; pregnancy (benzphetamine HCl); patients with anorexia nervosa, patients taking other centrally acting appetite-suppressant drugs (sibutramine).

Warnings

Blood pressure and pulse: Sibutramine substantially increases blood pressure in some patients.

Concurrent monoamine oxidase inhibitors: Do not use sibutramine concomitantly with MAOIs. There should be at least a 2-week interval after starting or stopping MAOIs before starting treatment with sibutramine.

Serotonin syndrome (sibutramine): The rare, but serious, constellation of symptoms also has been reported with the concomitant use of selective serotonin reuptake inhibitors and agents for migraine therapy (eg, sumatriptan, dihydroergotamine), certain opioids (eg, dextromethorphan, meperidine, pentazocine, fentanyl), lithium, or tryptophan. Because sibutramine inhibits serotonin reuptake, it should not be administered with other serotonergic agents.

Concomitant cardiovascular disease: Do not use sibutramine in patients with a history of coronary artery disease, CHF, arrhythmias, or stroke.

Glaucoma: Because sibutramine can cause mydriasis, use with caution in patients with narrow-angle glaucoma.

Tolerance: Tolerance to the anorectic effects may develop within a few weeks. If tolerance to the anorectic effect develops, do not exceed the recommended dose in an attempt to increase the effect; rather, discontinue the drug.

Other drugs: These agents should not be used in combination with other anorectic agents, including prescribed drugs (eg, SSRIs [eg, fluoxetine, sertraline, fluvoxamine, paroxetine]), *otc* preparations, and herbal products. When using CNS-active agents, consider the possibility of adverse interactions with alcohol.

Primary pulmonary hypertension (PPH): PPH, a rare, frequently fatal disease of the lungs, has been reported to occur in patients receiving certain anorectic agents. The initial symptom of PPH is usually dyspnea. Other initial symptoms include the following: Angina pectoris, syncope, or lower extremity edema. Advise patients to report immediately any deterioration in exercise tolerance. Discontinue treatment in patients who develop new, unexplained symptoms of dyspnea, angina pectoris, syncope, or lower extremity edema.

Valvular heart disease: Serious regurgitant cardiac valvular disease, primarily affecting the mitral, aortic, or tricuspid valves, has been reported in otherwise healthy people who had taken certain anorectic agents in combination with weight loss. The etiology of these valvulopathies has not been established and their course in individuals after the drugs are stopped is not known.

Pregnancy: (*Category* X – benzphetamine HCl; *category* C – sibutramine, phentermine, phendimetrazine; *category* B – diethylpropion).

Lactation: Safety for use in the nursing mother has not been established.

Children: Not recommended for use in children < 12 years of age. The safety and efficacy of sibutramine in pediatric patients < 16 years of age have not been established.

Precautions

Psychological disturbances: Psychological disturbances occurred in patients who received an anorectic agent together with a restrictive diet.

Cardiovascular disease: Use with caution and monitor blood pressure in patients with mild hypertension. Not recommended for patients with symptomatic cardiovascular disease, including arrhythmias.

Convulsions: Convulsions may increase in some epileptics receiving **diethylpropion**.

Seizures: Use **sibutramine** cautiously in patients with a history of seizures; discontinue in any patient who develops seizures.

Diabetes: Insulin requirements in diabetes mellitus may be altered in association with the use of anorexigenic drugs and the concomitant dietary restrictions.

PPH (sibutramine): Certain centrally acting weight loss agents that cause release of serotonin from nerve terminals have been associated with PPH.

Drug abuse and dependence: These drugs are chemically and pharmacologically related to the amphetamines and have abuse potential. Intense psychological or physical dependence and severe social dysfunction may be associated with long-term therapy or abuse. If this occurs, gradually reduce the dosage to avoid withdrawal symptoms.

Hazardous tasks: May produce dizziness, extreme fatigue, and depression after abrupt cessation of prolonged high dosage therapy; patients should observe caution while driving or performing other tasks requiring alertness.

Drug Interactions

Drugs that may affect anorexiants include MAO inhibitors, furazolidone, and SSRIs. Drugs that may be affected by anorexiants include guanethidine and TCAs. Drugs that may affect **sibutramine** include alcohol, cimetidine, erythromycin, ketoconazole, and other CYP3A inhibitors. Sibutramine may affect agents that may raise blood pressure or heart rate, CNS-active drugs, MAOIs, SSRIs, ergot alkaloids, lithium, certain opioids, $5HT_1$ receptor antagonists, and tryptophan.

Adverse Reactions

Adverse reactions may include the following: Palpitations; tachycardia; arrhythmias; hypertension or hypotension; fainting; overstimulation; nervousness; restlessness; dizziness; insomnia; weakness or fatigue; malaise; anxiety; tension; euphoria; elevated mood; drowsiness; depression; agitation; dysphoria; tremor; dyskinesia; dysarthria; confusion; incoordination; tremor; headache; change in libido; dry mouth; unpleasant taste; nausea; vomiting; abdominal discomfort; diarrhea; constipation; stomach pain; anorexia; increased appetite; dyspepsia; urticaria; rash; erythema; burning sensation; mydriasis; eye irritation; blurred vision; dysuria; polyuria; urinary frequency; impotence; menstrual upset; bone marrow depression; agranulocytosis; leukopenia; hair loss; ecchymosis; muscle pain; chest pain; excessive sweating; clamminess; chills; flushing; fever; myalgia; gynecomastia; back pain; flu syndrome; injury accident; asthenia; dysmenorrhea; arthralgia; rhinitis; pharyngitis; sinusitis; cough increase.

NARCOTIC AGONIST ANALGESICS

ALFENTANIL HCL
Injection: 500 mcg (as HCl)/mL (*c-II*) — *Alfenta* (Janssen)

CODEINE
Tablets: 15, 30, and 60 mg (as sulfate) (*c-II*)	Various
Tablets, soluble: 30 and 60 mg (as sulfate) (*c-II*)	Various
Solution, oral: 15 mg/5 mL (as phosphate) (*c-II*)	Various
Injection: 30 and 60 mg (as phosphate) (*c-II*)	Various

FENTANYL
Injection: 0.05 mg base (as citrate)/mL (*c-II*) — Various, *Sublimaze* (Taylor)

FENTANYL TRANSDERMAL SYSTEM
Patch: 25 mcg/hr, 50 mcg/hr, 75 mcg/hr, and 100 mcg/hr (*c-II*) — *Duragesic-25, Duragesic-50[1], Duragesic-75[1], Duragesic-100[1]* (Janssen)

FENTANYL TRANSMUCOSAL SYSTEM
Lozenges: 100, 200, 300, and 400 mcg (*c-II*)	*Fentanyl Oralet* (Abbott)
Lozenge on a stick: 200, 400, 600, 800, 1200, and 1600 mcg (*c-II*)	*Actiq* (Abbott)

HYDROMORPHONE HCL
Tablets: 1, 2, 3, 4, and 8 mg (*c-II*)	Various, *Dilaudid* (Knoll)
Liquid: 5 mg/5 mL (*c-II*)	Various, *Dilaudid* (Knoll)
Suppositories: 3 mg (*c-II*)	Various, *Dilaudid* (Knoll)
Injection: 1 mg/mL, 2 mg/mL, 4 mg/mL, and 10 mg/mL (*c-II*)	Various, *Dilaudid* (Knoll), *Dilaudid-HP* (Knoll)
Powder for injection, lyophilized: 250 mg (10 mg/mL after reconstitution)	*Dilaudid-HP* (Knoll)

LEVOMETHADYL ACETATE HCL
Solution: 10 mg/mL (*c-II*) — ORLAAM (Roxane)

LEVORPHANOL TARTRATE
Tablets: 2 mg (*c-II*) — *Levo-Dromoran* (ICN), *Levorphanol Tartrate* (Roxane)

MEPERIDINE HCl
Tablets: 50 and 100 mg (*c-II*)	Various, *Demerol* (Sanofi-Synthelabo, Abbott)
Syrup: 50 mg/5 mL (*c-II*)	
Injection: 25 mg/mL, 50 mg/mL, 75 mg/mL, and 100 mg/mL (*c-II*)	
Injection: 50 mg/mL, 75 mg/mL, and 100 mg/mL (*c-II*)	

METHADONE HCl
Tablets: 5 and 10 mg (*c-II*)	*Methadone HCl* (Roxane), *Methadose* (Mallinckrodt)
Dispersible Tablets: 40 mg (*c-II*)	*Methadone HCl Diskets[2]* (Eli Lilly), *Methadose[2]* (Mallinckrodt)
Oral Solution: 5 mg/5 mL and 10 mg/5 mL (*c-II*)	Various, *Methadone HCl* (Roxane)
Oral Concentrate: 10 mg/mL (*c-II*)	Various, *Methadone HCl[2]* (UDL), *Methadone HCl Intensol* (Roxane), *Methadose[2]* (Mallinckrodt)
Injection: 10 mg/mL (*c-II*)	*Dolophine HCl* (Roxane)
Powder: 50, 100, and 500 g	Various, *Methadose[2]* (Mallinckrodt)

MORPHINE SULFATE
Soluble Tablets: 10, 15, and 30 mg (*c-II*)	Various
Tablets: 15 and 30 mg (*c-II*)	Various, *MSIR* (Purdue Frederick)
Tablets, controlled-release: 15, 30, 60, 100, and 200 mg (*c-II*)	MS Contin (Purdue Frederick), *Oramorph SR* (Roxane)
Capsules: 15 and 30 mg (*c-II*)	*MSIR* (Purdue Frederick)
Capsules, sustained-release: 20, 30, 50, 60, 100 mg (*c-II*)	*Kadian* (AstraZeneca)
Solution: 10 mg/5 mL, 20 mg/5 mL, 20 mg/mL, and 100 mg/5 mL (*c-II*)	Various, *MSIR* (Purdue Frederick), *Roxanol* (Roxane), *Roxanol 100* (Roxane), *Roxanol T* (Roxane)
Rectal Suppositories: 5, 10, 20, and 30 mg (*c-II*)	Various, *RMS* (Upsher-Smith)
Injection: 0.5, 1, 2, 4, 5, 8, 10, 15, 25, and 50 mg/mL (*c-II*)	Various, *Astramorph PF* (AstraZeneca), *Duramorph* (Baxter), *Infumorph 200* (ESI Lederle)
Compounding powder	*Morphine Sulfate* (Paddock)

OPIUM	
Liquid: 10% (c-II)	Opium Tincture, Deodorized (Ranbaxy)
Liquid (camphorated tincture of opium): 2 mg morphine equiv./5 mL (c-III)	Paregoric (Various)
OXYCODONE HCl	
Tablets: 5 mg (c-II)	Various, Endocodone (Endo), M-oxy (Mallinckrodt), Percolone (Endo Labs), Roxicodone (Roxane)
Tablets, controlled-release: 10, 20, 40, 80, 160 mg² (c-II)	OxyContin (Purdue Pharma LP)
Tablets, immediate-release: 15 and 30 mg (c-II)	Roxicodone (Roxane)
Capsules, immediate release: 5 mg (c-II)	Various, OxyIR (Purdue Pharma LP)
Oral solution: 5 mg/5 mL (c-II)	Roxicodone (Roxane)
Solution, concentrate: 20 mg/mL (c-II)	OxyFAST (Purdue Pharma LP), Roxicodone Intensol (Roxane), Oxydose (Ethex)
OXYMORPHONE HCl	
Injection: 1 mg/mL and 1.5 mg/mL (c-II)	Numorphan (Endo Labs)
Suppositories: 5 mg (c-II)	Numorphan (Endo Labs)
PROPOXYPHENE HCl	
Capsules: 65 mg (as HCl) (c-IV)	Various, Darvon Pulvules (Eli Lilly)
PROPOXYPHENE NAPSYLATE	
Tablets: 100 mg (c-IV)	Darvon-N (Eli Lilly)
REMIFENTANIL HCl	
Powder for injection, lyophilized: 1 mg/mL (as HCl; after reconstitution) (c-II)	Ultiva (Abbott)
SUFENTANIL CITRATE	
Injection: 50 mcg (as citrate)/mL (c-II)	Various, Sufenta (Taylor)

[1] For use in opioid-tolerant patients only.
[2] For detoxification and maintenance only.

Indications

ALFENTANIL HCl: As an analgesic adjunct given in incremental doses in the maintenance of anesthesia with barbiturate/nitrous oxide/oxygen.

As an analgesic administered by continuous infusion with nitrous oxide/oxygen in the maintenance of general anesthesia.

As a primary anesthetic for induction of anesthesia in general surgery when endotracheal intubation and mechanical ventilation are required.

Analgesic component for monitored anesthesia care (MAC).

CODEINE: Relief of mild to moderate pain and for coughing induced by chemical or mechanical irritation of the respiratory system.

FENTANYL:

Pain – For analgesic action of short duration during anesthesia (premediaction, induction, maintenance) and in the immediate postoperative period (recovery room) as needed.

For use as a narcotic analgesic supplement in general or regional anesthesia.

For administration with a neuroleptic such as droperidol as an anesthetic premedication, for induction of anesthesia and as an adjunct in maintenance of general and regional anesthesia.

For use as an anesthetic agent with oxygen in selected high-risk patients (open heart surgery or certain complicated neurological or orthopedic procedures.

FENTANYL TRANSDERMAL SYSTEM:

Pain – Management of chronic pain in patients requiring opioid analgesia.

FENTANYL TRANSMUCOSAL SYSTEM:

Anesthesia (Fentanyl Oralet only) – Only indicated for use in a hospital setting 1) as an anesthetic premedication in the operating room setting or 2) to induce conscious sedation prior to a diagnostic or therapeutic procedure in other monitored anesthesia care settings in the hospital.

Breakthrough cancer pain (Actiq only) – Only indicated for the management of breakthrough cancer pain in patients with malignancies who are already receiving and are tolerant to opioid therapy for their underlying persistent cancer pain. Patients considered opioid-tolerant are those who are taking ≥ 60 mg morphine/day, 50 mcg transdermal fentanyl/hour, or an equianalgesic dose of another opioid for ≥ 1 week.

HYDROMORPHONE HCl: Relief of moderate to severe pain.

LEVOMETHADYL ACETATE HCl: Management of opiate dependence.

LEVORPHANOL TARTRATE:
> *Pain (Levorphanol Tartrate only)* – Management of pain where an opioid analgesic is appropriate.
> *Pain/Preoperative medication (Levo-Dromoran only)* – Management of moderate to severe pain or as a preoperative medication where an opioid analgesic is appropriate.

MEPERIDINE HCl:
> *Oral and parenteral* – Relief of moderate to severe pain.
> *Parenteral* – For preoperative medication, support of anesthesia and obstetrical analgesia.

METHADONE HCl: For relief of severe pain; detoxification and temporary maintenance treatment of narcotic addiction. Methadone is ineffective for the relief of general anxiety.

MORPHINE SULFATE:
> *Oral* –
>> *Immediate-release tablets/solution:* Relief of moderate to severe pain.
>> *Controlled/Extended/Sustained-release tablets:* Relief of moderate to severe pain in those who require opioid analgesics for more than a few days.
> *Parenteral* –
>> *IV:* Relief of severe pain; pain of MI; used preoperatively to sedate the patient and allay apprehension, facilitate anesthesia induction, and reduce anesthetic dosage; control postoperative pain; relieve anxiety and reduce left ventricular work by reducing preload pressure; treatment of dyspnea associated with acute left ventricular failure and pulmonary edema; produce anesthesia for open-heart surgery.
>> *SC/IM:* Relief of severe pain; relieve preoperative apprehension; preoperative sedation; control postoperative pain; supplement to anesthesia; analgesia during labor; acute pulmonary edema; allay anxiety.
>> *IV/Epidural/Intrathecal:* Management of pain not responsive to nonnarcotic analgesics (*Duramorph*, *Astramorph PF*; *Infumorph* for continuous epidural/intrathecal use only).
> *Rectal* – Severe acute and chronic pain.

OPIUM:
> *Diarrhea* – For treatment of diarrhea.
> *Unlabeled uses* –
>> *Neonatal abstinence syndrome:* Treatment of opioid-related drug withdrawal (neonates). Diluted opium tincture is the preferred treatment for neonatal withdrawal in newborns. Paregoric contains benzoic acid (an oxidative product of benzyl alcohol), usually camphor, and other ingredients that may have potential toxic effects.
>> *Management of short bowel syndrome:* Used to slow gastric emptying and delay bowel transit time in short bowel syndrome.

OXYCODONE HCl:
> *Pain* – Relief of moderate to severe pain.
>> *Immediate-release tablets:* Management of moderate to severe pain where use of an opioid analgesic is appropriate.
>> *Controlled-release tablets:* Management of moderate to severe pain when a continuous, around-the-clock analgesic is needed for an extended period of time. Not intended for use as a prn analgesic.
>>> Not indicated for pain in the immediate postoperative period (the first 12 to 24 hours following surgery), or if the pain is mild or not expected to persist for an extended period of time. Oxycodone controlled-release tablets are only indicated for postoperative use if the patient is already receiving the drug prior to surgery or if the postoperative pain is expected to be moderate to severe and persist

for an extended period of time. Individualize treatment, moving from parenteral to oral analgesics as appropriate.

Unlabeled uses – Postherpetic neuralgia (controlled-release).

OXYMORPHONE HCl: Relief of moderate to severe pain.

Parenterally for preoperative medication, support of anesthesia, obstetrical analgesia, and for relief of anxiety in patients with dyspnea associated with acute left ventricular failure and pulmonary edema.

PROPOXYPHENE (Dextropropoxyphene): Relief of mild to moderate pain.

REMIFENTANIL HCl:

General anesthesia – An analgesic agent for use during the induction and maintenance of general anesthesia for inpatient and outpatient procedures and for continuation as an analgesic into the immediate postoperative period under the direct supervision of an anesthesia practitioner in a postoperative anesthesia care unit or intensive care setting.

Monitored anesthesia care – An analgesic component of monitored anesthesia care.

SUFENTANIL CITRATE: Analgesic adjunct at dosages ≤ 8 mcg/kg to maintain balanced general anesthesia.

A primary anesthetic agent at dosages ≥ 8 mcg/kg to induce and maintain anesthesia with 100% oxygen in patients undergoing major surgical procedures, such as cardiovascular surgery or neurosurgical procedures in the sitting position, to provide favorable myocardial and cerebral oxygen balance or when extended postoperative ventilation is anticipated.

Pain – For analgesic action of short duration during anesthesia (premedication, induction, maintenance), and in the immediate postoperative period (recovery room) as needed.

For use as a narcotic analgesic supplement in general or regional anesthesia.

For administration with a neuroleptic such as droperidol as an anesthetic premedication, for induction of anesthesia and as an adjunct in maintenance of general and regional anesthesia.

For use as an anesthetic agent with oxygen in selected high-risk patients (open heart surgery or certain complicated neurological or orthopedic procedures).

Administration and Dosage

In obese patients (> 20% above ideal total body weight), determine dosage on the basis of lean body weight. Reduce dose in elderly or debilitated patients.

The most important factor to be considered in determining the appropriate dose is the extent of pre-existing opioid tolerance. Reduce initial doses in elderly or debilitated patients.

ALFENTANIL HCl:

Children < 12 years of age – Use is not recommended.

Alfentanil Dosage Range for Use During General Anesthesia				
Clinical status	≈ Duration of anesthesia	Induction (Initial dose)	Maintenance (Increments/ Infusion)	Total dose
Spontaneously breathing/ Assisted ventilation	≤ 30 min	8-20 mcg/kg	3-5 mcg/kg every 5-20 min or 0.5-1 mcg/kg/min	8-40 mcg/kg
Assisted or controlled ventilation				
Incremental injection (to attenuate response to laryngoscopy and intubation)	30-60 min	20-50 mcg/kg	5-15 mcg/kg every 5-20 min	≤ 75 mcg/kg
Continuous infusion[1] (to provide attenuation of response to intubation and incision)	> 45 min	50-75 mcg/kg	0.5-3 mcg/kg/min. Average infusion rate 1-1.5 mcg/kg/min	dependent on duration of procedure

Alfentanil Dosage Range for Use During General Anesthesia				
Clinical status	≈ Duration of anesthesia	Induction (Initial dose)	Maintenance (Increments/ Infusion)	Total dose
Anesthetic induction (give slowly [over 3 min]). Reduce concentration of inhalation agents by 30%-50% for initial hour)	> 45 min	130-245 mcg/kg	0.5-1.5 mcg/kg/min or general anesthetic	dependent on duration of procedure
MAC (for sedated and responsive spontaneously breathing patients)	≤ 30 min	3-8 mcg/kg	3-5 mcg/kg every 5-20 min or 0.25 to 1 mcg/kg/min	3-40 mcg/kg

[1] 0.5 to 3 mcg/kg/min with nitrous oxide/oxygen in general surgery. Following anesthetic induction dose, reduce infusion rate requirements by 30% to 50% for the first hour of maintenance. Vital sign changes that indicate response to surgical stress or lightening of anesthesia may be controlled by increasing rate to a max of 4 mcg/kg/min or administering bolus doses of 7 mcg/kg. If changes are not controlled after 3 bolus doses given over 5 minutes, use a barbiturate, vasodilator, or inhalation agent. Always adjust infusion rates downward in the absence of these signs until there is some response to surgical stimulation. Rather than an increase in infusion rate, administer 7 mcg/kg bolus doses of alfentanil or a potent inhalation agent in response to signs of lightening of anesthesia within the last 15 minutes of surgery. Discontinue infusion ≥ 10 to 15 minutes prior to the end of surgery.

CODEINE:
  Analgesic –
    Adults: 15 to 60 mg every 4 to 6 hours, orally, IM, IV or SC. Usual dose is 30 mg. Do not exceed 360 mg in 24 hours.
    Children (≥ 1 year of age): 0.5 mg/kg or 15 m² of body surface every 4 to 6 hours SC, IM or orally. Do not use IV in children
    Antitussive – (See also Respiratories chapter).
    Adults: 10 to 20 mg every 4 to 6 hours. Do not exceed 120 mg in 24 hours.
    Children (6 to 12 years of age): 5 to 10 mg orally every 4 to 6 hours. Do not exceed 60 mg in 24 hours.
    (2 to 6 years of age) – 2.5 to 5 mg orally every 4 to 6 hours. Do not exceed 30 mg in 24 hours.

FENTANYL:
  Premedication – 0.05 to 0.1 mg IM, 30 to 60 minutes prior to surgery.
  Adjunct to general anesthesia –
    Total low dosage: 0.002 mg/kg in small doses for minor, painful surgical procedures and postoperative pain relief; maintenance low dosage: Infrequently needed.
    Total low dosage: 0.002 to 0.02 mg/kg.
    Maintenance moderate dosage: 0.025 to 0.1 mg IV or IM when movement or changes in vital signs indicate surgical stress or lightening of analgesia.
    Total high dosage: 0.02 to 0.05 mg/kg. For "stress free" anesthesia. Use during open heart surgery and complicated neurosurgical and orthopedic procedures where surgery is prolonged and the stress response is detrimental.
    Maintenance high dosage: Ranging from 0.025 mg to half the initial loading dose.
    Adjunct to regional anesthesia – 0.05 to 0.1 mg IM or slowly IV over 1 to 2 minutes as required.
    Postoperatively (recovery room) – 0.05 to 0.1 mg IM for the control of pain, tachypnea, and emergence delirium; repeat dose in 1 to 2 hours as needed.
    Children (2 to 12 years) – For induction and maintenance, a reduced dose as low as 2 to 3 mcg/kg is recommended. Safety and efficacy in children < 2 years of age have not been established.
    General anesthetic: 0.05 to 0.1 mg/kg with oxygen and a muscle relaxant when attenuation of the responses to surgical stress is especially important. Up to 0.15 mg/kg may be necessary.

FENTANYL TRANSDERMAL SYSTEM:
  Application – Each system may be worn continuously for 72 hours. If analgesia for > 72 hours is required, apply a new system to a different skin site after removal of the previous transdermal system.

Dose selection – Maintain each patient at the lowest dose providing acceptable pain control. Unless the patient has pre-existing opioid tolerance, use the lowest dose, 25 mcg/hr, as the initial dose.

Upwards titration may be done no more frequently than 3 days after the initial dose; thereafter, it may be done no more frequently than every 6 days. For delivery rates in excess of 100 mcg/hr, multiple systems may be used.

Fentanyl Transdermal Dose Based on Daily Morphine Equivalence Dose[1]		
Oral 24 hour morphine (mg/day)	IM 24 hour morphine (mg/day)	Fentanyl transdermal (mcg/hr)
45-134	8-22	25
135-224	23-37	50
225-314	38-52	75
315-404	53-67	100
405-494	68-82	125
495-584	83-97	150
585-674	98-112	175
675-764	113-127	200
765-854	128-142	225
855-944	143-157	250
945-1034	158-172	275
1035-1124	173-187	300

[1] A 10 mg IM or 60 mg oral dose of morphine every 4 hours for 24 hours for 24 hours (total of 60 mg/day IM or 360 mg/day IM or 360 mg/day oral) was considered approximately equivalent to fentanyl transdermal 100 mcg/hr.

The majority of patients are adequately maintained with transdermal fentanyl administered every 72 hours. A small number of patients may require systems to be applied every 48 hours.

During the initial application, patients should use short-acting analgesics for the first 24 hours as needed until analgesic efficacy with the transdermal system is attained. Thereafter, some patients still may require periodic supplemental doses of other short-acting analgesics for breakthrough pain.

Dose titration – Base appropriate dosage increments on the daily dose of supplementary opioids, using the ratio of 90 mg/24 hours of oral morphine to a 25 mcg/hr increase in transdermal fentanyl dose.

Discontinuation – Upon system removal, it takes ≥ 17 hours for the fentanyl serum concentration to fall by 50% after system removal. Titrate the dose of the new analgesic based on the patient's report of pain until adequate analgesia has been attained. For patients requiring discontinuation of opioids, a gradual downward titration is recommended because it is not known at what dose level the opioid may be discontinued without producing the signs and symptoms of abrupt withdrawal.

FENTANYL TRANSMUCOSAL SYSTEM:

Fentanyl Oralet – Fentanyl transmucosal doses of 5 mcg/kg provide effects similar to usual doses of fentanyl given IM (0.75 to 1.25 mcg/kg). Larger doses have not been shown to increase efficacy. Adults should not receive doses > 5 mcg/kg (400 mcg), and most children not apprehensive at onset may be managed with the same 5 mcg/kg dose. Children apprehensive at onset and some younger children may need doses of 5 to 15 mcg/kg with an attendant increased risk of hypoventilation.

Children: Because of the excessive frequency of significant hypoventilation at higher doses, doses > 15 mcg/kg (maximum, 400 mcg) are contraindicated in children.

Adults: Because of the excessive frequency of significant hypoventilation at higher doses, doses > 5 mcg/kg (maximum, 400 mcg) are contraindicated in adults.

Vulnerable patients: Consider selection of a lower dose for vulnerable patients (eg, patients with head injury, cardiovascular or pulmonary disease, hepatic disease, liver dysfunction). If signs of excessive opioid effects appear before the unit is consumed, remove the dosage unit from the patient's mouth immediately.

Elderly: If fentanyl transmucosal is to be used in patients > 65 years of age, reduce the dose to 2.5 to 5 mcg/kg.

Administration: Begin administration of the unit 20 to 40 minutes prior to the anticipated need of desired effect. Patients typically take 10 to 20 minutes for complete consumption. Peak effect occurs ≈ 20 to 30 minutes after the start of administration.

Actiq – Use has not been established with opioid-tolerant children < 16 years of age. Keep out of the reach of children.

Open the foil package immediately prior to product use. Place the unit in the patient's mouth between the cheek and lower gum, moving it from one side to the other using the handle. Instruct the patient to suck, not chew, the lozenge. A unit dose, if chewed and swallowed, might result in lower peak concentrations and lower bioavailability.

Instruct the patient to consume the lozenge over a 15-minute period. Longer or shorter consumption times may produce less efficacy than reported in clinical trials. If signs of excessive opioid effects appear before the unit is consumed, remove the drug matrix from the patient's mouth immediately and decrease future doses.

Dose titration: Initial dose to treat episodes of breakthrough cancer pain should be 200 mcg.

Redosing within a single episode – Redosing may start 15 minutes after the previous unit has been completed (30 minutes after the start of the previous unit). Do not give > 2 units for each individual breakthrough cancer pain episode while patients are in the titration phase and consuming units which individually may be subtherapeutic.

Increasing the dose – Evaluate each new dose used over several episodes of breakthrough cancer pain (generally 1 to 2 days) to determine whether it provides adequate efficacy with acceptable side effects.

Daily limit – Once a successful dose has been found, instruct patients to limit consumption to ≤ 4 units/day. If consumption increases to > 4 units/day, reevaluate the dose of the long-acting opioid for persistent cancer pain.

Discontinuation – Recommend a gradual downward titration for discontinuation because it is not known at what dose level the opioid may be discontinued without producing the signs and symptoms of abrupt withdrawal.

Safety and handling – *Actiq* is supplied in individually sealed child-resistant foil pouches.

Disposal – Dispose all units remaining from a prescription as soon as they are no longer needed. Dispose all units immediately after use.

Storage/Stability – Protect from freezing and moisture. Do not store *Fentanyl Oralet* above 30°C (86°F) or *Actiq* above 25°C (77°F).

HYDROMORPHONE HCl:
Oral –
Tablet: 2 to 4 mg every 4 to 6 hours; ≥ 4 mg every 4 to 6 hours for more severe pain.

Liquid: 2.5 to 10 mg every 4 to 6 hours.

Parenteral – 1 to 2 mg SC or IM every 4 to 6 hours as needed. For severe pain, administer 3 to 4 mg every 4 to 6 hours as needed. May be given by slow IV injection over 2 to 5 minutes.

Rectal – 3 mg every 6 to 8 hours.

Children – Safety and efficacy have not been established.

LEVORPHANOL TARTRATE:
Oral – Recommended starting dose is 2 mg. Repeat in 6 to 8 hours (*Levo-Dromoran*) or 3 to 6 hours (*Levorphanol Tartrate*) as needed, provided the patient is assessed for signs of hypoventilation and excessive sedation.

Levo-Dromoran: If necessary, increase the dose to ≤ 3 mg every 6 to 8 hours, after adequate evaluation of the patient's response. Higher doses may be appropriate in opioid-tolerant patients. Adjust dosage according to the severity of the pain; the patient's age, weight, physical status, and underlying diseases; use of concomitant medications; and other factors.

The effective daily dosage range, depending on the severity of the pain, is 8 to 16 mg in 24 hours in the nontolerant patient. Total oral daily doses of > 6 to

12 mg in 24 hours are generally not recommended as starting doses in non-opioid-tolerant patients; lower total daily doses may be appropriate.

Levorphanol Tartrate: The effective daily dosage range, depending on the severity of the pain, is 8 to 16 mg in 24 hours in the nontolerant patient. Total oral daily doses of > 16 mg in 24 hours are generally not recommended as starting doses in non-opioid-tolerant patients

Chronic pain – Individualize dosage. Because there is incomplete cross-tolerance among opioids, when converting a patient from morphine to levorphanol, begin the total daily dose of oral levorphanol at ≈ $\frac{1}{15}$ to $\frac{1}{12}$ of the total daily dose of oral morphine that such patients had previously required, and then adjust the dose to the patient's clinical response. If a patient is to be placed on fixed-schedule dosing (round-the-clock) with this drug, take care to allow adequate time after each dose change (≈ 72 hours) for the patient to reach a new steady state before a subsequent dose adjustment to avoid excessive sedation because of drug accumulation.

Perioperative period (Levo-Dromoran) – Levorphanol has been used for analgesic action during premedication and the postoperative period. Factors to be considered in determining the dosage include age, body weight, physical status, underlying pathological condition, use of other drugs, type of anesthesia used, the surgical procedure involved, and the severity of pain.

Premedication (Levo-Dromoran) – Individualize the preoperative medication dose. Two mg levorphanol is approximately equivalent to 10 to 15 mg of morphine or 100 mg of meperidine.

LEVOMETHADYL ACETATE HCl:

Warning – Because of its potential for serious and possibly life-threatening proarrhythmic effects, reserve levomethadyl for use in the treatment of opiate-addicted patients who fail to show an acceptable response to other adequate treatments for opiate addiction, either because of insufficient effectiveness or the inability to achieve effective dose because of intolerable adverse effects from those drugs.

Cases of QT prolongation and serious arrhythmia (torsades de pointes) have been observed during postmarketing treatment with levomethadyl. Based on these reports, all patients should undergo a 12-lead ECG prior to administration to determine if a prolonged QT interval (QTc > 430 [male] or 450 [female] ms) is present. If there is a prolonged QT interval, do not administer levomethadyl. For patients in whom the potential benefit of treatment is felt to outweigh the risks of potentially serious arrhythmias, perform an ECG prior to treatment, 12 to 14 days after initiating treatment, and periodically thereafter, to rule out any alterations in the QT interval.

Administer levomethadyl with extreme caution to patients who may be at risk for development of prolonged QT syndrome (eg, CHF, bradycardia, use of a diuretic, cardiac hypertrophy, hypokalemia, hypomagnesemia).

Levomethadyl acetate HCl, used for the treatment of opiate addiction, shall be dispensed only by Opioid Treatment Programs certified by SAMHSA under 42 CFR Part 8, and registered by the Drug Enforcement Administration under 21. USC 823(g)(1). This does not preclude the maintenance or detoxification treatment of a patient who is hospitalized for medical conditions other than opiate addiction and who requires temporary maintenance for concurrent opiate addiction during the critical period of the patient's hospitalization.

Levomethadyl has no recommended uses outside of the treatment of opiate addiction.

Adjust the dose to achieve optimal therapeutic benefit with acceptable adverse opioid effects. Always dilute before administration and mix with diluent prior to dispensing. To avoid confusion between prepared doses of levomethadyl and methadone, use a different color liquid for dilution of each agent.

Dosing schedules – Usually administer 3 times/week, either on Monday, Wednesday, and Friday, or on Tuesday, Thursday, and Saturday. If withdrawal is a problem during the 72-hour interdose interval, the preceding dose may be increased. In some cases, an every-other-day schedule may be appropriate. The usual doses must not be given on consecutive days because of the risk of fatal overdose. No dose mentioned in this section is ever meant to be given as a daily dose.

Induction – The initial dose for street addicts should be 20 to 40 mg. Each subsequent dose, administered at 48- or 72-hour intervals, may be adjusted in increments of 5 to 10 mg until steady state is reached, usually within 1 or 2 weeks.

Patients dependent on methadone may require higher initial doses of levomethadyl. The suggested initial 3 times/week dose for such patients is 1.2 to 1.3 times the daily methadone maintenance dose being replaced. This initial dose should not exceed 120 mg; adjust subsequent doses, administered at 48- or 72-hour intervals, according to clinical response.

Most patients can tolerate the 72-hour interdose interval during the induction period. Some patients may require additional intervention. If additional opioids are required, and the patient is not eligible or appropriate for take-home doses of levomethadyl, give supplemental methadone in small doses rather than giving levomethadyl on 2 consecutive days.

In some cases, where the degree of tolerance is unknown, patients can be started on methadone to facilitate more rapid titration to an effective dose, then converted to levomethadyl after a few weeks of methadone therapy.

The crossover from methadone to levomethadyl should be accomplished in a single dose; complete transfer to levomethadyl is simpler and preferable to more complex regimens involving escalating doses of levomethadyl and decreasing doses of methadone.

Carefully titrate dosage to the individual; induction too rapid for the patient's level of tolerance may result in overdose. Serious hazards, as seen in association with all narcotic analgesics, are respiratory depression and, to a lesser degree, circulatory depression.

Maintenance – Most patients will be stabilized on doses in the range of 60 to 90 mg 3 times/week. Doses as low as 10 mg and as high as 140 mg 3 times/week have been given in clinical studies.

Supplemental dosing over the 72-hour interdose interval (weekend) is rarely needed. For example, if a patient on a Mon/Wed/Fri schedule complains of withdrawal on Sundays, the recommended dosage adjustment is to increase the Friday dose in 5 to 10 mg increments up to 40% over the Mon/Wed dose or to a maximum of 140 mg.

Most patients do not experience withdrawal during the 72-hour interdose interval after reaching pharmacological steady-state with or without adjustment of the Friday dose. If additional opioids are required, and the patient is not eligible or appropriate for take-home doses, give small doses of supplemental methadone rather than giving levomethadyl on 2 consecutive days.

If withdrawal symptoms persist after adjustment of dose, consideration may be given to every-other-day dosing if clinic hours permit. If the clinic is not open 7 days a week and every-other-day dosing is not practical, the patient's schedule may be adjusted so the 72-hour interval occurs during the week and the patient can come to the clinic to receive a supplemental dose of methadone.

The maximum *total* amount of levomethadyl recommended for any patient is 140-140-140 mg or 130-130-180 mg on a thrice-weekly schedule or 140 mg every other day.

Take-home doses – If it is determined that a patient is responsible in handling opioid drugs, then levomethadyl take-home doses are permitted. Refer to 42 CFR Part 8 for specific restrictions.

Reinduction after an unplanned lapse in dosing –

Following a lapse of 1 levomethadyl dose: 1) If a patient comes to the clinic to be dosed on the day following a missed scheduled dose (misses Monday, arrives Tuesday), administer the regular Monday dose on Tuesday, with the scheduled Wednesday dose administered on Thursday and the Friday dose given on Saturday. The patient's regular schedule may be resumed the following Monday (misses Wednesday, receives the regular dose on Thursday and Saturday, and returns to the regular Mon/Wed/Fri dosing schedule the next week).

2) If a patient misses 1 dose and comes to the clinic on the day of the next scheduled dose (misses Monday, arrives Wednesday), the usual dose will be well tolerated in most instances, although a reduced dose may be appropriate in selected cases.

Following a lapse of > 1 levomethadyl dose: Restart patients at an initial dose of 50% to 75% of their previous dose, followed by increases of 5 to 10 mg every dosing day (48- or 72-hour intervals) until their previous maintenance dose is achieved. Reinduct patients who have been off levomethadyl treatment for > 1 week.

Transfer from levomethadyl to methadone – Patients maintained on levomethadyl may be transferred directly to methadone. Because of the difference between the 2 compounds' metabolites and their pharmacological half-lives, it is recommended that methadone be started on a daily dose at 80% of the levomethadyl dose being replaced; the initial methadone dose must be given no sooner than 48 hours after the last levomethadyl dose. Subsequent increases or decreases of 5 to 10 mg in the daily methadone dose may be given to control symptoms of withdrawal or, less likely, symptoms of excessive sedation, in accordance with clinical observations.

Detoxification from levomethadyl – There is limited experience with detoxifying patients from levomethadyl in a systematic manner, and gradual reduction (5% to 10% a week) and abrupt withdrawal schedules have been used successfully.

MEPERIDINE HCl:

Relief of pain – While SC administration is suitable for occasional use, IM administration is preferred for repeated doses. If IV administration is required, decrease dosage and inject very slowly, preferably using a diluted solution. Meperidine is less effective when administered orally than when given parenterally. Reduce proportionately (usually by 25% to 50%) when administering concomitantly with phenothiazines and other tranquilizers.

Adults: 50 to 150 mg IM, SC, or orally every 3 to 4 hours, as necessary.

Children: 1.1 to 1.75 mg/kg (0.5 to 0.8 mg/lb) IM, SC, or orally up to adult dose, every 3 or 4 hours, as necessary.

Preoperative medication –

Adults: 50 to 100 mg IM or SC, 30 to 90 minutes before beginning anesthesia.

Children: 1.1 to 2.2 mg/kg (0.5 to 1 mg/lb) IM or SC, up to adult dose, 30 to 90 minutes before beginning anesthesia.

Support of anesthesia – Meperidine may be administered in repeated doses diluted to 10 mg/mL by slow IV injection, or by continuous IV infusion of solution diluted to 1 mg/mL.

Obstetrical analgesia – When pains become regular, administer 50 to 100 mg IM or SC; repeat at 1- to 3-hour intervals.

METHADONE HCl:

Warning – To treat narcotic addiction in detoxification or maintenance programs, methadone may be dispensed only by pharmacies and maintenance programs approved by the FDA and designated state authorities. Approved maintenance programs shall dispense and use methadone in oral form only and according to treatment requirements stipulated in Federal Methadone Regulations (21 CFR 291.505). Failure to abide by the requirements in these regulations may result in criminal prosecution, seizure of drug supply, revocation of program approval, and injunction precluding program operation.

Methadone, used as an analgesic, may be dispensed in any licensed pharmacy.

Note – If used to treat heroin dependence for > 3 weeks, the procedure passes from treatment of acute withdrawal syndrome (detoxification) to maintenance therapy. Maintenance may be undertaken only by approved methadone programs. This does not preclude maintenance addicts hospitalized for other conditions and who require temporary maintenance during the critical period of their stays or whose enrollment has been verified in a program approved for maintenance treatment with methadone.

Oral methadone is ≈ ½ as potent as parenteral. Oral administration results in a delay of onset, a lower peak, and an increased duration of analgesic effect. Duration of effect increases with repeated use because of cumulative effects.

Pain –

Adults: 2.5 to 10 mg IM, SC, or orally every 3 or 4 hours as necessary. Adjust dosage according to the severity of pain and patient response. For exceptionally severe pain, or in those tolerant of narcotic analgesia, it may be necessary to exceed the usual recommended dosage. Injection IM is preferred for repeated doses; SC use may cause local irritation.

Children: Not for analgesic use because of insufficient documentation.

Detoxification treatment – Detoxification treatment should not exceed 21 days and may not be repeated earlier than 4 weeks after completion of the preceding course.

Initially, 15 to 20 mg will often suppress withdrawal symptoms. When patients are physically dependent on high doses, 40 mg/day in single or divided doses is usually an adequate stabilizing dose. Continue stabilization for 2 to 3 days, then gradually decrease the dose on a daily basis or at 2-day intervals.

Maintenance treatment – Initial dosage should control abstinence symptoms following narcotic withdrawal, but should not cause sedation, respiratory depression, or other effects of acute intoxication. Adjust dosage as tolerated and required, up to 120 mg/day.

For a complete description of detoxification and maintenance regulations and dosage protocols, consult a local approved methadone program.

MORPHINE SULFATE: Morphine may suppress respiration in the elderly, those taking other CNS depressants, the very ill, and those patients with respiratory problems; therefore, lower doses may be required.

Oral –

Immediate-release: 5 to 30 mg (solution or tablets) every 4 hours or as directed by physician.

Controlled/Extended/Sustained-release: Swallow whole; do not break, chew, or crush. See below for sustained-release capsule administration.

Initial therapy – There has been no evaluation of controlled/extended/sustained-release morphine as an initial opioid analgesic in the management of pain. Because it may be more difficult to titrate a patient to adequate analgesia using a controlled/extended/sustained-release morphine, it is ordinarily advisable to begin treatment using an immediate-release morphine formulation.

The MS *Contin* 200 mg tablet is for use only in opioid-tolerant patients requiring daily morphine-equivalent dosages of ≥ 400 mg. Reserve this strength for patients who have already been titrated to a stable analgesic regimen using lower strengths of MS *Contin* or other opioids. If *Kadian* is chosen, start with 20 mg in those who do not have a proven tolerance to opioids. Increase at a rate ≤ 20 mg every other day. Individualize dosage.

Conversion from conventional immediate-release oral morphine to controlled/extended/sustained-release oral morphine – Give ½ the total daily oral morphine dose every 12 hours; ⅓ the total daily oral morphine requirement every 8 hours (MS *Contin* and extended-release tablets only); or the full daily morphine dose every 24 hours (*Kadian* only). Use the 15 mg tablet for initial conversion for patients whose total daily requirement is expected to be < 60 mg. The 30 mg tablet strength is recommended for patients with a daily morphine requirement of 60 to 120 mg. When the total daily dose is expected to be > 120 mg, the appropriate combination of tablet strengths should be employed.

Conversion from parenteral morphine or other opioids (parenteral or oral) to controlled/extended/sustained-release – Exercise particular care in the conversion process. Because of uncertainty about, and intersubject variation in, relative estimates of opioid potency and cross-tolerance, initial dosing regimens should be conservative; that is, an underestimation of the 24-hour oral morphine requirement is preferred to an overestimate. To this end, estimate initial individual doses conservatively. In patients whose daily morphine requirements are expected to be ≤ 120 mg/day, the 30 mg tablet strength is recommended for the initial titration period. Once a stable dose regimen is reached, the patient can be converted to the 60 or 100 mg tablet strength, or appropriate combination of tablet strengths, if desired.

Conversion from controlled/extended/sustained-release oral morphine to parenteral opioids – It is best to assume that the parenteral-to-oral potency is high. For example, to estimate the required 24-hour dose of morphine for IM use, one could employ a conversion of 1 mg morphine IM for every 6 mg of morphine as controlled-release tablet. Of course, the IM 24-hour dose would have to be divided by 6 and administered every 4 hours. This approach is recommended because it is least likely to cause overdose. For *Kadian*, initiate treatment at half the calculated equivalent parenteral dose. For example, to estimate the 24-hour dose of parenteral morphine for a patient taking *Kadian*, one would take the 24-hour *Kadian* dose, divide by an oral-to-parenteral conversion ratio of 3, divide the estimated 24-hour parenteral dose into 6 divided doses (for a 4-hour dosing interval), then halve this dose as an initial trial.

Conversion of sustained-release (Kadian) to other controlled-release oral forms – *Kadian* is not bioequivalent to other controlled-release formulations. Conversion from *Kadian* to the same total daily dose may lead to either excessive sedation at peak or inadequate analgesia at trough; observe closely and adjust dosage as appropriate.

Dosing adjustments – If signs of excessive opioid effects are observed early in a dosing interval, reduce the next dose. If this adjustment leads to inadequate analgesia (ie, "breakthrough" pain occurs late in the dosing interval), the dosing interval may be shortened. Alternatively, a supplemental dose of a short-acting analgesic may be given. As experience is gained, adjustments can be made to obtain an appropriate balance between pain relief, opioid side effects, and the convenience of the dosing schedule. It is recommended that the dosing interval never be extended beyond 12 hours because the administration of very large single doses may lead to acute overdose.

Sustained-release (Kadian): Capsules may be opened and the entire contents sprinkled on a small amount of applesauce immediately prior to ingestion. The pellets in the capsules should not be chewed, crushed, or dissolved because of risk of overdose.

Open the capsule and sprinkle entire contents over ≈ 10 mL of water and flush with swirling through a prewetted 16 French gastrostomy tube fitted with funnel at the port end. Additional aliquots of water are used to transfer all pellets and to flush the tube. Do not attempt the administration of pellets through a nasogastric tube.

May be given once or twice/day.

SC/IM – Prepare soluble tablets in sterile water and filter through a 0.22 micron membrane filter.

Adults: 10 mg (range, 5 to 20 mg)/70 kg every 4 hours as needed.

Children: 0.05 to 0.2 mg/kg every 4 hours as needed. Do not exceed 10 to 15 mg/dose.

IV –

Adults: 2 to 10 mg/70 kg of body weight. A strength of 2.5 to 15 mg of morphine may be diluted in 4 to 5 mL of Water for Injection. Administer slowly over 4 to 5 minutes. Rapid IV use increases the incidence of adverse reactions (see Warnings). Do not administer IV unless a narcotic antagonist is immediately available.

Continuous IV infusion: 0.1 to 1 mg/mL in 5% Dextrose in Water by controlled-infusion device; higher concentrations have been used.

Severe chronic pain associated with terminal cancer – Prior to initiation of the morphine infusion (in concentrations between 0.2 to 1 mg/mL), a loading dose of ≥ 15 mg of morphine sulfate may be administered by IV push to alleviate pain.

The infusion dosage range is 0.8 to 80 mg/hr, though doses up to 144 mg/hr have been used. Thus, for the 1 mg/mL solution, the infusion may be run from 0.8 to 80 mg/hr, and for a 0.5 mg/mL solution, the infusion may be run from 1.6 to 160 mL/hr.

A constant infusion rate must be maintained with an infusion pump in order to assure proper dosage control. Take care to avoid overdosage (respiratory depression) or abrupt cessation of therapy, which may give rise to withdrawal symptoms.

Open-heart surgery – Administer large doses (0.5 to 3 mg/kg) of morphine IV as the sole anesthetic or with a suitable anesthetic agent. The patients are given oxygen and cardiovascular function is not depressed by morphine, as long as adequate ventilation is maintained.

MI pain – 8 to 15 mg administered parenterally. For very severe pain, additional smaller doses may be given every 3 to 4 hours as needed.

Rectal – 10 to 30 mg every 4 hours as needed or as directed by physician.

Epidural (Duramorph, Astramorph PF) –

Adults: Initial injection of 5 mg in the lumbar region may provide satisfactory pain relief for up to 24 hours. If adequate pain relief is not achieved within 1 hour, carefully administer incremental doses of 1 to 2 mg at intervals sufficient to assess effectiveness. Give no more than 10 mg/24 hours.

For continuous infusion, an initial dose of 2 to 4 mg/24 hours is recommended. Further doses of 1 to 2 mg may be given if pain relief is not achieved initially.

Aged or debilitated patients: Administer with extreme caution (see Warnings). Doses < 5 mg may provide satisfactory pain relief for up to 24 hours.

Infumorph, Duramorph, Astramorph PF: Employ doses > 20 mg/day with caution because they may be associated with a higher likelihood of serious side effects. The starting dose must be individualized. The recommended initial epidural dose in patients who are not tolerant to opioids range from 3.5 to 7.5 mg/day. The usual starting dose for continuous epidural infusion, based upon limited data in patients who have some degree of opioid tolerance, is 4.5 to 10 mg/day. The dose requirements may increase significantly during treatment, frequently to 20 to 30 mg/day.

Intrathecal –

Adult: Intrathecal dosage is usually ¹⁄₁₀ that of epidural dosage. A single injection of 0.2 to 1 mg may provide satisfactory pain relief for up to 24 hours. (Caution: This is only 0.4 to 2 mL of the 0.5 mg/mL potency or 0.2 to 1 mL of the 1 mg/ mL potency.) Do not inject intrathecally > 2 mL of the 0.5 mg/mL potency or 1 mL of the 1 mg/mL potency. Use in lumbar area only. Repeated intrathecal injections are not recommended. A constant IV infusion of 0.6 mg/hr naloxone for 24 hours after intrathecal injection may reduce incidence of potential side effects.

Infumorph: Familiarize with the continuous microinfusion device. To minimize risk from glass or other particles, the product must be filtered through ≤ 5 micron microfilter before injecting into the microinfusion device. If dilution is required, 0.9% NaCl injection is recommended. Individualize the starting dose. The recommended initial lumbar intrathecal dose range in patients with no tolerance to opioids is 0.2 to 1 mg/day. The published range of doses for individuals who have some degree of opioid tolerance varies from 1 to 10 mg/day. Limited experience with continuous intrathecal infusion of morphine has shown that the daily doses have to be increased over time.

Aged or debilitated: Use extreme caution. Lower dose is usually satisfactory.

Repeat dosage: If pain recurs, consider alternative administration routes because experience with repeated doses by this route is limited.

Intraventricular – Currently available data indicate that this route of administration is effective in select patients with a short life expectancy and recalcitrant pain caused by head and neck malignancies and tumors (eg, superior sulcus tumors, breast carcinoma) that affect the brachial plexus. One to 2 doses/day are generally administered.

OPIUM:

Caution – Opium tincture contains 25 times more morphine than paregoric. Do not confuse opium tincture with paregoric; this may lead to an overdose of morphine.

Opium tincture –
    Adults: 0.6 mL (equiv. to 6 mg morphine) 4 times/day; maximum 6 mL/day.
Paregoric –
    Adults: 5 to 10 mL 1 to 4 times/day.
    Children: 0.25 to 0.5 mL/kg 1 to 4 times/day.

OXYCODONE HCl:
    Warning – Controlled-release oxycodone is an opioid agonist and a Schedule II controlled substance with an abuse liability similar to morphine.

    Oxycodone can be abused in a manner similar to other opioid agonists, legal or illicit. This should be considered when prescribing or dispensing oxycodone controlled-release tablets in situations where the physician or pharmacist is concerned about an increased risk of misuse, abuse, or diversion.

    Oxycodone controlled-release tablets are indicated for the management of moderate to severe pain when a continuous, around-the-clock analgesic is needed for an extended period of time.

    Oxycodone controlled-release tablets are not intended for use as a prn (as needed) analgesic.

    Oxycodone 80 and 160 mg controlled-release tablets are for use in opioid-tolerant patients only. These tablet strengths may cause fatal respiratory depression when administered to patients not previously exposed to opioids.

    Immediate-release tablets –
    Adults: 10 to 30 mg every 4 hours (5 mg every 6 hours for *OxyIR*, oxycodone immediate-release capsules, and *OxyFast*) as needed. Individualize dosage.

    OxyFAST 20 mg/mL solution is a highly concentrated solution. Take care in prescribing and dispensing this solution strength.

    Children: Not recommended for use in children.

    5 to 15 mg every 4 to 6 hours as needed for pain. Titrate the dose based upon the individual patient's response. Patients with chronic pain should have their dosage given on an around-the-clock basis to prevent the reoccurrence of pain rather than treating the pain after it has occurred. This dose can then be adjusted to an acceptable level of analgesia, taking into account side effects experienced by the patient.

    For control of severe chronic pain, administer on a regularly scheduled basis, every 4 to 6 hours, at the lowest dosage level that will achieve adequate analgesia.

    As with any potent opioid, it is critical to adjust the dosing regimen for each patient individually, taking into account the patient's prior analgesic treatment experience.

    Controlled-release tablets – Swallow tablets whole; do not break, chew, or crush. Taking broken, chewed, or crushed tablets could lead to the rapid release and absorption of a potentially fatal dose of oxycodone.

    One 160 mg tablet is comparable to two 80 mg tablets when taken on an empty stomach. However, with a high-fat meal there is a 25% greater peak plasma concentration following one 160 mg tablet. Use dietary caution when patients are initially titrated to 160 mg tablets.

    Take care to use low initial doses of controlled-release tablets in patients who are not already opioid tolerant, especially those who are receiving concurrent treatment with muscle relaxants, sedatives, or other CNS-active medications.

    Patients not already taking opioids (opioid näive): A reasonable starting dose for most patients who are opioid näive is 10 mg every 12 hours. If a nonopioid analgesic (eg, aspirin, acetaminophen, NSAID) is being provided, it may be continued.

    Patients currently on opioid therapy:
1.) Using standard conversion ratio estimates (see table below), multiply the mg/day of the previous opioids by the appropriate multiplication factors to obtain the equivalent total daily dose of oral oxycodone.
2.) Divide this 24-hour oxycodone dose in half to obtain the twice a day (every 12 hours) dose of controlled-release tablets.
3.) Round down to a dose that is appropriate for the tablet strengths available (10, 20, 40, 80, and 160 mg tablets).

4.) Discontinue all other around-the-clock opioid drugs when controlled-release tablet therapy is initiated.

No fixed conversion ratio is likely to be satisfactory in all patients, especially patients receiving large opioid doses. The recommended doses shown in the following table are only a starting point, and close observation and frequent titration are indicated until patients are stable in the new therapy.

Multiplication Factors for Converting the Daily Dose of Prior Opioids to the Daily Dose of Oral Oxycodone[1]		
Mg/day prior opioid × factor = mg/day oral oxycodone		
	Oral prior opioid	Parenteral prior opioid
Oxycodone	1	—
Codeine	0.15	—
Fentanyl TTS	see below	see below
Hydrocodone	0.9	—
Hydromorphone	4	20
Levorphanol	7.5	15
Meperidine	0.1	0.4
Methadone	1.5	3
Morphine	0.5	3

[1] To be used only for conversion to oral oxycodone. For patients receiving high-dose parenteral opioids, a more conservative conversion is warranted. For example, for high-dose parenteral morphine, use 1.5 instead of 3 as a multiplication factor.

Special instructions for 80 and 160 mg controlled-release tablets: For use in opioid-tolerant patients only.

Controlled-release tablets, 80 and 160 mg, are for use only in opioid-tolerant patients requiring daily oxycodone equivalent dosages of ≥ 160 mg for the 80 mg tablet and ≥ 320 mg for the 160 mg tablet. Take care in the prescribing of this tablet strength. Instruct patients against use by individuals other than the patient for whom it was prescribed, as such inappropriate use may have severe medical consequences.

Therapy cessation: When the patient no longer requires therapy with the controlled-release tablets, taper doses gradually over several days to prevent signs and symptoms of withdrawal in the physically dependent patient.

Conversion from controlled-release tablets to parenteral opioids: To avoid overdose, follow conservative dose conversion ratios. For patients receiving high-dose parenteral opioids, a more conservative conversion is warranted.

OXYMORPHONE HCl: Use smaller doses of oxymorphone than those recommended below for debilitated and elderly patients and those with severe liver disease.

IV – Initially, 0.5 mg.

SC or IM – Initially, 1 to 1.5 mg every 4 to 6 hours, as needed. For analgesia during labor, give 0.5 to 1 mg IM.

Rectal – 5 mg every 4 to 6 hours.

Safety for use in children < 12 years of age has not been established.

PROPOXYPHENE:
Warning –
Fatalities:

• Do not prescribe propoxyphene for patients who are suicidal or addiction-prone.

• Prescribe propoxyphene with caution for patients taking tranquilizers or antidepressant drugs and patients who use alcohol in excess.

• Tell patients not to exceed the recommended dose and to limit alcohol intake.

Propoxyphene products in excessive doses, either alone or in combination with other CNS depressants (including alcohol), are a major cause of drug-related deaths. Fatalities within the first hour of overdosage are not uncommon. In a survey of deaths caused by overdosage conducted in 1975, in ≈ 20% of fatal cases, death occurred within the first hour (5% within 15 minutes). Do not take propoxyphene in higher doses than those recommended by the physician. Judicious prescribing of propoxyphene is essential for safety. Consider nonnarcotic analgesics for depressed or suicidal patients. Do not prescribe propoxyphene for suicidal or addiction-prone patients. Caution patients about the concomitant use of propoxyphene products and alcohol because of potentially serious CNS-additive effects of these agents. Because of added CNS depressant effects, cautiously prescribe with concomitant sedatives, tranquilizers, muscle relaxants, antidepressants, or other CNS-depressant drugs. Advise patients of the additive depressant effects of these combinations.

Many propoxyphene-related deaths have occurred in patients with histories of emotional disturbances, suicidal ideation or attempts, or misuse of tranquilizers, alcohol, and other CNS-active drugs. Deaths have occurred as a consequence of the accidental ingestion of excessive quantities of propoxyphene alone or in combination with other drugs. Do not exceed the recommended dosage.

Because of differences in molecular weight, 100 mg of propoxyphene napsylate is required to supply propoxyphene equivalent to 65 mg of the HCl. In hepatic or renal impairment, reduce total daily dosage.

Propoxyphene HCl –
    Usual dose: 65 mg every 4 hours as needed. Do not exceed 390 mg/day.
Propoxyphene napsylate –
    Usual dose: 100 mg every 4 hours as needed. Do not exceed 600 mg/day.
Elderly – Propoxyphene metabolism rate may be reduced in some patients. Consider increased dosing interval.

REMIFENTANIL HCl: For IV use only. Individualize dosage.

Administer continuous infusions of remifentanil only by an infusion device. The injection site should be close to the venous cannula. Clear all IV tubing at the time of discontinuation of infusion.

During general anesthesia – Remifentanil is not recommended as the sole agent in general anesthesia because loss of consciousness cannot be assured and because of a high incidence of apnea, muscle rigidity, and tachycardia. Remifentanil is synergistic with other anesthetics and doses of thiopental, propofol, isoflurane, and midazolam have been reduced by up to 75% with the coadministration of remifentanil.

Remifentanil Dosing Guidelines - General Anesthesia and Continuing as an Analgesic into the Postoperative Care Unit or Intensive Care Setting			
Phase	Continuous IV infusion (mcg/kg/min)	Infusion dose range (mcg/kg/min)	Supplemental IV bolus dose (mcg/kg)
Induction of anesthesia (through intubation)	0.5 to 1[1]	NA[2]	NA[2]
Maintenance of anesthesia with:			
Nitrous oxide (66%)	0.4	0.1 - 2	1
Isoflurane (0.4 to 1.5 MAC)	0.25	0.05 - 2	1
Propofol (100 to 200 mcg/kg/min)	0.25	0.05 - 2	1
Continuation as an analgesic into the immediate postoperative period	0.1	0.025 - 0.2	not recommended

[1] An initial dose of 1 mcg/kg may be administered over 30 to 60 seconds.
[2] No data available.

During induction of anesthesia – Administer at an infusion rate of 0.5 to 1 mcg/kg/min with a hypnotic or volatile agent for the induction of anesthesia. If endotracheal intubation is to occur < 8 minutes after the start of infusion of remifentanil, then an initial dose of 1 mcg/kg may be administered over 30 to 60 seconds.

During maintenance of anesthesia – After endotracheal intubation, decrease the infusion rate of remifentanil in accordance with the dosing guidelines in the table above. Because of the rapid onset and short duration of action of remifentanil, the rate of administration during anesthesia can be titrated upward in 25% to 100% increments or downward in 25% to 50% decrements every 2 to 5 minutes to attain the desired level of μ-opioid effect. In response to light anesthesia or transient episodes of intense surgical stress, supplemental bolus doses of 1 mcg/kg may be administered every 2 to 5 minutes. At infusion rates > 1 mcg/kg/min, consider increases in the concomitant anesthetic agents to increase the depth of anesthesia.

Continuation as an analgesic into the immediate postoperative period under the direct supervision of an anesthesia practitioner – Remifentanil infusions may be continued into the immediate postoperative period for select patients for whom later transition to longer-acting analgesics may be desired. The use of bolus injections of remifentanil to treat pain during the postoperative period is not recommended. When used as an IV analgesic in the immediate postoperative period, administer remifentanil initially by continuous infusion at a rate of 0.1 mcg/kg/min. The infusion rate may be adjusted every 5 minutes in 0.025 mcg/kg/min increments to balance the patient's level of analgesia and respiratory rate. Infusion rates > 0.2 mcg/kg/min are associated with respiratory depression (respiratory rate < 8 breaths/min).

Individualization of dosage –

Elderly: Decrease the starting doses of remifentanil by 50% in elderly patients (> 65 years of age). Cautiously titrate to effect.

Children: The same doses (per kg) as adults are recommended for pediatric patients ≥ 2 years of age.

Obesity: Base the starting dose of remifentanil on ideal body weight (IBW) in obese patients (> 30% over their IBW).

SUFENTANIL CITRATE: In obese patients (> 20% above ideal total body weight), determine dosage on the basis of lean body weight. Reduce dosage in the elderly or debilitated. Monitor vital signs routinely.

For IV injection.

Adult dosage range: Total dosage –

1 to 2 mcg/kg: Administer with nitrous oxide/oxygen in patients undergoing general surgery ≤ 8 hours in which endotracheal intubation and mechanical ventilation are required. Expected duration of anesthesia is 1 to 2 hours.

Maintenance – 10 to 25 mcg (0.2 to 0.5 mL) as needed for surgical stress/ lightening of analgesia.

2 to 8 mcg/kg: Administer with nitrous oxide/oxygen in more complicated major surgical procedures. Expected duration of anesthesia is 2 to 8 hours.

Maintenance – 10 to 50 mcg (0.2 to 1 mL) for stress/lightening of analgesia.

8 to 30 mcg/kg (anesthetic doses): Administer with 100% oxygen and a muscle relaxant. Sufentanil produces sleep at dosages ≥ 8 mcg/kg and maintains a deep level of anesthesia without additional agents.

Maintenance – 0.5 to 10 mcg/kg for stress and lightening of anesthesia.

Epidural use in labor and delivery – 10 to 15 mcg administered with 10 mL bupivacaine 0.125% with or without epinephrine. Mix sufentanil and bupivacaine together before administration. Doses can be repeated twice (for a total of 3 doses) at ≥ 1-hour intervals until delivery.

Administer sufentanil by slow injection. Closely monitor respiration following each administration of an epidural injection of sufentanil.

Children (< 12 years of age) – For induction and maintenance of anesthesia in children undergoing cardiovascular surgery, a dose of 10 to 25 mcg/kg administered with 100% oxygen is recommended. Supplemental dosages of up to 25 to 50 mcg are recommended for maintenance.

Actions

Pharmacology:

Narcotic Agonist Comparative Pharmacology[1]							
Drug	Analgesic	Antitussive	Constipation	Respiratory depression	Sedation	Emesis	Physical dependence
Phenanthrenes							
Codeine	+	+++	+	+	+	+	+
Hydrocodone	+	+++	nd[2]	+	nd[2]	nd[2]	+
Hydromorphone	++	+++	+	++	+	+	++
Levorphanol	++	++	++	++	++	+	++
Morphine	++	+++	++	++	++	++	++
Oxycodone	++	+++	++	++	++	++	++
Oxymorphone	++	+	++	+++	nd[2]	+++	+++
Phenylpiperidines							
Alfentanil	++	nd[2]	nd[2]	nd[2]	nd[2]	nd[2]	nd[2]
Fentanyl	++	nd[2]	nd[2]	+	nd[2]	+	nd[2]
Meperidine	++	+	+	++	+	nd[2]	++
Sufentanil	+++	nd[2]	nd[2]	nd[2]	nd[2]	nd[2]	nd[2]
Diphenylheptanes							
Levomethadyl	++	nd[2]	++	nd[2]	nd[2]	+	+
Methadone	++	++	++	++	+	+	+
Propoxyphene	+	nd[2]	nd[2]	+	+	+	+
Anilidopiperidines							
Remifentanil	+++	nd[2]	+	++	nd[2]	++	+

[1] Table adapted from Catalano RB. The medical approach to management of pain caused by cancer. *Semin Oncol* 1975;2:379-92 and Reuler JB, et al. The chronic pain syndrome: Misconceptions and management. *Ann Intern Med* 1980;93:588-96.

[2] nd = No data available.

Pharmacokinetics: Pharmacokinetic profiles are summarized in the table below using morphine as the standard. Data based on IM administration unless otherwise noted.

Pharmacokinetics of Narcotic Agonist Analgesics[1]						
Drug	Onset (minutes)	Peak (hours)	Duration[2] (hours)	t½ (hours)	Approximate equianalgesic doses[3] (mg)	
					Parenteral	Other
Alfentanil	immediate	nd[4]	nd[4]	1 to 2[5]	IM 0.4 to 0.8	nd[4]
Codeine	10 to 30	0.5 to 1	4 to 6	3	IM 120 to 130 SC 120	Oral 180 - 200[6]
Fentanyl	7 to 8	nd[4]	1 to 2	1.5 to 6	IM 0.1 to 0.2	Transdermal 25 mcg/hr
Hydrocodone	nd[4]	nd[4]	4 to 6	3.3 to 4.5	nd[4]	Oral 30
Hydromorphone	15 to 30	0.5 to 1	4 to 5	2 to 3	IM 1.3 to 1.5 SC 1 to 1.5	Oral 7.5
Levomethadyl	2 to 4 hrs	1.5 to 2	48 to 72	2 to 6 days	nd[4]	nd[4]
Levorphanol	30 to 90	0.5 to 1	6 to 8	11 to 16	IM 2 SC 2	Oral 4
Meperidine	10 to 45	0.5 to 1	2 to 4	3 to 4	IM 75 SC 75 to 100	Oral 300[6]
Methadone	30 to 60	0.5 to 1	4 to 6[7]	15 to 30	IM 10 SC 8 to 10	Oral 10 to 20
Morphine	15 to 60[8]	0.5 to 1	3 to 7	1.5 to 2	IM 10 SC 10	Oral 30 to 60
Oxycodone	15 to 30	1	4 to 6	nd[4]	IM 10 to 15 SC 10 to 15	Oral 30[6]
Oxymorphone	5 to 10	0.5 to 1	3 to 6	nd[4]	IM 1 SC 1 to 1.5	Rectal 5, 10

Pharmacokinetics of Narcotic Agonist Analgesics[1]						
Drug	Onset (minutes)	Peak (hours)	Duration[2] (hours)	t½ (hours)	Approximate equianalgesic doses[3] (mg)	
					Parenteral	Other
Propoxyphene (PO)	30 to 60	2 to 2.5	4 to 6	6 to 12	nd[4]	Oral 130[9]
Remifentanil	1	1 min	short[10]	≈ 3 to 10 min	nd[4]	nd[4]
Sufentanil	1.3 to 3[5]	nd[4]	nd[4]	2.5	IM 0.01 to 0.04	nd[4]

[1] Caution: Recommended doses do not apply for adult patients with body weight < 50 kg. Recommended doses do not apply to patients with renal or hepatic insufficiency or other conditions affecting drug metabolism and kinetics.

[2] After IV administration, peak effects may be more pronounced but duration is shorter. Duration of action may be longer with the oral route.

[3] Based on morphine 10 mg IM or SC. The initial dose of the new drug is given at ½ to ⅔ of the calculated dose because opioid-specific tolerance may occur, and the new drug may have more relative effectiveness (and more side effects) than the drug being discontinued.

[4] nd = No data available.

[5] Data based on IV administration.

[6] Starting doses lower (codeine, 30 mg; oxycodone, 5 mg; meperidine, 50 mg).

[7] Duration and half-life increase with repeated use because of cumulative effects.

[8] Data based on intrathecal or epidural administration.

[9] Starting doses lower (propoxyphene, 65 to 130 mg). In equimolar doses (100 mg of napsylate equals 65 mg of HCl).

[10] The duration of action does not increase with prolonged administration.

Contraindications

Hypersensitivity to narcotics; diarrhea caused by poisoning until the toxic material has been eliminated; acute bronchial asthma; upper airway obstruction.

Morphine, epidural, or intrathecal: Presence of infection at injection site; anticoagulant therapy; bleeding diathesis; parenterally administered corticosteroids within a 2-week period or other concomitant drug therapy or medical condition that would contraindicate the technique of epidural or intrathecal analgesia.

Morphine, injection: Heart failure secondary to chronic lung disease; cardiac arrhythmias; brain tumor; acute alcoholism; delirium tremens; idiosyncrasy to the drug. Because of its stimulating effect on the spinal cord, do not use morphine in convulsive states (eg, status epilepticus, tetanus, strychnine poisoning).

Morphine, immediate release oral solution: Respiratory insufficiency; heart failure secondary to chronic lung disease; cardiac arrhythmias; increased intracranial or cerebrospinal pressure; head injuries; brain tumor; acute alcoholism; delirium tremens; convulsive disorders; after biliary tract surgery; suspected surgical abdomen; surgical anastomosis; idiosyncrasy to the drug; concomitantly with monoamine oxidase inhibitors (MAOIs) or within 14 days of such treatment.

Levorphanol: Acute alcoholism; bronchial asthma; increased intracranial pressure; respiratory depression; anoxia.

Meperidine: In patients taking MAOIs or in those who have received such agents within 14 days.

Hydromorphone injection: In patients not already receiving large amounts of parenteral narcotics; patients with respiratory depression in the absence of resuscitative equipment; status asthmaticus; use as obstetrical analgesia.

Fentanyl:
> *Transdermal* – Hypersensitivity to fentanyl and adhesives; in the management of acute or postoperative pain, including use in outpatient surgeries; in the management of mild or intermittent pain responsive to PRN or non-opioid therapy; in doses exceeding 25 mcg/hour at the initiation of opioid therapy; in children < 12 years of age or patient < 18 years of age who weigh < 50 kg, except in an authorized investigational research setting.

> *Transmucosal* – In children who weigh < 10 kg; treatment of acute or chronic pain (safety for use in these patients have not been established); doses > 15 mcg/kg in

children and > 5 mcg/kg in adults because of the excessive frequency of significant hypoventilation at higher doses; for use at home or in any other setting outside a hospital setting.

Opium: Opium tincture in children; diarrhea caused by poisoning until the toxic material has been eliminated.

Oxycodone: Hypercarbia; paralytic ileus.

Oxymorphone: Paralytic ileus; treatment of pulmonary edema secondary to a chemical respiratory irritant.

Remifentanil: Epidural or intrathecal administration.

Warnings

Respiratory depression: Narcotics may be expected to produce serious or potentially fatal respiratory depression if given in an excessive dose, too frequently, or in full dosage to compromised or vulnerable patients because the doses required to produce analgesia in the general clinical population may cause serious respiratory depression in vulnerable patients.

Reduce the initial dose by > 50% when the drug is given to patients with any condition affecting respiratory reserve or in conjunction with other drugs affecting the respiratory center. Individually titrate subsequent doses according to the patient's response. Respiratory depression can be reversed by naloxone, a specific antagonist.

Asthma and other respiratory conditions – Use with extreme caution in patients with acute asthma, bronchial asthma, chronic obstructive pulmonary disease, or cor pulmonale, a substantially decreased respiratory reserve, and with preexisting respiratory depression, hypoxia, or hypercapnia.

Excessive doses: These products given in excessive doses, either alone or in combination with other CNS depressants (including alcohol), are a major cause of drug-related deaths.

Suicide: Do not prescribe propoxyphene for patients who are suicidal or addiction-prone.

Head injury and increased intracranial pressure: Narcotics may obscure the clinical course of patients with head injuries. The respiratory depressant effects and the capacity to elevate cerebrospinal fluid pressure may be markedly exaggerated in the presence of head injury, brain tumor, other intracranial lesions or a preexisting elevated intracranial pressure.

Parenteral therapy: Give by very slow IV injection, preferably as a diluted solution. The patient should be lying down. Rapid IV injection increases the incidence of adverse reactions. Use caution when injecting SC or IM in chilled areas or in patients with hypotension or shock because impaired perfusion may prevent complete absorption.

Limit epidural or intrathecal administration of **morphine** to the lumbar area.
Hydrochlorides of opium alkaloids – Do not administer IV.

Hypotensive effect: Narcotic analgesics may cause severe hypotension in individuals whose ability to maintain blood pressure has been compromised by a depleted blood volume, or coadministration of drugs such as phenothiazines or general anesthetics.

Renal/Hepatic function impairment: Renal and hepatic dysfunction may cause a prolonged duration and cumulative effect; smaller doses may be necessary.

Meperidine – In patients with renal dysfunction, normeperidine (an active metabolite of meperidine) may accumulate, resulting in increased CNS adverse reactions.

Pregnancy: Category C.

Labor – Narcotics cross the placental barrier and can produce depression of respiration and psycho-physiologic effects in the neonate.

Levomethadyl is not recommended for use in pregnancy. Current regulations mandate monthly pregnancy tests in female patients of childbearing potential who are using levomethadyl. If a patient becomes pregnant while on levomethadyl, transfer her to **methadone** for the remainder of the pregnancy.

Lactation: Most of these agents appear in breast milk, but effects on the infant may not be significant. Some recommend waiting 4 to 6 hours after use before nursing.

Children: Safety and efficacy of **sufentanil** in children < 2 years of age undergoing cardiovascular surgery have been documented in a limited number of cases. Safety and efficacy of **fentanyl** in children < 2 years of age are not established. Hypotension has occurred in neonates with respiratory distress syndrome on **alfentanil** 20 mcg/kg.

Do not use **oxycodone** in children; **propoxyphene** use is not recommended in children. **Methadone** is not recommended as an analgesic in children; documented clinical experience is insufficient to establish suitable dosage regimens. Safety of **oxymorphone** and **hydromorphone** is not established in children.

Precautions

Acute abdominal conditions: Narcotics may obscure diagnosis or clinical course.

Special risk patients: Exercise caution in elderly and debilitated patients and in those suffering from conditions accompanied by hypoxia or hypercapnia when even moderate therapeutic doses may dangerously decrease pulmonary ventilation. Also exercise caution in patients sensitive to CNS depressants, including those with cardiovascular disease; myxedema; convulsive disorders; increased ocular pressure; acute alcoholism; delirium tremens; cerebral arteriosclerosis; ulcerative colitis; fever; decreased respiratory reserve (eg, emphysema, severe obesity); hypothyroidism; kyphoscoliosis; Addison's disease; prostatic hypertrophy; urethral stricture; CNS depression; coma; gallbladder disease; recent GI or GU tract surgery; toxic psychosis.

Skeletal muscle rigidity: **Alfentanil**, **fentanyl**, and **sufentanil** may cause skeletal muscle rigidity, particularly of the truncal muscles. The incidence and severity of muscle rigidity is usually dose-related. Alfentanil, fentanyl, and sufentanil may produce muscular rigidity that involves all skeletal muscles, including those of the neck and extremities.

Supraventricular tachycardias: Use with caution in atrial flutter and other supraventricular tachycardias; vagolytic action may increase the ventricular response rate.

Seizures: Seizures may be aggravated or may occur in individuals without a history of convulsive disorders if dosage is substantially increased because of tolerance.

Suppressed cough reflex: Exercise caution when using narcotic analgesics postoperatively and in patients with pulmonary disease because cough reflex is suppressed.

Tolerance: Some patients develop tolerance to the narcotic analgesic. This may occur after days or months of continuous therapy. The dose generally needs to be increased to obtain adequate analgesia.

Cross-tolerance – Cross-tolerance is not complete. Switching to another narcotic agonist, starting with half the predicted equianalgesic dose, may circumvent the cross-tolerance.

Drug abuse and dependence: Narcotic analgesics have abuse potential. Psychological dependence and physical tolerance and dependence may develop upon repeated use. However, most patients who receive opiates for medical reasons do not develop dependence syndromes.

Infants born to mothers physically dependent on narcotics will also be physically dependent and may exhibit respiratory difficulties and withdrawal symptoms.

Acute abstinence syndrome (withdrawal) – Severity is related to the degree of dependence, the abruptness of withdrawal and the drug used. Generally, withdrawal symptoms develop at the time the next dose would ordinarily be given.

Do not use a narcotic antagonist to detect dependence. If a narcotic antagonist must be used for serious respiratory depression in a physically dependent patient, give with extreme care, using $\frac{1}{10}$ to $\frac{1}{5}$ the usual initial dose.

With morphine, cerebral and spinal receptors may develop tolerance/dependence independently, as a function of local dosage. Take care to avert withdrawal in those patients who have been maintained on parenteral/oral narcotics when epidural or intrathecal administration is considered. Withdrawal may occur following chronic epidural or intrathecal administration, as well as the development of tolerance to morphine by these routes.

Hazardous tasks: May produce drowsiness or dizziness; observe caution while driving or performing other tasks requiring alertness or physical dexterity.

Drug Interactions

Drug/Drug interactions: Drugs that may affect narcotic analgesics include amitriptyline, barbiturate anesthetics, protease inhibitors, cimetidine, chlorpromazine, erythromycin, hydantoins, diazepam, droperidol, and rifampin. Charcoal and cigarette smoking may also affect narcotic analgesics. Drugs that may be affected by narcotic analgesics include carbamazepine, warfarin, MAOIs, furazolidone, nitrous oxide, beta blockers, and calcium channel blockers.

Drug/Lab test interactions: Determinations of plasma amylase or lipase levels may be unreliable for 24 hours after narcotic administration.

Adverse Reactions

Major hazards – Respiratory depression; apnea; circulatory depression; respiratory arrest; coma; shock; cardiac arrest; hypoventilation. Most cases of serious or fatal adverse events involving **levorphanol** reported to the manufacturer or the FDA have involved either the administration of large initial doses or too frequent doses of the drug to non-opioid-tolerant patients, or the simultaneous administration of levorphanol with other drugs affecting respiration. Reduce the initial levorphanol dose by approximately > 50% when it is given to patients along with another drug affecting respiration.

Most frequent – Respiratory depression; skeletal muscle rigidity; apnea; bradycardia; lightheadedness; dizziness; sedation; nausea; vomiting; sweating. Symptoms are more prominent in ambulatory patients and in those without severe pain. Use lower doses in these patients. Some reactions may be alleviated if the ambulatory patient lies down.

NARCOTIC AGONIST-ANTAGONIST ANALGESICS

There are 2 types of narcotic agonist-antagonists: 1) Drugs which are antagonists at the μ receptor and are agonists at other receptors (ie, pentazocine), 2) partial agonists (ie, buprenorphine) that have limited agonist activity at the μ receptor. The narcotic agonist-antagonist analgesics are potent analgesic agents with a lower abuse potential than pure narcotic agonists. Because of their narcotic antagonist activity, these agents may precipitate withdrawal symptoms in those with opiate dependence.

Narcotic Agonist-Antagonist Pharmacokinetics							
Agonist/Antagonist		Onset (min)	Peak (min)	Duration (hrs)	$t^1/_2$ (hrs)	Equivalent dose[1] (mg)	Relative antagonist activity
Buprenorphine	IM	15	60	6	2.2-3.5	0.3	equipotent with naloxone
	IV[2]						
Butorphanol	IM	<10	30-60	3-4	2.5-4	2-3	30× pentazocine or $^1/_{40}$ naloxone
Dezocine	IM	≤ 30	30-150	2-4[3]	nd	10	greater than pentazocine
	IV	≤ 15			2.4[4]		
Nalbuphine	IM	< 15[5]	60	3-6	5	10	10× pentazocine
	IV	12-30[2]	30				
Pentazocine	IM	15-20[2]	15-60[1]	3	2.2-3.5	30	weak
	IV	12-30[2]	nd				
	oral	15-30[2]	60-180				

[1] Parenteral dose equivalent to 10 mg morphine.
[2] Time to onset and peak effect shorter.
[3] Dose related.
[4] For 10 or 20 mg dose; 1.7 hr for 5 mg dose.
[5] Also for subcutaneous administration.
* nd – no data

PENTAZOCINE

Injection: 30 mg (as lactate) per mL (c-iv)   *Talwin* (Sanofi Winthrop)
Tablets: 50 mg (as HCl) and 0.5 mg naloxone HCl (c-iv)   *Talwin NX* (Sanofi Winthrop)

Warning:
  Talwin Nx: Talwin Nx is intended for oral use only. Severe, potentially lethal reactions (eg, pulmonary emboli, vascular occlusion, ulceration and abscesses, withdrawal symptoms in narcotic-dependent individuals) may result from misuse of this drug by injection or in combination with other substances.

Indications
Oral and parenteral: Relief of moderate to severe pain.

Parenteral: For preoperative or preanesthetic medication; supplement to surgical anesthesia.

Administration and Dosage
Oral:
  Adults – Initially, 50 mg every 3 or 4 hours; increase to 100 mg if necessary. Do not exceed a total daily dosage of 600 mg. When anti-inflammatory or antipyretic effects are desired in addition to analgesia, aspirin can be administered concomitantly.
  Children (< 12 years of age) – Clinical experience is limited; use is not recommended.
  Pentazocine tablets are intended for oral use only. Severe, potentially lethal reactions may result from misuse by injection or when combined with other sub-

stances. Oral pentazocine tablets contain 0.5 mg naloxone, a narcotic antagonist, to aid in elimination of the abuse potential.

Parenteral:

> *Adults* – 30 mg IM, SC or IV; may repeat every 3 to 4 hours. Doses in excess of 30 mg IV or 60 mg IM or SC are not recommended. Do not exceed a total daily dosage of 360 mg.

> Use SC only when necessary; severe tissue damage is possible at injection sites. When frequent injections are needed, administer IM, constantly rotating injection sites.

> *Patients in labor* – A single 30 mg IM dose is most common. A 20 mg IV dose, given 2 or 3 times at 2- to 3-hour intervals, has resulted in adequate pain relief when contractions become regular.

> *Children (< 12 years of age)* – Clinical experience is limited; use is not recommended.

> *Admixture incompatibility* – Do not mix pentazocine in the same syringe with soluble barbiturates because precipitation will occur.

Actions

Pharmacology: Pentazocine, a potent analgesic, weakly antagonizes the effects of morphine, meperidine, and other opiates at the μ-opioid receptor.

> *Talwin NX* – *Talwin* NX tablets, which contain naloxone, produce analgesic effects when administered orally because naloxone has poor bioavailability.

Pharmacokinetics: Pentazocine is well absorbed from the GI tract and from SC and IM sites. Oral bioavailability is < 20%; concentrations in plasma coincide closely with onset, intensity and duration of analgesia. It is excreted via the kidney, < 5% unchanged.

Contraindications

Hypersensitivity to pentazocine, naloxone (in *Talwin* NX) or any product component.

Warnings

Tissue damage: Severe sclerosis of skin, SC tissues, and underlying muscle has occurred at injection sites following multiple doses of pentazocine lactate.

Head injury and increased intracranial pressure: Pentazocine can produce effects that may obscure the clinical course of head injury patients. Use with extreme caution and only if essential.

MI: Exercise caution in the IV use of pentazocine for patients with acute MI accompanied by hypertension or left ventricular failure. Use the oral form with caution in MI patients who have nausea or vomiting.

Acute CNS manifestations: Patients receiving therapeutic doses have experienced hallucinations (usually visual), disorientation, and confusion that have cleared spontaneously.

> Seizures have occurred with the use of pentazocine.

Renal/Hepatic function impairment: The drug is metabolized in liver and excreted by the kidney; administer with caution to patients with such impairment. Extensive liver disease predisposes to greater side effects and may be the result of decreased drug metabolism.

Pregnancy: Category C.

> *Labor* – Use with caution in women delivering premature infants.

Lactation: Safety for use in the nursing mother has not been established.

Children: Safety and efficacy in children < 12 years of age have not been established.

Precautions

Respiratory conditions: Use caution and low dosage in patients with respiratory depression, severely limited respiratory reserve, severe bronchial asthma, obstructive respiratory conditions, and cyanosis.

Biliary tract pressure elevation: Biliary tract pressure elevation generally occurs for varying periods following narcotic use. However, some evidence suggests pentazocine causes little or no elevation in biliary tract pressures.

Patients receiving narcotics: Pentazocine is a mild narcotic antagonist. Some patients previously given narcotics, including methadone for the daily treatment of narcotic dependence, have experienced withdrawal symptoms after receiving pentazocine.

Drug abuse and dependence: Exercise special care in prescribing to emotionally unstable patients and to those with history of drug abuse; closely supervise when therapy exceeds 4 or 5 days.

"*Ts and Blues*" – Injection IV of oral preparations of **pentazocine** (*Talwin*, "Ts") and **tripelennamine** (PBZ, "Blues"), an H_1-blocking antihistamine has become a common form of drug abuse as a "substitute" for heroin.

Hazardous tasks: May produce sedation, dizziness, and occasional euphoria; observe caution while driving or performing other tasks requiring alertness, coordination, or physical dexterity.

Drug Interactions

Drugs that may interact with pentazocine include alcohol and barbiturate anesthetics.

Adverse Reactions

Significant adverse reactions include nausea; dizziness or lightheadedness; drowsiness; vomiting; euphoria; constipation; cramps; abdominal distress; anorexia; diarrhea; dry mouth; taste alteration; sedation; headache; weakness or faintness; depression; disturbed dreams; insomnia; syncope; hallucinations; tremor; irritability; excitement; tinnitus; disorientation; confusion; blurred vision; focusing difficulty; nystagmus; diplopia; miosis; edema of the face; sweating; anaphylactic reaction; rash; urticaria; soft tissue induration; nodules; cutaneous depression; ulceration (sloughing); severe sclerosis of the skin and SC tissues; diaphoresis; stinging on injection; flushed skin; dermatitis; pruritus; toxic epidermal necrolysis; decrease in blood pressure; tachycardia; circulatory depression; shock; hypertension; respiratory depression; dyspnea; transient apnea in newborns whose mothers received parenteral pentazocine during labor; depression of white blood cells (especially granulocytes); urinary retention; paresthesia; chills; neuromuscular and psychiatric muscle tremors; alterations in rate or strength of uterine contractions during labor (parenteral form).

PENTAZOCINE COMBINATIONS

Tablets: 12.5 mg (as HCl) and 325 mg aspirin (*c-iv*)	*Talwin Compound Caplets* (Sanofi Winthrop)
Tablets: 25 mg (as HCl) and 650 mg acetaminophen (*c-iv*)	*Talacen Caplets* (Sanofi Winthrop)

Administration and Dosage

Adults:

Pentazocine and aspirin – 2 tablets 3 or 4 times/day.

Pentazocine and acetaminophen – 1 tablet every 4 hours, up to 6 tablets/day.

Children: Not recommended for children < 12 years of age.

NALBUPHINE HCl

Injection: 10 and 20 mg/mL (*Rx*)	Various, *Nubain* (DuPont)

Indications

Relief of moderate to severe pain.

For preoperative analgesia, as a supplement to balanced analgesia, to surgical and postsurgical anesthesia and for obstetrical analgesia during labor and delivery.

Administration and Dosage

Adults: Usual dose is 10 mg/70 kg administered SC, IM, or IV every 3 to 6 hours as necessary. Individualize dosage. In nontolerant individuals, the recommended single maximum dose is 20 mg, with a maximum total daily dose of 160 mg.

Patients dependent on narcotics: Patients dependent on narcotics may experience withdrawal symptoms upon the administration of nalbuphine. If unduly troublesome, control by slow IV administration of small increments of morphine until relief occurs. If the previous analgesic was morphine, meperidine, codeine or another narcotic with similar duration of activity, administer 25% the anticipated nalbuphine dose initially. Observe for signs of withdrawal. If untoward symptoms do not occur, progressively increase doses at appropriate intervals until analgesia is obtained.

Actions

Pharmacology: Nalbuphine is a potent analgesic with narcotic agonist and antagonist actions. Its analgesic potency is essentially equivalent to that of morphine and about 3 times that of pentazocine on a milligram basis.

Pharmacokinetics: Onset of action occurs within 2 to 3 minutes after IV administration, and in < 15 minutes following SC or IM injection. Nalbuphine is metabolized in the liver; plasma half-life is 5 hours. The duration of analgesic activity ranges from 3 to 6 hours. Approximately 7% is excreted unchanged in the urine.

Contraindications

Hypersensitivity to nalbuphine.

Warnings

Head injury and increased intracranial pressure: The possible respiratory depressant effects and the potential of potent analgesics to elevate cerebrospinal fluid pressure may be markedly exaggerated in the presence of head injury, intracranial lesions, or a preexisting increase in intracranial pressure.

Renal function impairment: The drug is metabolized in the liver and excreted by the kidneys; patients with renal or liver dysfunction may overreact to customary doses.

Pregnancy: Safe use in pregnancy has not been established.

Labor and delivery – May produce respiratory depression in the neonate. Use with caution in women delivering premature infants.

Children: Not recommended in patients < 18 years of age.

Precautions

Respiratory depression: At the usual adult dose of 10 mg/70 kg, nalbuphine causes respiratory depression approximately equal to that produced by equal doses of morphine. However, nalbuphine exhibits a ceiling effect; increases in dosage beyond 30 mg produce no further respiratory depression. Respiratory depression induced by nalbuphine can be reversed by naloxone.

MI: Use with caution in patients with MI who have nausea or vomiting.

Biliary tract surgery: Use with caution in patients about to undergo biliary tract surgery because it may cause spasm of the sphincter of Oddi.

Drug abuse and dependence: Nalbuphine's low abuse potential is less than codeine and propoxyphene. Psychological and physical dependence and tolerance may follow nalbuphine abuse.

Abrupt discontinuation after prolonged use has been followed by symptoms of narcotic withdrawal.

Hazardous tasks: May produce drowsiness. Observe caution while driving or performing other tasks requiring alertness, coordination or physical dexterity.

Drug Interactions

Drugs that may interact with nalbuphine HCl include barbiturate anesthetics.

Adverse Reactions

Adverse reactions occurring in ≥ 3% of patients include sedation; sweaty/clammy feeling; nausea; vomiting; dizziness; vertigo; dry mouth; headache.

BUPRENORPHINE HCL

Injection: 0.324 mg (equiv. to 0.3 mg buprenorphine) per mL (c-v)   *Buprenex* (Reckitt & Colman)

Indications
Relief of moderate to severe pain.

Administration and Dosage
Patients ≥ 13 years of age: 0.3 mg IM or slow IV, every 6 hours, as needed. Repeat once (up to 0.3 mg) if required, 30 to 60 minutes after initial dosage, giving consideration to previous dose pharmacokinetics; use thereafter only as needed. In high-risk patients (eg, elderly, debilitated, presence of respiratory disease) or in patients where other CNS depressants are present, such as in the immediate postoperative period, reduce dose by ≈ 50%. Exercise extra caution with the IV route of administration, particularly with the initial dose.

Occasionally, it may be necessary to give up to 0.6 mg. Data are insufficient to recommend single IM doses > 0.6 mg for long-term use.

IV compatibility: Buprenorphine is compatible with: Isotonic saline, Lactated Ringer's Solution, 5% Dextrose and 0.9% Saline, 5% Dextrose, scopolamine HBr, haloperidol, glycopyrrolate, droperidol, and hydroxyzine HCl.

IV incompatibility: Buprenorphine is incompatible with diazepam and lorazepam.

Actions
Pharmacology: Buprenorphine is a semisynthetic centrally acting opioid analgesic derived from thebaine; a 0.3 mg dose is approximately equivalent to 10 mg morphine in analgesic effects. Buprenorphine exerts its analgesic effect via high affinity binding of CNS opiate receptors.

Its narcotic antagonist activity is approximately equipotent to naloxone.

Cardiovascular – Buprenorphine may cause a decrease or, rarely, an increase in pulse rate and blood pressure in some patients.

Respiratory effects – A therapeutic dose of 0.3 mg buprenorphine can decrease respiratory rate similarly to an equianalgesic dose of morphine (10 mg).

Pharmacokinetics: Onset of analgesic effect occurs 15 minutes after IM injection, peaks in about 1 hour, and persists up to 6 hours. When given IV, the time to onset and peak is shortened.

Buprenorphine is metabolized by the liver and its clearance is related to hepatic blood flow.

Contraindications
Hypersensitivity to buprenorphine.

Warnings
Narcotic-dependent patients: Because of the narcotic antagonist activity of buprenorphine, use in physically dependent individuals may result in withdrawal effects. Buprenorphine, a partial agonist, has opioid properties that may lead to psychic dependence because of a euphoric component of the drug. The drug may not be substituted in acutely dependent narcotic addicts because of its antagonist component.

Respiratory effects: There have been occasional reports of clinically significant respiratory depression associated with buprenorphine.

Head injury/increased intracranial pressure: Buprenorphine may elevate cerebrospinal fluid (CSF) pressure; use with caution in head injury, intracranial lesions, and other states where CSF pressure may be increased. Buprenorphine can produce miosis and changes in consciousness levels that may interfere with patient evaluation.

Hepatic function impairment: Buprenorphine is metabolized by the liver; the activity may be altered in those individuals with impaired hepatic function.

Pregnancy: Category C.

Labor and delivery – Safety and efficacy have not been established.

Lactation: It is not known whether buprenorphine is excreted in breast milk.

Children: Safety and efficacy for use in children have not been established.

Precautions

Use with caution in the following: Elderly or debilitated; severe impairment of hepatic, pulmonary or renal function; myxedema or hypothyroidism; adrenal cortical insufficiency; CNS depression or coma; toxic psychoses; prostatic hypertrophy or urethral stricture; acute alcoholism; delirium tremens; or kyphoscoliosis. Naloxone may not be effective in reversing respiratory depression.

Biliary tract dysfunction: Buprenorphine increases intracholedochal pressure to a similar degree as other opiates; administer with caution.

Hazardous tasks: May cause dizziness or drowsiness; observe caution while driving or performing other tasks requiring alertness.

Drug Interactions

Drugs that may interact with buprenorphine HCl include barbiturate anesthetics; diazepam.

Adverse Reactions

Adverse reactions occurring in ≥ 3% of patients include sedation, dizziness/vertigo, headache, hypotension, nausea/vomiting, hypoventilation, miosis, sweating.

TRAMADOL HCl

Tablets: 50 mg (*Rx*)   *Ultram* (Ortho-McNeil)

Indications
Pain: Management of moderate to moderately severe pain.

Administration and Dosage
For the treatment of painful conditions, 50 to 100 mg can be administered as needed for relief every 4 to 6 hours, not to exceed 400 mg/day. For moderate pain, 50 mg may be adequate as the initial dose, and for more severe pain, 100 mg is usually more effective as the initial dose.

Elderly: Available data do not suggest that a dosage adjustment is necessary in elderly patients 65 to 75 years of age unless they also have renal or hepatic impairment. For elderly patients > 75 years old, < 300 mg/day in divided doses as above is recommended.

Renal function impairment: In all patients with Ccr < 30 mL/min, it is recommended that the dosing interval be increased to 12 hours, with a maximum daily dose of 200 mg. Because only 7% of an administered dose is removed by hemodialysis, dialysis patients can receive their regular dose on the day of dialysis.

Hepatic function impairment: The recommended dose for patients with cirrhosis is 50 mg every 12 hours.

Actions
Pharmacology: Tramadol is a centrally acting synthetic analgesic compound. Although its mode of action is not completely understood, from animal tests 2 complementary mechanisms appear applicable: Binding to µ-opioid receptors and inhibition of reuptake of norepinephrine and serotonin.

Onset of analgesia is evident within 1 hour after administration and reaches a peak in ≈ 2 to 3 hours.

Pharmacokinetics:

Absorption – Tramadol is rapidly and almost completely absorbed after oral administration.

Distribution – Binding to human plasma proteins is ≈ 20% and appears to be independent of concentration up to 10 mcg/mL.

Metabolism – Tramadol is extensively metabolized after oral administration. Approximately 30% of the dose is excreted in the urine as unchanged drug.

Excretion – The plasma elimination half-life of tramadol is ≈ 6 to 7 hours.

Contraindications
Hypersensitivity to tramadol; acute intoxication with alcohol, hypnotics, centrally acting analgesics, opioids, or psychotropic drugs.

Warnings
Seizure: Administration of tramadol may enhance the seizure risk in patients taking MAO inhibitors, neuroleptics, other drugs that reduce the seizure threshold, patients with epilepsy or patients otherwise at increased risk for seizure.

Anaphylactoid reactions: Serious and rarely fatal anaphylactoid reactions have been reported in patients receiving tramadol therapy. Other reported reactions include pruritus, hives, bronchospasm, and angioedema. Patients with a history of anaphylactoid reactions to codeine and other opioids may be at increased risk and therefore should not receive tramadol.

Concomitant CNS depressants: Use with caution and in reduced dosages when administering to patients receiving CNS depressants such as alcohol, opioids, anesthetic agents, phenothiazines, tranquilizers, or sedative hypnotics.

Concomitant MAO inhibitors: Use with great caution in patients taking MAO inhibitors.

Pregnancy: Category C.

Lactation: Tramadol is not recommended for obstetrical preoperative medication or for post-delivery analgesia in nursing mothers.

Children: Not recommended in children < 16 years of age.

Precautions

Increased intracranial pressure or head trauma: Use with caution in patients with increased intracranial pressure or head injury. Pupillary changes (miosis) from tramadol may obscure the existence, extent, or course of intracranial pathology.

Acute abdominal conditions: Tramadol may complicate the clinical assessment of patients with acute abdominal conditions.

Opioid dependence: Tramadol is not recommended for patients who are dependent on opioids.

Drug abuse and dependence: Do not use tramadol in opioid-dependent patients. Tramadol has been shown to reinitiate physical dependence in some patients that have been previously dependent on other opioids.

Drug Interactions

Drugs that may interact with tramadol include carbamazepine, MAO inhibitors, and quinidine.

Drug/Food interactions: Food does not affect rate or extent of absorption; tramadol can be administered without regard to meals.

Adverse Reactions

Adverse reactions occurring in ≥ 3% of patients include dizziness/vertigo; nausea; constipation; headache; somnolence; vomiting; pruritus; CNS stimulation; asthenia; sweating; dyspepsia; dry mouth; diarrhea; malaise; vasodilation; abdominal pain; anorexia; flatulence; rash; visual disturbance; urinary retention/frequency; menopausal symptoms; hypertonia.

ACETAMINOPHEN (N-Acetyl-P-Aminophenol, APAP)

ACETAMINOPHEN

Suppositories: 80, 120, 125, 300, 325, and 650 mg (otc)
Various, *Acetaminophen Uniserts* (Upsher-Smith), *Acephen* (G & W Labs), *Neopap* (PolyMedica)

Tablets, chewable: 80 mg (otc)
Various, *St. Joseph Aspirin-Free for Children* (Schering-Plough), *Tylenol, Children's, Tylenol, Junior Strength* (McNeil-CPC)

Capsules: 80, 160, and 500 mg (otc)
Various, *Feverall Sprinkle Caps* (Upsher-Smith), *Dapa Extra Strength* (Ferndale)

Granules: 80 mg (otc)
Snaplets-FR Granules (Baker Cummins)

Caplets: 160 mg (otc)
Junior Strength Panadol (Sterling Health)

Caplets, extended release: 650 mg (otc)
Tylenol Extended Relief (McNeil-CPC)

Tablets: 160, 325, 500, and 650 mg (otc)
Various, *Tylenol Regular Strength Tablets* (McNeil-CPC), *Aspirin Free Anacin Maximum Strength* (Whitehall)

Elixir: 80, 120, 130, 160, and 325 mg/5 mL (otc)
Various, *Ridenol* (RID), *Dolanex* (Lannett), *Oraphen-PD* (Great Southern), *Tylenol Children's* (McNeil-CPC)

Liquid: 160 mg/5 mL and 500 mg/15 mL (otc)
Various, *St. Joseph Aspirin-Free Fever Reducer for Children* (Schering-Plough), *Tylenol Extra Strength* (McNeil-CPC)

Solution: 100 mg/mL and 120 mg/2.5 mL (otc)
Various, *Tempra Drops* (Mead Johnson Nutritional), *Liquiprin Infants' Drops* (Menley & James)

Suspension: 80 mg/0.8 mL and 160 mg/5 mL (otc)
Tylenol Infants' Drops (McNeil-CPC), *Tylenol, Children's* (McNeil-CPC)

ACETAMINOPHEN, BUFFERED

Effervescent granules: 325 mg w/2.781 g sodium bicarbonate & 2.224 g citric acid/dose measure (otc)
Bromo Seltzer (Warner-Lambert)

Indications

An analgesic-antipyretic in the presence of aspirin allergy, hemostatic disturbances (including anticoagulant therapy), bleeding diatheses (eg, hemophilia), upper GI disease (eg, ulcer, gastritis, hiatus hernia), and gouty arthritis; variety of arthritic and rheumatic conditions involving musculoskeletal pain, as well as in other painful disorders; diseases accompanied by discomfort and fever such as the common cold, "flu" and other bacterial or viral infections.

Unlabeled uses: Prophylactic APAP use in children receiving DTP vaccination appears to decrease incidence of fever and injection site pain. A dose immediately following vaccination and every 4 to 6 hrs thereafter for 48 to 72 hrs is suggested.

Administration and Dosage

Oral:

    Adults – 325 to 650 mg every 4 to 6 hours, or 1 g 3 to 4 times/day. Do not exceed 4 g/day.

    Children – May repeat doses 4 or 5 times/day; do not exceed 5 doses in 24 hours.

Acetaminophen Dosage for Children			
Age	Dosage (mg)	Age (years)	Dosage (mg)
0-3 months	40	4-5	240
4-11 months	80	6-8	320
1-2 years	120	9-10	400
2-3 years	160	11	480

    A 10 mg/kg/dose schedule has also been recommended.

Suppositories:

    Adults – 650 mg every 4 to 6 hrs. Give no more than 6 in 24 hours.

    Children –

        (3 to 11 months of age): 80 mg every 6 hours.

        (1 to 3 years of age): 80 mg every 4 hours.

        (3 to 6 years of age): 120 to 125 mg every 4 to 6 hours. Give no more than 720 mg/24 hours.

(6 to 12 years of age): 325 mg every 4 to 6 hours. Give no more than 2.6 g/ 24 hours.

Actions

Pharmacology: The site and mechanism of the analgesic effect is unclear. APAP reduces fever by a direct action on the hypothalamic heat-regulating centers, which increases dissipation of body heat (via vasodilatation and sweating). APAP is almost as potent as aspirin in inhibiting prostaglandin synthetase in the CNS, but its peripheral inhibition of prostaglandin synthesis is minimal.

APAP does not inhibit platelet aggregation, affect prothrombin response, or produce GI ulceration.

Pharmacokinetics:

Absorption – Absorption of acetaminophen is rapid and almost complete from the GI tract.

Distribution – Usual analgesic doses produce total serum concentrations of 5 to 20 mcg/mL.

Metabolism/Excretion – Average elimination half-life is 1 to 3 hours; half-life is slightly prolonged in neonates (2.2 to 5 hours) and in cirrhotics.

Contraindications

Hypersensitivity to acetaminophen.

Warnings

Do not exceed recommended dosage. Consult physician for use in children < 3 years of age, or for oral use longer than 5 days (children), 10 days (adults) or 3 days for fever. Chronic excessive use (> 4 g/day) eventually may lead to transient hepatotoxicity. The kidneys may undergo tubular necrosis; the myocardium may be damaged.

Hepatic function impairment: Hepatotoxicity and severe hepatic failure occurred in chronic alcoholics following therapeutic doses. Caution chronic alcoholics to limit acetaminophen intake to ≤ 2 g/day.

Pregnancy: Acetaminophen crosses the placenta. It is routinely used during all stages of pregnancy; when used in therapeutic doses, it appears safe for short-term use.

Lactation: Acetaminophen is excreted in breast milk. No adverse effects in nursing infants were reported.

Precautions

If a sensitivity reaction occurs, discontinue use.

Severe or recurrent pain or high or continued fever may indicate serious illness. If pain persists for more than 5 days, if redness is present or in arthritic and rheumatic conditions affecting children < 12 years of age, consult physician immediately.

Drug Interactions

Drugs that may affect APAP include barbiturates, carbamazepine, hydantoins, isoniazid, rifampin, sulfinpyrazone, ethyl alcohol, and activated charcoal.

Drug/Lab test interactions: Acetaminophen may interfere with *Chemstrip bG, Dextrostix,* and *Visidex II* home blood glucose measurement systems; decreases of > 20% in mean glucose values may be noted. This effect appears to be drug-, concentration-, and system-dependent.

Adverse Reactions

Used as directed, acetaminophen rarely causes severe toxicity or side effects.

SALICYLATES

ASPIRIN
Tablets, chewable: 81 mg (otc)
Bayer Children's Aspirin (Glenbrook), St. Joseph Adult Chewable Aspirin (Schering-Plough)

Gum tablets: 227.5 mg (otc)
Aspergum (Schering-Plough)

Tablets: 325 and 500 mg (otc)
Various, Genuine Bayer Aspirin Tablets and Caplets (Glenbrook), Empirin (Burroughs Wellcome), Genprin (Goldline), Maximum Bayer Aspirin Tablets and Caplets (Glenbrook), Norwich Extra-Strength (Procter & Gamble Pharm.)

Tablets, enteric-coated: 325 mg (otc)
Various, Ecotrin Tablets and Caplets (GlaxoSmith-Kline), Regular Strength Bayer Enteric Coated Caplets (Sterling Health)

Tablets, enteric-coated: 81, 165, 500, 650, and 975 mg (otc)
Various, Bayer Low Adult Strength (GlaxoSmith-Kline), 1/2 Halfprin (Kramer), Ecotrin Maximum Strength Tablets and Caplets (GlaxoSmithKline), Extra Strength Bayer Enteric 500 Aspirin (Sterling Health), Easprin (Parke-Davis)

Tablets, timed-release: 650 mg (otc)
8-hour Bayer Timed-Release Caplets (Glenbrook)

Tablets, controlled-release: 800 mg (Rx)
ZORprin (Boots)

Suppositories: 120 mg, 200 mg, 300 mg, and 600 mg (otc)
Various

ASPIRIN (Acetylsalicylic Acid; ASA), BUFFERED
Tablets: 325 mg with buffers (otc)
Various, Bayer Buffered Aspirin (Sterling Health), Magnaprin (Rugby), Regular Strength Ascriptin (Aventis), Bufferin (Bristol-Myers), Asprimox (Invamed), Adprin-B (Pfeiffer), Asprimox Extra Protection for Arthritis Pain (Bristol-Myers), Buffex (Roberts Med.)

Tablets, coated: 500 mg with buffers (otc)
Extra Strength Adprin-B (Pfeiffer), Extra Strength Bayer Plus Caplets (Sterling Health), Ascriptin Extra Strength (Aventis), Cama Arthritis Pain Reliever (Sandoz), Arthritis Pain Formula (White-hall)

Tablets, effervescent: 325 and 500 mg with buffers (otc)
Alka-Seltzer with Aspirin, Alka-Seltzer Extra Strength with Aspirin (Miles)

CHOLINE SALICYLATE
Liquid: 870 mg/5 mL (otc)
Arthropan (Purdue Frederick)

MAGNESIUM SALICYLATE
Tablets: 325, 467, 500, 545, 580, and 600 mg (otc)
Original Doan's (Ciba Consumer), Backache Maximum Strength Relief (B-M Squibb), Extra Strength Doan's (Ciba Consumer), Magan (Adria), Bayer Select Maximum Strength Backache (Sterling Health), Mobidin (Ascher)

SALSALATE (Salicylsalicyclic Acid)
Capsules: 500 mg (Rx)
Amigesic (Amide), Disalcid (3M)

Tablets: 500 mg (Rx)
Various, Disalcid (3M), Salflex (Carnrick), Salsitab (Upsher-Smith)

750 mg (Rx)
Various, Disalcid (3M), Salsitab (Upsher-Smith), Salflex (Carnrick), Marthritic (Marnel)

SODIUM SALICYLATE
Tablets, enteric-coated: 325 mg and 650 mg (otc)
Various

SODIUM THIOSALICYLATE
Injection: 50 mg/mL (Rx)
Various, Rexolate (Hyrex)

SALICYLATE COMBINATIONS
Tablets: 500 mg salicylate (as 293 mg choline salicylate and 362 mg Mg salicylate), 750 mg salicylate (as 440 mg choline salicylate and 544 mg Mg salicylate), 1000 mg salicylate (as 587 mg choline salicylate, 725 mg salicylate) (Rx)
Choline Magnesium Trisalicylate (Sidmak), Tricosal (Invamed), Trilisate (Purdue Frederick)

Liquid: 500 mg salicylate (as 293 mg choline salicylate and 362 mg Mg salicylate) per 5 mL (Rx)
Trilisate (Purdue Frederick)

Warning:
Children and teenagers should not use salicylates for chickenpox or flu symptoms before a doctor is consulted about Reye's syndrome, a rare but serious illness.

Indications

Mild to moderate pain; fever; various inflammatory conditions such as rheumatic fever, rheumatoid arthritis and osteoarthritis.

Aspirin: Aspirin, for reducing the risk of recurrent transient ischemic attacks (TIAs) or stroke in men who have had transient ischemia of the brain because of fibrin platelet emboli. It has not been effective in women and is of no benefit for completed strokes.

To reduce the risk of death or nonfatal myocardial infarction (MI) in patients with previous infarction or unstable angina pectoris.

Administration and Dosage

ASPIRIN (*Acetylsalicylic Acid; ASA*):

Minor aches and pains – 325 to 650 mg every 4 hours as needed. Some extra strength (500 mg) products suggest 500 mg every 3 hours or 1000 mg every 6 hours.

Arthritis, other rheumatic conditions (eg, osteoarthritis) – 3.2 to 6 g/day in divided doses.

Juvenile rheumatoid arthritis: 60 to 110 mg/kg/day in divided doses (every 6 to 8 hours). When starting at lower doses (eg, 60 mg/kg/day), may increase by 20 mg/kg/day after 5 to 7 days, followed by 10 mg/kg/day after another 5 to 7 days.

Maintain a serum salicylate level of 150 to 300 mcg/mL.

Acute rheumatic fever –

Adults: 5 to 8 g/day, initially.

Children: 100 mg/kg/day for 2 weeks, then decreased to 75 mg/kg/day for 4 to 6 weeks.

Therapeutic salicylate level: Therapeutic salicylate levelis 150 to 300 mcg/mL.

Transient ischemic attacks in men – 1300 mg/day in divided doses (650 mg 2 times/day, or 325 mg 4 times/day). One study indicated that a dose of 300 mg/day is as effective as the larger dose and may be associated with fewer side effects.

MI prophylaxis – 300 or 325 mg/day. This use applies to solid oral doseforms (buffered and plain) and to buffered aspirin in solution.

Children –

Analgesic/antipyretic dosage: 10 to 15 mg/kg/dose every 4 hours (see table), up to 60 to 80 mg/kg/day.

Recommended Aspirin Dosage in Children					
Age (years)	Weight		Dosage (mg every 4 hours)	No. of 81 mg tablets (every 4 hours)	No. of 325 mg tablets (every 4 hours)
	lbs	kg			
2-3	24-35	10.6-15.9	162	2	½
4-5	36-47	16-21.4	243	3	
6-8	48-59	21.5-26.8	324	4	1
9-10	60-71	26.9-32.3	405	5	
11	72-95	32.4-43.2	486	6	1½
12-14	≥ 96	≥ 43.3	648	8	2

Kawasaki disease (mucocutaneous lymph node syndrome): For acute febrile period, 80 to 180 mg/kg/day; very high doses may be needed to achieve therapeutic levels. After the fever resolves, dosage may be adjusted to 10 mg/kg/day.

ASPIRIN, BUFFERED: The addition of small amounts of antacids may decrease GI irritation and increase the dissolution and absorption rates of these products. Dosing is the same as with unbuffered aspirin.

CHOLINE SALICYLATE: Has fever GI side effects than aspirin.

Adults and children (> 12 years of age) – 870 mg every 3 to 4 hours; maximum 6 times/day. Rheumatoid arthritis patients may start with 5 to 10 mL, up to 4 times/day.

MAGNESIUM SALICYLATE: A sodium free salicylate derivative that may have a low incidence of GI upset. The product labeling and dosage are expressed as magnesium salicylate anhydrous. The possibility of magnesium toxicity exists in people with renal insufficiency.

Usual dose is 650 mg every 4 hours or 1090 mg, 3 times a day. May increase to 3.6 to 4.8 g/day in 3 or 4 divided doses.

Safety and efficacy for use in children have not been established.

SALSALATE (Salicylsalicylic Acid): After absorption, the drug is partially hydrolyzed into two molecules of salicylic acid. Insoluble in gastric secretions, it is not absorbed until it reaches the small intestine.

Usual adult dose is 3000 mg/day given in divided doses.

SODIUM SALICYLATE: Less effective than an equal dose of aspirin in reducing pain or fever. Patients hypersensitive to aspirin may be able to tolerate sodium salicylate. Each gram contains 6.25 mEq sodium.

Usual dose – 325 to 650 mg every 4 hours.

SODIUM THIOSALICYLATE: Intramuscular administration is preferred.

Acute gout – 100 mg every 3 to 4 hours for 2 days, then 100 mg/day until asymptomatic.

Muscular pain, musculoskeletal disturbances – 50 to 100 mg/day or on alternate days.

Rheumatic fever – 100 to 150 mg every 4 to 8 hours for 3 days, then reduce to 100 mg twice/day. Continue until patient is aymptomatic.

Actions

Pharmacology: Salicylates have analgesic, antipyretic, anti-inflammatory, and antirheumatic effects. Salicylates lower elevated body temperature through vasodilation of peripheral vessels, thus enhancing dissipation of excess heat. The anti-inflammatory and analgesic activity may be mediated through inhibition of the prostaglandin synthetase enzyme complex.

Aspirin – Aspirin differs from the other agents in this group in that it more potently inhibits prostaglandin synthesis, has greater anti-inflammatory effects and irreversibly inhibits platelet aggregation.

Irreversible inhibition of platelet aggregation (aspirin) – Single analgesic aspirin doses prolong bleeding time. Aspirin (no other salicylates) inhibits platelet aggregation for the life of the platelet (7 to 10 days).

Low doses of aspirin inhibit platelet aggregation and may be more effective than higher doses. Larger doses inhibit cyclooxygenase in arterial walls, interfering with prostacyclin production, a potent vasodilator and inhibitor of platelet aggregation.

Pharmacokinetics:

Absorption/Distribution – Salicylates are rapidly and completely absorbed after oral use. Bioavailability is dependent on the dosage form, presence of food, gastric emptying time, gastric pH, presence of antacids or buffering agents and particle size. Bioavailability of some enteric coated products may be erratic. Absorption from rectal suppositories is slower, resulting in lower salicylate levels. Protein binding of salicylates is concentration-dependent.

Metabolism/Excretion – Salicylic acid is eliminated by renal excretion.

Contraindications

Hypersensitivity to salicylates or nonsteroidal anti-inflammatory drugs (NSAIDs). Use extreme caution in patients with history of adverse reactions to salicylates. Cross-sensitivity may exist between aspirin and other NSAIDs that inhibit prostaglandin synthesis, and aspirin, and tartrazine. Aspirin cross-sensitivity does not appear to occur with sodium salicylate, salicylamide, or choline salicylate. Aspirin hypersensitivity is more prevalent in those with asthma, nasal polyposis, chronic urticaria.

In hemophilia, bleeding ulcers and hemorrhagic states.

Magnesium salicylate: Magnesium salicylate in advanced chronic renal insufficiency because of Mg^{++} retention.

Warnings

Otic effects: Discontinue use if dizziness, ringing in ears (tinnitus), or impaired hearing occurs. Tinnitus probably represents blood salicylic acid levels reaching or exceeding the upper limit of the therapeutic range.

Use in surgical patients: Avoid aspirin, if possible, for 1 week prior to surgery because of the possibility of postoperative bleeding.

Hypersensitivity reactions: Aspirin intolerance, manifested by acute bronchospasm, generalized urticaria/angioedema, severe rhinitis, or shock occurs in 4% to 19% of asthmatics. Symptoms occur within 3 hours after ingestion. Have epinephrine 1:1000 immediately available.

Foods – Foods may contribute to a reaction. Some foods with 6 mg/100 g salicylate include curry powder, paprika, licorice, Benedictine liqueur, prunes, raisins, tea, and gherkins. A typical American diet contains 10 to 200 mg/day salicylate.

Hepatic function impairment: Use caution in liver damage, preexisting hypoprothrombinemia, and vitamin K deficiency.

Pregnancy: Category D (aspirin); *Category C* (salsalate, magnesium salicylate). Avoid use during pregnancy, especially in third trimester.

Lactation: Salicylates are excreted in breast milk in low concentrations.

Children: Safety and efficacy of **magnesium salicylate** or **salsalate** have not been established. Administration of **aspirin** to children (including teenagers) with acute febrile illness has been associated with the development of Reye's syndrome. Dehydrated febrile children appear more prone to salicylate intoxication.

Precautions

Renal effects: Use with caution in chronic renal insufficiency; aspirin may cause a transient decrease in renal function, and may aggravate chronic kidney diseases (rare). In patients with renal impairment, take precautions when administering **magnesium salicylate**.

GI effects: Use caution in those intolerant to salicylate because of GI irritation, and in gastric ulcers, peptic ulcer, mild diabetes, gout, erosive gastritis, or bleeding tendencies. **Salsalate** and **choline salicylate** may cause less GI irritation than aspirin.

Although fecal blood loss is less with enteric coated aspirin than with uncoated, give enteric coated aspirin with caution to patients with GI distress, ulcer, or bleeding problems.

Hematologic effects: Aspirin interferes with hemostasis. Avoid use if patients have severe anemia, history of blood coagulation defects, or take anticoagulants.

Long-term therapy: To avoid potentially toxic concentrations, warn patients on long-term therapy not to take other salicylates (nonprescription analgesics, etc).

Salicylism: Salicylism may require dosage adjustment.

Controlled-release aspirin: Controlled-release aspirin, because of its relatively long onset of action, is not recommended for antipyresis or short-term analgesia. Not recommended in children > 12 years of age; contraindicated in all children with fever accompanied by dehydration.

Drug Interactions

Drugs that may affect aspirin include activated charcoal, ammonium chloride, ascorbic acid or methionine, antacids and urinary alkalinizers, carbonic anhydrase inhibitors, corticosteroids, and nizatidine. Drugs that may be affected by aspirin include alcohol, ACE inhibitors, anticoagulants (oral), beta-adrenergic blockers, heparin, loop diuretics, methotrexate, nitroglycerin, NSAIDs, probenecid and sulfinpyrazone, spironolactone, sulfonylureas and exogenous insulin, and valproic acid.

Drug/Lab test interactions: Salicylates compete with thyroid hormone for binding sites on thyroid binding pre-albumin and possibly thyroid binding globulin resulting in increases in **protein bound iodine**. Salicylates probably do not interfere with T_3 resin uptake.

Serum uric acid – Serum uric acid levels are elevated by salicylate levels < 10 mg/dL and decreased by levels > 10 mg/dL.

Salicylates in moderate to large (anti-inflammatory) doses cause false-negative readings for **urine glucose** by the glucose oxidase method and false-positive readings by the copper reduction method.

Salicylates in the urine interfere with **5-HIAA** determinations by fluorescent methods, but not by the nitrosonaphthol colorimetric method.

Salicylates in the urine interact with **urinary ketone** determinations by the ferric chloride (Gerhardt) method producing a reddish color.

Large doses may decrease urinary excretion of **phenolsulfonphthalein**.

Salicylates in the urine result in falsely elevated **vanillylmandelic acid (VMA)** with most tests, but falsely decrease VMA determinations by the Pisano method.

Adverse Reactions

Adverse reactions include the following: Hives; rashes; angioedema; nausea, dyspepsia (5% to 25%); heartburn; epigastric discomfort; anorexia; massive GI bleeding; occult blood loss; potentiation of peptic ulcer; persistent iron deficiency anemia; prolongation of bleeding time; leukopenia; thrombocytopenia; purpura; decreased plasma iron concentration; shortened erythrocyte survival time; fever; thirst; dimness of vision.

Miscellaneous:
Mild *"salicylism"* – Mild "salicylism" may occur after repeated use of large doses and consists of dizziness, tinnitus, difficulty hearing, nausea, vomiting, diarrhea, mental confusion, CNS depression, headache, sweating, hyperventilation, and lassitude. Salicylate serum concentrations correlate with pharmacological actions and adverse effects observed.

DIFLUNISAL

Tablets: 250 mg and 500 mg (*Rx*)   Various, *Dolobid* (Merck)

Indications

Acute or long-term symptomatic treatment of mild to moderate pain, rheumatoid arthritis, and osteoarthritis.

Administration and Dosage

Mild to moderate pain: Initially, 1 g, followed by 500 mg every 8 to 12 hours. A lower dosage may be appropriate; for example, 500 mg initially, followed by 250 mg every 8 to 12 hours.

Osteoarthritis/rheumatoid arthritis: 500 mg to 1 g/day in 2 divided doses. Individualize dosage. Do not exceed maintenance doses higher than 1.5 g/day.

Actions

Pharmacology: Diflunisal, a salicylic acid derivative, is a nonsteroidal, peripherally acting, nonnarcotic analgesic with anti-inflammatory and antipyretic properties. Chemically, it differs from aspirin and is not metabolized to salicylic acid. Its mechanisms are unknown. Diflunisal is a prostaglandin synthetase inhibitor.

Pharmacokinetics: Diflunisal is rapidly and completely absorbed following oral administration; peak plasma concentrations occur between 2 to 3 hours, producing significant analgesia within 1 hour and maximum analgesia within 2 to 3 hours. The first dose tends to have a slower onset of pain relief than other drugs achieving comparable peak effects. Time required to achieve steady state increases with dosage, from 3 to 4 days with 125 mg twice/day to 7 to 9 days with 500 mg twice/day. An initial loading dose shortens the time to reach steady-state levels.

Contraindications

Hypersensitivity to diflunisal.

Patients in whom acute asthmatic attacks, urticaria, or rhinitis are precipitated by aspirin or other nonsteroidal anti-inflammatory drugs.

Warnings

Peptic ulceration: Peptic ulceration and GI bleeding have been reported. Fatalities occurred rarely.

Renal function impairment: Because diflunisal is eliminated primarily by the kidneys, monitor patients with significant renal impairment; use a lower daily dosage.

Pregnancy: Category C.

Lactation: Diflunisal is excreted in breast milk. Because of the potential for adverse reactions in nursing infants, discontinue either nursing or the drug.

Children: Use in children < 12 years of age is not recommended.

Precautions

Platelet function: Platelet function and bleeding time are inhibited by diflunisal at higher doses.

Ophthalmologic effects: Ophthalmologic effects have been reported with these agents.

Peripheral edema: Peripheral edema has been observed. Use with caution in patients with compromised cardiac function, hypertension, or other conditions predisposing to fluid retention.

Acetylsalicylic acid: Acetylsalicylic acid has been associated with Reye's syndrome. Because diflunisal is a salicylic acid derivative, the possibility of its association with Reye's syndrome cannot be excluded.

Drug Interactions

Drug interactions with diflusinol include acetaminophen; anticoagulants, oral; hydrochlorothiazide; indomethacin; sulindac.

Adverse Reactions

Adverse reactions that occur in ≥ 3% include nausea, dyspepsia, GI pain, diarrhea, vomiting, headache, rash, fatigue/tiredness, tinnitus.

DICLOFENAC SODIUM AND MISOPROSTOL

Tablets: 50 mg diclofenac sodium/200 mcg misoprostol and   *Arthrotec* (Searle)
75 mg diclofenac sodium/200 mcg misoprostol (*Rx*)

Warning:
This product, because of the abortifacient property of the misoprostol component, is contraindicated in women who are pregnant. Advise patients of the abortifacient property and warn not to give the drug to others. Do not use in women with childbearing potential unless the patient requires nonsteroidal anti-inflammatory drug (NSAID) therapy and is at high risk of developing gastric or duodenal ulceration or of developing complications from gastric or duodenal ulcers associated with the use of the NSAID. In such patients, this drug may be prescribed if the patient:

- had a negative pregnancy test within 2 weeks prior to beginning therapy,
- is capable of complying with effective contraceptive measures,
- has received oral and written warnings of the hazards of misoprostol, the risk of possible contraception failure, and the danger to other women of childbearing potential should the drug be taken by mistake, and
- will begin using this product only on the second or third day of the next normal menstrual period.

Indications
Arthritis patients at high risk of ulcers: Treatment of the signs and symptoms of osteoarthritis or rheumatoid arthritis in patients at high risk of developing NSAID-induced gastric and duodenal ulcers and their complications.

Administration and Dosage
Swallow tablets whole; do not chew, crush, or dissolve. May take with meals to minimize GI effects. Avoid co-adminstration with magnesium-containing antacids.

Osteoarthritis: The recommended dose is 50 mg diclofenac/200 mcg misoprostol 3 times/day. For patients who experience intolerance, 50 mg/200 mcg or 75 mg/200 mcg twice/day can be used, but are less effective in preventing ulcers.

Rheumatoid arthritis: Recommended dose is 50 mg diclofenac/200 mcg misoprostol 3 or 4 times/day. For patients who experience intolerance, 50 mg/200 mcg or 75 mg/200 mcg twice/day can be used, but are less effective in preventing ulcers.

Special dosing considerations: For gastric ulcer prevention, 200 mcg 3 and 4 times/day are therapeutically equivalent but more protective than the twice daily regimen. For duodenal ulcer prevention, 4 times/day is more protective than the 2 or 3 times/day regimens. However, the 4 times/day regimen is less well tolerated.

Dosages may be individualized using the separate products (misoprostol and diclofenac), after which the patient may be changed to the appropriate diclofenac/misoprostol dose. If clinically indicated, misoprostol co-therapy with diclofenac/misoprostol, or use of the individual components to optimize the misoprostol dose or frequency of administration, may be appropriate. The total dose of misoprostol should not exceed 800 mcg/day, and do not administer > 200 mcg of misoprostol at any one time. Doses of diclofenac > 150 mg/day in osteoarthritis or > 225 mg/day in rheumatoid arthritis are not recommended.

Actions
Pharmacology: This product is a combination containing diclofenac sodium, a nonsteroidal anti-inflammatory drug (NSAID) with analgesic properties, and misoprostol, a GI mucosal protective prostaglandin E_1 analog.

Pharmacokinetics: The pharmacokinetics following oral administration of a single dose or multiple doses of diclofenac/misoprostol to healthy subjects under fasted conditions are similar to the pharmacokinetics of the 2 individual components. Food decreases the multiple-dose bioavailability profile of both formulations.

Contraindications

Hypersensitivity to diclofenac or to misoprostol or other prostaglandins. Do not give to patients who have experienced asthma, urticaria, or other allergic-type reactions after taking aspirin or other NSAIDs.

Warnings

Pregnancy: Category X.

Lactation: Diclofenac sodium is found in milk of breastfeeding mothers. Because of the potential for serious adverse reactions in nursing infants, this product is not recommended for breastfeeding mothers.

Children: Safety and efficacy in patients < 18 years of age have not been established.

Adverse Reactions

Adverse reactions reported in ≥ 3% of patients include abdominal pain, diarrhea, dyspepsia, nausea, and flatulence.

NONSTEROIDAL ANTI-INFLAMMATORY AGENTS

CELECOXIB

Capsules: 100 and 200 mg (*Rx*)	*Celebrex* (Searle)

DICLOFENAC

Tablets: 50 mg (as potassium) (*Rx*)	Various, *Cataflam* (Novartis)
Tablets, delayed-release: 25, 50, and 75 mg (as sodium) (*Rx*)	Various, *Voltaren* (Novartis)
Tablets, extended-release: 100 mg (as sodium) (*Rx*)	*Voltaren-XR* (Novartis)

ETODOLAC

Capsules: 200 and 300 mg (*Rx*)	Various, *Lodine* (Wyeth-Ayerst)
Tablets: 400 and 500 mg (*Rx*)	Various, *Lodine* (Wyeth-Ayerst)
Tablets, extended-release: 400, 500, and 600 mg	*Lodine XL* (Wyeth-Ayerst)

FENOPROFEN CALCIUM

Capsules: 200 and 300 mg (*Rx*)	Various, *Nalfon Pulvules* (Ranbaxy)
Tablets: 600 mg (*Rx*)	Various

FLURBIPROFEN

Tablets: 50 and 100 mg (*Rx*)	Various, *Ansaid* (Pharmacia)

IBUPROFEN

Tablets: 100 mg (*otc*)	*Junior Strength Motrin* (McNeil)
200 mg (*otc*)	Various, *Advil* (Whitehall-Robins), *Genpril* (Goldline), *Haltran* (Lee Pharm), *Maximum Strength Midol* (Bayer), *Menadol* (Rugby), *Motrin IB* (McNeil), *Nuprin* (Bristol-Myers Squibb)
400, 600, and 800 mg (*Rx*)	Various, *Motrin* (Pharmacia)
Tablets, chewable: 50 and 100 mg (*otc*)	*Children's Advil* (Whitehall-Robins), *Children's Motrin* (McNeil), *Jr. Strength Motrin* (McNeil), *Jr. Strength Advil* (Whitehall-Robins)
Capsules: 200 mg (*otc*)	*Advil Liqui-Gels* (Whitehall-Robins)
Suspension: 100 mg/5 mL (*Rx*)	*Children's Advil* (Wyeth-Ayerst)
100 mg/5 mL (*otc*)	Various, *Children's Motrin* (McNeil-CPC), *PediaCare Fever* (Pharmacia)
100 mg/2.5 mL (*otc*)	*Pediatric Advil Drops* (Wyeth-Ayerst)
Oral drops: 40 mg/mL (*otc*)	*Infants' Motrin* (McNeil), *PediaCare Fever* (Pharmacia)

INDOMETHACIN

Capsules: 25 and 50 mg (*Rx*)	Various, *Indocin* (Merck)
Capsules, sustained-release: 75 mg (*Rx*)	Various, *Indocin SR* (Forte Pharma)
Oral suspension: 25 mg/5 mL (*Rx*)	*Indocin* (Merck)
Suppositories: 50 mg (*Rx*)	*Indocin* (Merck)

KETOPROFEN

Tablets: 12.5 mg (*otc*)	*Orudis KT* (Whitehall-Robins)
Capsules: 25, 50, and 75 mg (*Rx*)	Various, *Orudis* (Wyeth-Ayerst)
Capsules, extended release: 100, 150, and 200 mg (*Rx*)	*Oruvail* (Wyeth-Ayerst)

KETOROLAC TROMETHAMINE

Tablets: 10 mg (*Rx*)	Various, *Toradol* (Roche)
Injection: 15 and 30 mg/mL (*Rx*)	*Toradol* (Roche)

MECLOFENAMATE SODIUM

Capsules: 50 and 100 mg (as sodium) (*Rx*)	Various

MEFENAMIC ACID

Capsules: 250 mg (*Rx*)	*Ponstel* (Parke-Davis)

MELOXICAM

Tablets: 7.5 mg (*Rx*)	*Mobic* (Boehringer Ingelheim/Abbott)

NABUMETONE

Tablets: 500 and 750 mg (*Rx*)	*Relafen* (GlaxoSmithKline)

NAPROXEN

Tablets: 200 mg (as naproxen sodium) (*otc*)	Various, *Aleve* (Bayer)
250 and 500 mg (as naproxen sodium) (*Rx*)	Various, *Anaprox* (Roche)
250, 375, and 500 mg (*Rx*)	Various, *Naprosyn* (Roche)
Tablets, delayed-release: 375 and 500 mg (*Rx*)	Various, *EC-Naprosyn* (Roche)

Tablets, controlled-release: 375 (412.5 mg naproxen sodium) and 500 mg (550 mg naproxen sodium) (*Rx*)	*Naprelan* (Carnrick Laboratories)
Suspension: 125 mg/5 mL (*Rx*)	Various, *Naprosyn* (Roche)
OXAPROZIN	
Tablets: 600 mg (*Rx*)	*Daypro* (Searle)
PIROXICAM	
Capsules: 10 and 20 mg (*Rx*)	Various, *Feldene* (Pfizer)
ROFECOXIB	
Tablets: 12.5 and 25 mg (*Rx*)	*Vioxx* (Merck)
Suspension: 12.5 mg/5 mL, 25 mg/5 mL (*Rx*)	*Vioxx* (Merck)
SULINDAC	
Tablets: 150 and 200 mg (*Rx*)	Various, *Clinoril* (Merck)
TOLMETIN SODIUM	
Tablets: 200 and 600 mg (as sodium) (*Rx*)	Various, *Tolectin 200 or 600* (McNeil)
Capsules: 400 mg (as sodium) (*Rx*)	Various, *Tolectin DS* (McNeil)
VALDECOXIB	
Tablets: 10 and 20 mg (*Rx*)	*Bextra* (Searle)

Indications

NSAIDs: Summary of Indications

Indications (✓-Labeled, X-Unlabeled)	Celecoxib	Diclofenac potassium	Diclofenac sodium/Diclofenac sodium XR	Etodolac	Fenoprofen	Flurbiprofen	Ibuprofen	Indomethacin	Indomethacin SR	Ketoprofen	Ketoprofen SR	Ketorolac	Meclofenamate	Mefenamic acid	Meloxicam	Nabumetone	Naproxen	Oxaprozin	Piroxicam	Rofecoxib	Sulindac	Tolmetin	Valdecoxib
Rheumatoid arthritis (RA)	✓	✓	✓	✓	✓	✓	✓	✓	✓	✓	✓		✓			✓	✓	✓	✓		✓	✓	✓
Osteoarthritis (OA)	✓	✓	✓	✓	✓	✓	✓	✓	✓	✓	✓		✓		✓	✓	✓	✓	✓	✓	✓	✓	✓
Ankylosing spondylitis		✓	✓[1]	X		X		✓	✓								✓				✓		
Mild to moderate pain		✓		✓	✓		✓			✓			✓	✓[6]			✓			✓			
Moderately severe acute pain												✓[5]											
Primary dysmenorrhea		✓			X	X	✓			✓			✓	✓			✓		X	✓	X		✓
Juvenile RA		X	X	X			✓			X							✓		X			✓	
Tendinitis				X				✓	✓								✓				✓		
Bursitis				X				✓	✓								✓				✓		
Acute painful shoulder			X	X		X		✓	✓												✓		
Acute gout				X				✓									✓				✓		
Fever							✓[2]																
Sunburn								X[3]															

NSAIDs: Summary of Indications

Indications / ✓-Labeled / X- Unlabeled	Celecoxib	Diclofenac potassium	Diclofenac sodium/ Diclofenac sodium XR	Etodolac	Fenoprofen	Flurbiprofen	Ibuprofen	Indomethacin	Indomethacin SR	Ketoprofen	Ketoprofen SR	Ketorolac	Meclofenamate	Mefenamic acid	Meloxicam	Nabumetone	Naproxen	Oxaprozin	Piroxicam	Rofecoxib	Sulindac	Tolmetin	Valdecoxib
Migraine																							
Abortive (acute attack)						X	X					X	X	X			X						
Prophylactic					X		X	X		X			X				X						
Menstrual					X			X		X			X	X			X						
Cluster headache								X															
Polyhydramnios								X															
Acne vulgaris, resistant							X																
Menorrhagia													X										
Premenstrual syndrome														X			X						
Cystoid macular edema								X³															
Closure of persistent patent ductus arteriosus								✓⁴															

1 Sodium only, not sodium XR.
2 In children only.
3 Topical formulation.
4 IV formulation only.
5 Therapy not to exceed 5 days.
6 Therapy not to exceed 1 week.

Rheumatoid arthritis (RA) (except **ketorolac, mefenamic acid,** *,* **meloxicam,** *and* **rofecoxib**) *and osteoarthritis (OA) (except ketorolac and mefenamic acid):* Relief of signs and symptoms; treatment of acute flares and exacerbation; long-term management.

Concomitant therapy – Concomitant therapy with other second-line drugs (eg, gold salts) demonstrates additional therapeutic benefit. Whether they can be used with partially effective doses of corticosteroids for a "steroid-sparing" effect and result in greater improvement is not established.

Use with salicylates is not recommended; greater benefit is not achieved, and the potential for adverse reactions is increased. The use of aspirin with nonsteroidal anti-inflammatory agents (NSAIDs) may cause a decrease in blood levels of the nonaspirin drug.

Juvenile RA (**tolmetin, naproxen**) – For the treatment of juvenile RA.

*Mild to moderate pain (***diclofenac potassium, etodolac, fenoprofen, ibuprofen, ketoprofen, ketorolac, meclofenamate, mefenamic acid, naproxen, naproxen sodium, rofecoxib**): Post-extraction dental pain, postsurgical episiotomy pain, and soft tissue athletic injuries.

Primary dysmenorrhea: **Diclofenac potassium, ibuprofen, ketoprofen, mefenamic acid, naproxen, naproxen sodium, rofecoxib.**

Idiopathic heavy menstrual blood loss: **Meclofenamate sodium.**

Familial adenomatous polyposis (FAP) (**Celecoxib**): To reduce the number of adenomatous colorectal polyps in FAP as an adjunct to usual care (eg, endoscopic surveillance, surgery). It is not known whether there is a clinical benefit from a reduction in the number of colorectal polyps in FAP patients. It also is not known whether the effects of celecoxib treatment will persist after celecoxib is discontinued. The efficacy and safety of celecoxib treatment in patients with FAP > 6 months have not been studied.

Administration and Dosage
CELECOXIB: Seek the lowest dose for each patient. Safety and efficacy in children < 18 years of age have not been evaluated.

Osteoarthritis – Recommended oral dosage is 200 mg/day administered as a single dose or as 100 mg twice a day.

Rheumatoid arthritis – Recommended oral dosage is 100 to 200 mg twice a day.

FAP – Continue usual medical care for FAP patients while on celecoxib. To reduce the number of adenomatous colorectal polyps in patients with FAP, the recommended oral dose is 400 mg /day. Take with food.

DICLOFENAC:
Osteoarthritis – 100 to 150 mg/day in divided doses (50 mg twice/day or 3 times/day [diclofenac sodium or potassium] or 75 mg twice/day [diclofenac sodium]). Dosages > 200 mg/day have not been studied.

Rheumatoid arthritis – 150 to 200 mg/day in divided doses (50 mg 3 or 4 times/day [diclofenac sodium or potassium] or 75 mg twice/day [diclofenac sodium]). Dosages > 225 mg/day of the delayed-release diclofenac sodium formulation and dosages > 200 mg/day of immediate-release diclofenac potassium formulation are not recommended.

Ankylosing spondylitis – 100 to 125 mg/day as 25 mg 4 times/day, with an extra 25 mg dose at bedtime, if necessary. Dosages > 125 mg/day have not been studied.

Analgesia and primary dysmenorrhea (diclofenac potassium only) – Recommended starting dose is 50 mg 3 times/day. In some patients, an initial dose of 100 mg followed by 50 mg doses will provide better relief. After the first day, when the maximum recommended dose may be 200 mg, the total daily dose should generally not exceed 150 mg.

ETODOLAC:
Osteoarthritis – Initially 600 to 1200 mg/day in divided doses, followed by adjustment in the range of 600 to 1200 mg/day in divided doses (400 mg 2 or 3 times/day; 300 mg 2, 3, or 4 times/day; 200 mg 3 or 4 times/day). Do not exceed 1200 mg/day.

Patients ≤ 60 kg: Do not exceed 20 mg/kg.

Analgesia –

Acute pain: 200 to 400 mg every 6 to 8 hrs. Do not exceed 1200 mg/day.

Patients ≤ 60 kg: Do not exceed 20 mg/kg.

FENOPROFEN: Do not exceed 3.2 g/day. If GI upset occurs, take with meals or milk.

Rheumatoid arthritis and osteoarthritis – 300 to 600 mg 3 or 4 times/day.

Mild to moderate pain – 200 mg every 4 to 6 hours, as needed.

FLURBIPROFEN:

Rheumatoid arthritis and osteoarthritis – Initial recommended total daily dose is 200 to 300 mg; administer in divided doses 2, 3, or 4 times/day. The largest recommended single dose in a multiple-dose daily regimen is 100 mg. Doses > 300 mg/day are not recommended.

IBUPROFEN:

Adults – Do not exceed 3.2 g/day. If GI upset occurs, take with meals or milk.

Rheumatoid arthritis and osteoarthritis: 1.2 to 3.2 g/day (300 mg 4 times/day or 400, 600, or 800 mg 3 or 4 times/day).

Mild to moderate pain: 400 mg every 4 to 6 hours, as necessary.

Primary dysmenorrhea: 400 mg every 4 hours, as necessary.

OTC use (minor aches and pains, dysmenorrhea, fever reduction): 200 mg every 4 to 6 hours while symptoms persist. If pain or fever do not respond to 200 mg, 400 mg may be used. Do not exceed 1.2 g in 24 hours. Do not take for pain for > 10 days or for fever for > 3 days, unless directed.

Children –

Juvenile arthritis: Usual dose is 30 to 40 mg/kg/day in 3 or 4 divided doses; 20 mg/kg/day may be adequate for milder disease. Doses > 50 mg/kg/day are not recommended.

Fever reduction/pain relief in children 6 months to 12 years of age: Adjust dosage on the basis of the initial temperature level. If baseline temperature is ≤ 39.2°C (102.5°F), recommended dose is 5 mg/kg; if baseline temperature is > 39.2°C (102.5°F), recommended dose is 10 mg/kg. Duration of fever reduction is longer with the higher dose. Maximum daily dosage is 40 mg/kg.

INDOMETHACIN:

Moderate to severe rheumatoid arthritis (including acute flares of chronic disease), ankylosing spondylitis, and osteoarthritis – 25 mg 2 or 3 times/day. If this is well tolerated, increase the daily dose by 25 or 50 mg (if required by continuing symptoms) at weekly intervals until a satisfactory response is obtained or until a daily dose of 150 to 200 mg is reached. Doses above this amount generally do not increase the effectiveness of the drug.

In patients who have persistent night pain or morning stiffness, giving a large portion, up to a maximum of 100 mg of the total daily dose at bedtime, may help to relieve pain. The total daily dose should not exceed 200 mg.

In acute flares of chronic rheumatoid arthritis, it may be necessary to increase the dosage by 25 or 50 mg/day.

Acute painful shoulder (bursitis or tendinitis) – 75 to 150 mg daily in 3 or 4 divided doses. Discontinue the drug after inflammation has been controlled for several days. Usual course of therapy is 7 to 14 days.

Acute gouty arthritis – 50 mg 3 times/day until pain is tolerable, then rapidly reduce the dose to complete cessation of the drug. Definite relief of pain usually occurs within 2 to 4 hours. Tenderness and heat usually subside in 24 to 36 hours, and swelling gradually disappears in 3 to 5 days. Do not use sustained release form.

Sustained-release form – Do not crush. The 75 mg sustained-release capsule can be taken once a day as an alternative to the 25 mg capsule 3 times/day. In addition, one 75 mg sustained-release capsule twice/day can be substituted for the 50 mg capsule 3 times/day. Do not use sustained-release form in acute gouty arthritis.

Children – Efficacy in children ≤ 14 years of age has not been established except in circumstances that warrant the risk. When using in children ≥ 2 years of age, closely monitor liver function. Suggested starting dose is 2 mg/kg/day in divided doses. Do not exceed 4 mg/kg/day or 150 to 200 mg/day, whichever is less.

KETOPROFEN: Take with antacids, food, or milk to minimize adverse GI effects.

Rheumatoid arthritis and osteoarthritis – Do not exceed 300 mg/day for regular-release formulation or 200 mg/day for extended-release capsules.

Daily dose: 150 to 300 mg divided into 3 or 4 doses.

Starting dose: 75 mg 3 times/day or 50 mg 4 times/day. Reduce initial dose to ½ to ⅓ in elderly or debilitated patients or those with impaired renal function.

Mild to moderate pain, primary dysmenorrhea – 25 to 50 mg every 6 to 8 hours as needed. Give smaller dosages initially to smaller patients, the elderly and those with renal or liver disease. Doses > 50 mg may be given, but doses > 75 mg do not display added therapeutic effects. Do not exceed 300 mg/day.

OTC –

Adults: 12.5 mg with a full glass of liquid every 4 to 6 hours. If pain or fever persists after 1 hour, follow with 12.5 mg. With experience, some patients may find an initial dose of 25 mg will give better relief. Do not exceed 25 mg in a 4 to 6 hour period or 75 mg in a 24-hour period.

Children: Do not give to those < 16 years of age unless directed by a physician.

KETOROLAC TROMETHAMINE: The combined duration of ketorolac IV/IM and oral is not to exceed 5 days. Oral use is only indicated as combination therapy to IV/IM.

IV/IM – When administering IV/IM, the IV bolus must be given over no less than 15 seconds. Give IM administration slowly and deeply into the muscle.

Single-dose treatment: Limit following regimen to single administration use only

   IM dosing –

      < 65 years of age: One 60 mg dose.

      ≥ 65 years of age, renal impairment, or < 50 kg (110 lbs): One 30 mg dose.

   IV dosing –

      < 65 years of age: One 30 mg dose.

      ≥ 65 years of age, renal impairment, or < 50 kg (110 lbs): One 15 mg dose.

Multiple-dose treatment:

      < 65 years of age – The recommended dose is 30 mg every 6 hours. The maximum daily dose should not exceed 120 mg.

      ≥ 65 years of age, renal impairment, or < 50 kg (110 lbs) – The recommended dose is 15 mg every 6 hours. The maximum daily dose for these populations should not exceed 60 mg.

Oral – Indicated only as continuation therapy to ketorolac IV/IM.

Transition from IV/IM to oral:

      < 65 years of age – 20 mg as a first oral dose for patients who received 60 mg IM single dose, 30 mg single IV dose or 30 mg multiple dose IV/IM followed by 10 mg every 4 to 6 hours, not to exceed 40 mg/24 hours.

      ≥ 65 years of age, renal impairment, or < 50 kg (110 lbs) – 10 mg as a first oral dose for patients who received a 30 mg IM single dose, 15 mg IV single dose, or 15 mg multiple dose IV/IM followed by 10 mg every 4 to 6 hours, not to exceed 40 mg/24 hours.

MECLOFENAMATE SODIUM:

Mild to moderate pain – 50 mg every 4 to 6 hours. Doses of 100 mg may be required for optimal pain relief. Do not exceed daily dosage of 400 mg.

Excessive menstrual blood loss and primary dysmenorrhea – 100 mg 3 times daily for up to 6 days, starting at the onset of menstrual flow.

Rheumatoid arthritis and osteoarthritis –

Usual dosage: 200 to 400 mg/day in 3 or 4 equal doses.

Initial dosage: Initiate at lower dosage; increase as needed to improve response. Do not exceed 400 mg/day.

Children – Safety and efficacy in children < 14 years of age are not established.

MEFENAMIC ACID:

Acute pain –

Adults (≥ 14 years of age): 500 mg, then 250 mg every 6 hours, as needed, usually not to exceed 1 week. Give with food.

Primary dysmenorrhea – 500 mg, then 250 mg every 6 hours. Start with the onset of bleeding and associated symptoms. Should not be necessary for > 2 to 3 days.

Children – Safety and efficacy in children < 14 years have not been established.

MELOXICAM:

Osteoarthritis – Use the lowest dosage for each patient. For treatment of osteoarthritis, the recommended starting and maintenance dose is 7.5 mg once/day. Some patients may receive additional benefit by increasing the dose to 15 mg once/day. The maximum recommended dose is 15 mg/day. Meloxicam may be taken without regard to meals.

NABUMETONE: Recommended starting dose is 1000 mg as a single dose with or without food. Some patients may obtain more symptomatic relief from 1500 to 2000 mg/day. Nabumetone can be given either once or twice/day. Dosages > 2000 mg/day have not been studied.

NAPROXEN:

Rx – Do not exceed 1.25 g/day naproxen (1.375 g/day naproxen sodium).

Rheumatoid arthritis, osteoarthritis, ankylosing spondylitis, pain, dysmenorrhea, acute tendinitis, and bursitis:

Naproxen – 250 to 500 mg twice/day. May increase to 1.5 g/day for limited periods.

Delayed release naproxen (EC-Naprosyn) – 375 to 500 mg twice/day. Do not break, crush, or chew tablets.

Controlled release (Naprelan) – 750 mg or 1500 mg once/day. Do not exceed 1000 mg/day.

Naproxen sodium – 275 to 550 mg twice/day. May increase to 1.65 g for limited periods.

Juvenile arthritis:

Naproxen only (not naproxen sodium) – Total daily dose is ≈ 10 mg/kg in 2 divided doses.

Suspension: Use the following as a guide:

Naproxen Suspension: Children's Dose	
Child's weight	Dose
13 kg (29 lb)	2.5 mL (0.5 tsp) bid
25 kg (55 lb)	5 mL (1 tsp) bid
38 kg (84 lb)	7.5 mL (1.5 tsp) bid

Acute gout:

Naproxen – 750 mg, followed by 250 mg every 8 hours until attack subsides.

Naproxen sodium – 825 mg, then 275 mg every 8 hours until attack subsides.

Controlled release (Naprelan) – 1000 to 1500 mg once/day on the first day followed by 1000 mg once/day until the attack has subsided.

Mild to moderate pain, primary dysmenorrhea, acute tendinitis, and bursitis:

Naproxen – 500 mg, followed by 250 mg every 6 to 8 hours. Do not exceed a 1.25 g total daily dose. Thereafter, total daily dose should not exceed 1000 mg.

Naproxen sodium – 550 mg, followed by 275 mg every 6 to 8 hours. Do not exceed a 1.375 g total daily dose.

Controlled release (Naprelan) – 1000 mg once daily. For patients requiring greater analgesic benefit, 1500 mg/day may be used for a limited period.

Children: Safety and efficacy in children < 2 years of age have not been established.

OTC –

Adults: 200 mg with a full glass of liquid every 8 to 12 hours while symptoms persist. With experience, some patients may find that an initial dose of 400 mg followed by 200 mg 12 hours later, if necessary, will give better relief. Do not exceed 600 mg in 24 hours unless otherwise directed.

Elderly (> 65 years of age): Do not take > 200 mg every 12 hours.

Children: Do not give to children < 12 years of age except under the advice and supervision of a physician.

OXAPROZIN:
>*Rheumatoid arthritis* – 1200 mg once/day.
>
>*Osteoarthritis* – 1200 mg once/day. For patients of low body weight or with milder disease, an initial dosage of 600 mg once a day may be appropriate.
>
>*Maximum dose* – 1800 mg/day (or 26 mg/kg, whichever is lower) in divided doses.

PIROXICAM: Initiate and maintain at a single daily dose of 20 mg. May divide daily dose. Do not assess effect of therapy for 2 weeks.
>*Children* – Use in children has not been established.

ROFECOXIB: Use the lowest effective dose for each patient.
>*OA* – The recommended starting dose is 12.5 mg once/day. The maximum recommended daily dose is 25 mg.
>
>*Acute pain and primary dysmenorrhea* – The recommended initial dose is 50 mg once/day. Use of rofecoxib for > 5 days in the management of pain has not been studied.
>
>*Tablets* – May be taken with or without food.

SULINDAC: Administer twice a day with food. The usual maximum dosage is 400 mg/day. Dosages above 400 mg/day are not recommended.
>*Osteoarthritis, rheumatoid arthritis, and ankylosing spondylitis* – Initial dosage is 150 mg twice a day.
>
>*Acute painful shoulder (acute subacromial bursitis/supraspinatus tendinitis); acute gouty arthritis* – 200 mg twice/day. After satisfactory response, reduce dosage accordingly.
>
>*Children* – Safety and efficacy have not been established.

TOLMETIN SODIUM:
>*Adults* –
>>*Rheumatoid arthritis and osteoarthritis:* Initially, 400 mg 3 times/day; preferably include dose on arising and at bedtime. Control is usually achieved at doses of 600 to 1800 mg/day generally in 3 divided doses. Doses > 1800 mg/day are not recommended.
>
>*Children* –
>>(≥ 2 years of age): Initially, 20 mg/kg/day in 3 or 4 divided doses. When control is achieved, usual dosage ranges from 15 to 30 mg/kg/day. Doses > 30 mg/kg/day are not recommended.

VALDECOXIB:
>*Osteoarthritis/Adult rheumatoid arthritis* – 10 mg once/day.
>
>*Primary dysmenorrhea* – 20 mg twice/day, as needed.

Actions

Pharmacology: Nonsteroidal anti-inflammatory drugs have analgesic, antipyretic, and anti-inflammatory activities. Major mechanism is believed to be inhibition of cyclooxygenase activity and prostaglandin synthesis.

Two COX isoenzymes have been identified: COX-1 and COX-2. Inhibition of COX-1 activity is considered a major contributor to NSAID GI toxicity. The function of the COX-2 isoenzyme is induced during pain and inflammatory stimuli.

Many NSAIDs inhibit both COX-1 and COX-2. Most NSAIDs are mainly COX-1 selective (eg, **aspirin, ketoprofen, indomethacin, piroxicam, sulindac**). Others are considered slightly selective for COX-1 (eg, **ibuprofen, naproxen, diclofenac**) and others may be considered slightly selective for COX-2 (eg, **etodolac, nabumetone**). The mechanism of action of **celecoxib** and **rofecoxib** is primarily selective inhibition of COX-2.

Pharmacokinetics:

Pharmacokinetic Parameters/Maximum Dosage Recommendations of NSAIDs

NSAID	Bioavail-ability (%)	Half-life (hours)	Volume of distr-ibution	Clearance	Peak (hours)	Protein binding (%)	Renal elimina-tion (%)	Fecal elimina-tion (%)
Acetic acids								
Diclofenac	50 to 60	2	0.1 to 0.2 L/kg	350 mL/min	2	> 99	65	-
Indomethacin	98	4.5	0.29 L/kg	0.084 L/hr/kg	2	90	60	33
Sulindac	90	7.8	NS[1]	≈2.71 L/hr	2 to 4	> 93	50	25
Tolmetin	NS[1]	2 to 7	NS[1]	NS[1]	0.5 to 1	NS[1]	≈ 100	-
COX-2 inhibitors								
Celecoxib	NS[1]	11	400 L	27.7 L/hr	3	97	27	57
Rofecoxib	93	17	91 L	120 to 141 mL/min	2 to 3	87	72	14
Fenamates								
Meclofenamate	≈ 100	1.3	23 L	206 mL/min	0.5 to 2	> 99	70	30
Mefenamic acid	NS[1]	2	1.06 L/kg	21.23 L/hr	2 to 4	> 90	52	20
Naphthylalkanones								
Nambumetone	> 80	22.5	0.1 to 0.2 L/kg	26.1 mL/min	9 to 12	> 99	80	9
Oxicams								
Piroxicam	NS[1]	50	0.15 L/kg	0.002 to 0.003 L/kg/hr	3 to 5	98.5	NS[1]	NS[1]
Meloxicam	89	15 to 20	10 L	7 to 9 mL/min	4 to 5	99.4	50	50
Propionic acids								
Fenoprofen	NS[1]	3	NS[1]	NS[1]	2	99	90	-
Flurbiprofen	NS[1]	5.7	0.1 to 0.2 L/kg	1.13 L/hr	≈ 1.5	> 99	> 70	-
Ibuprofen	> 80	1.8 to 2	0.15 L/kg	≈3 to 3.5 L/hr	1 to 2	99	45 to 79	-
Ketoprofen	90	2.1	0.1 L/kg	6.9 L/hr	0.5 to 2	> 99	80	-
Ketoprofen ER	90	5.4	0.1 L/kg	6.8 L/hr	6 to 7	> 99	80	-
Naproxen	95	12 to 17	0.16 L/kg	0.13 mL/min/kg	2 to 4	> 99	95	-
Oxaprozin	95	42 to 50	10 to 12.5 L	0.25 to 0.34 L/hr	3 to 5	> 99	65	35
Pyranocarboxylic acid								
Etodolac	≥ 80	7.3	0.362 L/kg	47 mL/hr/kg	≈ 1.5	> 99	72	16
Pyrrolizine carboxylic acid								
Ketorolac	100	5 to 6	≈ 0.2 L/kg	≈ 0.025 L/hr/kg	2 to 3	99	91	6

[1] NS = Not studied.

Contraindications

NSAID hypersensitivity: Because of potential cross-sensitivity to other NSAIDs, do not give these agents to patients in whom aspirin or other NSAIDs have induced symptoms of asthma, rhinitis, urticaria, nasal polyps, angioedema, bronchospasm, and other symptoms of allergic or anaphylactoid reactions.

Fenoprofen or mefenamic acid: Preexisting renal disease.

Mefenamic acid: Active ulceration or chronic inflammation of either the upper or lower GI tract.

Indomethacin suppositories: History of proctitis or recent rectal bleeding.

Celecoxib: Hypersensitivity to sulfonamides.

Ketorolac: Active peptic ulcer disease; recent GI bleeding or perforation; history of peptic ulcer disease or GI bleeding; advanced renal impairment or patients at risk for renal failure because of volume depletion; labor and delivery; nursing mothers; previously demonstrated hypersensitivity to ketorolac tromethamine; as prophylactic analgesic before any major surgery; intraoperatively when hemostasis is critical because of the increased risk of bleeding; suspected or confirmed cerebrovascular bleeding, hemorrhagic diathesis, incomplete hemostasis and those at high risk of bleeding; for neuraxial (epidural or intrathecal) administration; concomitant use with probenecid.

Warnings

Ketorolac tromethamine: Ketorolac is indicated for the short-term (up to 5 days) management of moderately severe acute pain that requires analgesia at the opioid level. It is not indicated for minor or chronic painful conditions. Increasing the dose beyond the label recommendations will not provide better efficacy but will result in increasing risk of developing serious adverse events.

GI effects – Ketorolac should not be used in active peptic ulcer disease, recent GI bleeding or perforation, a history of peptic ulcer disease or GI bleeding.

Renal effects – Ketorolac is contraindicated in patients with advanced renal impairment and in patients at risk for renal failure because of volume depletion.

Risk of bleeding – Ketorolac inhibits platelet function and is therefore contraindicated in patients with suspected or confirmed cerebrovascular bleeding, hemorrhagic diathesis, incomplete hemostasis, and those at high risk of bleeding.

Ketorolac is contraindicated as prophylactic analgesia before any major surgery and is contraindicated intra-operatively when hemostasis is critical because of the increased risk of bleeding.

Hypersensitivity – Hypersensitivity reactions, ranging from bronchospasm to anaphylactic shock, have occurred.

Intrathecal or epidural administration – Ketorolac is contraindicated for intrathecal or epidural administration because of its alcohol content.

Labor, delivery, and lactation – Use in labor and delivery and lactation is contraindicated.

Concomitant use with NSAIDs – Ketorolac is contraindicated in patients currently receiving aspirin or other NSAIDs because of the cumulative risk of inducing serious NSAID-related side effects; ketorolac is also contraindicated with the concomitant use of probenecid.

Administration and dosage – Ketorolac (oral) is indicated only as continuation therapy to ketorolac IV/IM; the combined duration of use of IV/IM and oral is not to exceed 5 days because of the increased risk of serious adverse events.

Special populations – Adjust dosage for patients ≥ 65 years of age, for patients < 50 kg (110 lbs) and for patients with moderately elevated serum creatinine. IV/IM doses are not to exceed 60 mg/day in these patients.

GI effects: Serious GI toxicity such as bleeding, ulceration, and perforation can occur at any time, with or without warning symptoms, in patients treated chronically with NSAID therapy. Higher doses of **meloxicam** (eg, 30 mg/day) were associated with increased risk of serious GI effects. Do not exceed daily doses of 15 mg.

CNS effects: **Indomethacin** may aggravate depression or other psychiatric disturbances, epilepsy, and parkinsonism. Some of these agents may also cause headaches (highest incidence with fenoprofen, indomethacin, and ketorolac).

Renal effects: Acute renal insufficiency, interstitial nephritis, hyperkalemia, hyponatremia, and renal papillary necrosis, and other medullary changes may occur.

Hypersensitivity reactions: A potentially fatal apparent hypersensitivity syndrome has occurred with **sulindac**. Severe hypersensitivity reactions with fever, rashes, abdominal pain, headache, nausea, vomiting, signs of liver damage, and meningitis have occurred in **ibuprofen** patients, especially those with systemic lupus erythematosus (SLE) or other collagen diseases.

Renal function impairment: NSAID metabolites are eliminated primarily by kidneys; use with caution. In cases of advanced kidney disease, treatment with **piroxicam** and **meloxicam** is not recommended.

Hepatic function impairment: Dose reduction may be needed with **naproxen**. Reduce the daily recommended dose of **celecoxib** capsules in patients with moderate hepatic impairment (Child Pugh Class II) by $\approx$ 50%.

Elderly: Age appears to increase the possibility of adverse reactions to NSAIDs. The risk of serious ulcer disease is increased; this risk appears to increase with dose. **Ketorolac** is cleared more slowly by the elderly; use caution and reduce dosage.

Pregnancy: *Category* B (ketoprofen, naproxen, flurbiprofen, diclofenac). *Category* C (etodolac, ketorolac, mefenamic acid, meloxicam, nabumetone, oxaprozin, tolmetin, piroxicam, rofecoxib, celecoxib). Avoid during pregnancy, especially in the third trimester.

Lactation: Most NSAIDs are excreted in breast milk. In general, do not use in nursing mothers because of effects on infant's cardiovascular system.

Children: **Mefenamic acid** and **meclofenamate** are not recommended in children < 14 years of age. **Indomethacin** is not recommended in children $\leq$ 14 years of age, except in circumstances that warrant the risk. Safety and efficacy of **meloxicam** have not been established in children < 18 years of age. **Tolmetin** and **naproxen** are the only agents labeled for juvenile rheumatoid arthritis. Safety and efficacy of tolmetin in infants < 2 years of age are not established. Safety and efficacy of other NSAIDs in children are not established.

Precautions

Steroid dosage: If reduced or eliminated during therapy, reduce slowly and observe patient closely for evidence of adverse effects, including adrenal insufficiency and exacerbation of symptoms.

Porphyria: Avoid the use of NSAIDs in patients with hepatic porphyria.

Platelet aggregation: NSAIDs can inhibit platelet aggregation; the effect is quantitatively less and of shorter duration than that seen with aspirin. These agents prolong bleeding time (within normal range) in healthy subjects.

Hematologic effects: Decreased hemoglobin or hematocrit levels have rarely required discontinuation.

Aseptic meningitis: Aseptic meningitis with fever and coma has been observed on rare occasions in patients on NSAIDs therapy, although it is probably more likely to occur in patients with SLE.

Cardiovascular effects: May cause fluid retention and peripheral edema.

Ophthalmologic effects: Effects include blurred or diminished vision, scotomata, changes in color vision, corneal deposits, and retinal disturbances, including maculas.

Infection: NSAIDs may mask the usual signs of infection.

Hepatic effects: Borderline liver function test elevations may occur in $\approx$ 15% of patients and may progress, remain essentially unchanged, or become transient with continued therapy.

Pancreatitis: Pancreatitis has occurred in patients receiving **sulindac**.

Auditory effects: Perform periodic auditory function tests during chronic **fenoprofen** therapy in patients with impaired hearing.

Dermatologic effects: Promptly discontinue **mefenamic acid** if rash occurs. A combination of dermatologic and allergic signs and symptoms suggestive of serum sickness have occasionally occurred in conjunction with the use of **piroxicam**.

Concomitant therapy: Do not use **naproxen sodium** and **naproxen** concomitantly; both drugs circulate as naproxen anion.

Do not use **diclofenac** immediate-release, delayed-release, and extended-release tablets concomitantly with other diclofenac-containing products because they also circulate in plasma as diclofenac anion.

Photosensitivity: Photosensitivity may occur.

Drug Interactions

Drugs that affect NSAIDs include cholestyramine, cimetidine, colestipol, diflunisal, DMSO, fluconazole, phenobarbital, probenecid, rifampin, ritonavir, salicylates, and sucralfate.

Drugs that may be affected by NSAIDs include aminoglycosides, anticoagulants, ACE inhibitors, beta blockers, cyclosporine, digoxin, dipyridamole, hydantoins, lithium, loop diuretics, methotrexate, penicillamine, potassium-sparing diuretics, sympathomimetics, and thiazide diuretics.

Drug/Lab test interactions: Naproxen use may result in increased urinary values for 17-ketogenic steroids. Although 17-hydroxycorticosteroid measurements (Porter-Silber test) do not appear to be artificially altered, temporarily discontinue naproxen therapy 72 hours before **adrenal function tests** are performed.

Naproxen – Naproxen may interfere with some urinary assays of 5-hydroxy indole-acetic acid.

Tolmetin – Tolmetin metabolites in urine give positive tests for proteinuria using acid precipitation tests (eg, sulfosalicylic acid).

Mefenamic acid – A false-positive reaction for urinary bile, using the *diazo tablet test*, may result.

Fenoprofen – Amerlex-M kit assay values of total and free triiodothyronine in patients on fenoprofen have been reported as falsely elevated.

Celecoxib – During the controlled clinical trials, there was an increased incidence of hyperchloremia in patients receiving celecoxib compared with patients on placebo. Other laboratory abnormalities that occurred more frequently in patients receiving celecoxib included hypophosphatemia and elevated BUN. These laboratory abnormalities were also seen in patients who received comparator NSAIDs in these studies. The clinical significance of these abnormalities has not been established.

Oxaprozin – False-positive urine immunoassay screening tests for benzodiazepines have been reported in patients taking oxaprozin. This is because of the lack of specificity of the screening tests. False-positive test results may be expected for several days following discontinuation of oxaprozin therapy.

NSAIDs by decreasing platelet adhesion and aggregation, can prolong bleeding time ≈ 3 to 4 minutes.

Drug/Food interactions: Administration of **tolmetin** with milk decreased total tolmetin bioavailability by 16%. When tolmetin was taken immediately after a meal, peak plasma concentrations were reduced by 50%, while total bioavailability was again decreased by 16%. Peak concentration of **etodolac** is reduced by ≈ ½ and the time to peak is increased by 1.4 to 3.8 hours following administration with food; however, the extent of absorption is not affected. Food may reduce the rate of absorption of **oxaprozin,** but the extent is unchanged.

Adverse Reactions

Cardiovascular: CHF; hypotension; hypertension (**rofecoxib, ketorolac**); palpitations; arrhythmias; tachycardia; vasodilation; peripheral edema; fluid retention.

CNS: Dizziness (**mefenamic acid, meloxicam, piroxicam, flurbiprofen, diclofenac, fenoprofen, rofecoxib**); headache (**ketorolac, fenoprofen, indomethacin, diclofenac, flurbiprofen, meclofenamate, meloxicam, nabumetone, naproxen, tolmetin, ketoprofen, sulindac, celecoxib, rofecoxib, mefenamic acid, piroxicam, ibu-**

profen); somnolence/drowsiness (**fenoprofen, naproxen**); asthenia (**tolmetin, etodolac**); malaise (**etodolac**); fatigue (**indomethacin**); insomnia (**meloxicam**).

Dermatologic: Rash/dermatitis, including maculopapular type (**ibuprofen, sulindac, meclofenamate, oxaprozin, nabumetone, mefenamic acid, meloxicam**); desquamation; angioneurotic edema; ecchymosis; petechiae; purpura; alopecia; pruritus (**nabumetone, naproxen**); eczema; skin discoloration; hyperpigmentation; skin irritation; peeling; skin eruptions (**naproxen**).

GI: Common GI adverse reactions include the following: Nausea; vomiting; diarrhea; constipation; abdominal distress/cramps/pain; dyspepsia; flatulence; anorexia; stomatitis.

> *Ulcer* – Gastric or duodenal ulcer with bleeding or perforation (**mefenamic acid**).
> *Bleeding* – Occult blood in the stool (**fenoprofen**).
> *Hepatic* – Elevated liver enzymes (**piroxicam, mefenamic acid**).
> *Other* – Gastritis (**etodolac**); pyrosis (**meclofenamate**); heartburn (**naproxen, meclofenamate, ibuprofen, rofecoxib, mefenamic acid, piroxicam**); epigastric discomfort (**rofecoxib**); GI distress (**tolmetin**); epigastric pain (**ibuprofen, rofecoxib**); indigestion (**ibuprofen**); GI tract fullness (**ibuprofen**); GI pain (**sulindac**); gross bleeding (**mefenamic acid**).

Hematologic: Neutropenia; eosinophilia; leukopenia; pancytopenia; thrombocytopenia; agranulocytosis; granulocytopenia; aplastic anemia; hemolytic anemia; epistaxis; menorrhagia; hemorrhage; bruising; hemolysis, ecchymosis (**naproxen**).

Metabolic: Decreased or increased appetite; weight decrease or increase (**tolmetin**); glycosuria; hyperglycemia; hypoglycemia; hyperkalemia; hyponatremia; flushing or sweating.

Renal: Urinary tract infection (**flurbiprofen, meloxicam**); elevated BUN (**ketoprofen**); hematuria; cystitis; azotemia; nocturia; proteinuria; polyuria; dysuria; urinary frequency; pyuria; oliguria; anuria.

Respiratory: Dyspnea (**naproxen**); upper respiratory tract infection (**rofecoxib, celecoxib, meloxicam**); pharyngitis; bronchospasm; rhinitis; shortness of breath.

Special senses: Blurred vision; photophobia; amblyopia; swollen, dry, or irritated eyes; conjunctivitis; iritis; reversible loss of color vision; hearing disturbances or loss; ear pain; change in taste (metallic or bitter); diplopia; tinnitus.

Miscellaneous: Edema (**flurbiprofen, naproxen, meloxicam**); lower extremity edema (**rofecoxib**); thirst; pyrexia (fever and chills); sweating; breast changes; gynecomastia; muscle cramps; facial edema; menstrual disorders; impotence; vaginal bleeding; influenza-like disease/symptoms (**meloxicam**).

SULFASALAZINE

Tablets: 500 mg (*Rx*)	Various, *Azulfidine* (Pharmacia)
Tablets, delayed-release: 500 mg (*Rx*)	*Azulfidine EN-tabs* (Pharmacia)

For complete prescribing information, refer to the monograph in the GI chapter.

Indications

Rheumatoid arthritis (RA; enteric-coated tablets): Treatment of patients with RA who have responded inadequately to salicylates or other nonsteroidal anti-inflammatory drugs (NSAIDs).

Juvenile rheumatoid arthritis (JRA; enteric-coated tablets): In the treatment of pediatric patients ≥ 6 years of age with polyarticular-course JRA who have responded inadequately to salicylates or other NSAIDs.

Ulcerative colitis: In the treatment of mild to moderate ulcerative colitis, and as adjunctive therapy in severe ulcerative colitis; for the prolongation of the remission period between acute attacks of ulcerative colitis (refer to the sulfasalazine monograph in the GI chapter).

Unlabeled uses: Psoriatic arthritis (2 g/day).

Administration and Dosage

Give the drug in evenly divided doses over each 24-hour period; intervals between nighttime doses should not exceed 8 hours, with administration after meals recommended when feasible. Swallow tablets whole; do not crush or chew. Experience suggests that with daily dosages of ≥ 4 g, the incidence of adverse effects tends to increase.

Some patients may be sensitive to treatment with sulfasalazine. Various desensitization-like regimens have been reported to be effective. These regimens suggest starting with a total daily dose of 50 to 250 mg initially, and doubling it every 4 to 7 days until the desired therapeutic level is achieved. If the symptoms of sensitivity recur, discontinue sulfasalazine. Do not attempt desensitization in patients who have a history of agranulocytosis, or who have experienced an anaphylactoid reaction while previously receiving sulfasalazine.

Rheumatoid arthritis:
Adults – 2 g daily in 2 evenly divided doses. It is advisable to initiate therapy with a lower dosage (eg, 0.5 to 1 g/day) to reduce possible GI intolerance. A suggested dosing schedule is given below.

Adult RA Sulfasalazine Dosing Schedule		
	Number of delayed-release tablets	
Week of treatment	Morning	Evening
1	—	1
2	1	1
3	1	2
4	2	2

A therapeutic response has been observed as early as 4 weeks after starting treatment, but treatment for 12 weeks may be required in some patients before clinical benefit is noted. Give consideration to increasing the daily dose to 3 g if the clinical response after 12 weeks is inadequate. Careful monitoring is recommended for doses > 2 g/day.

JRA-polyarticular course:
Children ≥ 6 years of age – 30 to 50 mg/kg of body weight daily in 2 evenly divided doses. Typically, the maximum dose is 2 g/day. To reduce possible GI intolerance, begin with a quarter to a third of the planned maintenance dose and increase weekly until reaching the maintenance dose at 1 month.

Adverse Reactions

Adverse reactions occurring in ≥ 3% of patients with RA include the following: Nausea, dyspepsia, rash, headache, abdominal pain, vomiting, fever, dizziness, stomatitis, pruritus, abnormal liver function tests, and leukopenia. One report showed a 10% rate of immunoglobulin suppression, which was slowly reversible and rarely accompanied by clinical findings.

AGENTS FOR GOUT

In addition to the agents in this section, sulindac and indomethacin (see Nonsteroidal Anti-inflammatory Agents monograph) and phenylbutazone and oxyphenbutazone (see individual monographs) are indicated for the treatment of gout.

PROBENECID

Tablets: 0.5 g (*Rx*)

Various, *Benemid* (Merck), *Probalan* (Lannett)

Indications

Hyperuricemia: Treatment of hyperuricemia associated with gout and gouty arthritis.

Plasma levels: Adjuvant to therapy with penicillins or cephalosporins, for elevation and prolongation of plasma levels of the antibiotic.

Administration and Dosage

Gout: Do not start therapy until an acute gouty attack has subsided. However, if an acute attack is precipitated during therapy, probenecid may be continued. Give full therapeutic doses of colchicine or other appropriate therapy to control the acute attack.

Adults – 0.25 g twice/day for 1 week; 0.5 g twice/day thereafter. Gastric intolerance may indicate overdosage, and may be reduced by decreasing dosage.

Renal impairment – Some degree of renal impairment may be present in patients with gout. A daily dosage of 1 g may be adequate. However, if necessary, the daily dosage may be increased by 0.5 g increments every 4 weeks within tolerance (usually not > 2 g/day) if symptoms of gouty arthritis are not controlled or the 24 hour urate excretion is not > 700 mg. Probenecid may not be effective in chronic renal insufficiency, particularly when the glomerular filtration rate is ≤ 30 mL/minute.

Urinary alkalinization – Urates tend to crystallize out of an acid urine; therefore, a liberal fluid intake is recommended, as well as sufficient sodium bicarbonate (3 to 7.5 g/day) or potassium citrate (7.5 g/day) to maintain an alkaline urine; continue alkalization until the serum uric acid level returns to normal limits and tophaceous deposits disappear. Thereafter, urinary alkalization and the restriction of purine-producing foods may be relaxed.

Maintenance therapy – Continue the dosage that maintains normal serum uric acid levels. When there have been no acute attacks for ≥ 6 months and serum uric acid levels have remained within normal limits, decrease the daily dosage by 0.5 g every 6 months. Do not reduce the maintenance dosage to the point where serum uric acid levels increase.

Penicillin or cephalosporin therapy: The PSP excretion test may be used to determine the effectiveness of probenecid in retarding penicillin excretion and maintaining therapeutic levels. The renal clearance of PSP is reduced to about the normal rate when dosage of probenecid is adequate.

Adults – 2 g/day in divided doses. Reduce dosage in older patients in whom renal impairment may be present. Not recommended in conjunction with penicillin or a cephalosporin in the presence of known renal impairment.

Children (2 to 14 years of age) – Initial dose 25 mg/kg or 0.7 g/m². Maintenance dose 40 mg/kg/day or 1.2 g/m², divided into 4 doses. For children weighing > 50 kg (110 lb), use the adult dosage. Do not use in children < 2 years of age.

Gonorrhea (uncomplicated) – Give probenecid as a single 1g dose immediately before or with 4.8 million units penicillin G procaine, aqueous, divided into at least 2 doses.

Neurosyphilis – Aqueous procaine penicillin G, 2 to 4 million units/day IM plus probenecid 500 mg 4 times/day, both for 10 to 14 days.†

Pelvic inflammatory disease (PID) – Cefoxitin 2 g IM plus probenecid, 1 g orally in a single dose concurrently.

† CDC 1993 Sexually Transmitted Diseases Treatment Guidelines. *MMWR.* 1993;42 (No. RR-14).

Actions

Pharmacology: A uricosuric and renal tubular blocking agent, probenecid inhibits the tubular reabsorption of urate, thus increasing the urinary excretion of uric acid and decreasing serum uric acid levels.

Probenecid also inhibits the tubular secretion of most penicillins and cephalosporins and usually increases plasma levels by any route the antibiotic is given.

Pharmacokinetics: Probenecid is well absorbed after oral administration and produces peak plasma concentrations in 2 to 4 hours. It is highly protein bound (85% to 95%). Probenecid is excreted in the urine primarily as metabolites.

Contraindications

Hypersensitivity to probenecid; children < 2 years of age; blood dyscrasias or uric acid kidney stones. Do not start therapy until an acute gouty attack has subsided.

Warnings

Exacerbation of gout: Exacerbation of gout following therapy with probenecid may occur; in such cases, colchicine or other appropriate therapy is advisable.

Salicylates: Use of salicylates is contraindicated in patients on probenecid therapy. Salicylates antagonize probenecid's uricosuric action.

Sulfa drug allergy: Probenecid is a sulfonamide; patients with a history of allergy to sulfa drugs may react to probenecid.

Hypersensitivity reactions: Rarely, severe allergic reactions and anaphylaxis have occurred. Most of these occur within several hours after readministration following prior use of the drug.

Renal function impairment: Dosage requirements may be increased in renal impairment. Probenecid may not be effective in chronic renal insufficiency, particularly when the glomerular filtration rate is ≤ 30 mL/minute. Probenecid is not recommended in conjunction with a penicillin in the presence of known renal impairment.

Pregnancy: Category B.

Children: Do not use in children < 2 years of age.

Precautions

Alkalinization of urine: Hematuria, renal colic, costovertebral pain, and formation of urate stones associated with use in gouty patients may be prevented by alkalization of urine and liberal fluid intake; monitor acid-base balance.

Peptic ulcer history: Use with caution.

Drug Interactions

Drugs that may affect probenecid include salicylates.

Drugs that may be affected by probenecid include acyclovir; allopurinol; barbiturates; benzodiazepines; clofibrate; dapsone; dyphylline; methotrexate; NSAIDs; pantothenic acid; penicillamine; rifampin; sulfonamides; sulfonylureas; zidovudine; salicylates.

Drug/Lab test interactions: A reducing substance may appear in the urine during therapy. Although this disappears with discontinuation, a false diagnosis of glycosuria may be made. Confirm suspected glycosuria by using a test specific for glucose.

Falsely high determination of **theophylline** has occurred in vitro using the Schack and Waxler technique, when therapeutic concentrations of theophylline and probenecid were added to human plasma.

Probenecid may inhibit the renal excretion of: **Phenolsulfonphthalein (PSP), 17-ketosteroids**, and **sulfobromophthalein (BSP)**.

Adverse Reactions

Adverse reactions may include headache; anorexia; nausea; vomiting; urinary frequency; hypersensitivity reactions; sore gums; flushing; dizziness; anemia; hemolytic anemia (possibly related to G-6-PD deficiency); nephrotic syndrome; hepatic necrosis; aplastic anemia; exacerbation of gout; uric acid stones with or without hematuria; renal colic or costovertebral pain.

ALLOPURINOL

Tablets: 100 and 300 mg (*Rx*) Various, *Zyloprim* (Prometheus)

Indications

Gout: Management of signs and symptoms of primary or secondary gout.

Malignancies: Management of patients with leukemia, lymphoma, and malignancies receiving therapy which causes elevations of serum and urinary uric acid. Discontinue allopurinol when the potential for overproduction of uric acid is no longer present.

Calcium oxalate calculi: Management of patients with recurrent calcium oxalate calculi whose daily uric acid excretion exceeds 800 mg/day (males) or 750 mg/day (females). Carefully assess therapy initially and periodically to determine that treatment is beneficial and that the benefits outweigh the risks.

Unlabeled uses: In a limited number of patients, the use of an allopurinol mouthwash (20 mg in 3% methylcellulose; 1 mg/mL) after fluorouracil administration prevented stomatitis, a major dose-limiting toxicity of fluorouracil. However, another report indicated that allopurinol mouthwash is not effective. Further study is needed.

Administration and Dosage

Control of gout and hyperuricemia: The average dose is 200 to 300 mg/day for mild gout and 400 to 600 mg/day for moderately severe tophaceous gout. Divide doses in excess of 300 mg. The minimum effective dose is 100 to 200 mg/day; the maximum recommended dose is 800 mg/day.

Children (6 to 10 years of age) – In secondary hyperuricemia associated with malignancy, give 300 mg/day; those < 6 years of age are generally given 150 mg/day. Evaluate response after approximately 48 hours of therapy and adjust dosage if necessary.

Another suggested dose is 1 mg/kg/day divided every 6 hours, to a maximum of 600 mg/day. After 48 hours of treatment, titrate dose according to serum uric acid levels.

Prevention of uric acid nephropathy during vigorous therapy of neoplastic disease: 600 to 800 mg/day for 2 to 3 days together with a high fluid intake. Similar considerations govern dosage regulation for maintenance purposes in secondary hyperuricemia.

To reduce the possibility of flare-up of acute gouty attacks: Start with 100 mg/day and increase at weekly intervals by 100 mg (without exceeding the maximum recommended dosage) until a serum uric acid level of ≤ 6 mg/dL is attained.

Serum uric acid levels: Normal serum urate levels are usually achieved in 1 to 3 weeks. The upper limit of normal is about 7 mg/dL for men and postmenopausal women and 6 mg/dL for premenopausal women. Do not rely on a single reading since estimation of uric acid may be difficult. By selecting the appropriate dose, and using uricosuric agents in certain patients, it is possible to reduce the serum uric acid level to normal and, if desired, to hold it as low as 2 to 3 mg/dL indefinitely.

Renal impairment: Accumulation of allopurinol and its metabolites can occur in renal failure; consequently, reduce the dose. With a Ccr of 10 to 20 mL/min, 200 mg/day is suitable. When the Ccr is < 10 mL/min, do not exceed 100 mg/day. With extreme renal impairment (Ccr < 3 mL/min) the interval between doses may also need to be increased. The correct dosage is best determined by using the serum uric acid level as an index.

Other suggested doses include: Ccr 60 mL/min, 200 mg/day; Ccr 40 mL/min, 15 mg/day; Ccr 20 mL/min, 100 mg/day; Ccr 10 mL/min, 100 mg on alternate days. Ccr < 10 mL/min, 100 mg 3 times a week.

Concomitant therapy: In patients treated with colchicine or anti-inflammatory agents, continue therapy while adjusting the allopurinol dosage until a normal serum uric acid level and freedom from acute attacks have been maintained for several months.

Replacement therapy: In transferring a patient from a uricosuric agent to allopurinol, gradually reduce the dose of the uricosuric agent over several weeks and gradually increase the dose of allopurinol until a normal serum uric acid level is maintained.

Recurrent calcium oxalate stones: For hyperuricosuric patients, 200 to 300 mg/day in single or divided doses. Adjust dose up or down depending upon the resultant control of the hyperuricosuria based upon subsequent 24 hour urinary urate determinations. Patients may also benefit from dietary changes such as reduction of animal protein, sodium, refined sugars, oxalate-rich foods and excessive calcium intake as well as increase in oral fluids and dietary fiber.

Actions
Pharmacology: Allopurinol inhibits xanthine oxidase, the enzyme responsible for the conversion of hypoxanthine to xanthine to uric acid. Allopurinol acts on purine catabolism, reducing the production of uric acid, without disrupting the biosynthesis of vital purines.

Administration generally results in a fall in both serum and urinary uric acid within 2 to 3 days. The magnitude of this decrease is dose-dependent. One week or more of treatment may be required before the full effects of the drug are manifested; likewise, uric acid may return to pretreatment levels slowly following cessation of therapy.

Pharmacokinetics: Allopurinol is $\approx$ 90% absorbed from the GI tract.

Effective xanthine oxidase inhibition is maintained over 24 hours with single daily doses. Allopurinol is cleared essentially by glomerular filtration; oxipurinol is reabsorbed in the kidney tubules in a manner similar to the reabsorption of uric acid.

Contraindications
Patients who have developed a severe reaction should not be restarted on the drug.

Warnings
Asymptomatic hyperuricemia: Generally, do not use to treat asymptomatic hyperuricemia. Treatment should be considered with persitent hyperuricemia characterized by a serum urate concentration of > 13 mg/dL. High serum urate may be nephrotoxic.

Hepatotoxicity: A few cases of reversible clinical hepatotoxicity have occurred; in some patients, asymptomatic rises in serum alkaline phosphatase or serum transaminase levels have been observed. If anorexia, weight loss or pruritus develop in patients on allopurinol, evaluation of liver function should be part of their diagnostic workup. Perform periodic liver function tests during early stages of therapy.

Hypersensitivity reactions: Discontinue at first appearance of skin rash or other signs of allergic reactions. In some instances, rash may be followed by more severe hypersensitivity reactions such as exfoliative, urticarial or purpuric lesions, or Stevens-Johnson syndrome, generalized vasculitis, irreversible hepatotoxicity and rarely, death.

Renal function impairment: Some patients with preexisting renal disease or poor urate clearance have increased BUN during allopurinol administration. Patients with impaired renal function require less drug and careful observation during the early stages of treatment; reduce dosage or discontinue therapy if increased abnormalities in renal function appear and persist.

Renal failure in association with allopurinol has been observed among patients with hyperuricemia secondary to neoplastic diseases. Concurrent conditions such as multiple myeloma and congestive myocardial disease were present. Renal failure is also frequently associated with gouty nephropathy and rarely with allopurinol-associated hypersensitivity reactions. Albuminuria has occurred among patients who developed clinical gout following chronic glomerulonephritis and chronic pyelonephritis.

In patients with severely impaired renal function or decreased urate clearance, the plasma half-life of oxipurinol is greatly prolonged. A dose of 100 mg/day or

300 mg twice a week, or less, may be sufficient to maintain adequate xanthine oxidase inhibition to reduce serum urate levels.

Pregnancy: Category C.

Lactation: Allopurinol and oxipurinol have been found in breast milk. Exercise caution when administering to a nursing woman.

Children: Allopurinol is rarely indicated for use in children, with the exception of those with hyperuricemia secondary to malignancy or to certain rare inborn errors of purine metabolism.

Precautions

Monitoring: Periodically determine liver and kidney function especially during the first few months of therapy. Perform BUN, serum creatinine, or Ccr and reassess the patient's dosage.

Acute attacks of gout: Acute attacks of gout have increased during the early stages of allopurinol administration when normal or subnormal serum uric acid levels have been attained; in general, give maintenance doses of colchicine prophylactically when allopurinol is begun. In addition, start patient at a low dose of allopurinol (100 mg/day) and increase at weekly intervals by 100 mg until a serum uric acid level of ≤ 6 mg/dL is attained without exceeding the maximum recommended dose. The attacks usually become shorter and less severe after several months of therapy.

Fluid intake: Fluid intake sufficient to yield a daily urinary output of at least 2 L and the maintenance of a neutral or slightly alkaline urine are desirable to avoid the theoretical possibility of formation of xanthine calculi under the influence of allopurinol therapy and to help prevent renal precipitation of urates in patients receiving concomitant uricosurics.

Drowsiness: Drowsiness has occurred occasionally. Patients should observe caution while driving or performing other tasks requiring alertness, coordination, or physical dexterity.

Bone marrow depression: Bone marrow depression has occurred in patients receiving allopurinol, most of whom received concomitant drugs with the potential for causing this reaction. This has occurred as early as 6 weeks to as long as 6 years after the initiation of therapy. Rarely, a patient may develop varying degrees of bone marrow depression, affecting one or more cell lines, while receiving allopurinol alone.

Drug Interactions

Drugs that may affect allopurinol include ACE inhibitors; aluminum salts; thiazide diuretics; uricosuric agents.

Drugs that may be affected by allopurinol include ampicillin; anticoagulants; cyclophosphamide; theophyllines; thiopurines.

Adverse Reactions

Adverse reactions may include skin rash; fever; chills; arthralgias; cholestatic jaundice; eosinophilia; mild leukocytosis; leukopenia; vesicular bullous dermatitis; eczematoid dermatitis; pruritus; urticaria; onycholysis; lichen planus; Stevens-Johnson syndrome; purpura; toxic epidermal necrolysis; nausea; vomiting; diarrhea; intermittent abdominal pain; gastritis; dyspepsia; increased alkaline phosphatase, AST and ALT; hepatomegaly; cholestatic jaundice; granulomatous hepatitis; hepatic necrosis; leukopenia; leukocytosis; eosinophilia; thrombocytopenia; headache; peripheral neuropathy; neuritis; paresthesia; somnolence; arthralgia; acute attacks of gout; ecchymosis; fever; myopathy; epistaxis; taste loss or perversion; renal failure; uremia; alopecia; hypersensitivity vasculitis; necrotizing angiitis.

COLCHICINE

Tablets: 0.5 mg (1/120 g) and 0.6 mg (1/100 g) (*Rx*)   *Colchicine* (Abbott)

Indications
Gout: Relieves pain of acute attacks, especially if adequate doses are given early in the attack. Many therapists use colchicine as interval therapy to prevent acute attacks. Recommended for regular prophylactic use between attacks and is often effective in aborting an attack when taken at the first sign of articular discomfort.

Administration and Dosage
Acute gouty arthritis: Begin at the first warning of an acute attack. Usual initial dose is 1 to 1.2 mg; follow with 0.5 to 1.2 mg every 1 to 2 hours, until pain is relieved, or nausea, vomiting, or diarrhea occurs. (Opiates may be needed to control diarrhea.) After ≥ 1 attacks, patients can often judge their requirements accurately enough to stop before the "diarrheal dose."

The total amount of colchicine needed to control pain and inflammation during an acute attack is 4 to 8 mg. Articular pain and swelling typically abate within 12 hours and are usually gone in 24 to 48 hours. Wait 3 days before initiating a second course to minimize the possibility of cumulative toxicity.

If ACTH is used to treat a gouty arthritis attack, give colchicine ≥ 1 mg/day, and continue for a few days after ACTH is withdrawn.

Prophylaxis during intercritical periods: To reduce the frequency and severity of paroxysms, administer continuously. If patients have < 1 attack/year, usual dose is 0.5 or 0.6 mg/day for 3 or 4 days a week; if > 1 attack/year, usual dose is 0.5 or 0.6 mg/day. Severe cases may require 1 to 1.8 mg/day.

Prophylaxis in patients undergoing surgery: In patients with gout, an attack may be precipitated by even a minor surgical procedure. Administer 0.5 or 0.6 mg 3 times/day for 3 days before and 3 days after surgery.

Prophylaxis or maintenance of recurrent or chronic gouty arthritis: 0.5 to 1 mg once or twice/day.

Actions
Pharmacology: The exact mechanism of action of colchicine in gout is not known. Colchicine apparently exerts its effect by reducing the inflammatory response to the deposited crystals and also by diminishing phagocytosis. Colchicine diminishes lactic acid production by leukocytes directly and by diminishing phagocytosis and thereby interrupts the cycle of urate crystal deposition and inflammatory response that sustains the acute attack.

Pharmacokinetics: Colchicine is rapidly absorbed after oral administration; peak plasma concentrations occur in 0.5 to 2 hours. High colchicine concentrations are found in the kidney, liver, and spleen. It is metabolized in the liver. Excretion occurs primarily by biliary and renal routes.

Contraindications
Hypersensitivity to colchicine; serious GI, renal, hepatic, or cardiac disorders; blood dyscrasias.

Warnings
Hepatic function impairment: Increased colchicine toxicity may occur.

Fertility impairment: Colchicine arrests cell division in animals and plants. It has adversely affected spermatogenesis in humans and in some animal species.

Elderly: Administer colchicine with great caution to elderly and debilitated patients.

Pregnancy: Category C.

Lactation: It is not known whether this drug is excreted in breast milk. Exercise caution when administering colchicine to a nursing woman.

Children: Safety and efficacy for use in children have not been established.

Precautions
Monitoring: Perform periodic blood counts in patients receiving long-term therapy.

GI effects: Vomiting, diarrhea, abdominal pain, and nausea may occur, especially with maximum doses. These may be particularly troublesome in the presence of peptic ulcer or spastic colon. At toxic doses, colchicine may cause severe diarrhea, generalized vascular damage, and renal damage with hematuria and oliguria. To avoid more serious toxicity, discontinue use when these symptoms appear, regardless of whether joint pain has been relieved.

Myopathy and neuropathy: Colchicine myoneuropathy appears to be a common cause of weakness in patients on standard therapy who have elevated plasma levels caused by altered renal function. It is often unrecognized and misdiagnosed as polymyositis or uremic neuropathy. Proximal weakness and elevated serum creatine kinase are generally present, and resolve in 3 to 4 weeks following drug withdrawal.

Malabsorption of vitamin B_{12}: Colchicine induces reversible malabsorption of vitamin B_{12}, apparently by altering the function of ileal mucosa.

Drug Interactions

Drug/Lab test interactions: Decreased **thrombocyte** values may be obtained. Colchicine may cause false-positive results when testing urine for **RBC** or **hemoglobin**.

Adverse Reactions

Adverse reactions may include bone marrow depression with aplastic anemia; agranulocytosis or thrombocytopenia (long-term therapy); peripheral neuritis; purpura; myopathy; loss of hair; reversible azoospermia; dermatoses; hypersensitivity; vomiting; diarrhea; abdominal pain; nausea; elevated alkaline phosphatase and AST.

AGENTS FOR MIGRAINE

In addition to the agents on the following pages, **propanolol** and **timolol** are indicated for migraine prophylaxis.

SEROTONIN 5-HT₁ RECEPTOR AGONISTS

ALMOTRIPTAN MALATE	
Tablets: 6.25 and 12.5 mg (*Rx*)	*Axert* (Pharmacia)
FROVATRIPTAN SUCCINATE	
Tablets: 2.5 mg (as base) (*Rx*)	*Frova* (Elan)
NARATRIPTAN	
Tablets: 1 and 2.5 mg (as HCl) (*Rx*)	*Amerge* (GlaxoSmithKline)
RIZATRIPTAN BENZOATE	
Tablets: 5 and 10 mg (*Rx*)	*Maxalt* (Merck)
Tablets, orally disintegrating: 5 and 10 mg (*Rx*)	*Maxalt-MLT* (Merck)
SUMATRIPTAN SUCCINATE	
Tablets: 25, 50, and 100 mg (as succinate) (*Rx*)	*Imitrex* (GlaxoSmithKline)
Injection: 12 mg/mL (as succinate) (*Rx*)	
Spray, nasal: 5 and 20 mg (*Rx*)	
ZOLMITRIPTAN	
Tablets: 2.5 and 5 mg (*Rx*)	*Zomig* (AstraZeneca)
Tablets, orally disintegrating: 2.5 mg (*Rx*)	*Zomig ZMT* (AstraZeneca)

Indications
Migraine: Acute treatment of migraine attacks with or without aura.

Cluster headache (sumatriptan injection only): Acute treatment of cluster headache episodes.

Not intended for the prophylactic therapy of migraine or for use in the management of hemiplegic or basilar migraine. Safety and efficacy have not been established for cluster headache, which is present in an older, predominantly male population (**almotriptan, frovatriptan, sumatriptan** tablets and spray, **zolmitriptan**).

Administration and Dosage
ALMOTRIPTAN: Doses of 6.25 and 12.5 mg were effective for the acute treatment of migraines in adults, with the 12.5 mg dose tending to be a more effective dose. Individuals may vary in response to doses of almotriptan. The choice of dose should therefore be made on an individual basis.

If the headache returns, the dose may be repeated after 2 hours, but do not give more than 2 doses within a 24-hour period. Controlled trials have not adequately established the effectiveness of a second dose if the initial dose is ineffective.

The safety of treating an average of > 4 headaches in a 30-day period has not been established.

Hepatic impairment – The maximum decrease expected in the clearance of almotriptan caused by hepatic impairment is 60%. Therefore, do not exceed the maximum daily dose of 12.5 mg over a 24-hour period, and use a starting dose of 6.25 mg.

Renal impairment – In patients with severe renal impairment, the clearance of almotriptan was decreased. Therefore, do not exceed the maximum daily dose of 12.5 mg over a 24-hour period, and use a starting dose of 6.25 mg.

FROVATRIPTAN: The recommended dosage is a single tablet (2.5 mg) taken orally with fluids.

If the headache recurs after initial relief, a second tablet may be taken, providing there is an interval of ≥ 2 hours between doses. The total daily dose of frovatriptan should not exceed 3 tablets (3 × 2.5 mg/day).

There is no evidence that a second dose of frovatriptan is effective in patients who do not respond to a first dose of the drug for the same headache.

The safety of treating an average of > 4 migraine attacks in a 30-day period has not been established.

NARATRIPTAN: Single doses of 1 and 2.5 mg taken with fluid were effective for the acute treatment of migraine in adults. A greater proportion of patients had headache response following a 2.5 mg dose than following a 1 mg dose. Individualize dosage, weighing the possible benefit of the 2.5 mg dose with the potential for a greater risk of adverse events. If the headache returns or if the patient has only partial response, the dose may be repeated once after 4 hours, for a maximum dose of 5 mg in a 24-hour period. There is evidence that doses of 5 mg do not provide a greater effect than 2.5 mg.

Renal/hepatic function impairment – The use of naratriptan is contraindicated in patients with severe renal impairment (Ccr < 15 mL/min) or severe hepatic impairment (Child-Pugh grade C) because of decreased clearance of the drug. In patients with mild to moderate renal or hepatic impairment, the maximum daily dose should not exceed 2.5 mg over a 24-hour period and a lower starting dose should be considered.

RIZATRIPTAN: Single doses of 5 and 10 mg were effective for the acute treatment of migraines in adults.

Redosing – Doses should be separated by at least 2 hours; no more than 30 mg should be taken in any 24-hour period.

Orally disintegrating tablets – Administration with liquid is not necessary. The orally disintegrating tablet is packaged in a blister within an outer aluminum pouch. Instruct patients not to remove the blister from the outer pouch until just prior to dosing. The blister pack should then be peeled open with dry hands and the orally disintegrating tablet placed on the tongue, where it will dissolve and be swallowed with saliva.

Phenylketonurics: Inform phenylketonuric patients that rizatriptan orally disintegrating tablets contain phenylalanine (a component of aspartame). Each 5 mg orally disintegrating tablet contains 1.05 mg phenylalanine, and each 10 mg orally disintegrating tablet contains 2.1 mg phenylalanine.

SUMATRIPTAN:

Oral – Single doses of 25, 50, or 100 mg tablets are effective for the acute treatment of migraine in adults. There is evidence that doses of 50 and 100 mg may provide a greater effect than 25 mg. Doses of 100 mg have not been proven to provide a greater effect than 50 mg. The choice of dose should be made on an individual basis, weighing the possible benefit of a higher dose with the potential for a greater risk of adverse events. If headache returns, or the patient has a partial response to the initial dose, additional doses may be taken at intervals of ≥ 2 hours up to a daily maximum of 200 mg. If headache returns following an initial treatment with the injection, additional doses of single tablets (≤ 100 mg/day) may be given with an interval of ≥ 2 hours between tablet doses.

Hepatic function impairment: Maximum single dose ≤ 50 mg.

MAO inhibitors: Because of the potential of MAO-A inhibitors to cause unpredictable elevations in the bioavailability of oral sumatriptan, their combined use is contraindicated.

The safety of treating an average of > 4 headaches in a 30-day period has not been established.

Injection – The maximum single adult dose is 6 mg injected SC.

Trials failed to show a clear benefit is associated with the administration of a second 6 mg dose in patients who have failed to respond to a first injection. The maximum recommended dose that may be given in 24 hours is two 6 mg injections separated by ≥ 1 hour. If side effects are dose-limiting, lower doses may be used. In patients receiving doses < 6 mg, use only the single-dose vial dosage form. An auto-injection device is available for use with 6 mg prefilled syringes to facilitate self-administration in patients in whom this dose is deemed necessary. With this device, the needle penetrates ≈ ¼ inch (5 to 6 mm). Because the injection is intended to be given subcutaneously, intramuscular or intravascular delivery should be avoided. Patients should be directed to use injection sites with an adequate skin and subcutaneous thickness to accommodate the length of the needle.

MAO inhibitors: Consider decreased doses of sumatriptan in patients receiving MAO inhibitors.

Intranasal – A single dose of 5, 10, or 20 mg administered in 1 nostril is effective for the acute treatment of migraine in adults. A greater proportion of patients had headache response following a 20 mg dose than following a 5- to 10-mg dose. Weigh the possible benefit of the 20 mg dose with the potential for a greater risk of adverse events. A 10 mg dose may be achieved by administering a single 5 mg dose in each nostril. There is evidence that doses > 20 mg do not provide a greater effect than 20 mg. If headache returns, the dose may be repeated once after 2 hours, not to exceed a total daily dose of 40 mg.

The safety of treating an average of > 4 headaches in a 30-day period has not been established.

ZOLMITRIPTAN: Initial recommended dose is ≤ 2.5 mg (achieved by manually breaking a 2.5 mg tablet in half). If the headache returns, the dose may be repeated after 2 hours, not to exceed 10 mg within a 24-hour period. Response is greater following the 2.5 or 5 mg dose compared with 1.25 mg, with little added benefit and increased side effects associated with the 5 mg dose.

Orally disintegrating tablets – A single dose of 2.5 mg was effective for the acute treatment of migraines in adults. If the headache returns, the dose may be repeated after 2 hours, not to exceed 10 mg within a 24-hour period. Trials have not adequately established the effectiveness of a second dose if the initial dose is ineffective.

Administration with a liquid is not necessary. The orally disintegrating tablet is packaged in a blister. Instruct patients not to remove the tablet from the blister until just prior to dosing. The blister pack should then be peeled open, and the orally disintegrating tablet placed on the tongue, where it will dissolve and be swallowed with the saliva. It is not recommended to break the orally disintegrating tablet.

On average, the safety of treating > 3 headaches in a 30-day period has not been established.

Actions

Pharmacology: **Naratriptan, rizatriptan, sumatriptan, frovatriptan, almotriptan**, and **zolmitriptan** are selective agonists for a vascular 5-hydroxytryptamine$_1$ (serotonin) receptor subtype. Use of 5-HT$_1$ agonists results in cranial vessel constriction and inhibition of pro-inflammatory neuropeptide release, which correlates with the relief of migraine.

Pharmacokinetics:

Pharmacokinetic Parameters of Triptans in Healthy Volunteers and in Patients with Migraine							
Drug	Dose and route of administration	T_{max} (hr)	C_{max} (mg/L)	Bioavailability (%)	t½ (hr)	AUC (mg/L•hr)	Plasma protein binding (%)
Sumatriptan	6 mg SC	0.17	72	96	2	90	14 to 21
	100 mg PO	1.5	54	14	2	158	
	20 mg IN	1.5	13	15.8	1.8	48	
	25 mg PR	1.5	27	19.2	1.8	78	
Zolmitriptan	2.5 mg PO	1.5	3.3/3.8[1]	39	2.3/2.6[1]	18/21[1]	25
	5 mg PO	1.5	10	46	3	42	
Naratriptan	2.5 mg PO	2	12.6	74	5.5	98	20
Rizatriptan	10 mg PO	1	19.8	40	2	50	14
Almotriptan	12.5 mg PO	2.5	49.5	80	3.1	266	
	25 mg PO	2.7	64	69	3.6	443	
Frovatriptan	2.5 mg PO	3	4.2/7[1]	29.6	25.7	94	≈ 15
	40 mg PO	5	24.7/53.4[1]	17.5	29.7	881	

† Adapted from *Drugs.* 2000;60:1267.
[1] Value for men and women, respectively.

Injection (Sumatriptan) – Following a 6 mg SC injection, distribution half-life was 15 minutes, terminal half-life was 115 minutes, and Vd central compartment was

50 L. The T_{max} or amount absorbed were not significantly altered by either the site or technique of injection (deltoid vs thigh).

Contraindications

Injectable preparations used IV, because of the potential to cause coronary vasospasm; patients with ischemic heart disease (angina pectoris, history of MI, silent MI, strokes, transient ischemic attacks [TIAs], or documented silent ischemia); Prinzmetal's variant angina or other significant underlying cardiovascular disease (see Warnings); patients with signs or symptoms consistent with ischemic heart disease or coronary artery vasospasm; patients with uncontrolled hypertension (**naratriptan, rizatriptan, sumatriptan,** and **zolmitriptan**); concurrent use of (or use within 24 hours of) ergotamine-containing preparations (or ergot-type medications such as dihydroergotamine or methysergide); concurrent MAO inhibitor therapy (or within 2 weeks of discontinuing an MAOI; see Drug Interactions); within 24 hours of another 5-HT₁ agonist; hypersensitivity to the product or any of its ingredients; management of hemiplegic or basilar migraine; ischemic bowel disease.

Naratriptan and sumatriptan: Cerebrovascular or peripheral vascular syndromes, severe hepatic impairment (Child-Pugh grade C); severe renal impairment (Ccr < 15 mL/min) (naratriptan only).

Frovatriptan: Peripheral vascular disease including but not limited to ischemic bowel disease.

Warnings

Use 5-HT₁ agonists only where a clear diagnosis of migraine has been established.

Risk of myocardial ischemia or infarction and other adverse cardiac events: Because of the potential of this class of compounds to cause coronary vasospasm, do not give these agents to patients with documented ischemic or vasospastic coronary artery disease.

It is recommended that patients who are intermittent long-term users of 5-HT₁ agonists who have or acquire risk factors predictive of CAD undergo periodic interval cardiovascular evaluation as they continue use.

Zolmitriptan – Patients with symptomatic Wolff-Parkinson-White syndrome or arrhythmias associated with other cardiac accessory conduction pathway disorders should not receive zolmitriptan.

Cardiac events and fatalities associated with 5-HT₁ agonists: Serious adverse cardiac events, including acute MI, life-threatening disturbances of cardiac rhythm, and death have been reported within a few hours following the administration of other 5-HT₁ agonists.

Cerebrovascular events and fatalities with 5-HT₁ agonists: Cerebral hemorrhage, subarachnoid hemorrhage, stroke, and other cerebrovascular events have been reported in patients treated with 5-HT₁ agonists, and some have resulted in fatalities. In a number of cases, it appears possible that the cerebrovascular events were primary, the agonist having been administered in the incorrect belief that the symptoms experienced were a consequence of migraine, when they were not. It should be noted that patients with migraine may be at increased risk of certain cerebrovascular events (eg, stroke, hemorrhage, TIA).

Other vasospasm-related events: Peripheral vascular ischemia and colonic ischemia with abdominal pain and bloody diarrhea have been reported with 5-HT₁ agonists.

Increases in blood pressure: Significant elevations in systemic blood pressure, including hypertensive crisis, have been reported on rare occasions in patients with and without a history of hypertension treated with 5-HT₁ agonists.

Local irritation: Approximately 5% noted irritation in the nose and throat after using **sumatriptan nasal spray.** The symptoms were transient and, in ≈ 60% of the cases, resolved in < 2 hours.

Hypersensitivity reactions: Hypersensitivity reactions have occurred on rare occasions, and severe anaphylaxis/anaphylactoid reactions have occurred. Such reactions can be life-threatening or fatal. Refer to Management of Acute Hypersensitivity Reactions.

Renal function impairment: Use **rizatriptan** and **sumatriptan** with caution in dialysis patients because of a decrease in the clearance.

Hepatic function impairment: Administer with caution to patients with diseases that may alter the absorption, metabolism, or excretion of drugs. The bioavailability may be markedly increased in patients with liver disease.

Elderly: Pharmacokinetics in the elderly are similar to those seen in younger adults.

Pregnancy: Category C.

Lactation: **Sumatriptan** is excreted in breast milk. **Zolmitriptan, naratriptan, almotriptan, frovatriptan,** and **rizatriptan** are excreted in rat milk.

Children: Safety and efficacy in children have not been established. 5-HT$_1$ receptor agonists are not recommended in patients < 18 years of age.

Precautions

Chest, jaw, or neck tightness: Chest, jaw, or neck tightness is relatively common after 5-HT$_1$ agonist administration, and atypical sensations over the precordium (tightness, pressure, heaviness) have occurred, but has only rarely been associated with ischemic ECG changes.

Seizures: There have been rare reports of seizures following **sumatriptan** use.

Binding to melanin-containing tissues: Accumulation in melanin-rich tissues (such as the eye) could occur over time, raising the possibility that toxicity in these tissues could occur after extended use.

Corneal opacities: **Sumatriptan, naratriptan,** and **almotriptan** cause corneal opacities and defects in dogs, raising the possibility that these changes may occur in humans.

Phenylketonurics: **Rizatriptan** and **zolmitriptan** orally disintegrating tablets contain phenylalanine (a component of aspartame). Each 5 mg rizatriptan orally disintegrating tablet contains 1.05 mg phenylalanine, and each 10 mg orally disintegrating tablet contains 2.1 mg phenylalanine. Each 2.5 mg zolmitriptan orally disintegrating tablet contains 2.81 mg phenylalanine.

Photosensitivity: Photosensitization may occur. Caution patients to take protective measures against exposure to sunlight or ultraviolet light until tolerance is determined.

Drug Interactions

Drugs that may affect 5-HT$_1$ receptor agonists include the following: Cimetidine, ergot-containing drugs, MAO inhibitors, ketoconazole, sibutramine, other 5-HT$_1$ receptor agonists, and propranolol. SSRIs may be affected by 5-HT$_1$ receptor agonists.

Adverse Reactions

Adverse reactions occurring in ≥ 3% of patients include the following: Paresthesia, warm/cold sensation, warm/hot sensation, miscellaneous sensations, asthenia, dizziness, drowsiness, fatigue, headache, myasthenia, somnolence, vertigo, miscellaneous CNS effects, chest pain/pressure, heaviness, neck/throat/jaw pain/pressure, pain in specified/unspecified locations, skeletal pain/pressure, dry mouth, dyspepsia, nausea.

METHYSERGIDE MALEATE

Tablets: 2 mg (Rx)   *Sansert* (Sandoz)

Warning:
   Retroperitoneal fibrosis, pleuropulmonary fibrosis, and fibrotic thickening of cardiac valves may occur in patients receiving long-term methysergide therapy.
   Reserve this drug for prophylaxis in patients whose vascular headaches are frequent or severe and uncontrollable and who are under close medical supervision.

Indications
   Vascular headache:
      Prevention or reduction – Prevention or reduction of intensity and frequency in
      patients suffering from one or more severe vascular headaches per week or from vas-
      cular headaches that are so severe that preventive therapy is indicated, regard-
      less of the frequency of the attack.
      Prophylaxis – Prophylaxis of vascular headache. Not for management of acute attacks.

Administration and Dosage
   Adults: 4 to 8 mg/day; take with meals. There must be a drug free interval of 3 to
   4 weeks after every 6 month course of treatment.

Actions
   Pharmacology: Methysergide is a semisynthetic ergot derivative. It has no intrinsic vasoconstrictor properties and its mechanism of action has not been established. It
   inhibits or blocks the effects of serotonin.
      Allow 1 to 2 days for the protective effects to develop; following termination,
   1 to 2 days are required before the effects subside.

Contraindications
   Pregnancy; peripheral vascular disease; severe arteriosclerosis; severe hypertension;
   coronary artery disease; phlebitis or cellulitis of the lower limbs; pulmonary disease; collagen diseases or fibrotic processes; impaired liver or renal function; valvular heart disease; debilitated states; serious infections.

Warnings
   Prolonged therapy: With long-term, uninterrupted administration, retroperitoneal fibrosis or
   related conditions have occurred. Continuous administration should not exceed 6 months.
      Pleuropulmonary fibrosis – Pleuropulmonary fibrosis, a similar nonspecific fibrotic pro-
   cess limited to pleural and immediately subjacent pulmonary tissues, usually presents
   with dyspnea, chest tightness/pain, pleural friction rubs, and pleural effusion.
      Cardiac fibrosis – Nonrheumatic fibrotic thickenings of the aortic root and of the aor-
   tic and mitral valves usually present clinically with cardiac murmurs and dyspnea.
      Other fibrotic complications – Fibrotic plaques simulating Peyronie's disease.
   Pregnancy: Category X.
   Lactation: Ergot derivatives in breast milk have caused symptoms of ergotism.
   Children: Not recommended for use in children.

Drug Interactions
   Beta blockers may interact with methysergine maleate.

Adverse Reactions
   Adverse reactions may include encroachment of retroperitoneal fibrosis on the aorta;
   inferior vena cava and their common iliac branches; intrinsic vasoconstriction of
   large and small arteries which may present with chest pain, abdominal pain or cold,
   numb, painful extremities with or without paresthesias and diminished or absent
   pulses; postural hypotension; tachycardia; nausea; vomiting; diarrhea; heartburn;
   abdominal pain; constipation; insomnia; drowsiness; mild euphoria; dizziness;
   ataxia; weakness; lightheadedness; hyperesthesia; facial flush; telangiectasia;
   increased hair loss; peripheral edema; neutropenia; eosinophilia; arthralgia; myalgia; weight gain.

ERGOTAMINE DERIVATIVES

ERGOTAMINE TARTRATE	
Tablets, sublingual: 2 mg (Rx)	*Ergomar* (Lotus)
DIHYDROERGOTAMINE	
Injection: 1 mg per mL (Rx)	*D.H.E. 45* (Sandoz)

Indications

Headache: To abort or prevent vascular headaches such as migraine, migraine variant, and cluster headache (histaminic cephalalgia).

Dihydroergotamine: Dihydroergotamine is used when rapid control is desired or when other routes of administration are not feasible.

Administration and Dosage

ERGOTAMINE: Initiate therapy as soon as possible after the first symptoms of an attack. Place 1 tablet under the tongue; take subsequent doses at 30 minute intervals if necessary. Do not exceed 3 tablets/24 hours. Do not exceed 10 mg/week.

DIHYDROERGOTAMINE:

IM – Inject 1 mg at first sign of headache; repeat at 1 hour intervals to a total of 3 mg. For optimal results, adjust the dose for several headaches to determine the minimal effective dose; use this dose at the onset of subsequent attacks.

IV – Where more rapid effect is desired, administer IV to a maximum of 2 mg. Do not exceed 6 mg/week.

Actions

Pharmacology: Ergotamine has partial agonist or antagonist activity against tryptaminergic, dopaminergic and alpha-adrenergic receptors, depending upon their site; it is a highly active uterine stimulant. It constricts peripheral and cranial blood vessels and depresses central vasomotor centers.

Ergotamine reduces extracranial blood flow, causes a decline in the amplitude of pulsation in the cranial arteries and decreases hyperperfusion of the basilar artery territory. Ergotamine is a potent emetic that stimulates the chemoreceptor trigger zone.

Dihydroergotamine, a hydrogenated derivative of ergotamine, differs mainly in its degree of activity. It has less vasoconstrictive action than ergotamine, is 12 times less active as an emetic and has less oxytocic effect.

Pharmacokinetics:

Absorption/Distribution – GI absorption of ergotamine is incomplete and erratic; following oral administration, peak blood levels are reached in ≈ 2 hours.

Onset of action occurs in 15 to 30 minutes following IM administration of dihydroergotamine and persists for 3 to 4 hours.

Metabolism/Excretion – Ergotamine is metabolized by the liver; 90% of the metabolites are excreted in the bile. Although plasma half-life is about 2 hours, ergotamine has long-lasting effects which may be caused by tissue storage.

Contraindications

Pregnancy (ergotamine's powerful uterine stimulant actions may cause fetal harm); hypersensitivity to ergot alkaloids; peripheral vascular disease (eg, thromboangiitis obliterans, leutic arteritis, severe arteriosclerosis, thrombophlebitis, Raynaud's disease); hepatic or renal impairment; severe pruritus; coronary artery disease; hypertension; sepsis; malnutrition.

Warnings

Pregnancy: Category X.

Lactation: Ergotamine is secreted into breast milk and has caused symptoms of ergotism (eg, vomiting, diarrhea) in the infant. Excessive dosing or prolonged administration may inhibit lactation.

Children: Safety and efficacy for use in children have not been established.

Precautions

Prolonged administration: Avoid prolonged administration or excessive dosage because of the danger of ergotism and gangrene.

Drug abuse and dependence: Patients who take ergotamine for extended periods of time may become dependent upon it and require progressively increasing doses for relief of vascular headaches and for prevention of dysphoric effects which follow withdrawal.

Drug Interactions

Drugs that may interact with ergot alkaloids include beta blockers, macrolides, nitrates, vasodilators, and caffeine.

Adverse Reactions

Nausea and vomiting (10%) may be relieved by atropine or phenothiazine antiemetics.

Miscellaneous: Numbness and tingling of fingers and toes; muscle pain in the extremities; pulselessness; weakness in the legs; precordial distress and pain; transient tachycardia or bradycardia; localized edema; itching.

Large doses – Large doses raise arterial pressure, produce coronary vasoconstriction, and slow the heart by both a direct action and a vagal effect.

ISOMETHEPTENE MUCATE/DICHLORALPHENAZONE/ ACETAMINOPHEN

Capsules: 65 mg isometheptene mucate, 100 mg dichloral-phenazone, 325 mg APAP (*Rx*)	Various, *Isocom* (Nutripharm), *Isopap* (Geneva), *Midchlor* (Schein), *Midrin* (Carnrick), *Migratine* (Major)

Indications

For relief of tension and vascular headaches.

Based on a review of this drug (isometheptene mucate) by the National Academy of Sciences-National Research Council or other information, FDA has classified the other indication as "possibly" effective in the treatment of migraine headache. Final classification of the less-than-effective indication requires further investigation.

Administration and Dosage

Migraine headache: Usual dosage is 2 capsules at once followed by 1 capsule every hour until relieved, up to 5 capsules within a 12 hour period.

Tension headache: Usual dosage is 1 or 2 capsules every 4 hours, up to 8 capsules/day.

Actions

Pharmacology: Isometheptene mucate acts by constricting dilated cranial and cerebral arterioles, thus reducing the stimuli that lead to vascular headaches.

Pharmacokinetics: Dichloralphenazone, a mild sedative, reduces the patient's emotional reaction to the pain of both vascular and tension headaches.

Acetaminophen raises the threshold to painful stimuli, thus exerting an analgesic effect against all types of headaches.

Contraindications

Glaucoma; severe cases of renal disease; hypertension; organic heart disease; hepatic disease; MAO inhibitor therapy.

Precautions

Observe caution: Observe caution in hypertension, peripheral vascular disease, and after recent cardiovascular attacks.

Drug Interactions

Drugs that may interact include MAO inhibitors.

Adverse Reactions

Adverse reactions may include transient dizziness and skin rash.

ANTIEMETIC/ANTIVERTIGO AGENTS

CHLORPROMAZINE

Tablets: 10, 25, 50, 100, and 200 mg (*Rx*)
Various, *Thorazine* (GlaxoSmithKline)

Capsules, sustained release: 30, 75, 150, 200, and 300 mg (*Rx*)
Thorazine Spansules (GlaxoSmithKline)

Syrup: 10 mg/5 mL (*Rx*)
Chlorpromazine HCl (Geneva), *Thorazine* (GlaxoSmithKline)

Concentrate: 30 and 100 mg/mL (*Rx*)
Various, *Thorazine* (GlaxoSmithKline)

Suppositories (as base): 25 and 100 mg (*Rx*)
Thorazine (GlaxoSmithKline)

Injection: 25 mg/mL (*Rx*)
Various, *Ormazine* (Hauck), *Thorazine* (GlaxoSmithKline)

PERPHENAZINE

Tablets: 2, 4, 8, and 16 mg (*Rx*)
Various, *Trilafon* (Schering)

Concentrate: 16 mg/5 mL (*Rx*)
Trilafon (Schering)

Injection: 5 mg/mL (*Rx*)
Trilafon (Schering)

TRIFLUPROMAZINE

Injection: 10 and 20 mg/mL (*Rx*)
Vesprin (Princeton)

PROCHLORPERAZINE

Tablets (as maleate): 5, 10, and 25 mg (*Rx*)
Various, *Compazine* (GlaxoSmithKline)

Capsules, sustained release: 10, 15, and 30 mg (*Rx*)
Compazine Spansules (GlaxoSmithKline)

Suppositories: 2.5, 5, and 25 mg (*Rx*)
Various, *Compazine* (GlaxoSmithKline)

Syrup: 5 mg/5 mL (*Rx*)
Compazine (GlaxoSmithKline)

Injection (as edisylate): 5 mg/mL (*Rx*)
Various, *Prochlorperazine* (Wyeth-Ayerst), *Compazine* (GlaxoSmithKline)

THIETHYLPERAZINE

Tablets: 10 mg (*Rx*)

Suppositories: 10 mg (*Rx*)
Norzine (Purdue Frederick), *Torecan* (Roxane)

Injection: 5 mg/mL (*Rx*)

METOCLOPRAMIDE

Tablets: 5 mg (*Rx*)
Various, *Reglan* (Robins)

Tablets: 10 mg (*Rx*)
Various, *Clopra* (Quantum), *Maxolon* (GlaxoSmithKline), *Octamide* (Adria), *Reclomide* (Major), *Reglan* (Robins)

Syrup: 5 mg/5 mL (*Rx*)
Various, *Reglan* (Robins), *Maxolon* (GlaxoSmithKline)

Concentrated solution: 10 mg/mL (*Rx*)
Metoclopramide Intensol (Roxane)

Injection: 5 mg/mL (*Rx*)
Various, *Octamide PFS* (Adria), *Reglan* (Robins)

Administration and Dosage

CHLORPROMAZINE HCl:

Adults –

Nausea and vomiting:

Oral – 10 to 25 mg every 4 to 6 hours, as needed; increase if necessary.

Rectal – 50 to 100 mg every 6 to 8 hours, as needed.

IM – 25 mg. If no hypotension occurs, give 25 to 50 mg every 3 to 4 hours, as needed, until vomiting stops. Then switch to oral dosage.

Intractable hiccoughs: Orally, 25 to 50 mg 3 or 4 times/day. If symptoms persist 2 to 3 days, give 25 to 50 mg IM. If still persistent, use slow IV infusion with patient flat in bed. Give 25 to 50 mg in 500 to 1000 mL saline. Monitor blood pressure.

Children –

Nausea and vomiting: Do not use in children < 6 months of age except where potentially lifesaving. Do not use in conditions for which specific children's dosages have not been established. The activity following IM use may last 12 hours.

Oral – 0.25 mg/lb (0.55 mg/kg) every 4 to 6 hours.

Rectal – 0.5 mg/lb (1.1 mg/kg) every 6 to 8 hours, as needed.

IM – 0.25 mg/lb (0.55 mg/kg) every 6 to 8 hours, as needed.

Maximum IM dosage –

Children up to 5 years of age: 40 mg/day.

Children 5 to 12 years of age: 75 mg/day, except in severe cases.

PERPHENAZINE:

Oral – 8 to 16 mg/day in divided doses; occasionally, 24 mg may be necessary. Early dosage reduction is desirable.

IM – Give to seated or recumbent patient; observe patient for a short period afterward.

Adults: 5 mg repeated every 6 hours as necessary. Do not exceed 15 mg in ambulatory or 30 mg in hospitalized patients. For severe conditions, an initial dose of 10 mg may be given. Place patients on oral therapy as soon as possible, usually within 24 hours. In general, reserve higher dosages for hospitalized patients.

Children (> 12 years of age): The lowest adult dose (5 mg). Pediatric dose not established.

IV – Use only when necessary to control severe vomiting, intractable hiccoughs or acute conditions such as violent retching during surgery. Limit use to recumbent hospitalized adults in doses not exceeding 5 mg. Give as a diluted solution by either fractional injection or slow drip infusion. In the surgical patient, slow infusion is preferred. When administered in divided doses, dilute to 0.5 mg/mL (1 mL mixed with 9 mL saline solution) and give not more than 1 mg per injection at not less than 1 to 2 minute intervals. Discontinue as soon as symptoms are controlled. Do not exceed 5 mg.

TRIFLUPROMAZINE HCl:

Adults –

IM (range): 5 to 15 mg repeated every 4 hours, up to 60 mg maximum daily dose.

Elderly or debilitated – 2.5 mg; maximum daily dose, 15 mg.

IV (range): 1 mg, up to 3 mg total daily dose.

Children (over 2½ years of age) –

IM: 0.2 to 0.25 mg/kg; maximum 10 mg/day. The duration of activity following IM administration may last up to 12 hours. Do not administer IV.

PROCHLORPERAZINE: Do not crush or chew sustained release preparations.

Adults: Control of severe nausea and vomiting –

Oral: Usually, 5 or 10 mg, 3 or 4 times/day; *sustained release* -15 mg on arising or 10 mg every 12 hours.

Rectal: 25 mg twice/day.

IM: Initially, 5 to 10 mg. If necessary, repeat every 3 or 4 hours. Do not exceed 40 mg/day.

SC: Do not administer SC because of local irritation.

Adult surgery: Control of severe nausea and vomiting – Total parenteral dosage should not exceed 40 mg/day. Hypotension may occur if the drug is given IV or by infusion.

IM: 5 to 10 mg, 1 to 2 hours before induction of anesthesia (may repeat once in 30 minutes), or to control acute symptoms during and after surgery (may repeat once).

IV injection: 5 to 10 mg, 15 to 30 minutes before induction of anesthesia, or to control acute symptoms during or after surgery. Repeat once if necessary. Prochlorperazine may be administered either undiluted or diluted in isotonic solution, but do not exceed 10 mg in a single dose of the drug. Do not exceed 5 mg/mL/min. Do not use bolus injection.

IV infusion: 20 mg/L of isotonic solution. Do not dilute in less than 1 L of isotonic solution. Add to IV infusion 15 to 30 minutes before induction.

Children (over 20 pounds or 2 years of age): Control of severe nausea and vomiting –

Oral or rectal: More than one day of therapy is seldom necessary.

9.1 to 13.2 kg – 2.5 mg 1 or 2 times/day (not to exceed 7.5 mg/day).

13.6 to 17.7 kg – 2.5 mg 2 or 3 times/day (not to exceed 10 mg/day).

18.2 to 38.6 kg – 2.5 mg 3 times/day or 5 mg twice/day (not to exceed 15 mg/day).

IM: 0.06 mg/lb (0.132 mg/kg). Give by deep IM injection. Control is usually obtained with one dose. Duration of action may be 12 hours. Subsequent doses may be given if necessary.

PROMETHAZINE:
  Oral and rectal –
    Motion sickness: The average adult dose is 25 mg twice/day. Take the initial dose 1 hour before travel, and repeat 8 to 12 hours later, if necessary. On succeeding days, administer 25 mg on arising and again before the evening meal. For children, administer 12.5 to 25 mg twice/day.
    Nausea and vomiting: The average dose for active therapy in children or adults is 25 mg. Repeat as necessary in doses of 12.5 to 25 mg at 4 to 6 hour intervals.
      Children – 0.25 to 0.5 mg/kg every 4 to 6 hours rectally, as needed. Do not use in children < 2 years of age. Adjust dose based on age, weight, and severity of condition.
  Parenteral – Administer preferably by deep IM injection. Proper IV administration is well tolerated, but hazardous. When used IV, give in a concentration no greater than 25 mg/mL, and at a rate not to exceed 25 mg/min; it is preferable to inject through an appropriate site in tubing of an IV infusion set.
    Motion sickness: 12.5 to 25 mg; may repeat as necessary 3 or 4 times a day.
    Nausea and vomiting: 12.5 to 25 mg; do not repeat more frequently than every 4 hours. For postoperative nausea and vomiting, administer IM or IV.
      In children < 12 years of age, do not exceed half the adult dose. As an adjunct to premedication, use 0.5 mg/lb (1.1 mg/kg) with an equal dose of narcotic or barbiturate and the appropriate dose of an atropine-like drug. Do not use in premature infants or neonates or in vomiting of unknown etiology in children.

THIETHYLPERAZINE MALEATE: Do not use IV (may cause severe hypotension).
    When used for nausea or vomiting associated with anesthesia and surgery, administer by deep IM injection at, or shortly before, termination of anesthesia.
  Adults –
    Oral and rectal: 10 to 30 mg/day in divided doses.
    IM: 2 mL, 1 to 3 times/day.
  Children – Dosage not determined. Not recommended in children < 12 years of age.

THIETHYLPERAZINE: Do not use IV (may cause severe hypotension). Use of this drug has not been studied following intracardiac or intracranial surgery.
    When used for nausea or vomiting associated with anesthesia and surgery, administer by deep IM injection at, or shortly before, termination of anesthesia.
  Adults –
    Oral and Rectal: 10 to 30 mg/day in divided doses.
    IM: 2 mL, 1 to 3 times/day.
  Children – Dosage not determined. Not recommended in children < 12 years of age.

METOCLOPRAMIDE:
  Prevention of chemotherapy-induced emesis – For doses in excess of 10 mg, dilute injection in 50 mL of a parenteral solution (Dextrose 5% in Water, Sodium Chloride Injection, Dextrose 5% in 0.45% Sodium Chloride, Ringer's or Lactated Ringer's Injection). Infuse slowly IV over not less than 15 minutes, 30 minutes before beginning cancer chemotherapy; repeat every 2 hours for 2 doses, then every 3 hours for 3 doses.
      The initial 2 doses should be 2 mg/kg if highly emetogenic drugs such as cisplatin or dacarbazine are used alone or in combination. For less emetogenic regimens, 1 mg/kg/dose may be adequate.
      Metoclopramide may have some potential value (10 mg orally or IV 30 minutes before each meal and at bedtime) in nausea and vomiting of a variety of etiologies (uncontrolled studies report 80% to 90% efficacy), including emesis during pregnancy and labor (5 to 10 mg orally or 5 to 20 mg IV or IM, 3 times a day).

Actions

  Pharmacology: Drug-induced vomiting (eg, drugs, radiation, metabolic disorders) is generally stimulated through the chemoreceptor trigger zone (CTZ), which in turn stimulates the vomiting center (VC) in the brain. Nausea of motion sickness is initiated by stimulation of labyrinthine mechanism of the ear, which sends impulses to CTZ. VC may also be stimulated directly by GI irritation, motion sickness, vestibular neuritis.

The following table indicates manufacturers' recommended uses for agents in this group. Several of these are indicated for uses other than as antiemetic/antivertigo agents.

Recommended Uses for Antiemetic/Antivertigo Agents			
	Indications		
Drug	Nausea and Vomiting	Motion Sickness	Vertigo
ANTIDOPAMINERGICS			
Phenothiazines Chlorpromazine [1]	✔		
Triflupromazine	✔		
Perphenazine [1]	✔		
Prochlorperazine	✔		
Promethazine[2]	✔	✔	
Thiethylperazine	✔		
Other Metoclopramide	✔		
ANTICHOLINERGICS			
Antihistamines Cyclizine	✔	✔	
Meclizine	✔	✔	✔[3]
Buclizine	✔	✔	
Diphenhydramine		✔	
Dimenhydrinate	✔	✔	✔
Other Trimethobenzamide	✔		
Scopolamine		✔	
MISCELLANEOUS			
Miscellaneous Diphenidol	✔		✔
Benzquinamide	✔		
Phosphorated Carbohydrate Solution	✔		
Hydroxyzine HCl	✔[4]		
Corticosteroids	✔[4]		
Cannabinoids	✔		

[1] Also indicated for relief of intractable hicoughs.
[2] For complete listing of promethazine products refer to Antihistamine Product Pages.
[3] Classified "possibly effective" by the FDA.
[4] This is an *unlabeled* use.

Warnings

Children: Not recommended for uncomplicated vomiting in children; limit use to prolonged vomiting of known etiology.

Children with acute illnesses (eg, chickenpox, CNS infections, measles, gastroenteritis) or dehydration seem to be much more susceptible to neuromuscular reactions, particularly dystonias, than are adults. Do not use dimenhydrinate in children under 2 years of age unless directed by a doctor.

Severe emesis – Severe emesis should not be treated with an antiemetic drug alone; where possible, establish cause of vomiting. Direct primary emphasis toward restoration of body fluids and electrolyte balance, and relief of fever and causative disease process. Avoid overhydration which may result in cerebral edema.

CYCLIZINE AND MECLIZINE

CYCLIZINE

Tablets: 50 mg (as HCl) (*otc*)	*Marezine* (Himmel)

MECLIZINE

Tablets: 12.5, 25, and 50 mg (*Rx*)	Various, *Antivert* (Roerig), *Ru-Vert*-M (Solvay), *Dramamine II* (Pharmacia)
Tablets, chewable: 25 mg (*Rx*)	Various
Tablets, chewable: 25 mg (*otc*)	Various, *Bonine* (Leeming)
Capsules: 25 mg (*Rx*)	Various, *Meni-D* (Seatrace)
Capsules: 30 mg (*otc*)	*Vergon* (Marnel)

Indications

Motion sickness, vestibular system disease: Prevention and treatment of nausea, vomiting, and dizziness of motion sickness.

Meclizine is "possibly effective" for the management of vertigo associated with diseases affecting the vestibular system.

Administration and Dosage

CYCLIZINE:

Oral –

Adults: 50 mg taken ½ hour before departure; repeat every 4 to 6 hours. Do not exceed 200 mg/day.

Children (6 to 12 years of age): 25 mg, up to 3 times/day.

Parenteral – For IM use only. Not recommended for use in children.

Adults: 50 mg every 4 to 6 hours, as necessary.

MECLIZINE:

Motion sickness – Take an initial dose of 25 to 50 mg, 1 hour prior to travel. May repeat dose every 24 hours for the duration of the journey.

Vertigo – 25 to 100 mg/day in divided doses.

Actions

Pharmacology: Cyclizine and meclizine have antiemetic, anticholinergic, and antihistaminic properties.

Cyclizine and meclizine have an onset of action of 30 to 60 minutes, depending on dosage; their duration of action is 4 to 6 hours and 12 to 24 hours, respectively.

Contraindications

Hypersensitivity to cyclizine or meclizine.

Warnings

Pregnancy: Category B. Meclizine presents the lowest risk of teratogenicity and is the drug of first choice in treating nausea and vomiting during pregnancy.

Lactation: Safety for use in the nursing mother has not been established.

Children: Safety and efficacy for use in children have not been established. Not recommended for use in children < 12 years of age.

Precautions

Hazardous tasks: May produce drowsiness; patients should observe caution while driving or performing other tasks requiring alertness.

Because of the anticholinergic action of these agents, use with caution and with appropriate monitoring in patients with glaucoma, obstructive disease of the GI or GU tract, and in elderly males with possible prostatic hypertrophy. These drugs may have a hypotensive action, which may be confusing or dangerous in postoperative patients.

May have additive effects with alcohol and other CNS depressants (eg, hypnotics, sedatives, tranquilizers, antianxiety agents); use with caution.

Adverse Reactions

Adverse reactions include the following: Hypotension; palpitations; tachycardia; drowsiness; restlessness; excitation; nervousness; insomnia; euphoria; blurred vision; diplopia; vertigo; tinnitus; auditory and visual hallucinations (particularly when dosage recommendations are exceeded); urticaria; rash; dry mouth; anorexia; nausea; vomiting; diarrhea; constipation; cholestatic jaundice (cyclizine); urinary frequency; difficult urination; urinary retention; dry nose and throat.

BUCLIZINE HCl

Tablets: 50 mg (*Rx*)   *Bucladin-S Softabs* (Stuart)

Indications
For the control of nausea, vomiting, and dizziness of motion sickness.

Administration and Dosage
Tablets can be taken without swallowing water. Place tablet in mouth and allow to dissolve, or chew or swallow whole.

Adults: A 50 mg dose usually alleviates nausea. In severe cases, 150 mg/day may be taken. Usual maintenance dose is 50 mg, 2 times/day. In prevention of motion sickness, take 50 mg at least hour before beginning travel. For extended travel, a second 50 mg dose may be taken after 4 to 6 hours.

Actions
Pharmacology: Acts centrally to suppress nausea and vomiting.

Contraindications
Hypersensitivity to buclizine HCl; pregnancy (see Warnings).

Warnings
Pregnancy: Clinical data are not adequate to establish safety in early pregnancy.

Children: Safety and efficacy for use in children have not been established.

Adverse Reactions
Drowsiness, dry mouth, headache, and jitteriness.

DIPHENHYDRAMINE

For complete prescribing information and product availability, see Antihistamines group monograph.

Indications
Treatment and prophylaxis (oral only) of motion sickness.

Administration and Dosage
Oral: Adults – 25 to 50 mg 3 or 4 times/day.

Children > 20 lbs (9.1 kg) – 12.5 to 25 mg 3 or 4 times/day (5 mg/kg/24 hr, or 150 mg/m^2/24 hr. Do not exceed 300 mg.

Give first dose 30 minutes before exposure to motion and repeat before meals and upon retiring for the duration of journey.

Parenteral: For use only when the oral form is impractical.

Adults – 10 to 50 mg IV or deep IM; 100 mg if required. Maximum daily dosage is 400 mg.

Children – 5 mg/kg/24 hrs or 150 mg/m^2/24 hr, in 4 divided doses, IV or deep IM. Maximum daily dosage is 300 mg.

DIMENHYDRINATE

Tablets: 50 mg (*Rx*)	*Dimetabs* (Jones Medical)
Tablets: 50 mg (*otc*)	Various, *Calm-X* (Republic Drug), *Dramamine* (Pharmacia), *Triptone Caplets* (Commerce)
Tablets, chewable: 50 mg (*otc*)	*Dramamine* (Pharmacia)
Capsules: 50 mg (*otc*)	*Vertab* (UAD)
Injection: 50 mg/mL (*Rx*)	Various, *Dinate* (Seatrace), *Dramamine* (Pasadena), *Dymenate* (Keene), *Hydrate* (Hyrex)
Liquid: 12.5 mg/4 mL (*otc*)	Various, *Dramamine* (Pharmacia),
Liquid: 12.5 mg/5 mL (*otc*)	*Children's Dramamine* (Pharmacia)
Liquid: 15.62 mg/5 mL (*Rx*)	*Dramamine* (Pharmacia)

Indications

For the prevention and treatment of nausea, vomiting, dizziness, or vertigo of motion sickness.

Administration and Dosage

Adults:

Oral – 50 to 100 mg every 4 to 6 hours. Do not exceed 400 mg in 24 hours.

IM – 50 mg, as needed.

IV – 50 mg in 10 mL Sodium Chloride Injection given over 2 minutes. Do not inject intra-arterially.

Children:

Oral (6 to 12 years of age) – 25 to 50 mg every 6 to 8 hours; do not exceed 150 mg in 24 hours.

Oral (2 to 6 years of age) – Up to 12.5 to 25 mg every 6 to 8 hours; do not exceed 75 mg in 24 hours.

IM – 1.25 mg/kg or 37.5 mg/m^2 4 times/day; do not exceed 300 mg/day.

Children (under 2 years of age): Only on advice of a physician.

Actions

Pharmacology: Dimenhydrinate consists of equimolar proportions of diphenhydramine and chlorotheophylline.

Pharmacokinetics: Dimenhydrinate has a depressant action on hyperstimulated labyrinthine function. The precise mode of action is not known. The antiemetic effects are believed to be caused by the diphenhydramine, an antihistamine also used as an antiemetic agent.

Contraindications

Neonates; patients hypersensitive to dimenhydrinate or its components.

Note: Most IV products contain Benzyl Alcohol, which has been associated with a fatal "gasping syndrome" in premature infants and low birth weight infants.

Warnings

Pregnancy: Category B.

Lactation: Small amounts of dimenhydrinate are excreted in breast milk.

Children: For infants and children especially, an overdose of antihistamines may cause hallucinations, convulsions, or death. Mental alertness may be diminished. In the young child, dimenhydrinate may produce excitation. Do not give to children under 2 years of age unless directed by a physician.

Precautions

Use with caution in conditions which might be aggravated by anticholinergic therapy (eg, prostatic hypertrophy, stenosing peptic ulcer, pyloroduodenal obstruction, bladder neck obstruction, narrow angle glaucoma, bronchial asthma, cardiac arrhythmias).

Drug Interactions

Drugs that may interact with dimenhydrinate may include CNS depressants and antibiotics.

Adverse Reactions

Adverse reactions may include drowsiness; confusion; nervousness; restlessness; headache; insomnia (especially in children); tingling, heaviness and weakness of hands; vertigo; dizziness; lassitude; excitation; nausea; vomiting; diarrhea; epigastric distress; constipation; anorexia; blurring of vision; diplopia; palpitations; hypotension; tachycardia; anaphylaxis; photosensitivity; urticaria; drug rash; hemolytic anemia; difficult or painful urination; nasal stuffiness; tightness of chest; wheezing; thickening of bronchial secretions; dryness of mouth, nose, and throat.

TRIMETHOBENZAMIDE HCl

Capsules: 100 mg (*Rx*)	*Tigan* (Roberts), *Trimazide* (Major)
Capsules: 250 mg (*Rx*)	Various, *Tigan* (Roberts)
Pediatric suppositories: 100 mg (*Rx*)	Various, *Pediatric Triban* (Great Southern), *Tebamide* (G&W Labs), *T-Gen* (Goldline), *Tigan* (Roberts), *Trimazide* (Major)
Suppositories: 200 mg (*Rx*)	Various, *Tebamide* (G&W), *T-Gen* (Goldline), *Tigan* (Roberts), *Triban* (Great Southern), *Trimazide* (Major)
Injection: 100 mg/mL (*Rx*)	Various, *Pediatric Triban* (Great Southern), *Ticon* (Hauck), *Tigan* (Roberts)

Indications

Control of nausea and vomiting.

Administration and Dosage

Oral:

    Adults – 250 mg, 3 or 4 times/day.

    Children (30 to 90 lbs; 13.6 to 40.9 kg) – 100 to 200 mg, 3 or 4 times/day.

Rectal:

    Adults – 200 mg, 3 or 4 times/day.

    Children (30 to 90 lbs; 13.6 to 40.9 kg) – 100 to 200 mg, 3 or 4 times/day.

    (< 30 lbs) – 100 mg, 3 or 4 times/day. Do not use in premature or newborn infants.

Injection: For IM use only.

    Adults – 200 mg 3 or 4 times/day. Pain, stinging, burning, redness, and swelling may develop at injection site.

Actions

Pharmacokinetics: Mechanism is obscure, but may be mediated through the chemoreceptor trigger zone; direct impulses to vomiting center are not inhibited.

Contraindications

Hypersensitivity to trimethobenzamide, benzocaine or similar local anesthetics; parenteral use in children; suppositories in premature infants or neonates.

Warnings

Pregnancy: Safety for use has not been established.

Lactation: Safety for use in the nursing mother has not been established.

Precautions

Encephalitides, gastroenteritis, dehydration, electrolyte imbalance (especially in children and the elderly or debilitated), and CNS reactions have occurred when used during acute febrile illness.

Exercise caution when giving the drug with alcohol and other CNS-acting agents such as phenothiazines, barbiturates, and belladonna derivatives.

Adverse Reactions

Adverse reactions may include: Hypersensitivity reactions; parkinson-like symptoms; hypotension or pain following IM injection; blood dyscrasias; blurred vision; coma; convulsions; depression; diarrhea; disorientation; dizziness; drowsiness; headache; jaundice; muscle cramps; opisthotonos; allergic-type skin reactions.

DRONABINOL

Gelatin capsules: 2.5, 5, and 10 mg (c-III)   *Marinol* (Roxane)

Indications

Antiemetic: Treatment of nausea and vomiting associated with cancer chemotherapy in patients not responding adequately to conventional antiemetic treatment.

Appetite stimulation: Treating anorexia associated with weight loss in AIDS patients.

Administration and Dosage

Antiemetic: Initially, give 5 mg/m^2 1 to 3 hours prior to the administration of chemotherapy, then every 2 to 4 hours after chemotherapy is given, for a total of 4 to 6 doses/day. If the 5 mg/m^2 dose is ineffective, and there are no significant side effects, increase the dose by 2.5 mg/m^2 increments to a maximum of 15 mg/m^2 per dose. Use caution, however, as the incidence of disturbing psychiatric symptoms increases significantly at this maximum dose. Administration with phenothiazines may improve efficacy (vs either drug alone) without additional toxicity.

Appetite stimulation: Initially, give 2.5 mg twice/day before lunch and supper. For patients who cannot tolerate 5 mg/day, reduce dosage to 2.5 mg/day as a single evening or bedtime dose. When adverse reactions are absent or minimal and further therapeutic effect is desired, increase to 2.5 mg before lunch and 5 mg before supper (or 5 mg at lunch and 5 mg after supper). Although most patients respond to 2.5 mg twice/day, 10 mg twice/day has been tolerated in about 50% of patients. The dosage may be increased to a maximum of 20 mg/day in divided doses. Use caution in escalating the dosage because of the increased frequency of dose-related adverse reactions at higher dosages.

Actions

Pharmacology: Dronabinol is the principal psychoactive substance present in *Cannabis sativa* L (marijuana). The mechanism of action is unknown.

Cannabinoids have complex CNS effects, including central sympathomimetic activity.

Pharmacokinetics:

Absorption/Distribution – Following oral administration, dronabinol is almost completely absorbed (90% to 95%). It has an onset of action of ≈ 0.5 to 1 hour and peak effect at 2 to 4 hours. Duration for psychoactive effects is 4 to 6 hours, but the appetite stimulant effect may continue for ≥ 24 hours after administration.

Metabolism/Excretion – Dronabinol undergoes extensive first-pass hepatic metabolism.

Biliary excretion is the major route of elimination. Extended use at the recommended doses may cause accumulation of toxic amounts of dronabinol and its metabolites.

Contraindications

Hypersensitivity to dronabinol, marijuana, or sesame oil.

Warnings

Tolerance: Following 12 days of dronabinol, tolerance to the cardiovascular and subjective effects developed at doses ≤ 210 mg/day. An initial tachycardia induced by dronabinol was replaced successively by normal sinus rhythm and then bradycardia. A fall in supine blood pressure, made worse by standing, was also observed initially. Within days, these effects disappeared, indicating development of tolerance. Tachyphylaxis and tolerance did not, however, appear to develop to the appetite stimulant effect.

Patient supervision: Because of individual variation, determine clinically the period of patient supervision required.

Elderly: Use caution because the elderly are generally more sensitive to the psychoactive effects. In antiemetic studies, no difference in tolerance or efficacy was apparent in patients > 55 years of age.

Pregnancy: Category B.

Lactation: Dronabinol is concentrated and excreted in breast milk; nursing mothers should not use dronabinol.

Children: Not recommended for AIDS-related anorexia in children because it has not been studied in this population. Dosage for chemotherapy-induced emesis is the same as in adults. Use caution in children because of the psychoactive effects.

Precautions

Hypertension or heart disease: Use with caution since dronabinol may cause a general increase in central sympathomimetic activity.

Psychiatric patients: In manic, depressive, or schizophrenic patients, symptoms of these disease states may be exacerbated by the use of cannabinoids.

Drug abuse and dependence: Dronabinol is highly abusable. Limit prescriptions to the amount necessary for a single cycle of chemotherapy.

A withdrawal syndrome consisting of irritability, insomnia, and restlessness was observed in some subjects within 12 hours following abrupt withdrawal of dronabinol. The syndrome reached its peak intensity at 24 hours when subjects exhibited hot flashes, sweating, rhinorrhea, loose stools, hiccoughs, and anorexia. The syndrome was essentially complete within 96 hours. EEG changes following discontinuation were consistent with a withdrawal syndrome. Several subjects reported impressions of disturbed sleep for several weeks after discontinuing high doses.

Hazardous tasks: Because of its profound effects on mental status, warn patients not to drive, operate complex machinery, or engage in any activity requiring sound judgment and unimpaired coordination while receiving treatment. Effects may persist for a variable and unpredictable period of time.

Drug Interactions

Drugs that may be affected by dronabinol include amphetamines, cocaine, sympathomimetics, anticholinergics, antihistamines, tricyclic antidepressants, alcohol, sedatives, hypnotics, psychomimetics, disulfiram, fluoxetine, and theophylline.

Adverse Reactions

Adverse reactions occurring in ≥ 3% of patients include euphoria, nausea, vomiting, dizziness, paranoid reaction, and somnolence.

5-HT₃ RECEPTOR ANTAGONISTS

ONDANSETRON	
Tablets: 4, 8, 24 mg (as HCl dihydrate) (*Rx*)	*Zofran* (GlaxoSmithKline)
Solution, oral: 4 mg/5 mL (5 mg as HCl) (*Rx*)	
Injection: 2 mg/mL and 32 mg/50 mL (pre-mixed) (as HCl dihydrate) (*Rx*)	
Tablets, orally disintegrating: 4 and 8 mg (as base) (*Rx*)	*Zofran ODT* (GlaxoSmithKline)
GRANISETRON	
Tablets: 1 mg (1.12 mg as HCl) (*Rx*)	*Kytril* (GlaxoSmithKline)
Injection: 1 mg/mL (1.12 mg/mL as HCl) (*Rx*)	
DOLASETRON	
Tablets: 50 and 100 mg (*Rx*)	*Anzemet* (Aventis)
Injection: 20 mg/mL (*Rx*)	
ALOSETRON HCl	
Tablets: 1 mg (1.124 mg alosetron HCl equiv. to 1 mg alosetron) (*Rx*)	*Lotronex* (GlaxoSmithKline)

Indications

Antiemetic: Prevention of nausea and vomiting associated with initial and repeat courses of emetogenic cancer therapy, including high-dose cisplatin; prevention of postoperative nausea or vomiting (**ondansetron** and **dolasetron**); treatment of postoperative nausea or vomiting (**dolasetron injection**); prevention of nausea and vomiting associated with radiotherapy in patients receiving either total body irradiation, single high-dose fraction or daily fractions to the abdomen (**oral ondansetron** and **granisetron**).

Irritable bowel syndrome (IBS): For the treatment of IBS in women whose predominant bowel syndrome is diarrhea (**alosetron**). The safety and efficacy of alosetron in men have not been established.

Unlabeled uses:

Granisetron – Acute nausea and vomiting following surgery (1 to 3 mg IV).

Dolasetron – Radiotherapy-induced nausea and vomiting (40 mg IV or 0.3 mg/kg IV).

Administration and Dosage

ONDANSETRON:

Prevention of nausea/vomiting associated with cancer chemotherapy –

Parenteral: The recommended IV dosage is three 0.15 mg/kg doses or a single 32 mg dose. With the 3 dose regimen, the first dose is infused over 15 minutes beginning 30 minutes before the start of emetogenic chemotherapy. Subsequent doses are administered 4 and 8 hours after the first dose. The single 32 mg dose is infused over 15 minutes beginning 30 minutes before the start of emetogenic chemotherapy.

Children – On the basis of the limited available information, the dosage in children 4 to 18 years of age should be three 0.15 mg/kg doses (see above). Little information is available about dosage in children ≤ 3 years of age.

Oral (moderately emetogenic cancer chemotherapy): Recommended dose is 8 mg twice/ day. Administer the first dose 30 minutes before the start of emetogenic chemotherapy, with a subsequent dose 8 hours after the first dose. Administer 8 mg twice a day (every 12 hours) for 1 to 2 days after completion of chemotherapy.

Children – For patients ≥ 12 years of age, dosage is same as adults; for children 4 to 11 years, use 4 mg 3 times a day. Give the first dose 30 min before chemotherapy, with subsequent doses 4 and 8 hours after the first dose. Give 4 mg 3 times a day (every 8 hours) for 1 to 2 days after completion of chemotherapy.

Prevention of nausea and vomiting associated with radiotherapy (oral) – 8 mg 3 times/day.

Total body irradiation: 8 mg 1 to 2 hours before each fraction of radiotherapy administered each day.

Single high-dose fraction radiotherapy to the abdomen: 8 mg 1 to 2 hours before radiotherapy, with subsequent doses every 8 hours after the first dose for 1 to 2 days after completion of radiotherapy.

Daily fractionated radiotherapy to the abdomen: 8 mg 1 to 2 hours before radiotherapy, with subsequent doses every 8 hours after the first dose for each day radiotherapy is given.

Children: There is no experience with tablets or oral solution use in the prevention of radiation-induced nausea and vomiting in children.

Prevention of postoperative nausea or vomiting –

Parenteral: Immediately before induction of anesthesia, or postoperatively if the patient experiences nausea or vomiting shortly after surgery, administer 4 mg undiluted IV in not less than 30 seconds, preferably over 2 to 5 minutes. Alternatively, 4 mg undiluted may be administered IM as a single injection in adults. In patients who do not achieve adequate control of postoperative nausea and vomiting following a single, prophylactic, preinduction, IV dose of ondansetron 4 mg, administration of a second IV dose of 4 mg ondansetron postoperatively does not provide additional control of nausea and vomiting.

Children – Patients 2 to 12 years of age weighing ≤ 40 kg may receive 0.1 mg/ kg IV; give a single 4 mg dose for those weighing > 40 kg. Administer over ≥ 30 seconds, preferably over 2 to 5 minutes.

Oral: 16 mg given as a single dose 1 hour before induction of anesthesia.

Children: There is no experience in children for use of tablets or oral solution.

Prevention of nausea and vomiting associated with highly emetogenic cancer chemotherapy (oral) – The recommended adult oral dosage is 24 mg administered 30 minutes before the start of single-day highly emetogenic chemotherapy, including cisplatin ≥ 50 mg/ m². Multi-day, single-dose administration of 24 mg has not been studied. Efficacy of the 32 mg single dose beyond 24 hrs in these patients has not been established.

Children: There is no experience with the use of 24 mg tablets.

Hepatic function impairment – Do not exceed an 8 mg oral dose. For IV use, a single maximum daily dose of 8 mg infused over 15 minutes beginning 30 minutes before the start of emetogenic chemotherapy is recommended.

GRANISETRON:

IV – The recommended dosage is 10 mcg/kg infused IV over 5 minutes, beginning within 30 minutes before initiation of chemotherapy, and only on the day(s) chemotherapy is given.

Children: The recommended dose in children 2 to 16 years of age is 10 mcg/kg. Children < 2 years of age have not been studied.

Elderly, renal, or hepatic function impairment: No dosage adjustment is recommended.

Oral – 2 mg once/day or 1 mg twice/day. In the 2 mg once/day regimen, two 1 mg tablets are given up to 1 hour before chemotherapy. In the 1 mg twice/day regimen, give the first dose up to 1 hour before chemotherapy and the second dose 12 hours after the first. Either regimen is administered only on the day(s) chemotherapy is given. Continued treatment while not on chemotherapy has not been found to be useful.

Radiation (either total body irradiation or fractionated abdominal radiation): 2 mg once/day. Two 1 mg tablets are taken within 1 hour of radiation.

Children: There is no experience with oral granisetron in the prevention of radiation-induced nausea and vomiting in pediatric patients.

Elderly, renal/hepatic function impairment: No dosage adjustment is recommended.

DOLASETRON:

Cardiac effects – Administer dolasetron with caution in patients who have or may develop prolongation of cardiac conduction intervals, particularly QT_c.

Infusion rate – Dolasetron injection can be safely infused IV as rapidly as 100 mg/30 seconds or diluted in a compatible IV solution to 50 mL and infused over a period of up to 15 minutes.

Chemotherapy-induced nausea and vomiting, prevention –

IV:

Adults – 1.8 mg/kg as a single dose ≈ 30 minutes before chemotherapy. Alternatively, for most patients a fixed dose of 100 mg can be administered over 30 seconds.

Children (2 to 16 years of age) – 1.8 mg/kg as a single dose ≈ 30 minutes before chemotherapy, up to a maximum of 100 mg.

Oral:

Adults – 100 mg within 1 hour before chemotherapy.

Children (2 to 16 years of age) – 1.8 mg/kg within 1 hour before chemotherapy, up to a maximum of 100 mg.

Postoperative nausea or vomiting, prevention/treatment –

IV:

Adults – 12.5 mg as a single dose ≈ 15 minutes before the cessation of anesthesia or as soon as nausea or vomiting presents.

Children (2 to 16 years of age) – 0.35 mg/kg as a single dose ≈ 15 minutes before the cessation of anesthesia or as soon as nausea or vomiting presents, up to a maximum of 12.5 mg.

Oral (prevention only) –

Adults: 100 mg 2 hours before surgery.

Children (2 to 16 years of age): 1.2 mg/kg within 2 hours before surgery, up to a maximum of 100 mg.

ALOSETRON:

Usual adult dose – 1 mg taken orally twice/day with or without food for up to 1 year. Individual patients who experience constipation may need to interrupt treatment.

Actions

Pharmacology: Selective 5-hydroxytryptamine$_3$ (5-HT$_3$) receptor antagonists are antinauseant and antiemetic agents with little or no affinity for other serotonin receptors, alpha- or beta-adrenergic, dopamine-D$_2$, histamine-H$_1$, benzodiazepine, picrotoxin, or opioid receptors.

Pharmacokinetics: The elimination half-lives of these drugs range from 4 to 8 hours. Elimination is primarily via hepatic metabosim. Plasma concentrations of **alosetron** are 30% to 50% lower and less variable in men compared with women given the same dose. Plasma protein binding is 65% for **granisetron** and 70% to 76% for **ondansetron**.

Contraindications

Hypersensitivity to the drug or components of the product; markely prolonged QTc or atrioventricular Block II to III (**dolasetron**); patients receiving class I or III antiarrhythmic agents (**dolasetron**).

Warnings

Acute ischemic colitis: Acute ischemic colitis was infrequent (0.1% to 1%) in patients receiving **alosetron** in 3-month clinical trials.

Constipation: Constipation is a frequent and dose-related side effect of treatment with **alosetron**. Do not use alosetron in IBS patients who are currently constipated or whose predominant bowel symptom is constipation.

Postoperatively: Routine prophylaxis is not recommended for patients in whom there is little expectation that nausea or vomiting will occur postoperatively. In patients where nausea or vomiting must be avoided postoperatively, IV **ondansetron** is recommended even where the incidence of postoperative nausea or vomiting is low. For patients who have postoperative nausea or vomiting, ondansetron may be given to prevent further episodes.

Cardiac effects: Acute, usually reversible, ECG changes (PR and QTc prolongation; QRS widening) caused by **dolasetron** have been observed. Dolasetron appears to prolong both depolarization and, to a lesser extent, repolarization time. The magnitude and frequency of the ECG changes increased with dose. These ECG interval prolongations usually returned to baseline within 6 to 8 hours, but in some patients were present at 24 hour follow up.

Administer dolasetron with caution in patients who have or may develop prolongation of cardiac conduction intervals, particularly QTc. These include patients with hypokalemeia or hypomagnesemia, patients taking diuretics with potential for inducing electrolyte abnormalities, patients with congential QT syndrome, patients taking antiarrhythmic drugs or other drugs that lead to QT prolongation and cumulative high dose anthracycline therapy.

Peristalsis: Ondansetron does not stimulate gastric or intestinal peristalsis. Do not use instead of nasogastric suction. Use in abdominal surgery may mask a progressive ileus or gastric distension.

Hypersensitivity reactions: Rare cases of hypersensitivity reactions, sometimes severe, have occurred.

Hepatic function impairment: Increased exposure to alosetron is likely to occur in patients with hepatic insufficiency.

Pregnancy: Category B.

Lactation: It is not known whether 5-HT₃ antagonists are excreted in breast milk.

Children:

Granisetron – Safety and efficacy of the injection in children < 2 years of age have not been established. Safety and efficacy of the oral doseform in children have not been established.

Ondansetron – Little information is available about dosage in children ≤ 3 years of age.

Dolasetron – Safety and efficacy in children < 2 years of age have not been established. See Adminstration and Dosage for use in children ≥ 2 years of age.

Alosetron – Safety and efficacy in pediatric patients have not been established.

Precautions

Benzyl alcohol: Some of these products contain benzyl alcohol, which has been associated with a fatal "gasping syndrome" in premature infants.

Drug Interactions

Inducers or inhibitors of P450 enzymes may change the clearance and, hence, the half-life of 5-HT$_3$ antagonists. No dosage adjustment is recommended for patients on these drugs. **Dolasetron** may be affected by atenolol, cimetidine, and rifampin. **Ondansetron** may be affected by rifampin. **Alosetron** inhibits N-acetyltransferase which may affect drugs such as isoniazid, procainide, and hydralazine.

Drug/Food interactions: **Alosetron** absorption is decreased by ≈ 25% by coadministration with food, with a mean delay in time to peak concentration of 15 minutes.

Adverse Reactions

Adverse reactions occurring in ≥ 3% of patients:

Ondansetron: Anxiety/agitation; dizziness; drowsiness/sedation; malaise/fatigue; fever/pyrexia; gynecological disorder; hypoxia; injection site reaction; pruritus; urinary retention; hypotension; headache; chills/shivering; abdominal pain; constipation; diarrhea; increased AST and ALT; arrhythmias; wound problem; musculoskeletal pain; extrapyramidal syndrome.

Granisetron: Asthenia; headache; abdominal pain; constipation; diarrhea; nausea/vomiting; increased AST and ALT; somnolence; CNS stimulation; decreased appetite; leukopenia; shivers; anemia; alopecia; thrombocytopenia.

Dolasetron: Bradycardia/tachycardia; hypotension; dizziness; headache; malaise/fatigue; abdominal pain; dyspepsia; fever/pyrexia; pruritis; increased AST and ALT.

Alosetron: Hypertension; sleep disorders; abdominal pain; constipation; nausea; GI docomfort/pain; GI gaseous symptoms; viral GI infections; dyspeptic symptoms.

MEPROBAMATE

| Tablets: 200, 400, and 600 mg (c-iv) | Various, *Equanil* (Wyeth-Ayerst), *Miltown* (Wallace) |

Indications

Management of anxiety disorders or short-term relief of the symptoms of anxiety.

Administration and Dosage

Adults: 1.2 to 1.6 g/day in 3 to 4 divided doses; do not exceed 2.4 g/day.

Children: 100 to 200 mg 2 or 3 times/day.

Actions

Pharmacology: Meprobamate has selective effects at multiple sites in the CNS, including the thalamus and limbic system. It also appears to inhibit multineuronal spinal reflexes. Meprobamate is mildly tranquilizing, and has some anticonvulsant and muscle relaxant properties.

Pharmacokinetics:

Absorption/Distribution – Meprobamate is well absorbed from the GI tract; peak plasma concentrations are reached within 1 to 3 hours.

Metabolism/Excretion – The liver metabolizes 80% to 92% of the drug; the remainder is excreted unchanged in the urine. Excretion is mainly renal (90%), with < 10% appearing in feces.

Contraindications

Acute intermittent porphyria; allergic or idiosyncratic reactions to meprobamate or related compounds.

Warnings

Hypersensitivity reactions: Usually seen between the first to fourth dose in patients having no previous exposure to the drug.

Renal function impairment: Use with caution to avoid accumulation, since meprobamate is metabolized in the liver and excreted by the kidney.

Elderly: To avoid oversedation, use lowest effective dose.

Pregnancy: Category D.

Lactation: Meprobamate is excreted into breast milk at concentrations 2 to 4 times that of maternal plasma.

Children: Do not administer to children < 6 years of age. The 600 mg tablet is not intended for use in children.

Precautions

Epilepsy: May precipitate seizures in epileptic patients.

Drug abuse and dependence: Physical and psychological dependence and abuse may occur. Abrupt discontinuation after prolonged and excessive use may precipitate a recurrence of pre-existing symptoms or withdrawal syndrome characterized by anxiety, anorexia, insomnia, vomiting, ataxia, tremors, muscle twitching, confusional states, and hallucinations. Generalized seizures occur in about 10% of cases and are more likely to occur in people with CNS damage or preexistent or latent convulsive disorders. Onset of withdrawal symptoms usually occurs within 12 to 48 hours after drug discontinuation; symptoms usually cease in the next 12 to 48 hours.

When excessive dosage has continued for weeks or months, reduce gradually over a period of 1 or 2 weeks rather than stopping abruptly.

Hazardous tasks: May produce drowsiness, dizziness, or blurred vision; patients should observe caution while driving or performing other tasks requiring alertness.

Drug Interactions

Alcohol: Acute ingestion may result in a decreased clearance of meprobamate through inhibition of hepatic metabolic systems; enhanced CNS depressant effects may occur.

Adverse Reactions

Adverse reactions may include drowsiness; ataxia; dizziness; slurred speech; headache; vertigo; weakness; impairment of visual accommodation; euphoria; overstimulation; paradoxical excitement; nausea; vomiting; diarrhea; palpitations; tachycardia; various arrhythmias; syncope; hypotensive crises; allergic/idiosyncratic reactions; leukopenia; acute nonthrombocytopenic purpura; petechiae; ecchymoses; eosinophilia; peripheral edema; fever; hyperpyrexia; chills; angioneurotic edema; bronchospasm; oliguria; anuria; anaphylaxis; erythema multiforme; exfoliative dermatitis; stomatitis; proctitis; Stevens-Johnson syndrome; bullous dermatitis; paresthesias; agranulocytosis; aplastic anemia; thrombocytopenic purpura.

BENZODIAZEPINES

OXAZEPAM	
Capsules: 10, 15, and 30 mg (c-iv)	Various, *Serax* (Wyeth-Ayerst)
Tablets: 15 mg (c-iv)	Various, *Serax* (Wyeth-Ayerst)
PRAZEPAM	
Capsules: 5, 10, and 20 mg (c-iv)	Various, *Centrax* (Parke-Davis)
Tablets: 5 or 10 mg (c-iv)	Various, *Centrax* (Parke-Davis)
LORAZEPAM	
Tablets: 0.5, 1, and 2 mg (c-iv)	Various, *Ativan* (Wyeth-Ayerst)
Concentrated oral solution: 2 mg/mL (c-iv)	*Lorazepam Intensol* (Roxane)
Injection: 2 or 4 mg/mL (c-iv)	Various, *Ativan* (Wyeth-Ayerst)
ALPRAZOLAM	
Tablets: 0.25, 0.5, 1, and 2 mg (c-iv)	Various, *Xanax* (Pharmacia)
Oral solution: 0.5 mg/5 mL (c-iv)	*Alprazolam* (Roxane)
Intensol solution: 1 mg/mL (c-iv)	*Alprazolam* (Roxane)
CHLORDIAZEPOXIDE	
Capsules: 5, 10, and 25 mg (c-iv)	Various, *Librium* (Roche)
Tablets: 10 or 25 mg (c-iv)	*Libritabs* (Roche)
Powder for injection: 100 mg (c-iv)	*Librium* (Roche)
DIAZEPAM	
Tablets: 2, 5, and 10 mg (c-iv)	Various, *Valium* (Roche), *Dizac* (Ohmeda)
Oral solution: 5 mg/5 mL (c-iv)	Various
Oral solution, intensol: 5 mg/mL (c-iv)	*Diazepam Intensol* (Roxane)
Injection: 5 mg/mL (c-iv)	Various, *Valium* (Roche)
CLORAZEPATE DIPOTASSIUM	
Capsules: 3.75, 7.5, and 15 mg (c-iv)	Various
Tablets: 3.75, 7.5, and 15 mg (c-iv)	Various, *Tranxene* (Abbott)
Tablets: 11.25 and 22.5 mg (c-iv)	*Tranxene-SD Half Strength* (Abbott), *Tranxene-SD* (Abbott)

Indications

Anxiety: For the management of anxiety disorders or for the short-term relief of the symptoms of anxiety. Anxiety or tension associated with the stress of everyday life usually does not require treatment with an antianxiety agent.

Administration and Dosage

OXAZEPAM:

Mild to moderate anxiety, with associated tension, irritability, agitation, or related symptoms of functional origin or secondary to organic disease – 10 to 15 mg 3 or 4 times/day.

Severe anxiety syndromes, agitation, or anxiety associated with depression – 15 to 30 mg 3 or 4 times/day.

Older patients with anxiety, tension, irritability and agitation – Initial dosage is 10 mg 3 times/day. If necessary, increase cautiously to 15 mg 3 or 4 times/day.

Alcoholics with acute inebriation, tremulousness, or anxiety on withdrawal – 15 to 30 mg 3 or 4 times/day.

Children (6 to 12 years of age) – Dosage is not established.

PRAZEPAM: The usual dose is 30 mg/day administered in divided doses. Adjust dosage gradually within the range of 20 to 60 mg/day.

Elderly – Initiate treatment at 10 to 15 mg/day in divided doses.

May also be administered as a single daily dose at bedtime. The starting dose is 20 mg/night. The optimum dose ranges from 20 to 40 mg.

LORAZEPAM:

Oral – 2 to 6 mg/day (varies from 1 to 10 mg/day) given in divided doses; take the largest dose before bedtime.

Anxiety: Initial dose, 2 to 3 mg/day given 2 or 3 times/day.

Insomnia caused by anxiety or transient situational stress: 2 to 4 mg at bedtime.

Elderly or debilitated patients: Initial dose, 1 to 2 mg/day in divided doses.

IM – 0.05 mg/kg up to a maximum of 4 mg. For optimum effect, administer at least 2 hours before operative procedure.

IV – Initial dose is 2 mg total or 0.044 mg/kg (0.02 mg/lb), whichever is smaller. This will sedate most adults; ordinarily, do not exceed in patients > 50 years of age. If a greater lack of recall would be beneficial, doses as high as 0.05 mg/kg up to a total of 4 mg may be given. For optimum effect, give 15 to 20 minutes before the procedure.

Children (< 18 years of age) – Parenteral use is not recommended.

ALPRAZOLAM: Reduce gradually when terminating or decreasing daily dose. Decrease by no more than 0.5 mg every 3 days.

Anxiety disorders – Initial dose is 0.25 to 0.5 mg 3 times/day. Titrate to max total dose of 4 mg/day in divided doses.

Elderly or debilitated patients – 0.25 mg, given 2 or 3 times/day. Gradually increase if needed and tolerated.

Panic disorder – Initial dose is 0.5 mg 3 times/day. Depending on response, increase dose at intervals of 3 to 4 days in increments of no more than 1 mg/day.

Successful treatment has required doses > 4 mg/day; in controlled studies, doses in the range of 1 to 10 mg/day were used.

CHLORDIAZEPOXIDE:

Oral –

Mild to moderate anxiety: 5 or 10 mg 3 or 4 times/day.

Severe anxiety: 20 or 25 mg 3 or 4 times/day.

Geriatric patients or patients with debilitating disease: 5 mg 2 to 4 times/day.

Preoperative apprehension and anxiety: On days preceding surgery, 5 to 10 mg 3 or 4 times/day.

Acute alcohol withdrawal: 50 to 100 mg; repeat as needed (up to 300 mg/day). Parenteral form usually used initially. Reduce to maintenance levels.

Children: Initially, 5 mg 2 to 4 times/day (may be increased in some children to 10 mg 2 or 3 times/day). Not recommended in children under 6 years of age.

A dosage of 0.5 mg/kg/day every 6 to 8 hours in children > 6 years of age has also been recommended.

Parenteral – Use lower doses (25 to 50 mg) for elderly or debilitated patients and for older children. A dosage of 0.5 mg/kg/day every 6 to 8 hours IM in children > 12 years of age has also been recommended. Acute symptoms may be rapidly controlled by parenteral administration; subsequent treatment, if necessary, may be given orally. While 300 mg may be given during a 6 hour period, do not exceed this dose in any 24 hour period. Not recommended in children < 12 years of age.

Acute alcohol withdrawal: 50 to 100 mg IM or IV initially; repeat in 2 to 4 hours if necessary.

Acute or severe anxiety: 50 to 100 mg IM or IV initially; then 25 to 50 mg 3 or 4 times/day if necessary.

Preoperative apprehension/anxiety: 50 to 100 mg IM 1 hour prior to surgery.

DIAZEPAM:

Oral –

Management of anxiety disorders and relief of symptoms of anxiety (depending upon severity of symptoms): 2 to 10 mg 2 to 4 times/day.

Acute alcohol withdrawal: 10 mg 3 or 4 times during the first 24 hours; reduce to 5 mg 3 or 4 times/day, as needed.

Adjunct in skeletal muscle spasm: 2 to 10 mg 3 or 4 times/day.

Adjunct in convulsive disorders: 2 to 10 mg 2 to 4 times/day.

Elderly patients or in the presence of debilitating disease: 2 to 2.5 mg 1 or 2 times/day initially; increase gradually as needed and tolerated.

Children: 1 to 2.5 mg 3 or 4 times/day initially; increase gradually as needed and tolerated. Not for use in children under 6 months. For sedation or muscle relaxation, a dosage of 0.12 to 0.8 mg/kg/24 hours divided 3 to 4 times a day has been recommended.

Oral, sustained release – Do not crush or chew sustained release formula

Whenever oral diazepam 5 mg 3 times a day would be considered appropriate dosage, one 15 mg sustained release capsule daily may be used.

Management of anxiety disorders and relief of symptoms of anxiety: 15 to 30 mg/day, depending upon severity of symptoms.

Adjunct in skeletal muscle spasm: 15 to 30 mg/day.

Oral, solution – Dosage same as oral tablets.

Intensol: The **Intensol** is a concentrated oral solution as compared to standard oral liquid medications. It is recommended that the **Intensol** be mixed with liquid or semisolid food such as water, juices, soda or soda-like beverages, applesauce, and puddings. Use only the calibrated dropper provided with the product.

Parenteral –

Children: Administer slowly over 3 minutes. Do not exceed 0.25 mg/kg. After an interval of 15 to 30 minutes, the initial dose can be repeated.

Moderate anxiety disorders and symptoms of anxiety: 2 to 5 mg IM or IV. Repeat in 3 to 4 hours if necessary.

Severe anxiety disorders and symptoms of anxiety: 5 to 10 mg IM or IV. Repeat in 3 to 4 hours if necessary.

Acute alcohol withdrawal: 10 mg IM or IV initially; then 5 to 10 mg in 3 to 4 hours if necessary.

Endoscopic procedures:

IV – 10 mg or less is usually adequate; up to 20 mg may be used, especially when concomitant narcotics are omitted.

IM – 5 to 10 mg 30 minutes prior to procedure if IV route cannot be used.

Muscle spasm: 5 to 10 mg IM or IV initially; then 5 to 10 mg in 3 to 4 hours if necessary. Tetanus may require larger doses.

Status epilepticus and severe recurrent convulsive seizures: The IV route is preferred; administer slowly. Use the IM route if IV administration is impossible. Administer 5 to 10 mg initially; repeat if necessary at 10 to 15 minute intervals up to maximum dose of 30 mg. If necessary, repeat therapy in 2 to 4 hours. A dose of 0.2 to 0.5 mg/kg every 15 to 30 minutes for 2 to 3 doses (maximum dose, 30 mg).

Infants (over 30 days of age) and children (under 5 years of age): Inject 0.2 to 0.5 mg slowly every 2 to 5 minutes up to a maximum of 5 mg; 0.2 to 0.5 mg/kg/dose every 15 to 30 minutes for 2 to 3 doses (maximum dose, 5 mg) has been recommended.

Neonates: 0.5 to 1 mg/kg/dose every 15 to 30 minutes for 2 to 3 doses has been suggested.

Preoperative medication: 10 mg IM before surgery.

Cardioversion: 5 to 15 mg IV, 5 to 10 minutes prior to procedure.

Tetanus:

Infants (over 30 days of age) – 1 to 2 mg IM or IV slowly, repeated every 3 to 4 hours as necessary.

Children (≥ 5 years of age) – 5 to 10 mg repeated every 3 to 4 hours may be required.

Sedation or muscle relaxation:

Children – 0.04 to 0.2 mg/kg/dose every 2 to 4 hours, maximum of 0.6 mg/kg within an 8 hour period.

Adults – 2 to 10 mg/dose every 3 to 4 hours as needed.

HALAZEPAM: The usual dose is 20 to 40 mg 3 or 4 times a day. The optimal dosage usually ranges from 80 to 160 mg/day.

Elderly (≥ 70 years of age) or debilitated patients – 20 mg once or twice/day.

CHLORAZEPATE DIPOTASSIUM:

Symptomatic relief of anxiety – 30 mg/day in divided doses. Adjust gradually within the range of 15 to 60 mg/day.

Elderly or debilitated patients: Initiate treatment at a dose of 7.5 to 15 mg/day.

Maintenance therapy: Give the 22.5 mg tablet in a single daily dose as an alternate dosage form for patients stabilized on 7.5 mg 3 times/day. Do not use to initiate therapy. The 11.25 mg tablet may be administered as a single dose every 24 hours.

Symptomatic relief of acute alcohol withdrawal –

Day 1: 30 mg initially, followed by 30 to 60 mg in divided doses.

Day 2: 45 to 90 mg in divided doses.

Day 3: 22.5 to 45 mg in divided doses.

Day 4: 15 to 30 mg in divided doses.

Thereafter, gradually reduce the dose to 7.5 to 15 mg once/day. Discontinue drug as soon as patient's condition is stable.

The maximum recommended total daily dose is 90 mg. Avoid excessive reductions in the total amount of drug administered on successive days.

Actions

Pharmacology: Benzodiazepines appear to potentiate the effects of gamma-aminobutyrate (GABA) (ie, they facilitate inhibitory GABA neurotransmission) and other inhibitory transmitters by binding to specific benzodiazepine receptor sites.

Pharmacokinetics:

Benzodiazepine Pharmacokinetics						
Drug	Dosage range (mg/day)[1]	Peak plasma level (hrs)[1]	Elimination t½ (hr)	Metabolites	Speed of onset[1]	Protein binding
Alprazolam	0.75-4	1-2	6.3-26.9	Alpha-hydroxy-alprazolam; Benzophenone	inter-mediate	80%
Chlordiazepoxide	15-100	0.5-4	5-30	Desmethyl chlordiazepoxide;[2] Demoxepam; Desmethyldiazepam	inter-mediate	96%
Clonazepam	1.5-20	1-2	18-50	Inactive 7–amino or 7-acetylamino derivatives[2]	inter-mediate	97%
Clorazepate	15-60	1-2	40-50	Desmethyldiazepam	fast	97%-98%
Diazepam	4-40	0.5-2	20-80	Desmethyldiazepam;[2] nordiazepam	very fast	98%
Halazepam	60-160	1-3	14	Desmethyldiazepam;[2] 3-hydroxyhalazepam	slow	97%
Lorazepam	2-4	2-4	10-20	Inactive glucuronide conjugate	inter-mediate	85%
Oxazepam	30-120	2-4	5-20	Inactive glucuronide conjugate	slow	87%

[1] Oral administration.
[2] Major metabolite.
[3] Nordiazepam (active metabolite).

Contraindications

Hypersensitivity to benzodiazepines; psychoses; acute narrow-angle glaucoma; patients with clinical or biochemical evidence of significant liver disease (clonazepam); intra-arterial use (lorazepam injection); children < 6 months of age, lactation (diazepam); coadministration with ketoconazole and itraconazole caused by inhibition of cytochrome P450 3A.

Warnings

Psychiatric disorders: These agents are not intended for use in patients with a primary depressive disorder or psychosis, nor in those psychiatric disorders in which anxiety is not a prominent feature.

Renal function impairment: Observe usual precautions in the presence of impaired renal or hepatic function to avoid accumulation of these agents.

Elderly: The initial dose should be small and dosage increments made gradually, in accordance with the response of the patient, to preclude ataxia or excessive sedation.

Pregnancy: Category D.

Lactation: Benzodiazepines are excreted in breast milk (**lorazepam** not known). Chronic **diazepam** use in nursing mothers reportedly caused infants to become lethargic and to lose weight; do not give to nursing mothers.

Children:
   Chlordiazepoxide – Chlordiazepoxide is not recommended in children < 6 years of age (oral) or 12 years of age (injectable).
   Halazepam, prazepam, alprazolam – Safety and efficacy for use in patients < 18 years of age have not been established.
   Lorazepam – Do not use in patients < 18 years of age (injection); safety and efficacy for use in patients < 12 years old are not established (oral).
   Clorazepate – Not recommended for use in patients < 9 years of age.
   Diazepam – Not for use in children < 6 months of age (oral); safety and efficacy have not been established in the neonate (≤ 30 days of age; injectable).

Precautions

Monitoring: Because of isolated reports of neutropenia and jaundice, perform periodic blood counts, and liver function tests during long-term therapy.

Suicide: In those patients in whom depression accompanies anxiety, suicidal tendencies may be present, and protective measures may be required.

Paradoxical reactions: Excitement, stimulation, and acute rage have occurred in psychiatric patients and hyperactive aggressive children. These reactions may be secondary to relief of anxiety and usually appear in the first 2 weeks of therapy.

Multiple seizure type: When used in patients in whom several different types of seizure disorders coexist, **clonazepam** may increase the incidence or precipitate the onset of generalized tonic-clonic (grand mal) seizures.

Chronic respiratory disease: **Clonazepam** may produce an increase in salivation. Use with caution in patients if increased salivation causes respiratory difficulty.

Drug abuse and dependence: Prolonged use of therapeutic doses can lead to dependence. Withdrawal syndrome has occurred after as little as 4 to 6 weeks of treatment. It is more likely if the drug was short-acting (eg, alprazolam), if it was taken regularly for > 3 months and if it was abruptly discontinued. Higher dosages may not be a factor affecting withdrawal.
   Parenteral administration – Parenteral (IM or IV) therapy is indicated primarily in acute states. Keep patients under observation, preferably in bed, for up to 3 hours.

Hazardous tasks: May produce drowsiness or dizziness; observe caution while driving or performing other tasks requiring alertness.

Drug Interactions

Drugs that may affect benzodiazepines include cimetidine, oral contraceptives, disulfiram, fluoxetine, isoniazid, ketoconazole, metoprolol, propoxyphene, propranolol, valproic acid, alcohol, barbiturates, narcotics, antacids, probenecid, ranitidine, rifampin, scopolamine, and theophyllines.

Drugs that may be affected by benzodiazepines include digoxin, levodopa, neuromuscular blocking agents, and phenytoin.

Adverse Reactions

Cardiovascular: Bradycardia; tachycardia; cardiovascular collapse; hypertension; hypotension; palpitations; edema.

CNS: Sedation and sleepiness; depression; lethargy; apathy; fatigue; hypoactivity; light-headedness; memory impairment; disorientation; anterograde amnesia; restlessness; confusion; crying; sobbing; delirium; headache; slurred speech; stupor; seizures; coma; syncope; rigidity; tremor; vertigo; dizziness; euphoria; nervousness; irritability; difficulty in concentration; agitation; inability to perform complex mental functions; unsteadiness; ataxia; incoordination; weakness; vivid dreams.

Dermatologic: Urticaria; pruritus; skin rash; dermatitis; hair loss; hirsutism; ankle and facial edema.

GI: Constipation; diarrhea; dry mouth; sore gums; nausea; anorexia; change in appetite; vomiting; difficulty in swallowing; increased salivation; gastritis.

GU: Incontinence; changes in libido; urinary retention; menstrual irregularities.

Ophthalmic: Visual disturbances; diplopia; nystagmus.

Psychiatric: Behavior problems; hysteria; psychosis; suicidal tendencies.

Respiratory: Respiratory disturbances; nasal congestion.

Miscellaneous: Depressed hearing; auditory disturbances; hiccoughs; fever; diaphoresis; paresthesias; muscular disturbance; gynecomastia; galactorrhea; leukopenia; blood dyscrasias including agranulocytosis; anemia; thrombocytopenia; eosinophilia; increase or decrease in body weight; dehydration; joint pain.

BUSPIRONE HCl

Tablets: 5 and 10 mg (*Rx*)	*BuSpar* (Mead Johnson Pharm)

Indications

Management of anxiety disorders or short-term relief of symptoms of anxiety.

Administration and Dosage

Initial dose: 15 mg/day (5 mg 3 times a day).

To achieve an optimal therapeutic response, increase the dosage 5 mg/day, at intervals of 2 to 3 days, as needed. Do not exceed 60 mg/day. Divided doses of 20 to 30 mg/day have been commonly used.

Actions

Pharmacology: Mechanism of action is unknown. It differs from benzodiazepines in that it does not exert anticonvulsant or muscle relaxant effects. It also lacks prominent sedative effects associated with more typical anxiolytics. Buspirone has effects on serotonin, dopamine, and norephinephrine.

Pharmacokinetics: Buspirone is rapidly absorbed and undergoes extensive first-pass metabolism. Approximately 95% of buspirone is plasma protein bound. In a single dose study, 29% to 63% of the dose was excreted in the urine within 24 hours.

Contraindications

Hypersensitivity to buspirone HCl.

Warnings

Renal/Hepatic function impairment: Because buspirone is metabolized by the liver and excreted by the kidneys, do not use in patients with severe hepatic or renal impairment.

Elderly: No unusual adverse age-related phenomena have been identified.

Pregnancy: Category B.

Lactation: The extent of the excretion in breast milk of buspirone or its metabolites is not known.

Children: Safety and efficacy for use in children < 18 years of age are not known.

Precautions

Interference with cognitive and motor performance: Buspirone is less sedating than other anxiolytics and does not produce significant functional impairment. However, its CNS effect may not be predictable. Therefore, caution patients about driving or using complex machinery until they are certain that buspirone does not affect them adversely.

Withdrawal reactions: Withdraw patients from their prior treatment gradually before starting buspirone, especially patients who have been using a CNS depressant chronically.

Dopamine receptor binding: Buspirone can bind to central dopamine receptors.

Monitoring: Patients have been treated for several months without ill effect. If used for extended periods, periodically reassess the usefulness of the drug.

Drug Interactions
Drugs that may interact with buspirone include alcohol, haloperidol, monoamine oxidase inhibitors, and trazodone.

Drug/Food interactions: Administration with food may decrease the rate of absorption, but it may increase the bioavailability by decreasing the first-pass metabolism.

Adverse Reactions
Adverse reactions occurring in ≥ 3% of patients include dizziness, drowsiness, nervousness, insomnia, lightheadedness, nausea, dry mouth, headache, and fatigue.

HYDROXYZINE

Tablets: 10, 25, 50, and 100 mg (as HCl) (*Rx*)	Various, *Atarax* (Roerig)
Syrup: 10 mg/5 mL (as HCl) (*Rx*)	Various, *Atarax* (Roerig)
Capsules: 25, 50, and 100 mg (as pamoate equivalent to HCl) (*Rx*)	Various, *Vistaril* (Pfizer)
Oral suspension: 25 mg/5 mL (as pamoate equiv. to HCl) (*Rx*)	*Vistaril* (Pfizer)
Injection: 25 and 50 mg/mL (as HCl) (*Rx*)	Various, *Vistaril* (Pfizer), *Hyzine-50* (Hyrex), *Quiess* (Forest)

Indications
Symptomatic relief of anxiety and tension associated with psychoneurosis and as an adjunct in organic disease states in which anxiety is manifest.

Management of pruritus caused by allergic conditions such as chronic urticaria, atopic and contact dermatoses and in histamine-mediated pruritus.

As a sedative when used as premedication and following general anesthesia.

IM only: For the acutely disturbed or hysterical patient; the acute or chronic alcoholic with anxiety withdrawal symptoms or delirium tremens; allay anxiety; adjunctive therapy in asthma.

Antiemetic (parenteral only) – In controlling nausea and vomiting (excluding nausea and vomiting of pregnancy). As pre- and postoperative and pre- and postpartum adjunctive medication to control emesis.

Analgesia, adjunctive therapy (parenteral only) – As pre- and postoperative and pre- and postpartum adjunctive medication to permit reduction in narcotic dosage.

Administration and Dosage
Parenteral: Hydroxyzine is for deep IM administration only and may be given without further dilution. Avoid IV, SC, or intra-arterial administration (see Warnings). Inject well within the body of a relatively large muscle. In adults, the preferred site is the upper outer quadrant of the buttock or the midlateral thigh. In children, inject into the midlateral muscles of the thigh. In infants and small children, use the periphery of the upper outer quadrant of the gluteal region only when necessary, such as in burn patients, in order to minimize the possibility of sciatic nerve damage.

Use the deltoid area only if well developed, and then only with caution to avoid radial nerve injury. Do not inject into the lower and mid-third of the upper arm.

Start patients on IM therapy when indicated. Maintain on oral therapy whenever practicable. Adjust dosage according to patient's response.

Anxiety –
  Adults: 50 to 100 mg 4 times a day.

Pruritus –
  Adults: 25 mg 3 or 4 times a day.

Sedative (as premedication and following general anesthesia) –
  Adults: 50 to 100 mg.
  Children: 0.6 mg/kg.

Antiemetic/Analgesia, adjunctive therapy (parenteral only) –
  Adults: 25 to 100 mg IM as pre- and postoperative/pre- and postpartum adjunctive medication to permit reduction of narcotic dosage. Reduce dosage of concomitant CNS depressants by 50%.

  Children: 1.1 mg/kg (0.5 mg/lb) IM to control emesis or as pre- and postoperative adjunctive medication to permit reduction of narcotic dosage. Reduce dosage of concomitant CNS depressants by 50%.

Oral:

  Anxiety – The efficacy of hydroxyzine as an antianxiety agent for long-term use (> 4 months) has not been assessed; periodically reevaluate its usefulness.
    Adults: 50 to 100 mg 4 times a day.
    Children (> 6 years of age): 50 to 100 mg/day in divided doses.
    Children (< 6 years of age): 50 mg/day in divided doses.

  Pruritus –
    Adults: 25 mg 3 or 4 times/day.
    Children (> 6 years of age): 50 to 100 mg/day in divided doses.
    Children (< 6 years of age): 50 mg/day in divided doses.

  Sedative (as premedication and following general anesthesia) –
    Adults: 50 to 100 mg.
    Children: 0.6 mg/kg.

Actions

Pharmacology: Hydroxyzine is not a cortical depressant; its action may be caused by suppressing activity in subcortical areas of CNS.

  Bronchodilator activity, antihistaminic, and analgesic effects have been confirmed. Hydroxyzine has antispasmodic properties, and an antiemetic effect has been demonstrated.

Pharmacokinetics: Oral hydroxyzine is rapidly absorbed from the GI tract; clinical effects are usually noted within 15 to 30 minutes after administration. Mean elimination half-life is 3 hours; half-life may be longer in elderly patients. Hydroxyzine is mainly metabolized by the liver.

Contraindications

Hypersensitivity to hydroxyzine; early pregnancy, lactation.

Hydroxyzine injection is for IM use only. Do not inject SC, IV or intra-arterially.

Warnings

Administration: For deep IM administration only; avoid SC, IV or intra-arterial injection. Tissue necrosis has been associated with SC or intra-arterial injection; hemolysis has occurred following IV administration. .

Hypersensitivity reactions: Hypersensitivity reactions have occurred.

Pregnancy: Do not use in pregnancy.

Lactation: It is not known whether this drug is excreted in breast milk.

Precautions

ECG changes: ECG abnormalities, particularly alterations in T-waves.

Porphyria: May exacerbate porphyria and is considered unsafe in porphyric patients.

Hazardous tasks: May produce drowsiness.

Drug Interactions

Drugs that may interact with hydroxyzine include CNS depressants.

Adverse Reactions

Adverse reactions may include dry mouth; drowsiness; involuntary motor activity, including rare instances of tremor and convulsions; hypersensitivity reactions, including wheezing, dyspnea, and chest tightness.

DOXEPIN HCl

Doxepin is a tricyclic antidepressant which also has antianxiety effects. The following is an abbreviated monograph for doxepin. For complete information, refer to the Tricyclic Antidepressants monograph.

Indications

For the treatment of psychoneurotic patients with depression or anxiety; depression or anxiety associated with alcoholism or organic disease; psychotic depressive disorders with associated anxiety including involutional depression and manic-depressive disorders.

The target symptoms of psychoneurosis that respond to doxepin include anxiety, tension, depression, somatic symptoms and concerns, insomnia, guilt, lack of energy, fear, apprehension, and worry.

Administration and Dosage

The total daily dosage may be given on a divided or once-a-day dosage schedule. If the once-a-day schedule is employed, the maximum recommended dose is 150 mg/day, given at bedtime.

Not recommended in children < 12 years of age.

Mild to moderate severity: Start with 75 mg/day. The optimum dose range is 75 to 150 mg/day.

More severely ill: Gradual increase to 300 mg/day may be necessary. Additional therapeutic effect is rarely obtained by exceeding a dose of 300 mg/day.

Very mild symptoms or emotional symptoms accompanying organic disease: Some of these patients have been controlled on doses as low as 25 to 50 mg/day.

Dilution the oral concentrate: Dilute the oral concentrate with 120 mL of liquid (eg, water, milk and orange, grapefruit, tomato, prune, or pineapple juices) just prior to administration; not compatible with a number of carbonated beverages. For patients on methadone maintenance taking oral doxepin, mix the concentrate with methadone and lemonade, orange juice, water, and sugar water. *Do not mix with grape juice.* Preparation and storage of bulk dilutions are not recommended.

ANTIDEPRESSANTS

Antidepressant Pharmacologic and Pharmacokinetic Parameters								
	Major side effects			Amine uptake blocking activity					
0 - none + - slight ++ - moderate +++ - high ++++ - very high +++++ - highest	Anticholinergic	Sedation	Orthostatic hypotension	Norepinephrine	Serotonin	Half-life (hours)	Therapeutic plasma level (ng/mL)	Time to reach steady state (days)	Dose range (mg/day)
Tricyclics - Tertiary Amines									
Amitriptyline	++++	++++	++	++	++++	31-46	110-250[1]	4-10	50-300
Clomipramine	+++	+++	++	++	+++++	19-37	80-100	7-14	25-250
Doxepin	++	+++	++	+	++	8-24	100-200[1]	2-8	25-300
Imipramine	++	++	+++	++[2]	++++	11-25	200-350[1]	2-5	30-300
Trimipramine	++	+++	++	+	+	7-30	180[1]	2-6	50-300
Tricyclics - Secondary Amines									
Amoxapine[3]	+++	++	+	+++	++	8[4]	200-500	2-7	50-600
Desipramine	+	+	+	++++	++	12-24	125-300	2-11	25-300
Nortriptyline	++	++	+	++	+++	18-44	50-150	4-19	30-100
Protriptyline	+++	+	+	++++	++	67-89	100-200	14-19	15-60
Phenethylamine									
Venlafaxine	0	0	0	+++	+++	5-11 [1]	-	3-4	75-375
Tetracyclic									
Maprotiline	++	++	+	+++	0/+	21-25	200-300[1]	6-10	50-225
Mirtazapine	++	+++	++	+++	+++	20-40	-	5	15-45
Triazolopyridine									
Trazodone	+	++++	++	0	+++	4-9	800-1600	3-7	150-600
Aminoketone									
Bupropion[5]	++	++	+	0/+	0/+	8-24	-	1.5-8	200-450
Selective Serotonin Reuptake Inhibitors									
Citalopram	0/+	0/+	0/+	0/+	++++	33	-	7	20-60
Fluoxetine	0/+	0/+	0/+	0/+	+++++	1-16 days[1]	-	2-4 weeks	20-80
Fluvoxamine	0/+	0/+	0	0/+	+++++	15.6	-	≈ 7	50-300
Paroxetine	0	0/+	0	0/+	+++++	10-24	-	7-14	10-50
Sertraline	0	0/+	0	0/+	+++++	1-4 days[1]	-	7	50-200
Monoamine Oxidase Inhibitors									
Tranylcypromine	+	+	0	-	-	2.4-2.8	-	-	30-60
Phenelzine	+	+	+	-	-	-	-	-	45-90
Miscellaneous									
Nefazodone	0/+	++	+	0/+	+++++	2-4	-	4-5	200-600

[1] Parent compound plus active metabolite.
[2] Via desipramine, the major metabolite.
[3] Also blocks dopamine receptors.
[4] 30 hours for major metabolite 8-hydroxyamoxapine.
[5] Inhibits dopamine uptake.

TRICYCLIC COMPOUNDS

AMITRIPTYLINE	
Tablets: 10, 25, 50, 75, 100, and 150 mg (*Rx*)	Various, *Elavil* (Zeneca)
Injection: 10 mg/mL (*Rx*)	*Elavil* (Zeneca)
NORTRIPTYLINE HCl	
Capsules: 10, 25, 50, and 75 mg (*Rx*)	Various, *Aventyl HCl Pulvules* (Eli Lilly), *Pamelor* (Novartis)
Solution: 10 mg (as base)/5 mL (*Rx*)	*Aventyl HCl* (Eli Lilly), *Pamelor* (Novartis)
IMIPRAMINE HCl	
Tablets: 10, 25, and 50 mg (*Rx*)	Various, *Tofranil* (Novartis)
IMIPRAMINE PAMOATE	
Capsules: 75, 100, 125, and 150 mg (as imipramine HCl equivalent) (*Rx*)	*Tofranil-PM* (Novartis)
DOXEPIN HCl	
Capsules: 10, 25, 50, 75, 100, and 150 mg (*Rx*)	Various, *Sinequan* (Roerig)
Oral concentrate: 10 mg/mL (*Rx*)	Various, *Sinequan* (Roerig)
TRIMIPRAMINE MALEATE	
Capsules: 25, 50, and 100 mg (*Rx*)	*Surmontil* (Wyeth)
AMOXAPINE	
Tablets: 25, 50, 100, and 150 mg (*Rx*)	Various, *Asendin* (Lederle)
DESIPRAMINE HCl	
Tablets: 10, 25, 50, 75, 100, and 150 mg (*Rx*)	Various, *Norpramin* (Aventis)
PROTRIPTYLINE HCl	
Tablets: 5 and 10 mg (*Rx*)	Various, *Vivactil* (Merck)
CLOMIPRAMINE HCl	
Capsules: 25, 50, and 75 mg (*Rx*)	Various, *Anafranil* (Novartis)

Indications

Relief of symptoms of depression (except clomipramine). The activating properties of **protriptyline** make it particularly suitable for withdrawn and anergic patients.

Agents with significant sedative action may be useful in depression associated with anxiety and sleep disturbances. The activating properties of **protriptyline** make it particularly suitable for withdrawn and anergic patients.

Amoxapine: Relief of depressive symptoms in patients with neurotic or reactive depressive disorders and endogenous and psychotic depression; depression accompanied by anxiety or agitation.

Doxepin: Treatment of psychoneurotic patients with depression or anxiety; depression or anxiety associated with alcoholism (not to be taken concomitantly with alcohol); depression or anxiety associated with organic disease (the possibility of drug interaction should be considered if the patient is receiving other drugs concomitantly); psychotic depressive disorders with associated anxiety including involutional depression and manic-depressive disorders. The target symptoms of psychoneurosis that respond particularly well to doxepin include anxiety, tension, depression, somatic symptoms and concerns, sleep disturbances, guilt, lack of energy, fear, apprehension, and worry.

Imipramine: Treatment of enuresis in children ≥ 6 years of age as temporary adjunctive therapy.

Clomipramine: Only for treatment of Obsessive-Compulsive Disorder (OCD).

Administration and Dosage

Plasma levels: Determination of plasma levels may be useful in identifying patients who appear to have toxic effects and may have excessively high levels, or those in whom lack of absorption or noncompliance is suspected. Make adjustments in dosage according to patient's clinical response and not based on plasma levels.

Adolescent, elderly, and outpatients: Initiate therapy at a low dosage and increase gradually. Most antidepressant drugs have a lag period of 10 days to 4 weeks before a therapeutic reponse is noted. Increasing the dose will not shorten this period but rather increase the incidence of adverse reactions. Following remission, maintenance medication may be required for a longer time at the lowest dose that will maintain remission. Continue maintenance therapy ≥ 3 months to decrease the possibility of relapse.

AMITRIPTYLINE HCl:

Outpatients – 75 mg/day in divided doses. May increase to 150 mg/day. Alternatively, initiate therapy with 50 to 100 mg at bedtime. Increase by 25 to 50 mg as necessary, to a total of 150 mg/day.

Hospitalized patients: Hospitalized patients may require 100 mg/day initially. Gradually increase to 200 to 300 mg, if necessary.

Adolescent and elderly patients – 10 mg 3 times a day with 20 mg at bedtime may be satisfactory in adolescent and elderly patients who cannot tolerate higher doses.

Maintenance – 40 to 100 mg/day. Total daily dosage may be given in a single dose, preferably at bedtime.

IM – Do not administer IV. Initially, 20 to 30 mg IM, 4 times a day. The effects may be more rapid with IM than with oral administration.

Children – Not recommended for children < 12 years of age.

AMOXAPINE: Amoxapine is not recommended for patients < 16 years of age.

Usual effective dose range is 200 to 300 mg/day. If no response is seen at 300 mg, increase dosage, depending upon tolerance, to 400 mg/day. Hospitalized patients refractory to antidepressant therapy and who have no history of convulsive seizures may have dosage cautiously increased up to 600 mg/day in divided doses.

Adults – Initially, 50 mg 2 or 3 times/day. Depending upon tolerance, increase dosage to 100 mg 2 or 3 times/day by the end of the first week. Increase above 300 mg/day only if 300 mg/day has been ineffective for at least 2 weeks. Once an effective dosage is established, the drug may be given in a single bedtime dose (not to exceed 300 mg). If the total daily dosage exceeds 300 mg, give in divided doses.

Elderly patients – Initially, 25 mg 2 or 3 times a day. If tolerated, dosage may be increased by the end of the first week to 50 mg 2 or 3 times a day. Although 100 to 150 mg/day may be adequate for many elderly patients, some may require higher dosage; carefully increase up to 300 mg/day. Once an effective dosage is established, give amoxapine in a single bedtime dose, not to exceed 300 mg.

CLOMIPRAMINE HCl: Administer in divided doses with meals to reduce GI side effects. After titration, the total daily dose may be given once/day at bedtime to minimize daytime sedation.

Adults – Initiate at 25 mg/day and gradually increase, as tolerated, to approximately 100 mg during the first 2 weeks. Thereafter, the dosage may be increased gradually over the next several weeks to a maximum of 250 mg/day.

Children and adolescents – Initiate at 25 mg/day and gradually increase during the first 2 weeks, as tolerated, to a daily maximum of 3 mg/kg or 100 mg, whichever is smaller. Thereafter, the dosage may be increased to a daily maximum of 3 mg/kg or 200 mg, whichever is smaller.

DESIPRAMINE HCl: Not recommended for use in children < 12 years of age.

Adults – 100 to 200 mg/day. Initial therapy may be given in divided doses or as a single daily dose. In more severely ill patients, gradually increase to 300 mg/day, if necessary. Do not exceed 300 mg/day.

Elderly and adolescents – 25 to 100 mg/day. Dosages > 150 mg not recommended.

DOXEPIN HCl: Not recommended for use in children < 12 years of age.

Mild to moderate anxiety or depression – Initially, 75 mg/day. Usual optimum dosage is 75 to 150 mg/day. Alternatively, the total daily dosage, up to 150 mg, may be given at bedtime.

Mild symptomatology or emotional symptoms accompanying organic disease – 25 to 50 mg/day as often as effective.

More severe anxiety or depression – Higher doses (eg, 50 mg 3 times/day) may be required; if necessary, gradually increase to 300 mg/day.

Oral concentrate – Dilute oral concentrate with ≈ 120 mL of water, milk or fruit juice prior to administration. Do not mix with carbonated beverages.

IMIPRAMINE HCl:

    Depression –

     · *Hospitalized patients:* Initially, 100 orally in divided doses; gradually increase to 200 mg/day, as required. If no response occurs after 2 weeks, increase to 250 to 300 mg/day. Administer the total daily dosage once/day at bedtime.

    Outpatients: Initially, 75 mg/day, increased to 150 mg/day. Do not exceed 200 mg/day. Give once/day, preferably at bedtime.

    Maintenance – 50 to 150 mg/day or lowest dose that will maintain remission.

    Adolescent and elderly patients: Initially, 30 to 40 mg/day orally; it is generally not necessary to exceed 100 mg/day.

    Childhood enuresis (≥ 6 years of age) – Initially, 25 mg/day 1 hour before bedtime. If no satisfactory response in 1 week, increase up to 50 mg/night if < 12; up to 75 mg/night if > 12. A dose > 75 mg/day does not enhance efficacy and increases side effects. Do not exceed 2.5 mg/kg/day. In early night bedwetters, it may be more effective given earlier and in divided amounts (25 mg midafternoon and bedtime).

IMIPRAMINE PAMOATE:

    Hospitalized patients – Initiate therapy at 100 to 150 mg/day; may be increased to 200 mg/day. If there is no response after 2 weeks, increase dosage to 250 to 300 mg/day.

    Outpatients – Initiate therapy at 75 mg/day. If necessary, dosage may be increased to 200 mg/day.

    Adult maintenance dosage – The usual maintenance dose is 75 to 150 mg/day.

    Adolescent and geriatic patients – Initiate therapy in these age groups with imipramine HCl at a total daily dosage of 25 to 50 mg because imipramine pamoate does not come in these strengths. Dosage may be increased according to response and tolerance, but it is generally unnecessary to exceed 100 mg/day in these patients. Imipramine pamoate capsules may be used when total daily dosage is established at ≥ 75 mg.

NORTRIPTYLINE:

    Adults – 25 mg 3 or 4 times/day; begin at a low level and increase as required. Total daily dose can be given at bedtime. Doses above 150 mg/day are not recommended.

    Elderly and adolescent patients – 30 to 50 mg/day in divided doses or once/day. Not recommended for use in children.

PROTRIPTYLINE HCl: Not recommended for use in children.

    Adults – 15 to 40 mg/day divided into 3 or 4 doses. May increase to 60 mg/day. Dosages above 60 mg/day are not recommended. Make any increases in the morning dose.

    Adolescent and elderly patients – Initially, 5 mg 3 times/day; increase gradually, if necessary. In elderly patients, monitor the cardiovascular system closely if dose exceeds 20 mg/day.

TRIMIPRAMINE MALEATE: Not recommended for use in children.

    Adult outpatients – Initially, 75 mg/day in divided doses; increase to 150 mg/day. Do not exceed 200 mg/day. The total dosage requirement may be given at bedtime.

    Adult hospitalized patients – Initially, 100 mg/day in divided doses, increased gradually in a few days to 200 mg/day depending upon individual response and tolerance. If improvement does not occur in 2 to 3 weeks, increase to a maximum dose of 250 to 300 mg/day.

    Adolescent and elderly patients – Initially, 50 mg/day, with gradual increments up to 100 mg/day.

    Maintenance – Maintenance medication may be required at the lowest dose that will maintain remission (range 50 to 150 mg/day). Administer as a single bedtime dose.

Actions

Pharmacology: The tricyclic antidepressants (TCAs), structurally related to the pheno-thiazine antipsychotic agents, possess 3 major pharmacologic actions in varying degrees: Blocking of the amine pump, sedation, and peripheral and central anticho-linergic action. In contrast to phenothiazines, which act on dopamine receptors, TCAs inhibit reuptake of norepinephrine or serotonin (5-hydroxytryptamine, 5-HT) at the presynaptic neuron. Amoxapine, a metabolite of loxapine, retains some of the postsynaptic dopamine receptor-blocking action of neuroleptics.

Other pharmacological effects – Clinical effects, in addition to antidepressant effects, include sedation, anticholinergic effects, mild peripheral vasodilator effects and pos-sible "quinidine-like" actions.

Pharmacokinetics:

Absorption/Distribution – The TCAs are well absorbed from the GI tract with peak plasma concentrations occurring in 2 to 4 hours; they undergo a significant first-pass effect. They are highly bound (> 90%) to plasma proteins, are lipid soluble and are widely distributed in tissues, including the CNS.

Metabolism/Excretion – Metabolism of TCAs occurs in the liver by demethylation, hydroxylation and glucuronidation, and it varies for each patient. Some intermedi-ate active metabolites include:

Amitriptyline ➡ nortriptyline
Amoxapine ➡ 7 hydroxy and 8 hydroxyamoxapine
Clomipramine ➡ desmethylclomipramine
Doxepin ➡ desmethyldoxepin
Imipramine ➡ desipramine

Because of the long half-life, a single daily dose may be given. Up to 2 to 4 weeks may be required to achieve maximal clinical response.

Contraindications

Prior sensitivity to any tricyclic drug. Not recommended for use during the acute recovery phase following myocardial infarction. Concomitant use of monoamine oxidase inhibitors (MAOIs) is generally contraindicated.

Doxepin: Patients with glaucoma or a tendency for urinary retention.

Cross-sensitivity may occur among the dibenzazepines (**clomipramine, desipramine, imipramine, nortriptyline,** and **trimipramine**). In addition, dibenzoxepines (**doxe-pin, amoxapine**) may produce cross-sensitivity.

Warnings

Tardive dyskinesia: Tardive dyskinesia, a syndrome consisting of potentially irreversible, involuntary, dyskinetic movements may develop in patients treated with neurolep-tics (eg, antipsychotics). Amoxapine is not an antipsychotic, but it has substan-tive neuroleptic activity.

Neuroleptic malignant syndrome (NMS): NMS is a potentially fatal condition reported in association with antipsychotic drugs and with **amoxapine**.

Hyperthermia has occurred with **clomipramine**; most cases occurred when it was used with other drugs (eg, neuroleptics) and may be examples of an NMS.

Seizure disorders: Because TCAs lower the seizure threshold, use with caution in patients with a history of seizures or other predisposing factors (eg, brain damage of vary-ing etiology, alcoholism, concomitant drugs known to lower the seizure threshold). However, seizures have occurred both in patients with and without a history of sei-zure disorders. Seizure was identified as the most significant risk of **clomipramine** use.

Anticholinergic effects: Use with caution in patients with a history of urinary retention, urethral or ureteral spasm; narrow-angle glaucoma, angle-closure glaucoma, or increased intraocular pressure.

Cardiovascular disorders: Use with extreme caution in patients with cardiovascular disor-ders because of the possibility of conduction defects, arrhythmias, CHF, sinus tachy-cardia, MI, strokes, and tachycardia. These patients require cardiac surveillance at all dose levels of the drug. In high doses, TCAs may produce arrhythmias, sinus tachycardia, conduction defects, and prolonged conduction time. Tachycardia and postural hypotension may occur more frequently with **protriptyline**.

Hyperthyroid patients: Hyperthyroid patients or those receiving thyroid medication require close supervision because of the possibility of cardiovascular toxicity, including arrhythmias.

Psychiatric patients: Schizophrenic or paranoid patients may exhibit a worsening of psychosis with TCA therapy, and manic-depressive patients may experience a shift to a hypomanic or manic phase; this may also occur when switching antidepressants and withdrawing them. In overactive or agitated patients, increased anxiety or agitation may occur. Paranoid delusions, with or without associated hostility, may be exaggerated. Reduction of TCA dosage and concomitant antipsychotic therapy may be necessary.

The possibility of suicide in depressed patients remains during treatment and until significant remission occurs. Patients should not have easy access to large quantities of the drug; prescribe small quantities of TCAs.

Mania/Hypomania: Hypomanic or manic episodes may occur, particularly in patients with cyclic disorders. Such reactions may necessitate discontinuation of the drug.

MAOIs: Do not give MAOIs with or immediately following TCAs. Allow at least 14 days to elapse between MAOI discontinuation and TCA institution. Some TCAs have been used safely and successfully with MAOIs. Initiate TCA cautiously with gradual dosage increase until achieving optimum response.

Rash: Antidepressant drugs can cause skin rashes or "drug fever" in susceptible individuals. They are more likely to occur during the first few days of treatment but may also occur later. Discontinue if rash or fever develop.

Renal/Hepatic function impairment: Use with caution and in reduced doses in patients with hepatic impairment; metabolism may be impaired, leading to drug accumulation. Use with caution in patients with significantly impaired renal function.

Elderly: Be cautious in dose selection for an elderly patient, usually starting at the low end of the dosing range. Elderly patients may be sensitive to the anticholinergic side effects of TCAs.

Elderly patients taking **amitriptyline** may be at increased risk for falls; start on low doses of amitriptyline and observe closely.

Pregnancy: (*Category D* - amitriptyline, imipramine, nortriptyline; *Category C* - amoxapine, clomipramine, desipramine, doxepin, protriptyline, trimipramine).

Lactation: These agents are excreted into breast milk in low concentrations.

Children: Not recommended for patients < 12 years of age. Safety and efficacy are not established for **amoxapine** in children < 16 years of age or **trazodone** or **clomipramine** in children < 10 years of age. The safety and efficacy of **imipramine** as temporary adjunctive therapy for nocturnal enuresis in pediatric patients < 6 years of age have not been established. The safety of the drug for long-term, chronic use as adjunctive therapy for nocturnal enuresis in pediatric patients ≥ 6 years of age has not been established. Safety and efficacy are not established in the pediatric age group for **trimipramine, nortriptyline, protriptyline**, and **desipramine**.

Do not exceed 2.5 mg/kg/day of **imipramine**.

Precautions

Monitoring: Perform baseline and periodic leukocyte and differential counts and liver function studies. Fever or sore throat may signal serious neutrophil depression; discontinue therapy if there is evidence of pathological neutropenia.

Monitor ECG – Monitor ECG prior to initiation of large doses of TCAs and at appropriate intervals thereafter.

Electroconvulsive therapy: Electroconvulsive therapy with coadministration of TCAs may increase the hazards of therapy.

Elective surgery: Discontinue therapy for as long as possible before elective surgery.

Blood sugar levels: Elevated and lowered blood sugar levels have occurred.

Sexual dysfuntion: Sexual dysfuntion was markedly increased in male patients with OCD taking clomipramine (42% ejaculatory failure, 20% impotence) compared to placebo. Sexual dysfunction also occurs with other TCAs.

Weight changes: Weight gain occurred in 18% of patients receiving **clomipramine**. Some patients had weight gain in excess of 25% of their initial body weight. Weight gain also occurs with other TCAs.

Serotonin syndrome: Some TCAs inhibit neuronal reuptake of serotonin and can increase synaptic serotonin levels (eg, **clomipramine, amitriptyline**). Either therapeutic or excessive doses of these drugs, in combination with other drugs that also increase synaptic serotonin levels (such as MAOIs), can cause a serotonin syndrome consisting of tremor, agitation, delirium, rigidity, myoclonus, hyperthermia, and obtundation.

Hazardous tasks: May impair mental or physical abilities required for the performance of potentially hazardous tasks.

Photosensitivity: Photosensitization (photoallergy or phototoxicity) may occur.

Drug Interactions

P450 system: Concomitant use of TCAs with other drugs metabolized by cytochrome P450 2D6 may require lower doses than those usually prescribed for either the TCA or the other drug.

Drugs that may affect tricyclic compounds include barbiturates, carbamazepine, charcoal, cimetidine, haloperidol, histamine H_2-antagonists, MAO inhibitors, rifamycins, SSRIs, smoking, and valproic acid.

Drugs that may be affected by tricyclic compounds include anticholinergics, carbamazepine, clonidine, dicumarol, grepafloxacin, guanethidine, levodopa, quinolones, sparfloxacin, and sympathomimetics.

Adverse Reactions

Sedation and anticholinergic effects are reported most frequently.

Withdrawal symptoms – Although not indicative of addiction, abrupt cessation after prolonged therapy may produce nausea, headache, vertigo, nightmares, and malaise. Gradual dosage reduction may produce, within 2 weeks, transient symptoms including irritability, restlessness, dreams, and sleep disturbance.

Enuretic children – Consider adverse reactions reported with adult use. Most common are nervousness, sleep disorders, tiredness, and mild GI disturbances. These usually disappear with continued therapy or dosage reduction.

Cardiovascular:

General – Arrhythmias; changes in AV conduction; ECG changes (most frequently with toxic doses); flushing; heart block; hot flushes; hypertension; hypotension; orthostatic hypotension; palpitations; precipitation of CHF; premature ventricular contractions; stroke; sudden death; syncope; tachycardia.

Desipramine – Hypertensive episodes during surgery. There have been reports of sudden death in children.

CNS:

General – Agitation; akathisia; alterations in EEG patterns; anxiety; ataxia; coma; confusion (especially in the elderly); disorientation; disturbed concentration; dizziness; drowsiness; dysarthria; exacerbation of psychosis; excitement; excessive appetite; extrapyramidal symptoms including abnormal involuntary movements and tardive dyskinesia; fatigue; hallucinations; delusions; headache; hyperthermia; hypomania; incoordination; insomnia; mania; nervousness; neuroleptic malignant syndrome; nightmares; numbness; panic; paresthesias of extremities; peripheral neuropathy; restlessness; tremors; seizures; tingling; weakness.

GU: Gynecomastia and testicular swelling in the male; breast enlargement, menstrual irregularity and galactorrhea in the female; increased or decreased libido; painful ejaculation; impotence; nocturia; urinary frequency.

GI: Nausea and vomiting; anorexia; epigastric distress; diarrhea; flatulence; dysphagia; increased salivation; stomatitis; glossitis; parotid swelling; abdominal cramps; pancreatitis; black tongue.

Hematologic: Bone marrow depression including agranulocytosis; eosinophilia; purpura; thrombocytopenia; leukopenia.

   Clomipramine – Anemia; leukemoid reaction; lymphadenopathy; lymphoma-like disorder.

Hypersensitivity:
   General – Cross-sensitivity with other TCAs; drug fever; edema (general or of face and tongue); itching; petechiae; photosensitization; pruritus; rash; urticaria; vasculitis.

Respiratory:
   General – Exacerbation of asthma.

Special senses: Tinnitus; abnormal lacrimation.

Miscellaneous:
   General – Alopecia; fever; hyperthermia; hyperpyrexia; local edema; nasal stuffiness; increased perspiration; proneness to falling; weight gain or loss.

   Clomipramine – Abnormal skin odor; arthralgia; back pain; chest pain; chills; dependent edema; general edema; fever; halitosis; increased susceptibility to infection; malaise; muscle weakness; myalgia; pain; thirst; withdrawal syndrome.

TETRACYCLIC COMPOUNDS

MAPROTILINE	
Tablets: 25, 50, and 75 mg (*Rx*)	Various
MIRTAZAPINE	
Tablets: 15, 30, and 45 mg (*Rx*)	*Remeron* (Organon)
Tablets, orally disintegrating: 15, 30, and 45 mg (*Rx*)	*Remeron SolTab* (Organon)

Indications
Depression: Treatment of depression.

Administration and Dosage
MAPROTILINE HCl: May be given as a single daily dose or in divided doses. Therapeutic effects are sometimes seen within 3 to 7 days, although as long as 2 to 3 weeks are usually necessary before improvement is observed.

   Initial adult dosage –
   Mild to moderate depression: An initial dose of 75 mg/day is suggested for outpatients. In some patients, especially the elderly, an initial dose of 25 mg/day may be used. Because of the long half-life of maprotiline, maintain initial dosage for 2 weeks. The dosage may then be increased gradually in 25 mg increments, as required and tolerated. Most patients respond to a dose of 150 mg/day, but doses as high as 225 mg/day may be required.

   Severe depression: Give hospitalized patients an initial daily dose of 100 to 150 mg, which may be gradually increased, as required and tolerated. Most hospitalized patients with moderate to severe depression respond to a daily dosage of 150 mg, although doses as high as 225 mg may be required. Do not exceed 225 mg/day.

   Maintenance – Dosage may be reduced to 75 to 150 mg/day with adjustment depending on therapeutic response.

   Elderly – In general, lower doses are recommended for patients > 60 years of age. Doses of 50 to 75 mg/day are satisfactory as maintenance therapy for elderly patients who do not tolerate higher amounts.

   Maprotiline is not recommended for patients < 18 years of age.

MIRTAZAPINE:
   Initial treatment – The recommended starting dose for mirtazapine is 15 mg/day administered in a single dose, preferably in the evening prior to sleep. Patients not responding to the initial 15 mg dose may benefit from dosage increases up to a maximum of 45 mg/day. Do not change dose at intervals of < 1 or 2 weeks.

Maintenance/Extended treatment – Treatment for acute episodes of depression should continue for ≥ 6 months.

Switching to or from a monoamine oxidase inhibitor (MAOI) – At least 14 days should elapse between discontinuation of an MAOI and initiation of therapy with mirtazapine. In addition, allow at least 14 days after stopping mirtazapine before starting an MAOI.

Elderly and renal/hepatic function impairment – The clearance of mirtazapine is reduced in elderly patients and in patients with moderate to severe renal or hepatic impairment.

Administration of orally disintegrating tablets – Open tablet blister pack with dry hands and place tablet on tongue. The tablet will disintegrate rapidly on the tongue and can be swallowed with saliva. Use the tablet immediately after removal from the blister; it cannot be scored. No water is needed. Do not attempt to split the tablet. Use orally disintegrating tablets immediately upon opening individual tablet blisters.

Actions

Pharmacology: Tetracyclics enhance central noradrenergic and serotonergic activity. They do not inhibit monoamine oxidase. Although maprotiline and mirtazapine are in the same chemical class, they each affect different neurotransmitters and thus have different side effect profiles. Maprotiline primarily acts by blocking reuptake of norepinephrine at nerve endings.

Mirtazapine is a potent antagonist of $5\text{-}HT_2$ and $5\text{-}HT_3$ receptors. It is a potent antagonist of histamine (H_1) receptors and a moderate antagonist at muscarinic receptors.

Pharmacokinetics:

Maprotiline – The mean time to peak is 12 hours. The elimination half-life averages 43 hours. Binding to serum proteins is ≈ 88%. Maprotiline is metabolized in the liver and excreted via the bile.

Mirtazapine – Mirtazapine is rapidly and completely absorbed following oral administration and has a half-life of ≈ 20 to 40 hours, with females of all ages exhibiting significantly longer elimination half-lives than males (37 vs 26 hours). Steady-state plasma levels of mirtazapine are attained within 5 days. Mirtazapine is ≈ 85% bound to plasma protein.

Metabolism/Excretion: Mirtazapine has an absolute bioavailability of ≈ 50%. It is eliminated predominantly via urine (75%) with 15% in feces.

Contraindications

Hypersensitivity to maprotiline or mirtazapine; coadministration with monamine oxidase inhibitors (MAOIs).

Maprotiline: Known or suspected seizure disorders; during acute phase of MI.

Warnings

Anticholinergic properties: Maprotiline should be administered with caution in patients with increased intraocular pressure, history of urinary retention, or history of narrow-angle glaucoma because of the drug's anticholinergic properties.

Monoamine oxidase inhibitors (MAOIs): Do not give tetracyclics with MAOIs. Allow a minimum of 14 days to elapse after discontinuation of MAOIs before starting a tetracyclic.

Seizures: Seizures are rare. The risk of seizures may be increased when tetracyclics are taken concomitantly with phenothiazines, when the dosage of benzodiazepines is rapidly tapered in patients receiving tetracyclics or when the recommended dosage of the tetracyclic is exceeded.

Cardiovascular: Use with caution in patients with a history of MI and angina because of the possibility of conduction defects, arrhythmia, MI, strokes, and tachycardia. Use with caution in patients predisposed to hypotension.

Electroshock therapy: Avoid concurrent administration of maprotiline with electroshock therapy because of the lack of experience in this area.

Agranulocytosis: In clinical trials, two patients treated with mirtazapine developed agranulocytosis and a third patient developed severe neutropenia. All 3 patients recovered after mirtazapine was stopped.

Renal/Hepatic function impairment: Use mirtazapine with caution in patients with impaired renal and hepatic function.

Elderly: Oral clearance was reduced in the elderly compared with the younger subjects. Caution is indicated in administering mirtazapine to elderly patients.

Pregnancy: Category B (maprotiline); Category C (mirtazapine).

Lactation:

> *Maprotiline* – Maprotiline is excreted in breast milk. At steady state, the concentration in milk corresponds closely to the concentrations in whole blood.
>
> *Mirtazapine* – It is not known if mirtazapine is excreted in breast milk.

Children: Safety and efficacy in children (< 18 years of age for **maprotiline**) have not been established.

Precautions

Monitoring: Discontinue **maprotiline** if there is evidence of pathological neutrophil depression. Perform leukocyte and differential counts in patients who develop fever and sore throat during therapy.

Somnolence: Somnolence was reported in 54% of patients treated with mirtazapine.

Dizziness: Dizziness was reported in 7% of patients treated with mirtazapine.

Increased appetite/Weight gain: Appetite increase was reported in 17% of patients treated with mirtazapine. In some trials, weight gain of ≥ 7% of body weight occurred in 7.5% of patients treated.

Cholesterol/Triglycerides: Nonfasting cholesterol increases to ≥ 20% above the upper limits of normal and nonfasting triglyceride increases to ≥ 500 mg/dL were observed.

Mania/Hypomania: Use carefully in patients with a history of mania/hypomania.

Suicidal ideation: Closely supervise high-risk patients during initial drug therapy.

Elective surgery: Prior to elective surgery, discontinue **maprotiline** for as long as possible, because little is known about the interaction between maprotiline and general anesthetics.

Orthostatic hypotension: Orthostatic hypotension was infrequently observed in clinical trials with depressed patients.

Lab test abnormalities: Clinically significant ALT elevations (≥ 3 times the upper limit of the normal range) were observed in 2% of patients exposed to mirtazapine.

Hazardous tasks: Caution patients about engaging in hazardous activities until they are reasonably certain that tetracyclics do not adversely affect their ability to engage in such activities.

Drug Interactions

Drugs that may affect maprotiline include thyroid hormones, benzodiazepines, and phenothiazines. Drugs that may be affected by maprotiline include anticholinergics, guanethidine, and sympathomimetics. Drugs that may be affected by mirtazapine include alcohol and diazepam.

Adverse Reactions

Adverse reactions include asthenia; flu syndrome; dry mouth; constipation; increased appetite; weight gain; abnormal dreams; anxiety; dizziness; drowsiness; headache; nervousness; somnolence; abnormal thinking; tremor; weakness and fatigue; blurred vision.

TRAZODONE HCl

Tablets: 50 and 100 mg (*Rx*)	Various, *Desyrel* (Mead Johnson)
Tablets: 150 and 300 mg (*Rx*)	Various, *Desyrel Dividose* (Mead Johnson)

Indications
Treatment of depression.

Administration and Dosage
Initiate dosage at a low level and increase gradually. Drowsiness may require the administration of a major portion of the daily dose at bedtime or a reduced dosage. Take shortly after a meal or light snack.

Adults: An initial dose is 150 mg/day in divided doses. This may be increased by 50 mg/day every 3 to 4 days. The maximum dose for outpatients usually should not exceed 400 mg/day in divided doses. Inpatients or more severely depressed subjects may be given up to, but not in excess of, 600 mg/day in divided doses.

Maintenance: Keep dosage at the lowest effective level. Once an adequate response has been achieved, dosage may be gradually reduced with subsequent adjustment depending on response.

Actions
Pharmacology: Trazodone is not a monoamine oxidase inhibitor and does not stimulate the CNS. In animals, it selectively inhibits serotonin uptake by brain synaptosomes and potentiates the behavioral changes induced by the serotonin precursor, 5–hydroxytryptophan.

Pharmacokinetics:
   Absorption/Distribution – Trazodone is well absorbed after oral administration. Peak plasma levels occur in ≈ 1 hour when taken on an empty stomach or in 2 hours when taken with food.
   Metabolism/Excretion – Trazodone is extensively metabolized in the liver and is a CYP3A4 substrate. Elimination is biphasic, with a half-life of 3 to 6 hours and 5 to 9 hours, respectively, and is unaffected by food.

Contraindications
Hypersensitivity to trazodone; initial recovery phase of MI.

Warnings
Preexisting cardiac disease: Not recommended for use during the initial recovery phase of MI. Trazodone may be arrhythmogenic in some patients. Arrhythmias identified include isolated PVCs, ventricular couplets, and short episodes (3 to 4 beats) of ventricular tachycardia. Closely monitor patients with preexisting cardiac disease, particularly for cardiac arrhythmias.

Priapism: Patients with prolonged or inappropriate penile erection should discontinue use immediately and consult a physician or go to an emergency room. Priapism of the clitoris has also occurred.

Pregnancy: Category C.

Lactation: The drug may be excreted in breast milk.

Children: Safety and efficacy for use in children < 18 years of age are not established.

Precautions
Suicide: The possibility of suicide in seriously depressed patients is inherent in the illness and may persist until significant remission occurs.

Hypotension: Hypotension, including orthostatic hypotension and syncope, has occurred.

Elective surgery: There is little known about the interaction between trazodone and general anesthetics; therefore, prior to elective surgery, discontinue trazodone for as long as clinically feasible.

Electroconvulsive therapy: Avoid concurrent administration with electroconvulsive therapy because of the absence of experience in this area.

Lab test abnormalities: Discontinue the drug in any patient whose white blood cell count or absolute neutrophil count falls below normal levels. White blood cell and differential counts are recommended for patients who develop fever and sore throat (or other signs of infection) during therapy.

Hazardous tasks: May produce drowsiness, dizziness, or blurred vision.

Drug Interactions
Trazodone may affect CNS depressants (alcohol, barbiturates), digoxin, monoamine oxidase inhibitors, phenytoin, and warfarin. Trazodone may be affected by carbamazepine, phenothiazines, and SSRIs.

Adverse Reactions
Adverse reactions occurring in ≥ 3% of patients include: Hypotension, syncope, tachycardia/palpitations, anger/hostility, confusion, dizziness/lightheadedness, drowsiness, excitement, fatigue, headache, incoordination, insomnia, nervousness, nightmares/vivid dreams, tremors, abdominal/gastric disorder, constipation, diarrhea, dry mouth, nausea/vomiting, blurred vision, allergic skin condition/edema, aches/pains, decreased appetite, nasal/sinus congestion, weight gain/loss.

BUPROPION HCl

Tablets: 75 and 100 mg (*Rx*)	*Wellbutrin* (GlaxoSmithKline)
Tablets, sustained-release: 100 and 150 mg	*Wellbutrin SR* (GlaxoSmithKline)

Indications
Depression: Treatment of depression. Effectiveness of bupropion in long-term use (> 6 weeks) has not been evaluated.

Administration and Dosage
General: It is particularly important to administer bupropion in a manner most likely to minimize the risk of seizure (see Warnings). Do not exceed dose increases of 100 mg/day in a 3-day period. Gradual escalation of dosage also is important to minimize agitation, motor restlessness, and insomnia often seen during the initial days of treatment. If necessary, these effects may be managed by temporary reduction of dose or the short-term administration of an intermediate- to long-acting sedative-hypnotic. A sedative-hypnotic usually is not required beyond the first week of treatment. Insomnia also may be minimized by avoiding bedtime doses. If distressing, untoward effects supervene, stop dose escalation.

Bupropion immediate-release: Do not exceed dose increases of 100 mg/day in a 3-day period. No single dose of bupropion should exceed 150 mg. Administer 3 times/day, preferably with at least 6 hours between successive doses.

Adults – 300 mg/day, given 3 times/day. Begin dosing at 200 mg/day, given as 100 mg twice/day. Based on clinical response, this dose may be increased to 300 mg/day, given as 100 mg 3 times/day no sooner than 3 days after beginning therapy.

Bupropion Dosage Regimen					
			Number of tablets		
Treatment day	Total daily dose	Tablet strength	Morning	Midday	Evening
1	200 mg	100 mg	1	0	1
4	300 mg	100 mg	1	1	1

Increasing the dosage > 300 mg/day – An increase in dosage, up to a maximum of 450 mg/day given in divided doses of not more than 150 mg each may be considered for patients in whom no clinical improvement is noted after several weeks of treatment at 300 mg/day. Dosing above 300 mg/day may be accomplished using the 75 or 100 mg tablets. The 100 mg tablets must be administered 4 times/day with at least 4 hours between successive doses in order not to exceed the limit of 150 mg in a single dose. Discontinue in patients who do not demonstrate an adequate response after an appropriate period of 450 mg/day.

Maintenance – Use the lowest dose that maintains remission. Although it is not known how long the patient should remain on bupropion, acute episodes of depression generally require several months or longer of treatment.

Bupropion sustained-release (SR): The usual adult target dosage is 300 mg/day given as 150 mg twice/day. Begin dosing with 150 mg/day given as a single daily dose in the morning. If the 150 mg initial dose is adequately tolerated, increase to 300 mg/day given as 150 mg twice/day as early as day 4 of dosing. Allow ≥ 8 hours between successive doses.

Increasing the dosage > 300 mg/day – As with other antidepressants, the full antidepressant effect of the SR formula may not be evident until > 4 weeks of treatment. Consider an increase in dosage to the maximum of 400 mg/day given as 200 mg twice/day for patients in whom no clinical improvement is noted after several weeks of 300 mg/day treatment.

Maintenance – The lowest dose that maintains remission is recommended.

Hepatic impairment: Use bupropion with extreme caution in patients with severe hepatic cirrhosis. The dose should not exceed 75 mg once a day (100 mg every day or 150 mg every other day for bupropion SR) in these patients. Use bupropion with caution in patients with hepatic impairment (including mild to moderate hepatic cirrhosis) and consider a reduced frequency or dose in patients with mild to moderate hepatic cirrhosis.

Renal impairment: Use bupropion with caution in patients with renal impairment and consider a reduced frequency or dose.

Actions

Pharmacology: The mechanism of the antidepressant effect of bupropion is not known. Bupropion does not inhibit monoamine oxidase. It is a weak blocker of the neuronal uptake of serotonin and norepinephrine; it also inhibits the neuronal reuptake of dopamine to some extent.

Pharmacokinetics:

Absorption/Distribution – Following oral administration, peak plasma concentrations are usually achieved within 2 hours for buproprion and 3 hours for bupropion SR, followed by a biphasic decline. The half-life of the second (postdistributional) phase of buproprion ranges 8 to 24 hours and mean elimination half-life for bupropion SR is 21 hours.

Contraindications

Hypersensitivity to the drug; seizure disorder; current or prior diagnosis of bulimia or anorexia nervosa (because of a higher incidence of seizures noted in such patients treated with bupropion); concurrent administration of a monoamine oxidase inhibitor (MAOI; at least 14 days should elapse between discontinuation of an MAOI and initiation of treatment with bupropion); contraindicated in patients being treated with other bupropion products (eg, for smoking cessation) because of the incidence of dose-dependent seizures.

Warnings

Seizures: Bupropion is associated with seizures in ≈ 0.4% of patients treated at doses between 300 and 450 mg/day. This incidence of seizures may exceed that of other marketed antidepressants by as much as 4-fold. The estimated seizure incidence increases almost 10-fold between 450 and 600 mg/day. Given the wide variability among individuals and their capacity to metabolize and eliminate drugs, this disproportionate increase in seizure incidence with dose incrementation calls for caution in dosing.

Recommendations for reducing seizure risk – (1) The total daily dose does not exceed 450 mg (400 mg SR); (2) the daily dose is administered 3 times/day, with each single dose not to exceed 150 mg to avoid high peak concentrations of bupropion or its metabolites (twice/day for SR tablets with each single dose not to exceed 200 mg to avoid high peak concentrations of bupropion and its metabolites); and (3) the rate of incrementation of dose is very gradual.

Use extreme caution when: (1) Administered to patients with a history of seizure, cranial trauma, or other predisposition toward seizure; (2) circumstances associated with an increased seizure risk include excessive use of alcohol; abrupt withdrawal from alcohol or other sedatives; addiction to opiates, cocaine, or stimulants; use of *otc* stimulants and anorectics; and diabetes treated with oral hypogly-cemics or insulin; or (3) prescribed with other agents (eg, antipsychotics, other antidepressants, theophylline, systemic steroids) or treatment regimens (eg, abrupt discontinuation of a benzodiazepine) that lower seizure threshold.

Hepatotoxicity: In animals receiving large doses of bupropion chronically, there was an increased incidence of hepatic hyperplastic nodules, hepatocellular hypertrophy, and histologic changes with laboratory tests that suggested mild hepatocellular injury.

Hypersensitivity reactions: Anaphylactoid reactions characterized by symptoms such as pru-ritus, urticaria, angioedema, and dyspnea requiring medical treatment have been reported. In addition, there have been rare spontaneous postmarketing reports of erythema multiforme, Stevens-Johnson syndrome, and anaphylactic shock associ-ated with bupropion.

Renal/Hepatic function impairment: Initiate treatment of patients with renal or hepatic impairment at reduced dosage.

Half-lives of the metabolites are prolonged by cirrhosis and the metabolites accu-mulate to levels 2 to 3 times those in healthy individuals.

Elderly: Because elderly patients are more likely to have decreased renal function, take care in dose selection; it may be useful to monitor renal function (see Precautions, Administration and Dosage).

Pregnancy: Category B.

Lactation: Bupropion and its metabolites are secreted in breast milk.

Children: Safety and efficacy in children < 18 years of age have not been established.

Precautions

CNS symptoms: A substantial proportion of patients experience some degree of increased restlessness, agitation, anxiety, and insomnia, especially shortly after initiation of treatment.

Neuropsychiatric phenomena: Patients have shown a variety of neuropsychiatric signs and symptoms including delusions, hallucinations, psychotic episodes, confusion, and paranoia.

Activation of psychosis or mania: Antidepressants can precipitate manic episodes in bipolar manic depressive patients during the depressed phase of their illness and may acti-vate latent psychosis in other susceptible patients.

Altered appetite and weight: A weight loss of > 5 pounds occurred in 28% of patients treated with immediate-release formulation of bupropion. In patients treated with bupro-pion SR, 2.7% gained > 5 lbs and 15% lost > 5 lbs.

Suicide: The possibility of a suicide attempt is inherent in depression and may persist until significant remission occurs. Accordingly, write prescriptions for the smallest number of tablets consistent with good patient management.

Heart disease: Exercise care in patients with a recent history of MI or unstable heart dis-ease.

Drug abuse and dependence: Studies in healthy volunteers, subjects with a history of mul-tiple drug abuse, and depressed patients showed some increase in motor activity and agitation/excitement. In individuals experienced with drugs of abuse, a single dose of 400 mg bupropion produced mild amphetamine-like activity as compared with placebo.

Hazardous tasks: Advise patients that bupropion may impair ability to perform tasks requiring judgment or motor and cognitive skills.

Drug Interactions

Drugs that may interact with bupropion include MAOIs and levodopa, ritonavir, carbamazepine, TCAs, and nicotine replacement products.

CYP450: Exercise care when administering drugs known to affect hepatic drug metabo-lizing enzyme systems (eg, carbamazepine, cimetidine, phenobarbital, phenytoin).

In vitro studies indicate that bupropion is primarily metabolized to hydroxybupropion by the cytochrome P450 2B6 isoenzyme. Therefore, the potential exists for a drug interaction between bupropion and drugs that affect the cytochrome P450 2B6 metabolism (eg, orphenadrine, cyclophosphamide).

Approach with caution coadministration of bupropion with drugs that are metabolized by the cytochrome P450 2D6 (CYP2D6) isoenzyme, including certain antidepressants, antipsychotics, beta blockers, and Type 1C antiarrhythmics and initiate coadministration at the lower end of the dose range of the concomitant medication. If bupropion is added to the treatment regimen of a patient already receiving a drug metabolized by CYP2D6, consider the need to decrease the dose of the original medication, particularly for those concomitant medications with a narrow therapeutic index.

Use caution during coadministration of bupropion and agents (eg, antipsychotics, other antidepressants, theophylline, systemic steroids) or treatment regimens (eg, abrupt discontinuation of benzodiazepines) that lower seizure threshold. Use low initial dosing and small gradual dose increases.

Adverse Reactions

Adverse reactions occurring in ≥ 3% of patients include constipation; nausea/vomiting; anorexia; diarrhea; appetite increase; dyspepsia; menstrual complaints; impotence; dry mouth; headache/migraine; excessive sweating; tremor; sedation; akinesia/bradykinesia; sensory disturbance; impaired sleep quality; increased salivary flow; auditory disturbance; blurred vision; gustatory disturbance; dizziness; tachycardia; cardiac arrythmias; hypertension; palpitations; rash; confusion; hostility; disturbed concentration; decreased libido; upper respiratory complaints; fatigue; arthritis; agitation; flushing; hot flashes; insomnia; nervousness; somnolence; irritability; memory decreased; anxiety; pruritus; weight loss/gain; abdominal pain; urinary frequency; myalgia; arthralgia; pharyngitis; sinusitis; tinnitus; taste perversion; amblyopia; infection; chest pain; pain.

VENLAFAXINE

Tablets: 25, 37.5, 50, 75, and 100 mg (*Rx*)	*Effexor* (Wyeth Labs)
Capsules, extended-release: 37.5, 75, and 150 mg	*Effexor* XR (Wyeth Labs)

Indications

Depression: Treatment of depression.

Anxiety: Treatment of generalized anxiety disorder (GAD) (venlafaxine ER).

Administration and Dosage

Venlafaxine immediate-release:

> *Depression* –

>> *Initial treatment:* The recommended starting dose is 75 mg/day, administered in 2 or 3 divided doses, taken with food. Depending on tolerability and the need for further clinical effect, the dose may be increased to 150 mg/day. If needed, further increase the dose up to 225 mg/day. When increasing the dose, make increments of up to 75 mg/day at intervals of ≥ 4 days. Certain patients, including more severely depressed patients, may respond more to higher doses, up to a maximum of 375 mg/day, generally in 3 divided doses.

>> *Discontinuing venlafaxine* – When discontinuing venlafaxine after > 1 week of therapy, it is generally recommended that the dose be tapered to minimize the risk of discontinuation symptoms. Patients who have received venlafaxine for ≥ 6 weeks should have their dose tapered gradually over a 2-week period.

>> *Maintenance/Continuation/Extended treatment* – It is not known whether the dose needed for maintenance is identical to the dose needed to achieve an initial response. Periodically assess patients to determine the need for maintenance treatment and the appropriate dose for such treatment.

Venlafaxine extended-release:
   Depression –
      Initial treatment: The recommended starting dosage for venlafaxine extended-release is 75 mg/day administered in a single dose with food either in the morning or evening at approximately the same time each day. Swallow capsule whole; do not divide, crush, chew, or place in water. For some new patients, it may be desirable to start at 37.5 mg/day for 4 to 7 days to allow them to adjust to the medication before increasing to 75 mg/day. Patients not responding to the initial 75 mg/day dosage may benefit from dose increases to a maximum of ≈ 225 mg/day. Dose increases should be in increments of up to 75 mg/day as needed and should be made at intervals of ≥ 4 days because steady-state plasma levels of venlafaxine and the major metabolite are achieved in most patients by 4 days.

      GAD – For most patients, the recommended starting dose is 75 mg/day, administered in a single dose. For some patients, it may be desirable to start at 37.5 mg/day for 4 to 7 days to allow new patients to adjust to the medication before increasing to 75 mg/day. Although a dose-response relationship for effectiveness in GAD was not clearly established in fixed-dose studies, certain patients not responding to the initial 75 mg/day dose may benefit from dose increases to a maximum of ≈ 225 mg/day. Dose increases should be increments of up to 75 mg/day, as needed, and should be made at intervals of not less than 4 days.

      Discontinuing venlafaxine ER – When discontinuing treatment after > 1 week of therapy, taper the dose to minimize the risk of discontinuation symptoms. In clinical trials, tapering was achieved by reducing the daily dose by 75 mg at 1-week intervals. Individualization of tapering may be necessary.

   Renal/Hepatic function impairment: It is recommended that the total daily dose be reduced by 50% in patients with moderate hepatic impairment and by 25% to 50% in patients with mild to moderate renal impairment. It is recommended that the total daily dose be reduced by 50% and the dose be withheld until the dialysis treatment is completed (4 hours) in patients undergoing hemodialysis.

   Switching patients from immediate-release to extended-release venlafaxine: Depressed patients currently treated at a therapeutic dose with venlafaxine may be switched to the extended-release form at the nearest equivalent dose (mg/day; eg, 37.5 mg venlafaxine 2 times/day to 75 mg venlafaxine ER once daily). However, individual dosage adjustments may be necessary.

   Switching patients to or from a monoamine oxidase inhibitor (MAOI): At least 14 days should elapse between discontinuation of an MAOI and initiation of therapy with venlafaxine. In addition, allow ≥ 7 days after stopping venlafaxine before starting an MAOI.

Actions
   Pharmacology: Venlafaxine is chemically unrelated to other available antidepressant agents. Venlafaxine and its active metabolite, O-desmethylvenlafaxine (ODV), are potent inhibitors of neuronal serotonin and norepinephrine reuptake and weak inhibitors of dopamine reuptake.

   Pharmacokinetics: Venlafaxine is well absorbed (at least 92%) and extensively metabolized in the liver. ODV is the only major active metabolite. Renal elimination of venlafaxine and its metabolites is the primary route of excretion. Venlafaxine ER provides a slower rate of absorption but the same extent of absorption compared with the immediate-release tablet.

Contraindications
   Hypersensitivity to venlafaxine or any ingredients of the product; concomitant use in patients taking monoamine oxidase inhibitors (MAOIs).

Warnings
   MAO inhibitors: Because venlafaxine is an inhibitor of norepinephrine and serotonin reuptake, it is recommended that venlafaxine not be used in combination with an MAOI. Allow at least 7 days after stopping venlafaxine before starting an MAOI.

Sustained hypertension: There is a dose-dependent increase in the incidence of sustained hypertension for venlafaxine from 3% for doses < 100 mg/day up to 13% for doses > 300 mg/day.

Renal/Hepatic function impairment: In patients with renal impairment (GFR, 10 to 70 mL/min) or cirrhosis of the liver, a lower dose may be necessary.

Elderly: No overall differences in effectiveness, safety, or response were observed between elderly and younger patients.

Pregnancy: Category C.

Lactation: Venlafaxine and ODV are excreted in breast milk.

Children: Safety and efficacy in patients < 18 years of age for immediate-release or ER venlafaxine have not been established.

Precautions

Anxiety and insomnia: Anxiety, nervousness, and insomnia were reported for venlafaxine-treated patients, and led to drug discontinuation.

Appetite/Weight changes: Anorexia was reported for venlafaxine-treated patients. A dose-dependent weight loss often was noted in patients treated for several weeks.

Mania/Hypomania: Hypomania or mania has occurred in patients treated with venlafaxine.

Seizures: Seizures have been reported in venlafaxine-treated patients.

Suicide: The possibility of a suicide attempt is inherent in depression and may persist until significant remission occurs.

Hyponatremia: Hyponatremia and the syndrome of inappropriate antidiuretic hormone secretion (SIADH) may occur with venlafaxine.

Mydriasis: Mydriasis has been reported; monitor patients with raised intraocular pressure or those at risk of acute narrow angle glaucoma.

Abnormal bleeding: There have been reports of abnormal bleeding (most commonly ecchymosis) associated with venlafaxine treatment.

Concomitant illness: Caution is advised in administering venlafaxine to patients with diseases or conditions that could affect hemodynamic responses or metabolism.

Cardiac patients: Venlafaxine has not been evaluated in patients with a recent history of MI or unstable heart disease.

Drug abuse and dependence: Carefully evaluate patients for history of drug abuse and follow such patients closely, observing them for signs of misuse or abuse of venlafaxine.

Hazardous tasks: Caution patients about operating hazardous machinery, including automobiles, until they are reasonably certain that venlafaxine therapy does not adversely affect their ability to engage in such activities.

Drug Interactions

Drugs that may affect venlafaxine include cimetidine and MAOIs. Avoid alcohol. Drugs that may be affected by venlafaxine include desipramine, haloperidol, St. John's wort, trazodone, sibutramine, and sumatriptan.

Venlafaxine is metabolized to its active metabolite, ODV, by cytochrome $P4502D_6$. Therefore, the potential exists for a drug interaction between venlafaxine and drugs that inhibit this isoenzyme.

Adverse Reactions

Adverse reactions occurring in $\geq 3\%$ of patients include nausea; somnolence; insomnia; dizziness; abnormal ejaculation/orgasm; blurred vision; vasodilation; dry mouth; nervousness; anxiety; tremor; abnormal dreams; hypertonia; paresthesia; headache; asthenia; infection; chills; yawning; sweating; rash; constipation; anorexia; diarrhea; vomiting; dyspepsia; flatulence; impotence; urinary frequency; increased blood pressure/hypertension; decreased libido; agitation; depression; weight loss; pharyngitis.

NEFAZODONE HCl

Tablets: 50, 100, 150, 200, and 250 mg (*Rx*)	*Serzone* (Bristol-Myers Squibb)

Indications
Depression: Treatment of depression.

Administration and Dosage
Initial treatment: Recommended starting dose is 200 mg/day, administered in 2 divided doses. In clinical trials, the effective dose range was generally 300 to 600 mg/day. Increase doses in increments of 100 to 200 mg/day, again on a twice/day schedule, at intervals of no less than 1 week.

Elderly/Debilitated patients: The recommended initial dose is 100 mg/day on a twice/day schedule.

Actions
Pharmacology: Nefazodone is an antidepressant with a chemical structure unrelated to available antidepressant agents. The mechanism of action is unknown. Nefazodone inhibits neuronal uptake of serotonin and norepinephrine.

Pharmacokinetics:

Absorption/Distribution – Nefazodone is rapidly and completely absorbed, but is subject to extensive metabolism so that its absolute bioavailability is low (about 20%) and variable. Nefazodone is widely distributed in body tissues, including the CNS.

Metabolism/Excretion – Nefazodone is extensively metabolized after oral administration by < 1% is excreted unchanged in urine.

The mean half-life of nefazodone ranged between 11 and 24 hours. Nefazodone is extensively (> 99%) bound to human plasma proteins in vitro.

Contraindications
Coadministration with cisapride and pimozide; hypersensitivity to nefazodone or other phenylpiperazine antidepressants.

Warnings
Long-term use: The effectiveness of nefazodone in long-term use (ie, for more than 6 to 8 weeks) has not been systematically evaluated.

Serious interactions:

MAO inhibitors – Because nefazodone is an inhibitor of both serotonin and norepinephrine reuptake, it is recommended that nefazodone not be used in combination with an MAOI, or within 14 days of discontinuing treatment with an MAOI. Allow at least 1 week after stopping nefazodone before starting an MAOI.

Triazolobenzodiazepines – Triazolam and alprazolam, metabolized by cytochrome P450 3A4, have revealed substantial and clinically important increases in plasma concentrations of these compounds when administered concomitantly with nefazodone. If triazolam is coadministered with nefazodone, a 75% reduction in the initial triazolam dosage is recommended. For many patients (eg, the elderly), it is recommended that triazolam not be used in combination with nefazodone. No dosage adjustment is required for nefazodone.

Cisapride/pimozide – Cisapride and pimozide are metabolized by the cytochrome P450 3A4 isozyme; inhibitors of 3A4 can block the metabolism of these drugs, resulting in increased plasma concentrations of parent drug, which is associated with QT prolongation and with rare cases of serious cardiovascular adverse events, including death, principally because of ventricular tachycardia of the torsades de pointes type. In vitro, nefazodone inhibits 3A4. Consequently, it is recommended that nefazodone not be used in combination with cisapride or pimozide.

Hepatic function impairment: Rare cases of severe idiosyncratic hepatocellular injury have occurred. It is suggested that routine liver chemistries be obtained prior to initiating therapy and monitored routinely throughout the course of treatment. Obtain liver function tests for patients at the first symptoms suggestive of hepatic dysfunction (eg, nausea, vomiting, abdominal pain, fatigue, anorexia, dark urine).

Pregnancy: Category C.

Lactation: It is not known whether nefazodone or its metabolites are excreted in breast milk.

Children: Safety and efficacy in individuals < 18 years of age have not been established.

Precautions

Postural hypotension: Use nefazodone with caution in patients with known cardiovascular or cerebrovascular disease that could be exacerbated by hypotension and conditions that would predispose patients to hypotension.

Mania/hypomania: As with all antidepressants, use nefazodone cautiously in patients with a history of mania.

Suicide: The possibility of a suicide attempt is inherent in depression and may persist until significant remission occurs.

Seizures: Rare occurrences of convulsions (including grand mal seizures) following nefazodone administration have been reported since market introduction. A causal relationship to nefazodone has not been established.

Priapism: If patients present with prolonged or inappropriate erections, they should discontinue therapy immediately and consult their physicians.

Elective surgery: Little is known about the potential for interaction between nefazodone and general anesthetics; therefore, prior to elective surgery, discontinue nefazodone for as long as clinically feasible.

Bradycardia: Sinus bradycardia was observed in nefazodone patients. Treat patients with a recent MI or unstable heart disease with caution.

Hepatic cirrhosis: In patients with cirrhosis of the liver, the AUC values of nefazodone and its metabolite HO-NEF were increased by $\approx 25\%$.

Drug abuse and dependence: Carefully evaluate patients for a history of drug abuse and follow such patients closely, observing them for signs of misuse or abuse of nefazodone.

Hazardous tasks: Caution patients about operating hazardous machinery, including automobiles, until they are reasonably certain that nefazodone therapy does not adversely affect their ability to engage in such activities.

Drug Interactions

Drugs that affect nefazadone include sibutramine, buspirone and propranolol. Nefazodone may affect alcohol, benzodiazepines, buspirone, carbamazepine, cisapride, digoxin, haloperidol, HMG-CoA reductase inhibitors, MAOIs, pimozide, propranolol, St. Johns wort, and trazodone.

Potential interaction with drugs that inhibit or are metabolized by cytochrome P450 (3A4 and 2D6) isozymes: Caution is indicated in the combined use of nefazodone with any drugs known to be metabolized by the 3A4 isozyme (in particular, cisapride or pimozide).

Drugs highly bound to plasma protein: Administration to a patient taking another drug that is highly protein bound may cause increased free concentrations of the other drug, potentially resulting in adverse events. Conversely, adverse effects could result from displacement of nefazodone by other highly bound drugs.

Drug/Food interactions: Food delays absorption of nefazodone and decreases the bioavailability by $\approx 20\%$.

Adverse Reactions

Adverse reactions occurring in $\geq 3\%$ of patients include nausea; headache; asthenia; flu syndrome; dry mouth; nausea; constipation; dyspepsia; diarrhea; increased appetite; peripheral edema; pharyngitis; cough; blurred vision; abnormal vision; somnolence; dizziness; insomnia; lightheadedness; confusion; memory impairment; paresthesia; vasodilation; concentration decreased; postural hypotension; infection; abnormal dreams.

SELECTIVE SEROTONIN REUPTAKE INHIBITORS

CITALOPRAM HBr
Tablets: 20 and 40 mg (*Rx*)   *Celexa* (Forest Pharmaceuticals)
Solution, oral: 10 mg/5 mL *Rx*

FLUOXETINE HCl
Tablets: 10 mg (*Rx*)   *Prozac* (Dista)
Capsules, delayed release: 90 mg (*Rx*)   *Prozac Weekly* (Eli Lilly)
Pulvules: 10, 20, and 40 mg (*Rx*)   *Prozac* (Dista), *Sarafem* (Eli Lilly)
Solution, oral: 20 mg/5 mL (*Rx*)   *Prozac* (Dista)

FLUVOXAMINE MALEATE
Tablets: 25, 50, and 100 mg (*Rx*)   Various, *Luvox* (Solvay)

PAROXETINE HCl
Tablets: 10, 20, 30, and 40 mg (*Rx*)   *Paxil* (GlaxoSmithKline)
Suspension: 10 mg/5 mL (*Rx*)

SERTRALINE HCl
Tablets: 25, 50, 100 mg (*Rx*)   *Zoloft* (Roerig)
Oral concentrate: 20 mg/mL (*Rx*)

Indications

Depression: Fluoxetine, paroxetine, sertraline, citalopram.

Obsessive-Compulsive disorder (OCD): Fluoxetine, fluvoxamine, sertraline, paroxetine.

Post-traumatic stress disorder (PTSD): Sertraline.

Bulimia nervosa: Fluoxetine.

Panic disorder: Sertraline, paroxetine.

Premenstrual dysphoric disorder (PMDD): Fluoxetine.

Social anxiety disorder, generalized anxiety disorder: Paroxetine.

Unlabeled uses:
   Fluoxetine – Alcoholism (40 to 80 mg/day); anorexia nervosa (20 to 80 mg/day); attention-deficit hyperactivity disorder (20 to 60 mg/day); bipolar II affective disorder (20 to 80 mg/day); borderline personality disorder (5 to 80 mg/day); narcolepsy (20 to 40 mg/day); kleptomania (60 to 80 mg/day); migraine, chronic daily headaches, and tension-type headache (20 mg every other day to 40 mg/day); post-traumatic stress disorder (10 to 80 mg/day); schizophrenia (20 to 60 mg/day); trichotillomania (20 to 80 mg/day); levodopa-induced dyskinesia (40 mg/day); social phobia (10 to 60 mg/day); chronic rheumatoid pain (20 mg/day); panic disorder (10 to 70 mg/day); diabetic peripheral neuropathy (5 to 40 mg/day).
   Fluvoxamine – Fluvoxamine is being investigated in the treatment of the following: Depression; autism; panic disorder; social phobia; generalized anxiety disorder; post-traumatic stress disorder; premenstrual dysphoric disorder.
   Paroxetine – Bipolar depression in conjunction with lithium; premenstrual dysphoric disorder; chronic headache; premature ejaculation; fibromyalgia syndrome; diabetic neuropathy; post-traumatic stress disorder.
   Sertraline – Social phobia; premenstrual dysphoric disorder.
   Citalopram – Alcoholism treatment; panic disorder (20 to 30 mg/day); premenstrual dysphoria (as intermittent administration); social phobia; trichotillomania.

Administration and Dosage
   CITALOPRAM HBr:
      Initial therapy – 20 mg once/day in the morning or evening with or without food. Dose increases should usually occur in increments of 20 mg at intervals of no less than 1 week. Doses > 40 mg/day are not recommended.
      Maintenance therapy – Antidepressant efficacy is maintained for periods of ≤ 24 weeks following 6 or 8 weeks of initial treatment (32 weeks total). Periodically re-evaluate the long-term usefulness of the drug for the individual patient if citalopram is used for extended periods.

Elderly/Hepatic function impairment – 20 mg/day is the recommended dose for most elderly patients and patients with hepatic impairment, with titration to 40 mg/day only for nonresponding patients.

Renal impairment – Use with caution in patients with severe renal impairment.

FLUOXETINE HCl:

Depression –

Initial: 20 mg/day in the morning. Consider a dose increase after several weeks if no clinical improvement is observed. Administer doses > 20 mg/day on a once (morning) or twice (eg, morning and noon) daily schedule. Do not exceed a maximum dose of 80 mg/day.

Weekly dosing: Initiate 7 days after the last 20 mg/day dose. If satisfactory response is not maintained, consider reestablishing a daily dosing regimen.

Maintenance: Optimal duration of fluoxetine therapy remains speculative. Acute episodes of depression generally require several months or longer of sustained pharmacological therapy.

Obsessive-Compulsive disorder –

Initial: 20 mg/day in the morning. Consider a dose increase after several weeks if insufficient clinical improvement is observed. Administer doses > 20 mg/day on a once (morning) or twice (morning and noon) daily schedule. A dose range of 20 to 60 mg/day is recommended; however, doses of up to 80 mg/day have been well tolerated. Do not exceed 80 mg/day.

Maintenance: Patients have been continued on therapy for an additional 6 months without loss of benefit.

Bulimia nervosa –

Initial: The recommended dose is 60 mg/day, administered in the morning. For some patients it may be advisable to titrate up to this target dose over several days. Fluoxetine doses > 60 mg/day have not been systematically studied in patients with bulimia.

Maintenance: Patients have been continued on therapy for an additional 6 months without loss of benefit. However, make dosage adjustments to maintain the patient on the lowest effective dosage, and periodically reassess the patient to determine the need for treatment.

PMDD –

Initial: 20 mg/day. Do not exceed a maximum dose of 80 mg/day.

Maintenance/Continuation: Systemic evaluation has shown that its efficacy is maintained for periods ≤ 6 months at a dose of 20 mg/day. Reassess patients periodically to determine the need for continued treatment.

Hepatic function impairment – Use a lower or less frequent dosage.

Special risk patients – Consider a lower or less frequent dosage for patients, such as the elderly, with concurrent disease or on multiple medications.

Switching patients to a TCA – Dosage of TCA may need to be reduced, and plasma TCA concentrations may need to be monitored temporarily when fluoxetine is coadministered or has been recently discontinued.

FLUVOXAMINE MALEATE:

Initial therapy – Recommended starting dose is 50 mg as a single bedtime dose. Increase dose in 50 mg increments every 4 to 7 days, as tolerated, until maximum therapeutic benefit is achieved, not to exceed 300 mg/day. It is advisable to give total daily doses > 100 mg in 2 divided doses; if doses are unequal, give larger dose at bedtime.

Pediatric therapy – In patients 8 to 17 years of age, the starting dose is 25 mg as a single daily dose at bedtime. Increase the dose in 25 mg increments every 4 to 7 days as tolerated, until maximum therapeutic benefit is achieved (not to exceed 200 mg/day). Divide total daily doses > 50 mg into 2 doses. If the 2 divided doses are not equal, give the larger dose at bedtime.

Maintenance therapy – Although efficacy has not been documented > 10 weeks in controlled trials, OCD is a chronic condition; it is reasonable to consider continuation for a responding patient.

Elderly/Hepatic function impairment – These patients have been observed to have decreased fluvoxamine clearance. It may be appropriate to modify initial dose and subsequent titration.

PAROXETINE HCl:

Depression –

Initial dose: 20 mg/day. Administer as a single daily dose, usually in the morning. Usual range is 20 to 50 mg/day. Some patients not responding to a 20 mg dose may benefit from dose increases, in 10 mg/day increments, up to a maximum of 50 mg/day. Dose changes should occur at intervals of at least 1 week.

Maintenance therapy: It is generally agreed that acute episodes of depression require several months or longer of sustained pharmacologic therapy. Efficacy has been maintained for period up to 1 year with doses that averaged about 30 mg.

OCD –

Initial: 20 mg/day. Administer as a single daily dose, usually in the morning. Start with 20 mg/day and may be increased in 10 mg/day increments. Dose changes should occur at intervals of at least 1 week. Usual range is 20 to 60 mg/day. The maximum dosage should not exceed 60 mg/day.

Maintenance therapy: Patients have been continued on therapy for 6 months without loss of benefit. However, make dosage adjustments to maintain the patient on the lowest effective dosage, and periodically reassess the patient to determine the need for treatment.

Panic disorder –

Initial: 20 mg/day; the recommended target dose is 40 mg/day. Administer as a single daily dose, usually in the morning. Start with 10 mg/day and may be increased in 10 mg/day increments. Dose changes should occur at intervals of at least 1 week. Usual range is 10 to 60 mg/day. The maximum dosage should not exceed 60 mg/day.

Maintenance therapy: Long-term maintenance of efficacy has been demonstrated for 3 months. Make dosage adjustments to maintain the patient on the lowest effective dosage, and reassess the patients periodically to determine the need for continued treatment.

Social anxiety disorder –

Initial: 20 mg/day administered as a single daily dose with or without food, usually in the morning. Usual range is 20 to 60 mg/day. Available information does not suggest any additional benefit for doses > 20 mg/day.

Maintenance: Although the efficacy beyond 12 weeks of dosing has not been demonstrated in controlled clinical trials, social anxiety disorder is recognized as a chronic condition, and it is reasonable to consider continuation of treatment for a responding patient. Make dosage adjustments to maintain the patient on the lowest effective dosage, and periodically reassess patients to determine the need for continued treatment.

Generalized anxiety disorder –

Initial: 20 mg/day administered as a single daily dose with or without food, usually in the morning. Usual range is 20 to 50 mg/day. Change doses in 10 mg/day increments and at intervals of ≥ 1 week. There is not sufficient evidence to suggest a greater benefit to doses > 20 mg/day.

Maintenance: Although efficacy beyond 8 weeks of dosing has not been established, generalized anxiety disorder is recognized as a chronic condition and it is reasonable to consider continuation of treatment to a responding patient. Make dosage adjustments to maintain the patient on the lowest effective dosage and periodically assess patients to determine the need for continued treatment.

Elderly or debilitated or patients with severe renal or hepatic impairment – The recommended initial dose is 10 mg/day. Increases may be made if indicated. Do not exceed 40 mg/day.

SERTRALINE HCl:

Adults –

Initial treatment:

Depression and OCD – 50 mg once/day.

Panic disorder and PTSD – 25 mg once/day. After 1 week, increase the dose to 50 mg once/day.

While a relationship between dose and effect for depression, OCD, PTSD, or panic disorder has not been established, patients were dosed in a range of 50 to 200 mg/day in the clinical trials. Consequently, patients not responding to a 50 mg dose may benefit from dose increases up to a maximum of 200 mg/day. Given the 24-hour elimination half-life of sertraline, dose changes should not occur at intervals of < 1 week.

Maintenance/Continuation/Extended treatment –

Depression: It is generally agreed that acute episodes of depression require several months or longer of sustained pharmacologic therapy. Whether the dose of antidepressant needed to induce remission is identical to the dose needed to maintain or sustain euthymia is unknown. Systematic evaluation of sertraline has shown that the antidepressant efficacy is maintained for a period of ≤ 44 weeks following 8 weeks of open-label acute treatment (52 weeks total) at doses of 50 to 200 mg/day (mean dose, 70 mg/day).

OCD, panic disorder: Although the efficacy of sertraline beyond 10 to 12 weeks of dosing for OCD and panic disorder has not been documented in controlled trials, all are chronic conditions and it is reasonable to consider continuation of a responding patient. Dosage adjustments may be needed to maintain the patient on the lowest effective dosage, and patients should be periodically reassessed to determine the need for continued treatment.

PTSD: It is generally agreed that PTSD requires several months or longer of sustained pharmacological therapy beyond response to initial treatment.

Long-term use – Systematic evaluation of sertraline has demonstrated that its efficacy in PTSD is maintained for periods of up to 28 weeks following 24 weeks of treatment at a dose of 50 to 200 mg/day. It is not known whether the dose of sertraline needed for maintenance treatment is identical to the dose needed to achieve an initial response. The physician who elects to use sertraline for extended periods should periodically reevaluate the long-term usefulness of the drug for the individual patient.

Children –

OCD: Initiate dosage with 25 mg once/day for children (6 to 12 years of age) and 50 mg once/day in adolescents (13 to 17 years of age) in the morning or evening. While a relationship between dose and effect has not been established for OCD, patients were dosed in a range of 25 to 200 mg/day in trials for pediatric patients 6 to 17 years of age with OCD. Patients not responding to an initial dose of 25 or 50 mg/day may benefit from dose increases up to a maximum of 200 mg/day. For children with OCD, take into account the generally lower body weights compared with adults when increasing the dose to avoid excess dosing. Given the 24-hour elimination half-life, dose changes should not occur at intervals of < 1 week.

Hepatic function impairment – Give a lower or less-frequent dosage in patients with hepatic impairment. Use with caution in these patients.

Oral concentrate – Dilute prior to use with 4 oz. (½ cup) of water, ginger ale, lemon/lime soda, lemonade, or orange juice only. Administer the dose immediately after mixing; do not mix in advance.

Actions

Pharmacology: These agents are potent and selective inhibitors of neuronal serotonin reuptake and they also have a weak effect on norepinephrine and dopamine neuronal reuptake.

Pharmacokinetics:

SSRIs	Time to peak plasma concentration (hr)	Peak plasma concentration (ng/mL)	Half-life (hrs)	Protein binding (%)	Time to reach steady state (days)	Primary route of elimination	Bioavailability (%)
Citalopram	2-4	120 to 150 nmol/L	≈ 35	≈ 80	≈ 7	35% renal, 65% fecal	≈ 80
Fluoxetine	6-8	15-55	1 to 384[1]	≈ 94.5	≈ 28	hepatic	94
Fluvoxamine	3-8	88-546	13.6-15.6	≈ 80	≈ 7	≈94% renal	53
Paroxetine	5.2	61.7	21	≈ 93-95	≈10	64% renal, 36% fecal	100[2]
Sertraline	4.5-8.4	20-55	26-104[1]	98	7	40%-45% renal, 40%-45% fecal	nd[*]

[1] t½ includes the active metabolite.
[2] The bioavailability of 25 mg paroxetine CR is not affected by food.
[*] nd = no data

Contraindications

Hypersensitivity to SSRIs; in combination with an MAO inhibitor, or within 14 days of discontinuing an MAOI; coadministration of **fluvoxamine** with cisapride.

Warnings

Long-term use: The effectiveness of long-term use of SSRIs for OCD, panic disorder, and bulimia has not been systematically evaluated. However, the long-term use of SSRIs for depression has been evaluated and demonstrated to maintain antidepressant response for up to 1 year.

MAO Inhibitors: It is recommended that SSRIs not be used in combination with an MAOI, or within 14 days of discontinuing treatment with an MAOI. Allow ≥ 2 weeks after stopping the SSRIs before starting an MAOI.

Platelet function: Altered platelet function or abnormal results from laboratory studies in patients taking **fluoxetine, paroxetine,** or **sertraline** have occurred.

Rash and accompanying events: Seven percent of patients taking **fluoxetine** have developed a rash or urticaria; ≈ 33% were withdrawn from treatment. Most patients improved promptly with discontinuation of fluoxetine or adjunctive treatment with antihistamines or steroids; all patients recovered completely. Several other patients have had systemic syndromes suggestive of serum sickness.

Systemic events, possibly related to vasculitis, have developed in patients with rash. Although rare, these events may be serious, involving lung, kidney, or liver. Death has been associated with the events.

Renal function impairment: Use of a lower or less-frequent dose of **fluoxetine** for renally impaired patients is not routinely necessary.

Reduce the initial dosage of **paroxetine** in patients with severe renal impairment.

Use **sertraline** with caution in patients with severe renal impairment.

No adjustment of of **citalopram** dosage for such patients is recommended.

No adjustment of **fluvoxamine** is recommended.

Hepatic function impairment: SSRIs are extensively metabolized by the liver. Use with caution in patients with severe liver impairment.

Elderly: The disposition of single doses of **fluoxetine** in healthy elderly subjects (≥ 65 years of age) did not differ significantly from that in younger normal subjects. Clearance of **fluvoxamine** is decreased by ≈ 50% in elderly patients. A lower starting dose of **paroxetine** is recommended. Sertraline plasma clearance may be lower. In 2 pharmacokinetic studies, **citalopram** AUC was increased by 23% and

30%, respectively, in elderly subjects as compared with younger subjects, and its half-life was increased by 30% and 50%, respectively.

Pregnancy: Category C.

Lactation: **Fluoxetine, fluvoxamine, citalopram,** and **paroxetine** are excreted in breast milk. It is not known whether **sertraline** or its metabolites are excreted in breast milk.

Children: Safety and efficacy in children (< 18 years of age) have not been established.

Precautions

Anxiety, nervousness, and insomnia: Anxiety, nervousness, and insomnia occurred in 4% to 28% of patients treated with an SSRI.

Altered appetite and weight: Significant weight loss, especially in underweight depressed patients, has occurred. Approximately 3% to 9% of patients treated with an SSRI experienced anorexia during initial therapy.

Mania/hypomania: Activation of mania/hypomania occurred infrequently in ≈ 0.1% to 2.2% of patients taking SSRIs. Use cautiously in patients with a history of mania.

Seizures: Seizures have occurred with **fluoxetine** (0.1%), **fluvoxamine** (0.2%), **paroxetine** (0.1%), **sertraline** (0.2%), and **citalopram** (0.3%). These percentages appear similar to the rate associated with other antidepressants. Use with care in patients with history of seizures. Discontinue therapy if seizures occur.

Suicide: The possibility of a suicide attempt is inherent in depression and may persist until significant remission occurs.

MI: SSRIs have not been systematically evaluated in patients with a recent history of MI or unstable heart disease. The ECGs of patients who received SSRIs in clinical trials were evaluated and the data indicate that they are not associated with the development of clinically significant ECG abnormalities.

Concomitant illness: Use caution in patients with diseases or conditions that could affect metabolism or hemodynamic responses.

Electroconvulsive therapy (ECT): There are no clinical studies establishing the benefit of the combined use of ECT and SSRIs. Rare prolonged seizure in patients on **fluoxetine** has occurred.

Hyponatremia: Several cases of SSRI-induced hyponatremia (some with serum sodium < 110 mmol/L) have occurred. The hyponatremia appeared to be reversible when the drug was discontinued. The majority of these occurrences have been in older patients and in patients taking diuretics or who were otherwise volume-depleted.

Diabetes: **Fluoxetine** may alter glycemic control. Hypoglycemia has occurred during therapy, and hyperglycemia has developed following discontinuation of the drug. The dosage of insulin or the sulfonylurea may need to be adjusted when fluoxetine is started or discontinued.

Uricosuric effect: **Sertraline** is associated with a mean decrease in serum uric acid of ≈ 7%. The clinical significance of this weak uricosuric effect is unknown, and there have been no reports of acute renal failure with sertraline.

Drug abuse and dependence: Before staring an SSRI, carefully evaluate patients for history of drug abuse and follow such patients closely, observing them for signs of misuse or abuse.

Hazardous tasks: SSRIs may cause dizziness or drowsiness. Patients should be instructed to observe caution while driving or performing tasks requiring alertness, coordination, or physical dexterity.

Photosensitivity: Photosensitization may occur.

Drug Interactions

Drugs highly bound to plasma protein: Because SSRIs are highly bound to plasma protein, administration to a patient taking another drug that is highly protein-bound may cause increased free concentrations of the other drug, potentially resulting in adverse events. Conversely, adverse effects could result from displacement of SSRIs by other highly bound drugs.

P450 system: Concomitant use of SSRIs with drugs metabolized by cytochrome $P4502D_6$ may require lower doses than usually prescribed for either **paroxetine** or the other drug since paroxetine may significantly inhibit the activity of this isozyme.

Hepatic metabolism of **citalopram** occurs primarily through cytochrome P450 3A4 and 2C19 isoenzymes. Inhibitors of 3A4 (eg, azole antifungals, macrolide antibiotics) and 2C19 (eg, omeprazole) would be expected to increase plasma citalopram levels. Inducters of 3A4 (eg, carbamazepine) would be expected to decrease citalopram levels.

Serotonin syndrome: The serotonin syndrome is a rare complication of therapy with serotonergic drugs. When this problem occurs with SSRIs, it is most commonly in the setting of other concurrent medications that increase serotonin by different mechanisms.

Drugs that may affect selective serotonin reuptake inhibitors include azole antifungals, cimetidine, cyproheptadine, lithium, MAO inhibitors, phenytoin, smoking, L-tryptophan, barbiturates, and macrolides.

Drugs that may be affected by selective serotonin reuptake inhibitors include phenytoin, alcohol, tricyclic antidepressants, nonsedating antihistamines, cyclosporine, haloperidol, pimozide, sumatriptan, benzodiazepines, beta blockers, buspirone, carbamazepine, clozapine, diltiazem, digoxin, lithium, methadone, procyclidine, theophylline, tolbutamide, warfarin, phenothiazines, St. John's wort, sympathomimetics, and tacrine.

Drug/Food interactions: In one study following a single dose of **sertraline** with and without food, sertraline AUC was slightly increased and C_{max} was 25% greater. Time to reach peak plasma level decreased from 8 hours post-dosing to 5.5 hours.

Food does not appear to affect systemic bioavailability of **fluoxetine** although it may delay absorption. **Fluvoxamine** and **citalopram** bioavailability is not affected by food. Thus, fluoxetine, fluvoxamine, and citalopram may be given with or without food.

Adverse Reactions

Commonly observed –

SSRIs Adverse Reactions (%) (≥ 3% in at least one agent)					
Adverse reaction	Citalopram	Fluoxetine	Fluvoxamine	Paroxetine	Sertraline
Cardiovascular					
Palpitations	—	2	3	2-3	≥ 1
Vasodilatation	—	3	3	3-4	—
Chest pain		1.3	—	3	≥ 1
CNS					
Insomnia	15	20	21	13-24	16-28
Somnolence	18	13	22	19-24	13-15
Nervousness	—	13	12	6-9	6
Anxiety	4	13	5	5	4
Dizziness	—	10	11	12-14	13
Tremor	8	10	5	8-11	5-11
Libido decreased	2	4	2	3-9	1-11
Myoclonus/twitching	—	0.1-1	≥ 1	3	0.1-1
Agitation	3	≥ 1	2	5	6
Paresthesia	≥ 1	—	—	4	3
Hypertonia	0.1- 1	0.1-1	2	—	≥ 1
Fatigue	5	—	—	—	12
Concentration, decreased	≥ 1	—	—	3	—
Abnormal dreams	—	5	—	4	0.1-1
Abnormal thinking	—	4	—	0.1-1	—
Depersonalization	0.1-1	0.1-1	0.1-1	3	3

SSRIs Adverse Reactions (%) (≥ 3% in at least one agent)					
Adverse reaction	Citalopram	Fluoxetine	Fluvoxamine	Paroxetine	Sertraline
Dermatologic					
Sweating, excessive	11	8	7	9-14	5-8
Rash	≥ 1	4	—	3	23
Pruritus	≥ 1	3	—	≥ 1	0.1 to 1
GI					
Nausea	21	23	40	23-26	26-30
Vomiting	4	3	5	—	4
Decreased appetite	—	—	—	6-9	—
Diarrhea/loose stools	8	12	11	10-12	18-24
Dyspepsia	5	8	10	2	6-10
Dry mouth	20	10	14	18	15
Anorexia	4	11	6	6	3-11
Constipation	—	4.5	10	8-16	6-8
Abdominal pain	3	3.4	—	4	—
Flatulence	≥ 1	3	4	4	3
Increased appetite	—	≥ 1	—	2-4	≥ 1
Tooth disorder/caries	—	—	3	< 0.1	0.1-1
GU					
Sexual dysfunction/impotence/ anorgasmia	3	—	2	5-8	≥ 1
Urinary frequency	—	≥ 1	3	2-3	2
Urinary tract infection	—	—	0.1-1	2	—
Abnormal ejaculation	6	—	8	21-23	7-19
Male genital disorders, others	—	—	—	10	—
Urination disorder/retention	0.1-1	0.1-1	1	3	0.1-1
Female genital disorders	—	—	—	2-9	—
Menstrual disorder	3	—	0.1-1	—	0.1-1
Respiratory					
Upper respiratory tract infection	5	—	9	—	0.1-1
Pharyngitis	—	5	—	—	—
Sinusitis	3	—	≥ 1	—	0.1-1
Rhinitis	5	—	—	3	≥ 1
Yawn	2	—	2	4	≥ 1
Special senses					
Vision disturbances/blurred vision/abnormal vision	≥ 1	3	—	4	4
Taste perversion/change	≥ 1	≥ 1	3	2	3
Amblyopia	—	—	3	—	—
Miscellaneous					
Headache	—	21	22	18	26
Asthenia	—	12	14	14-22	≥ 1
Flu syndrome	—	5	3	—	—
Back pain	—	2	—	3	≥ 1
Accidental injury	—	4	≥ 1	—	—
Myalgia	2	5	—	2	≥ 1

[1] Data are pooled from different studies and are not necessarily comparable.

MONOAMINE OXIDASE INHIBITORS

ISOCARBOXAZID	
Tablets: 10 mg (Rx)	Marplan (Hoffman-La Roche)
PHENELZINE	
Tablets: 15 mg (as sulfate) (Rx)	Nardil (Parke-Davis)
TRANYLCYPROMINE	
Tablets: 10 mg (as sulfate) (Rx)	Parnate (GlaxoSmithKline)

Indications

Depression: In general, the MAOIs appear to be indicated in patients with atypical (exogenous) depression, and in some patients unresponsive to other antidepressive therapy. They are rarely a drug of first choice.

Administration and Dosage

ISOCARBOXAZID:

Initial dosage – 10 mg twice/day. Increase dosage by 10 mg every 2 to 4 days to achieve a dosage of 40 mg by the end of the first week. Increase by increments of up to 20 mg/week, to a maximum recommended dosage of 60 mg/day. Daily dosage should be divided into 2 to 4 doses.

Maintenance dosage – After maximum clinical response is achieved, attempt to reduce the dosage slowly over a period of several weeks without jeopardizing therapeutic response. Beneficial effect may not be seen in some patients for 3 to 6 weeks. If no response is obtained by then, discontinue therapy.

Because of the limited experience with systematically monitored patients receiving isocarboxazid at the higher end of the currently recommended dose range of up to 60 mg/day, caution is indicated in patients for whom a dose of 40 mg/day is exceeded.

PHENELZINE:

Initial dose – 15 mg 3 times a day.

Early phase treatment – Increase dosage to ≥ 60 mg/day at a fairly rapid pace consistent with patient tolerance. It may be necessary to increase dosage up to 90 mg/day to obtain sufficient MAO inhibition. Many patients do not show a clinical response until treatment at 60 mg has been continued for at least 4 weeks.

Maintenance dose – After maximum benefit is achieved, reduce dosage slowly over several weeks. Maintenance dose may be as slow as 15 mg/day or every other day; continue for as long as required.

TRANYLCYPROMINE: The usual effective dosage is 30 mg/day in divided doses. If there is no improvement after 2 weeks, increase dosage in 10 mg/day increments of 1 to 3 weeks. Dosage range may be extended to a maximum of 60 mg/day from the usual 30 mg/day. Withdrawal from tranylcypromine should be gradual.

Actions

Pharmacology: These drugs are non-selective MAOIs and cause an increase in the concentration of endogenous epinephrine, norepinephrine, and serotonin (5HT) in storage sites throughout the nervous system.

Pharmacokinetics: Phenelzine and tranylcypromine are well absorbed orally. The clinical effects of phenelzine may continue for ≤ 2 weeks after discontinuation of therapy. When tranylcypromine is withdrawn, MAO activity is recovered in 3 to 5 days (possibly up to 10 days), although the drug is excreted in 24 hours.

Contraindications

Hypersensitivity to these agents; pheochromocytoma; CHF; a history of liver disease or abnormal liver function tests; severe impairment of renal function; confirmed or suspected cerebrovascular defect; cardiovascular disease; hypertension; history of headache; in patients over 60 because of the possibility of existing cerebral sclerosis with damaged vessels; coadministration with other MAOIs; dibenzazepine-related agents including tricyclic antidepressants, carbamazepine, and cyclobenzaprine; buproprion; SSRIs; buspirone; sympathomimetics; meperidine; dextromethorphan; anesthetic agents; CNS depressants; antihypertensives; caffeine; cheese or other foods with high tyramine content (see Warnings and Drug Interactions).

Warnings

Hypertensive crises: The most serious reactions involve changes in blood pressure; it is inadvisable to use these drugs in elderly or debilitated patients or in the presence of hypertension, cardiovascular, or cerebrovascular disease. Not recommended in patients with frequent or severe headaches because headache during therapy may be the first symptom of a hypertensive reaction.

Warning to the patient – Warn all patients against eating foods with high tyramine or tryptophan content and for 2 weeks after discontinuing MAOIs. Also warn patients against drinking alcoholic beverages and against self-medication with certain proprietary agents such as cold, hay fever, or weight reduction preparations containing sympathomimetic amines while undergoing therapy. Instruct patients not to consume excessive amounts of caffeine in any form and to report promptly the occurrence of headache or other unusual symptoms.

Concomitant antidepressants: In patients receiving a selective serotonin reuptake inhibitor (SSRIs) in combination with an MAOI, there have been reports of serious, sometimes fatal, reactions including hyperthermia, rigidity, myoclonus, autonomic instability with possible rapid fluctuations of vital signs, and mental status changes that include extreme agitation progressing to delirium and coma. It is recommended that SSRIs not be used in combination with an MAOI, or within 14 days of an MAOI. Allow ≥ 2 weeks after stopping the SSRIs before starting an MAOI. Allow ≥ 5 weeks after stopping fluoxetine before starting an MAOI.

MAOIs should not be administered together with or immediately following tricyclic antidepressants (TCAs). At least 14 days should elapse between the discontinuation of the MAOIs and the institution of a TCA. Some TCAs have been used safely and successfully in combination with MAOIs.

Withdrawal: Withdrawal may be associated with nausea, vomiting, and malaise.

Coexisting symptoms: **Tranylcypromine** and **isocarboxazid** may aggravate coexisting symptoms in depression, such as anxiety and agitation.

Renal function impairment: Observe caution in patients with impaired renal function because there is a possibility of cumulative effects in such patients.

Elderly: Older patients may suffer more morbidity than younger patients during and following an episode of hypertension or malignant hyperthermia with MAOI use. Use with caution in the elderly.

Pregnancy: Category C.

Lactation: Safety for use during lactation has not been established. **Tranylcypromine** is excreted in breast milk.

Children: Not recommended for patients < 16 years of age.

Precautions

Hypotension: Follow all patients for symptoms of postural hypotension. Blood pressure usually returns to pretreatment levels rapidly when the drug is discontinued or the dosage is reduced.

Hypomania: Hypomania has been the most common severe psychiatric side effect reported. This has been largely limited to patients in whom disorders characterized by hyperkinetic symptoms coexist with, but are obscured by, depressive affect.

Diabetes: There is conflicting evidence as to whether MAOIs affect glucose metabolism or potentiate hypoglycemic agents. Consider this if used in diabetics.

Epilepsy: The effect of MAOIs on the convulsive threshold may vary. Do not use with metrizamide; discontinue MAOI ≥ 48 hours prior to myelography and resume ≥ 24 hours postprocedure.

Hepatic complications: Perform periodic liver function tests, such as bilirubins, alkaline phosphatase, or transaminases during therapy; discontinue at the first sign of hepatic dysfunction or jaundice.

Myocardial ischemia: MAOIs may suppress anginal pain that would otherwise serve as a warning of myocardial ischemia.

Hyperthyroid patients: Use **tranylcypromine** and **isocarboxazid** cautiously because of increased sensitivity to pressor amines.

Switching MAOIs: In several case reports, hypertensive crisis, cerebral hemorrhage and death have possibly resulted from switching from one MAOI to another without a waiting period. However, in other patients no adverse reactions occurred. Nevertheless, a waiting period of 10 to 14 days is recommended when switching from one MAOI to another.

Drug abuse and dependence: There have been reports of drug dependency in patients using doses of **tranylcypromine** and **isocarboxazid** significantly in excess of the therapeutic range.

Drug Interactions

Drugs that may affect MAOIs include dibenzazepine-related entities, disulfiram, methylphenidate, metrizamide, and sulfonamide.

Drugs that may be affected by MAOIs include anesthetics, antidepressants, antidiabetic agents, barbiturates, beta blockers, bupropion, buspirone, carbamazepine, cyclobenzapine, dextromethorphan, guanethidine, levodopa, meperidine, methyldopa, rauwolfia alkaloids, sulfonamide, sumatriptan, sympathomimetics, thiazide diuretics, and L-tryptophan.

Drug/Food interactions: Warn all patients against eating foods with a high **tyramine** content. Hypertensive crisis may result (see Warnings).

Adverse Reactions

Cardiovascular: Orthostatic hypotension, associated in some patients with falling; disturbances in cardiac rate and rhythm.

CNS: Dizziness; vertigo; headache; overactivity; hyperreflexia; tremors; muscle twitching; mania; hypomania; jitteriness; confusion; memory impairment; sleep disturbances including hypersomnia and insomnia; weakness; myoclonic movements; fatigue; drowsiness; restlessness; overstimulation including increased anxiety, agitation and manic symptoms.

GI: Constipation; nausea; diarrhea; abdominal pain.

Miscellaneous: Edema; dry mouth; blurred vision; hyperhidrosis; elevated serum transaminases; minor skin reactions such as skin rashes; anorexia; weight changes.

ANTIPSYCHOTIC AGENTS

Actions
Pharmacology:

Select Dosage and Pharmacologic Parameters of Antipsychotics							
Antipsychotic agent	Approx. equiv. dose (mg)	Adult daily dosage range (mg)	Sedation	Extrapyramidal symptoms	Anticholinergic effects	Orthostatic hypotension	Weight gain	Therapeutic plasma concentration (ng/mL)
Conventional (typical) agents								
Phenothiazines:								
Aliphatic								
Chlorpromazine	100	30 to 800	+++	++	++	+++		30 to 500
Promazine	200	40 to 1200	++	++	+++	++		
Triflupromazine	25	60 to 150	+++	++	+++	++		
Piperazine								
Fluphenazine	2	0.5 to 40	+	+++	+	+		0.5 to 3
Perphenazine	10	12 to 64	++	++	+	+		0.8 to 1.2
Prochlorperazine	15	15 to 150	++	+++	+	+		
Trifluoperazine	5	2 to 40	+	+++	+	+		
Piperidines								
Mesoridazine	50	30 to 400	+++	+	+++	++		
Thioridazine	100	150 to 800	+++	+	+++	+++		
Thioxanthenes:								
Thiothixene	4	8 to 30	+	+++	+	++		2 to 57
Phenylbutylpiperadines:								
Butyrophenone								
Haloperidol	2	1 to 15	+	+++	+	+		5 to 12
Diphenylbutylpiperadine								
Pimozide	0.3 to 0.5	1 to 10	++	+++	++	+		
Dihydroindolones:								
Molindone	10	15 to 225	++	++	+	+		
Dibenzepine:								
Dibenzoxazepines								
Loxapine	15	20 to 250	+	++	+	+		
Novel (atypical) agents								
Dibenzepines:								
Dibenzodiazepine								
Clozapine	50	300 to 900	+++	+	+++	++	++	
Thienbenzodiazepine								
Olanzapine		5 to 20	+++	+	+++	++	++	
Dibenzothiazepine								
Quetiapine		50 to 800	++	+	0	++	+	
Benzisoxazoles:								
Risperidone		4 to 16	+	+ to ++[1]	0	+	+	

+++ = High incidence of side effects   ++ = Moderate incidence of side effects   + = Low incidence of side effects.
[1] At doses > 10 mg/day, risperidone's EPS profile is similar to typical antipsychotics.

The exact mode of action is not fully understood. Antipsychotics block postsynaptic dopamine receptors in the basal ganglia, hypothalamus, limbic system, brain stem, and medulla.

Pharmacokinetics:
Absorption – Oral absorption tends to be erratic and variable. Peak plasma levels are seen 2 to 6 hours after oral use.

Distribution – These agents are widely distributed in tissues; CNS concentrations exceed those in plasma. They are highly bound to plasma proteins (91% to 99%).

Metabolism – Extensive biotransformation occurs in the liver.

Excretion – One-half of the excretion of these agents occurs via the kidneys and the other half occurs through enterohepatic circulation. Elimination half-lives range from 10 to ≥ 20 hours.

Contraindications

Comatose or severely depressed states; hypersensitivity (cross-sensitivity between phenothiazines may occur); presence of large amounts of other CNS depressants; bone marrow depression; blood dyscrasias; circulatory collapse (thioxanthenes); subcortical brain damage; Parkinson's disease (**haloperidol**); liver damage; cerebral arteriosclerosis; coronary artery disease; severe hypotension or hypertension; pediatric surgery (**prochlorperazine**); myeloproliferative disorders; history of clozapine-induced agranulocytosis or severe granulocytopenia (**clozapine**); treatment of simple tics or tics other than those associated with Tourette's disorder; drug-induced motor and phonic tics until it is determined whether the tics are caused by drugs or Tourette's disorder; patients with congenital long QT syndrome or history of cardiac arrhythmias; administration with other drugs that prolong the QT interval; patients receiving the azole antifungal agents itraconazole and ketoconazole; patients receiving the macrolide antibiotics clarithromycin, erythromycin, azithromycin, and dirithromycin (**pimozide**).

Warnings

Tardive dyskinesia (TD): TD, a syndrome consisting of potentially irreversible, involuntary dyskinetic movements, may develop in patients treated with neuroleptic drugs. Both the risk of developing TD and the likelihood that it will become irreversible are increased as duration of treatment and total cumulative dose administered increase.

Neuroleptic malignant syndrome (NMS): NMS is a rare idiosyncratic combination of EPS, hyperthermia, and autonomic disturbance. Onset may be hours to months after drug initiation, but once started, proceeds rapidly over 24 to 72 hours. It is most commonly associated with **haloperidol** and depot **fluphenazines**, but has occurred with **thiothixene, clozapine,** and **thioridazine** and may occur with other agents. NMS is potentially fatal, and requires intensive symptomatic treatment and immediate discontinuation of neuroleptic treatment.

CNS effects: These agents may impair mental or physical abilities, especially during the first few days. Drowsiness may occur during the first or second week, after which it generally disappears. If troublesome, lower the dosage. Caution patients against activities requiring alertness (eg, operating vehicles or machinery).

Antiemetic effects: Drugs with antiemetic effect can obscure signs of toxicity of other drugs, or mask symptoms of disease (eg, brain tumor, intestinal obstruction, Reye's syndrome). They can suppress the cough reflex; aspiration of vomitus is possible.

Agranulocytosis: Agranulocytosis, defined as a granulocyte count of < 500/mm³, occurs in association with **clozapine** use at a cumulative incidence at 1 year of ≈ 1.3%. This reaction could prove fatal if not detected early and therapy interrupted.

Serum cholesterol: Decreased serum cholesterol occurs. **Chlorpromazine** may raise plasma cholesterol.

Cardiovascular: Use with caution in patients with cardiovascular disease or mitral insufficiency. Increased pulse rates occur in most patients.

Orthostatic hypotension – Can occur, especially during intial titration in association with rapid dose escalation, and may represent a continuing risk in some patients.

Carefully watch patients who are undergoing surgery, and who are on large doses of phenothiazines, for hypotensive phenomena. The hypotensive effects may occur after the first injection of the antipsychotic, occasionally after subsequent injections, and rarely after the first oral dose. Recovery is usually spontaneous and symptoms disappear within 0.5 to 2 hours.

Tachycardia – Tachycardia, which may be sustained, has also been observed.

ECG changes: A minority of **clozapine** patients experience ECG repolarization changes similar to those seen with other antipsychotic drugs, including S-T segment depression and flattening or inversion of T waves, which all normalize after discontinuation of clozapine.

Risperidone appears to lengthen the QT interval in some patients. Other drugs that prolong the QT interval have been associated with the occurrence of torsades de pointes.

Ophthalmic: Use with caution in patients with a history of glaucoma. During prolonged therapy, ocular changes may occur; these include particle deposition in the cornea and lens, progressing in more severe cases to star-shaped lenticular opacities. Pigmentary retinopathy occurs most frequently in patients receiving **thioridazine** dosages > 1 g/day.

Cataracts – Lens changes have also been observed in patients taking **quetiapine** during long-term treatment. Examination of the lens by methods adequate to detect cataract formation, such as slit-lamp exam, is recommended at initiation of treatment or shortly thereafter, and at 6-month intervals.

Seizure disorders: These drugs can lower the convulsive threshold and may precipitate seizures. Use cautiously in patients with a history of epilepsy and only when absolutely necessary.

GI dysmotility: Adynamic ileus occasionally occurs with **phenothiazine** therapy and, if severe, can result in complications and death. Esophageal dysmotility and aspiration have been associated with antipsychotic drug use. Aspiration pneumonia is a common cause of morbidity and mortality in elderly patients, in particular those with advanced Alzheimer's dementia. Use **quetiapine** cautiously in patients at risk for aspiration pneumonia.

Adynamic ileus: Adynamic ileus occasionally occurs with phenothiazine therapy and, if severe, can result in complications and death. Use **quetiapine** cautiously in patients at risk for aspiration pneumonia.

Sudden death: Previous brain damage or seizures may be predisposing factors; avoid high doses in known seizure patients.

Priapism: Priapism has been reported with many of the antipsychotic agents.

Hepatic effects: Jaundice usually occurs between the second and fourth weeks of treatment and is regarded as a hypersensitivity reaction.

Renal function impairment: Administer cautiously to those with diminished renal function.

Hepatic function impairment: Use with caution in patients with impaired hepatic function. Patients with a history of hepatic encephalopathy caused by cirrhosis have increased sensitivity to the CNS effects of antipsychotic drugs (ie, impaired cerebration and abnormal slowing of the EEG). Dosage adjustments may be necessary in patients receiving **quetiapine** who are hepatically impaired.

Carcinogenesis: Neuroleptic drugs (except **promazine**) elevate prolactin levels which persist during chronic use. Tissue culture experiments indicate ≈ ⅓ of human breast cancers are prolactin-dependent in vitro, a factor of potential importance if use of these drugs is contemplated in a patient with previously detected breast cancer.

Elderly: Dosages in the lower range are sufficient for most elderly patients. Monitor response and adjust dosage accordingly. Increase dosage gradually in elderly patients.

Pregnancy: Category C. (Category B, clozapine).

Lactation: **Chlorpromazine** and **haloperidol** have been detected in breast milk. Safety for use in the nursing mother has not been established.

Children: In general, these products are not recommended for children < 12 years of age. **Loxapine** is not recommended in children < 16 years of age.

Precautions

Monitoring: Periodic assessment of transaminases is recommended in patients with significant hepatic disease (**olanzapine**).

Anticholinergic effects: Most antipsychotic agents are associated with constipation, dry mouth, and tachycardia, all adverse events possibly related to cholinergic antagonism. Anticholinergic effects of **clozapine** are very potent. Use caution in patients with clinically significant prostatic hypertrophy, narrow-angle glaucoma or a history of paralytic ileus. **Olanzapine** exhibits in vitro muscarinic receptor affinity and was associated with constipation, dry mouth, and tachycardia.

Dysphagia: Esophageal dysmotility and aspiration have been associated with antipsychotic drug use.

Cholesterol: Decreased serum cholesterol has occurred with some agents; however, **chlorpromazine** and **quetiapine** may raise plasma cholesterol.

Concomitant conditions: Use with caution in patients: Exposed to extreme heat or phosphorus insecticides; in a state of alcohol withdrawal; with dermatoses or other allergic reactions to phenothiazine derivatives because of the possibility of cross-sensitivity; who have exhibited idiosyncrasy to other centrally acting drugs.

Hematologic: Various blood dyscrasias have occurred.

Myelography: Discontinue phenothiazines at least 48 hours before myelography because of the possibility of seizures; do not resume therapy for at least 24 hours postprocedure.

Thyroid: Severe neurotoxicity (rigidity, inability to walk or talk) may occur in patients with thyrotoxicosis who are also receiving antipsychotics.

Hyperpyrexia: A significant, not otherwise explained rise in body temperature may indicate intolerance to antipsychotics.

ECT: Reserve concurrent use with electroconvulsive treatment for those patients for whom it is essential; the hazards may be increased.

Abrupt withdrawal: These drugs are not known to cause psychic dependence and do not produce tolerance or addiction. However, following abrupt withdrawal of high dose therapy, symptoms such as gastritis, nausea, vomiting, dizziness, headache, tachycardia, insomnia, and tremulousness have occurred. These symptoms can be reduced by gradual reduction of the dosage (one suggestion is 10% to 25% every 2 weeks) or by continuing antiparkinson agents for several weeks after the antipsychotic is withdrawn.

Suicide: Suicide possibility in depressed patients remains during treatment and until significant remission occurs. This type of patient should not have access to large quantities of the drug.

Cutaneous pigmentation changes/photosensitivity: Rare instances of skin pigmentation have occurred, primarily in females on long-term, high dose therapy. Photosensitization may occur; caution patients against exposure to ultraviolet light or undue exposure to sunlight during phenothiazine therapy. These effects occur most commonly with **chlorpromazine** (3%).

Drug abuse and dependence: Evaluate patients for history of drug abuse, and observe such patients closely for signs of **risperidone** misuse or abuse (eg, development of tolerance, increases in dose, drug-seeking behavior).

Drug Interactions

Drugs that may affect phenothiazines include aluminum salts, anorexiants, anticholinergics, barbiturates, charcoal, lithium, meperidine, methyldopa, metrizamide, and propranolol.

Drugs that may be affected by phenothiazines include barbiturate anesthetics, bromocriptine, norepinephrine, epinephrine, guanethidine, phenytoin, propranolol, TCAs, and valproic acid.

Drugs that may affect the antipsychotics include carbamazepine, cimetidine, fluoxetine, methyldopa, phenytoin, and clozapine.

Drugs that may be affected by antipsychotics include dopamine agonists, levodopa, antiarrhythmics, phenothiazines, lorazepam, thioridazine, anticholinergics, and antihypertensives.

Drug/Lab test interactions: An increase in cephalin flocculation sometimes accompanied by alterations in other liver function tests has occurred in patients receiving **fluphenazine** enanthate who have had no clinical evidence of liver damage.

Phenothiazines may discolor the urine pink to red-brown.

False-positive pregnancy tests have occurred, but are less likely to occur when a serum test is used.

An increase in protein bound iodine, not attributable to an increase in thyroxine, has been noted.

Adverse Reactions

Typical antipsychotic agents –

CNS effects: Headache; weakness; tremor; staggering gait; twitching; tension; jitteriness; fatigue; slurring; insomnia; vertigo; drowsiness (80%, usually lasts 1 week); akinesia; ataxia; pseudoparkinsonism; akathesia; dystonias; cerebral edema; exacerbation of psychotic symptoms including hallucinations; catatonic-like states; lethargy; restlessness; hyperactivity; agitation; nocturnal confusion; toxic confusional states; bizarre dreams; depression; euphoria; excitement; paranoid reactions.

Autonomic: Dry mouth; nasal congestion; nausea; vomiting; paresthesia; anorexia; pallor; flushed facies; salivation; perspiration; constipation; fecal impaction; diarrhea; urinary retention, frequency or incontinence; bladder paralysis; polyuria; enuresis; priapism; ejaculation inhibition; male impotence (not reported with **molindone**).

Heatstroke/Hyperpyrexia – Heatstroke/Hyperpyrexia induced by neuroleptics has occurred.

Hepatic – Jaundice usually occurs between the second and fourth weeks of therapy and is regarded as a hypersensitivity reaction.

Hematologic – Eosinophilia; leukopenia; leukocytosis; anemia; tendency toward lymphomonocytosis; thrombocytopenia; granulocytopenia; aplastic anemia; hemolytic anemia; thrombocytopenic or nonthrombocytopenic purpura; agranulocytosis; pancytopenia.

Agranulocytosis – Most cases occurred between therapy weeks 4 and 10. Watch for sudden appearance of sore mouth, gums, throat, or other signs of infection.

Cardiovascular – Hypotension; postural hypotension; hypertension; tachycardia (especially with rapid increase in dosage); bradycardia; cardiac arrest; circulatory collapse; syncope; lightheadedness; faintness; dizziness.

Cardiovascular effects are generally attributable to the piperidine phenothiazines > aliphatic > piperazines (see table).

Hypersensitivity – Urticarial (5%), maculopapular hypersensitivity reactions; pruritus; dry skin; erythema; photosensitivity; eczema; asthma; rashes, including acneiform; hair loss; exfoliative dermatitis.

Endocrine – Lactation and moderate breast engorgement in females; galactorrhea; mastalgia; amenorrhea; menstrual irregularities; gynecomastia in males on large doses; changes in libido; hyperglycemia or hypoglycemia; hyponatremia; glycosuria; raised plasma cholesterol levels; pituitary tumor correlated with hyperprolactinemia. Resumption of menses in previously amenorrheic women has been reported with **molindone**. Initially, heavy menses may occur.

Ophthalmic – Glaucoma; photophobia; blurred vision; miosis; mydriasis; ptosis; star-shaped lenticular opacities; epithelial keratopathies; pigmentary retinopathy.

Respiratory – Laryngospasm; bronchospasm; increased depth of respiration; dyspnea.

Miscellaneous – Increases in appetite and weight (excessive weight gain has not occurred with **molindone**); dyspepsia; peripheral or facial edema; suppression of cough reflex (with potential for aspiration or asphyxia); enlarged parotid glands; polyphagia; polydipsia; systemic lupus; erythematous-like syndrome.

Atypical antipsychotic agents:

Cardiovascular – Chest pain/angina; hypertension; hypotension; postural hypotension; tachycardia.

CNS – Aggressive reaction; agitation; akathesia; anxiety; confusion; disturbed sleep/nightmares; dizziness; headache; insomnia; personality disorder; restlessness; rigidity; seizures (convulsions); somnolence/drowsiness; syncope; tremor.

Dermatologic – Dry skin; rash.

GI – Abdominal pain; constipation; dry mouth; dyspepsia; nausea; vomiting.

Hematologic/Lymphatic – Leukopenia/decreased WBC/neutropenia.

Respiratory – Coughing; pharyngitis; rhinitis; upper respiratory tract infection.

Miscellaneous – Arthralgia; asthenia; back pain; fever; muscle pain; sweating; visual disturbances; weight gain; joint pain; extremity pain (other than joint); amblyopia; hypertonia.

PHENOTHIAZINE AND THIOXANTHENE DERIVATIVES

PHENOTHIAZINE DERIVATIVES
CHLORPROMAZINE HCl

Tablets: 10, 25, 50, 100, and 200 mg (*Rx*)	Various, *Thorazine* (GlaxoSmithKline)
Capsules, sustained release: 30, 75, and 150 mg (*Rx*)	*Thorazine Spansules* (GlaxoSmithKline)
Syrup: 10 mg/5 mL (*Rx*)	*Thorazine* (GlaxoSmithKline)
Concentrate: 30 mg/mL and 100 mg/mL (*Rx*)	Various, *Thorazine* (GlaxoSmithKline)
Suppositories (as base): 25 and 100 mg (*Rx*)	*Thorazine* (GlaxoSmithKline)
Injection: 25 mg/mL (*Rx*)	Various, *Thorazine* (GlaxoSmithKline)

FLUPHENAZINE

Tablets: 1, 2.5, 5, and 10 mg (*Rx*)	Various, *Permitil* (Schering), *Prolixin* (Apothecon)
Elixir: 2.5 mg/5 mL (*Rx*)	*Prolixin* (Apothecon)
Concentrate: 5 mg/mL (*Rx*)	Various, *Prolixin* (Apothecon)
Injection: 2.5 mg/mL and 25 mg/mL (*Rx*)	Various, *Prolixin* (Apothecon) Various, *Prolixin Decanoate* (Apothecon)

MESORIDAZINE

Tablets: 10, 25, 50, and 100 mg (*Rx*)	*Serentil* (Boehringer Ingelheim)
Concentrate: 25 mg/mL (*Rx*)	*Serentil* (Boehringer Ingelheim)
Injection: 25 mg/mL (*Rx*)	*Serentil* (Boehringer Ingelheim)

PERPHENAZINE

Tablets: 2, 4, 8, and 16 mg (*Rx*)	Various, *Trilafon* (Schering)
Concentrate: 16 mg/5 mL (*Rx*)	*Trilafon* (Schering)
Injection: 5 mg/mL (*Rx*)	*Trilafon* (Schering)

PROCHLORPERAZINE

Tablets: 5, 10, and 25 mg (*Rx*)	Various, *Compazine* (GlaxoSmithKline)
Capsules, sustained release: 10 and 15 mg (*Rx*)	*Compazine* (GlaxoSmithKline)
Suppositories: 2.5, 5, and 25 mg (*Rx*)	*Compazine* (GlaxoSmithKline)
Syrup: 5 mg/5 mL (*Rx*)	*Compazine* (GlaxoSmithKline)
Injection: 5 mg/mL (*Rx*)	Various, *Compazine* (GlaxoSmithKline)

PROMAZINE HCl

Tablets: 25 and 50 mg (*Rx*)	Various, *Sparine* (Wyeth-Ayerst)
Injection: 25 mg/mL and 50 mg/mL (*Rx*)	Various

TRIFLUPROMAZINE HCl

Injection: 10 mg/mL and 20 mg/mL (*Rx*)	*Vesprin* (Apothecon)

THIORIDAZINE HCl

Tablets: 10, 15, 25, 50, 100, 150, and 200 mg (*Rx*)	Various, *Mellaril* (Novartis)
Concentrate: 30 mg/mL and 100 mg/mL (*Rx*)	Various, *Mellaril* (Novartis)
Suspension: 25 mg/5 mL and 100 mg/5 mL (*Rx*)	*Mellaril-S* (Novartis)

TRIFLUOPERAZINE	
Tablets: 1, 2, 5, and 10 mg (*Rx*)	Various, *Stelazine* (GlaxoSmithKline)
Concentrate: 10 mg/mL (*Rx*)	Various, *Stelazine* (GlaxoSmithKline)
Injection: 2 mg/mL (*Rx*)	Various, *Stelazine* (GlaxoSmithKline)

THIOXANTHENE DERIVATIVES

THIOTHIXENE	
Capsules: 1, 2, 5, 10, and 20 mg (*Rx*)	Various, *Navane* (Roerig)
Concentrate: 5 mg/mL (*Rx*)	Various, *Navane* (Roerig)

Indications

Chlorpromazine HCl:

Psychotic disorders – Management of manifestations of psychotic disorders; control of the manifestations of the manic type of manic-depressive illness.

Behavioral disorders, pediatric – Treatment of severe behavioral problems in children marked by combativeness or explosive hyperexcitable behavior (out of proportion to immediate provocations), and in the short-term treatment of hyperactive children who show excessive motor activity with accompanying conduct disorders consisting of some or all of the following symptoms: Impulsivity, difficulty sustaining attention, aggressivity, mood lability and poor frustration tolerance.

Surgery – Relief of restlessness and apprehension prior to surgery.

Tetanus – An adjunct in treatment of tetanus.

Acute intermittant porphyria – Treatment of acute intermittent porphyria.

Emesis – Also indicated for the control of nausea and vomiting and relief of intractable hiccoughs (see Antiemetic/Antivertigo Agents).

Fluphenazine:

Psychotic disorders – Management of manifestations of psychotic disorders; esterified formulations (enanthate and decanoate) are indicated for patients requiring prolonged and parenteral neuroleptic therapy (eg, chronic schizophrenics).

Mesoridazine:

Schizophrenia – Reduces the severity of emotional withdrawal, conceptual disorganization, anxiety, tension, hallucinatory behavior, suspiciousness and blunted affect.

Behavioral problems in mental deficiency and chronic brain syndrome – Reduces hyperactivity and uncooperativeness associated with mental deficiency and chronic brain syndrome.

Alcoholism (acute and chronic) – Ameliorates anxiety, tension, depression, nausea and vomiting in acute and chronic alcoholics without producing hepatic dysfunction or hindering the functional recovery of the impaired liver.

Psychoneurotic manifestations – Reduces the symptoms of anxiety and tension and prevalent symptoms often associated with neurotic components of many disorders. It also benefits personality disorders in general.

Perphenazine:

Psychotic disorders – Management of manifestations of psychotic disorders.

Emesis (IV only) – To control severe nausea and vomiting and intractable hiccoughs (see Antiemetic/Antivertigo Agents).

Prochlorperazine:

Psychotic disorders – Management of manifestations of psychotic disorders.

Anxiety – Short-term treatment of generalized nonpsychotic anxiety; however, prochlorperazine is not the drug of choice for this indication.

Emesis – To control severe nausea and vomiting (see Antiemetic/Antivertigo Agents).

Promazine HCl:

Psychotic disorders – Management of the manifestations of psychotic disorders.

Trifluoperazine HCl:

Psychotic disorders – Management of manifestations of psychotic disorders.

Anxiety – Short-term treatment of nonpsychotic anxiety (not the drug of choice in most patients).

Thoridazine HCl:
  Psychotic disorders – Management of manifestations of psychotic disorders and short-term treatment of moderate to marked depression with variable degrees of anxiety in adults.

  Psychoneurotic manifestations – Treatment of multiple symptoms such as agitation, anxiety, depressed mood, tension, sleep disturbances and fears in the geriatric patient.

  Behavioral disorders, pediatric – Treatment of severe behavioral problems in children marked by combativeness or explosive hyperexcitable behavior (out of proportion to immediate provocations) and in the short-term treatment of hyperactive children who show excessive motor activity with accompanying conduct disorders consisting of some or all of the followng symptoms: Impulsivity, difficulty sustaining attention, aggressivity, mood lability and poor frustration tolerance.

Thiothixene:
  Psychotic disorders – Management of manifestations of psychotic disorders.

Administration and Dosage
  CHLORPROMAZINE:
    Adults –
      Concentrate: Add desired dosage to ≥ 60 mL of diluent just prior to administration. Suggested vehicles are tomato or fruit juice, milk, simple syrup, orange syrup, carbonated beverages, coffee, tea, or water. Semisolid foods (eg, soups, puddings) may also be used.
      Sustained release capsules: Do not crush or chew. Swallow whole.
      Injection: Do not inject SC. Inject IM slowly, deep into upper outer quadrant of buttock. Use the IV route only for severe hiccoughs, surgery, and tetanus.
      Outpatients: For prompt control of severe symptoms 25 mg IM; if necessary, repeat in 1 hour. Give subsequent oral doses of 25 to 50 mg 3 times/day.
        The usual initial oral dose is 10 mg 3 or 4 times/day or 25 mg 2 or 3 times/day. For more serious cases, give 25 mg 3 times/day. After 1 or 2 days, increase daily dosage by 20 to 50 mg semiweekly, until patient becomes calm and cooperative. Continue optimum dosage for 2 weeks, then gradually reduce to maintenance level; 200 mg per day is not unusual.
      Psychotic disorders:
        Acutely manic or disturbed –
          IM: 25 mg initially. If necessary, give an additional 25 to 50 mg injection in 1 hour. Increase gradually over several days (up to 400 mg every 4 to 6 hours in severe cases) until patient is controlled. Patient usually becomes quiet and cooperative within 24 to 48 hours. Substitute oral dosage and increase until the patient is calm; 500 mg/day is usually sufficient. While gradual increases to 2000 mg or more/day may be necessary, little therapeutic gain is achieved by exceeding 1000 mg/day for extended periods.
        Less acutely disturbed –
          Oral: 25 mg 3 times/day. Increase gradually until effective dose is reached, usually 400 mg/day.
      Behavioral disorders, pediatric: Chlorpromazine should generally not be used in children < 6 months old except where potentially lifesaving. It should not be used in conditions for which specific children's dosages have not been established.
        Outpatients –
          Oral: 0.5 mg/kg (0.25 mg/lb) every 4 to 6 hours, as needed.
          Rectal: 1 mg/kg (0.5 mg/lb) every 6 to 8 hours, as needed.
          IM: 0.5 mg/kg (0.25 mg/lb) every 6 to 8 hours, as needed.
        Hospitalized patients –
          Oral: Start with low doses and increase gradually. In severe behavior disorders or psychotic conditions, 50 to 100 mg/day, or in older children, 200 mg or more daily may be necessary. There is little evidence that improvement in severely disturbed mentally retarded patients is enhanced by doses > 500 mg/day.
          IM: *Up to 5 years of age:* Do not exceed 40 mg/day.

5 to 12 years of age – Do not exceed 75 mg/day, except in unmanageable cases.

Surgery:

Adults –

Preoperative: 25 to 50 mg orally 2 to 3 hours before surgery or 12.5 to 25 mg IM 1 to 2 hours before surgery.

Intraoperative (to control acute nausea and vomiting):

IM – 12.5 mg. Repeat in ½ hour if necessary and if no hypotension occurs.

IV – 2 mg per fractional injection at 2-minute intervals. Do not exceed 25 mg (dilute 1 mg/mL with saline).

Children –

Preoperative: 0.5 mg/kg (0.25 mg/lb) orally 2 to 3 hours before operation or 0.5 mg/kg (0.25 mg/lb) IM 1 to 2 hours before operation.

Intraoperative (administer only to control acute nausea and vomiting):

IM – 0.25 mg/kg (0.125 mg/lb); repeat in ½ hour if needed, and if no hypotension occurs.

IV – 1 mg per fractional injection at 2 minute intervals; do not exceed IM dosage. Always dilute to 1 mg/mL with saline.

Tetanus:

Adults – 25 to 50 mg IM 3 or 4 times/day, usually with barbiturates. For IV use, 25 to 50 mg diluted to at least 1 mg/mL and administered at a rate of 1 mg/minute.

Children (IM or IV) – 0.5 mg/kg (0.25 mg/lb) every 6 to 8 hours. When given IV, dilute to at least 1 mg/mL and administer at a rate of 1 mg per 2 minutes. In children up to 23 kg (50 lbs), do not exceed 40 mg/day; 23 to 45 kg (50 to 100 lbs), do not exceed 75 mg/day, except in severe cases.

Acute intermittent porphyria: 25 to 50 mg orally or 25 mg IM 3 or 4 times/day until patient can take oral therapy.

Admixture compatibility: A mixture of chlorpromazine, hydroxyzine and meperidine in the same glass or plastic syringe is stable for 1 year when stored at refrigeration (4°C; 39°F) or room temperature (25°C; 77°F). The combination was unstable at higher temperatures.

A precipitate or discoloration may occur when chlorpromazine is admixed with morphine, meperidine or other products preserved with cresols.

FLUPHENAZINE HCl:

Oral –

Adults: Initially 0.5 to 10 mg/day in divided doses administered at 6 to 8 hour intervals. In general, a daily dose in excess of 3 mg is rarely necessary. Use doses in excess of 20 mg with caution. When symptoms are controlled, reduce dosage gradually to daily maintenance doses of 1 to 5 mg, often given as a single daily dose.

Geriatric patients – Starting dose is 1 to 2.5 mg/day, adjusted according to response.

IM *(fluphenazine HCl) –* The average starting dose is 1.25 mg IM (fluphenazine HCl). The initial total daily dosage may range from 2.5 to 10 mg, divided and given at 6 to 8 hour intervals. In general, the parenteral dose is ≈ ⅓ to ½ the oral dose. Use dosages exceeding 10 mg/day IM with caution.

Esterified formulations (enanthate and decanoate formulations): Administer IM or SC. Use a dry syringe and needle of at least 21 gauge. A wet needle or syringe may cause the solution to become cloudy. Initiate with 12.5 to 25 mg. Determine subsequent injections and dosage interval in accordance with patient response. Do not exceed 100 mg. If doses > 50 mg are needed, increase succeeding doses cautiously in 12.5 mg increments.

Significantly more injection site leakage has occurred after IM administration compared to SC use; consider this possibility with nonresponders to IM therapy.

Initially, treat patients who have never taken phenothiazines with a shorter-acting form of the drug before administering the enanthate or decanoate. This helps to determine the response to fluphenazine and to establish appropriate dosage. The equivalent dosage of fluphenazine HCl to the longer-acting forms is not known; exercise caution when switching from shorter-acting forms to the enanthate.

No precise formula can be given to convert to use of fluphenazine decanoate. However, in a controlled multicenter study, 20 mg fluphenazine HCl daily was equivalent to 25 mg decanoate every 3 weeks. This is an approximate conversion ratio of 0.5 mL (12.5 mg) decanoate every 3 weeks for every 10 mg fluphenazine HCl daily.

Severely agitated patients – Treat initially with a rapid-acting phenothiazine such as fluphenazine HCl injection. When acute symptoms subside, administer 25 mg of the enanthate or decanoate; adjust subsequent dosage as necessary.

"Poor risk" patients – "Poor risk" patients (known phenothiazine hypersensitivity or with disorders predisposing to undue reactions): Initiate cautiously oral or parenteral fluphenazine HCl. When appropriate dosage is established, give equivalent dose of enanthate or decanoate.

PERPHENAZINE:
 Psychotic disorders –
  Oral: Moderately disturbed nonhospitalized patients: 4 to 8 mg 3 times/day; reduce as soon as possible to minimum effective dosage.
   Hospitalized patients – 8 to 16 mg 2 to 4 times/day; avoid dosages > 64 mg/day.
  IM: Use when rapid effect and prompt control are required or when oral administration is not feasible. Administer by deep IM injection to a seated or recumbent patient; observe patient for a short period after administration. Therapeutic effect usually occurs in 10 minutes and is maximal in 1 to 2 hours. The average duration of effect is 6 hours, occasionally, 12 to 24 hours.
   Initial dose – 5 mg every 6 hours. The total daily dosage should not exceed 15 mg in ambulatory patients or 30 mg in hospitalized patients. Initiate oral therapy as soon as possible, generally within 24 hours. However, patients have been maintained on parenteral therapy for several months. Use equal or higher dosage when the patient is transferred to oral therapy after receiving the injection.
   While 5 mg IM has a definite tranquilizing effect, it may be necessary to use 10 mg to initiate therapy in severely agitated states. Most patients are controlled and oral therapy can be instituted within a maximum of 24 to 48 hours. Acute conditions (hysteria, panic reaction) often respond well to a single dose, whereas in chronic conditions, several injections may be required.
  Children: Pediatric dosage has not been established. Children > 12 years of age may receive the lowest limit of the adult dosage.
  Elderly: Administer one-third to one-half the adult dose.

PROCHLORPERAZINE: Administration SC is not advisable because of local irritation. Individualize dosage. Begin with the lowest recommended dosage.
 Psychotic disorders – Although response ordinarily is seen within 1 to 2 days, longer treatment is usually required before maximal improvement is observed.
  Oral:
   Adults – In mild conditions, give 5 or 10 mg 3 or 4 times/day. In moderate to severe conditions, for hospitalized or adequately supervised patients, give 10 mg 3 or 4 times/day. Increase dosage gradually until symptoms are controlled or side effects become bothersome. When dosage is increased by small increments every 2 or 3 days, side effects either do not occur or are easily controlled. Some patients respond to 50 to 75 mg/day. In more severe disturbances, optimum dosage is 100 to 150 mg/day.
   Children – 2.5 mg 2 or 3 times/day. Do not give > 10 mg on first day. Increase dosage according to patient response.
  IM:
   Adults – For immediate control of severely disturbed adults, inject an initial dose of 10 to 20 mg deeply into the upper outer quadrant of the buttock. Many patients respond shortly after the first injection. If necessary, repeat every 2 to 4 hours (or in resistant cases, every hour) to gain control. More than 3 or 4 doses

are seldom necessary. After control is achieved, switch patient to the oral drug at the same dosage level or higher. If prolonged parenteral therapy is needed, give 10 to 20 mg every 4 to 6 hours.

Children < 12 years of age – 0.03 mg/kg (0.06 mg/lb) by deep IM injection. After control is achieved, usually after 1 dose, switch to oral form at same dosage level or higher.

Rectal:

Children 2 to 5 years of age – Do not exceed 20 mg total daily dose.

Children 6 to 12 years of age – Do not exceed 25 mg total daily dose.

Anxiety –

Oral: 5 mg 3 or 4 times/day; 15 mg (sustained release) on arising, or 10 mg (sustained release) every 12 hours. Do not administer > 20 mg/day or for > 12 weeks.

Elderly – Lower doses are sufficient for most elderly patients. Since they appear more susceptible to hypotension and neuromuscular reactions, observe patients closely. Monitor response and adjust dosage accordingly; increase dosage gradually.

Children – Do not use in children < 20 lbs (9.1 kg) or < 2 years of age. Do not use in pediatric surgery. Children seem more prone to develop extrapyramidal reactions, even on moderate doses. Use the lowest effective dose. Occasionally, the patient may react to the drug with signs of restlessness and excitement; if this occurs, do not administer additional doses. Use with caution in children with acute illnesses or dehydration. Do not use in conditions for which children's dosages are not established.

Compatibility – Do not mix prochlorperazine injection with other agents in the syringe. Do not dilute with any diluent containing parabens as a preservative.

PROMAZINE: Injection IM is preferred. Because of increased potential of orthostatic hypotension, reserve parenteral administration for bedfast patients, although acute states in ambulatory patients may also be treated by IM injection, provided proper precautions are taken. Give IM injections deep into large muscle masses (eg, gluteal region). IV administration is not recommended.

Adults – In the management of severely agitated patients, administer initial doses of 50 to 150 mg IM, depending on the degree of excitation. Once control is obtained, administer orally. The oral or IM dose is 10 to 200 mg at 4 to 6 hour intervals. Maintenance dosage may range from 10 to 200 mg given at 4 to 6 hour intervals.

Do not exceed a total daily dose of 1000 mg, since higher doses have not yielded greater results.

Children (> 12 years of age) – In acute episodes of chronic psychotic disease, 10 to 25 mg may be given every 4 to 6 hours.

MESORIDAZINE:

Mesoridazine Dosage Guidelines		
Disease state	Initial oral dose	Optimum total dosage range (mg/day)
Schizophrenia	50 mg tid	100-400
Behavior problems in mental deficiency and chronic brain syndrome	25 mg tid	75-300
Alcoholism	25 mg bid	50-200
Psychoneurotic manifestations	10 mg tid	30-150

IM administration – For most patients, 25 mg initially. May repeat dose in 30 to 60 minutes, if necessary. The usual optimum dosage range is 25 to 200 mg/day.

Concentrate – Concentrate may be diluted just prior to administration with distilled water, acidified tap water or orange or grape juice. Do not prepare and store bulk dilutions.

THIORIDAZINE:

Psychotic manifestations – Usual initial dose is 50 to 100 mg 3 times/day; increase gradually to a maximum of 800 mg/day, if necessary, to control symptoms; then reduce gradually to the minimum maintenance dose. Total daily dosage ranges from 200 to 800 mg divided into 2 to 4 doses.

Psychoneurotic manifestations – Usual initial dose is 25 mg 3 times/day. Dosage ranges from 10 mg 2 to 4 times/day in milder cases, to 50 mg 3 or 4 times/day for more severely disturbed patients. Total daily dosage ranges from 20 to 200 mg.

Behavioral disorders, pediatric – Not recommended for children < 2 years of age. For children aged 2 to 12, the dosage ranges from 0.5 mg to a maximum of 3 mg/kg/day.

Moderate disorders: 10 mg 2 or 3 times/day is the usual starting dose.

Hospitalized, severely disturbed or psychotic children: 25 mg 2 or 3 times/day.

TRIFLUPROMAZINE:
Psychotic disorders – 60 mg IM, up to a maximum of 150 mg/day.

Children: The recommended IM dosage range is 0.2 to 0.25 mg/kg, up to a maximum total dose of 10 mg/day. Do not administer to children < 2.5 years of age.

TRIFLUOPERAZINE:
Psychotic disorders – 2 to 5 mg orally twice/day. Most patients will show optimum response with 15 or 20 mg/day, although a few may require ≥ 40 mg/day. Optimum therapeutic dosage levels should be reached within 2 or 3 weeks.

IM (for prompt control of severe symptoms) – 1 to 2 mg by deep injection every 4 to 6 hours, as needed. More than 6 mg/24 hours is rarely necessary.

Children 6 to 12 years of age – Adjust dosage to the weight of the child and severity of symptoms. These dosages are for children, aged 6 to 12, who are hospitalized or under close supervision.

Oral: Initial dose is 1 mg once or twice/day. While it is usually not necessary to exceed 15 mg/day, older children with severe symptoms may require higher doses.

IM: There has been little experience in children. However, if it is necessary to achieve rapid control of severe symptoms, administer 1 mg once or twice a day.

Elderly patients – Usually, lower dosages are sufficient.

Treatment of nonpsychotic anxiety – 1 or 2 mg twice/day. Do not administer > 6 mg/day or for > 12 weeks.

THIOTHIXENE:
Oral – Not recommended in children < 12 years of age.

Mild conditions: Initially 2 mg 3 times/day. If indicated, an increase to 15 mg/day is often effective.

Severe conditions: Initially 5 mg twice/day. Optimal is 20 to 30 mg/day. If indicated, 60 mg/day is often effective. Exceeding 60 mg/day rarely increases response.

PHENYLBUTYLPIPERADINE DERIVATIVES

HALOPERIDOL
Tablets: 0.5, 1, 2, 5, 10, and 20 mg (*Rx*) — Various, *Haldol* (McNeil)
Concentrate: 2 mg/mL (*Rx*) — Various, *Haldol* (McNeil)
Injection: 5 mg/mL, 50 mg/mL, and 100 mg/mL (*Rx*) — Various, *Haldol* (McNeil), *Haldol Decanoate 50* (McNeil), *Haldol Decanoate 100* (McNeil)

PIMOZIDE
Tablets: 2 mg (*Rx*) — *Orap* (Gate)

Indications
Haloperidol:
Psychotic disorder – Psychotic disorder management; haloperidol decanoate is a long-acting parenteral antipsychotic for patients requiring prolonged parenteral neuroleptic therapy (eg, chronic schizophrenia).

Tourette's – For the control of tics and vocal utterances in children and adults with Tourette's disorder.

Behavioral problems – Behavioral problems in children with combative, explosive hyperexcitability that cannot be accounted for by immediate provocation.

Hyperactivity – For short-term treatment of hyperactive children who show excessive motor activity with accompanying conduct disorders consisting of impulsivity, difficulty sustaining attention, aggression, mood lability or poor frustration tolerance.

Pimozide:

Tourette's – For the suppression of severely compromising motor and phonic tics in patients with Tourette's disorder who have failed to respond satisfactorily to standard treatment.

Unlabeled uses:

Haloperidol – IM or IV for acute psychiatric situations at 2 to 30 mg, approximately every 60 minutes, at a rate of 5 mg/min; for intractable hiccoughs at 1.5 mg orally 3 times/day or 3 to 15 mg IM or IV in divided doses. Suggested doses for children 3 to 6 years old include: Agitation and hyperkinesia - 0.01 to 0.03 mg/kg/day orally; infantile autism - 0.5 to 4 mg/day.

Administration and Dosage

HALOPERIDOL: Individualize dosage. Children, debilitated, or geriatric patients and those with a history of adverse reactions to neuroleptic drugs may require less haloperidol.

Psychotic disorders –

Adults: Initial dosage range: Moderate symptoms or geriatric or debilitated patients: 0.5 to 2 mg given 2 or 3 times/day; severe symptoms or chronic or resistant patients: 3 to 5 mg 2 or 3 times/day. To achieve prompt control, higher doses may be required.

Patients who remain severely disturbed or inadequately controlled may require dosage adjustment. Daily dosages up to 100 mg may be necessary. Infrequently, doses > 100 mg have been used for severely resistant patients; however, safety of prolonged administration of such doses has not been demonstrated.

Children (3 to 12 years of age): Do not use in children < 3 years of age. Initial dose is 0.5 mg/day (25 to 50 mcg/kg/day). If required, increase in 0.5 mg increments each 5 to 7 days up to 0.15 mcg/kg/day or until therapeutic effect is obtained. Total dose may be divided and given 2 or 3 times/day. The dose in this age group has not been well established.

IM administration: 2 to 5 mg for prompt control of the acutely agitated patient with moderately severe to very severe symptoms. Depending on response, administer subsequent doses as often as every 60 minutes, although 4- to 8-hour intervals may be satisfactory.

The safety and efficacy of IM administration in children have not been established.

The oral form should replace the injectable as soon as feasible. For an approximation of the total daily dose required, use the parenteral dose administered in the preceding 24 hours; carefully monitor the patient for the first several days. Give the first oral dose within 12 to 24 hours following the last parenteral dose.

Tourette's –

Adults: A starting dose of 0.5 to 1.5 mg 3 times/day by mouth has been suggested; up to about 10 mg/day may be needed. Requirements vary considerably and the dose must be very carefully adjusted to obtain the optimum response.

Children (3 to 12 years of age): 0.05 to 0.075 mg/kg/day. Severely disturbed psychotic children may require higher doses.

Behavioral disorders/Hyperactivity –

Children (3 to 12 years of age): 0.05 to 0.075 mg/kg/day. Severely disturbed psychotic children may require higher doses.

In severely disturbed, nonpsychotic children or in hyperactive children with conduct disorders, short-term administration may suffice. There is little evidence that behavior improvement is further enhanced by dosages > 6 mg/day.

Haloperidol decanoate injection – Administer by deep IM injection. A 21-gauge needle is recommended. The maximum volume per injection site should not exceed 3 mL. The recommended interval between doses is 4 weeks. Do not administer IV.

For patients previously maintained on low doses of antipsychotics (eg, up to the equivalent of 10 mg/day oral haloperidol), it is recommended that the initial dose of haloperidol decanoate be 10 to 15 times the previous daily dose in oral haloperidol equivalents; limited clinical experience suggests that lower initial doses may be adequate. Express the dose in terms of its haloperidol content. The preferred approach to determining the minimum effective dose is to begin with lower initial doses and to adjust the dose upward as needed. The initial dose of haloperidol decanoate should not exceed 100 mg regardless of previous antipsychotic dose requirements. Haloperidol decanoate has been effectively administered at monthly intervals in several clinical studies.

Elderly/Debilitated – Lower initial doses and more gradual adjustment are recommended. Clinical experience with haloperidol decanoate at doses > 450 mg/month has been limited.

PIMOZIDE: Introduce the drug slowly and gradually. Perform ECG at baseline and periodically thereafter, especially during dosage adjustment.

Tourette's –

Adults:

Initial dose – 1 to 2 mg/day in divided doses. Thereafter, increase dose every other day.

Maintenance dose – < 0.2 mg/kg/day or 10 mg/day, whichever is less. Do not exceed 0.2 mg/kg/day or 10 mg/day.

Children (> 12 years of age): Although Tourette's disorder most often has its onset between the ages of 2 and 15 years, information on the use and efficacy of pimozide in patients < 12 years of age is limited.

Initiate at a dose of 0.05 mg/kg preferably taken once at bedtime; dose may be increased every third day to a maximum of 0.2 mg/kg, not to exceed 10 mg/day.

Gradual withdrawal – Periodically attempt to reduce dosage to see if tics persist. Increases of tic intensity and frequency may represent a transient, withdrawal-related phenomenon rather than a return of symptoms. Allow 1 or 2 weeks to elapse before concluding that an increase in tic manifestations is caused by the underlying disease rather than drug withdrawal.

MOLINDONE HCl

Tablets: 5, 10, 25, 50, and 100 mg *(Rx)*
Concentrate: 20 mg/mL *(Rx)*

Moban (Gate)

Indications
Psychotic disorders: Management of manifestations of psychotic disorders.

Administration and Dosage
Initial dosage: 50 to 75 mg/day, increased to 100 mg/day in 3 or 4 days. Individualize dosage; patients with severe symptoms may require up to 225 mg/day.

Start elderly and debilitated patients on lower dosage.

Maintenance therapy:
Mild – 5 to 15 mg 3 or 4 times/day;
Moderate – 10 to 25 mg 3 or 4 times/day;
Severe – 225 mg/day may be required.

DIBENZAPINE DERIVATIVES

LOXAPINE	
Capsules: 5, 10, 25, and 50 mg (*Rx*)	Various, *Loxitane* (Lederle)
Concentrate: 25 mg/mL (*Rx*)	*Loxitane C* (Lederle)
Injection: 50 mg/mL (*Rx*)	*Loxitane IM* (Lederle)
CLOZAPINE	
Tablets: 25 and 100 mg (*Rx*)	Various, *Clozaril* (Novartis)
OLANZAPINE	
Tablets: 2.5, 5, 7.5, 10, 15, and 20 mg (*Rx*)	*Zyprexa* (Eli Lilly)
Tablets, orally disintegrating: 5 and 10 mg (*Rx*)	*Zyprexa Zydis* (Eli Lilly)
QUETIAPINE FUMARATE	
Tablets: 25, 100, 200, and 300 mg (*Rx*)	*Seroquel* (Astra Zeneca)

Warning:

Clozapine: Because of the significant risk of agranulocytosis, a potentially life-threatening adverse event, reserve clozapine for use in the treatment of severely ill schizophrenic patients who fail to show an acceptable response to adequate courses of standard antipsychotic drug treatment, either because of insufficient effectiveness or the inability to achieve an effective dose because of intolerable adverse effects from those drugs. Consequently, before initiating treatment with clozapine, it is strongly recommended that a patient be given at least two trials, each with a different standard antipsychotic drug product, at an adequate dose and for an adequate duration. Patients who are being treated with clozapine must have a baseline white blood cell (WBC) and differential count before initiation of treatment, and a WBC count every week throughout treatment and for 4 weeks after the discontinuation of clozapine.

Indications

Clozapine:

> *Psychotic disorders* – Management of severely ill schizophrenic patients who fail to respond adequately to standard antipsychotic drug treatment.

Loxapine:

> *Psychotic disorders* – Management of the manifestations of psychotic disorders.

Olanzapine:

> *Schizophrenia* – Treatment of schizophrenia.

> *Bipolar mania* – Short-term treatment of acute manic episodes associated with Bipolar I disorder.

Quetiapine fumarate:

> *Schizophrenia* – Treatment of schizophrenia.

Administration and Dosage

LOXAPINE:

> *Oral* – Individualize dosage. Administer in divided doses, 2 to 4 times/day.

> *Initial dosage:* 10 mg twice/day. In severely disturbed patients, up to 50 mg/day may be desirable. Increase dosage fairly rapidly over the first 7 to 10 days until psychotic symptoms are controlled. The usual range is 60 to 100 mg/day. Dosage > 250 mg/day is not recommended.

> *Maintenance therapy:* Reduce dosage to the lowest level compatible with control of symptoms; usual range is 20 to 60 mg/day.

> IM: For prompt symptomatic control in the acutely agitated patient and in patients whose symptoms render oral medication temporarily impractical.

> Administer IM (not IV) in 12.5 to 50 mg doses at intervals of 4 to 6 hours or longer. Many patients respond satisfactorily to twice/day dosage. Once control is achieved, institute oral medication, usually within 5 days.

CLOZAPINE: Clozapine is available only through the *Clozaril* Patient Management System, a program that combines WBC testing, patient monitoring, pharmacy and drug distribution services, all linked to compliance with required safety monitoring. Do not dispense more than a 1–week supply. For more information, call (800) 448-5938.

Initial – 25 mg once or twice/day, and then continued with daily dosage increments of 25 to 50 mg/day, if well tolerated, to achieve a target dose of 300 to 450 mg/day by the end of 2 weeks. Make subsequent dosage increments no more than once or twice weekly, in increments not to exceed 100 mg. Cautious titration and a divided dosage schedule are necessary to minimize the risks of hypotension, seizure, and sedation.

In a multicenter study, patients were titrated during the first 2 weeks up to a maximum dose of 500 mg/day, on a 3 times/day basis, and were then dosed in a total daily dose range of 100 to 900 mg/day, on a 3 times/day basis thereafter, with clinical response and adverse effects as guides to correct dosing.

Clozapine Therapy Guidelines Based on WBC and Granulocyte Count		
WBC Count (mm^3)	Granulocyte Count (mm^3)	Guidelines
< 3500, or history of myelo-proliferative disorder, or previous clozapine-induced agranulocytosis or granulocytopenia		Do not initiate treatment.
< 3500, or > 3500 with a substantial drop from baseline, following initiation of treatment		Repeat WBC and differential counts. Symptoms of infection: Lethargy, weakness, fever, sore throat.
3000 to 3500 on subsequent counts	> 1500	Perform twice weekly WBC and differential counts.
< 3000	< 1500	Interrupt therapy, monitor for flu-like symptoms or other symptoms of infection. May resume therapy if no signs of infection develop, WBC count > 3000 and granulocyte count > 1500. However, continue twice weekly WBC and differential counts until WBC returns to 3500.
< 2000	< 1000	Consider bone marrow aspiration to ascertain granulopoietic status. If granulopoiesis is deficient, consider protective isolation. If infection develops, perform cultures and institute antibiotics. Do not rechallenge with clozapine since agranulocytosis may develop with a shorter latency.

Dose adjustment – Continue daily dosing on a divided basis to an effective and tolerable dose level. While many patients may respond adequately at doses between 300 to 600 mg/day, it may be necessary to raise the dose to the 600 to 900 mg/day range. Do not exceed 900 mg/day. The mean and median clozapine doses are approximately 600 mg/day.

Because of the possibility of increased adverse reactions at higher doses, particularly seizures, give patients adequate time to respond to a given dose level before escalation to a higher dose.

Because of the significant risk of agranulocytosis and seizure, events which both present a continuing risk over time, avoid the extended treatment of patients failing to show an acceptable level of clinical response.

Maintenance – Continue clozapine at the lowest level needed to maintain remission. Periodically reassess patients to determine the need for maintenance treatment.

Discontinuation – In the event of planned termination of clozapine therapy, gradual reduction in dose is recommended over a 1 to 2 week period. However, should a patient's medical condition require abrupt discontinuation (eg, leukopenia), carefully observe the patient for the recurrence of psychotic symptoms.

Reinitiation of treatment – Follow the original dosage build-up guidelines. However, certain additional precautions seem prudent. Reexposure of a patient might enhance the risk of an untoward event's occurrence and increase its severity. Patients discontinued for WBC counts < 2000 per mm^3 or a granulocyte count < 1000 per mm^3 must not be restarted on clozapine. (See Warnings.)

Clozapine is available only through the *Clozaril* Patient Management System, a program that combines WBC testing, patient monitoring, pharmacy, and drug distribution services, all linked to compliance with required safety monitoring. Do not dispense more than a 1-week supply.

OLANZAPINE:

Schizophrenia – Initial dose is 5 to 10 mg/day without regard to meals with a target dose of 10 mg/day within several days of initiation. Adjust dosage at 5 mg increments in intervals not < 1 week if indicated.

Antipsychotic efficacy was demonstrated in a dose range of 10 to 15 mg/day in clinical trials. However, increases in efficacy were not demonstrated in doses > 10 mg/day. Doses > 10 mg/ day are recommended only after clinical assessment. The safety of doses > 20 mg/day has not been evaluated in clinical trials.

Maintenance treatment: Periodically reassess patients to determine the need for maintenance treatment.

Bipolar mania – Initial dose is 10 to 15 mg/day without regard to meals. Adjust dosage at 5 mg increments in intervals > 24 hours if indicated.

Short-term (3 to 4 weeks) antimanic efficacy was demonstrated in a dose range of 5 to 20 mg/ day in clinical trials. The safety of doses > 20 mg/day has not been evaluated.

Maintenance treatment: Data is not available to support the use of olanzapine in long-term treatment (beyond 3 to 4 weeks). However, it is generally agreed that pharmacological treatment beyond an acute response in mania is desirable, both for maintenance of the initial response and for prevention of new manic episodes.

Dosing in special populations – The recommended starting dose is 5 mg in patients who are debilitated, who have a predisposition to hypotensive reactions, who otherwise exhibit a combination of factors that may result in slower metabolism of olanzapine (eg, nonsmoking female patients ≥ 65 years of age), or who may be more pharmacodynamically sensitive to olanzapine.

Administration of orally disintegrating tablets – Peel back foil on blister; do not push tablet through foil. Using dry hands, remove from the foil and place the entire tablet in the mouth. The tablet will disintegrate with or without liquid.

QUETIAPINE FUMARATE:

Usual dose – Initial dose of 25 mg twice/day, with increases in increments of 25 to 50 mg twice/day or three times/day on the second and third day, as tolerated, to a target dose range of 300 to 400 mg/day by the fourth day, given twice or three times a day. Further dosage adjustments, if indicated, should generally occur at intervals of ≥ 2 days. Dose increments/decrements of 25 to 50 mg twice/day are recommended. Antipsychotic efficacy was demonstrated in a dose range of 150 to 750 mg/day. The safety of doses > 800 mg/day has not been evaluated in clinical trials.

Maintenance – Unknown; however, the effectiveness of maintenance treatment is well established for many other antipsychotic drugs. Continue quetiapine in responding patients, but at the lowest dose needed to maintain remission. Periodically reassess patients.

Special populations – Consider a slower rate of dose titration and a lower target dose in the elderly, patients with hepatic impairment, debilitated patients or those who have a predisposition to hypotensive reactions. Perform dose escalation with caution.

Reinitiation of treatment in patients previously discontinued – When restarting patients who have had an interval of < 1 week off quetiapine, titration of quetiapine is not required and the maintenance dose may be reinitiated. For patients who have been off quetiapine for > 1 week, follow the initial titration schedule.

BENZISOXAZOLE DERIVATIVES

ZIPRASIDONE HCl
Capsules: 20, 40, 60, and 80 mg (*Rx*)   Geodon (Pfizer)

Indications
Ziprasidone:
> *Schizophrenia* – When deciding among the alternative treatments available for this condition, consider ziprasidone's greater capacity to prolong the QT/QTc interval compared with several other antipsychotic drugs. Prolongation of the QTc interval is associated in some other drugs with the ability to cause torsade de pointes-type arrhythmia, a potentially fatal polymorphic ventricular tachycardia, and sudden death. In many cases, this would lead to the conclusion that other drugs should be tried first. Whether ziprasidone will cause torsade de pointes or increase the rate of sudden death is not yet known.

Administration and Dosage
Ziprasidone:
> *Initial treatment* – Administer ziprasidone capsules at an initial daily dose of 20 mg twice/day with food. In some patients, daily dosage subsequently may be adjusted on the basis of individual clinical status up to 80 mg twice/day. Dosage adjustments, if indicated, should generally occur at intervals of ≥ 2 days, as steady state is achieved within 1 to 3 days. In order to ensure use of the lowest effective dose, observe patients for improvement for several weeks before upward dosage adjustment.

> *Maintenance treatment* – While there is no body of evidence available to answer the question of how long a patient should be treated with ziprasidone, systematic evaluation of ziprasidone has shown that its efficacy in schizophrenia is maintained for periods of ≤ 52 weeks at a dose of 20 to 80 mg twice/day. No additional benefit was demonstrated for doses > 20 mg twice/day.

RISPERIDONE

Tablets: 0.25, 0.5, 1, 2, 3, and 4 mg (*Rx*)   Risperdal (Janssen)
Oral solution: 1 mg/mL (*Rx*)

Indications
Psychotic disorders: Management of the manifestations of psychotic disorders.

Administration and Dosage
Initial dose: Initial dose is 1 mg twice/day (day 1), increasing by 1 mg twice/day as tolerated (on days 2 and 3), up to a target dose of 3 mg twice/day (by day 3). Further dosage adjustments at 1 to 2 mg increments may be made at intervals of > 1 week. Risperidone is safe and effective up to 8 mg as a once/day administration. Although not indicated, studies suggest patients are more likely to continue on risperidone if the titration period was longer (6 days vs 3 days).

> Mix oral solution with 3 to 4 oz of water, coffee, orange juice, or lowfat milk; not compatible with cola or tea.

> Antipsychotic efficacy was demonstrated in a dose range of 4 to 16 mg/day in the clinical trials supporting efficacy of risperidone; however, maximal effect was generally seen in a range of 4 to 8 mg/day. Doses > 6 mg/day for twice-a-day dosing were not demonstrated to be more effective than lower doses, were associated with more extrapyramidal symptoms and other adverse effects, and are not generally recommended. In a single study supporting daily dosing, the efficacy results were generally stronger for 8 mg than for 4 mg. The safety of doses > 16 mg/day has not been evaluated in clinical trials.

Special populations: The recommended initial dose is 0.5 mg twice/day in patients who are elderly, debilitated, have severe renal or hepatic impairment, are predisposed to hypotension, or in whom hypotension would pose a risk. Use dosage increases in these patients in increments of 0.5 mg twice/day. Adjust dose at increments of 0.5 mg twice/day, with dosage increases > 1.5 mg twice/day occurring at intervals of > 1 week.

Once/day dosing in the elderly or debilitated may occur after the patient has been titrated on a twice/day regimen for 2 to 3 days at the target dose.

Reinitiation of treatment: When restarting patients who have had an interval off risperidone, follow the initial 3-day dose titration schedule.

Maintenance therapy: It is recommended that responding patients be continued on risperidone, but at the lowest dose needed to maintain remission. Periodically reassess patients to determine the need for maintenance treatment.

Reinitiation of treatment: When restarting patients who have had an interval off risperidone, follow the initial 3-day dose titration schedule.

Switching from other antipsychotics: When switching from other antipsychotics to risperidone, immediate discontinuation of the previous antipsychotic treatment upon initiation of risperidone therapy is recommended when medically appropriate. In all cases, minimize the period of overlapping antipsychotic administration. When switching patients from depot antipsychotic, initiate risperidone therapy in place of the next scheduled injection. Periodically reevaluate the need for continuing existing EPS medications.

LITHIUM

Capsules: 150 mg lithium carbonate (4.06 mEq lithium) (*Rx*)	*Lithium Carbonate* (Roxane)
Capsules: 300 mg lithium carbonate (8.12 mEq lithium) (*Rx*)	Various, *Eskalith* (SKB), *Lithonate* (Solvay Pharm.)
Capsules: 600 mg lithium carbonate (16.24 mEq lithium) (*Rx*)	*Lithium Carbonate* (Roxane)
Tablets: 300 mg lithium carbonate (8.12 mEq lithium) (*Rx*)	Various, *Eskalith* (GlaxoSmithKline), *Lithane* (Miles Pharm.), *Lithotabs* (Solvay Pharm.)
Tablets, slow release: 300 mg lithium carbonate (8.12 mEq lithium) (*Rx*)	*Lithobid* (Ciba)
Tablets, controlled release: 450 mg lithium carbonate (12.18 mEq lithium) (*Rx*)	*Eskalith CR* (GlaxoSmithKline)
Syrup: 8 mEq lithium (as citrate equivalent to 300 mg lithium carbonate) per 5 mL (*Rx*)	Various

---

Warning:
Toxicity is closely related to serum lithium levels and can occur at therapeutic doses. Facilities for serum lithium determinations are required to monitor therapy.

Indications

Mania: For the treatment of manic episodes of manic-depressive illness. Maintenance therapy prevents or diminishes the frequency and intensity of subsequent manic episodes in those manic-depressive patients with a history of mania.

Unlabeled uses: Lithium carbonate (300 to 1000 mg/day) has improved the neutrophil count in patients with cancer chemotherapy-induced neutropenia, in children with chronic neutropenia, and in AIDS patients receiving zidovudine.

Administration and Dosage

Individualize dosage according to both serum levels and clinical response.

Serum lithium levels: Draw blood samples immediately prior to the next dose (8 to 12 hours after the previous dose) when lithium concentrations are relatively stable. Do not rely on serum levels alone.

Acute mania: Optimal patient response is usually established and maintained with 600 mg 3 times/day or 900 mg twice/day for the slow release form. Such doses normally produce an effective serum lithium level ranging between 1 and 1.5 mEq/L.

Determine serum levels twice weekly during the acute phase, and until the serum level and clinical condition of the patient have been stabilized.

Long-term use: The desirable serum levels are 0.6 to 1.2 mEq/L. Dosage will vary, but 300 mg 3 to 4 times/day will usually maintain this level. Monitor serum levels in uncomplicated cases on maintenance therapy during remission every 2 to 3 months.

Actions
Pharmacology: Lithium alters sodium transport in nerve and muscle cells, and effects a shift toward intraneuronal catecholamine metabolism. The specific mechanism in mania is unknown, but it affects neurotransmitters associated with affective disorders. Its antimanic effects may be the result of increases in norepinephrine reuptake and increased serotonin receptor sensitivity.

Pharmacokinetics:

Absorption/Distribution – Lithium is readily absorbed from the GI tract. Peak serum levels occur in 0.5 to 3 hours and absorption is complete within 8 hours. Onset of action is slow (5 to 14 days). Until the desired therapeutic effect is attained, maintain a steady-state serum level of 0.8 to 1.4 mEq/L, then slowly decrease the lithium dose to a maintenance level. The therapeutic serum level range is from 0.4 to 1 mEq/L.

Excretion – About 95% of the lithium dose is eliminated by the kidney.

Warnings
High-risk patients: The risk of lithium toxicity is very high in patients with significant renal or cardiovascular disease, severe debilitation, dehydration, or sodium depletion, or in patients receiving diuretics. Undertake treatment with extreme caution.

Encephalopathic syndrome: Encephalopathic syndrome has occurred in a few patients given lithium plus a neuroleptic. In some instances, irreversible brain damage occurred. Monitor closely for evidence of neurologic toxicity.

Renal function impairment: Morphologic changes with glomerular and interstitial fibrosis and nephron atrophy have occurred in patients on chronic lithium therapy. The relationship between such changes and renal function has not been established.

Acquired nephrogenic diabetes insipidus – Acquired nephrogenic diabetes insipidus unresponsive to vasopressin has been associated with chronic lithium administration. Polydipsia and polyuria occur frequently. The mechanism is thought to be the decreased response of the renal tubules to the antidiuretic hormone causing decreased reabsorption of water. Impairment of the concentrating ability of the kidneys is reversed when lithium therapy is discontinued. Management may involve decreasing the dose, discontinuing lithium, or the cautious use of a thiazide diuretic or amiloride. Monitor the patient's renal status.

Elderly: The decreased rate of excretion in the elderly contributes to a high incidence of toxic effects. Use lower doses and more frequent monitoring.

Pregnancy: Category D.

Lactation: Lithium is excreted in breast milk. Do not nurse during lithium therapy.

Children: Safety and efficacy for use in children < 12 years old have not been established.

Precautions
Infection: Concomitant infection with elevated temperature may necessitate a temporary reduction or cessation of medication.

Hazardous tasks: Observe caution while driving or performing other tasks requiring alertness.

Tolerance of lithium: Tolerance of lithium is greater during the acute manic phase and decreases when manic symptoms subside.

Hypothyroidism: Hypothyroidism may occur with long-term lithium administration. Patients may develop enlargement of thyroid gland and increased thyroid-stimulating hormone levels.

Sodium depletion: Lithium decreases renal sodium reabsorption, which could lead to sodium depletion. Therefore, the patient must maintain a normal diet (including salt) and an adequate fluid intake (2500 to 3000 mL).

Parameters to monitor: Perform the following laboratory tests prior to and periodically during lithium therapy: Serum creatinine; complete blood count; urinalysis; sodium and potassium; fasting glucose; electrocardiogram; and thyroid function tests. Check lithium serum levels twice weekly until dosage is stabilized. Once steady state has been reached, monitor the level weekly. Once the patient is on maintenance therapy, the level may be checked every 2 to 3 months.

Drug Interactions

Drugs that may affect lithium include acetazolamide, carbamazepine, fluoxetine, haloperidol, loop diuretics, methyldopa, NSAIDs, osmotic diuretics, theophyllines, thiazide diuretics, urinary alkalinizers, and verapamil.

Drugs that may be affected by lithium include phenothiazines, sympathomimetics, iodide salts, neuromuscular blocking agents, and tricyclic antidepressants.

Adverse Reactions

Adverse reactions may include arrhythmia; hypotension; peripheral circulatory collapse; bradycardia; sinus node dysfunction with severe bradycardia; ECG changes; tremor; muscle hyperirritability; ataxia; choreoathetotic movements; hyperactive deep tendon reflexes; pseudotumor cerebri; euthyroid goiter; hypothyroidism; EEG changes; blackout spells; epileptiform seizures; slurred speech; dizziness; vertigo; incontinence of urine or feces; somnolence; psychomotor retardation; restlessness; confusion; stupor; coma; acute dystonia; downbeat nystagmus; blurred vision; startled response; hypertonicity; slowed intellectual functioning; hallucinations; poor memory; tongue movements; tics; tinnitus; cog wheel rigidity; anorexia; nausea; vomiting; diarrhea; dry mouth; gastritis; salivary gland swelling; abdominal pain; excessive salivation; flatulence; indigestion; albuminuria; oliguria; glycosuria; decreased Ccr; symptoms of nephrogenic diabetes; drying and thinning of hair; anesthesia of skin; chronic folliculitis; xerosis cutis; alopecia; exacerbation of psoriasis; acne; angioedema; fatigue; lethargy; sleepiness; dehydration; weight loss; transient scotomata; impotence; sexual dysfunction; dysgeusia; taste distortion; tightness in chest; hypercalcemia; hyperparathyroidism; salty taste; swollen lips; swollen, painful joints; fever; polyarthralgia; dental caries; leukocytosis; headache; transient hyperglycemia; generalized pruritus with or without rash; cutaneous ulcers; worsening of organic brain syndromes; excessive weight gain; edematous swelling of ankles or wrists; thirst or polyuria, sometimes resembling diabetes insipidus; metallic taste; painful discoloration of fingers and toes and coldness of the extremities.

DEXMETHYLPHENIDATE HCl

Tablets: 2.5, 5, and 10 mg (*c-ii*)   *Focalin* (Novartis)

Warning:
> *Drug dependence:* Give dexmethylphenidate cautiously to patients with a history of drug dependence or alcoholism. Chronic, abusive use can lead to marked tolerance and psychological dependence with varying degrees of abnormal behavior. Frank psychotic episodes can occur, especially with parenteral abuse. Careful supervision is required during drug withdrawal from abusive use because severe depression may occur. Withdrawal following chronic therapeutic use may unmask symptoms of the underlying disorder that may require follow-up.

Indications
Attention deficit hyperactivity disorder (ADHD): For the treatment of ADHD. Dexmethylphenidate is indicated as an integral part of a total treatment program for ADHD that may include other measures (eg, psychological, educational, social) for patients with this syndrome. Drug treatment may not be indicated for all patients. Stimulants are not intended for use in the patient who exhibits symptoms secondary to environmental factors or other primary psychiatric disorders, including psychosis.

Administration and Dosage
Administer twice/day, at least 4 hours apart, with or without food.

Individualize dosage according to the needs and responses of the patient.

Patients new to methylphenidate: The recommended starting dose of dexmethylphenidate for patients who are not currently taking racemic methylphenidate or for patients who are on stimulants other than methylphenidate is 5 mg/day (2.5 mg twice/day).

Dosage may be adjusted in 2.5 to 5 mg increments to a maximum of 20 mg/day (10 mg twice/day). In general, dosage adjustments may proceed at approximately weekly intervals.

Patients currently using methylphenidate: For patients currently using methylphenidate, the recommended starting dose of dexmethylphenidate is half the dose of racemic methylphenidate. The maximum recommended dose is 20 mg/day (10 mg twice/day).

Dose reduction and discontinuation: If paradoxical aggravation of symptoms or other adverse events occur, reduce the dosage, or, if necessary, discontinue the drug.

If improvement is not observed after appropriate dosage adjustment over a 1-month period, discontinue the drug.

Actions
Pharmacology: Dexmethylphenidate HCl is a CNS stimulant. It is the more pharmacologically active enantiomer of the *d*- and *l*-enantiomers and is thought to block the reuptake of norepinephrine and dopamine into the presynaptic neuron and increase the release of these monoamines into the extraneuronal space.

Pharmacokinetics:
> *Absorption* – Dexmethylphenidate HCl is readily absorbed following oral administration. In patients with ADHD, plasma dexmethylphenidate concentrations increase rapidly, reaching a maximum in the fasted state at ≈ 1 to 1.5 hours postdose.

> *Distribution* – Plasma dexmethylphenidate concentrations in children decline exponentially following oral administration.

> *Metabolism* – Dexmethylphenidate is metabolized primarily to *d*-α-phenyl-piperidine acetic acid (also known as *d*-ritalinic acid) by de-esterification. This metabolite has little or no pharmacological activity.

> In vitro studies showed that dexmethylphenidate did not inhibit cytochrome P450 isoenzymes.

Excretion – The mean plasma elimination half-life of dexmethylphenidate is ≈ 2.2 hours.

Contraindications

Patients with marked anxiety, tension, and agitation, because the drug may aggravate these symptoms; hypersensitivity to methylphenidate or other components of the product; patients with glaucoma, motor tics, or a family history or diagnosis of Tourette's syndrome; during treatment with monoamine oxidase inhibitors (MAOIs), and also within a minimum of 14 days following discontinuation of an MAOI (hypertensive crises may result).

Warnings

Depression: Do not use dexmethylphenidate to treat severe depression.

Fatigue: Do not use dexmethylphenidate for the prevention or treatment of normal fatigue states.

Long-term suppression of growth: Although a causal relationship has not been established, suppression of growth (eg, weight gain, height) has been reported with long-term stimulant use in children.

Psychosis: In psychotic children, administration of methylphenidate may exacerbate symptoms of behavior disturbance and thought disorder.

Seizures: Methylphenidate may lower the convulsive threshold in patients with history of seizures, in patients with prior EEG abnormalities in the absence of a history of seizures, and, very rarely, in the absence of a history of seizures and no prior EEG evidence of seizures. In the presence of seizures, discontinue the drug.

Hypertension and other cardiovascular conditions: Use cautiously in patients with hypertension. Monitor blood pressure at appropriate intervals in all patients taking dexmethylphenidate, especially those with hypertension. Caution is indicated in treating patients whose underlying medical conditions might be compromised by increases in blood pressure or heart rate (eg, pre-existing hypertension, heart failure, recent MI, hyperthyroidism).

Visual disturbance: Difficulties with accommodation and blurring of vision have been reported.

Carcinogenesis: In a lifetime carcinogenicity study carried out in B6C3F1 mice, racemic methylphenidate caused an increase in hepatocellular adenomas and, in males only, an increase in hepatoblastomas at a daily dose of ≈ 60 mg/kg/day. The significance to these results to humans is unknown.

Pregnancy: Category C.

Lactation: It is not known whether dexmethylphenidate is excreted in human milk.

Children: The safety and efficacy of dexmethylphenidate in children < 6 years of age have not been established.

Precautions

Monitoring: Periodic CBC, differential, and platelet counts are advised during prolonged therapy.

Drug Interactions

Drugs that may be affected by dexmethylphenidate or racemic methylphenidate include antihypertensive agents, pressor agents, coumarin anticoagulants, anticonvulsants, tricyclic antidepressants, selective serotonin reuptake inhibitors, and clonidine.

Adverse Reactions

Adverse reactions occurring in ≥ 5% of patients include abdominal pain, anorexia, fever, and nausea.

Adverse reactions with other methylphenidate HCl products – Nervousness and insomnia are the most common adverse reactions reported with other methylphenidate products. In children, loss of appetite, abdominal pain, weight loss during prolonged therapy, insomnia, and tachycardia may occur more frequently; however, any of the other adverse reactions listed below also may occur.

METHYLPHENIDATE HCl

Tablets: 5, 10, and 20 mg *(c-II)*	Various, *Ritalin* (Novartis), *Methylin* (Mallinckrodt)
Tablets, extended-release: 10 mg *(c-II)*	*Metadate ER* (Medeva), *Methylin ER* (Mallinckrodt)
18 mg *(c-II)*	*Concerta* (Alza)
20 mg *(c-II)*	Various, *Metadate ER* (Medeva), *Methylin ER* (Mallinckrodt)
36 and 54 mg *(c-II)*	*Concerta* (Alza)
Tablets, sustained release: 20 mg *(c-II)*	Various, *Ritalin-SR* (Novartis)
Capsules, extended-release: 20 mg *(c-II)*	*Metadate CD* (Celltech)

Indications
Attention deficit disorders (ADD)/attention deficit hyperactivity disorders (ADHD): As part of a total treatment program in children with a behavioral syndrome characterized by moderate to severe distractibility, short attention span, hyperactivity, emotional lability, and impulsivity.

Narcolepsy (Ritalin, Ritalin SR): Treatment of narcolepsy.

Administration and Dosage
Adults: Individualize dosage. Administer in divided doses 2 or 3 times/day, preferably 30 to 45 minutes before meals. Average dose is 20 to 30 mg/day. Dosage ranges from 10 to 15 mg/day to 40 to 60 mg/day. Patients who are unable to sleep if medication is taken late in the day should take the last dose before 6 pm.

Children (≥ 6 years of age): Start with small doses (eg, 5 mg before breakfast and lunch) with gradual increments of 5 to 10 mg weekly. Daily dosage > 60 mg is not recommended. If improvement is not observed after dosage adjustment over 1 month, discontinue use. If paradoxical aggravation of symptoms or other adverse effects occurs, reduce dosage or discontinue the drug.

Discontinue periodically to assess condition. Improvement may be sustained when the drug is either temporarily or permanently discontinued. Drug treatment should not be indefinite and usually may be discontinued after puberty.

All patients: Sustained-release (SR) tablets have a duration of ≈ 8 hours and may be used in place of regular tablets when the 8-hour dosage of the SR tablets corresponds to the titrated 8-hour dosage of the regular tablets. SR tablets must be swallowed whole, never crushed or chewed.

Concerta: Administer orally once/day in the morning with or without food.

Patients new to methylphenidate – The recommended starting dose for patients who are not currently taking methylphenidate or for patients who are on stimulants other than methylphenidate is 18 mg once/day. Dosage may be adjusted in 18 mg increments at weekly intervals to a maximum of 54 mg/day taken once/day in the morning.

Patients currently using methylphenidate – Dosage may be adjusted in 18 mg increments at weekly intervals to a maximum of 54 mg/day taken once/day in the morning.

Recommended Dose Conversion from Methylphenidate Regimens to *Concerta*	
Previous methylphenidate daily dose	Recommended *Concerta* dose
5 mg methylphenidate twice/day or 5 mg methylphenidate 3 times/day or 20 mg methylphenidate SR	18 mg every morning
10 mg methylphenidate twice/day or 10 mg methylphenidate 3 times/day or 40 mg methylphenidate SR	36 mg every morning
15 mg methylphenidate twice/day or 15 mg methylphenidate 3 times/day or 60 mg methylphenidate SR	54 mg every morning

In other methylphenidate regimens, use clinical judgment when selecting the starting dose. Daily dosage > 54 mg is not recommended.

Metadate CD: Administer once/day in the morning before breakfast.

Initial treatment – 20 mg once/day. Adjust dosage in weekly 20 mg increments to a maximum of 60 mg/day taken once/day in the morning, depending upon tolerability and degree of efficacy. Daily dosage > 60 mg is not recommended.

Maintenance/Extended treatment: There is no evidence as to how long the patient with ADHD should be treated. Pharmacological treatment of ADHD may be needed for extended periods. Periodically re-evaluate the long-term usefulness of the drug for the individual patient with trials off medication to assess the patient's functioning without pharmacotherapy. Improvement may be sustained when the drug is either temporarily or permanently discontinued.

Dose reduction and discontinuation: If paradoxical aggravation of symptoms or other adverse events occur, reduce dosage or discontinue the drug.

If improvement is not observed after appropriate dosage adjustment over a 1-month period, discontinue the drug.

Actions

Pharmacology: Methylphenidate is a mild cortical stimulant with CNS actions similar to the amphetamines. The exact mechanism of action is not fully understood.

Pharmacokinetics: Rapidly and well absorbed from the GI tract, methylphenidate achieves peak blood levels in 1 to 3 hours. Peak plasma levels occur in children in 4.7 hours for the SR tablets and 1.9 hours for the regular tablets. Plasma half-life ranges from 1 to 3 hours, but pharmacologic effects persist up to 4 to 6 hours.

Contraindications

Marked anxiety, tension, and agitation because the drug may aggravate these symptoms; hypersensitivity to methylphenidate; glaucoma.

Patients with motor tics or with a family history or diagnosis of Tourette's syndrome.

Severe depression of either exogenous or endogenous origin; prevention or treatment of normal fatigue states.

Warnings

Do not use for severe depression of exogenous or endogenous origin. Do not use for the prevention or treatment of normal fatigue states.

Seizure disorders: Methylphenidate may lower the seizure threshold in patients with a history of seizures, with prior EEG abnormalities in absence of seizures and, very rarely, in the absence of history of seizures and no prior EEG evidence of seizures.

GI obstruction: Because the *Concerta* tablet is nondeformable and does not appreciably change in shape in the GI tract, do not administer to patients with pre-existing severe GI narrowing (pathologic or iatrogenic; for example, small bowel inflammatory disease, "short gut" syndrome because of adhesions or decreased transit time, past history of peritonitis, cystic fibrosis, chronic intestinal pseudo-obstruction, or Meckel's diverticulum). There have been rare reports of obstructive symptoms in patients with known strictures in association with the ingestion of other drugs in nondeformable controlled-release formulations. Because of the controlled-release design of the tablet, only use *Concerta* in patients who are able to swallow the tablet whole.

Hypertension: Use cautiously; monitor blood pressure in all patients, especially those with hypertension.

Severe depression: Do not use methylphenidate for severe depression of either exogenous or endogenous origin.

Fatigue: Do not use methylphenidate for the prevention or treatment of normal fatigue states.

Long-term suppression of growth: Suppression of growth has been reported with long-term use in children. Interrupt treatment for patients who are not growing or gaining weight as expected.

Psychosis: Methylphenidate may exacerbate symptoms of behavior disturbances and thought disorder.

Visual disturbances: Visual disturbances have been encountered rarely. Difficulties with accommodation and blurring of vision have been reported.

Pregnancy: Category C.

Lactation: The amount of methylphenidate excreted in breast milk is unknown.

Children: Do not use in children < 6 years of age because safety and efficacy have not been established. In psychotic children, the drug may exacerbate symptoms of behavior disturbance and thought disorder. Precipitation of Tourette's syndrome has been reported.

Safety and efficacy of long-term use in children are not established. Although a causal relationship has not been established, suppression of growth (eg, weight gain or height) has been reported with long-term use of stimulants in children. Carefully monitor patients on long-term therapy.

Precautions

Patients with an element of agitation may react adversely; discontinue therapy if necessary.

Perform periodic CBC, differential, and platelet counts during prolonged therapy.

Acute stress: When symptoms are associated with acute stress reactions, treatment with methylphenidate usually is not indicated.

Drug abuse and dependence: Give cautiously to emotionally unstable patients, such as those with a history of drug dependence or alcoholism, because such patients may increase dosage on their own initiative.

Drug Interactions

Drugs that may affect methyphenidate include monoamine oxidase inhibitors (MAOIs). Drugs that may be affected by methylphenidate HCl include guanethidine, anticonvulsants, selective serotonin reuptake inhibitors (SSRIs), and tricyclic antidepressants (TCAs).

Adverse Reactions

Adverse reactions may include skin rash; urticaria; fever; arthralgia; exfoliative dermatitis; erythema multiforme with necrotizing vasculitis; thrombocytopenic purpura; dizziness; headache; dyskinesia; drowsiness; Tourette's syndrome; toxic psychosis; blood pressure and pulse changes; tachycardia; angina; cardiac arrhythmias; palpitations; anorexia; nausea; abdominal pain; weight loss; nervousness; insomnia; leukopenia; anemia; hair loss; loss of appetite; abdominal pain.

PEMOLINE

Tablets: 18.75, 37.5, and 75 mg (c-iv)

Tablets, chewable: 37.5 mg (c-iv)

Pemoline (Apothecon), *Cylert* (Abbott),
PemADD (Mallinckrodt)
Cylert (Abbott), *PemADD CT* (Mallinckrodt)

Warning:

Because of its association with life-threatening hepatic failure, pemoline should not ordinarily be considered as first-line drug therapy for attention deficit hyperactivity disorder (ADHD). Because pemoline provides an observable symptomatic benefit, patients who fail to show substantial clinical benefit within 3 weeks of completing dose titration should be withdrawn from therapy.

Since pemoline's marketing in 1975, 15 cases of acute hepatic failure have been reported to the FDA. While the absolute number of reported cases is not large, the rate of reporting ranges from 4 to 17 times the rate expected in the general population. This estimate may be conservative because of underreporting and because the long latency between initiation of pemoline treatment and the occurrence of hepatic failure may limit recognition of the association. If only a portion of actual cases were recognized and reported, the risk could be substantially higher.

Of the 15 cases reported as of December 1998, 12 resulted in death or liver transplantation, usually within 4 weeks of the onset of signs and symptoms of liver failure. The earliest onset of heptic abnormalities occurred 6 months after initiation of pemoline. Although some reports described dark urine and nonspecific prodromal symptoms (eg, anorexia, malaise, GI symptoms), in other reports it was not clear if any prodromol symptoms preceded the onset of jaundice.

Initiate treatment with pemoline only in individuals without liver disease and with normal baseline liver function tests. It is not clear if baseline and periodic liver function testing are predictive of these instances of acute liver failure; however, it is generally believed that early detection of drug-induced hepatic injury along with immediate withdrawal of the suspect drug enhances the likelihood for recovery. Accordingly, the following liver monitoring program is recommended: Determine serum ALT levels at baseline and every 2 weeks thereafter. If pemoline therapy is discontinued and then restarted, perform liver function test monitoring at baseline and reinitiate at the frequency above.

Discontinue pemoline if serum ALT is increased to a clinically significant level or any increase ≥ 2 times the upper limit of normal, or if clinical signs and symptoms suggest liver failure.

The physician who elects to use pemoline should obtain written informed consent from the patient prior to initiation of pemoline therapy.

Indications

ADHD: As part of a total treatment program in children with a behavioral syndrome characterized by moderate to severe distractibility, short attention span, hyperactivity, emotional lability, and impulsivity.

Administration and Dosage

Administer as a single dose each morning. Recommended starting dose is 37.5 mg/day. Gradually increase at 1-week intervals using increments of 18.75 mg until desired response is obtained. Mean effective doses range from 56.25 to 75 mg/day. Maximum recommended dose is 112.5 mg/day.

Clinical improvement is gradual; significant benefit may not be evident until week 3 or 4 of administration.

Interrupt drug administration occasionally to determine if there is a recurrence of behavioral symptoms sufficient to require continued therapy.

Actions

Pharmacology: Pemoline is a CNS stimulant. Although structurally dissimilar to the amphetamines and methylphenidate, it has pharmacologic activity similar to that of other stimulants but with minimal sympathomimetic effects. Although the exact mechanism of action is unknown, pemoline may act through dopaminergic mechanisms.

Pharmacokinetics: Pemoline is rapidly absorbed from the GI tract. Approximately 50% is protein bound. Peak serum levels occur within 2 to 4 hours after ingestion of a single dose. The serum half-life is ≈ 12 hours. Steady state is reached in ≈ 2 to 3 days. The drug is widely distributed throughout body tissues, including the brain. Pemoline is metabolized by the liver and primarily excreted by the kidneys. Approximately 50% is excreted unchanged and only minor fractions are present as metabolites.

Contraindications

Known hypersensitivity or idiosyncrasy to pemoline; hepatic insufficiency.

Warnings

Renal function impairment: Administer with caution to patients with significantly impaired renal function.

Pregnancy: Category B.

Lactation: It is not known whether pemoline is excreted in breast milk. Exercise caution when administering pemoline to a nursing woman.

Children: Safety and efficacy in children < 6 years of age have not been established.

In psychotic children, administration may exacerbate symptoms of behavior disturbance and thought disorder. CNS stimulants, including pemoline, can precipitate motor and phonic tics and Tourette's syndrome. Therefore, clinical evaluation for tics and Tourette's syndrome in children and their families should precede use of stimulants.

Chronic administration may be associated with growth inhibition; therefore, monitor growth during treatment. Long-term effects in children have not been well established.

Treatment is not indicated in all cases of ADHD; consider therapy only in light of complete history and evaluation of the child. The decision to prescribe pemoline should depend on the assessment of the chronicity and severity of the child's symptoms and their appropriateness for his or her age, and not depend solely on the presence of ≥ 1 of the behavioral characteristics.

Precautions

Hepatic effects: See Black Box Warning.

Drug abuse and dependence: The pharmacologic similarity of pemoline to other psychostimulants with known dependence liability suggests that psychological or physical dependence might occur. There have been isolated reports of transient psychotic symptoms occurring in adults following the long-term misuse of excessive oral doses. Give with caution to emotionally unstable patients who may increase the dosage on their own initiative.

Drug Interactions

Carefully monitor patients receiving pemoline with other drugs, especially drugs with CNS activity.

Decreased seizure threshold has been reported in patients receiving pemoline concomitantly with antiepileptic medications.

Adverse Reactions

Most frequent – Insomnia usually occurs early in therapy prior to optimum therapeutic response; it is often transient or responds to dosage reduction.

CNS: Convulsive seizures; Tourette's syndrome; hallucinations; dyskinetic movements of tongue, lips, face, and extremities; abnormal oculomotor function (eg, nystagmus, oculogyric crisis); mild depression; dizziness; increased irritability; headache; drowsiness.

GI: Stomachache; nausea. Anorexia with weight loss may occur during the first weeks. In most cases it is transient; weight gain usually resumes within 3 to 6 months.

Hepatic: Hepatic dysfunction including elevated liver enzymes, hepatitis, jaundice, and fatal hepatic failure has occurred. Elevated liver enzymes are not rare and appear reversible upon drug discontinuance. Most patients with elevated liver enzymes were asymptomatic.

Miscellaneous: Growth suppression with long-term use of stimulants in children; skin rashes; aplastic anemia (rare).

TACRINE HCI (Tetrahydroaminoacridine; THA)

Capsules: 10, 20, 30, and 40 mg (*Rx*)   *Cognex* (Parke-Davis)

Indications

Alzheimer's disease: Treatment of mild to moderate dementia of the Alzheimer's type.

Administration and Dosage

The rate of dose escalation may be slowed if a patient is intolerant to the recommended titration schedule. However, it is not advisable to accelerate the dose incrementation plan. Following initiation of therapy, or any dosage increase, observe patients carefully for adverse effects. Take between meals whenever possible; however, if minor GI upset occurs, take with meals to improve tolerability. Taking tacrine with meals can be expected to reduce plasma levels ≈ 30% to 40%.

Initiation of treatment: The initial dose of tacrine is 40 mg/day (10 mg 4 times/day). Maintain this dose for ≥ 4 weeks with every other week monitoring of transaminase levels beginning at week 4 of therapy. It is important that the dose not be increased during this period because of the potential for delayed onset of transaminase elevations.

Dose titration: Following 4 weeks of treatment at 40 mg/day (10 mg 4 times/day), increase the dose to 80 mg/day (20 mg 4 times/day), providing there are no significant transaminase elevations and the patient is tolerating treatment. Titrate patients to higher doses (120 and 160 mg/day in divided doses on a 4 times/day schedule) at 4-week intervals on the basis of tolerance.

Dose adjustment: Monitor serum transaminase levels (specifically ALT) every other week from at least week 4 to week 16 following initiation of treatment, after which monitoring may be decreased to every 3 months. For patients who develop ALT elevations > 2 times the upper limit of normal (ULN), the dose and monitoring regimen should be modified as described in the table below.

A full monitoring and dose titration sequence must be repeated in the event that a patient suspends treatment with tacrine for > 4 weeks.

Recommended Tacrine Dose and Monitoring Regimen Modification in Response to Transaminase Elevations	
Transaminase levels	Treatment and monitoring regimen
≤ 2 × ULN	Continue treatment according to recommended titration and monitoring schedule.
> 2 to ≤ 3 × ULN	Continue treatment according to recommended titration. Monitor transaminase levels weekly until levels return to normal limits.
> 3 to ≤ 5 × ULN	Reduce the daily dose by 40 mg/day. Monitor ALT levels weekly. Resume dose titration and every other week monitoring when transaminase levels return to within normal limits.
> 5 × ULN	Stop treatment. Monitor the patient closely for signs and symptoms associated with hepatitis and follow transaminase levels until within normal limits (see Rechallenge).

Experience is limited in patients with ALT > 10 × ULN. The risk of rechallenge must be considered against demonstrated clinical benefit. Patients with clinical jaundice confirmed by a significant elevation in total bilirubin (> 3 mg/dL) or those exhibiting clinical signs or symptoms of hypersensitivity (eg, rash or fever) in association with ALT elevations should immediately and permanently discontinue tacrine and not be rechallenged.

Rechallenge: Patients who are required to discontinue treatment because of transaminase elevations may be rechallenged once transaminase levels return to within normal limits. Rechallenge of patients exposed to transaminase elevations < 10 × ULN has not resulted in serious liver injury. However, because experience in the rechallenge of patients who had elevations > 10 × ULN is limited, the risks associated with the rechallenge of these patients are not well characterized. Carefully and frequently (weekly) monitor serum ALT when rechallenging such patients. If rechallenged, give patients an initial dose of 40 mg/day (10 mg 4 times/day) and monitor transaminase levels weekly. If, after 6 weeks on 40 mg/day, the patient is tolerating the dosage with no unacceptable elevations in transaminases, recommended dose titration and transaminase monitoring may be resumed.

Continue weekly monitoring of ALT levels for a total of 16 weeks, after which monitoring may be decreased to monthly for 2 months and every 3 months thereafter.

Actions

Pharmacology: Tacrine is a centrally acting reversible cholinesterase inhibitor, commonly referred to as THA.

Pharmacokinetics:

Absorption – Maximal plasma concentrations occur within 1 to 2 hours.

Distribution – Mean volume of distribution of tacrine is ≈ 349 L. Tacrine is ≈ 55% bound to plasma proteins.

Metabolism – Tacrine is extensively metabolized by the cytochrome P450 system.

Excretion – The elimination half-life is ≈ 2 to 4 hours.

Contraindications

Hypersensitivity to tacrine or acridine derivatives; patients previously treated with tacrine who developed treatment-associated jaundice; a serum bilirubin > 3 mg/dL; signs or symptoms of hypersensitivity (eg, rash or fever) in association with ALT elevations.

Warnings

Anesthesia: Tacrine is likely to exaggerate succinylcholine-type muscle relaxation during anesthesia.

Cardiovascular conditions: Tacrine may have vagotonic effects on the heart rate.

GI disease/dysfunction: Tacrine is an inhibitor of cholinesterase and may be expected to increase gastric acid secretion caused by increased cholinergic activity. Therefore, closely monitor patients at increased risk for developing ulcers for symptoms of active or occult GI bleeding.

Hepatic effects: Prescribe with care in patients with current evidence or history of abnormal liver function indicated by significant abnormalities in serum transaminase, bilirubin, and gamma-glutamyl transpeptidase levels.

The incidence of transaminase elevations is higher among females. There are no other known predictors of the risk of hepatocellular injury.

GU effects: Cholinomimetics may cause bladder outflow obstruction.

Neurological conditions:

Seizures – Cholinomimetics are believed to have some potential to cause generalized convulsions; however, seizure activity may also be a manifestation of Alzheimer's disease.

Cognitive function – Worsening of cognitive function has been reported following abrupt discontinuation of tacrine or after a large reduction in total daily dose (≥ 80 mg/day).

Pulmonary conditions: Because of its cholinomimetic action, use tacrine with care in patients with a history of asthma.

Hepatic disease: Although studies in patients with liver disease have not been done, it is likely that functional hepatic impairment will reduce the clearance of tacrine and its metabolites.

Pregnancy: Category C.

Lactation: It is not known whether this drug is excreted in breast milk.

Children: There are no adequate and well controlled trials to document the safety and efficacy of tacrine in any dementing illness occurring in children.

Precautions

Monitoring: Monitor serum transaminase levels (specifically ALT) every other week from at least week 4 to week 16 following initiation of treatment, after which monitoring may be decreased to every 3 months. Repeat a full monitoring sequence in the event that a patient suspends treatment with tacrine for > 4 weeks. If transaminase elevations occur, modify the dose (see Administration and Dosage).

Continue to monitor ALT levels weekly for a total of 16 weeks, then decrease to monthly for 2 months and to every 3 months thereafter.

Hematology: Decreased absolute neutrophil counts (ANC) < 500 to 1500/mcL have been reported rarely. The total clinical experience in > 12,000 patients does not indicate a clear association between tacrine treatment and serious white blood cell abnormalities.

Drug Interactions

Drugs that may be affected by tacrine include anticholinergics, cholinomimetics, cholinesterase inhibitors, and theophylline.

Drugs that may affect tacrine include cimetidine.

Tacrine is primarily eliminated by hepatic metabolism via cytochrome P450 drug metabolizing enzymes. Drug interactions may occur when it is given concurrently with agents such as theophylline that undergo extensive metabolism via cytochrome P450 IA2.

Adverse Reactions

Adverse reactions occurring in ≥ 3% of patients include elevated transaminases; nausea; vomiting; diarrhea; dyspepsia; myalgia; headache; fatigue; chest pain; weight decrease; agitation; depression; abnormal thinking; anxiety; anorexia; abdominal pain; flatulence; constipation; dizziness; confusion; ataxia; insomnia; somnolence; urinary incontinence; urinary tract infection; urination frequency; rash; facial flushing; coughing; upper respiratory tract infection; rhinitis.

RIVASTIGMINE

Capsules: 1.5, 3, 4.5, 6 mg (as tartrate) (*Rx*)	*Exelon* (Novartis)
Solution: 2 mg/mL (as tartrate) (*Rx*)	*Exelon* (Novartis)

Indications

Alzheimer's dementia: For the treatment of mild to moderate dementia of the Alzheimer's type.

Administration and Dosage

The recommended starting dose of rivastigmine is 1.5 mg twice a day. If dose is well tolerated, after a minimum of 2 weeks of treatment, the dose may be increased to 3 mg twice a day. Subsequent increases to 4.5 and 6 mg twice/day should be attempted after a minimum of 2 weeks at the previous dose. If adverse effects (eg, nausea, vomiting, abdominal pain, loss of appetite) cause intolerance during treatment, instruct the patient to discontinue treatment for several doses and then restart at the same or next lower dose level. If treatment is interrupted for longer than several days, reinitiate treatment with the lowest daily dose and titrate as described above. The maximum dose is 6 mg twice/day (12 mg/day).

Take with food in divided doses in the morning and evening.

Oral solution: Each dose of rivastigmine may be swallowed directly from the syringe or first mixed with a small glass of water, cold fruit juice, or soda. Instruct patients to stir and drink the mixture.

Rivastigmine oral solution and capsules may be interchanged at equal doses.

Storage/Stability: When rivastigmine oral solution is combined with cold fruit juice or soda, the mixture is stable at room temperature for ≤ 4 hours.

Actions

Pharmacology: While the precise mechanism of rivastigmine's action is unknown, it is postulated to exert its therapeutic effect by enhancing cholinergic function. This is accomplished by increasing the concentration of acetylcholine through reversible inhibition of its hydrolysis by cholinesterase. If this proposed mechanism is correct, rivastigmine's effect may lessen as the disease process advances and fewer cholinergic neurons remain functionally intact.

Pharmacokinetics:

    Absorption – Rivastigmine is rapidly and completely absorbed with an absolute bioavailability of ≈ 36% (3 mg dose). Peak plasma concentrations are reached in ≈ 1 hour.

    Distribution – Rivastigmine is widely distributed throughout the body with a volume of distribution in the range of 1.8 to 2.7 L/kg.

    Rivastigmine is ≈ 40% bound to plasma proteins.

    Metabolism – Rivastigmine is rapidly and extensively metabolized, primarily via cholinesterase-mediated hydrolysis to the decarbamylated metabolite.

    Excretion – The elimination half-life is ≈ 1.5 hours, with most elimination as metabolites via the urine.

Contraindications

Hypersensitivity to rivastigmine, other carbamate derivatives, or other components of the formulation.

Warnings

GI effects: Rivastigmine is associated with significant GI adverse reactions, including nausea and vomiting, anorexia, and weight loss.

Weight loss: In the controlled trials, ≈ 26% of women on high doses of rivastigmine (> 9 mg/day) had weight loss of ≥ 7% of their baseline weight compared with 6% in the placebo-treated patients. Approximately 18% of the males in the high dose group experienced a similar degree of weight loss compared with 4% in placebo-treated patients. It is not clear how much of the weight loss was associated with anorexia, nausea, vomiting, and diarrhea associated with drug administration.

Anorexia: In the controlled clinical trials, of the patients treated with a rivastigmine dose of 6 to 12 mg/day, 17% developed anorexia compared with 3% of the placebo patients. Neither the time course nor the severity of the anorexia is known.

Peptic ulcers/GI bleeding: Because of their pharmacological action, cholinesterase inhibitors may be expected to increase gastric acid secretion caused by increased cholinergic activity. Therefore, monitor patients closely for symptoms of active or occult GI bleeding, especially those at increased risk for developing ulcers (eg, those with a history of ulcer disease or those receiving concurrent nonsteroidal anti-inflammatory drugs [NSAID]). Clinical studies of rivastigmine have shown no significant increase, relative to placebo, in the incidence of either peptic ulcer disease or GI bleeding.

Anesthesia: Rivastigmine, as a cholinesterase inhibitor, is likely to exaggerate succinylcholine-type muscle relaxation during anesthesia.

Cardiovascular effects: Drugs that increase cholinergic activity may have vagotonic effects on heart rates (eg, bradycardia). The potential for this action may be particularly important in patients with "sick sinus syndrome" or other supraventricular cardiac conduction conditions.

Urinary obstruction: Drugs that increase cholinergic activity may cause urinary obstruction.

Seizures: Drugs that increase cholinergic activity are believed to have some potential for causing seizures. However, seizure activity also may be a manifestation of Alzheimer's disease.

Pulmonary effects: Like other drugs that increase cholinergic activity, use with care in patients with a history of asthma or obstructive pulmonary disease.

Pregnancy: Category B.

Lactation: It is not known whether rivastigmine is excreted in breast milk.

Drug Interactions

Drugs that may interfere with rivastigmine include anticholinergics and cholinomimetics and other cholinesterase inhibitors.

Adverse Reactions

Adverse reactions occurring in ≥ 3% of patients include the following: Dizziness; headache; insomnia; confusion; depression; anxiety; somnolence; hallucination; tremor; aggressive reaction; nausea; vomiting; diarrhea; anorexia; abdominal pain; dyspepsia; constipation; flatulence; accidental trauma; fatigue; urinary tract infection; asthenia; malaise; rhinitis; increased sweating; hypertension; influenza-like symptoms; syncope; weight decrease.

GALANTAMINE HBr

Tablets: 4, 8, and 12 mg (*Rx*)   *Reminyl* (Janssen)

Indications

Alzheimer's disease: Treatment of mild to moderate dementia of the Alzheimer's type.

Administration and Dosage

Dosage: 16 to 32 mg/day given twice/day. As the dose of 32 mg/day is less well tolerated than lower doses and does not provide increased effectiveness, the recommended dose range is 16 to 24 mg/day given twice/day.

Starting dose is 4 mg twice/day (8 mg/day). After a minimum of 4 weeks of treatment, if well tolerated, increase the dose to 8 mg twice/day (16 mg/day). Attempt a further increase to 12 mg twice/day (24 mg/day) only after a minimum of 4 weeks at the previous dose.

Administer galantamine twice/day, preferably with morning and evening meals.

Inform patients and caregivers that if therapy has been interrupted for several days or longer, the patient should be restarted at the lowest dose and the dose escalated to the current dose.

The abrupt withdrawal of galantamine in those patients who had been receiving doses in the effective range was not associated with an increased frequency of adverse events in comparison with those continuing to receive the same doses of that drug. However, the beneficial effects of galantamine are lost when the drug is discontinued.

Hepatic impairment: Galantamine plasma concentrations may be increased in patients with moderate to severe hepatic impairment. In patients with moderately impaired hepatic function, the dose generally should not exceed 16 mg/day. The use of galantamine in patients with severe hepatic impairment is not recommended.

Renal impairment: For patients with moderate renal impairment, the dose generally should not exceed 16 mg/day. In patients with severe renal impairment (Ccr < 9 mL/min), the use of galantamine is not recommended.

Actions

Pharmacology: Galantamine, a tertiary alkaloid extracted from daffodil bulbs, is a competitive and reversible inhibitor of acetylcholinesterase. While the precise mechanism of galantamine's action is unknown, it may exert its therapeutic effect by enhancing cholinergic function. This is accomplished by increasing the concentration of acetylcholine through reversible inhibition of its hydrolysis by cholinesterase.

Pharmacokinetics:

Absorption/Distribution – Galantamine is rapidly and completely absorbed with time-to-peak concentration in $\approx$ 1 hour. Bioavailability of the tablet was the same as the bioavailability of an oral solution (90%). Food did not affect the AUC of galantamine but C_{max} decreased by 25% and T_{max} was delayed by 1.5 hours.

The plasma protein binding of galantamine is 18% at therapeutically relevant concentrations.

Metabolism/Excretion – Galantamine is metabolized by hepatic cytochrome P450 enzymes, glucuronidated, and excreted unchanged in the urine. In vitro studies indicated that cytochrome CYP2D6 and CYP3A4 were the major cytochrome P450 isoenzymes involved in the metabolism of galantamine, and inhibitors of both pathways modestly increase oral bioavailability of galantamine.

After IV or oral administration, $\approx$ 20% of the dose was excreted as unchanged galantamine in the urine in 24 hours, representing a renal clearance of $\approx$ 65 mL/min, about 20% to 25% of the total plasma clearance of $\approx$ 300 mL/min.

Galantamine has a terminal elimination half-life of $\approx$ 7 hours (range, 4.4 to 10) and pharmacokinetics are linear over the range of 8 to 32 mg/day.

Special populations –

CYP2D6 poor metabolizers: Approximately 7% of the normal population has a genetic variation that leads to reduced levels of activity of the CYP2D6 isozyme. They are referred to as poor metabolizers. After a single oral dose of 4 or 8 mg galantamine, CYP2D6 poor metabolizers demonstrated a similar C_{max} and $\approx$ 35% AUC increase of unchanged galantamine compared with extensive metabolizers. Dosage adjustment is not necessary in patients identified as poor metabolizers as the dose of drug is individually titrated to tolerability.

Contraindications

Known hypersensitivity to galantamine or to any excipients used in the formulation.

Warnings

Pregnancy: Category B.

Lactation: It is not known whether galantamine is excreted in breast milk. Galantamine has no indication for use in nursing mothers.

Children: There are no adequate and well-controlled trials documenting the safety and efficacy of galantamine in any illness occurring in children. Therefore, the use of galantamine in children is not recommended.

Precautions

Special risk:

Anesthesia – Galantamine, as a cholinesterase inhibitor, is likely to exaggerate the neuromuscular blockade effects of succinylcholine-type and similar neuromuscular blocking agents during anesthesia.

Cardiovascular conditions – Because of their pharmacological action, cholinesterase inhibitors have vagotonic effects on the sinoatrial and atrioventricular nodes, leading to bradycardia and AV block. These actions may be particularly important to patients with supraventricular cardiac conduction disorders or to patients taking other drugs concomitantly that significantly slow heart rate. However, postmarketing surveillance of marketed anticholinesterase inhibitors has shown that bradycardia and all types of heart block have been reported in patients with and without known underlying cardiac conduction abnormalities. Therefore, consider all patients to be at risk for adverse effects on cardiac conduction.

Patients treated with galantamine $\geq$ 24 mg/day using the recommended dosing schedule showed a dose-related increase in risk of syncope.

GI conditions – Through their primary action, cholinomimetics may increase gastric acid secretion because of increased cholinergic activity. Therefore, monitor patients closely for symptoms of active or occult GI bleeding, especially those with an increased risk for developing ulcers (eg, those with a history of ulcer disease or patients using concurrent nonsteroidal anti-inflammatory drugs [NSAIDs]).

Galantamine has been shown to produce nausea, vomiting, diarrhea, anorexia, and weight loss. In patients who experienced nausea, the median duration was 5 to 7 days.

GU – Although this was not observed in clinical trials with galantamine, cholinomimetics may cause bladder outflow obstruction.

Neurological conditions –

Seizures: Cholinesterase inhibitors are believed to have some potential to cause generalized convulsions.

Pulmonary conditions: Because of its cholinomimetic action, prescribe galantamine with care to patients with a history of severe asthma or obstructive pulmonary disease.

Drug Interactions

Galantamine may interact with succinylcholine or bethanechol, cimetidine, ketoconazole, paroxetine, and erythromycin.

Adverse Reactions

The most frequent adverse reactions leading to discontinuation of galantamine therapy included nausea, dizziness, vomiting, anorexia, and syncope.

Adverse events occurring in ≥ 5% of galantamine patients and ≥ 2 times placebo include nausea, diarrhea, anorexia, vomiting, and weight decrease. Other adverse events occurring in ≥ 3% of patients receiving galantamine include dizziness, headache, depression, insomnia, somnolence, tremor, abdominal pain, dyspepsia, urinary tract infection, hematuria, fatigue, rhinitis, and anemia.

DONEPEZIL HCl

Tablets: 5 and 10 mg (*Rx*)   *Aricept* (Eisai/Pfizer)

Indications

Alzheimer's disease: The treatment of mild to moderate dementia of the Alzheimer's type.

Administration and Dosage

The dosages of donepezil are 5 and 10 mg once per day in the evening, just prior to retiring.

The higher dose of 10 mg did not provide a statistically significant clinical benefit greater than that of 5 mg. Do not increase to 10 mg until patients have been on a daily dose of 5 mg for 4 to 6 weeks.

Donepezil may be taken with or without food.

Actions

Pharmacology: Donepezil enhances cholinergic function. This increase in cholinergic function is accomplished by increasing the concentration of acetylcholine through reversible inhibition of its hydrolysis by acetylcholinesterase (AChE). If this proposed mechanism of action is correct, donepezil's effect may lessen as the disease process advances and fewer cholinergic neurons remain functionally intact.

Pharmacokinetics:

Absorption – Donepezil is well absorbed with a relative oral bioavailability of 100% and reaches peak plasma concentrations in 3 to 4 hours.

Distribution – Following multiple dose administration, steady state is reached within 15 days. Donepezil is ≈ 96% bound to human plasma proteins.

Metabolism – Donepezil is excreted in urine. It is metabolized by CYP 450 isoenzyme 2D6 and 3A4 and undergoes glucuronidation.

Excretion – The elimination half-life of donepezil is ≈ 70 hours and the mean apparent plasma clearance is 0.13 L/hr/kg.

Contraindications

Hypersensitivity to donepezil or to piperidine derivatives.

Warnings

Anesthesia: Donepezil, as a cholinesterase inhibitor, is likely to exaggerate succinyl-choline-type muscle relaxation during anesthesia.

Cardiovascular: Cholinesterase inhibitors may have vagotonic effects on heart rate (eg, bradycardia). The potential for this action may be particularly important to patients with "sick sinus syndrome" or other supraventricular cardiac conduction conditions. Syncopal episodes have occurred in association with the use of donepezil.

GI: Through their primary action, cholinesterase inhibitors may be expected to increase gastric acid secretion because of increased cholinergic activity. Therefore, monitor patients closely for symptoms of active or occult GI bleeding, especially those at increased risk for developing ulcers.

GU: Cholinomimetics may cause bladder outflow obstruction.

Seizures: Cholinomimetics may have some potential to cause generalized convulsions. However, seizure activity also may be a manifestation of Alzheimer's disease.

Pulmonary: Prescribe cholinesterase inhibitors with care for patients with a history of asthma or obstructive pulmonary disease.

Pregnancy: Category C.

Lactation: It is not known whether donepezil is excreted in breast milk.

Children: There are no adequate and well controlled tirals to document the safety and efficacy of donepezil in any illness occurring in children.

Drug Interactions

Drugs that may affect donepezil are ketoconazole and quinidine. Drugs that may be affected by donepezil include anticholinergics, cholinometics/cholinesterase inhibitors, NSAIDs, furosemide, digoxin, warfarin, theophylline, and cimetidine.

Adverse Reactions

Adverse reactions that may occur in ≥ 3% of patients include headache, whole body pain, fatigue, nausea, diarrhea, vomiting, anorexia, muscle cramps, insomnia, dizziness, depression, abnormal dreams, ecchymosis, and weight decrease.

AMPHETAMINES

Amphetamine, dextroamphetamine, and methamphetamine also are indicated for attention deficit disorders in children, as part of a total treatment program. For complete prescribing information on the amphetamines for this and other uses, consult the general amphetamine monograph.

ERGOLOID MESYLATES (Dihydrogenated Ergot Alkaloids, Dihydroergotoxine)

Tablets, sublingual: 0.5 mg (*Rx*)	Various, *Gerimal* (Rugby), *Hydergine* (Sandoz)
Tablets, oral: 0.5 mg (*Rx*)	Various
Tablets, sublingual: 1 mg (*Rx*)	Various, *Gerimal* (Rugby), *Hydergine* (Sandoz)
Tablets, oral: 1 mg (*Rx*)	Various, *Gerimal* (Rugby), *Hydergine* (Sandoz)
Capsules, liquid: 1 mg (*Rx*)	*Hydergine LC* (Sandoz)
Liquid: 1 mg/mL (*Rx*)	*Hydergine* (Sandoz)

Indications

Age-related mental capacity decline: Individuals > 60 years of age who manifest signs and symptoms of an idiopathic decline in mental capacity. Patients who respond suffer from some process related to aging or have some underlying dementing condition.

Administration and Dosage

The usual starting dose is 1 mg 3 times/day. Alleviation of symptoms usually is gradual; results may not be observed for 3 to 4 weeks. Doses up to 4.5 to 12 mg/day have been used. Up to 6 months of treatment may be necessary to determine efficacy, using doses of ≥ 6 mg/day. Do not chew or crush sublingual tablets.

Actions

Pharmacology: Ergoloid mesylates contain equal proportions of dihydroergocornine mesylate, dihydroergocristine mesylate, and dihydroergocryptine mesylate.

The mechanism by which ergoloid mesylates produce mental effects is unknown.

Pharmacokinetics: Ergoloid mesylates are rapidly absorbed from the GI tract; peak plasma concentrations are achieved within 0.6 to 3 hours. The liquid capsule has a 12% greater bioavailability than the oral tablet. The mean half-life of unchanged ergoloid in plasma is about 2.6 to 5.1 hours.

Contraindications

Hypersensitivity to ergoloid mesylates.

Acute or chronic psychosis, regardless of etiology.

Precautions

Before prescribing: Before prescribing ergoloid mesylates, exclude the possibility that the patient's signs and symptoms arise from a potentially reversible and treatable condition. Exclude delirium and dementiform illness secondary to systemic disease, primary neurological disease, or primary disturbance of mood.

Reassessment: Periodically reassess the diagnosis and the benefit of current therapy to the patient.

Adverse Reactions

Adverse reactions may include sublingual irritation; transient nausea and GI disturbances.

SEDATIVES/HYPNOTICS, NONBARBITURATE

To facilitate comparison, the products are divided into the following 2 groups: Miscellaneous nonbarbiturates and benzodiazepines. Although sedative doses can be given, these agents primarily are intended to be hypnotics.

In the table below, some pharmacokinetic properties of the nonbarbiturate sedative/hypnotics are compared. Do not use this table to predict exact duration of effect, but use as a guide in drug selection.

Nonbarbiturate Sedative/Hypnotics Pharmacokinetic Parameters							
Drug	Adult oral dose		Onset (min)	Duration of action (hrs)	Half-life (hrs)	Protein binding (%)	Urinary excretion, unchanged (%)
	Hypnotic	Sedative					
Miscellaneous nonbarbiturates							
Chloral hydrate	0.5 to 1 g	250 mg tid pc	30	nd	7 to 10[1]	35-41	nd
Ethchlorvynol	500 mg	100 to 200 mg bid or tid	15 to 60	5	10 to 20[2]	nd	40[3]
Paraldehyde	10 to 30 mL	5 to 10 mL	10 to 15	8 to 12	3.4 to 9.8	nd	small
Propiomazine	nd	10 to 20 mg	nd	nd	nd	nd	nd
Benzodiazepines							
Estazolam	1 to 2 mg	na	nd	nd	10 to 24	93	< 5
Flurazepam	15 to 30 mg	na	17	7 to 8	150 to 100[4]	97	< 1[4]
Quazepam	15 mg	na	nd	nd	25 to 41	> 95	trace
Temazepam	15 to 30 mg	na	nd	nd	10 to 17	98	1.5
Triazolam	0.125 to 0.5 mg	na	nd	nd	1.5 to 5.5	90	2

[1] Trichloroethanol, the principal metabolite.
[2] In acute use, half-life of the distribution phase (1 to 3 hours) is more appropriate.
[3] Free and conjugated forms of the major metabolite, secondary alcohol of ethchlorvynol.
[4] Active metabolite, desalkylflurazepam.
na = Not applicable.
nd = No data.

ZOLPIDEM TARTRATE

Tablets: 5 and 10 mg (c-iv)   *Ambien* (Searle)

Indications
Insomnia: Short-term treatment.

Administration and Dosage
Adults: Individualize dosage. Usual dose is 10 mg immediately before bedtime.
Downward dosage adjustment may be necessary when given with agents having known CNS-depressant effects because of the potentially additive effects.

Elderly or debilitated patients: Elderly or debilitated patients may be especially sensitive to the effects of zolpidem. Patients with hepatic insufficiency do not clear the drug as rapidly as healthy individuals. An initial 5 mg dose is recommended in these patients.

Maximum dose: The total dose should not exceed 10 mg.

Actions
Pharmacology: Zolpidem is a nonbenzodiazepine hypnotic. While zolpidem is a hypnotic agent with a chemical structure unrelated to benzodiazepines, barbiturates, or other drugs with known hypnotic properties, it interacts with a GABA-BZ receptor complex and shares some of the pharmacological properties of the benzodiazepines.

Pharmacokinetics: The pharmacokinetic profile is characterized by rapid absorption from the GI tract and a short elimination half-life. Zolpidem is converted to inactive metabolites that are eliminated primarily by renal excretion.

Warnings

Duration of therapy: Generally limit hypnotics to 7 to 10 days of use; re-evaluate the patient if they are to be taken for > 2 to 3 weeks. Do not prescribe in quantities exceeding a 1 month supply.

Psychiatric/Physical disorder: Because sleep disturbances may be the presenting manifestation of a physical or psychiatric disorder, initiate symptomatic treatment of insomnia only after a careful evaluation of the patient.

Abrupt discontinuation: Following the rapid dose decrease or abrupt discontinuation of sedative/hypnotics, signs and symptoms similar to those associated with withdrawal from other CNS-depressant drugs have occurred.

CNS-depressant effects: Zolpidem, like other sedative/hypnotic drugs, has CNS-depressant effects. Because of the rapid onset of action, only ingest immediately prior to going to bed. Zolpidem had additive effects when combined with alcohol; therefore, do not take with alcohol.

Renal function impairment: Data in end-stage renal failure patients repeatedly treated with zolpidem did not demonstrate drug accumulation or alterations in pharmacokinetic parameters. No dosage adjustment in renally impaired patients is required; however, closely monitor these patients.

Hepatic function impairment: Modify dosing accordingly in patients with hepatic insufficiency.

Elderly: Closely monitor these patients. Impaired motor or cognitive performance after repeated exposure or unusual sensitivity to sedative/hypnotic drugs is a concern in the treatment of elderly or debilitated patients.

Pregnancy: Category B.

Lactation: The use of zolpidem in nursing mothers is not recommended.

Children: Safety and efficacy in children < 18 years of age have not been established.

Precautions

Respiratory depression: Although preliminary studies did not reveal respiratory depressant effects at hypnotic doses in healthy individuals, observe caution if zolpidem is prescribed to patients with compromised respiratory function, since sedative/hypnotics have the capacity to depress respiratory drive.

Depression: As with other sedative/hypnotic drugs, administer zolpidem with caution to patients exhibiting signs or symptoms of depression. Suicidal tendencies may be present in such patients and protective measures may be required. Intentional overdosage is more common in this group of patients; therefore, prescribe the least amount of drug that is feasible for the patient at any one time.

Drug abuse and dependence: Sedative/hypnotics have produced withdrawal signs and symptoms following abrupt discontinuation. These reported symptoms range from mild dysphoria and insomnia to a withdrawal syndrome that may include abdominal and muscle cramps, vomiting, sweating, tremors, and convulsions. Zolpidem does not reveal any clear evidence for withdrawal syndrome.

Because individuals with a history of addiction to, or abuse of, drugs or alcohol are at risk of habituation and dependence, they should be under careful surveillance when receiving zolpidem or any other hypnotic.

Drug Interactions

Drug/Food interactions: For faster sleep onset, do not administer with or immediately after a meal.

Adverse Reactions

Adverse reactions occurring in ≥ 3% of patients include dizziness; drugged feelings; headache; allergy; back pain; headache; drowsiness; dizziness; lethargy; nausea; dyspepsia; diarrhea; myalgia; arthralgia; upper respiratory tract infection; sinusitis; pharyngitis; dry mouth.

ZALEPLON

Capsules: 5 and 10 mg (c-ɪv)	*Sonata* (Wyeth-Ayerst)

Indications
Insomnia: Short-term treatment of insomnia.

Administration and Dosage
The recommended dose of zaleplon for most nonelderly adults is 10 mg. For certain low-weight individuals, 5 mg may be a sufficient dose. Although the risk of certain adverse events associated with zaleplon appears to be dose dependent, the 20 mg dose has been shown to be adequately tolerated and may be considered for the occasional patient who does not benefit from a trial of a lower dose. Doses > 20 mg have not been adequately evaluated and are not recommended. Hypnotics should generally be limited to 7 to 10 days of use, and re-evaluation of the patient is recommended if they are to be taken for > 2 to 3 weeks.

Take zaleplon immediately before bedtime or after going to bed and experiencing difficulty falling asleep. Taking it with or immediately after a heavy, high-fat meal results in slower absorption and would be expected to reduce the effect of zaleplon on sleep latency.

Elderly/Debilitated: Elderly and debilitated patients appear to be more sensitive to the effects of hypnotics; therefore, the recommended dose for these patients is 5 mg. Doses > 10 mg are not recommended.

Hepatic function impairment: Treat patients with mild to moderate hepatic impairment with zaleplon 5 mg because of reduced clearance. Do not use in patients with severe hepatic impairment.

Renal function impairment: No dose adjustment is necessary in patients with mild to moderate renal impairment.

Concomitant cimetidine – Give an initial dose of 5 mg to patients concomitantly taking cimetidine (see Drug Interactions).

Actions
Pharmacology: Zaleplon is a nonbenzodiazepine hypnotic. Zaleplon has a chemical structure unrelated to benzodiazepines, barbiturates, or other drugs with known hypnotic properties.

Zaleplon binds selectively to the brain omega$_1$ receptor situated on the alpha subunit of the GABA$_A$ receptor complex and potentiates t-butyl-bicyclophosphorothionate (TBPS) binding.

Pharmacokinetics:

Absorption – Zaleplon is rapidly and almost completely absorbed following oral administration. Peak plasma concentrations are attained within ≈ 1 hour after oral administration.

Distribution – Zaleplon is a lipophilic compound with a volume of distribution of ≈ 1.4 L/kg following IV administration, indicating substantial distribution into extravascular tissues.

Metabolism – After oral administration, zaleplon is extensively metabolized with < 1% of the dose excreted unchanged in urine.

Excretion – Following oral or IV administration, zaleplon is rapidly eliminated with a mean half-life of ≈ 1 hour.

Contraindications
None known.

Warnings
Duration of therapy: Because sleep disturbances may be the presenting manifestation of a physical or psychiatric disorder, initiate symptomatic treatment of insomnia only after careful evaluation of the patient. The failure of insomnia to remit after 7 to 10 days of treatment may indicate the need for evaluation of a primary psychiatric or medical illness. Do not prescribe zaleplon in quantities exceeding a 1-month supply.

Abnormal thinking/behavior changes: A variety of abnormal thinking and behavior changes have been reported to occur in association with the use of sedatives/hypnotics.

Rapid dose decrease/discontinuation: Following rapid dose decrease or abrupt discontinuation of sedatives/hypnotics, there have been reports of signs and symptoms similar to those associated with withdrawal from other CNS-depressant drugs.

CNS effects: Zaleplon, like other hypnotics, has CNS-depressant effects. Caution patients receiving zaleplon against engaging in hazardous occupations requiring complete mental alertness or motor coordination (eg, operating machinery or driving a motor vehicle) after ingesting the drug, including potential impairment of the performance of such activities that may occur the day following zaleplon ingestion. Zaleplon, as well as other hypnotics, may produce additive CNS-depressant effects when coadministered with other psychotropic medications, anticonvulsants, antihistamines, ethanol, and other drugs that produce CNS depression. Do not take zaleplon with alcohol.

Hepatic function impairment: Zaleplon is metabolized primarily by the liver and undergoes significant presystemic metabolism. Consequently, the oral clearance of zaleplon was reduced by 70% and 87% in compensated and decompensated cirrhotic patients, respectively.

Elderly: Impaired motor or cognitive performance after repeated exposure or unusual sensitivity to sedative/hypnotic drugs is a concern in the treatment of elderly or debilitated patients.

Pregnancy: Category C.

Lactation: Because the effects of zaleplon on a nursing infant are not known, it is recommended that nursing mothers not take zaleplon.

Children: The safety and efficacy have not been established.

Precautions

Timing of drug administration: Take zaleplon immediately before bedtime or after going to bed and experiencing difficulty falling asleep. As with all sedatives/hypnotics, taking zaleplon while ambulatory may result in short-term memory impairment, hallucinations, impaired coordination, dizziness, and lightheadedness.

Respiratory effects: Although preliminary studies did not reveal respiratory depressant effects at hypnotic doses of zaleplon in healthy subjects, observe caution if zaleplon is prescribed to patients with compromised respiratory function because sedatives/hypnotics have the capacity to depress respiratory drive.

Depression: As with other sedative/hypnotic drugs, administer zaleplon with caution to patients exhibiting signs or symptoms of depression. Suicidal tendencies may be present in such patients and protective measures may be required. Intentional overdosage is more common in this group of patients; therefore, prescribe the least amount of the drug that is feasible for the patient at any one time.

Drug abuse and dependence:

Abuse – Two studies assessed the abuse liability of zaleplon at doses of 25, 50, and 75 mg in subjects with known histories of sedative drug abuse. The results of these studies indicate that zaleplon has an abuse potential similar to benzodiazepine and benzodiazepine-like hypnotics.

Drug Interactions

Drugs that induce CYP3A4: CYP3A4 is a minor metabolizing enzyme of zaleplon. The CYP3A4-inducer rifampin reduced zaleplon C_{max} and AUC by $\approx$ 80%.

Cimetidine: Cimetidine inhibits aldehyde oxidase and CYP3A4, the primary and secondary enzymes, respectively, responsible for zaleplon metabolism. Use an initial dose of 5 mg for patients concomitantly treated with cimetidine.

Drug/Food interactions: The effects of zaleplon on sleep onset may be reduced if it is taken with or immediately after a high-fat/heavy meal.

Adverse Reactions

Adverse effects occurring in ≥ 3% of patients include the following: Amnesia; anxiety; dizziness; paresthesia; somnolence; dyspepsia; nausea; eye pain; abdominal pain; asthenia; headache; myalgia; dysmenorrhea.

BENZODIAZEPINES

ESTAZOLAM	
Tablets: 1 and 2 mg (*c-iv*)	*ProSom* (Abbott)
FLURAZEPAM HCl	
Capsules: 15 and 30 mg (*c-iv*)	Various, *Dalmane* (Roche)
QUAZEPAM	
Tablets: 7.5 and 15 mg (*c-iv*)	*Doral* (Wallace)
TEMAZEPAM	
Capsules: 7.5, 15, and 30 mg (*c-iv*)	Various, *Restoril* (Sandoz)
TRIAZOLAM	
Tablets: 0.125 and 0.25 mg (*c-iv*)	Various, *Halcion* (Pharmacia)

Indications

Insomnia: Insomnia characterized by difficulty in falling asleep, frequent nocturnal awakenings, or early morning awakening. Can be used for recurring insomnia or poor sleeping habits and in acute or chronic medical situations requiring restful sleep.

Administration and Dosage

ESTAZOLAM:

    Adults – 1 mg at bedtime; however, some patients may need a 2 mg dose.

    Elderly – If healthy, 1 mg at bedtime; initiate increases with particular care.

    Debilitated or small elderly patients – Consider a starting dose of 0.5 mg, although this is only marginally effective in the overall elderly population.

FLURAZEPAM:

    Adults – 30 mg before bedtime. In some patients, 15 mg may suffice.

    Elderly or debilitated – Initiate with 15 mg until individual response is determined.

QUAZEPAM:

    Adults – Initiate at 15 mg until individual responses are determined; may reduce to 7.5 mg in some patients.

    Elderly or debilitated – Attempt to reduce nightly dosage after the first 1 or 2 nights.

TEMAZEPAM:

    Adults – Give 15 to 30 mg before bedtime.

    Elderly or debilitated – Initiate with 15 mg until individual response is determined.

TRIAZOLAM:

    Adults – 0.125 to 0.5 mg before bedtime.

    Elderly or debilitated – 0.125 to 0.25 mg. Initiate with 0.125 mg until individual response is determined.

Actions

Pharmacology: **Estazolam, flurazepam, quazepam, temazepam,** and **triazolam** are benzodiazepine derivatives useful as hypnotics. Benzodiazepines are believed to potentiate gamma aminobutyric acid (GABA) neuronal inhibition.

Pharmacokinetics:

		Select Benzodiazepine (Hypnotic) Pharmacokinetic Parameters			
Drug	Usual adult oral dose (mg)	Time to peak plasma levels (hrs)	Half-life (hrs)	Protein binding (%)	Urinary excretion, unchanged (%)
Estazolam	1 to 2	2	8 to 28	93	< 5
Flurazepam	15 to 30	0.5 to 1 (7.6 to 13.6)[1]	2 to 3 (47 to 100)[1]	97	< 1
Quazepam	7.5 to 15	2 (1 to 2)	41 (47 to 100)[1]	> 95	trace
Temazepam	15 to 30	1.2 to 1.6	3.5 to 18.4 (9 to 15)	96	0.2
Triazolam	0.125 to 0.5	1 to 2	1.5 to 5.5	78 to 89	2

[1] N-desalkylflurazepam, active metabolite.

Contraindications

Hypersensitivity to other benzodiazepines; pregnancy (see Warnings); established or suspected sleep apnea (**quazepam**).

Concurrent use with ketoconazole, itraconazole, and nefazodone, medications that significantly impair the oxidative metabolism of **triazolam** mediated by cytochrome P450 3A (CYP3A).

Warnings

Anterograde amnesia: Anterograde amnesia of varying severity and paradoxical reactions has occurred following therapeutic doses of **triazolam**. Although this effect generally occurred with a dose of 0.5 mg, it has also been reported with 0.125 and 0.25 mg doses. This effect may occur with some other benzodiazepines, but data suggest that it may occur at a higher rate with triazolam. Cases of "traveler's amnesia" have been reported by individuals who have taken triazolam to induce sleep while traveling.

Renal/Hepatic function impairment: Observe usual precautions under these conditions. Abnormal liver function tests as well as blood dyscrasias have been reported with benzodiazepines.

Elderly: The risk of developing oversedation, dizziness, confusion, or ataxia increases substantially with larger doses of benzodiazepines in elderly and debilitated patients. Initiate with lowest effective dose.

Pregnancy: Category X (estazolam, quazepam, temazepam, triazolam, flurazepam).

Lactation: Safety for use in the nursing mother has not been established.

Children:

Flurazepam – Not for use in children < 15 years of age.

Estazolam, quazepam, temazepam, triazolam – Not for use in children < 18 years of age.

Precautions

Monitoring: When **triazolam** or **estazolam** treatment is protracted, obtain periodic blood counts, urinalysis, and blood chemistry analyses.

Depression: Administer with caution in severely depressed patients or in those in whom there is evidence of latent depression or suicidal tendencies. Signs or symptoms of depression may be intensified by hypnotic drugs.

Sleep disorder: Rebound sleep disorder, which is characterized by recurrence of insomnia to levels worse than before treatment began, may occur following abrupt withdrawal of triazolam, usually during the first 1 to 3 nights. Gradual rather than abrupt discontinuation of the drug may help avoid this syndrome.

Nocturnal sleep: Disturbed nocturnal sleep may occur for the first or second night after discontinuing use.

Morning insomnia: Early morning insomnia, or early morning awakenings, appears to be more common with the use of short half-life agents (**temazepam, triazolam**) than agents with intermediate or long half-lives (**estazolam, flurazepam, quazepam**). However, daytime sleepiness appears to be more prevalent with the long half-life agents.

Respiratory depression and sleep apnea: Observe caution. In patients with compromised respiratory function, respiratory depression and sleep apnea have occurred.

Drug abuse and dependence: Withdrawal symptoms following abrupt discontinuation of benzodiazepines have occurred in patients receiving excessive doses over extended periods of time. Gradual withdrawal is preferred.

Hazardous tasks: Observe caution while driving or performing tasks requiring alertness.

Drug Interactions
Drugs that may affect benzodiazepines include alcohol/CNS depressants, cimetidine, oral contraceptives, disulfiram, isoniazid, probenecid, rifampin, smoking, theophyllines, and macrolides.

Drugs that may be affected by benzodiazepines include digoxin, neuromuscular blocking agents (nondepolarizing), and phenytoin.

Adverse Reactions
Adverse reactions include the following: Palpitations; chest pains; tachycardia; headache; nervousness; apprehension; irritability; confusion; euphoria; relaxed feeling; weakness; tremor; lack of concentration; coordination disorders; confusional states/memory impairment; depression; dreaming/nightmares; insomnia; paresthesia; restlessness; tiredness; dysesthesia; heartburn; nausea; vomiting; diarrhea; constipation; GI pain; anorexia; taste alterations; dry mouth; body/joint pain; tinnitus; GU complaints; cramps/pain; congestion.

Estazolam: Other adverse reactions reported only for estazolam include the following: Somnolence (42%); asthenia (11%); hypokinesia (8%); hangover (3%); cold symptoms, lower extremity/back/abdominal pain (1% to 3%).

SEDATIVES AND HYPNOTICS, BARBITURATES

AMOBARBITAL SODIUM

Powder for injection: (c-II)	*Amytal Sodium* (Lilly)

APROBARBITAL

Elixir: 40 mg/5 mL (c-III)	*Alurate* (Roche)

BUTABARBITAL SODIUM

Tablets: 15, 30, 50, and 100 mg (c-III)	Various, *Butisol Sodium* (Wallace)
Elixir: 30 mg/5 mL (c-III)	Various, *Butisol Sodium* (Wallace)

MEPHOBARBITAL

Tablets: 32, 50, and 100 mg (c-IV)	*Mebaral* (Sanofi Winthrop)

PENTOBARBITAL SODIUM

Capsules: 50 and 100 mg (c-II)	Various, *Nembutal Sodium* (Abbott)
Suppositories: 30, 60, 120, and 200 mg (c-III)	*Nembutal Sodium* (Abbott)
Injection: 50 mg/mL (c-II)	*Pentobarbital Sodium* (Wyeth-Ayerst), *Nembutal Sodium* (Abbott)

PHENOBARBITAL

Tablets: 15, 16, 30, 60, and 100 mg (c-IV)	Various, *Solfoton* (ECR Pharm.)
Capsules: 16 mg (c-IV)	*Solfoton* (ECR Pharm.)
Elixir: 15 mg/5 mL and 20 mg/5 mL (c-IV)	Various
Injection: 30, 60, 65, and 130 mg/mL (c-IV)	Various, *Luminal Sodium* (Sanofi Winthrop)

SECOBARBITAL SODIUM

Capsules: 100 mg (c-II)	Various, *Seconal Sodium Pulvules* (Lilly)
Injection: 50 mg/mL (c-II)	*Secobarbital Sodium* (Wyeth-Ayerst)

ORAL COMBINATIONS

Capsules: 50 mg amobarbital sodium and 50 mg secobarbital sodium; 100 mg amobarbital sodium and 100 mg secobarbital sodium (c-II)	*Tuinal 100 mg Pulvules*, *Tuinal 200 mg Pulvules* (Lilly)

The following general discussion of the barbiturates refers to their use as sedative-hypnotic agents and as anticonvulsants.

Indications

Sedation: Although traditionally used as nonspecific CNS depressants for daytime sedation, the barbiturates have generally been replaced by the benzodiazepines.

Hypnotic: Short-term treatment of insomnia, because barbiturates appear to lose their effectiveness in sleep induction and maintenance after 2 weeks. If insomnia persists, seek alternative therapy (including nondrug) for chronic insomnia.

Preanesthetic: Used as preanesthetic sedatives.

Anticonvulsant (mephobarbital, phenobarbital): Treatment of partial and generalized tonic-clonic and cortical focal seizures.

Acute convulsive episodes: Emergency control of certain acute convulsive episodes (eg, those associated with status epilepticus, cholera, eclampsia, meningitis, tetanus, and toxic reactions to strychnine or local anesthetics).

Administration and Dosage

IM injection: IM injection of the sodium salts should be made deeply into a large muscle. Do not exceed 5 mL at any one site because of possible tissue irritation. Monitor patient's vital signs.

IV: Restrict to conditions in which other routes are not feasible, either because the patient is unconscious or resists, or because prompt action is imperative. Slow IV injection is essential; observe patients carefully during administration.

Rectal administration: Rectally administered barbiturates are absorbed from the colon and are used occasionally in infants for prolonged convulsive states, or when oral or parenteral administration may be undesirable.

Elderly/Debilitated: Reduce dosage because these patients may be more sensitive to barbiturates.

Hepatic/Renal function impairment: Reduce dosage.

MEPHOBARBITAL:

Sedative –
Adults: 32 to 100 mg 3 or 4 times/day. Optimum dose is 50 mg 3 or 4 times/day.

Children: 16 to 32 mg 3 or 4 times/day.

Epilepsy –
Adults: Average dose is 400 to 600 mg/day.
Children (< 5 years of age): 16 to 32 mg 3 or 4 times/day.
Children (> 5 years of age): 32 to 64 mg 3 or 4 times/day.

Take at bedtime if seizures generally occur at night, and during the day if attacks are diurnal. Start treatment with a small dose and gradually increase over 4 or 5 days until optimum dosage is determined.

Combination drug therapy – May be used in combination with phenobarbital, in alternating courses or concurrently. When the two are used at the same time, the dose should be ≈ ½ the amount of each used alone. The average daily dose for an adult is 50 to 100 mg phenobarbital and 200 to 300 mg mephobarbital. May also be used with phenytoin. When used concurrently, a reduced dose of phenytoin is advisable, but the full dose of mephobarbital may be given. Satisfactory results have been obtained with an average daily dose of 230 mg phenytoin plus about 600 mg mephobarbital.

AMOBARBITAL SODIUM: The maximum single dose for an adult is 1 g.

Sedative – The usual adult dosage is 30 to 50 mg 2 or 3 times/day.

Hypnotic – The usual adult dose is 65 to 200 mg.

IM – The average IM dose ranges from 65 to 500 mg.

IV – Do not exceed the rate of 50 mg/min. Ordinarily, 65 to 500 mg may be given to a child 6 to 12 years of age.

APROBARBITAL:

Sedative – 40 mg 3 times/day.

Mild insomnia – 40 to 80 mg before retiring.

Pronounced insomnia – 80 to 160 mg before retiring.

BUTABARBITAL SODIUM:

Adults –
Daytime sedation: 15 to 30 mg 3 or 4 times/day.
Bedtime hypnotic: 50 to 100 mg
Preoperative sedation: 50 to 100 mg, 60 to 90 minutes before surgery.

Children –
Preoperative sedation: 2 to 6 mg/kg/day (maximum 100 mg).

PENTOBARBITAL SODIUM:

Oral –
Adults:
Sedation – 20 mg 3 or 4 times/day.
Hypnotic – 100 mg at bedtime.
Children:
Sedation/Preanesthetic – 2 to 6 mg/kg/day (maximum 100 mg), depending on age, weight, and degree of sedation desired.
Hypnotic – Base dosage on age and weight.

Rectal – Do not divide suppositories.
Adults: 120 to 200 mg.
Children:
12 to 14 years of age (36.4 to 50 kg; 80 to 110 lbs) – 60 or 120 mg.
5 to 12 years of age (18.2 to 36.4 kg; 40 to 80 lbs) – 60 mg.
1 to 4 years of age (9 to 18.2 kg; 20 to 40 lbs) – 30 or 60 mg.
2 months to 1 year of age (4.5 to 9 kg; 10 to 20 lbs) – 30 mg.

Parenteral –
IV: Initially administer 100 mg in the 70 kg adult. Reduce dosage proportionally for pediatric or debilitated patients. At least 1 minute is necessary to determine the full effect. If needed, additional small increments of the drug may be given to a total of 200 to 500 mg for healthy adults.

IM: The usual adult dosage is 150 to 200 mg; children's dosage frequently ranges from 2 to 6 mg/kg as a single IM injection, not to exceed 100 mg.

PHENOBARBITAL:

Anticonvulsant – In infants and children, a loading dose of 15 to 20 mg/kg produces blood levels of ≈ 20 mcg/mL shortly after administration.

Oral –

Adults:

Sedation – 30 to 120 mg/day in 2 to 3 divided doses. A single dose of 30 to 120 mg may be given at intervals; frequency is determined by response. It is generally considered that no more than 400 mg should be given during a 24-hour period.

Hypnotic – 100 to 200 mg.

Anticonvulsant – 60 to 100 mg/day.

Children:

Anticonvulsant – 3 to 6 mg/kg/day.

Sedation – 8 to 32 mg.

Hypnotic – Determined by age and weight.

Parenteral –

Adults:

Sedation – 30 to 120 mg/day IM or IV in 2 to 3 divided doses.

Preoperative sedation – 100 to 200 mg, IM only, 60 to 90 minutes before surgery.

Hypnotic – 100 to 320 mg IM or IV.

Acute convulsions – 200 to 320 mg IM or IV, repeat 6 hours as necessary.

Children:

Preoperative sedation – 1 to 3 mg/kg IM or IV.

Anticonvulsant – 4 to 6 mg/kg/day for 7 to 10 days to blood level of 10 to 15 mcg/mL, or 10 to 15 mg/kg/day, IV or IM.

Status epilepticus – 15 to 20 mg/kg IV over 10 to 15 minutes. It is imperative to achieve therapeutic levels as rapidly as possible. When given IV, it may require ≥ 15 minutes to attain peak levels in the brain.

SECOBARBITAL SODIUM:

Oral –

Adults:

Preoperative sedation – 200 to 300 mg 1 to 2 hours before surgery.

Bedtime hypnotic – 100 mg.

Children: For preoperative sedation, 2 to 6 mg/kg (maximum 100 mg).

Parenteral –

Adults:

Hypnotic – Usual dose is 100 to 200 mg IM or 50 to 250 mg IV.

Preoperative sedation – For light sedation, 1 mg/kg (0.5 to 0.75 mg/lb) IM, 10 to 15 minutes before procedure.

Dentistry – In patients who are to receive nerve blocks, 100 to 150 mg IV.

Children:

Preoperative sedation – 4 to 5 mg/kg IM.

Status epilepticus – 15 to 20 mg/kg IV over 15 minutes.

Actions

Pharmacology: These agents depress the sensory cortex, decrease motor activity, alter cerebellar function, and produce drowsiness, sedation, and hypnosis.

Barbiturates have little analgesic action at subanesthetic doses and may increase the reaction to painful stimuli. All barbiturates exhibit anticonvulsant activity in anesthetic doses. However, only phenobarbital and mephobarbital are effective as oral anticonvulsants in subhypnotic doses.

Pharmacokinetics:

Pharmacokinetics of Sedatives and Hypnotic Barbiturates						
		Half-Life (hrs)		Oral dosage range (mg)		Onset (minutes)	Duration (hours)
Barbiturate		Range	Mean	Sedative[1]	Hypnotic		
Long-acting	Mephobarbital	11 to 67	34	32 to 200	—	30 to ≥ 60	10 to 16
	Phenobarbital	53 to 118	79	30 to 120	100 to 320		
Intermediate	Amobarbital[2]	16 to 40	25	—	—	45 to 60	6 to 8
	Aprobarbital	14 to 34	24	120	40 to 160		
	Butabarbital	66 to 140	100	45 to 120	50 to 100		
Short-acting	Pentobarbital	15 to 50	≈[3]	40 to 120	100	10 to 15	3 to 4
	Secobarbital	15 to 40	28	—	100		

[1] Total daily dose; administered in 2 to 4 divided doses.
[2] Available as injection only.
[3] May follow dose-dependent kinetics. Mean t½ is 50 hours for 50 mg and 22 hours for 100 mg.

Contraindications

Barbiturate sensitivity; manifest or latent porphyria; marked impairment of liver function; severe respiratory disease when dyspnea or obstruction is evident; nephritic patients; patients with respiratory disease where dyspnea or obstruction is present; intra-arterial administration; SC administration; previous addiction to the sedative/hypnotic group.

Warnings

Habit forming: Tolerance or psychological and physical dependence may occur with continued use. Administer with caution, if at all, to patients who are mentally depressed, have suicidal tendencies or a history of drug abuse. Limit prescribing and dispensing to the amount required for the interval until the next appointment.

Withdrawal symptoms – Withdrawal symptoms can be severe and may cause death.

Treatment of dependence – Treatment of dependence consists of cautious and gradual withdrawal of the drug that takes an extended period of time.

IV administration: Too rapid administration may cause respiratory depression, apnea, laryngospasm, or vasodilation with fall in blood pressure. Parenteral solutions of barbiturates are highly alkaline. Therefore, use extreme care to avoid perivascular extravasation or intra-arterial injection.

Phenobarbital sodium – Phenobarbital sodium may be administered IM or IV as an anticonvulsant for emergency use. When administered IV, it may require ≥ 15 minutes before reaching peak concentrations in the brain.

Pain: Exercise caution when administering to patients with acute or chronic pain, because paradoxical excitement could be induced or important symptoms could be masked.

Seizure disorders: Status epilepticus may result from abrupt discontinuation, even when administered in small daily doses in the treatment of epilepsy.

Effects on vitamin D: Barbiturates may increase vitamin D requirements, possibly by increasing the metabolism of vitamin D via enzyme induction.

Renal function impairment: Barbiturates are excreted either partially or completely unchanged in the urine and are contraindicated in impaired renal function.

Hepatic function impairment: Barbiturates are metabolized primarily by hepatic microsomal enzymes. Administer with caution and initially in reduced doses.

Elderly: May produce marked excitement, depression, and confusion.

Pregnancy: Category D.

Lactation: Exercise caution when administering to the nursing mother because small amounts are excreted in breast milk.

Children: In some people, especially children, barbiturates repeatedly produce excitement rather than depression. Barbiturates may produce irritability, excitability, inappropriate tearfulness, and aggression in children. Safety and efficacy of amobarbital (children < 6 years of age) and aprobarbital have not been established.

Precautions

Monitoring: During prolonged therapy, perform periodic laboratory evaluation of organ systems, including hematopoietic, renal, and hepatic systems.

Special risk patients: Untoward reactions may occur in the presence of fever, hyperthyroidism, diabetes mellitus, and severe anemia. Use with caution.

Use **mephobarbital** with caution in myasthenia gravis and myxedema.

Drug Interactions

Drugs that may affect barbiturates include alcohol, charcoal, chloramphenicol, MAO inhibitors, rifampin, and valproic acid. Drugs that may be affected by barbiturates include acetaminophen, anticoagulants, beta blockers, carbamazepine, chloramphenicol, clonazepam, oral contraceptives, corticosteroids, digitoxin, doxorubicin, doxycycline, felodipine, fenoprofen, griseofulvin, hydantoins, methoxyflurane, metronidazole, narcotics, phenmetrazine, phenylbutazone, quinidine, theophylline, and verapamil.

Adverse Reactions

Adverse reactions may include somnolence; agitation; confusion; hyperkinesia; ataxia; CNS depression; nightmares; nervousness; psychiatric disturbance; hallucinations; insomnia; anxiety; dizziness; abnormal thinking; headache; fever (especially with chronic phenobarbital use); hypoventilation; apnea; bradycardia; hypotension; syncope; nausea; vomiting; constipation; liver damage, particularly with chronic phenobarbital use; skin rashes; angioedema (particularly following chronic phenobarbital use).

ANTICONVULSANTS

	Anticonvulsants: Indications and Pharmacokinetics					
	Drug	Labeled indications	Protein binding (%)	Metabolism/ Excretion	t½ (hrs)	Therapeutic serum levels (mcg/mL)
Barbiturates	Phenobarbital[1] (PB)	Status epilepticus Epilepsy, all forms Tonic-clonic	40 to 60	Liver; 25% eliminated unchanged in urine	53 to 140	15 to 40
Hydantoins	Phenytoin	Tonic-clonic Psychomotor	≈90	Liver; renal excretion. < 5% excreted unchanged	Dose-dependent[2]	5 to 20
	Mephenytoin	Tonic-clonic Psychomotor Focal Jacksonian	nd	Liver	95 (active metabolite)	nd
	Ethotoin	Tonic-clonic Psychomotor	nd	Liver; renal excretion of metabolites	3 to 9[3]	15 to 50
Succinimides	Ethosuximide	Absence	0	Liver; 25% excreted unchanged in urine	30 (children 7 to 9 yrs) 40 to 60 (adults)	40 to 100
	Methsuximide	Absence	nd	Liver; < 1% excreted unchanged in urine	<2 (40, active metabolite)	nd
	Phensuximide	Absence	nd	Urine, bile	8 (active metabolite)	nd
Sulfonamides	Zonisamide	Partial[4]	40	Accetylation and reduction; excreted in urine	63	nd
Oxazolidinediones	Trimethadione	Absence	0	Demethylated to dimethadione; 3% excreted unchanged	6 to 13 days (dimethadione)	≥ 700 (dimethdione)
Benzodiazepines	Clonazepam	Absence Myoclonic Akinetic	50 to 85	5 metabolites identified; urine is major excretion route	18 to 60	20 to 80 ng/mL
	Clorazepate	Partial[4]	97	Hydrolyzed in stomach to desmethyldiazepam (active); metabolized in liver, renally excreted	30 to 100	nd
	Diazepam	Status epilepticus[4] Epilepsy, all forms[4]	97 to 99	Liver, active metabolites	20 to 50	nd

Anticonvulsants: Indications and Pharmacokinetics						
	Drug	Labeled indications	Protein binding (%)	Metabolism/ Excretion	t½ (hrs)	Therapeutic serum levels (mcg/mL)
Miscellaneous	Primidone	Tonic-clonic Psychomotor Focal	20 to 25	Metabolized to PB and PEMA, both active	5 to 15 (primidone) 10 to 18 (PEMA) 53 to 140 (PB)	5 to 12 (primidone) 15 to 40 (PB)
	Valproic acid	Absence	80 to 94	Liver; excreted in urine	5 to 20	50 to 150
	Carbamazepine	Tonic-clonic Mixed Psychomotor	≈ 75	Liver to active 10, 11-epoxide. 72% excreted in urine, 28% in feces	18 to 54 (initial) 10 to 20[5] ≈ 6 (10, 11-epoxide)	4 to 12
	Phenacemide	Severe mixed psychomotor	nd	Liver	nd	nd
	Felbamate[6]	Partial (adults) Partial/generalized assoc. with Lennox-Gastaut syndrome (children)	22 to 25	40% to 50% unchanged in urine, 40% as unidentified metabolites and conjugates	20 to 23	nd[7]
	Oxcarbazepine	Partial	40	Reduced to 10-monohydroxy metabolite (active); excreted in urine (80%)	2; 9 (MHD)	nd[7]
	Lamotrigine	Partial (adults)	≈ 55	Glucuronic acid conjugation to inactive metabolites; 94% excreted in urine, 2% in feces	≈ 33[5]	nd

[1] Other barbiturates are also used as anticonvulsants. See Sedatives/Hypnotics section.
[2] Exhibits dose-dependent, nonlinear pharmacokinetics.
[3] Below 8 mcg/mL; > 8 mcg/mL, t½ not defined because of dose-dependent, nonlinear pharmacokinetics.
[4] Recommended for adjunctive use.
[5] Undergoes autoinduction. Half-life after repeated doses.
[6] Because of cases of aplastic anemia, it has been recommended that the use of this drug be discontinued unless, in the judgment of the physician, continued therapy is warranted.
[7] Value of monitoring blood levels not established.

HYDANTOINS

PHENYTOIN SODIUM, PARENTERAL
Injection: 50 mg/mL (*Rx*)　　　　　　　Various, *Dilantin* (Parke-Davis)

PHENYTOIN, ORAL
Tablets, chewable: 50 mg (*Rx*)　　　　　*Dilantin Infatab* (Parke-Davis)
Oral suspension: 30 and 125 mg/5 mL (*Rx*)　*Dilantin-30 or -125* (Parke-Davis)

PHENYTOIN SODIUM, ORAL, PROMPT
Capsules: 30 and 100 mg (*Rx*)　　　　　Various, *Diphenylan Sodium* (Lannett)

PHENYTOIN SODIUM, EXTENDED
Capsules: 30 and 100 mg (*Rx*)　　　　　*Dilantin Kapseals* (Parke-Davis)

PHENYTOIN SODIUM WITH PHENOBARBITAL
Capsules: 100 mg/16 and 32 mg (*Rx*)　　*Dilantin with Phenobarbital Kapseals* (Parke-Davis)

MEPHENYTOIN
Tablets: 100 mg (*Rx*)　　　　　　　　　*Mesantoin* (Sandoz)

ETHOTOIN
Tablets: 250 and 500 mg (*Rx*)　　　　　*Peganone* (Abbott)

FOSPHENYTOIN SODIUM
Injection: 150 mg (100 mg phenytoin) and 750 mg (500 mg phenytoin) (*Rx*)　*Cerebyx* (Parke-Davis)

Indications

Control of grand mal and psychomotor seizures.

Phenytoin: To prevent and treat seizures occurring during or following neurosurgery.
   Parenteral – For the control of status epilepticus of the grand mal type.

Mephenytoin: For patients refractory to less toxic anticonvulsants; focal and Jacksonian seizures.

Administration and Dosage

PHENYTOIN SODIUM, PARENTERAL:

Status epilepticus – In adults, administer loading dose of 10 to 15 mg/kg slowly. Follow by maintenance doses of 100 mg orally or IV every 6 to 8 hours. For neonates and children, oral absorption of phenytoin is unreliable; IV loading dose is 15 to 20 mg/kg in divided doses of 5 to 10 mg/kg.

Neurosurgery (prophylactic dosage) – 100 to 200 mg IM at $\approx$ 4 hour intervals during surgery and the postoperative period.

PHENYTOIN AND PHENYTOIN SODIUM, ORAL: Phenytoin sodium contains 92% phenytoin. Phenytoin and phenytoin sodium prompt are not for once/day dosing. Phenytoin sodium extended may be used for once/day dosing.

Loading dose – An oral loading dose of phenytoin may be used in adults who require rapid steady-state serum levels and where IV administration is not possible.

Initially, 1 g of phenytoin capsules is divided into 3 doses (400 mg, 300 mg, 300 mg) and administered at intervals of 2 hours. Normal maintenance dosage is then instituted 24 hours after the loading dose, with frequent serum level determinations.

Adults – Adults who have recieved no previous treatment may be started on 100 mg (125 mg suspension) 3 times/day. Satisfactory maintenance dosage is 300 to 400 mg/day. An increase to 600 mg/day (625 mg/day suspension) may be necessary.

Pediatric – Initially, 5 mg/kg/day in 2 or 3 equally divided doses with subsequent dosage individualized to a maximum of 300 mg/day. Daily maintenance dosage is 4 to 8 mg/kg. Children over 6 years may require the minimum adult dose (300 mg/day). If the daily dosage cannot be divided equally, give the larger dose before retiring.

Single daily dosage – In adults, if seizure control is established with divided doses of three 100 mg extended phenytoin sodium capsules daily, once/daydosage with 300 mg may be considered; patient compliance is essntial on a once/day regimen. Only extended phenytoin sodium capsules are recommended once/day.

Bioavailability – Because of the potential bioavailability differences between products, brand interchange is not recommended. Dosage adjustments may be required when switching from the extended to the prompt products.

MEPHENYTOIN: Start with 50 or 100 mg/day during the first week and therafter increase the daily dose by 50 or 100 mg at weekly intervals.

Adults – The average dose ranges from 200 to 600 mg/day. In some instances, as much as 800 mg/day may be required to obtain full seizure control.

Children – Children usually require from 100 to 400 mg/day.

ETHOTOIN: Administer in 4 to 6 divided doses/day. Take after food; space doses as evenly as practical.

Adults – The initial daily dose should be $\leq$ 1 g, with subsequent gradual dosage increases over several days. The usual adult maintenance dose is 2 to 3 g/day; < 2 g/day is ineffective in most adults.

Pediatric – Initial dose should not exceed 750 mg/day. The usual maintenance dose in children ranges from 500 mg to 1 g/day, although occasionally 2 g or rarely 3 g/day may be necessary.

FOSPHENYTOIN: The dose, concentration in dosing solutions and infusion rate of IV fosphenytoin is expressed as phenytoin sodium equivalents (PE) to avoid the need to perform molecular weight-based adjustments when coverting between fosphenytoin and phenytoin sodium doses. Prescribe and dipense fosphenytoin in PEs. Fosphenytoin has important differences in administration from those for parenteral phenytoin sodium.

Dilute fosphenytoin in 5% Dextrose or 0.9% Saline Solution for Injection to a concentration ranging from 1.5 to 25 mg PE/mL.

Status epilepticus – The loading dose 15 to 20 mg PE/kg administered at 100 to 150 mg PE/min.

Because the full antiepileptic effect of phenytoin, whether given as fosphenytoin or parenteral phenytoin, is not immediate, other measures, including concomitant administration of an IV benzodiazepine, will usually be necessary for control of status epilepticus.

Nonemergent and maintenance dosing –

Loading dose: 10 to 20 mg PE/kg given IV or IM.

Maintenance dose: 4 to 6 mg PE/kg/day.

Because if the risk of hypotension, administer at a rate of ≤ 150 mg PE/min.

Continuously monitor the electrocardiogram, blood pressure, and respiratory function and observe the patient throughout the period of maximal serum phenytoin concentrations, ≈ 10 to 20 minutes after the end of the infusion.

Renal/Hepatic function impairment – Because of an increased fraction of unbound phenytoin in patients with renal or hepatic disease, or in those with hypoalbuminemia, interpret total phenytoin plasma concentrations with caution. Unbound phenytoin concentrations may be more useful in these patients. After IV administration, fosphenytoin clearance to phenytoin may be increased without a similar increase in phenytoin clearance. This has the potential to increase the frequency and severity of adverse events.

Elderly – Age does not have a significant impact on the pharmacokinetics of fosphenytoin following administration. Phenytoin clearance is decreased slightly in elderly patients and lower or less frequent dosing may be required.

Actions

Pharmacology: The primary site of action of hydantoins appears to be the motor cortex, where spread of seizure activity is inhibited. Possibly by promoting sodium efflux from neurons, hydantoins tend to stabilize the threshold against hyperexcitability.

Pharmacokinetics:

Absorption/Distribution – Phenytoin is slowly absorbed from the small intestine. Rate and extent of absorption varies and is dependent on the product formulation. Bioavailability may differ among products of different manufacturers. Administration IM results in precipitation of phenytoin at the injection site, resulting in slow and erratic absorption, which may continue for up to 5 days or more. Plasma protein binding is 87% to 93% and is lower in uremic patients and neonates. Volume of distribution averages 0.6 L/kg.

Phenytoin's therapeutic plasma concentration is 10 to 20 mcg/mL, although many patients achieve complete seizure control at lower serum concentrations.

Metabolism/Excretion – Phenytoin is metabolized in the liver and excreted in the urine. The metabolism of phenytoin is capacity-limited and shows saturability. Elimination is exponential (first-order) at plasma concentrations < 10 mcg/mL, and plasma half-life ranges from 6 to 24 hours.

Contraindications

Hypersensitivity to hydantoins.

Ethotoin: Hepatic abnormalities or hematologic disorders.

Phenytoin: Because of its effect on ventricular automaticity, do not use phenytoin in sinus bradycardia, sino-atrial block, second- and third-degree AV block, or in patients with Adams-Stokes syndrome.

Warnings

Withdrawal: Abrupt withdrawal in epileptic patients may precipitate status epilepticus.

Other seizures: Hydantoins are not indicated in seizures caused by hypoglycemia or other metabolic causes.

Mephenytoin: Use only if safer anticonvulsants have failed after an adequate trial.

Phenytoin: Use with caution in hypotension and severe myocardial insufficiency.

Hypersensitivity reactions: Phenytoin hypersensitivity reactions are not typical; they may present as one of many different syndromes (eg, lymphoma, hepatitis, Stevens-Johnson syndrome) and may include such symptoms as fever, rash, arthralgias, or lymphadenopathy.

Hepatic function impairment: Biotransformation of hydantoins occurs in the liver; elderly patients or those with impaired liver function or severe illness may show early signs of toxicity.

    Induced abnormalities – Phenytoin-induced hepatitis is one of the more commonly reported hypersensitivity syndromes.

Pregnancy: There is an association between use of anticonvulsant drugs by women with epilepsy and an elevated incidence of birth defects in children born to these women. The great majority of mothers receiving anticonvulsant medication deliver normal infants.

Lactation: These drugs are excreted in breast milk.

Precautions

Hematologic effects: Perform blood counts and urinalyses when therapy is begun and at monthly intervals for several months thereafter. Blood dyscrasias have occurred.

Dermatologic effects: Discontinue these drugs if a skin rash appears. If the rash is exfoliative, purpuric, or bullous, do not resume use.

Lymph node hyperplasia: Lymph node hyperplasia has been associated with hydantoins, and may represent a hypersensitivity reaction.

Hyperglycemia: Hyperglycemia, resulting from the drug's inhibitory effect on insulin release, has occurred. Hydantoins also may raise blood sugar levels in hyperglycemic people.

Cardiovascular: Death from cardiac arrest has occurred after too-rapid IV administration, sometimes preceded by marked QRS widening. Administer cautiously in the presence of advanced AV block. Do not exceed an IV infusion rate of 50 mg/min.

Osteomalacia: Osteomalacia has been associated with phenytoin therapy.

Acute intermittent porphyria: Administer hydantoins cautiously to patients with acute intermittent porphyria.

Drug Interactions

Increased hydantoin effects:

Hydantoin Drug Interactions: Increased Hydantoin Effects			
Inhibit metabolism		Displace anticonvulsant	Unknown
Amiodarone	Metronidazole	Salicylates	Chlorpheniramine
Benzodiazepines	Miconazole	Tricyclic antidepressants	Ibuprofen
Chloramphenicol	Omeprazole	Valproic acid	Phenothiazines
Cimetidine	Phenacemide		
Disulfiram	Phenylbutazone		
Ethanol	Succinimides		
(acute ingestion)	Sulfonamides		
Fluconazole	Trimethoprim		
Isoniazid	Valproic acid		

Decreased hydantoin effects:

Hydantoin Drug Interactions: Decreased Hydantoin Effects		
Increase metabolism	Decrease absorption	Unknown
Barbiturates Carbamazepine Diazoxide Ethanol (chronic ingestion) Rifampin Theophylline	Antacids Charcoal Sucralfate	Antineoplastics Folic acid Influenza virus vaccine Loxapine Nitrofurantoin Pyridoxine

Hydantoin Drug Interactions: Decreased Effects of Other Drugs		
Increased metabolism by phenytoin		Other
Acetaminophen Amiodarone Carbamazepine Cardiac glycosides Corticosteroids Dicumarol Disopyramide Doxycycline Estrogens	Haloperidol Methadone Metyrapone Mexiletine Oral contraceptives Quinidine Theophylline Valproic acid	Cyclosporine Dopamine Furosemide Levodopa Levonorgestrel Mebendazole Nondepolarizing muscle relaxants Phenothiazines Sulfonylureas

Drugs that may be affected by hydantoins include lithium, meperidine, primidone, and warfarin.

Drug/Lab test interactions: Phenytoin may interfere with the **metyrapone** and the 1 mg **dexamethasone** tests.

Drug/Food interactions: Several case reports and single-dose studies suggest that enteral nutritional therapy may decrease phenytoin concentrations; however, this has not been substantiated.

Adverse Reactions

Cardiovascular:

Phenytoin IV – Cardiovascular collapse; CNS depression; hypotension (when the drug is administered rapidly IV).

CNS: Nystagmus; ataxia; dysarthria; slurred speech; mental confusion; dizziness; insomnia; transient nervousness; motor twitchings; diplopia; fatigue; irritability; drowsiness; depression; numbness; tremor; headache.

Dermatologic: Manifestations sometimes accompanied by fever have included scarlatiniform, morbilliform, maculopapular, urticarial, and nonspecific rashes; a morbilliform rash is the most common.

Endocrine: Diabetes insipidus; hyperglycemia.

GI: Nausea; vomiting; diarrhea; constipation.

GU: Urinary retention; oliguria; dysuria; vaginitis; albuminuria; genital edema; kidney failure; polyuria; urethral pain; urinary incontinence; vaginal moniliasis.

Hematologic: Hematopoietic complications, some fatal, include thrombocytopenia, leukopenia, granulocytopenia, agranulocytosis, and pancytopenia. Macrocytosis and megaloblastic anemia usually respond to folic acid therapy. Eosinophilia; monocytosis; leukocytosis; simple anemia; hemolytic anemia; aplastic anemia; ecchymosis.

Respiratory: Pneumonia; pharyngitis; sinusitis; hyperventilation; rhinitis; apnea; aspiration pneumonia; asthma; dyspnea; atelectasis; increased cough/sputum; epistaxis; hypoxia; pneumothorax; hemoptysis; bronchitis; chest pain; pulmonary fibrosis.

Special senses: Tinnitus; diplopia; taste perversion; amblyopia; deafness; visual field defect; eye pain; conjunctivitis; photophobia; hyperacusis; mydriasis; parosmia; ear pain; taste loss.

Lab test abnormalities: Phenytoin may decrease serum thyroxine and free thyroxine concentrations.

Miscellaneous: Polyarthropathy; hyperglycemia; weight gain; chest pain; edema; fever; photophobia; conjunctivitis; gynecomastia.

Gingival hyperplasia – Gingival hyperplasia occurs frequently with phenytoin.

ZONISAMIDE

Capsules: 100 mg (Rx) | *Zonegran* (Elan)

Indications
Epilepsy: Adjunctive therapy in the treatment of partial seizures in adults with epilepsy.

Administration and Dosage
Adults > 16 years of age: Individualize dose starting with 100 mg/day. The dose may be increased after 2 weeks to 200 mg/day. Additional dose increases to 300 and 400 mg/day may be made in ≥ 2 weeks to achieve steady state at each dose level. Administer zonisamide once or twice/day, except during the 100 mg dosage initiation. Zonisamide may be taken with or without food. Swallow the capsules whole. Use caution in patients with renal or hepatic disease.

Although the regimen described is one that has been shown to be tolerated, the prescriber may wish to prolong the duration of treatment at the lower doses in order to fully assess the effects of zonisamide at steady state, noting that many of the side effects of zonisamide are more frequent at doses of ≥ 300 mg/day. Although there is some evidence of greater response at doses > 100 to 200 mg/day, the increase appears small, and formal dose-response studies have not been conducted. Evidence from controlled trials suggest that zonisamide doses > 100 to 600 mg/day are effective, but there is no suggestion of increasing response > 400 mg/day. There is little experience with doses > 600 mg/day.

Discontinuation of therapy: Abrupt withdrawal of zonisamide in patients with epilepsy may precipitate increased seizure frequency or status epilepticus. Gradually reduce dose of zonisamide.

Actions
Pharmacology: The precise mechanism(s) of action is unknown.

In vitro pharmacological studies suggest that zonisamide blocks sodium channels and reduces voltage-dependent, transient inward currents (T-type Ca^{2+} currents), consequently stabilizing neuronal membranes and suppressing neuronal hypersynchronization. Zonisamide does not appear to potentiate the synaptic activity of GABA. In vivo microdialysis studies demonstrated that zonisamide facilitates dopaminergic and serotonergic neurotransmission.

Pharmacokinetics: Peak plasma concentrations (range, 2 to 5 mcg/mL) in healthy volunteers occur within 2 to 6 hours. The apparent volume of distribution of zonisamide is ≈ 1.45 L/kg. At concentrations of 1 to 7 mcg/mL, it is ≈ 40% bound to human plasma proteins. The elimination half-life of zonisamide in plasma is ≈ 63 hours. The elimination half-life in red blood cells is ≈ 105 hours. Zonisamide is excreted primarily in urine.

Contraindications
Hypersensitivity to sulfonamides or zonisamide.

Warnings
Hypersensitivity reactions: Fatalities have occurred, although rarely, as a result of severe reactions to sulfonamides (zonisamide is a sulfonamide) including Stevens-Johnson syndrome (SJS), toxic epidermal necrolysis (TEN), fulminant hepatic necrosis, agranulocytosis, aplastic anemia, and other blood dyscrasias. Such reactions may occur when a sulfonamide is readministered regardless of the route of administration.

Renal function impairment: Zonisamide was associated with a statistically significant 8% mean increase from the baseline of serum creatinine and blood urea nitrogen (BUN). The increase appeared to persist over time but was not progressive; this has been interpreted as an effect on glomerular filtration rate (GFR). The decrease in GFR appeared within the first 4 weeks of treatment. There is no information about reversibility, after drug discontinuation, of the effects of GFR after long-term use. Discontinue zonisamide in patients who develop acute renal failure or a clinically significant sustained increase in the creatinine/BUN concentration. Do not use zonisamide in patients with renal failure (estimated GFR < 50 mL/min), as there has been insufficient experience concerning drug dosing and toxicity.

Fertility impairment: The effect of zonisamide on human fertility is unknown.

Elderly: Use caution in selecting a dose for an elderly patient, usually starting at the low end of the dosing range.

Pregnancy: Category C.

Lactation: It is not known whether zonisamide is excreted in breast milk.

Children: Safety and efficacy of zonisamide in pediatric patients have not been established. Zonisamide is not approved for pediatric use.

Precautions

Lab test abnormalities: Monitor renal function periodically.

Zonisamide was associated with an increase in serum alkaline phosphatase, with a mean increase of $\approx$ 7% over the baseline.

Hazardous tasks: Zonisamide may produce drowsiness, especially at higher doses. Advise patients not to drive a car or operate other complex machinery until they have gained experience on zonisamide.

Drug Interactions

CYP 450: Drugs that induce liver enzymes such as phenytoin, carbamazepine, or phenobarbital increase the metabolism and clearance of zonisamide and decrease its half-life. Concurrent medication with drugs that either induce or inhibit CYP3A4 would be expected to alter serum concentrations of zonisamide. Zonisamide is not expected to interfere with the metabolism of other drugs that are metabolized by cytochrome P450 isozymes.

Drug/Food interactions: The time to maximum concentration of zonisamide is delayed in the presence of food, but no effect on bioavailability occurs.

Adverse Reactions

The most commonly observed adverse events associated with the use of zonisamide were somnolence, anorexia, dizziness, headache, nausea, and agitation/irritability.

The adverse events most commonly associated with discontinuation were somnolence, fatigue, or ataxia (6%); anorexia (3%); difficulty concentrating (2%); difficulty with memory, mental slowing, nausea/vomiting (2%); and weight loss (1%). Many of these adverse events were dose-related.

Adverse reactions occurring in ≥ 3% of patients include the following: Agitation/irritability; anxiety; ataxia; confusion; depression; difficulty concentrating; difficulty with memory; dizziness; fatigue; headache; insomnia; mental slowing; nystamus; paresthesia; somnolence; tiredness; abdominal pain; anorexia; diarrhea; dyspepsia; nausea; diplopia; speech abnormalities; flu syndrome; rash; weight loss.

CLONAZEPAM

Tablets: 0.5, 1, and 2 mg (c-iv)   *Klonopin* (Roche)

For complete prescribing information, refer to the Benzodiazepine monograph in the Antianxiety Agents section.

Indications
Used alone or as adjunctive treatment of the Lennox-Gastaut syndrome (petit mal variant), akinetic, and myoclonic seizures. It may be useful in patients with absence (petit mal) seizures who have failed to respond to succinimides.

Administration and Dosage
Adults: Initial dose should not exceed 1.5 mg/day in 3 divided doses. Increase in increments of 0.5 to 1 mg every 3 days until seizures are adequately controlled or until side effects preclude any further increase. Individualize maintenance dosage. Maximum recommended dosage is 20 mg/day.

Infants and children (≤ 10 years or 30 kg): To minimize drowsiness, the initial dose should be between 0.01 to 0.03 mg/kg/day, not to exceed 0.05 mg/kg/day, given in 2 or 3 divided doses. Increase dosage by not more than 0.25 to 0.5 mg every third day until a daily maintenance dose of 0.1 to 0.2 mg/kg has been reached, unless seizures are controlled or side effects preclude further increase. When possible, divide the daily dose into 3 equal doses. If doses are not equally divided, give the largest dose at bedtime.

CLORAZEPATE DIPOTASSIUM

Tablets: 3.75, 7.5, 11.25, 15, and 22.5 mg (c-iv)   Various, *Tranxene-T* (Abbott)

For complete prescribing information, refer to the Benzodiazepine monograph in the Antianxiety Agents section.

Indications
Partial seizures: As adjunctive therapy in the management of partial seizures.

Alcohol withdrawal: Symptomatic relief of anxiety and for the symptomatic relief of acute alcohol withdrawal (see monograph in the Antianxiety Agents section).

Administration and Dosage
Adults and children (> 12 years of age): The maximum initial dose is 7.5 mg 3 times/day. Increase dosage by no more than 7.5 mg every week and do not exceed 90 mg/day.

Children: Maximum initial dose is 7.5 mg 2 times/day. Increase by ≤ 7.5 mg every week; do not exceed 60 mg/day. Not recommended in patients < 9 years of age.

DIAZEPAM

Tablets: 2, 5, and 10 mg (c-iv)	Various, *Valium* (Roche)
Solution (intensol): 5 mg/mL (c-iv)	*Diazepam Intensol* (Roxane)
Solution: 5 mg/5 mL (c-iv)	*Diazepam* (Roxane)
Injection: 5 mg/mL (c-iv)	Various, *Valium* (Roche), *Dizac Emulsified* (Ohmeda)
Gel, rectal: 2.5 mg (pediatric), 5 mg (pediatric), 10 mg (pediatric and adult), 15 mg (adult), and 20 mg (adult) (c-iv)	*Diastat* (Athena)

For complete prescribing information, refer to the Benzodiazepine monograph in the Antianxiety Agents section.

Indications

Oral: May be used adjunctively in convulsive disorders; it is not proven useful as sole therapy.

Parenteral: Adjunct in status epilepticus and severe recurrent convulsive seizures.

Rectal: For selected, refractory patients on stable regimens of anti-epileptic agents who require intermittent use of diazepam to control bouts of increased seizure activity.

Administration and Dosage

Oral (tablets, oral solution, and Intensol): Adults – 2 to 10 mg 2 to 4 times/day.

    Elderly or debilitated patients – 2 to 2.5 mg once or twice/day initially.

    Children – Not for use in children < 6 months of age. Give 1 to 2.5 mg 3 or 4 times/day initially; increase gradually as needed and tolerated.

Intensol preparation: Mix with liquid or semi-solid food such as water, juices, soda, applesauce, and puddings. Consume the entire amount immediately. Do not store.

Parenteral:

    Adults – Do not administer diazepam emulsified injection IM. Initially 5 to 10 mg. May be repeated at 10 to 15 minute intervals up to a maximum dose of 30 mg if necessary. Therapy may be repeated in 2 to 4 hours; however, residual active metabolites may persist.

    Children ≥ 5 years of age – 1 mg every 2 to 5 minutes up to a maximum of 10 mg. Repeat in 2 to 4 hours if necessary.

    Infants > 30 days of age and children < 5 years of age – 0.2 to 0.5 mg slowly every 2 to 5 minutes up to a maximum of 5 mg. Safety and efficacy of parenteral diazepam has not been established in the neonate (≤ 30 days of age).

    Admixture incompatibility – Do not mix or dilute with other solutions or drugs in syringe or infusion flask. Diazepam interacts with plastic containers and administration sets, significantly decreasing availability of drug delivered.

Rectal: 0.2 to 0.5 mg/kg depending on age.

    2 to 5 years of age – 0.5 mg/kg.

    6 to 11 years of age – 0.3 mg/kg.

    ≥ 12 years of age – 0.2 mg/kg.

Calculate the recommended dose by rounding upward to the next available unit dose. A second dose, when required, may be given 4 to 12 hours after the first dose. Do not treat > 5 episodes per month or > 1 episode every 5 days.

    Elderly and debilitated – Adjust dosage downward to reduce ataxia or oversedation.

Diazepam Rectal Dosing Based on Age and Weight			
2 to 5 years of age weight (kg)	6 to 11 years of age weight (kg)	≥ 12 years of age weight (kg)	Dose (mg)
6 to 11	10 to 18	14 to 27	5
12 to 22	19 to 37	28 to 50	10
23 to 33	38 to 55	51 to 75	15
34 to 44	56 to 74	76 to 111	20

A 2.5 mg supplemental dose may be given for patients requiring more precise dose titration or as a partial replacement dose for patients who may expel a portion of the first dose.

LAMOTRIGINE

Tablets: 25, 100, 150, and 200 mg (*Rx*)

Tablets, chewable: 2, 5, and 25 mg (*Rx*)

Lamictal (GlaxoSmithKline)

Lamictal Chewable Dispersible Tablets (Glaxo-SmithKline)

Warning:

Serious rashes requiring hospitalization and discontinuation of treatment have been reported in association with lamotrigine use. The incidence of these rashes, which include Stevens-Johnson syndrome, is ≈ 1% in pediatric patients (< 16 years of age) and 0.3% in adults.

Rare cases of toxic epidermal necrolysis or rash-related death have occurred, but their numbers are too few to permit a precise estimate of the rate.

Because the rate of serious rash is greater in pediatric patients than in adults, it bears emphasis that lamotrigine is approved only for use in pediatric patients < 16 years of age who have seizures associated with the Lennox-Gastaut syndrome (see Indications).

Other than age, no factors have been identified that are known to predict the risk of occurrence or the severity of rash associated with lamotrigine. It is suggested, yet to be proven, that the risk of rash may also be increased by 1) coadministration of lamotrigine with valproic acid (VPA), 2) exceeding the recommended initial dose of lamotrigine, or 3) exceeding the recommended dose escalation for lamotrigine. However, cases have been reported in the absence of these factors.

Nearly all cases of life-threatening rashes associated with lamotrigine have occurred within 2 to 8 weeks of treatment initiation. However, isolated cases have been reported after prolonged treatment (eg, 6 months). Accordingly, duration of therapy cannot be relied upon as a means to predict the potential risk heralded by the first appearance of a rash.

Although benign rashes also occur with lamotrigine, it is not possible to predict reliably which rashes will prove to be life-threatening. Accordingly, discontinue lamotrigine at the first sign of rash, unless the rash is clearly not drug-related. Discontinuation of treatment may not prevent a rash from becoming life-threatening or permanently disabling or disfiguring.

Indications

Epilepsy: Adjunctive therapy in the treatment of partial seizures in adults with epilepsy and as adjunctive therapy in the generalized seizures of Lennox-Gastaut syndrome in pediatric and adult patients.

Indicated for conversion to monotherapy in adults with partial seizures who are receiving treatment with a single enzyme-inducing AED.

Safety and efficacy have not been established as initial monotherapy, for conversion to monotherapy from non-enzyme-inducing AEDs (eg, valproate), or for simultaneous conversion to monotherapy from ≥ 2 concomitant AEDs.

Administration and Dosage

Adjunctive therapy: For dosing guidelines below, enzyme-inducing antiepileptic drugs (EIAEDs) include phenytoin, carbamazepine, phenobarbital, and primidone.

Lamictal added to AED regimen containing VPA and EIAEDs – The effect of AEDs other than EIAEDs and VPA on the metabolism of lamotrigine is not currently known. Therefore, no specific dosing guidelines can be provided in that situation. Conservative starting doses and dose escalations (as with comcomitant VPA) would be prudent; maintenance dosing would be expected to fall between the maintenance dose with VPA and the maintenance dose without VPA, but with an EIAED. Smaller starting doses and slower dose escalations than those used in clinical trials are recommended because of the suggestions that the risk of rash may be decreased by smaller starting doses and slower dose escalations. It may take several weeks to months to achieve an individualized maintenance dose. It is likely that patients 2 to 6 years of age will require a maintenance dose at the higher end of the maintenance dose range.

Lamotrigine added to AEDs other than EIAEDs and VPA – The effect of AEDs other than EIAEDs and VPA on the metabolism of lamotrigine cannot be predicted. Therefore, no specific dosing guidelines can be provided in that situation. Exercise conservative starting doses and dose escalations (as with concomitant VPA). Maintenance dosing would be expected to fall between the maintenance dose with VPA and the maintenance dose when added to EIAEDs without VPA.

Patients 2 to 12 years of age:

Lamotrigine Added to an AED Regimen Containing VPA in Patients 2 to 12 Years of Age			
Weeks 1 and 2	0.15 mg/kg/day in 1 or 2 divided doses, rounded down to the nearest whole tablet.		
Weeks 3 and 4	0.3 mg/kg/day in 1 or 2 divided doses, rounded down to the nearest whole tablet.		
Weight-based dosing can be achieved by using the following guide:			
If the patient's weight is:		Give this daily dose using the most appropriate combination of lamotrigine 2 and 5 mg tablets	
Greater than	And less than	Weeks 1 and 2	Weeks 3 and 4
6.7 kg	14 kg	2 mg every other day	2 mg every day
14.1 kg	27 kg	2 mg every day	4 mg every day
27.1 kg	34 kg	4 mg every day	8 mg every day
34.1 kg	40 kg	5 mg every day	10 mg every day
Usual maintenance dose: 1 to 5 mg/kg/day (maximum 200 mg/day in 1 or 2 divided doses). To achieve the usual maintenance dose, increase subsequent doses every 1 to 2 weeks as follows: Calculate 0.3 mg/kg/day, round this amount down to the nearest whole tablet, and add this amount to the previously administered daily dose.			

The smallest available strength of lamotrigine chewable dispersible tablets is 2 mg. Administer only whole tablets. If the calculated dose cannot be achieved using whole tablets, round down to the nearest whole tablet.

Lamotrigine Added to EIAEDs (Without Valproic Acid) in Patients 2 to 12 Years of Age	
Weeks 1 and 2	0.6 mg/kg/day in 2 divided doses, rounded down to the nearest 5 mg.
Weeks 3 and 4	1.2 mg/kg/day in 2 divided doses, rounded down to the nearest 5 mg.
Usual maintenance dose: 5 to 15 mg/kg/day (maximum 400 mg/day in 2 divided doses). To achieve the usual maintenance dose, increase subsequent doses every 1 to 2 weeks as follows: Calculate 1.2 mg/kg/day, round this amount down to the nearest 5 mg, and add this amount to the previously administered daily dose.	

Patients > 12 years of age: Recommended dosing guidelines for lamotrigine added to valproic acid and guidelines for lamotrigine added to EIAEDs are summarized in the tables below.

Lamotrigine Added to AED Regimen Containing Valproic Acid in Patients > 12 Years of Age	
Weeks 1 and 2	25 mg every other day
Weeks 3 and 4	25 mg every day
Usual maintenance dose: 100 to 400 mg/day (1 or 2 divided doses). To achieve maintenance, doses may be increased by 25 to 50 mg/day every 1 to 2 weeks. The usual maintenance dose in patients adding lamotrigine to valproic acid alone ranges from 100 to 200 mg/day.	

Lamotrigine Added to EIAEDs (Without Valproic Acid) in Patients > 12 Years of Age	
Weeks 1 and 2	50 mg/day
Weeks 3 and 4	100 mg/day in 2 divided doses
Usual maintenance dose: 300 to 500 mg/day (in 2 divided doses). To achieve maintenance, increase doses by 100 mg/day every 1 to 2 weeks.	

Conversion from a single EIAED to monotherapy with lamotrigine in patients ≥ 16 years of age: The goal of the transition regimen is to effect the conversion to monotherapy with lamotrigine under conditions that ensure adequate seizure control while mitigating the risk of serious rash associated with the rapid titration of lamotrigine.

The recommended maintenance dose of lamotrigine as monotherapy is 500 mg/day given in 2 divided doses.

The conversion regimen involves first titrating lamotrigine to the target dose (500 mg/day in 2 divided doses) while maintaining the dose of the EIAED at a fixed level.

Withdraw concomitant EIAED by 20% decrements each week over a 4-week period.

Because of an increased risk of rash, do not exceed the recommended initial dose and subsequent dose escalations (see Warning Box).

Usual maintenance dose: In patients receiving multi-drug regimens employing EIAEDs without valproic acid, maintenance doses of adjunctive lamotrigine as high as 700 mg/day have been used. In patients receiving valproic acid alone, maintenance doses of adjunctive lamotrigine as high as 200 mg/day have been used.

Renal function impairment: Base initial doses on the patient's AED regimen (see above); reduced maintenance doses may be effective for patients with significant renal function impairment. Use with caution in these patients.

Hepatic function impairment: Generally, reduce initial, escalation, and maintenance doses by ≈ 50% in patients with moderate (Child-Pugh Grade B) and 75% in patients with severe (Child-Pugh Grade C) hepatic impairment. Adjust escalation and maintenance doses according to clinical response.

Discontinuation strategy: For patients receiving lamotrigine in combination with other AEDs, consider a re-evaluation for all AEDs in the regimen if a change in seizure control or an appearance or worsening of adverse experiences is observed.

If a decision is made to discontinue therapy with lamotrigine, a stepwise reduction of dose over ≥ 2 weeks (≈ 50% per week) is recommended unless safety concerns require a more rapid withdrawal (see Precautions).

Discontinuing an EIAED prolongs the half-life of lamotrigine; discontinuing valproic acid shortens the half-life of lamotrigine.

Target plasma levels: A therapeutic plasma concentration range has not been established for lamotrigine. Base dosing of lamotrigine on therapeutic response.

Administration of chewable dispersible tablets: Swallow lamotrigine chewable dispersible tablets whole, chewed, or dispersed in water or diluted fruit juice. If chewed, consume a small amount of water or diluted fruit juice to aid in swallowing.

To disperse chewable dispersible tablets, add the tablets to a small amount of liquid (1 teaspoon or enough to cover the medication). Approximately 1 minute later, when the tablets are completely dispersed, swirl the solution and consume the entire quantity immediately. Do not attempt to administer partial quantities of the dispersed tablets.

Actions

Pharmacology: Lamotrigine is chemically unrelated to existing AEDs. The precise mechanism(s) by which lamotrigine exerts its anticonvulsant action are unknown.

Pharmacokinetics:

Absorption/Distribution – Lamotrigine is rapidly and completely absorbed after oral administration.

Metabolism/Excretion – Lamotrigine is eliminated more rapidly in patients who have been taking hepatic EIAEDs.

Following multiple administrations (150 mg twice a day) to healthy volunteers taking no other medications, lamotrigine induced its own metabolism resulting in a 25% decrease (25.4 hours) in half-life and a 37% increase (0.58 mL/min/kg) in plasma clearance at steady state compared with values obtained in the same volunteers following a single dose.

Contraindications

Hypersensitivity to the drug or its components.

Warnings

Hypersensitivity reactions: Hypersensitivity reactions, some fatal or life-threatening, also have occurred. Some reactions have included clinical features of multiorgan dysfunction such as hepatic abnormalities and evidence of disseminated intravascular coagulation. It is important to note that early manifestations of hypersensitivity (eg, fever, lymphadenopathy) may be present even though a rash is not evident.

Withdrawal seizures: Do not abruptly discontinue AEDs because of the possibility of increasing seizure frequency. Unless safety concerns require a more rapid withdrawal, taper the dose of lamotrigine over a period of at least 2 weeks.

Organ failure: Fatalities associated with multi-organ failure and various degrees of hepatic failure have been reported during premarketing development. These cases occurred in association with other serious events (eg, status epilepticus, overwhelming sepsis), making it impossible to identify the initiating cause.

Addition of lamotrigine to a multidrug regimen that includes valproic acid: Because valproic acid reduces the clearance of lamotrigine, the dosage of lamotrigine in the presence of valproic acid is less than half of that required in its absence.

Dermatologic: Use caution, especially in pediatric patients.

There is evidence that the inclusion of valproate in a multidrug regimen increases the risk of serious, potentially life-threatening rash.

Renal/Hepatic function impairment: Use with caution.

Elderly: Exercise caution in dose selection for elderly patients.

Pregnancy: Category C.

Lactation: Preliminary data indicate that lamotrigine passes into breast milk.

Children: In pediatric patients, lamotrigine is only indicated as adjunctive therapy for the generalized seizures of Lennox-Gastaut syndrome. Safety and efficacy for other uses in patients < 16 years of age have not been established.

Precautions

Monitoring: The value of monitoring plasma concentrations of lamotrigine has not been established. Because of the possible pharmacokinetic interactions between lamotrigine and other AEDs being taken concomitantly, monitoring of the plasma levels of lamotrigine and concomitant AEDs may be indicated, particularly during dosage adjustments.

Status epilepticus: Valid estimates of the incidence of treatment-emergent status epilepticus among lamotrigine-treated patients are difficult to obtain. At a minimum, 7 of 2343 adult patients had episodes that could unequivocally be described as status epilepticus. In addition, variably defined episodes of seizure exacerbation (eg, seizure clusters, seizure flurries) were reported.

Melanin-containing tissues: Lamotrigine binds to melanin and may cause toxicity in these tissues after extended use. Be aware of the possibility of long-term ophthalmologic effects.

Special risk: Caution is advised when using lamotrigine in patients with diseases or conditions that could affect metabolism or elimination of the drug, such as renal or hepatic function impairment (see Warnings) or cardiac function impairment.

Photosensitivity: Photosensitization (photoallergy or phototoxicity) may occur.

Drug Interactions

Drugs that may affect lamotrigine include carbamazepine, acetaminophen, folate inhibitors, phenobarbital, primidone, phenytoin, valproic acid, rifamycins, and succinimides.

Drugs that may be affected by lamotrigine include carbamazepine and valproic acid.

Adverse Reactions

Approximiately 11% of the 3378 adult patients who received lamotrigine in premarketing clinical trials discontinued treatment because of an adverse experience.

Adverse reactions occurring in ≥ 3% of patients include rash; ataxia; blurred vision; diplopia; dizziness; nausea; vomiting; headache; fever; abdominal pain; diarrhea; dyspepsia; constipation; somnolence; incoordination; insomnia; tremor; depression; anxiety; convulsion; irritability; rhinitis; pharyngitis; cough increased; pruritus; vision abnormality; dysmenorrhea; vaginitis; tooth disorder; speech disorder; flu syndrome; eczema; anorexia; urinary tract infection; pneumonia; infection; accidental injury; flu syndrome; asthenia; hemorrhage.

With Lennox-Gastaut syndrome, 3.8% of patients on lamotrigine discontinued because of adverse experiences. The most common adverse experience that led to discontinuation was rash.

Approximately 10% of the 1136 pediatric patients with Lennox-Gastaut syndrome discontinued treatment because of an adverse experience. The adverse events most commonly associated with discontinuation were rash (3.9%), aggravated reaction (1.7%), and ataxia (0.9%).

LEVETIRACETAM

Tablets: 250, 500, and 750 mg (*Rx*)   *Keppra* (UCB Pharma)

Indications

Epilepsy: Adjunctive therapy in the treatment of partial onset seizures in adults with epilepsy.

Administration and Dosage

Initiate treatment with 1000 mg/day, given as twice/day dosing (500 mg twice per day). Additional dosing increments may be given (1000 mg/day additional every 2 weeks) to a maximum recommended daily dose of 3000 mg. Long-term experience at doses > 3000 mg/day is relatively minimal, and there is no evidence that doses > 3000 mg/day confer additional benefit.

Give orally with or without food.

Renal function impairment: Individualize dosing according to the patient's renal function status. Recommended doses and adjustment for dose are shown in the following table. To use this dosing table, an estimate of the patient's Ccr in mL/min is needed.

Levetiracetam Dosing Adjustment Regimen for Patients with Impaired Renal Function			
Group	Ccr (mL/min)	Dosage (mg)	Frequency
Normal	> 80	500 to 1500	q 12 h
Mild	50-80	500 to 1000	q 12 h
Moderate	30-50	250 to 750	q 12 h
Severe	< 30	250 to 500	q 12 h
ESRD patients using dialysis	—	500 to 1000[1]	q 12 h

[1] Following dialysis, a 250 to 500 mg supplemental dose is recommended.

Hepatic function impairment: No dose adjustment is needed for patients with hepatic impairment.

Actions

Pharmacology: Levetiracetam is chemically unrelated to other antiepileptic drugs. The precise mechanism by which levetiracetam exerts its antiepileptic effect is unknown.

Pharmacokinetics: Absorption is rapid, with peak plasma concentrations occurring in ≈ 1 hour following oral administration in fasted subjects. Steady state is achieved after 2 days of multiple twice/day dosing. Levetiracetam is not extensively metabolized. Levetiracetam is eliminated from the systemic circulation by renal excretion.

Contraindications

Hypersensitivity to the drug or any of its ingredients.

Warnings

CNS effects:

Somnolence – In controlled trials of patients with epilepsy, 14.8% of levetiracetam-treated patients reported somnolence compared with 8.4% of placebo patients.

Asthenia – In controlled trials of patients with epilepsy, 14.7% of levetiracetam-treated patients reported asthenia vs 9.1% with placebo.

Coordination difficulties – A total of 3.4% of levetiracetam-treated patients experienced coordination difficulties (reported as either ataxia, abnormal gait, or incoordination) vs 1.6% with placebo.

Somnolence, asthenia, and coordination difficulties occurred most frequently within the first 4 weeks of treatment.

Psychotic symptoms – In controlled trials of patients with epilepsy, 5 (0.7%) of levetiracetam-treated patients experienced psychotic symptoms compared with 1 (0.2%) placebo patient. A total of 13.3% of levetiracetam patients experienced other behavioral symptoms (eg, agitation, hostility, anxiety, apathy, emotional lability, depersonalization, depression) compared with 6.2% of placebo patients.

In addition, 4 (0.5%) levetiracetam-treated patients attempted suicide vs 0% with placebo.

Withdrawal seizure: Withdraw antiepileptic drugs, including levetiracetam, gradually to minimize the potential of increased seizure frequency.

Renal function impairment: Take caution in dosing patients with moderate and severe renal impairment and patients undergoing hemodialysis. Reduce dosage in patients with impaired renal function receiving levetiracetam, and give supplemental doses to patients after dialysis (see Actions and Administration and Dosage).

Elderly: No overall differences in safety were observed between subjects ≥ 65 years of age and younger subjects. There were insufficient numbers of elderly subjects in controlled trials of epilepsy to adequately assess the effectiveness of levetiracetam in these patients.

Pregnancy: Category C.

Lactation: It is not known whether this drug is excreted in breast milk. Use caution when levetiracetam is administered to a nursing woman.

Children: Safety and efficacy in patients < 16 years of age have not been established.

Precautions

Hematologic effects: Minor but statistically significant decreases compared with placebo in total mean RBC count ($0.03 \times 10^6/mm^2$), mean hemoglobin (0.09 g/dL), and mean hematocrit (0.38%), were seen in levetiracetam-treated patients in controlled trials.

A total of 3.2% of treated and 1.8% of placebo patients had ≥ 1 possibly significant (≤ $2.8 \times 10^9/L$) decreased WBC, and 2.4% of treated and 1.4% of placebo patients had ≥ 1 possibly significant (≤ $1 \times 10^9/L$) decreased neutrophil count. Of the treated patients with a low neutrophil count, all but one rose toward or to baseline with continued treatment. No patient was discontinued secondary to low neutrophil counts.

Hazardous tasks: Patients should use caution while driving or performing other tasks requiring alertness, coordination or physical dexterity.

Drug Interactions

Antiepileptic drugs (AEDs): Potential drug interactions between levetiracetam and existing AEDs (phenytoin, carbamazepine, valproic acid, phenobarbital, lamotrigine, gabapentin, and primidone) were assessed by evaluating the serum concentrations of levetiracetam and these AEDs during placebo-controlled clinical studies. These data indicate that levetiracetam does not influence the plasma concentration of existing AEDs and that these AEDs do not influence the pharmacokinetics of levetiracetam.

Drug/Food interactions: Food does not affect the extent of absorption of levetiracetam, but it decreases C_{max} by 20% and delays T_{max} by 1.5 hours.

Adverse Reactions

The most frequently reported adverse events associated with the use of levetiracetam in combination with other AEDs were somnolence, asthenia, infection, and dizziness.

Adverse reactions occurring in $\geq$ 3% of patients include the following: Somnolence; dizziness; depression; nervousness; ataxia; vertigo; pharyngitis; rhinitis; asthenia; headache; infection; pain; anorexia.

Adverse reactions most commonly associated with discontinuation or dose reduction of levetiracetam in patients with epilepsy include somnolence and convulsion.

PRIMIDONE

Tablets: 50 mg (*Rx*)	*Mysoline* (Wyeth-Ayerst)
Tablets: 250 mg (*Rx*)	Various, *Mysoline* (Wyeth-Ayerst)
Oral Suspension: 250 mg/5 mL (*Rx*)	*Mysoline* (Wyeth-Ayerst)

Indications

Epilepsy: For control of grand mal, psychomotor, or focal epileptic seizures, either alone or with other anticonvulsants. It may control grand mal seizures refractory to other anticonvulsants.

Unlabeled uses: Benign familial tremor (essential tremor, 750 mg/day).

Administration and Dosage

Individualize dosage.

Adults and children (> 8 years of age): Patients who have received no previous treatment may be started on primidone according to the following regimen:

Days 1 to 3 – 100 to 125 mg at bedtime.

Days 4 to 6 – 100 to 125 mg twice/day.

Days 7 to 9 – 100 to 125 mg 3 times/day.

Day 10 – maintenance – 250 mg 3 to 4 times/day. If required, increase dose to 250 mg 5 to 6 times/day, but do not exceed doses of 500 mg 4 times/day (2 g/day).

Children (< 8 years of age): The following regimen may be used to initiate therapy:

Days 1 to 3 – 50 mg at bedtime.

Days 4 to 6 – 50 mg twice/day.

Days 7 to 9 – 100 mg twice/day.

Day 10 – maintenance – 125 to 250 mg 3 times/day, or 10 to 25 mg/kg/day in divided doses.

Patients already receiving other anticonvulsants: Start primidone at 100 to 125 mg at bedtime; gradually increase to maintenance level as the other drug is gradually decreased. When therapy with primidone alone is the objective, the transition should not be completed in < 2 weeks.

Bioequivalence: Bioequivalence problems have been documented for primidone products marketed by different manufacturers. Brand interchange is not recommended unless comparative bioavailability data are available.

Actions

Pharmacology: Primidone's mechanism of antiepileptic action is not known.

Primidone and its 2 metabolites, phenobarbital and phenylethylmalonamide (PEMA) have anticonvulsant activity.

Pharmacokinetics: Primidone is readily absorbed from the GI tract. Phenobarbital appears in plasma after several days of continuous therapy. Therapeutic plasma concentrations are 5 to 12 mcg/mL for primidone and 15 to 40 mcg/mL for phenobarbital. PEMA and phenobarbital have longer half-lives (10 to 18 hours and 53 to 140 hours, respectively) and accumulate with chronic use. About 40% of primidone is excreted unchanged in the urine.

Contraindications
Porphyria; hypersensitivity to phenobarbital.

Warnings
Status epilepticus: Abrupt withdrawal of antiepileptic medication may precipitate status epilepticus.

Therapeutic efficacy: Therapeutic efficacy of a dosage regimen takes several weeks to assess.

Pregnancy: The effects of primidone in pregnancy are unknown.

Lactation: Primidone appears in breast milk in substantial quantities.

Precautions
Monitoring: Because therapy generally extends over prolonged periods, perform complete blood counts and a sequential multiple analysis test every 6 months.

Hazardous tasks: Patients should use caution while driving or performing other tasks requiring alertness, coordination, or physical dexterity.

Drug Interactions
Drugs that may affect primidone include acetazolamide, carbamazepine, hydantoins, isoniazid, nicotinamide, and succinimides.

Drugs that may be affected by primidone include carbamazepine.

Adverse Reactions
Adverse reactions may include ataxia, vertigo, fatigue, hyperirritability, emotional disturbances, diplopia, nystagmus, drowsiness, personality deterioration with mood changes, paranoia, nausea, anorexia, vomiting, megaloblastic anemia, thrombocytopenia, impotence, morbilliform or maculopapular skin eruptions, crystalluria.

VALPROIC ACID and DERIVATIVES

Capsules: 250 mg (valproic acid) (*Rx*)	Various, *Depakene* (Abbott)
Syrup: 250 mg (as sodium valproate)/5 mL (*Rx*)	Various, *Depakene* (Abbott)
Tablets, delayed release: 125, 250, and 500 mg (as divalproex sodium) (*Rx*)	*Depakote* (Abbott)
Tablets, extended-release: 500 mg	*Depakote ER* (Abbott)
Capsules, sprinkle: 125 mg (as divalproex sodium) (*Rx*)	*Depakote* (Abbott)
Injection: 5 mL (as valproate acid) (*Rx*)	*Depacon* (Abbott)

Warning:

Hepatotoxicity: Hepatic failure resulting in fatalities has occurred in patients receiving valproic acid and its derivatives. Children < 2 years of age are at a considerably increased risk of developing fatal hepatotoxicity, especially those on multiple anticonvulsants, those with congenital metabolic disorders, those with severe seizure disorders accompanied by mental retardation, and those with organic brain disease. In this patient group, use with extreme caution and as a sole agent. Weigh benefits of seizure control against risks. Above this age group, the incidence of fatal hepatotoxicity decreases considerably in progressively older patient groups. These incidents usually have occurred during the first 6 months of treatment. Serious or fatal hepatotoxicity may be preceded by nonspecific symptoms such as loss of seizure control, malaise, weakness, lethargy, facial edema, anorexia, jaundice, and vomiting. Monitor patients closely for appearance of these symptoms. Perform liver function tests prior to therapy and at frequent intervals thereafter, especially during the first 6 months.

Teratogenicity: Valproate can produce teratogenic effects such as neural tube defects (eg, spina bifida). Accordingly, the use of divalproex sodium in women of childbearing potential requires that the benefits of its use be weighed against the risk of injury to the fetus. This is especially important when the treatment of a spontaneously reversible condition not ordinarily associated with permanent injury or risk of death (eg, migraine) is contemplated (see Warnings and Patient Information). An information sheet describing the teratogenic potential of valproate is available for patients.

Pancreatitis: Cases of life-threatening pancreatitis have been reported in children and adults receiving valproate. Some of the cases have been described as hemorrhagic with a rapid progression from initial symptoms to death. Cases have been reported shortly after initial use as well as after several years of use. Warn patients and guardians that abdominal pain, nausea, vomiting, or anorexia can be symptoms of pancreatitis that require prompt medical evaluation. If pancreatitis is diagnosed, discontinue valproate ordinarily. Initiate alternative treatment for the underlying medical condition as clinically indicated.

Indications

Epilepsy: For use as sole and adjunctive therapy in the treatment of simple and complex absence seizures and adjunctively in patients with multiple seizure types that include absence seizures; as monotherapy and adjunctive therapy in the treatment of patients with complex partial seizures that occur either in isolation or in association with other types of seizures (divalproex sodium, valproate sodium injection).

Valproate sodium injection is indicated as an IV alternative in patients for whom oral administration of valproate products is temporarily not feasible.

Mania (divalproex sodium delayed-release tablets): Manic episodes associated with bipolar disorder.

Migraine (divalproex sodium delayed-release and extended-release tablets): As prophylaxis of migraine headaches.

Unlabeled uses: May be effective in patients with intractable status epilepticus who have not responded to other therapies (adults: 200 to 1200 mg every 6 hours rectally with phenytoin and phenobarbital; children: 15 to 20 mg/kg).

Administration and Dosage

Oral products: Bedtime administration may minimize effects of CNS depression. GI irritation may be minimized by taking with food or by slowly increasing the dose. Delayed-release divalproex sodium may reduce the incidence of irritative GI effects.

Sprinkle capsules: May swallow whole or open capsule and sprinkle entire contents on a small amount (teaspoonful) of soft food such as applesauce or pudding. Swallow drug/food mixture immediately; do not chew. Do not store for future use.

Injection: For IV use only. Administer as a 60-minute infusion ($\leq$ 20 mg/min) with the same frequency as the oral products. Rapid infusion of valproate has been associated with an increase in adverse events. Use of valproate sodium injection for periods of > 14 days has not been studied. Switch patients to oral valproate products as soon as it is clinically feasible.

Extended-release tablets: Extended-release tablets are intended for once/day oral administration. Swallow whole and do not crush or chew. The recommended starting dose is 500 mg once/day for 1 week, thereafter increasing to 1000 mg once/day. Although doses other than 1000 mg once/day have not been evaluated in patients with migraines, the effective dose range of delayed-released tablets in these patients is 500 to 1000 mg/day. As with other valproate products, individualize doses of the extended-release tablets and adjust the dose as necessary. The extended-release tablets are not bioequivalent to the delayed-release tablets. If a patient requires smaller dose adjustments than that available with the extended-release tablets, use the delayed-release tablets instead.

Conversion from valproic acid to divalproex sodium: In patients previously receiving valproic acid, initiate divalproex sodium at the same total daily dose and dosing schedule. After the patient is stabilized on divalproex sodium, administration 2 or 3 times/day may be used in selected patients.

Conversion from oral products to injection: When switching from oral products, the total daily dose of valproate sodium injection should be equivalent to the total daily dose of the oral product. Closely monitor patients receiving doses near the maximum recommended daily dose of 60 mg/kg/day, particularly those not receiving enzyme-inducing drugs. If the total daily dose exceeds 250 mg, give in a divided regimen.

Elderly: Reduce the starting dose because of a decrease in unbound clearance of valproate; base therapeutic dose on clinical response.

Complex partial seizures:

    Monotherapy – Adults and children $\geq$ 10 years of age.

    Initiate therapy at 10 to 15 mg/kg/day; increase by 5 to 10 mg/kg/week until seizures are controlled or side effects preclude further increases. The maximum recommended dosage is 60 mg/kg/day. If the total daily dose is > 250 mg, give in divided doses. *Depacon* has not been studied systematically as initial therapy.

    Conversion to monotherapy: Initiate therapy at 10 to 15 mg/kg/day. The dosage should be increased by 5 to 10 mg/kg/week to achieve optimal clinical response. Ordinarily, optimal clinical response is achieved at daily doses < 60 mg/kg/day. If satisfactory clinical response has not been achieved, measure plasma levels to determine whether or not they are in the usually accepted therapeutic range (50 to 100 mcg/mL). Concomitant antiepilepsy drug (AED) dosage can ordinarily be reduced by $\approx$ 25% every 2 weeks. This reduction may be started at initiation of therapy or delayed by 1 to 2 weeks if there is a concern that seizures are likely to occur with a reduction. The speed and duration of withdrawal of the concomitant AED can be highly variable; monitor patients closely during this period for increased seizure frequency.

    Adjunctive therapy – Divalproex sodium may be added to the patient's regimen at a dosage of 10 to 15 mg/kg/day. The dosage may be increased by 5 to 10 mg/kg/week to achieve optimal clinical response. Ordinarily, optimal clinical response is achieved at daily doses < 60 mg/kg/day. If satisfactory clinical response has not been achieved, measure plasma levels to determine whether or not they are in the usually accepted therapeutic range (50 to 100 mcg/mL). No recommendation regarding the safety of valproate for use at doses > 60 mg/kg/day can be made. If the total daily dose exceeds 250 mg, administer in divided doses.

Simple and complex absence seizures: The recommended initial dose is 15 mg/kg/day, increasing at 1 week intervals by 5 to 10 mg/kg/day until seizures are controlled or side effects preclude further increase. The maximum recommended dosage is 60 mg/kg/day. If the total daily dose is > 250 mg, give in divided doses.

In epileptic patients previously receiving valproic acid therapy, initiate divalproex sodium at the same daily dose and dosing schedule. After the patient is stabilized on divalproex tablets, a dosing schedule of 2 or 3 times a day may be elected in selected patients.

Mania (divalproex sodium delayed-release tablets): 750 mg/day in divided doses; increase as rapidly as possible to achieve the lowest therapeutic dose that produces the desired clinical effect or the desired range of plasma concentrations.

Migraine (divalproex sodium delayed-release tablets): 250 mg orally twice/day. Some patients may benefit from doses up to 1000 mg/day.

Therapeutic serum levels: Therapeutic serum levels for most patients will range from 50 to 100 mcg/mL; however, a good correlation has not been established between daily dose, serum level and therapeutic effect.

Actions

Pharmacology: This group includes valproic acid, sodium valproate (the sodium salt) and divalproex sodium, a stable coordination compound containing equal proportions of valproic acid and sodium valproate. Regardless of form, dosage is expressed as valproic acid equivalents.

Valproic acid is chemically unrelated to other drugs used to treat seizure disorders. Although the mechanism of action is not established, its activity may be related to increased brain levels of gamma-aminobutyric acid (GABA).

Pharmacokinetics: Valproic acid is rapidly absorbed orally. Peak levels after IV administration of valproate sodium occur at the end of the 1-hour infusion. The absolute bioavailability of divalproex extended-release (ER) tablets administered as a single dose after a meal was ≈ 90% relative to IV infusion. Maximum valproate plasma concentrations in these studies were achieved on average 7 to 14 hours after the ER dose intake. The ER tablets are not bioequivalent to the delayed-release tablets. Valproate is rapidly distributed and primarily metabolized in liver.

Contraindications

Hepatic disease or significant hepatic dysfunction; hypersensitivity to valproic acid.

Warnings

Pancreatitis: Cases of life-threatening pancreatitis have been reported in children and adults receiving valproate. Some of the cases have been described as hemorrhagic with rapid progression from initial symptoms to death. Some cases have occurred shortly after initial use as well as after several years of use.

Thrombocytopenia: The frequency of thrombocytopenia may be dose-related. The probability of thrombocytopenia increases significantly at total trough valproate plasma concentrations > 110 mcg/mL in females and 135 mcg/mL in males.

Acute head injuries: A study evaluating the effect of IV valproate in the prevention of post-traumatic seizures in patients with acute head injuries found a higher incidence of death in valproate treatment groups compared to the IV phenytoin treatment group. Until further information is available, it seems prudent not to use valproate sodium injection in patients with acute head trauma for the prophylaxis of posttraumatic seizures.

Hepatotoxicity: See Warning Box.

Long-term use: Safety and effectiveness for long-term use in mania (> 3 weeks) have not been systematically evaluated in clinical trials.

Discontinuation: Do not abruptly discontinue in patients in whom the drug is administered to prevent major seizures because of the strong possibility of precipitating status epilepticus with attendant hypoxia and threat to life.

Elderly: In elderly patients, increase dosage more slowly and with regular monitoring for fluid and nutritional intake, dehydration, somnolence, and other adverse events. Consider dose reductions or discontinuation of valproate in patients with decreased food or fluid intake and in patients with excessive somnolence (see Administration and Dosage).

A reduced starting dose will be required (see Administration and Dosage).

Pregnancy: Category D.

Lactation: Concentrations of valproic acid in breast milk are 1% to 10% of serum concentrations. Exercise caution when administering to a nursing woman.

Children: See Warning Box. The safety and efficacy of divalproex sodium for the treatment of acute mania has not been studied in individuals < 18 years of age.

Experience has indicated that pediatric patients < 2 years of age are at a considerably increased risk of developing fatal hepatotoxicity. When divalproex sodium is used in this patient group, it should be used with extreme caution and as a sole agent. Above 2 years of age, experience in epilepsy has indicated that the incidence of fatal hepatoxicity decreases considerably in progressively older patient groups.

Divalproex sodium extended-release tablets are not recommended in children.

Migraine – The safety and efficacy of divalproex sodium for the prophylaxis of migraines has not been studied in individuals < 16 years of age.

Precautions

Hematologic effects: Thrombocytopenia, inhibition of the secondary phase of platelet aggregation and abnormal coagulation parameters have occurred; determine platelet counts and bleeding time before initiating therapy, at periodic intervals and prior to surgery.

Hyperammonemia: Hyperammonemia, with or without lethargy or coma, may occur in the absence of abnormal liver function tests. If clinically significant symptoms occur, modify therapy or discontinue the drug.

Suicidal ideation: Suicidal ideation may be a manifestation of certain psychiatric disorders, and may persist until significant remission of symptoms occurs.

Hazardous tasks: Patients should use caution while driving or performing other tasks requiring alertness, coordination, or physical dexterity.

Drug Interactions

Drugs that may affect valproic acid include charcoal, chlorpromazine, cimetidine, clonazepam, felbamate, rifampin, salicylates, carbamazepine, erythromycin, lamotrigine, cholestyramine, phenobarbital, and phenytoin. Drugs that may be affected by valproic acid include alcohol and other CNS depressants, benzodiazepines, carbamazepine, clonazepam, clozapine, ethosuximide, diazepam, lamotrigine, phenytoin, phenobarbital, primidone, tolbutamide, warfarin, tricyclic antidepressants, and zidovudine.

Drug/Lab test interactions: Valproic acid is partially eliminated in the urine as a keto-metabolite, which may lead to a false interpretation of the urine ketone test. There have been reports of altered thyroid function tests associated with valproic acid.

Adverse Reactions

Adverse event	Tablets Migraine	Adjunctive therapy for complex partial seizures	High-dose[2]	Low-dose[2]	Extended-release[1] Migraine	Injection
CNS						
Asthenia	20	27	21	10	-	-
Somnolence	17	27	30	18	7	1.7
Dizziness	12	25	18	13	-	5.2
Tremor	9	25	57	19	-	0.6
Ataxia	-	8	-	-	-	-
Nystagmus	-	8	7	1	-	-
Emotional lability	-	6	-	-	-	-
Abnormal thinking	-	6	-	-	-	-
Amnesia	-	5	-	-	-	-
Euphoria	-	-	-	-	-	0.9
Hypesthesia	-	-	-	-	-	0.6
Nervousness	-	-	11	7	-	0.9
Paresthesia	-	-	-	-	-	0.9
Insomnia	-	-	15	9	-	-
Amnesia	-	-	7	4	-	-
Depression	-	-	5	4	-	-
GI						
Nausea	31	48	34	26	15	3.2
Dyspepsia	13	8	11	10	7	-
Diarrhea	12	13	23	19	7	0.9
Vomiting	11	27	23	15	7	1.3
Abdominal pain	9	23	12	9	7	1.1
Increased appetite	6	-	-	-	-	-
Constipation	-	5	-	-	-	-
Anorexia	-	12	11	4	-	-
Hemic/Lymphatic						
Thrombocytopenia	-	-	24	1	-	-
Ecchymosis	-	-	5	4	-	-
Respiratory						
Flu syndrome	-	12	-	-	-	-
Infection	-	12	20	13	-	-
Bronchitis	-	5	-	-	-	-
Rhinitis	-	5	-	-	-	-
Pharyngitis	-	-	8	2	-	0.6
Dyspnea	-	-	5	1	-	-
Special senses						
Diplopia	-	16	-	-	-	-
Amblyopia/Blurred vision	-	12	8	4	-	-
Taste perversion	-	-	-	-	-	1.9
Tinnitus	-	-	7	1	-	-
Miscellaneous						
Weight gain	8	-	9	4	-	-
Back pain	8	-	-	-	-	-
Alopecia	7	6	24	13	-	-
Fever	-	6	-	-	-	-
Weight loss	-	6	-	-	-	-
Chest pain	-	-	-	-	-	1.7
Injection site inflammation	-	-	-	-	-	0.6
Headache	-	31	-	-	-	4.3

Adverse Events Reported by ≥ 5% (%)						
	Tablets				Extended-release[1]	
		Epilepsy				
Adverse event	Migraine	Adjunctive therapy for complex partial seizures	High-dose[2]	Low-dose[2]	Migraine	Injection
Miscellaneous (cont.)	-	-	-	-	-	-
Weight gain						
Injection site pain	-	-	-	-	-	2.6
Injection site reaction	-	-	-	-	-	2.4
Pain (unspecified)	-	-	-	-	-	1.3
Vasodilation	-	-	-	-	-	0.9
Sweating	-	-	-	-	-	0.9
Peripheral edema	-	-	8	3	-	-
Infection	-	-	-	-	15	-

- = No data available.
[1] n = 122.
[2] Monotherapy for complex partial seizures.

Mania: The following additional adverse events were reported (> 1% to 5%).

Cardiovascular – Hypertension; hypotension; palpitations; postural hypotension; tachycardia; vascular anomaly; vasodilation.

CNS – Abnormal dreams; abnormal gait; agitation; ataxia; catatonic reaction; confusion; dysarthria; hallucinations; hypertonia; hypokinesia; insomnia; paresthesia; reflexes increased; tardive dyskinesia; thinking abnormalities; vertigo; amnesia; nervousness; speech disorder; hypertonia.

Dermatologic – Alopecia; discoid lupus erythematosis; dry skin; furunculosis; maculopapular rash; seborrhea; pruritus.

GI – Anorexia; fecal incontinence; flatulence; gastroenteritis; glossitis; periodontal abscess; dry mouth; flatulence; GI disorder (unspecified); stomatitis; tooth disorder.

GU – Dysuria; urinary incontinence; cystitis; metrorrhagia; vaginal bleeding.

Metabolic/Nutritional – Edema; peripheral edema.

Musculoskeletal – Arthralgia; arthrosis; leg cramps; twitching.

Respiratory – Dyspnea; rhinitis; sinusitis; increased cough; pharyngitis.

Special senses – Abnormal vision; amblyopia; conjunctivitis; deafness; dry eyes; ear disorder; ear pain; eye pain; tinnitus; taste perversion.

Miscellaneous – Chest pain; chills; chills and fever; cyst; fever; infection; neck pain; neck rigidity; fever; face edema; accidental injury; viral infection; malaise; ecchymosis.

CARBAMAZEPINE

Tablets, chewable: 100 mg (*Rx*)	Various, *Tegretol* (Geigy)
Tablets: 200 mg (*Rx*)	Various, *Epitol* (Lemmon), *Tegretol* (Geigy)
Tablets, extended release: 100, 200, and 400 mg (*Rx*)	*Tegretol-XR* (Novartis)
Capsules, extended release: 200 and 300 mg (*Rx*)	*Carbatrol* (Athena Neurosciences)
Suspension: 100 mg/5 mL (*Rx*)	*Tegretol* (Novartis)

> **Warning:**
> Aplastic anemia and agranulocytosis have been reported in association with carbamazepine therapy. The risk of developing these reactions is 5 to 8 times greater than in the general population. Consider discontinuation of the drug if any evidence of significant bone marrow depression develops.

Indications

Epilepsy: Partial seizures with complex symptoms. Patients with these seizures appear to show greatest improvement. Generalized tonic-clonic seizures; mixed seizure patterns or other partial or generalized seizures.

Trigeminal neuralgia: Treatment of pain associated with true trigeminal neuralgia and glossopharyngeal neuralgia.

Unlabeled uses: Management of alcohol (200 mg 4 times/day up to 1000 mg/day), cocaine, and benzodiazepine withdrawal (200 mg twice/day up to 800 mg/day).

Nonneuritic pain syndromes (eg, central pain states, painful neuromas, phantom limb pain; 100 mg twice/day initial, 600 to 1400 mg/day maintenance).

Neurogenic or central diabetes insipidus; it is generally ineffective for nephrogenic diabetes insipidus (200 mg 2 or 3 times/day).

Hereditary and nonhereditary chorea in children (15 to 25 mg/kg/day).

Restless legs syndrome (100 to 300 mg at bedtime).

Administration and Dosage

Conversion from conventional tablets to extended-release tablets: Extended-release carbamazapine is for twice/day administration. Administer the same total daily mg dose of extended-release carbamazepine. Swallow extended-release carbamazepine tablets whole; never crush or chew. Inspect extended-release carbamazepine tablets for chips or cracks; do not consume damaged tablets. Extended-release carbamazepine tablet coating is not absorbed and is excreted in the feces; these coatings may be noticeable in the stool.

Epilepsy:

Initial –

Adults and children (> 12 years of age): 200 mg twice/day (100 mg 4 times/day of suspension). Increase at weekly intervals by ≤ 200 mg/day using a 3 or 4 times/day regimen (2 times/day with extended release) until the best response is obtained. Do not exceed 1000 mg/day in children 12 to 15 years of age or 1200 mg/day in patients > 15 years of age. Doses ≤ 1600 mg/day have been used in adults.

Children (6 to 12 years of age): 100 mg twice/day (50 mg 4 times/day of suspension). Increase at weekly intervals gradually by adding ≤ 100 mg/day using a 3 or 4 times/day regimen (2 times/day with extended release) until the best response is obtained. Do not exceed 1000 mg/day.

Children (< 6 years of age): 10 to 20 mg/kg/day 2 or 3 times/day (4 times/day with suspension). Increase weekly to achieve optimal clinical response administered 3 or 4 times/day.

Maintenance –

Adults and children (> 12 years of age): Adjust to minimum effective level, usually 800 to 1200 mg/day.

Children (6 to 12 years of age): Adjust to minimum effective level, usually 400 to 800 mg/day. May also be calculated on basis of 20 to 30 mg/kg/day, in divided doses 3 or 4 times/day.

Children (< 6 years of age): Ordinarily, optimal clinical response is achieved at daily doses < 35 mg/kg. If satisfactory clinical response has not been achieved, measure plasma levels to determine whether or not they are in the therapeutic range. No recommendation regarding the safety of carbamazepine for use at doses > 35 mg/kg/24 hours can be made.

Combination therapy – When added to existing anticonvulsant therapy, do so gradually while other anticonvulsants are maintained or gradually decreased, except phenytoin, which may have to be increased.

Trigeminal neuralgia:

Initial – 100 mg twice/day on the first day (50 mg 4 times/day of suspension). May increase by up to 200 mg/day using 100 mg increments every 12 hours (50 mg 4 times/day of suspension) as needed. Do not exceed 1200 mg/day.

Maintenance – Control of pain can usually be maintained with 400 to 800 mg/day (range 200 to 1200 mg/day). Attempt to reduce the dose to the minimum effective level or to discontinue the drug at least once every 3 months.

Actions

Pharmacology: Carbamazepine's mechanism of action is unknown. It appears to act by reducing polysynaptic responses and blocking the post–tetanic potentiation.

Pharmacokinetics:

Absorption/Distribution – Both the suspension and tablet deliver equivalent amounts of drug to the systemic circulation; however, the suspension is absorbed somewhat faster than the tablet. Carbamazepine is 76% bound to plasma proteins.

Metabolism/Excretion – Carbamazepine is metabolized in the liver to the 10,11-epoxide, which also has anticonvulsant activity. It may induce its own metabolism. Initial half-life ranges from 25 to 65 hours and decreases to 12 to 17 hours with repeated doses.

Contraindications

History of bone marrow depression; hypersensitivity to carbamazepine and tricyclic antidepressants; concomitant use of monoamine oxidase (MAO) inhibitors. Discontinue MAO inhibitors for a minimum of 14 days before carbamazepine administration.

Warnings

Minor pain: This drug is not a simple analgesic. Do not use for the relief of minor aches or pains.

Dermatologic: Severe dermatologic reactions, including toxic epidermal necrolysis (Lyell's syndrome) and Stevens-Johnson syndrome, have been reported with carbamazepine. These reactions have been extremely rare; however, a few fatalities have been reported.

Hematologic: Patients with a history of adverse hematologic reaction to any drug may be particularly at risk.

Glaucoma: Carbamazepine has shown mild anticholinergic activity; therefore, use with caution in patients with increased intraocular pressure.

CNS effects: Because of the drug's relationship to other tricyclic compounds, the possibility of activating latent psychosis, confusion, or agitation in elderly patients may occur.

Pregnancy: Category D.

Lactation: Concentration of carbamazepine in milk is ≈ 60% of the maternal plasma concentration.

Children: The safety of carbamazepine in pediatric patients has been studied ≤ 6 months.

Precautions

Hyponatremia: Hyponatremia has been reported in association with carbamazepine use, either alone or in combination with other drugs.

Absence seizures: Absence seizures (petit mal) do not appear to be controlled by carbamazepine.

Special risk patients: Prescribe carbamazepine only after benefit-to-risk appraisal in patients with a history of the following: Cardiac, hepatic, or renal damage; adverse hematologic reaction to other drugs; interrupted courses of therapy with the drug.

Laboratory tests: Perform baseline liver function tests and periodic evaluations. Obtain baseline and periodic eye examinations (slit lamp, funduscopy, and tonometry), urinalysis, and BUN determinations.

Obtain complete pretreatment hematological testing as a baseline. Repeat these tests at monthly intervals during the first 2 months and, thereafter, obtain yearly or every-other-year CBC, white cell differential, and platelet count.

Hazardous tasks: May produce drowsiness, dizziness or blurred vision; patients should observe caution while driving or performing other tasks requiring alertness.

Drug Interactions

Drugs that can increase carbamazepine serum levels include cimetidine, danazol, diltiazem, erythromycin, clarithromycin, fluoxetine, isoniazid, niacinamide, proproxyphene, ketaconazole, itraconazole, verapamil, and valproate.

Drugs that can decrease carbamazepine serum levels include cisplatin, doxorubicin, felbamate, rifampin, phenobarbital, primidone, and theophylline.

The serum levels of oral contraceptives, haloperidol, bupropion, anticoagulants, felbamate, valproic acid, felodipine, tricyclic antidepressants, and lamotrigine can be lowered by carbamazepine.

Drug/Lab test interactions:

Thyroid function – Thyroid function tests show decreased values with carbamazepine.

Pregnancy tests – Interference with some pregnancy tests has been reported.

Adverse Reactions

Adverse reactions may include dizziness; drowsiness; unsteadiness; nausea; vomiting; aplastic anemia; leukopenia; agranulocytosis; eosinophilia; leukocytosis; thrombocytopenia; pancytopenia; bone marrow depression; fever and chills; dyspnea; pneumonitis; pneumonia; pulmonary eosinophilia; asthma; abnormal liver function tests; cholestatic/hepatocellular jaundice; hepatitis; urinary frequency; acute urinary retention; oliguria with hypertension; renal failure; azotemia; impotence; albuminuria; glycosuria; elevated BUN; microscopic deposits in urine; disturbances of coordination; confusion; headache; fatigue; blurred vision; visual hallucinations; speech disturbances; abnormal involuntary movements; peripheral neuritis and paresthesias; depression with agitation; talkativeness; tinnitus; hyperacusis; behavioral changes in children; paralysis; cerebral arterial insufficiency; pruritic and erythematous rashes; urticaria; Stevens-Johnson syndrome; photosensitivity reactions; alterations in pigmentation; exfoliative dermatitis; alopecia; diaphoresis; erythema multiforme and nodosum; purpura; aggravation of disseminated lupus erythematosus; toxic epidermal necrolysis; gastric distress; abdominal pain; diarrhea; constipation; anorexia; dryness of mouth or pharynx; glossitis and stomatitis; CHF; hypotension; syncope and collapse; edema; primary thrombophlebitis; recurrence of thrombophlebitis; aggravation of coronary artery disease; arrhythmias; AV block; adenopathy or lymphadenopathy; cardiovascular complications that have resulted in fatalities; transient diplopia; oculomotor disturbances; nystagmus; scattered, punctate cortical lens opacities; conjunctivitis; aching joints; muscles; leg cramps; inappropriate antidiuretic hormone secretion syndrome (SIADH).

GABAPENTIN

Capsules: 100, 300, and 400 mg (*Rx*)
Tablets: 600 and 800 mg (*Rx*)
Solution, oral: 250 mg/5 mL (*Rx*)

Neurontin (Parke-Davis)

Indications
Epilepsy: Adjunctive therapy in the treatment of partial seizures with and without secondary generalization in patients > 12 years of age with epilepsy. Also indicated as adjunctive therapy for partial seizures in children 3 to 12 years of age.

Administration and Dosage
Recommended for add-on therapy in patients ≥ 3 years of age, taken with or without food.

Patients > 12 years of age: The effective dose is 900 to 1800 mg/day in divided doses (3 times/day) using 300 or 400 mg capsules or 600 or 800 mg tablets. The starting dose is 300 mg 3 times/day. If necessary, the dose may be increased using 300 or 400 mg capsules or 600 or 800 mg tablets 3 times/day up to 1800 mg/day. Dosages up to 2400 mg/day have been well tolerated in long-term clinical studies. Doses of 3600 mg/day also have been administered to a small number of patients for a relatively short duration, and have been well tolerated. The maximum time between doses in the 3 times/day schedule should not exceed 12 hours.

Pediatric patients 3 to 12 years of age: The starting dose should range from 10 to 15 mg/kg/day in 3 divided doses, and the effective dose reached by upward titration over a period of ≈ 3 days. The effective dose of gabapentin in patients ≥ 5 years of age is 25 to 35 mg/kg/day and given in divided doses (3 times/day). The effective dose in pediatric patients 3 and 4 years of age is 40 mg/kg/day and given in divided doses (3 times/day). Gabapentin may be administered as the oral solution, capsule, tablet, or using combinations of these formulations. Dosages up to 50 mg/kg/day have been well tolerated in a long-term clinical study. The maximum time interval between doses should not exceed 12 hours.

It is not necessary to monitor gabapentin plasma concentrations to optimize therapy. Further, because there are no significant pharmacokinetic interactions with other commonly used anti-epileptic drugs, the addition of gabapentin does not alter the plasma levels of these drugs appreciably.

If gabapentin is discontinued or an alternate anticonvulsant medication is added to the therapy, this should be done gradually over a minimum of 1 week.

Renal function impairment:

Gabapentin Dosage Based on Renal Function		
Ccr (mL/min)	Total daily dose (mg/day)	Dose regimen (mg)
> 60	1200	400 tid
30 to 60	600	300 bid
15 to 30	300	300 qd
< 15	150	300 qod[1]
Hemodialysis	—	200 to 300[2]

[1] Every other day.
[2] Loading dose of 300 to 400 mg in patients who have never received gabapentin, then 200 to 300 mg gabapentin following each 4 hours of hemodialysis.

Use of gabapentin in patients < 12 years of age with compromised renal function has not been studied.

Actions
Pharmacology: Gabapentin is an oral antiepileptic agent. The mechanism by which it exerts its anticonvulsant action is unknown.

Pharmacokinetics: Gabapentin bioavailability is not dose-proportional. It circulates largely unbound (< 3%) to plasma protein and is eliminated from the systemic circulation by renal excretion as unchanged drug; it is not appreciably metabolized.

Contraindications
Hypersensitivity to the drug or its ingredients.

Warnings
Neuropsychiatric adverse events (3 to 12 years of age): Gabapentin use in pediatric patients with epilepsy 3 to 12 years of age is associated with the occurrence of CNS-related adverse events.

Among the gabapentin-treated patients, most of the events were mild to moderate in intensity.

Withdrawal-precipitated seizure: Antiepileptic drugs should not be abruptly discontinued because of the possibility of increasing seizure frequency.

Status epilepticus: In the placebo controlled studies, the incidence of status epilepticus in patients receiving gabapentin was 0.6% vs 0.5% with placebo.

Sudden and unexplained deaths: During the course of premarketing development of gabapentin, 8 sudden and unexplained deaths were recorded among 2203 patients.

Elderly: No systematic studies in geriatric patients have been conducted. Adverse clinical events reported among 59 gabapentin-exposed patients > 65 years of age did not differ in kind from those reported for younger individuals.

Pregnancy: Category C.

Lactation: Gabapentin is secreted into breast milk.

Children: Safety and efficacy in children < 3 years of age has not been established.

Drug Interactions
Drugs that may affect gabapentin include antacids and cimetidine. Drugs that may be affected by gabapentin include oral contraceptives.

Drug/Lab test interactions: Because false-positive readings were reported with the *Ames N-Multistix SG* dipstick test for urinary protein when gabapentin was added to other antiepileptic drugs, the more specific sulfosalicylic acid precipitation procedure is recommended to determine the presence of urine protein.

Adverse Reactions
Adverse reactions occurring in ≥ 3% of patients include somnolence, weight gain, hostility, emotional lability, nausea/vomiting, bronchitis, viral infections, fever, dizziness, ataxia, fatigue, nystagmus, rhinitis, diplopia, amblyopia, and tremor.

TIAGABINE HCl

Tablets: 4, 12, 16, and 20 mg *(Rx)*	*Gabitril Filmtabs* (Abbott)

Indications
Partial seizures: Adjunctive therapy for treatment of partial seizures.

Administration and Dosage
Tiagabine is given orally and should be taken with food.

Children (12 to 18 years of age): Initiate tiagabine at 4 mg once/day. Modification of concomitant antiepilepsy drugs is not necessary, unless clinically indicated. The total daily dose of tiagabine may be increased by 4 mg at the beginning of week 2. Thereafter, the total daily dose of may be increased by 4 to 8 mg at weekly intervals until clinical response is achieved or up to 32 mg/day. Give the total daily dose in 2 to 4 divided doses. Doses > 32 mg/day have been tolerated in a small number of adolescent patients for a relatively short duration.

Adults and children > 18 years of age: Initiate tiagabine at 4 mg once/day. Modification of concomitant antiepilepsy drugs is not necessary, unless clinically indicated. The total daily dose of tiagabine may be increased by 4 to 8 mg at weekly intervals until clinical response is achieved or up to 56 mg/day. Give the total daily dose in 2 to 4 divided doses. Doses > 56 mg/day have not been systematically evaluated in adequate well controlled trials.

Experience is limited in patients taking total daily doses > 32 mg/day using twice/ day dosing. A typical dosing titration regimen for patients taking enzyme-inducing antiepilepsy drugs (EIAEDs) is provided.

Typical Dosing Titration Regimen of Tiagabine for Patients Taking EIAEDs		
Week	Initiation and titration schedule	Total daily dose
Week 1	Initiate at 4 mg once/day	4 mg/day
Week 2	Increase total daily dose by 4 mg	8 mg/day (in 2 divided doses)
Week 3	Increase total daily dose by 4 mg	12 mg/day (in 3 divided doses)
Week 4	Increase total daily dose by 4 mg	16 mg/day (in 2 to 4 divided doses)
Week 5	Increase total daily dose by 4 to 8 mg	20 to 24 mg/day (in 2 to 4 divided doses)
Week 6	Increase total daily dose by 4 to 8 mg	24 to 32 mg/day (in 2 to 4 divided doses)
Usual adult maintenance dose	32 to 56 mg/day in 2 to 4 divided doses	

Actions

Pharmacology: The precise mechanism by which tiagabine exerts its antiseizure effect is unknown, although it is believed that it blocks GABA uptake into presynaptic neurons, permitting more GABA to be available for receptor binding on the surfaces of postsynaptic cells.

Pharmacokinetics:

Absorption/Distribution – Absorption of tiagabine is rapid and nearly complete (> 95%), with an absolute oral bioavailability of ≈ 90%. Following multiple dosing, steady state is achieved within 2 days. Tiagabine is 96% bound to plasma proteins.

Metabolism/Excretion – Tiagabine is likely to be metabolized primarily by the P450 3A (CYP3A) isoform, although contributions to the metabolism of tiagabine from CYP 1A2, CYP 2D6, or CYP 2C19 have not been excluded. Approximately 2% of an oral dose of tiagabine is excreted unchanged, with 25% and 63% of the remaining dose excreted into the urine and feces, respectively, primarily as metabolites.

Contraindications

Hypersensitivity to the drug or its ingredients.

Warnings

Withdrawal seizures: Do not abruptly discontinue antiepilepsy drugs (AEDs) because of the possibility of increasing seizure frequency. Withdraw tiagabine gradually to minimize the potential for increased seizure frequency, unless safety concerns require a more rapid withdrawl.

EEG abnormalities: Patients with a history of spike and wave discharges on EEG have been reported to have exacerbations of their EEG abnormalities associated with these cognitive/neuropsychiatric events. This raises the possibility that these clinical events may, in some cases, be a manifestation of underlying seizure activity.

Status epilepticus: Among the patients treated with tiagabine across all epilepsy studies (controlled and uncontrolled), 5% had some form of status epilepticus. Of the 5%, 57% of patients experienced complex partial status epilepticus. A critical risk factor for status epilepticus was the presence of the condition history; 33% of patients with a history of status epilepticus had recurrence during tiagabine treatment.

Sudden unexpected death in epilepsy (SUDEP): There have been as many as 10 cases of SUDEP during the clinical development of tiagabine among 2531 patients with epilepsy (3831 patient-years of exposure).

The rate is within the range of estimates for the incidence of SUDEP not receiving tiagabine. The estimated SUDEP rates in patients receiving tiagabine are similar to those observed in patients receiving other AEDs, chemically unrelated to tiagabine, who underwent clinical testing in similar populations at about the same time. This evidence suggests that the SUDEP rates reflect population rates, not a drug effect.

Hepatic function impairment: Because the clearance of tiagabine is reduced in patients with liver disease ($\approx$ 60%), dosage reduction or longer dosing intervals may be necessary in these patients.

Pregnancy: Category C.

Lactation: Tiagabine or its metabolites are excreted in the milk of rats. Use in women who are nursing only if the benefits clearly outweigh the risks.

Children: Safety and efficacy in children < 12 years of age have not been established.

Precautions

Concomitant EIAED: Virtually all experience with tiagabine has been obtained in patients receiving $\geq$ 1 concomitant EIAED. Use in noninduced patients (eg, patients receiving valproate monotherapy) may require lower doses or a slower dose titration of tiagabine for clinical response. Patients taking a combination of inducing and noninducing drugs (eg, carbamazepine and valproate) should be considered to be induced.

Generalized weakness: Moderately severe to incapacitating generalized weakness has been reported following administration of tiagabine in $\approx$ 1% of patients with epilepsy. The weakness resolved in all cases after a reduction in dose or discontinuation of tiagabine.

Ophthalmic effects: Although no specific recommendations for periodic ophthalmologic monitoring exists, be aware of the possibility of long-term ophthalmologic effects.

Therapeutic drug monitoring: Because of the potential for pharmacokinetic interactions between tiagabine and drugs that induce or inhibit hepatic metabolizing enzymes, it may be useful to obtain plasma levels of tiagabine before and after changes are made in the therapeutic regimen.

Drug Interactions

Drugs that may affect tiagabine include valproate, carbamazepine, phenytoin, and phenobarbital. Valproate may be affected by tiagabine.

Drug/Food interactions: A high-fat meal decreases the rate, but not the extent (AUC), of tiagabine absorption.

Adverse Reactions

Adverse reactions that occurred in $\geq$ 3% of patients include abdominal pain; pain (unspecified); dizziness; asthenia; somnolence; nervousness; tremor; insomnia; difficulty with concentration/attention; ataxia; confusion; speech disorder; difficulty with memory; parasthesia; depression; emotional lability; abnormal gait; nausea; diarrhea; vomiting; pharyngitis; cough increased; rash.

TOPIRAMATE

Tablets: 25, 100, and 200 mg (*Rx*)	*Topamax* (Ortho-McNeil)[*]
Capsules, sprinkle: 15 and 25 mg (*Rx*)	

Indications

Partial onset seizures: Adjunctive therapy for partial onset seizure treatment in adults and children 2 to 16 years of age.

Tonic-clonic seizures: Adjunctive therapy for primary generalized tonic-clonic seizures in adults and children 2 to 16 years of age.

Seizures associated with Lennox-Gastaut syndrome: Adjunctive therapy in patients $\geq$ 2 years of age with seizures associated with Lennox-Gastaut syndrome.

Administration and Dosage

Topiramate is effective in adults and pediatric patients $\geq$ 2 years of age with partial onset seizures or primary generalized tonic-clonic seizures and in patients $\geq$ 2 years of age with seizures associated with Lennox-Gastaut syndrome. Doses > 400 mg/day (600, 800, and 1000 mg/day) have not been shown to improve responses. Doses > 1600 mg/day have not been studied.

Because of the bitter taste, do not break tablets.

Topiramate can be taken without regard to meals.

Adults (≥ 17 years of age): The recommended total daily dose as adjunctive therapy is 400 mg/day in 2 divided doses. It is recommended that therapy be initiated at 25 to 50 mg/day followed by titration to an effective dose in increments of 25 to 50 mg/week. Titrating in increments of 25 mg/week may delay the time to reach an effective dose.

Pediatric patients (2 to 16 years of age): The recommended total daily dose as adjunctive therapy is ≈ 5 to 9 mg/kg/day in 2 divided doses. Begin titration at ≤ 25 mg (based on a range of 1 to 3 mg/kg/day) nightly for the first week. Then increase the dosage at 1- or 2-week intervals by increments of 1 to 3 mg/kg/day (administered in 2 divided doses) to achieve optimal clinical response. Guide dose titration by clinical outcome.

Sprinkle capsules: Swallow whole or administer by carefully opening the capsule and sprinkling the entire contents on a small amount (teaspoon) of soft food. Swallow this drug/food mixture immediately; do not chew. Do not store for future use.

Hepatic function impairment: In hepatically impaired patients, topiramate plasma concentrations may be increased. Administer with caution.

Renal function impairment: In renally impaired subjects (Ccr < 70 mL/min/1.73 m²), 50% of the usual adult dose is recommended. Such patients will require a longer time to reach steady state at each dose.

Hemodialysis: Topiramate is cleared by hemodialysis 4 to 6 times greater than a healthy individual; a prolonged period of dialysis may cause topiramate levels to fall below that required to maintain an anti-seizure effect.

Actions

Pharmacology: Topiramate is a sulfamate-substituted monosaccharide with a broad spectrum of antiepileptic activity. The precise mechanism by which topiramate exerts its antiseizure effect is unknown.

Pharmacokinetics:

Absorption/Distribution – Absorption of topiramate is rapid, with peak plasma concentrations occurring at ≈ 2 hours following a 400 mg oral dose. The relative bioavailability of topiramate from the tablet formulation is ≈ 80% compared with a solution. The bioavailability of topiramate is not affected by food.

Steady state is reached in ≈ 4 days in patients with normal renal function. Topiramate is 13% to 17% bound to human plasma proteins over the concentration range of 1 to 250 mcg/mL.

Metabolism/Excretion – Topiramate is not extensively metabolized and is primarily eliminated unchanged in the urine (≈ 70% of an administered dose). The mean plasma elimination half-life is 21 hours after single or multiple doses. Overall, plasma clearance is ≈ 20 to 30 mL/min following oral administration.

Bioequivalency – The sprinkle formulation is bioequivalent to the immediate-release tablet formulation and, therefore, may be substituted as therapeutically equivalent.

Contraindications

A history of hypersensitivity to any component of this product.

Warnings

Acute myopia and secondary angle closure glaucoma: A syndrome consisting of acute myopia associated with secondary angle closure glaucoma has been reported in patients receiving topiramate. Symptoms include acute onset of decreased visual acuity or ocular pain. Ophthalmologic findings can include myopia, anterior chamber shallowing, ocular hyperemia (redness), and increased intraocular pressure. Mydriasis may or may not be present. This syndrome may be associated with supraciliary effusion resulting in anterior displacement of the lens and iris, with secondary angle closure glaucoma. Symptoms typically occur within 1 month of initiating topiramate therapy. In contrast to primary narrow angle glaucoma, which is rare before 40 years of age, secondary angle closure glaucoma associated with topiramate has been reported in pediatric patients as well as adults. The primary treatment to reverse symptoms is discontinuation of topiramate as rapidly as possible, according to the judgment of the treating physician. Other measures, in conjunction with discontinuation of topiramate, may be helpful.

Withdrawal: Withdraw antiepileptic drugs, including topiramate, gradually to minimize the potential of increased seizure frequency.

CNS-related adverse events:

    Adults – Adverse events most often associated with the use of topiramate were CNS-related. The most significant of these can be classified into 2 general categories: 1) Psychomotor slowing, difficulty with concentration, and speech or language problems, in particular, word-finding difficulties, and 2) somnolence or fatigue.

    Children – The incidences of cognitive/neuropsychiatric adverse events in pediatric patients generally were lower than previously observed in adults. These events included psychomotor slowing, difficulty with concentration/attention, speech disorders/related speech problems, and language problems. The most frequently reported neuropsychiatric events in this population were somnolence and fatigue.

Pregnancy: Category C.

Lactation: Topiramate is excreted in the milk of lactating rats. It is not known if topiramate is excreted in human breast milk. Weigh the potential benefit to the mother against the potential risk to the infant.

Children: Safety and efficacy in children < 2 years of age have not been established.

Precautions

Kidney stones: A total of 1.5% patients exposed to topiramate during its development reported the occurrence of kidney stones; an incidence ≈ 2 to 4 times that expected in a similar, untreated population. Kidney stones also have been reported in pediatric patients.

    An explanation for the association of topiramate and kidney stones may lie in the fact that topiramate is a weak carbonic anhydrase inhibitor. Carbonic anhydrase inhibitors (eg, acetazolamide, dichlorphenamide) promote stone formation by reducing urinary citrate excretion and by increasing urinary pH. The concomitant use of topiramate with other carbonic anhydrase inhibitors or potentially in patients on a ketogenic diet may create a physiological environment that increases the risk of kidney stone formation and should be avoided.

    Increased fluid intake increases urinary output, lowering substance concentration involved in stone formation. Hydration is recommended to reduce new stone formation.

Paresthesia: Paresthesia, an effect associated with the use of other carbonic anhydrase inhibitors, appears to be a common effect of topiramate.

Drug Interactions

Topiramate has demonstrated inhibitory effect on the cytochrome $P4502C_{meph}$. Antiepileptic drug interactions with topiramate include phenytoin (minimal change to 25% increase in plasma concentration, with a 48% decrease in topiramate concentration), carbamazepine (40% decrease in topiramate concentration), valproic acid (11% decrease in plasma concentration, with a 14% decrease in topiramate concentration). Plasma concentration changes of clinical significance were not noted with phenobarbital, primidone, or CBZ epoxide, an active metabolite of carbamazepine. Other drugs that may interact with topiramate include alcohol or CNS depressants, carbonic anhydrase inhibitors, contraceptives or oral estrogens, and digoxin.

Adverse Reactions

Adverse reactions occurring in ≥ 3% of adult patients include somnolence, dizziness, ataxia, psychomotor slowing, speech disorders/related speech problems, nervousness, nystagmus, paresthesia, difficulty with memory, tremor, confusion, difficulty with concentration/attention, depression, language problems, abnormal coordination, agitation, mood problems, aggressive reaction, apathy, emotional lability, cognitive problems, abnormal gait, nausea, dyspepsia, anorexia, abdominal pain, constipation, dry mouth, breast pain, urinary tract infection, weight decrease, rhinitis, pharyngitis, sinusitis, diplopia, abnormal vision, fatigue, asthenia, back pain, chest pain, influenza-like symptoms, leg pain, hot flushes, allergy.

Adverse reactions occurring in ≥ 3% of pediatric patients include somnolence, insomnia, ataxia, nervousness, difficulty with memory, confusion, difficulty with concentration/attention, aggressive reaction, abnormal gait, hyperkinesia, personality disorder (behavior problems), skin disorder, nausea, anorexia, constipation, gastroenteritis, increased saliva, urinary incontinence, weight decrease, pneumonia, fatigue, injury, purpura, epistaxis, viral infection.

MAGNESIUM SULFATE

Injection: 12.5% (1 mEq/mL) and 50% (4 mEq/mL) (*Rx*)   Various

Indications

Seizure: Seizure prevention and control in severe pre-eclampsia or eclampsia without producing deleterious CNS depression in the mother or infant, and in convulsions associated with abnormally low levels of plasma magnesium as a contributing factor.

Acute nephritis in children: Acute nephritis in children to control hypertension, encephalopathy, and convulsions.

Hypomagnesemia: Magnesium deficiency, prevention and correction in total parenteral nutrition.

Unlabeled uses: In asthmatic patients who respond poorly to β-agonists, IV magnesium sulfate (1.2 g) may be a beneficial adjunct for treatment of acute exacerbations of moderate to severe asthma.

Administration and Dosage

Individualize dosage. Monitor the patient's clinical status to avoid toxicity. Discontinue as soon as the desired effect is obtained. Repeat doses are dependent on continuing presence of the patellar reflex and adequate respiratory function.

IM: 4 to 5 g of a 50% solution every 4 hours as necessary.

IV: 4 g of a 10% to 20% solution, not exceeding 1.5 mL/min of a 10% solution.

IV infusion: 4 to 5 g in 250 mL of 5% Dextrose or Sodium Chloride, not exceeding 3 mL/min.

Pediatric: IM - 20 to 40 mg/kg in a 20% solution; repeat as necessary.

Actions

Pharmacology: Magnesium prevents or controls convulsions by blocking neuromuscular transmission and decreasing the amount of acetylcholine liberated at the end plate by the motor nerve impulse.

One gram of magnesium sulfate provides 8.12 mEq of magnesium.

Pharmacokinetics: With IV use, the onset of anticonvulsant action is immediate and lasts about 30 minutes. With IM use, onset occurs in 1 hour and persists for 3 to 4 hours. Effective anticonvulsant serum levels range from 2.5 or 3 to 7.5 mEq/L. Magnesium is excreted by the kidney.

Contraindications

Do not give in toxemia of pregnancy during the 2 hours preceding delivery.

Warnings

IV use: IV use in eclampsia is reserved for immediate control of life-threatening convulsions.

Renal function impairment: Because magnesium is excreted by the kidneys, parenteral use in the presence of renal insufficiency may lead to magnesium intoxication. Use with caution.

Pregnancy: Category A. When administered by continuous IV infusion (especially for > 24 hours preceding delivery) to control convulsions in toxemic mothers, the newborn may show signs of magnesium toxicity, including neuromuscular or respiratory depression.

Precautions
Monitoring: Monitor serum magnesium levels and clinical status to avoid overdosage.

Urine output: Maintain at a level of 100 mL every 4 hours.

Drug Interactions
Drugs that may interact with magnesium sulfate include neuromuscular blockers.

Adverse Reactions
Adverse reactions may include magnesium intoxication; flushing; sweating; hypotension; depressed reflexes; flaccid paralysis; hypothermia; circulatory collapse; cardiac depression; CNS depression; respiratory paralysis; hypocalcemia; tetany.

OXCARBAZEPINE

OXCARBAZEPINE
Tablets: 150, 300, and 600 mg (Rx)   Trileptal (Novartis)

Indications
Epilepsy: For use as monotherapy or adjunctive therapy in the treatment of partial seizures in adults with epilepsy and as adjunctive therapy in the treatment of partial seizures in children 4 to 16 years of age with epilepsy.

Administration and Dosage
Oxcarbazepine may be taken with or without food.

Withdrawal of antiepileptic drugs (AEDs): Withdraw gradually to minimize the potential of increased seizure frequency.

Adults:
Adjunctive therapy (600 mg/day twice/day) – If clinically indicated, the dose may be increased by a maximum of 600 mg/day at approximately weekly intervals; the recommended daily dose is 1200 mg/day. Daily doses > 1200 mg/day show somewhat greater effectiveness in controlled trials, but most patients were not able to tolerate the 2400 mg/day dose, primarily because of CNS effects. Observe and monitor closely the plasma levels of the concomitant AEDs during the period of oxcarbazepine titration, especially at oxcarbazepine doses > 1200 mg/day.

Conversion to monotherapy (600 mg/day twice/day) – Patients receiving concomitant AEDs may be converted to monotherapy by initiating treatment with oxcarbazepine at 600 mg/day twice/day while simultaneously initiating the reduction of the concomitant AED dose. Withdraw the concomitant AEDs over 3 to 6 weeks, while reaching the maximum dose of oxcarbazepine in ≈ 2 to 4 weeks. Oxcarbazepine may be increased as clinically indicated by a maximum increment of 600 mg/day at approximate weekly intervals to achieve the recommended daily dose of 2400 mg/day. A daily dose of 1200 mg/day has been shown to be effective in patients in whom monotherapy has been initiated with oxcarbazepine.

Initiation of monotherapy (600 mg/day twice/day) – Increase by 300 mg/day every third day to a dose of 1200 mg/day. Controlled trials in these patients examined the effectiveness of a 1200 mg/day dose; a dose of 2400 mg/day has been shown to be effective in patients converted from other AEDs to oxcarbazepine monotherapy.

Pediatric patients 4 to 16 years of age:
Adjunctive therapy – 8 to 10 mg/kg not to exceed 600 mg/day twice/day. Achieve the target maintenance dose of oxcarbazepine over 2 weeks, according to patient weight, using the following table.

Oxcarbazepine Target Maintenance Doses for Pediatric Patients	
Patient weight (kg)	Target maintenance dose (mg/day)
20 to 29	900
29.1 to 39	1200
> 39	1800

In the clinical trial, in which the intention was to reach these target doses, the median daily dose was 31 mg/kg with a range of 6 to 51 mg/kg.

Renal function impairment (Ccr < 30 mL/min): Initiate therapy at ½ the usual starting dose (300 mg/day) and increase slowly to achieve the desired clinical response.

Actions

Pharmacology: Oxcarbazepine activity is primarily exerted through the 10-monohydroxy metabolite (MHD) of oxcarbazepine. The precise mechanism by which oxcarbazepine and MHD exert their antiseizure effect is unknown.

Pharmacokinetics:

Absorption – Following oral administration of oxcarbazepine, it is completely absorbed and extensively metabolized to its pharmacologically active MHD metabolite.

Distribution – Approximately 40% of MHD is bound to serum proteins, predominantly to albumin.

Metabolism – Oxcarbazepine is rapidly reduced by cytosolic enzymes in the liver to its MHD, which is primarily responsible for the pharmacological effect of oxcarbazepine. MHD is metabolized further by conjugation with glucuronic acid.

Excretion – The half-life of the parent drug is ≈ 2 hours, while the half-life of MHD is ≈ 9 hours.

Contraindications

Known hypersensitivity to oxcarbazepine or any of its components.

Warnings

Hyponatremia: Clinically significant hyponatremia generally occurred during the first 3 months of treatment with oxcarbazepine, although there were patients who first developed a serum sodium < 125 mmol/L > 1 year after initiation of therapy. Most patients who developed hyponatremia were asymptomatic, but patients in the clinical trials were frequently monitored and some had their oxcarbazepine dose reduced or discontinued or had their fluid intake restricted for hyponatremia. When oxcarbazepine was discontinued, normalization of serum sodium generally occurred within a few days without additional treatment.

Measure serum sodium levels for patients during maintenance treatment with oxcarbazepine.

History of hypersensitivity reaction to carbamazepine: Approximately 25% to 30% of patients who have had hypersensitivity reactions to carbamazepine will experience a hypersensitivity reaction with oxcarbazepine.

Hepatic function impairment: The pharmacokinetics of oxcarbazepine and MHD have not been evaluated in severe hepatic impairment. Adjust dose in renally impaired patients.

Carcinogenesis: In mice, a dose-related increase in the incidence of hepatocellular adenomas was observed with oxcarbazepine.

There was an increase in the incidence of benign testicular interstitial cell tumors and granular cell tumors in the cervix and vagina in rats.

Mutagenesis: Oxcarbazepine increased mutation frequencies in the Ames test in vitro in the absence of metabolic activation in 1 of 5 bacterial strains. Oxcarbazepine and MHD produced increases in chromosomal aberrations and polyploidy in the Chinese hamster ovary assay in vitro in the absence of metabolic activation.

Fertility impairment: In a fertility study in rats, estrous cyclicity was disrupted and numbers of corpora lutea, implantations, and live embryos were reduced in females receiving the highest dose ($\approx$ 2 times the maximum recommended human dose on a mg/m^2 basis).

Elderly: Following administration of single (300 mg) and multiple (600 mg/day) doses of oxcarbazepine to elderly volunteers (60 to 82 years of age), the maximum plasma concentrations and AUC values of MHD were 30% to 60% higher than in younger volunteers (18 to 32 years of age).

Pregnancy: Category C.

Lactation: Oxcarbazepine and its active metabolite MHD are excreted in human breast milk.

Children: After a single-dose administration of 5 to 15 mg/kg of oxcarbazepine, the dose-adjusted AUC values of MHD were 30% to 40% lower in children < 8 years of age than in children > 8 years of age. The clearance in children > 8 years of age approaches that of adults.

Oxcarbazepine has been shown to be effective as adjunctive therapy for partial seizures in patients 4 to 16 years of age.

Precautions

CNS effects: Psychomotor slowing, difficulty with concentration, and speech or language problems; somnolence or fatigue; and coordination abnormalities, including ataxia and gait disturbances.

Lab test abnormalities: Serum sodium levels < 125 mmol/L have been observed in patients treated with oxcarbazepine. Experience from clinical trials indicates that serum sodium levels return toward normal when the oxcarbazepine dosage is reduced or discontinued or when the patient was treated conservatively (eg, fluid restriction).

Laboratory data from clinical trials suggest that oxcarbazepine use was associated with decreases in T_4, without changes in T_3 or TSH.

Drug Interactions

Cytochrome P450: Oxcarbazepine inhibits CYP2C19 and induces CYP3A4/5 with potentially important effects on plasma concentrations of other drugs.

Strong inducers of cytochrome P450 enzymes (ie, carbamazepine, phenytoin, phenobarbital) have been shown to decrease the plasma levels of MHD (29% to 40%).

Cimetidine, erythromycin, and dextropropoxyphene had no effect on the pharmacokinetics of MHD. Results with warfarin show no evidence of interaction with either single or repeated doses of oxcarbazepine.

Drugs that may be affected by oxcarbazepine include felodipine, oral contraceptives, phenobarbital, and phenytoin. Drugs that may affect oxcarbazepine include carbamazepine, phenobarbital, phenytoin, valproic acid, and verapamil.

Adverse Reactions

Adverse reactions that occurred in $\geq$ 3% of patients were as follows: Headache; dizziness; somnolence; anxiety; ataxia; nystagmus; abnormal gait; insomnia; tremor; amnesia; convulsions aggravated; emotional lability; hypoesthesia; nervousness; abnormal coordination; speech disorder; confusion; dysmetria; abnormal thinking; rash; nausea; vomiting; abdominal pain; anorexia; dry mouth; diarrhea; dyspepsia; constipation; urinary tract infection; hyponatremia; back pain; rhinitis; upper respiratory tract infection; coughing; bronchitis; pharyngitis; epistaxis; chest infection; sinusitis; diplopia; vertigo; taste perversion; abnormal vision; fatigue; fever; asthenia; falling down (nos); infection viral.

Adjunctive therapy/monotherapy in adults previously treated with other AEDs – The most commonly observed ($\geq$ 5%) adverse experiences seen in association with oxcarbazepine and substantially more frequent than in placebo-treated patients were the following: Dizziness, somnolence, diplopia, fatigue, nausea, vomiting, ataxia, abnormal vision, abdominal pain, tremor, dyspepsia, abnormal gait.

Approximately 23% of these 1537 adult patients discontinued treatment because of an adverse experience. The adverse experiences most commonly associated with discontinuation were the following: Dizziness (6.4%), diplopia (5.9%), ataxia (5.2%), vomiting (5.1%), nausea (4.9%), somnolence (3.8%), headache (2.9%), fatigue (2.1%), abnormal vision (2.1%), tremor (1.8%), abnormal gait (1.7%), rash (1.4%), hyponatremia (1%).

Adjunctive therapy/monotherapy in pediatric patients previously treated with other AEDs – The most commonly observed (≥ 5%) adverse experiences seen in association with oxcarbazepine in pediatric patients were similar to those seen in adults.

Approximately 11% of the 456 pediatric patients discontinued treatment because of an adverse experience. The adverse experiences most commonly associated with discontinuation were the following: Somnolence (2.4%); vomiting (2%); ataxia (1.8%); diplopia, dizziness (1.3%); fatigue, nystagmus (1.1%).

CYCLOBENZAPRINE HCl

Tablets: 10 mg (*Rx*)	Various, *Flexeril* (Merck)

Indications
Musculoskeletal conditions: Adjunct to rest and physical therapy for relief of muscle spasm associated with acute painful musculoskeletal conditions.

Unlabeled uses: Cyclobenzaprine (10 to 40 mg/day) appears to be a useful adjunct in the management of the fibrositis syndrome.

Administration and Dosage
Give 10 mg 3 times/day (range, 20 to 40 mg/day in divided doses). Do not exceed 60 mg/day. Do not use longer than 2 or 3 weeks.

Actions
Pharmacology: Cyclobenzaprine, structurally related to the tricyclic antidepressants (TCAs), relieves skeletal muscle spasm of local origin without interfering with muscle function. It is ineffective in muscle spasm caused by CNS disease. The net effect is a reduction of tonic somatic motor activity, influencing both gamma and alpha motor systems.

Pharmacokinetics: Cyclobenzaprine is well absorbed after oral administration, but there is a large intersubject variation in plasma levels. The onset of action occurs in 1 hour with a duration of 12 to 24 hours. It is highly bound to plasma proteins, extensively metabolized and excreted primarily via the kidneys. Elimination half-life is 1 to 3 days.

Contraindications
Hypersensitivity to cyclobenzaprine; concomitant use of monoamine oxidase (MAO) inhibitors or within 14 days after their discontinuation; acute recovery phase of MI and in patients with arrhythmias, heart block, or conduction disturbances or CHF; hyperthyroidism.

Warnings
Spasticity: Cyclobenzaprine is not effective in the treatment of spasticity associated with cerebral or spinal cord disease, or in children with cerebral palsy.

Duration: Use only for short periods (up to 2 or 3 weeks); effectiveness for more prolonged use is not proven.

Similarity to TCAs: Cyclobenzaprine is closely related to the TCAs. In short-term studies for indications other than muscle spasm associated with acute musculoskeletal conditions, and usually at doses greater than those recommended, some of the more serious CNS reactions noted with the TCAs have occurred.

Pregnancy: Category B.

Lactation: It is not known whether cyclobenzaprine is excreted in breast milk.

Children: Safety and efficacy in children < 15 years of age have not been established.

Precautions
Anticholinergic effects: Because of its anticholinergic action, use with caution in patients with a history of urinary retention, angle-closure glaucoma, and increased intraocular pressure.

Hazardous tasks: May impair mental or physical abilities required for performance of hazardous tasks; patients should observe caution while driving or performing other tasks requiring alertness, coordination, and physical dexterity.

Drug Interactions
Drugs that may interact with cyclobenzaprine HCl include MAO inhibitors and TCAs.

Adverse Reactions
Adverse reactions occurring in ≥ 3% of patients include drowsiness, dizziness, fatigue, tiredness, asthenia, blurred vision, headache, nervousness, confusion, dry mouth, nausea, constipation, dyspepsia, unpleasant taste, purpura, bone marrow depression, leukopenia, eosinophilia, thrombocytopenia, elevation and lowering of blood sugar levels, and weight gain or loss.

DIAZEPAM

Tablets: 2, 5, and 10 mg (c-iv)	Various, *Valium* (Roche)
Oral solution: 5 mg/5 mL (c-iv)	*Diazepam* (Roxane)
Concentrated oral solution: 5 mg/mL (c-iv)	*Diazepam Intensol* (Roxane)
Injection: 5 mg/mL (c-iv)	Various, *Valium* (Roche), *Zetran* (Hauck), *Dizac* (Ohmeda)

The following is an abbreviated monograph. For complete prescribing information, refer to the Benzodiazepines monograph in the Antianxiety Agents section.

Indications

An adjunct for the relief of skeletal muscle spasm caused by reflex spasm to local pathology (such as inflammation of the muscles or joints, or secondary to trauma); spasticity caused by upper motor neuron disorders; athetosis; stiff-man syndrome. Injectable diazepam may also be used as an adjunct in tetanus.

Also used as an antianxiety agent and an anticonvulsant.

Administration and Dosage

Oral: Individualize dosage for maximum beneficial effect.

Adults – 2 to 10 mg 3 or 4 times/day.

Geriatric or debilitated patients – 2 to 2.5 mg 1 or 2 times/day initially, increasing as needed and tolerated.

Children – 1 to 2.5 mg 3 or 4 times/day initially, increasing as needed and tolerated (not for use in children > 6 months of age).

Intensol – Dosages are same as those listed above. Mix with liquid or semi-solid food such as water, juices, soda or soda-like beverages, applesauce, and puddings. Stir in gently. Consume the entire mixture immediately. Do not store for future use.

Sustained release – 15 to 30 mg once/day.

Parenteral: Use lower doses (2 to 5 mg) and slow dosage increases for elderly or debilitated patients and when other sedatives are given. When acute symptoms are controlled with the injectable form, administer oral therapy if further treatment is required.

Neonates (≤ 30 days of age) – Safety and efficacy have not been established. Prolonged CNS depression has been observed in neonates, apparently because of inability to biotransform diazepam into inactive metabolites.

Children – Give slowly over 3 minutes in a dosage not to exceed 0.25 mg/kg. After a 15 to 30 minute interval, the initial dosage can be safely repeated. If relief is not obtained after a third administration, begin adjunctive therapy appropriate to the condition being treated.

IM: Inject deeply into the muscle.

IV: Inject slowly, taking at least 1 minute for each 5 mg (1 mL). Do not use small veins (ie, dorsum of hand or wrist). Avoid intra-arterial administration or extravasation. Do not mix or dilute with other solutions or drugs.

Adults – 5 to 10 mg, IM or IV initially, then 5 to 10 mg in 3 to 4 hours, if necessary. For tetanus, larger doses may be required.

Children – For tetanus in infants > 30 days of age, 1 to 2 mg IM or IV slowly; repeat every 3 to 4 hours as necessary. In children ≥ 5 years of age, 5 to 10 mg. Repeat every 3 to 4 hours if necessary to control tetanus spasms. Have respiratory assistance available.

Actions

Pharmacology: Major muscle relaxant actions occur in the following 2 proposed sites: At the spinal level resulting in enhancement of GABA-mediated presynaptic inhibition, and at supraspinal sites, probably in the brain stem reticular formation.

BACLOFEN

Tablets: 10 and 20 mg (*Rx*)   Various, *Lioresal* (Geigy)
Intrathecal: 10 mg/20 mL (500 mcg/mL) and 10 mg/5 mL   *Lioresal* (Medtronic)
(2000 mcg/mL) (*Rx*)

Indications

Oral: For the alleviation of signs and symptoms of spasticity resulting from multiple sclerosis, particularly for the relief of flexor spasms and concomitant pain, clonus and muscular rigidity. Patients should have reversible spasticity so that treatment will aid in restoring residual function.

May be of some value in patients with spinal cord injuries and other spinal cord diseases.

Intrathecal: Management of severe spasticity of spinal cord origin in patients who are unresponsive to oral baclofen therapy or experience intolerable CNS side effects at effective doses. Intended for use by the intrathecal route in single bolus test doses (via spinal catheter or lumbar puncture) and, for chronic use, only in implantable pumps approved by the FDA specifically for the administration of baclofen into the intrathecal space.

Intrathecal therapy may be considered an alternative to destructive neurosurgical procedures. Prior to implantation of a device for chronic intrathecal infusion, patients must show a response in a screening trial.

The efficacy as a treatment for spasticity of cerebral origin is not established.

Unlabeled uses:
Oral – Treatment of trigeminal neuralgia (50 to 60 mg/day).
Intrathecal – 25, 50, or 100 mcg appears to be beneficial in children for reducing spasticity in cerebral palsy.

Administration and Dosage

Oral: Individualize dosage. Start at a low dosage and increase gradually until the optimum effect is achieved (usually 40 to 80 mg/day).

The following dosage schedule is suggested: 5 mg 3 times/day for 3 days; 10 mg 3 times/day for 3 days; 15 mg 3 times/day for 3 days; 20 mg 3 times/day for 3 days. Thereafter, additional increases may be necessary, but the total daily dose should not exceed 80 mg/day (20 mg 4 times/day).

The lowest effective dose is recommended. If benefits are not evident after a reasonable trial period, withdraw the drug slowly.

Intrathecal: Refer to the manufacturer's manual for the implantable intrathecal infusion pump for specific instructions and precautions for programming the pump or refilling the reservoir.

Consult complete *Drug Facts and Comparisons* monograph and/or manufacturer product information for full intrathecal dosing information.

Dilution instructions –
Screening: Both strengths (10 mg/5 mL and 10 mg/20 mL) must be diluted with sterile preservative-free Sodium Chloride for Injection, USP to a 50 mcg/mL concentration for bolus injection into the subarachnoid space.

Maintenance: For patients who require concentrations other than 500 or 2000 mcg/mL, baclofen intrathecal must be diluted with sterile, preservative free Sodium Chloride for Injection, USP.

Delivery regimen – Baclofen intrathecal is most often administered in a continuous infusion mode immediately following implant. For those patients implanted with programmable pumps who have achieved relatively satisfactory control on continuous infusion, further benefit may be attained using more complex schedules of delivery.

Actions

Pharmacology: The precise mechanism of action is not known. Baclofen can inhibit both monosynaptic and polysynaptic reflexes at the spinal level, possibly by hyperpolarization of afferent terminals, although actions at supraspinal sites also may contribute to its clinical effect. Baclofen has CNS-depressant properties.

Pharmacokinetics:

Oral – Baclofen is rapidly and extensively absorbed. Absorption may be dose-dependent, being reduced with increasing doses. Peak serum levels are reached in ≈ 2 hours; half-life is 3 to 4 hours. It is excreted primarily by the kidney in unchanged form with intersubject variation in absorption or elimination.

Intrathecal –

Bolus: The onset of action is generally 0.5 to 1 hour after an intrathecal bolus dose. Peak spasmolytic effect is seen at ≈ 4 hours after dosing and effects may last 4 to 8 hours. Onset, peak response, and duration of action may vary with individual patients depending on the dose and severity of symptoms.

Continuous infusion: The antispastic action is first seen at 6 to 8 hours after initiation of continuous infusion. Maximum activity is observed in 24 to 48 hours. The mean CSF clearance was ≈ 30 mL/hour in 10 patients on continuous intrathecal infusion.

Contraindications

Hypersensitivity to baclofen.

Oral: Treatment of skeletal muscle spasm resulting from rheumatic disorders; stroke, cerebral palsy, and Parkinson's disease.

Intrathecal: IV, IM, SC, or epidural administration.

Warnings

Intrathecal administration: Because of the possibility of potentially life-threatening CNS depression, cardiovascular collapse, or respiratory failure, physicians must be adequately trained and educated in chronic intrathecal infusion therapy.

Infection: Patients should be infection-free prior to the screening trial with baclofen injection because the presence of a systemic infection may interfere with an assessment of the patient's response.

Patients should be infection-free prior to pump implantation because the presence of infection may increase the risk of surgical complications. Moreover, a systemic infection may complicate attempts to adjust the pump's dosing rate.

Abrupt drug withdrawal: Hallucinations and seizures have occurred on abrupt withdrawal. An isolated case of manic psychosis has been reported. Except in cases of serious adverse reactions, reduce dose slowly when drug is discontinued.

Stroke: Baclofen has not significantly benefited patients with stroke; they also have poor drug tolerance.

Renal function impairment: Because baclofen is primarily excreted unchanged through the kidneys, administer with caution to patients with impaired renal function. Dosage reduction may be necessary.

Pregnancy: Category C.

Lactation: In mothers treated with oral baclofen in therapeutic doses, the active substance passes into the breast milk. It is not known whether detectable levels of drug are present in breast milk of nursing mothers receiving intrathecal baclofen.

Children:

Oral – Safety for use in children < 12 years of age has not been established. Oral baclofen is not recommended for use in children.

Intrathecal – Safety in children < 4 years of age has not been established.

Precautions

Epilepsy: Monitor the clinical state and EEG at regular intervals because deterioration in seizure control and EEG changes have occurred in patients taking this drug.

Need for spasticity: Use with caution where spasticity is used to sustain upright posture and balance in locomotion, or whenever spasticity is utilized to obtain increased function.

Ovarian cysts: Ovarian cysts have been found by palpation in about 4% of multiple sclerosis patients treated with baclofen for up to 1 year. In most cases, these cysts disappeared spontaneously while patients continued to receive the drug. Ovarian cysts are estimated to occur spontaneously in ≈ 1% to 5% of the normal female population.

Psychotic disorders: Cautiously treat patients suffering from psychotic disorders, schizophrenia, or confusional states and keep under careful surveillance, because exacerbations of these conditions have been observed with oral administration.

Autonomic dysreflexia: Use with caution in patients with a history of autonomic dysreflexia. The presence of nociceptive stimuli or abrupt withdrawl may cause an autonomic dysreflexic episode.

Hazardous tasks: Because of the possibility of sedation, patients should observe caution while driving or performing other tasks requiring alertness, coordination, or physical dexterity.

Adverse Reactions
Adverse reactions occurring in ≥ 3% of patients include drowsiness, weakness of extremities, dizziness/lightheadedness, seizures, headache, nausea/vomiting, numbness/itching/tingling, hypotension, blurred vision, constipation, hypotonia, slurred speech, coma, lethargy/fatigue, confusion, insomnia, and urinary frequency.

DANTROLENE SODIUM

Capsules: 25, 50, and 100 mg (*Rx*)
Powder for injection: 20 mg/vial. Concentration following reconstitution is ≈ 0.32 mg/mL. In 70 mL vials. (*Rx*)

Dantrium (Procter & Gamble)
Dantrium Intravenous (Procter & Gamble)

Warning:
Dantrolene has a potential for hepatotoxicity. Do not use in conditions other than those recommended. The incidence of symptomatic hepatitis (fatal and nonfatal) reported in patients taking up to 400 mg/day is much lower than in those taking ≥ 800 mg/day. Even sporadic short courses of these higher dose levels within a treatment regimen markedly increased the risk of serious hepatic injury. Liver dysfunction, as evidenced by liver enzyme elevations, has been observed in patients exposed to the drug for varying periods of time. Overt hepatitis has been most frequently observed between the third and twelfth months of therapy. Risk of hepatic injury appears to be greater in females, in patients > 35 years of age, and in patients taking other medications in addition to dantrolene.

Monitor hepatic function, including frequent determinations of AST or ALT. If no observable benefit is derived from therapy after 45 days, discontinue use.

Use the lowest possible effective dose for each patient.

Indications
Spasticity:
    Oral – For the control of clinical spasticity resulting from upper motor neuron disorders such as spinal cord injury, stroke, cerebral palsy, or multiple sclerosis. It is of particular benefit to the patient whose functional rehabilitation has been retarded by the sequelae of spasticity. Such patients must have presumably reversible spasticity where relief of spasticity will aid in restoring residual function.

Malignant hyperthermia (MH):
    IV – Management of the fulminant hypermetabolism of skeletal muscle characteristic of MH crisis, along with appropriate supportive measures.
        Preoperatively, and sometimes postoperatively, to prevent or attenuate the development of clinical and laboratory signs of MH in individuals judged to be susceptible to MH.
    Oral – Preoperatively to prevent or attenuate the development of signs of MH in susceptible patients who require anesthesia or surgery. Currently accepted clinical practices in the management of such patients must still be adhered to (careful monitoring for early signs of MH, minimizing exposure to triggering mechanisms, and prompt use of IV dantrolene and indicated supportive measures if signs of MH appear).
        Following a MH crisis to prevent recurrence of MH.

Administration and Dosage

Exercise caution at meals on the day of administration because difficulty swallowing and choking has been reported.

Chronic spasticity: Titrate and individualize dosage. In view of the potential for liver damage in long-term use, discontinue therapy if benefits are not evident within 45 days.

Adults – Begin with 25 mg once/day, increase to 25 mg 2 to 4 times/day, then increase by increments of 25 mg up to as high as 100 mg 2 to 4 times/day if necessary. As most patients will respond to ≤ 400 mg/day, higher doses rarely are needed. Maintain each dosage level for 4 to 7 days to determine response. Adjust dosage to achieve maximal benefit without adverse effects.

Children – Use a similar approach. Start with 0.5 mg/kg twice/day; increase to 0.5 mg/kg, 3 or 4 times/day; then by increments of 0.5 mg/kg, up to 3 mg/kg, 2 to 4 times/day if necessary. Do not exceed doses higher than 100 mg 4 times/day.

MH:

Preoperative prophylaxis – Dantrolene may be given orally or IV to patients judged susceptible to MH as part of the overall patient management to prevent or attenuate development of clinical and laboratory signs of MH.

Oral – Give 4 to 8 mg/kg/day orally in 3 or 4 divided doses for 1 or 2 days prior to surgery, with last dose given ≈ 3 to 4 hours before scheduled surgery with a minimum of water. This dosage usually will be associated with skeletal muscle weakness and sedation (sleepiness or drowsiness) or excessive GI irritation (nausea or vomiting); adjust within the recommended dosage range to avoid incapacitation or excessive GI irritation.

IV – Dantrolene IV may decrease the grip strength and increase weakness of leg muscles, especially walking down stairs.

Treatment – As soon as the MH reaction is recognized, discontinue all anesthetic agents. Use of 100% oxygen is recommended. Administer dantrolene by continuous rapid IV push beginning at a minimum dose of 1 mg/kg, and continuing until symptoms subside or a maximum cumulative dose of 10 mg/kg has been reached. If the physiologic and metabolic abnormalities reappear, repeat the regimen. Administration should be continuous until symptoms subside.

Children – Dose is the same as for adults.

Postcrisis follow-up – Following a MH crisis, give 4 to 8 mg/kg/day orally, in 4 divided doses for 1 to 3 days to prevent recurrence. IV dantrolene may be used when oral administration is not practical. The IV dose must be individualized, starting with 1 mg/kg or more as the clinical situation dictates.

Actions

Pharmacology: In isolated nerve-muscle preparation, dantrolene produced relaxation by affecting contractile response of the skeletal muscle at a site beyond the myoneural junction and directly on the muscle itself. In skeletal muscle, the drug dissociates the excitation-contraction coupling, probably by interfering with the release of calcium from the sarcoplasmic reticulum.

MH – Dantrolene may prevent changes within the muscle cell that result in MH syndrome by interfering with calcium release from the sarcoplasmic reticulum to the myoplasm.

Pharmacokinetics:

Absorption/Distribution – Absorbtion after oral administration is incomplete (≈ 70%) and slow but consistent, and dose-related blood levels are obtained.

Metabolism – Dantrolene is found in measurable amounts in blood and urine. Mean half-life in adults is 9 hours after a 100 mg oral dose and 4 to 8 hours after IV administration. Because it is probably metabolized by hepatic microsomal enzymes, metabolism enhancement by other drugs is possible.

Contraindications

Oral: Active hepatic disease, such as hepatitis and cirrhosis; where spasticity is used to sustain upright posture and balance in locomotion or to obtain or maintain increased function; treatment of skeletal muscle spasm resulting from rheumatic disorders.

Warnings

Hepatic effects: Fatal and nonfatal liver disorders of an idiosyncratic or hypersensitivity type may occur. At the start of therapy, perform baseline liver function studies. If abnormalities exist, the potential for hepatotoxicity could be enhanced.

Perform liver function studies at appropriate intervals during therapy. If such studies reveal abnormal values, generally discontinue therapy. Some laboratory values may return to normal with continued therapy; others may not.

If symptoms of hepatitis accompanied by liver function test abnormalities or jaundice appear, discontinue therapy. If caused by dantrolene and detected early, abnormalities may revert to normal when the drug is discontinued. See Warning Box.

Long-term use: Safety and efficacy have not been established.

Continued long-term administration is justified if use of the drug: Significantly reduces painful or disabling spasticity such as clonus; significantly reduces the intensity or degree of nursing care required; rids the patient of any annoying manifestation of spasticity considered important by the patient.

Brief withdrawal for 2 to 4 days will frequently demonstrate exacerbation of the manifestations of spasticity and may serve to confirm a clinical impression.

In view of the potential for liver damage in long-term use, discontinue therapy if benefits are not evident within 45 days.

MH: IV use is not a substitute for previously known supportive measures. These measures include discontinuing the suspect triggering agents, attending to increased oxygen requirements, managing the metabolic acidosis, instituting cooling when necessary, attending to urinary output, and monitoring electrolyte imbalance.

Pregnancy: Category C (parenteral).

Lactation: Do not use in nursing women.

Children: Safety for use in children < 5 years of age has not been established.

Precautions

Extravasation: Because of the high pH of the IV formulation, prevent extravasation into the surrounding tissues.

Special risk: Use with caution in patients with impaired pulmonary function, particularly those with obstructive pulmonary disease; severely impaired cardiac function caused by myocardial disease; history of previous liver disease or dysfunction.

Hazardous tasks: Patients should use caution while driving or performing other tasks requiring alertness, coordination or physical dexterity.

Photosensitivity: Photosensitization may occur; therefore, caution patients to take protective measures against exposure to ultraviolet light or sunlight until tolerance is determined.

Drug Interactions

Drugs that may interact with dantrolene include clofibrate, estrogens, warfarin, and verapamil.

Avoid alcohol and other CNS depressants.

Adverse Reactions

Adverse reactions may include drowsiness; dizziness; weakness; general malaise; fatigue; diarrhea; constipation; GI bleeding; anorexia; dysphagia; gastric irritation; abdominal cramps; hepatitis; speech disturbance; seizure; headache; lightheadedness; visual disturbance; diplopia; taste alteration; insomnia; mental depression; confusion; increased nervousness; tachycardia; erratic blood pressure; phlebitis; increased urinary frequency; hematuria; crystalluria; difficult erection; urinary incontinence; nocturia; dysuria; urinary retention; abnormal hair growth; acne-like rash; pruritus; urticaria; eczematoid eruption; sweating; myalgia; backache; chills; fever; feeling of suffocation; excessive tearing; pleural effusion with pericarditis; severity: pulmonary edema developing during treatment of MH crisis; thrombophlebitis following IV dantrolene; urticaria; erythema; hepatitis; seizures; pleural effusion with pericarditis.

PARKINSON'S DISEASE

Parkinsonism is a neurological disease with a variety of origins characterized by tremor, rigidity, akinesia, and disorders of posture and equilibrium. The onset is slow and progressive, with symptoms advancing over months to years.

	Drug Therapy for Parkinsonism					
	Indications					
Drugs	Post-encephalitic	Arterio-sclerotic	Idiopathic	Drug/chemical induced	Adjunct to Levodopa/carbidopa	Usual daily dose range (mg)
Anticholinergics						
Procyclidine	✔	✔	✔	✔		7.5 to 20
Trihexyphenidyl	✔	✔	✔	✔	✔	1 to 15
Benztropine	✔	✔	✔	✔		0.5 to 6.5
Biperiden	✔	✔	✔	✔		2 to 8
Ethopropazine	✔	✔	✔	✔		50 to 600
Diphenhydramine	✔	✔	✔	✔		10 to 400
Dopaminergic Agents						
Levodopa	✔	✔	✔	✔[1]		500 to 8000
Carbidopa/Levodopa	✔		✔	✔[1]		10/100 to 200/2000
Amantadine	✔	✔	✔	✔		200 to 400
Bromocriptine	✔		✔			12.5 to 100
Pergolide					✔	1 to 5
Selegiline					✔	10
Pramipexole			✔			0.375 to 4.5
Ropinirole			✔			0.75 to 3

[1] Not effective in drug-induced extrapyramidal symptoms.

ANTICHOLINERGICS

PROCYCLIDINE
Tablets: 5 mg (*Rx*)   *Kemadrin* (GlaxoSmithKline)
TRIHEXYPHENIDYL HCl
Tablets: 2 and 5 mg (*Rx*)   Various, *Artane* (Lederle)
Capsules, sustained release: 5 mg (*Rx*)   *Artane Sequels* (Lederle)
Elixir: 2 mg/5 mL (*Rx*)   *Artane* (Lederle)
BENZTROPINE MESYLATE
Tablets: 0.5, 1, and 2 mg (*Rx*)   Various, *Cogentin* (Merck)
Injection: 1 mg/mL (*Rx*)   *Cogentin* (Merck)
BIPERIDEN
Tablets: 2 mg (*Rx*)   *Akineton* (Knoll)
Injection: 5 mg/mL (*Rx*)   *Akineton* (Knoll)
ETHOPROPAZINE HCl
Tablets: 10 and 50 mg (*Rx*)   *Parsidol* (Parke-Davis)

Indications
Adjunctive therapy in all forms of parkinsonism (postencephalitic, arteriosclerotic and idiopathic) and in the control of drug-induced extrapyramidal disorders.

Administration and Dosage
Give before or after meals, as determined by patient's reaction. Postencephalitic patients (more prone to excessive salivation) may prefer to take it after meals and may, in addition, require small amounts of atropine. If the mouth dries excessively, take before meals, unless it causes nausea. If taken after meals, thirst can be allayed by mint candies, chewing gum, or water.

PROCYCLIDINE:
Parkinsonism (for patients who have received no other therapy) – Initially, 2.5 mg 3 times/ day after meals. If well tolerated, gradually increase dose to 5 mg; administer 3 times/ day, and occasionally before retiring, if necessary. In some cases, smaller doses may be effective.

For drug-induced extrapyramidal symptoms – Begin with 2.5 mg 3 times/day; increase by 2.5 mg/day increments until the patient obtains relief of symptoms. Individualize dosage. In most cases, results will be obtained with 10 to 20 mg/day.

TRIHEXYPHENIDYL HCl:
Parkinsonism – Initially, administer 1 to 2 mg the first day; increase by 2 mg increments at intervals of 3 to 5 days, until a total of 6 to 10 mg is given daily. Many patients derive maximum benefit from a total daily dose of 6 to 10 mg; however, postencephalitic patients may require a total daily dose of 12 to 15 mg. Trihexyphenidyl is tolerated best if divided into 3 doses and taken at mealtimes. High doses may be divided into 4 parts, administered at mealtimes and at bedtime.

Concomitant use with levodopa: Trihexyphenidyl 3 to 6 mg/day in divided doses is usually adequate.

Drug-induced extrapyramidal disorders – Start with a single 1 mg dose. Daily dosage usually ranges between 5 to 15 mg, although reactions have been controlled on as little as 1 mg/day.

Sustained release – Do not use for initial therapy. Once patients are stabilized on conventional dosage forms, they may be switched to sustained release capsules on a milligram per milligram of total daily dose basis. Administer as a single dose after breakfast or in 2 divided doses 12 hours apart.

BENZTROPINE MESYLATE: Because there is not significant difference in onset of action after IV or IM injection, there is usually no need to use the IV route. In emergency situations, when the condition of the patients is alarming, 1 to 2 mL will normally provide quick relief.

Dosage titration – Because of cumulative action, initiate therapy with a low dose, increase in increments of 0.5 mg gradually at 5 or 6 day intervals to the smallest amount necessary for optimal relief. Maximum daily dose is 6 mg.

Dose intervals – Some patients experience greatest relief by taking the entire dose at bedtime; others react more favorably to divided doses, 2 to 4 times/day.

Pakinsonism – 1 to 2 mg/day, with a range of 0.5 to 6 mg/day, orally or parenterally.

Idiopathic parkinsonism: Start with 0.5 to 1 mg at bedtime; 4 to 6 mg/day may be required.

Postencephalitic parkinsonism: 2 mg/day in ≥ 1 dose. In highly sensitive patients, begin therapy with 0.5 mg at bedtime; increase as necessary.

Drug-induced extrapyramidal disorders – Administer 1 to 4 mg once or twice/day.

Acute dystonic reactions: 1 to 2 mL IM or IV usually relieves the condition quickly. After that, 1 to 2 mL orally 2 times/day usually prevents recurrence.

Extrapyramidal disorders which develop soon after initiating treatment with neuroleptic drugs are likely to be transient. A dosage of 1 to 2 mg orally 2 or 3 times a day usually provides relief within 1 or 2 days. After 1 or 2 weeks, withdraw drug to determine its continued need. If such disorders recur, reinstitute benztropine.

BIPERIDEN:
Parkinsonism – 2 mg 3 or 4 times/day, orally. Individualize dosage with dosing titrated to a maximum of 16 mg/24 hours.

Drug-induced extrapyramidal disorders –
Oral: 2 mg 1 to 3 times/day.
Parenteral: 2 mg IM or IV. Repeat every half-hour until symptoms are resolved, but do not give more than 4 consecutive doses per 24 hours.

ETHOPROPAZINE:
Initially – 50 mg once or twice/day; increase gradually, if necessary.
Mild to moderate symptoms – 100 to 400 mg/day.
Severe cases – Gradually increase to 500 or 600 mg or more daily.

DIPHENYDRAMINE:
> Oral –
>> Adults: 25 to 50 mg 3 to 4 times/day.
>> Children > 20 lbs (9 kg): 12.5 to 25 mg 3 or 4 times/day or 5 mg/kg/day. Do not exceed 300 mg/day or 150 mg/m²/day.
> Parenteral – Administer IV or deeply IM.
>> Adults: 10 to 50 mg; 100 mg if required. Maximum daily dosage is 400 mg.
>> Children: 5 mg/kg/day or 150 mg/m²/day.

Actions

Pharmacology: Anticholinergic agents reduce the incidence and severity of akinesia, rigidity, and tremor by ≈ 20%; secondary symptoms such as drooling are also reduced. In addition to suppressing central cholinergic activity, these agents also may inhibit the reuptake and storage of dopamine at central dopamine receptors, thereby prolonging the action of dopamine.

Pharmacokinetics:

Various Antiparkinson Anticholinergic Pharmacokinetic Parameters				
Anticholinergic	Time to peak concentration (hrs)	Peak concentration (mcg/L)	Half-life (hrs)	Oral bioavailability (%)
Benztropine[1]				
Biperiden	1 to 1.5	4 to 5	18.4 to 24.3	29
Diphenhydramine	2 to 4	65 to 90	4 to 15	50 to 72
Ethopropazine[1]				
Procyclidine	1.1 to 2	80	11.5 to 12.6	52 to 97
Trihexyphenidyl	1 to 1.3	87.2	5.6 to 10.2	≈ 100

[1] No data available.

Contraindications

Hypersensitivity to any component; glaucoma, particularly angle-closure glaucoma; pyloric or duodenal obstruction; stenosing peptic ulcers; prostatic hypertrophy or bladder neck obstructions; achalasia (megaesophagus); myasthenia gravis; megacolon.

Benztropine: Children < 3 years of age; use with caution in older children.

Warnings

Ophthalmic: Incipient narrow-angle glaucoma may be precipitated by these drugs.

Elderly: Geriatric patients, particularly > 60 years of age, frequently develop increased sensitivity to anticholinergic drugs and require strict dosage regulation. Occasionally, mental confusion and disorientation may occur; agitation, hallucinations, and psychotic-like symptoms may develop.

Pregnancy: Category C.

Lactation: An inhibitory effect on lactation may occur.

Children: Safety and efficacy for use in children have not been established.

Precautions

Concomitant conditions: Use caution in patients with tachycardia, cardiac arrhythmias, hypertension, hypotension, prostatic hypertrophy (particularly in the elderly), or any tendency toward urinary retention, liver or kidney disorders, and obstructive disease of the GI or GU tract.

CNS: When used to treat extrapyramidal reactions resulting from phenothiazines in psychiatric patients, antiparkinson agents may exacerbate mental symptoms and precipitate a toxic psychosis.

In addition, 19% to 30% of patients given anticholinergics develop depression, confusion, delusions, or hallucinations.

Tardive dyskinesia – Tardive dyskinesia may appear in some patients on long-term therapy with phenothiazines and related agents, or may occur after therapy has been discontinued.

Dry mouth: If dry mouth is so severe that swallowing or speaking is difficult, or if loss of appetite and weight occurs, reduce dosage or discontinue drug temporarily.

Abuse potential: Some patients may use these agents for mood elevations or psychedelic experiences. Cannabinoids, barbiturates, opiates, and alcohol may have additive effects with anticholinergics.

Hazardous tasks: May impair mental or physical abilities; patients should observe caution while driving or performing other tasks requiring alertness.

Drug Interactions

Drugs that may interact with anticholinergic antiparkinson agents include amantadine, digoxin, haloperidol, levodopa, and phenothiazines.

Adverse Reactions

Adverse reactions include the following: Tachycardia; palpitations; hypotension; disorientation; confusion; memory loss; hallucinations; psychoses; agitation; nervousness; delusions; delirium; paranoia; euphoria; excitement; lightheadedness; dizziness; headache; listlessness; depression; drowsiness; weakness; giddiness; paresthesia; heaviness of the limbs; dry mouth; nausea; vomiting; epigastric distress; constipation; development of duodenal ulcer; skin rash; urticaria; other dermatoses; blurred vision; mydriasis; diplopia; increased intraocular tension; angle-closure glaucoma; dilation of pupils; muscular weakness; muscular cramping; urinary retention; urinary hesitancy; dysuria; elevated temperature; flushing; numbness of fingers; decreased sweating, hyperthermia, heat stroke; difficulty in achieving or maintaining an erection.

LEVODOPA AND CARBIDOPA

Tablets: 10 mg carbidopa and 100 mg levodopa, 25 mg carbidopa and 100 mg levodopa, 25 mg carbidopa and 250 mg levodopa (*Rx*)	Various, *Sinemet* (DuPont)
Tablets, sustained release: 50 mg carbidopa and 200 mg levodopa, 25 mg carbidopa and 100 mg levodopa (*Rx*)	*Sinemet CR* (DuPont)

Indications

Treatment of symptoms of idiopathic Parkinson's disease (paralysis agitans), postencephalitic parkinsonism, and sympathetic parkinsonism that may follow injury to the nervous system by carbon monoxide and manganese intoxication.

Administration and Dosage

Patients not receiving levodopa:

Sinemet – 1 tablet of 25 mg carbidopa/100 mg levodopa 3 times/day or 10 mg carbidopa/100 mg levodopa 3 or 4 times/day. Dosage may be increased by 1 tablet every day or every other day, as necessary, until a dosage of 8 tablets a day is reached.

Tablets of the 2 ratios (eg, 1:4, 25/100 or 1:10, 10/100 and 25/250) may be given separately or combined as needed to provide the optimum dosage.

Provide at least 70 to 100 mg carbidopa per day. When more carbidopa is required, substitute one 25/100 tablet for each 10/100 tablet. When more levodopa is required, substitute the 25/250 tablet for the 25/100 or 10/100 tablet.

Sinemet CR – 1 tablet twice/day at intervals of not less than 6 hours. Doses and dosing intervals may be increased or decreased based on response. Most patients have been adequately treated with 2 to 8 tablets per day (divided doses) at intervals of 4 to 8 hours while awake. Higher doses ($\geq$ 12 tablets per day) and intervals < 4 hours have been used but are not usually recommended. If an interval of < 4 hours is used or if the divided doses are not equal, give the smaller doses at the end of the day.

Sinemet CR – Sinemet CR may be administered as whole or half tablets which should not be crushed or chewed.

Patients currently treated with levodopa: Levodopa must be discontinued at least 8 hours before therapy with levodopa/carbidopa. Substitute the combination drug at a dosage that will provide $\approx$ 25% of the previous levodopa dosage.

Sinemet – Suggested starting dosage is 1 tablet of 25 mg carbidopa/250 mg levodopa 3 or 4 times a day for patients taking > 1500 mg levodopa or 25 mg carbidopa/100 mg levodopa for patients taking < 1500 mg levodopa.

Sinemet CR – Usually 1 tablet twice/day.

Patients currently treated with conventional carbidopa/levodopa preparations: Substitute dosage with *Sinemet CR* at an amount that provides ≈ 10% more levodopa per day, although this may need to be increased to a dosage that provides up to 30% more levodopa per day. Use intervals of 4 to 8 hours while awake.

Guidelines for Initial Conversion from *Sinemet* to *Sinemet CR*	
Sinemet Total daily levodopa dose (mg)	*Sinemet CR* Suggested dosage regimen
300 to 400	1 tablet twice/day
500 to 600	1½ tablets twice/day or 1 tablet 3 times/day
700 to 800	Total of 4 tablets in ≥ 3 divided doses (eg, 1½ tablets am, 1½ tablets early pm, 1 tablet later pm)
900 to 1000	Total of 5 tablets in ≥ 3 divided doses (eg, 2 tablets am, 2 tablets early pm, 1 tablet later pm)

Combination therapy: Other antiparkinson drugs can be given concurrently; dosage adjustment may be necessary.

Sinemet – Sinemet (25/100 or 10/100) can be added to the dosage regimen of *Sinemet CR* in selected patients with advanced disease who need additional levodopa.

Actions

Pharmacology: These agents are used in combination because carbidopa inhibits decarboxylation of levodopa and makes more levodopa available for transport to the brain. There is less variation in plasma levodopa levels than with the conventional formulation. However, the sustained release form is less systemically bioavailable (70% to 75%) and may require increased daily doses to achieve the same level of symptomatic relief.

Pharmacokinetics: The half-life of levodopa may be prolonged following the sustained release form because of continuous absorption. In elderly subjects, the mean time to peak levodopa concentration was 2 hours for sustained-release vs 0.5 hours for conventional. The maximum concentration following the sustained-release form was about 35% of the conventional form.

Warnings

CNS effects: Certain adverse CNS effects (eg, dyskinesias) will occur at lower dosages and sooner during therapy with the sustained-release form.

Drug Interactions

Drug/Food interactions: Administration of a single dose of the sustained-release form with food increased the extent of levodopa availability by 50% and increased peak levodopa concentrations by 25%.

Adverse Reactions

In clinical trials, the adverse reaction profile of the sustained-release form did not differ substantially from that of the conventional form.

ENTACAPONE

Tablets: 200 mg   *Comtan* (Novartis)

Indications

Parkinson's disease: As an adjunct to levodopa/carbidopa to treat patients with idiopathic Parkinson's disease who experience the signs and symptoms of end-of-dose "wearing-off." The effectiveness of entacapone has not been systematically evaluated in patients with idiopathic Parkinson's disease who do not experience end-of-dose "wearing-off."

Administration and Dosage

The recommended dose of entacapone is one 200 mg tablet administered concomitantly with each levodopa/carbidopa dose to a maximum of 8 times/day (200 mg × 8 = 1600 mg/day). Clinical experience with daily doses > 1600 mg is limited.

Always administer entacapone in combination with levodopa/carbidopa. Entacapone has no antiparkinsonian effect of its own.

In clinical trials, the majority of patients required a decrease in daily levodopa dose if their daily dose of levodopa had been ≥ 800 mg, or if they had moderate or severe dyskinesias prior to treatment with entacapone.

Reducing the daily levodopa dose or extending the interval between doses may be necessary to optimize patient reponse. In clinical trials, the average reduction in the daily levodopa dose was ≈ 25% in those patients requiring a levodopa dose reduction. (More than 58% of patients with levodopa doses > 800 mg daily required such a reduction.)

Entacapone can be combined with the immediate- and sustained-release formulations of levodopa/carbidopa.

Entacapone may be taken with or without food.

Withdrawing patients from entacapone: Rapid withdrawal or abrupt reduction in the entacapone dose could lead to emergence of signs and symptoms of Parkinson's disease and may lead to hyperpyrexia and confusion, a symptom complex resembling neuroleptic malignant syndrome (see Precautions). Consider this syndrome in the differential diagnosis for any patient who develops a high fever or severe rigidity. If a decision is made to discontinue treatment with entacapone, monitor patients closely and adjust other dopaminergic agents as needed. Although tapering entacapone has not been evaluated, it seems reasonable to withdraw patients slowly if the decision to discontinue treatment is made.

Actions

Pharmacology: Entacapone is a selective and reversible inhibitor of catechol-O-methyltransferase (COMT), which alters the plasma pharmacokinetics of levodopa. When entacapone is given in conjunction with levodopa and an aromatic amino acid decarboxylase inhibitor (such as carbidopa), plasma levels of levodopa are greater and more sustained than after administration of levodopa and an aromatic amino acid decarboxylase inhibitor alone.

Pharmacokinetics: Entacapone is rapidly absorbed, with a T_{max} of ≈ 1 hour. The absolute bioavailability following oral administration is 35%. The plasma protein binding of entacapone is 98%, mainly to serum albumin. Entacapone is almost completely metabolized prior to excretion, with only a small amount (0.2% of dose) excreted in the urine.

Contraindications

Hypersensitivity to the drug or any of its ingredients.

Warnings

Hepatic function impairment: Treat hepatically impaired patients with with caution. The AUC and C_{max} of entacapone approximately doubled in patients with documented liver disease compared with controls.

Carcinogenesis: An increased incidence of renal tubular adenomas and carcinomas was found in male rats treated with the highest dose of entacapone.

Mutagenesis: Entacapone was mutagenic and clastogenic in the in vitro mouse lymphoma/thymidine kinase assay in the presence and absence of metabolic activation, and was clastogenic in cultured human lymphocytes in the presence of metabolic activation.

Pregnancy: Category C.

Lactation: It is not known whether entacapone is excreted in human breast milk.

Children: There is no identified potential use of entacapone in pediatric patients.

Precautions

Hypotension/Syncope: Dopaminergic therapy in patients with Parkinson's disease has been associated with orthostatic hypotension. Entacapone enhances levodopa bioavailability and, therefore, might be expected to increase the occurrence of orthostatic hypotension. However, in entacapone clinical trials, no differences from placebo were seen for measured orthostasis or symptoms of orthostasis.

Diarrhea: In clinical trials, diarrhea devloped in 10% and 4% of patients treated with 200 mg entacapone and placebo, respectively, and was regarded as severe in 1.3% of patients.

Hallucinations: Dopaminergic therapy in Parkinson's disease patients has been associated with hallucinations. In clinical trials, hallucinations developed in ≈ 4% of patients treated with 200 mg entacapone or placebo.

Dyskinesia: Entacapone may potentiate the dopaminergic side effects of levodopa and may cause or exacerbate pre-existing dyskinesia.

Dopaminergic therapy reactions: The events listed below are rare events known to be associated with the use of drugs that increase dopaminergic activity, although they are most often associated with the use of direct dopamine agonists:

 Rhabdomyolysis – Cases of severe rhabdomyolysis have been reported with entacapone use. The complicated nature of these cases makes it impossible to determine what role, if any, entacapone played in their pathogenesis.

 Hyperpyrexia and confusion –

  Tapering of dose: Cases of a symptom complex resembling neuroleptic malignant syndrome characterized by elevated temperature, muscular rigidity, altered consciousness, and elevated creatine phosphokinase (CPK) have been reported in association with the rapid dose reduction or withdrawal of other dopaminergic drugs.

  Prescribers should exercise caution when discontinuing entacapone treatment. When considered necessary, withdrawal should proceed slowly. Consider this syndrome in the differential diagnosis for any patient who develops a high fever or severe rigidity.

 Fibrotic complications – Cases of retroperitoneal fibrosis, pulmonary infiltrates, pleural effusion, and pleural thickening have been reported in some patients treated with ergot-derived dopaminergic agents. Although these adverse events are believed to be related to the ergoline structure of these compounds, whether other nonergot-derived drugs (eg, entacapone) that increase dopaminergic activity can cause them is unknown.

Renal toxicity: In a 1-year toxicity study, entacapone (plasma exposure 20 times that in humans receiving the MRDD of 1600 mg) caused an increased incidence of nephrotoxicity in male rats.

Biliary excretion: As most entacapone excretion is via the bile, exercise caution when drugs known to interfere with biliary excretion, glucuronidation, and intestinal beta-glucuronidase are given concurrently with entacapone (see Drug Interactions).

Lab test abnormalities: Entacapone is an iron chelator. The impact of entacapone on the body's iron stores is unknown; however, a tendency towards decreasing serum iron concentrations was noted in clinical trials. In a controlled clinical study, serum ferritin levels (as a marker of iron deficiency and subclinical anemia) were not changed with entacapone compared with placebo after 1 year of treatment and there was no difference in rates of anemia or decreased hemoglobin levels.

Drug Interactions

Entacapone inhibited the CYP isoenzymes 1A2, 2A6, 2C9, 2C19, 2D6, 2E1, and 3A only at very high concentrations and would not be expected to be inhibited in clinical use.

Monoamine oxidase (MAO) inhibitors: MAO and COMT are the 2 major enzyme systems involved in the metabolism of catecholamines. Do not treat patients concomitantly with entacapone and a nonselective MAO inhibitor.

 Entacapone can be taken concomitantly with a selective MAO-B inhibitor (eg, selegiline).

Drugs metabolized by COMT: Adminster drugs known to be metabolized by COMT (ie, iso-proterenol, epinephrine, norepinephrine, dopamine, dobutamine, methyldopa, apomorphine, isoetherine, bitolterol) with caution in patients receiving entacapone regardless of the route of administration (including inhalation), as their interaction may result in increased heart rates, arrhythmias, and excessive changes in blood pressure.

Drugs that interfere with biliary excretion of glucuronidation (erythromycin, rifampin, cholestyramine) might decrease entacapone elimination.

Drug/Food interactions: Food does not affect the pharmacokinetics of entacapone.

Adverse Reactions
Adverse reactions that occur in $\geq 3\%$ of patients include the following: Dyskinesias; dizziness; nausea; diarrhea; abdominal pain; urine discoloration; hyper- and hypokinesia; constipation; vomiting; dry mouth; back pain; fatigue; dyspnea.

AMANTADINE HCl

Capsules: 100 mg (*Rx*)	Various, *Symadine* (Solvay), *Symmetrel* (DuPont)
Syrup: 50 mg/5 mL (*Rx*)	*Symmetrel* (DuPont)

This is an abbreviated monograph. For full prescribing information, refer to the Antiviral Agents monograph.

Indications
Parkinson's disease/syndrome and drug-induced extrapyramidal reactions: Idiopathic Parkinson's disease (paralysis agitans); postencephalitic parkinsonism; arteriosclerotic parkinsonism; drug-induced extrapyramidal reactions; symptomatic parkinsonism following injury to the nervous system by carbon monoxide intoxication.

Administration and Dosage
Parkinson's disease: 100 mg twice/day when used alone. Onset of action is usually within 48 hrs. Initial dose is 100 mg/day for patients with serious associated medical illnesses or those receiving high doses of other antiparkinson drugs. After one to several weeks at 100 mg once/day, increase to 100 mg twice/day, if necessary. Patients whose responses are not optimal at 200 mg/day may occasionally benefit from an increase up to 400 mg/day in divided doses; supervise closely. Patients initially benefiting from amantadine often experience decreased efficacy after a few months. Benefit may be regained by increasing to 300 mg/day, or by temporary discontinuation for several weeks. Other antiparkinson drugs may be necessary.

Concomitant therapy – When amantadine and levodopa are initiated concurrently, the patient can exhibit rapid therapeutic benefits. Maintain the dose at 100 mg/day or twice/day, while levodopa is gradually increased to optimal benefit.

Renal function impairment: The following table is designed to yield steady-state plasma concentrations of 0.7 to 1 mcg/mL.

Suggested Dosage Guidelines for Amantadine in Impaired Renal Function		
Ccr (mL/min/1.73 m^2)	Estimated half-life (hours)	Suggested maintenance regimen[1]
100	11	100 mg twice a day or 200 mg/day
80	14	100 mg twice a day
60	19	200 mg alternated with 100 mg/day
50	23	100 mg/day
40	29	100 mg/day
30	40	200 mg twice weekly
20	66	100 mg 3 times weekly
10	178	200 mg alternated with 100 mg every 7 days
3 times weekly chronic hemodialysis	199	200 mg alternated with 100 mg every 7 days

[1] Loading dose on first day of 200 mg. Reproduced with permission from Horadam VW, Sharp JG, Smilack JD, et al. Pharmacokinetics of amantadine HCl in subjects with normal and impaired renal function. *Ann Intern Med.* 1981;94:454-458.

Drug-induced extrapyramidal reactions: 100 mg twice/day. Patients with suboptimal responses may benefit from 300 mg/day in divided doses.

Actions

Pharmacology: The exact mechanism of action is unknown, but amantadine is thought to release dopamine from intact dopaminergic terminals that remain in the substantia nigra of parkinson patients.

BROMOCRIPTINE MESYLATE

Tablets: 2.5 mg (*Rx*)	*Parlodel SnapTabs* (Sandoz)
Capsules: 5 mg (*Rx*)	*Parlodel* (Sandoz)

Indications

Parkinson's disease: Treatment of idiopathic or postencephalitic Parkinson's disease.

Administration and Dosage

Parkinson's disease: Initiate treatment at a low dosage and individualize; increase the daily dosage slowly until a maximum therapeutic response is achieved. If possible, maintain the dosage of levodopa during this introductory period.

Initially, use 1.25 mg (one-half of a 2.5 mg tablet) twice daily with meals. Assess dosage titrations every 2 weeks to ensure that the lowest dosage producing an optimal therapeutic response is not exceeded. If necessary, increase the dosage every 2 to 4 weeks by 2.5 mg/day with meals. If it is necessary to reduce the dose because of adverse reactions, reduce dose gradually in 2.5 mg increments. Usual range is 10 to 40 mg/day.

The safety of bromocriptine has not been demonstrated in dosages exceeding 100 mg/day.

Actions

Pharmacology: Bromocriptine, a dopamine agonist, may relieve akinesia, rigidity, and tremor in patients with Parkinson's disease. It produces its therapeutic effect by directly stimulating the dopamine receptors in the corpus striatum.

SELEGILINE HCl (L-Deprenyl)

Tablets: 5 mg (*Rx*)	*Eldepryl* (Somerset)

Indications

Parkinson's disease: Adjunct in the management of parkinsonian patients being treated with levodopa/carbidopa who exhibit deterioration in the quality of their response to this therapy.

Administration and Dosage

Parkinsonian patients receiving levodopa/carbidopa therapy who demonstrate a deteriorating response to this treatment: 10 mg per day administered as divided doses of 5 mg each taken at breakfast and lunch. There is no evidence that additional benefit will be obtained from the administration of higher doses.

After 2 to 3 days of treatment, attempt to reduce the dose of levodopa/carbidopa. A reduction of 10% to 30% appears typical. Further reductions of levodopa/carbidopa may be possible during continued selegiline therapy.

Actions

Pharmacology: Selegiline HCl is a levorotatory acetylenic derivative of phenethylamine. Although the mechanism of action is not fully understood, inhibition of monoamine oxidase (MAO) type B activity is of primary importance and selegiline may act through other mechanisms to increase dopaminergic activity.

Pharmacokinetics:

Absorption/Distribution – Selegiline is rapidly absorbed; $\approx$ 73% of a dose is absorbed; maximum plasma concentration occurs 0.5 to 2 hours following administration.

Metabolism/Excretion – The drug is rapidly metabolized. Over 48 hours, 45% of the dose appeared in the urine as metabolites. Unchanged selegiline is not detected in urine.

Contraindications
Hypersensitivity to the drug; use with meperidine.

Warnings
Maximum dose: Do not use at daily doses exceeding those recommended (10 mg/day) because of the risks associated with nonselective inhibition of MAO.

Pregnancy: Category C.

Lactation: It is not known whether selegiline is excreted in breast milk.

Children: The effects of selegiline in children have not been evaluated.

Precautions
Hypertensive crisis: In theory, because MAO-A of the gut is not inhibited, patients treated with selegiline at a dose of 10 mg/day can take medications containing pharmacologically active amines and consume tyramine-containing foods without risk of uncontrolled hypertension.

Levodopa side effects: Some patients given selegiline may experience an exacerbation of levodopa-associated side effects, presumably caused by the increased amounts of dopamine reacting with supersensitive postsynaptic receptors.

Drug Interactions
Drugs that may interact with selegiline include fluoxetine and meperidine.

Adverse Reactions
Adverse reactions occurring in $\geq$ 3% of patients include nausea, dizziness, lightheadedness, fainting, abdominal pain, confusion, hallucinations, depression, loss of balance, insomnia, orthostatic hypotension, increased akinetic involuntary movements, agitation, arrhythmias, bradykinesia, chorea, delusions, hypertension, new or increased angina pectoris, syncope, and dry mouth.

PERGOLIDE MESYLATE

Tablets: 0.05, 0.25, and 1 mg (*Rx*)　　　　　*Permax* (Athena Neurosciences)

Indications
Parkinson's disease: Adjunctive treatment to levodopa/carbidopa in the management of the signs and symptoms of Parkinson's disease.

Administration and Dosage
Initiate with a daily dose of 0.05 mg for the first 2 days. Gradually increase the dosage by 0.1 or 0.15 mg/day every third day over the next 12 days of therapy. The dosage may then be increased by 0.25 mg/day every third day until an optimal therapeutic dosage is achieved.

Pergolide is usually administered in divided doses 3 times/day. During dosage titration, the dosage of concurrent levodopa/carbidopa may be cautiously decreased.

In clinical studies, the mean therapeutic daily dosage of pergolide was 3 mg/day. The average concurrent daily dosage of levodopa/carbidopa (expressed as levodopa) was $\approx$ 650 mg/day. The efficacy of pergolide at doses above 5 mg/day has not been systematically evaluated.

Actions
Pharmacology: Pergolide mesylate is a potent dopamine receptor agonist at both D_1 and D_2 receptor sites. In Parkinson's disease, pergolide is believed to exert its therapeutic effect by directly stimulating postsynaptic dopamine receptors in the nigrostriatal system.

Pharmacokinetics: Following oral administration, ≈ 55% of the dose can be recovered from the urine and 5% from expired CO_2, suggesting that a significant fraction is absorbed. Pergolide is ≈ 90% bound to plasma proteins. The major route of excretion is via the kidney.

Contraindications

Hypersensitivity to pergolide or other ergot derivatives.

Warnings

Symptomatic hypotension: In clinical trials, ≈ 10% of patients taking pergolide with levodopa vs 7% taking placebo with levodopa experienced symptomatic orthostatic or sustained hypotension, especially during initial treatment. Increase the dosage in carefully adjusted increments over a period of 3 to 4 weeks.

Hallucinosis: Pergolide with levodopa caused hallucinosis in ≈ 14% of patients as opposed to 3% taking placebo with levodopa.

Pregnancy: Category B.

Lactation: It is not known whether this drug is excreted in breast milk.

Children: Safety and efficacy for use in children have not been established.

Precautions

Cardiac dysrhythmias: Exercise caution in patients prone to cardiac dysrhythmias. In a study comparing pergolide and placebo, patients on pergolide had significantly more episodes of atrial premature contractions and sinus tachycardia.

The use of pergolide in patients on levodopa may cause or exacerbate preexisting states of confusion and hallucinations or preexisting dyskinesia.

Drug Interactions

Drugs that may interact with pergolide mesylate include dopamine antagonists, metoclopramide, and drugs known to affect protein binding.

Adverse Reactions

Adverse reactions occurring in ≥ 3% of patients include pain, abdominal pain, injury, accident, headache, asthenia, chest pain, flu syndrome, postural hypotension, vasodilation, nausea, constipation, diarrhea, dyspepsia, anorexia, dry mouth, dyskinesia, dizziness, hallucinations, dystonia, confusion, somnolence, insomnia, anxiety, tremor, depression, rhinitis, dyspnea, rash, abnormal vision, peripheral edema, hallucinations, and confusion.

DOPAMINE RECEPTOR AGONISTS, NON-ERGOT

PRAMIPEXOLE
Tablets: 0.125, 0.25, 1, and 1.5 mg (*Rx*)   *Mirapex* (Pharmacia)
ROPINIROLE
Tablets: 0.25, 0.5, 1, 2, and 5 mg (*Rx*)   *Requip* (GlaxoSmithKline)

Indications

Parkinson's disease: For the treatment of the signs and symptoms of idiopathic Parkinson's disease.

Administration and Dosage

PRAMIPEXOLE: May take with food to reduce the occurrence of nausea.

Initial treatment – Increase gradually from a starting dose of 0.375 mg/day given in 3 divided doses every 5 to 7 days to 4.5 mg/day in patients with Ccr > 60 mL/min.

Maintenance treatment – Pramipexole is effective and well tolerated over a dosage range of 1.5 to 4.5 mg/day administered in equally divided doses 3 times/day with or without concomitant levodopa (≈ 800 mg/day). When pramipexole is used in combination with levodopa, consider a reduction of the levodopa dosage.

Discontinuation – Discontinue over a period of 1 week.

ROPINIROLE: Take 3 times/day, with or without food. Taking ropinirole with food may reduce the occurrence of nausea.

The recommended starting dose is 0.25 mg 3 times/day. Based on individual patient response, dosage should then be titrated in weekly increments as described in the table below. After week 4, if necessary, daily dosage may be increased by 1.5 mg/day on a weekly basis up to a dose of 9 mg/day, and then by ≤ 3 mg/day weekly to a total dose of 24 mg/day.

Ascending-Dose Schedule of Ropinirole		
Week	Dosage	Total daily dose
1	0.25 mg 3 times/day	0.75 mg
2	0.5 mg 3 times/day	1.5 mg
3	0.75 mg 3 times/day	2.25 mg
4	1 mg 3 times/day	3 mg

When ropinirole is administered as adjunct therapy to levodopa, the concurrent dose of levodopa may be decreased gradually as tolerated.

Discontinue ropinirole gradually over a 7-day period. Decrease the frequency of administration from 3 times/day to twice/day for 4 days. For the remaining 3 days, decrease the frequency to once/day prior to complete withdrawl of ropinirole.

Actions

Pharmacology: **Pramipexole** and **ropinirole** are non-ergot dopamine agonists for Parkinson's disease with high specificity at the D_2 subfamily of dopamine receptors, binding with higher affinity to D_3 than to D_2 or D_4 receptor subtypes.

The mechanism of action is believed to be related to its ability to stimulate dopamine receptors in the striatum.

Pharmacokinetics: Non-ergot dopamine agonists are rapidly absorbed. The absolute bioavailability is > 90%. Steady-state concentrations are achieved within 2 days of dosing. Terminal half-life is ≈ 8 hours in young healthy volunteers and ≈ 12 hours in elderly volunteers. Urinary excretion is the major route of elimination.

Contraindications

Hypersensitivity to the drug or any components of the product.

Warnings

Symptomatic hypotension: Patients require careful monitoring for signs and symptoms of orthostatic hypotension while being treated with dopaminergic agonists, especially during dose escalation.

Hallucinations: Hallucinations were observed in a greater number of patients receiving dopaminergics than placebo. Age appears to increase the risk of hallucination attributable to dopaminergics.

Renal function impairment: Excercise caution when prescribing to patients with renal insufficiency.

Elderly: Pramipexole total oral clearance was ≈ 30% lower in subjects > 65 years old compared with younger subjects, because of a decline in pramipexole renal clearance. The incidence of hallucinations appears to increase with age.

Pregnancy: Category C.

Lactation: It is not known whether these drugs are excreted in breast milk.

Children: Safety and efficacy have not been established.

Precautions

Monitoring: Monitor for signs and symptoms of orthostatic hypotension.

Dyskinesia: Dopamine receptor agonists may potentiate the dopaminergic side effects of levodopa and may cause or exacerbate pre-existing dyskinesia. Decreasing the dose of levodopa may ameliorate this side effect.

CNS effects: Use concomitant CNS depressants with caution because of the possible additive sedative effects.

Binding to melanin: Ropinirole binds to melanin-containing tissues in pigmented rats.

Drug Interactions

Drugs that may affect dopamine receptors agonists include cimetidine; estrogen; cipro-floxacin; drugs eliminated via renal excretion; inhibitors of CYP1A2 and dopa-mine antagonists. Drugs that may be affected by dopamine receptor agonists include levodopa.

Drug/Food interactions: **Pramipexole** and **ropinirole** T_{max} are increased by $\approx$ 1 and 2.5 hours, respectively, when taken food, although the extent of absorption is not affected.

Adverse Reactions

Adverse reactions occurring in $\geq$ 3% of patients with early Parkinson's disease (with-out levodopa) included the following: Increased sweating; dry mouth; flushing; syn-cope; orthostatic symptoms; hypertension; palpitations; dizziness; somnolence; insomnia; hallucinations (see Warnings); confusion; amnesia; hypesthesia; yawn-ing; nausea; constipation; vomiting; dyspepsia; abdominal pain; anorexia; flatulence; peripheral edema; pharyngitis; rhinitis; sinusitis; bronchitis; dyspnea; abnormal vision; eye abnormality; asthenia; fatigue; viral infection; pain; edema; urinary tract infection; chest pain; malaise; impotence; peripheral ischemia; increased alkaline phosphatase.

Adverse reactions occurring in $\geq$ 3% of patients with advanced Parkinson's disease (with levodopa) included the following: Postural hypotension; syncope; dyskine-sia; extrapyramidal syndrome; insomnia; dizziness; somnolence; hallucinations; head-ache; dream abnormalities; confusion; falls; dystonia; gait abnormalities/hypokinesia; hypertonia; amnesia; tremor/twitching; nervousness; paresthesia; aka-thisia; thinking abnormalities; paresis; nausea; constipation; abdominal pain; vomiting; diarrhea; urinary frequency; urinary tract infection; arthritis; twitching; pneumonia; dyspnea; rhinitis; accommodation abnormalities; vision abnormalities; accidental injury; asthenia; dry mouth; increased sweating; general edema; chest pain; malaise; increased drug level; pain.

DISULFIRAM

Tablets: 250 and 500 mg (*Rx*) Various, *Antabuse* (Wyeth-Ayerst)

Warning:
> Never give disulfiram to a patient in a state of alcohol intoxication or without the patient's full knowledge. Instruct the patient's relatives accordingly.

Indications
An aid in the management of selected chronic alcoholics who want to remain in a state of enforced sobriety.

Administration and Dosage
Do not administer until the patient has abstained from alcohol for at least 12 hours.

Initial dosage schedule: Administer a maximum of 500 mg/day in a single dose for 1 to 2 weeks. If a sedative effect is experienced, take at bedtime or decrease dosage.

Maintenance regimen: The average maintenance dose is 250 mg/day (range, 125 to 500 mg), not to exceed 500 mg/day.

Actions
Pharmacology: Disulfiram produces an intolerance to alcohol that results in a highly unpleasant reaction when the patient under treatment ingests even small amounts of alcohol. Disulfiram blocks oxidation of alcohol at the acetaldehyde stage by inhibiting aldehyde dehydrogenase. Accumulation of acetaldehyde produces the disulfiram-alcohol reaction. This reaction persists as long as alcohol is being metabolized.

Pharmacokinetics: Disulfiram is rapidly absorbed from the GI tract and eliminated slowly from the body. About 12 hours are required for its full action. Disulfiram is metabolized to diethyldithiocarbamate, which is oxidized to carbon disulfide and diethylamine. Ingestion of alcohol may produce unpleasant symptoms for 1 to 2 weeks after the last dose of disulfiram.

Contraindications
Severe myocardial disease or coronary occlusion; psychoses; hypersensitivity to disulfiram or to other thiuram derivatives used in pesticides and rubber vulcanization; patients receiving or who have recently received metronidazole, paraldehyde, alcohol, or alcohol-containing preparations.

Warnings
Disulfiram-alcohol reaction: Disulfiram plus alcohol, even small amounts, produces flushing, throbbing in head and neck, throbbing headaches, respiratory difficulty, nausea, copious vomiting, sweating, thirst, chest pain, palpitations, dyspnea, hyperventilation, tachycardia, hypotension, syncope, marked uneasiness, weakness, vertigo, blurred vision, and confusion. In severe reactions there may be respiratory depression, cardiovascular collapse, arrhythmias, MI, acute CHF, unconsciousness, convulsions, and death. The intensity of the reaction is proportional to the amounts of disulfiram and alcohol ingested.

Concomitant conditions: Because of the possibility of an accidental reaction, use with caution in patients with diabetes mellitus, hypothyroidism, epilepsy, cerebral damage, chronic and acute nephritis, or hepatic cirrhosis or insufficiency.

Pregnancy: Category C.

Precautions
Monitoring: Perform baseline and follow-up transaminase tests (10 to 14 days) to detect hepatic dysfunction resulting from therapy. Perform a CBC and SMA-12 test every 6 months.

Ethylene dibromide: Patients should not be exposed to ethylene dibromide or its vapors.

Drug Interactions
Drugs that may interact with disulfiram include alcohol, benzodazepines, caffeine, hydantoins, isoniazid, metronidazole, tricyclic antidepressants, and warfarin.

Adverse Reactions

Adverse reactions may include peripheral neuropathy; polyneuritis; optic or retrobulbar neuritis (with impaired vision, color perceptions and blindness); drowsiness; headache; restlessness; occasional skin eruptions; acneiform eruptions; allergic dermatitis; metallic or garlic-like aftertaste; hepatotoxicity resembling viral or alcoholic hepatitis; multiple cases of cholestatic and fulminant hepatitis; arthropathy; acetonemia; impotence.

NICOTINE

NICOTINE TRANSDERMAL	
Transdermal Systems (*otc*)	Various, *Habitrol* (Basel Pharm.), *Nicoderm CQ* (GlaxoSmithKline Consumer), *Nicotrol* (Pharmacia)
NICOTINE POLACRILEX	
Chewing gum: 2 and 4 mg nicotine (as polacrilex) (*otc*)	Various, *Nicorette* (GlaxoSmithKline Consumer)
NICOTINE INHALATION SYSTEM	
Inhaler: 4 mg delivered (10 mg/cartridge) (*Rx*)	*Nicotrol Inhaler* (Pharmacia)
NICOTINE NASAL SPRAY	
Spray pump: 0.5 mg nicotine/actuation (10 mg/mL) (*Rx*)	*Nicotrol NS* (Pharmacia)

Indications

As an aid to smoking cessation for the relief of nicotine withdrawal symptoms. Use as part of a comprehensive behavioral smoking-cessation program.

Administration and Dosage

Nicotine Replacement Pharmacotherapy			
Type of therapy	Dosage	Duration	Availability
Gum	< 24 cigarettes/day: 2 mg gum up to 24 pieces/day	up to 12 weeks	*otc*
	> 25 cigarettes/day: 4 mg gum up to 24 pieces/day		
Inhaler	6 to 16 cartridges/day	up to 6 months	Rx only
Transdermal patch	21 mg/24 hr 14 mg/24 hr 7 mg/24 hr	4 to 6 weeks then 2 weeks then 2 weeks	*otc*
	15 mg/16 hr	6 weeks	
Nasal spray	8 to 40 doses/day	3 to 6 months	Rx only

NICOTINE TRANSDERMAL SYSTEM:

Recommended Dosing Schedule of Transdermal Nicotine for Healthy Patients		
	Duration	
Dose	Per strength of patch	Entire course of therapy
Habitrol[1] 21 mg/day 14 mg/day 7 mg/day	First 4 weeks Next 2 weeks Last 2 weeks	8 weeks
Nicoderm[1] 21 mg/day 14 mg/day 7 mg/day	First 6 weeks Next 2 weeks Last 2 weeks	8 to 10 weeks
Nicotrol 15 mg/16 hrs	6 weeks	6 weeks

[1] Start with 14 mg/day for 6 weeks for patients who smoke < 10 cigarettes/day. Decrease dose to 7 mg/day for the final 2 weeks.

Habitrol, Nicoderm – After 24 hours, remove the used system and apply a new system to an alternate skin site. Skin sites should not be reused for at least a week. Caution patients not to continue to use the same system for > 24 hours.

Nicotrol – Each day apply a new system upon waking and remove at bedtime.

NICOTINE POLACRILEX (GUM): Advise patient to stop smoking completely when beginning to use the gum. If the patient smokes < 25 cigarettes/day, start with the 2 mg nicotine gum. If the patient smokes > 25 cigarettes/day, use according to the following 12-week schedule:

Nicotine Polacrilex Dosing Schedule		
Weeks 1 to 6	Weeks 7 to 9	Weeks 10 to 12
1 piece every 1 to 2 hours	1 piece every 2 to 4 hours	1 piece every 4 to 8 hours

Instruct patient to chew the gum slowly until it tingles, then park it between the cheek and gum. When the tingle is gone, instruct patient to begin chewing again until the tingle returns. Repeat the process until most of the tingle is gone ($\approx$ 30 minutes).

Advise patient not to eat or drink for 15 minutes before chewing the nicotine gum or while chewing a piece. To improve the chances of quitting, chew at least 9 pieces/day for the first 6 weeks. If there are strong and frequent cravings, use a second piece within the hour. However, do not continuously use 1 piece after another since this may cause hiccoughs, heartburn, nausea, or other side effects.

Do not use > 24 pieces/day. Stop using the nicotine gum at the end of 12 weeks. If there is still a need to use nicotine gum, have the patient contact a physician.

NICOTINE INHALATION SYSTEM: Patients should be encouraged to use at least 6 cartridges/day at least for the first 3 to 6 weeks of treatment. Additional doses may be needed to control the urge to smoke with a maximum of 16 cartridges/day for up to 12 weeks. The safety and efficacy of the continued use of the nicotine inhaler for periods > 6 months have not been studied and such use is not recommended.

NICOTINE NASAL SPRAY: Patients should be started with 1 or 2 doses/hour, which may be increased up to a maximum recommended dose of 40 mg (80 sprays, somewhat < ½ of the bottle) per day

Encourage patients to use at least the recommended minimum of 8 doses/day, as less is unlikely to be effective.

Actions

Pharmacology: Nicotine, the chief alkaloid in tobacco products, binds stereoselectively to acetylcholine receptors at the autonomic ganglia, in the adrenal medulla, at neuromuscular junctions, and in the brain.

Pharmacokinetics:

Nicotine Pharmacokinetics					
Parameter	Smoking	Gum	Transdermal	Nasal spray	Inhaler
Time to peak levels (hours)	ND[1]	0.25 to 0.5	2 to 12	0.25	0.25
Peak plasma level (ng/mL)	44	5 to 10	5 to 17	12	6
Half-life (hours)	15 to 20[2]	3 to 4	3 to 4	1 to 2	ND

[1] No data.
[2] Refers to cotinine, the primary plasma metabolite of nicotine.

Contraindications

Hypersensitivity to nicotine or any components of the products, including menthol.

Warnings

Nicotine risks: Nicotine from any source can be toxic and addictive. Smoking causes lung disease, cancer, and heart disease, and may adversely affect pregnant women or the fetus.

Renal/Hepatic function impairment: Anticipate some influence of hepatic impairment on drug kinetics (reduced clearance). Only severe renal impairment should affect clearance of nicotine or its metabolites from circulation.

Elderly: Nicotine **inhaler** and **nasal spray** therapy appeared to be as effective in elderly patients $\geq$ 60 years of age as in younger smokers.

Pregnancy: Category D (**inhaler, spray, transdermal patch**); *Category C* (**gum**). Nicotine is contraindicated in women who are or may become pregnant; advise patients to use contraceptive measures.

Lactation: Nicotine passes freely into breast milk and has the potential for serious adverse reactions in nursing infants.

Children: Safety and efficacy in children/adolescents < 18 years of age who smoke are not evaluated.

Precautions

General: Urge the patient to stop smoking completely when initiating nicotine replacement therapy. Inform patients that if they continue to smoke while using the product, they may experience adverse effects because of peak nicotine levels higher than those experienced from smoking alone. If there is a clinically significant increase in cardiovascular or other effects attributable to nicotine, the treatment should be discontinued. Physicians should anticipate that concomitant medications may need dosage adjustment (see Drug Interactions). Sustained use (> 6 months) of inhaler or nasal spray by patients who stop smoking has not been studied and is not recommended (see Drug Abuse and Dependence).

Bronchospastic disease: The **inhaler** and **nasal spray** have not been specifically studied in asthma or chronic pulmonary disease. Nicotine is an airway irritant and might cause bronchospasm.

Use of the **nasal spray** or **inhaler** in patients with severe reactive airway disease is not recommended.

Nasal disorders: Use of the **nasal spray** is not recommended in patients with known chronic nasal disorders (eg, allergy, rhinitis, nasal polyps, sinusitis) because such use has not been adequately studied.

Cardiovascular: Specifically, screen and evaluate patients with coronary heart disease, serious cardiac arrhythmias or vasospastic diseases before nicotine is prescribed. There have been occasional reports of tachyarrhythmias associated with nicotine use; therefore, if an increase in cardiovascular symptoms occurs, discontinue the drug.

Accelerated hypertension – Nicotine therapy constitutes a risk factor for development of malignant hypertension in patients with accelerated hypertension. **Inhaler** therapy should be used with caution in these patients and only when the benefits of including nicotine replacement in a smoking cessation program outweigh the risks.

Endocrine: Because of the action of nicotine on the adrenal medulla, use with caution in patients with hyperthyroidism, pheochromocytoma or insulin-dependent diabetes.

Oral/GI: Use caution in patients with oral or pharyngeal inflammation and in those with history of esophagitis or active or inactive peptic ulcer.

Dental problems: Dental problems might be exacerbated by chewing nicotine gum.

Drug abuse and dependence: Urge patients to stop smoking completely when initiating therapy. If patients smoke while using nicotine, they may experience adverse effects because of peak nicotine levels higher than those caused by smoking alone.

The nicotine **inhaler** is likely to have a low abuse potential based on slower absorption, smaller fluctuations, and lower blood levels of nicotine when compared with cigarettes. Nicotine **nasal spray** has a dependence potential intermediate between other nicotine-based therapies and cigarettes. To minimize risk of dependence, encourage patients to gradually withdraw or stop gum and inhaler usage at 3 months, transdermal nicotine after 4 to 8 weeks. Chronic consumption is toxic and addicting.

Drug Interactions

Smoking cessation, with or without nicotine substitutes, may alter response to concomitant medication in ex-smokers. Smoking may affect alcohol, benzodiazepines, beta-adrenergic blockers, caffeine, clozapine, fluvoxamine, olanzapine, tacrine, theophylline, clorazepate, lidocaine (oral), estradiol, flecanide, imipramine, heparin, insulin, mexiletine, opioids, propranolol, catecholamines, and cortisol.

Nasal spray: The extent of absorption and peak plasma concentration is slightly reduced in patients with the common cold/rhinitis. In addition, the time to peak concentration is prolonged. The use of a nasal vasoconstrictor such as xylometazoline in patients with rhinitis will further prolong the time to peak.

Adverse Reactions

Inhaler – Local irritation (mouth, throat); coughing; rhinitis; dyspepsia; headache; taste complaints; pain in jaw and neck; tooth disorders; sinusitis; influenza-like symptoms; pain; back pain; allergy; paresthesia; flatulence; fever; dizziness; anxiety; sleep disorder; depression; withdrawal syndrome; drug dependence; fatigue; myalgia; nausea; diarrhea; hiccough; chest discomfort; bronchitis; hypertension.

Nasal spray – Runny nose; throat irritation; watering eyes; sneezing; cough; nasal congestion; subjective comments related to the taste or usage of the dosage form; sinus irritation; transient epistaxis; eye irritation; transient changes in sense of smell; pharyngitis; paresthesias of the nose, mouth, or head; numbness of the nose or mouth; burning of the nose or eyes; earache; facial flushing; transient changes in sense of taste; hoarseness; nasal ulcer or blister; headache; back pain; dyspnea; nausea; arthralgia; menstrual disorder; palpitation; flatulence; tooth disorder; gum disorder; myalgia; abdominal pain; confusion; acne; dysmenorrhea.

Gum – Injury to mouth, teeth, or dental work; belching; increased salivation; mild jaw muscle ache; sore mouth or throat.

Transdermal – Erythema, pruritus, and burning at the application site.

BUPROPION HCl

Tablets, sustained release: 150 mg (*Rx*)	*Zyban* (GlaxoSmithKline)

Indications

Smoking cessation: An aid to smoking cessation treatment.

Administration and Dosage

The recommended and maximum dose of bupropion is 300 mg/day, given as 150 mg twice/day. Begin dosing at 150 mg/day given every day for the first 3 days, followed by a dose increase for most patients to the recommended usual dose of 300 mg/day. There should be an interval of $\geq$ 8 hours between successive doses. Do not give doses > 300 mg/day.

Initiate treatment with bupropion while the patient is still smoking because $\approx$ 1 week of treatment is required to achieve steady-state blood levels of bupropion. Patients should set a "target quit date" within the first 2 weeks of treatment with bupropion, generally in the second week. Continue treatment for 7 to 12 weeks; base duration of treatment on the relative benefits and risks for individual patients. If a patient has not made significant progress toward abstinence by week 7 of therapy with bupropion, it is unlikely that he or she will quit during that attempt; discontinue treatment. Dose tapering of bupropion is not required when discontinuing treatment. It is important that patients continue to receive counseling and support throughout treatment with bupropion and for a period of time thereafter.

Maintenance: Nicotine dependence is a chronic condition. Some patients may need continuous treatment. Systematic evaluation of bupropion 300 mg/day for maintenance therapy demonstrated that treatment for up to 6 months was effective. Whether to continue treatment with bupropion for periods > 12 weeks for smoking cessation must be determined for individual patients.

Combination treatment: Combination treatment with bupropion and nicotine transdermal system (NTS) may be prescribed for smoking cessation.

Hepatic function impairment: Use extreme caution in patients with severe hepatic cirrhosis. The dose should not exceed 150 mg every other day in these patients. Use bupropion with caution in patients with hepatic impairment (including mild to moderate hepatic cirrhosis) and consider a reduced frequency of dosing in patients with mild to moderate hepatic cirrhosis (see Warnings).

Renal function impairment: Use caution in patients with renal impairment and consider a reduced frequency of dosing (see Warnings).

Actions

Pharmacology: Bupropion is a nonnicotine aid to smoking cessation. The mechanism by which bupropion enhances the ability of patients to abstain from smoking is unknown. However, it is presumed that this action is mediated by noradrenergic or dopaminergic mechanisms.

Pharmacokinetics: Following oral administration to healthy volunteers, mean peak plasma concentrations were achieved within 3 hours. Bupropion is 84% bound to human plasma proteins in vitro. Bupropion is extensively metabolized with a mean elimination half-life of ≈ 21 hours.

Contraindications

Coadministration with a monoamine oxidase (MAO) inhibitor, *Wellbutrin*, *Wellbutrin SR* or any medications that contain bupropion; current or prior diagnosis of bulimia or anorexia nervosa, seizure disorders; patients who have shown an allergic response to bupropion or other ingredients in the formulation.

Warnings

Antidepressants: Bupropion is the active ingredient found in *Wellbutrin* and *Wellbutrin SR* used to treat depression. Do not use in combination with *Wellbutrin*, *Wellbutrin SR* or any other medication that contains bupropion.

Anorexia nervosa/bulimia: Do not give with current or prior diagnosis of bulimia or anorexia nervosa because of a higher incidence of seizures noted in patients treated for bulimia with the immediate-release formulation of bupropion.

Seizures: Because the use of bupropion is associated with a dose-dependent risk of seizures, do not prescribe doses > 300 mg/day for smoking cessation. The seizure rate associated with doses of sustained —release bupropion ≤ 300 mg/day is ≈ 0.1%.

Concomitant medications – Many medications (eg, antipsychotics, antidepressants, theophylline, systemic steroids) and treatment regimens (eg, abrupt discontinuation of benzodiazepines) are known to lower seizure threshold.

Reducing the risk of seizures – Retrospective analysis suggests that the risk of seizures may be minimized if the total daily dose of bupropion does not exceed 300 mg (the maximum recommended dose) and no single dose exceeds 150 mg.

Hypersensitivity reactions: Anaphylactoid reactions characterized by symptoms such as pruritus, urticaria, angioedema, and dyspnea requiring medical treatment have been reported at a rate of ≈ 1 to 3 per thousand in clinical trials of bupropion. In addition, there have been rare postmarketing reports of erythema multiformes, Stevens-Johnson syndrome, and anaphylactic shock associated with bupropion.

Renal function impairment: Use bupropion with caution in patients with renal impairment and consider a reduced frequency of dosing as bupropion and its metabolites may accumulate in such patients to a greater extent than usual.

Hepatic function impairment: Use with extreme caution in patients with severe hepatic cirrhosis. In these patients, a reduced frequency of dosing is required, as peak bupropion levels are substantially increased and accumulation is likely to occur in such patients to a greater extent than usual. The dose should not exceed 150 mg every other day.

Use with caution in patients with hepatic impairment (including mild to moderate hepatic cirrhosis) and consider reduced frequency of dosing in patients with mild to moderate hepatic cirrhosis.

Pregnancy: *Category B.*

To monitor fetal outcomes of pregnant women exposed to bupropion, the manufacturer maintains a bupropion pregnancy registry. Health care providers are encouraged to register patients by calling (800) 336-2176.

Lactation: Bupropion and its metabolites are secreted in breast milk.

Children: Safety and efficacy in patients < 18 years of age has not been established.

Precautions

Insomnia: In one trial, 29% of patients treated with 150 mg/day and 35% of patients treated with 300 mg/day experienced insomnia vs 21% with placebo.

Psychosis or mania: Antidepressants can precipitate manic episodes in bipolar disorder patients during the depressed phase of their illness and may activate latent psychosis in other susceptible individuals. The sustained-release formulation of bupropion is expected to pose similar risks. There were no reports of activation of psychosis or mania in clinical trials conducted in nondepressed smokers.

Cardiac effects: Hypertension, in some cases severe, requiring acute treatment, has been reported in patients receiving bupropion alone and in combination with nicotine replacement therapy. These events have been observed in both patients with and without evidence of pre-existing hypertension.

Use caution in patients with a recent history of MI or unstable heart disease. Bupropion was well tolerated in depressed patients who had previously developed orthostatic hypotension while receiving tricyclic antidepressants and was generally well tolerated in depressed patients with stable CHF. Bupropion was associated with a rise in supine blood pressure in the study of patients with CHF, resulting in discontinuation of treatment in 2 patients for exacerbation of baseline hypertension.

Drug abuse and dependence: Bupropion is likely to have a low abuse potential. There have been a few reported cases of drug dependence and withdrawal symptoms associated with the immediate-release formulation of bupropion.

Drug Interactions

Because bupropion is extensively metabolized, the coadministration of other drugs may affect its clinical activity. In particular, certain drugs may induce the metabolism of bupropion (eg, carbamazepine, phenobarbital, phenytoin) while other drugs may inhibit the metabolism of bupropion (eg, cimetidine, ritonavir).

Drugs that may increase the effects or side effects of bupropion include levodopa, MAOIs, ritonavir, antidepressants, antipsychotics, beta blockers, type IC antiarrhythmics.

Drugs that lower seizure threshold: Concurrent administration of bupropion and agents (eg, antipsychotics, antidepressants, theophylline, systemic steroids) or treatment regimens (eg, abrupt discontinuation of benzodiazepines) that lower seizure threshold should be undertaken only with extreme caution.

Drug/Food interactions: Food increased the C_{max} by 11%, the extent of absorption (AUC) by 17% and the mean time to peak concentration of bupropion.

Adverse Reactions

Adverse reactions occurring in $\geq$ 3% of patients include: Abdominal pain; insomnia; dream abnormality; anxiety; disturbed concentration; dizziness; nervousness; application site reaction; rash; pruritus; nausea; dry mouth; constipation; diarrhea; anorexia; myalgia; arthralgia; rhinitis; increased cough; pharyngitis; taste perversion.

Chapter 8

GASTROINTESTINAL AGENTS

Antacids, 665
Sucralfate, 668
Anticholinergics/Antispasmodics, 669
Histamine H_2 Antagonists, 674
Prostaglandins, 680
    Misoprostol, 680
Proton Pump Inhibitors, 682
Lipase Inhibitors, 686
    Orlistat, 686
GI Stimulants, 688
    Metoclopramide, 688
Laxatives, 692
Polyethylene Glycol-Electrolyte Solution, 699
Polyethylene Glycol Solution, 700
Antidiarrheals, 701
    Difenoxin and Atropine Sulfate, 701
    Diphenoxylate and Atropine Sulfate, 702
    Loperamide, 703
    Bismuth Subsalicylate, 705
Mesalamine, 706
Olsalazine, 708
Balsalazide, 709
Sulfasalazine, 710
Helicobacter Pylori Agents, 713
Mouth and Throat Products, 715
    Pilocarpine HCl, 715

ANTACIDS

MAGNESIA (Magnesium Hydroxide)
Tablets, chewable: 311 mg (*otc*)
Phillips' Chewable (Sterling Health)

Liquid: 400 mg/5 mL, 800 mg/5 mL (*otc*)
Various, *Phillips' Milk of Magnesia* (Sterling Health), *Phillips' Concentrated Milk of Magnesia* (Sterling Health)

ALUMINUM HYDROXIDE GEL
Tablets: 300, 500, 600 mg (*otc*)
Amphojel (Wyeth-Ayerst), *Alu-Tab* (3M Pharm)

Capsules: 400, 500 mg (*otc*)
Alu-Cap (3M Pharm), *Dialume* (Aventis)

Suspension: 320 mg/5 mL, 450 mg/5 mL, 675 mg/5 mL (*otc*)
Various, *Amphojel* (Wyeth-Ayerst)

Liquid: 600 mg/5 mL (*otc*)
Various, *AlternaGEL* (J & J-Merck)

ALUMINUM CARBONATE GEL, BASIC
Tablets: Equiv. to 608 mg dried aluminum hydroxide gel or 500 mg aluminum hydroxide (*otc*)
Basaljel (Wyeth-Ayerst)

Capsules: Equiv. to 608 mg dried aluminum hydroxide gel or 500 mg aluminum hydroxide (*otc*)
Basaljel (Wyeth-Ayerst)

Suspension: Equiv. to 400 mg aluminum hydroxide/5 mL (*otc*)
Basaljel (Wyeth-Ayerst)

CALCIUM CARBONATE
Tablets, chewable: 350, 420, 750, 850, 1000 mg (*otc*)
Amitone (Menley & James), *Mallamint* (Roberts), *Extra Strength Tums E-X* (GlaxoSmithKline), *Alka-Mints* (Bayer), *Tums Ultra* (GlaxoSmithKline), *Extra Strength Alkets Antacid* (Roberts Pharm), *Dicarbosil* (BIRA)

Tablets: 500, 600, 650, 1000, 1250 mg (*otc*)
Various, *Maalox Antacid Caplets* (Aventis)

Gum tablets: 500 mg (*otc*)
Chooz (Schering-Plough)

Suspension: 1250 mg/5 mL (*otc*)
Various

Lozenges: 600 mg (*otc*)
Mylanta (J & J-Merck)

MAGNESIUM OXIDE
Tablets: 400, 420, 500 mg (*otc*)
Various, *Mag-Ox 400* (Blaine), *Maox 420* (Kenneth A. Manne)

Capsules: 140 mg (*otc*)
Uro-Mag (Blaine)

MAGALDRATE
Suspension: 540 mg/5 mL (*otc*)
Riopan (Whitehall)

Liquid: 540 mg/5 mL (*otc*)
Various, *Iosopan* (Goldline)

SODIUM BICARBONATE
Tablets: 325, 520, 650 mg (*otc*)
Various, *Bell/ans* (C.S. Dent)

SODIUM CITRATE
Solution: 450 mg (*otc*)
Citra pH (ValMed)

Indications

Hyperacidity: Symptomatic relief of upset stomach associated with hyperacidity (heartburn, gastroesophageal reflux, acid indigestion, and sour stomach); hyperacidity associated with peptic ulcer and gastric hyperacidity.

Aluminum carbonate: Treatment, control, or management of hyperphosphatemia, or for use with a low phosphate diet.

Calcium carbonate: Treating calcium deficiency states.

Magnesium oxide: Treatment of magnesium deficiencies or magnesium depletion.

Unlabeled uses: Antacids with aluminum and magnesium hydroxides or aluminum hydroxide alone effectively prevent significant stress ulcer bleeding. Antacids also are effective in treatment and maintenance of duodenal ulcer, and may be effective in treating gastric ulcer. Antacids also are recommended, initially, for gastroesophageal reflux disease (GERD).

Aluminum hydroxide has been used to reduce phosphate absorption in hyperphosphatemia in patients with chronic renal failure.

Calcium carbonate also may be used to bind phosphate.

Administration and Dosage

MAGNESIA (Magnesium Hydroxide):

Antacid dose, adults, and children > 12 years of age –

Liquid: 5 to 15 mL up to 4 times daily with water.

Liquid, concentrated: 2.5 to 7.5 mL up to 4 times daily with water.

Tablets: 622 mg to 1244 mg up to 4 times daily.

ALUMINUM HYDROXIDE GEL:

Tablets/Capsules – 500 to 1500 mg 3 to 6 times daily, between meals and at bedtime.

Suspension – 5 to 30 mL as needed between meals and at bedtime or as directed.

ALUMINUM CARBONATE GEL, BASIC:

Antacid – 2 capsules or tablets or 10 mL of regular suspension (in water or fruit juice) as often as every 2 hours, up to 12 times daily.

CALCIUM CARBONATE: 0.5 to 1.5 g, as needed.

MAGNESIUM OXIDE:

Capsules – 140 mg 3 to 4 times daily.

Tablets – 400 to 800 mg/day.

MAGALDRATE (Aluminum Magnesium Hydroxide Sulfate):

Suspension/Liquid – 5 to 10 mL between meals and at bedtime.

SODIUM BICARBONATE: 0.3 to 2 g 1 to 4 times daily.

SODIUM CITRATE: 30 mL daily.

Actions

Pharmacology: Antacids neutralize gastric acidity, resulting in an increase in the pH of the stomach and duodenal bulb. Additionally, by increasing the gastric pH above 4, they inhibit the proteolytic activity of pepsin. Antacids do not "coat" the mucosal lining, but may have a local astringent effect. Antacids also increase the lower esophageal sphincter tone. Aluminum ions inhibit smooth muscle contraction, thus inhibiting gastric emptying.

Acid neutralizing capacity (ANC) – ANC is a consideration in selecting an antacid. It varies for commercial antacid preparations and is expressed as mEq/mL. Milliequivalents of ANC is defined by the mEq of HCl required to keep an antacid suspension at pH 3.5 for 10 minutes in vitro. An antacid must neutralize at least 5 mEq/dose. Also, any ingredient must contribute at least 25% of the total ANC of a given product to be considered an antacid.

Aluminum hydroxide and calcium-containing antacids may reduce LDL cholesterol and increase the HDL/LDL ratio.

Warnings

Sodium content: Sodium content of antacids may be significant. Patients with hypertension, CHF, marked renal failure, or those on restricted or low-sodium diets should use a low sodium preparation.

"Acid rebound": Antacids may cause dose-related rebound hyperacidity because they may increase gastric secretion or serum gastrin levels.

Milk-alkali syndrome: Milk-alkali syndrome, an acute illness with symptoms of headache, nausea, irritability, and weakness, or a chronic illness with alkalosis, hypercalcemia and, possibly, renal impairment, has occurred following the concurrent use of high-dose calcium carbonate and sodium bicarbonate.

Hypophosphatemia: Prolonged use of aluminum-containing antacids may result in hypophosphatemia in normophosphatemic patients if phosphate intake is not adequate.

Renal function impairment: Use magnesium-containing products with caution, particularly when > 50 mEq magnesium is given daily. Hypermagnesemia and toxicity may occur because of decreased clearance of the magnesium ion.

Prolonged use of aluminum-containing antacids in patients with renal failure may result in or worsen dialysis osteomalacia.

Pregnancy: If pregnant, consult a physician before using.

Precautions

   GI hemorrhage: Use aluminum hydroxide with care in patients who have recently suffered massive upper GI hemorrhage.

Drug Interactions

Drugs that may be affected by antacids include allopurinol, amphetamines, benzodiazepines, captopril, chloroquine, corticosteroids, dicumarol, diflunisal, digoxin, ethambutol, flecainide, fluoroquinolones, histamine H_2 antagonists, hydantoins, iron salts, isoniazid, ketoconazole, levodopa, lithium, methenamine, methotrexate, nitrofurantoin, penicillamine, phenothiazines, quinidine, salicylates, sodium polystyrene sulfonate, sulfonylureas, sympathomimetics, tetracyclines, thyroid hormones, ticlopidine, and valproic acid.

Adverse Reactions

   Magnesium-containing antacids – Laxative effect as saline cathartic, may cause diarrhea; hypermagnesemia in renal failure patients.

   Aluminum-containing antacids – Constipation (may lead to intestinal obstruction); aluminum-intoxication; osteomalacia and hypophosphatemia; accumulation of aluminum in serum, bone, and the CNS (aluminum accumulation may be neurotoxic); encephalopathy.

   Antacids – Dose-dependent rebound hyperacidity and milk-alkali syndrome.

SUCRALFATE

Tablets: 1 g (*Rx*)
Suspension: 1 g/10 mL (*Rx*)

Carafate (Aventis)

Indications

Duodenal ulcer: Short-term treatment (≤ 8 weeks) of active duodenal ulcer.

Tablets: Maintenance therapy for duodenal ulcer patients at reduced dosage after healing of acute ulcers.

Administration and Dosage

Active duodenal ulcer:

Adults – 1 g 4 times/day on an empty stomach (1 hour before meals and at bedtime).

Take antacids as needed for pain relief but not within ½ hour before or after sucralfate.

While healing with sucralfate may occur within the first 2 weeks, continue treatment for 4 to 8 weeks unless healing is demonstrated by X-ray or endoscopic examination.

Maintenance therapy (tablets only):

Adults – 1 g twice daily.

Actions

Pharmacology: Sucralfate, a basic aluminum salt of sulfated sucrose, is a polysaccharide with antipeptic activity. In the acidic medium of gastric juice, the aluminum ion splits off, leaving a highly polar anion that is essentially nonabsorbable. It exerts a local rather than systemic action. Sucralfate forms an ulcer-adherent complex with proteinaceous exudate. The ulcer-adherent complex covers the ulcer site and protects it against acid, pepsin, and bile salts. Sucralfate has minimal acid neutralizing capacity.

Pharmacokinetics: Sucralfate is minimally absorbed (3% to 5%) from the GI tract. Approximately 90% is excreted in the stool. The small amounts of the sulfated disaccharide absorbed are excreted primarily in the urine.

Warnings

Chronic renal failure/dialysis: During sucralfate administration, small amounts of aluminum are absorbed from the GI tract. Concomitant use with other aluminum-containing products may increase the total body burden of aluminum. Patients with normal renal function receiving these agents concomitantly adequately excrete aluminum in the urine. However, patients with chronic renal failure or receiving dialysis have impaired excretion of absorbed aluminum, and aluminum does not cross dialysis membranes. Aluminum accumulation and toxicity have occurred.

Pregnancy: Category B.

Lactation: It is not known whether this drug is excreted in breast milk.

Children: Safety and efficacy in children have not been established.

Drug Interactions

Drugs that may interact include aluminum-containing antacids, anticoagulants, digoxin, hydantoins, ketoconazole, quinidine, and quinolones.

Adverse Reactions

Adverse reactions in clinical trials were minor and rarely led to drug discontinuation. Constipation was the most frequent complaint (2%).

GASTROINTESTINAL ANTICHOLINERGICS/ANTISPASMODICS

ANISOTROPINE METHYLBROMIDE

Tablets: 50 mg (*Rx*) — Various

ATROPINE SULFATE

Injection: 0.05, 0.1, 0.3, 0.4, 0.5, 0.8, and1 mg/mL (*Rx*) — Various
Tablets: 0.4 mg (*Rx*) — *Atropine Sulfate* (Lilly), *Sal-Tropine* (Hope)
Tablets, soluble: 0.4 and 0.6 mg (*Rx*) — *Atropine Sulfate* (Lilly)

BELLADONNA

Liquids: 27 to 33 mg belladonna alkaloids/100 mL (*Rx*) — Various

CLIDINIUM BROMIDE

Capsules: 2.5 and 5 mg (*Rx*) — *Quarzan* (Roche)

DICYCLOMINE HCl

Capsules: 10 and 20 mg (*Rx*) — Various, *Bentyl* (Lakeside Pharm.)
Tablets: 20 mg (*Rx*) — Various, *Bentyl* (Lakeside Pharm.)
Syrup: 10 mg/5 mL (*Rx*) — Various, *Bentyl* (Lakeside Pharm.)
Injection: 10 mg/mL (*Rx*) — Various, *Bentyl* (Lakeside Pharm.)

GLYCOPYRROLATE

Tablets: 1 and 2 mg (*Rx*) — *Robinul* (Robins)
Injection: 0.2 mg/mL (*Rx*) — Various, *Robinul* (Robins)

LEVOROTATORY ALKALOIDS OF BELLADONNA

Tablets: 0.25 mg (*Rx*) — *Bellafoline* (Sandoz)

L-HYOSCYAMINE SULFATE

Tablets: 0.125 and 0.15 mg (*Rx*) — *Levsin* (Schwarz Pharma), *Gastrosed* (Roberts/ Hauck), *Cystospaz* (PolyMedica), *Donnamar* (Marnel), *ED-SPAZ* (Edwards)
Tablets, sublingual: 0.125 mg (*Rx*) — *Levsin/SL* (Schwarz Pharma), *A-Spas S/L* (Hyrex)
Tablets, extended release: 0.375 mg (*Rx*) — *Levbid* (Schwarz Pharma)
Capsules, timed release: 0.375 mg (*Rx*) — Various, *Cystospaz-M* (PolyMedica), *Levsinex Timecaps* (Schwarz Pharma)
Solution: 0.125 mg/mL (*Rx*) — *Levsin Drops* (Schwarz Pharma), *Gastrosed* (Roberts Hauck)
Elixir: 0.125 mg/5 mL (*Rx*) — *Levsin* (Schwarz Pharma)
Injection: 0.5 mg/mL (*Rx*) — *Levsin* (Schwarz Pharma)

METHSCOPOLAMINE BROMIDE

Tablets: 2.5 mg (*Rx*) — *Pamine* (Kenwood/Bradley)

MEPENZOLATE BROMIDE

Tablets: 25 mg (*Rx*) — *Cantil* (Aventis)

METHANTHELINE BROMIDE

Tablets: 50 mg (*Rx*) — *Banthine* (Schiapparelli Searle)

OXYPHENCYCLIMINE HCl

Tablets: 10 mg (*Rx*) — *Daricon* (GlaxoSmithKline)

PROPANTHELINE BROMIDE

Tablets: 7.5 and 15 mg (*Rx*) — Various, *Pro-Banthine* (Schiapparelli Searle)

SCOPOLAMINE HBr (Hyoscine HBr)

Injection: 0.3, 0.4, 0.86, and 1 mg/mL (*Rx*) — Various

TRIDIHEXETHYL CHLORIDE

Tablets: 25 mg (*Rx*) — *Pathilon* (Lederle)

Indications

Peptic ulcer: Adjunctive therapy for peptic ulcer. These agents suppress gastric acid secretion.

Other GI conditions: Functional GI disorders (diarrhea, pylorospasm, hypermotility, neurogenic colon), irritable bowel syndrome (spastic colon, mucous colitis), acute enterocolitis, ulcerative colitis, diverticulitis, mild dysenteries, pancreatitis, splenic flexure syndrome, and infant colic.

Biliary tract: For spastic disorders of the biliary tract. Given in conjunction with a narcotic analgesic.

Urogenital tract: Uninhibited hypertonic neurogenic bladder.

Bradycardia: **Atropine** is used in the suppression of vagally mediated bradycardias.

Preoperative medication: **Atropine, scopolamine, hyoscyamine,** and **glycopyrrolate** are used as preanesthetic medication to control bronchial, nasal, pharyngeal, and salivary secretions and to block cardiac vagal inhibitory reflexes during induction of anesthesia and intubation. Scopolamine is used for preanesthetic sedation and for obstetric amnesia.

Antidotes for poisoning by cholinergic drugs: Atropine is used for poisoning by organophosphorous insecticides, chemical warfare nerve gases, and as an antidote for mushroom poisoning caused by muscarine in certain species, such as *Amanita muscaria.*

Miscellaneous uses: Calming delirium; motion sickness (**scopolamine**); parkinsonism.

Unlabeled uses:

    Bronchial asthma – Atropine and related agents are effective in some patients with cholinergic-mediated bronchospasm.

    Glycopyrrolate may be effective in the treatment of bronchial asthma.

Administration and Dosage

ANISOTROPINE METHYLBROMIDE: 50 mg 3 times daily.

ATROPINE SULFATE:

    Adults – 0.4 to 0.6 mg.

    Children –

Atropine Dosage Recommendations in Children		
Weight		Dose
lb	kg	mg
7 to 16	3.2 to 7.3	0.1
16 to 24	7.3 to 10.9	0.15
24 to 40	10.9 to 18.1	0.2
40 to 65	18.1 to 29.5	0.3
65 to 90	29.5 to 40.8	0.4
> 90	40.8	0.4 to 0.6

    Hypotonic radiography – 1 mg IM.

    Surgery – Give SC, IM, or IV. The average adult dose is 0.5 mg (range, 0.4 to 0.6 mg). In children, it has been suggested to use a dose of 0.01 mg/kg to a maximum of 0.4 mg, repeated every 4 to 6 hours as needed. A recommended infant dose is 0.04 mg/kg (infants < 5 kg) or 0.03 mg/kg (infants > 5 kg), repeated every 4 to 6 hours as needed.

    Bradyarrhythmias – The usual IV adult dosage ranges from 0.4 to 1 mg every 1 to 2 hours as needed; larger doses, up to a maximum of 2 mg, may be required. In children, IV dosage ranges from 0.01 to 0.03 mg/kg.

    Poisoning – In anticholinesterase poisoning from exposure to insecticides, give large doses of at least 2 to 3 mg parenterally; repeat until signs of atropine intoxication appear.

BELLADONNA:

    Belladonna tincture –

        Adults: 0.6 to 1 mL 3 to 4 times daily.

        Children: 0.03 mL/kg (0.8 mL/m^2) 3 times daily.

CLIDINIUM BROMIDE:

    Adults – 2.5 to 5 mg 3 or 4 times daily before meals and at bedtime.

    Geriatric or debilitated patients – 2.5 mg 3 times daily before meals.

DICYCLOMINE HCl:

    Oral –

        Adults: The only oral dose shown to be effective is 160 mg/day in 4 equally divided doses. However, because of side effects, begin with 80 mg/day (in 4 equally divided doses). Increase dose to 160 mg/day unless side effects limit dosage.

    Parenteral – IM only. Not for IV use.

        Adults: 80 mg/day in 4 divided doses.

GLYCOPYRROLATE: Not recommended for children < 12 years of age for the management of peptic ulcer.

Oral – 1 mg 3 times daily or 2 mg 2 to 3 times daily.

   Maintenance: 1 mg 2 times daily.

Parenteral –

   Peptic ulcer: 0.1 to 0.2 mg IM or IV 3 or 4 times daily.

   Preanesthetic medication: 0.002 mg/lb (0.004 mg/kg) IM, 30 minutes to 1 hour prior to anesthesia. Children < 2 years of age may require up to 0.004 mg/lb. Children < 12 years of age, give 0.002 to 0.004 mg/lb IM.

   Intraoperative medication: Adults, 0.1 mg IV. Repeat as needed at 2- to 3-minute intervals. Children, give 0.002 mg/lb (0.004 mg/kg) IV, not to exceed 0.1 mg in a single dose; may be repeated at 2- to 3-minute intervals.

   Reversal of neuromuscular blockade: Adults and children, 0.2 mg for each 1 mg neostigmine or 5 mg pyridostigmine. Administer IV simultaneously.

L-HYOSCYAMINE SULFATE:

   Oral –

      Adults: 0.125 to 0.25 mg 3 or 4 times/day orally or sublingually; or 0.375 to 0.75 mg in sustained release form every 12 hours.

      Children: Individualize dosage according to weight.

   Parenteral – 0.25 to 0.5 mg SC, IM or IV, 2 to 4 times daily, as needed.

LEVOROTATORY ALKALOIDS OF BELLADONNA:

   Oral –

      Adults: 0.25 to 0.5 mg 3 times daily.

      Children (> 6 years of age): 0.125 to 0.25 mg 3 times daily.

METHSCOPOLAMINE BROMIDE: 2.5 mg 30 minutes before meals and 2.5 to 5 mg at bedtime.

MEPENZOLATE BROMIDE:

   Adults – 25 to 50 mg 4 times daily with meals and at bedtime.

   Children – Safety and efficacy have not been established.

METHANTHELINE BROMIDE:

   Adults – 50 to 100 mg every 6 hours.

   Pediatric –

      Newborns: 12.5 mg 2 times daily, then 12.5 mg 3 times daily.

      Infants (1 to 12 months of age): 12.5 mg 4 times daily, increased to 25 mg 4 times daily.

      Children (> 1 year of age): 12.5 to 50 mg 4 times daily.

OXPHENCYCLIMINE HCl:

   Adults – 5 to 10 mg 2 or 3 times daily, preferably in the morning and at bedtime. Some respond to 5 mg 2 times/day, while some may require higher dosage 3 times/day.

   Children – Not for use in children < 12 years of age.

PROPANTHELINE BROMIDE:

   Adults – 15 mg 30 minutes before meals and 30 mg at bedtime. For patients with mild manifestations, geriatric patients, or those of small stature, take 7.5 mg 3 times daily.

   Children –

      Peptic ulcer: Safety and efficacy have not been established.

      Antisecretory: 1.5 mg/kg/day divided 3 to 4 times daily.

      Antispasmodic: 2 to 3 mg/kg/day divided every 4 to 6 hours and at bedtime.

SCOPOLAMINE HBr (Hyoscine HBr): Give SC or IM; may give IV after dilution with Sterile Water for Injection.

   Adults – 0.32 to 0.65 mg.

   Children – 0.006 mg/kg. Maximum dosage, 0.3 mg.

TRIDIHEXETHYL CHLORIDE: 25 to 50 mg 3 or 4 times daily before meals and at bedtime. Bedtime dose, 50 mg.

Actions

Pharmacology: GI anticholinergics are used primarily to decrease motility (smooth muscle tone) in GI, biliary, and urinary tracts and for antisecretory effects. Antispasmodics, related compounds, decrease GI motility by acting on smooth muscle.

These agents inhibit the muscarinic actions of acetylcholine at postganglionic parasympathetic neuroeffector sites including smooth muscle, secretory glands, and CNS sites. Large doses may block nicotinic receptors at the autonomic ganglia and at the neuromuscular junction.

Pharmacokinetics:

Belladonna alkaloids – Belladonna alkaloids are rapidly absorbed after oral use. They readily cross the blood-brain barrier and affect the CNS.

Atropine – Atropine has a half-life of ≈ 2.5 hours; 94% of a dose is eliminated through the urine in 24 hours.

Quaternary anticholinergics – Synthetic or semisynthetic derivatives structurally related to the belladonna alkaloids, they are poorly and unreliably absorbed orally. Because they do not cross the blood-brain barrier, CNS effects are negligible. Duration of action is more prolonged than alkaloids.

Contraindications

Hypersensitivity: Hypersensitivity to anticholinergic drugs. Patients hypersensitive to belladonna or to barbiturates may be hypersensitive to **scopolamine.**

Ocular: Narrow-angle glaucoma; adhesions (synechiae) between the iris and lens.

Cardiovascular: Tachycardia; unstable cardiovascular status in acute hemorrhage; myocardial ischemia.

GI: Obstructive disease (eg, achalasia, pyloroduodenal stenosis or pyloric obstruction, cardiospasm); paralytic ileus; intestinal atony of the elderly or debilitated; severe ulcerative colitis; toxic megacolon complicating ulcerative colitis; hepatic disease.

GU: Obstructive uropathy (eg, bladder neck obstruction caused by prostatic hypertrophy); renal disease.

Musculoskeletal: Myasthenia gravis.

Atropine: Atropine is contraindicated in asthma patients.

Dicyclomine: Dicyclomine is contraindicated in infants < 6 months of age.

Warnings

Heat prostration: Heat prostration can occur with anticholinergic drug use (fever and heat stroke caused by decreased sweating) in the presence of a high environmental temperature.

Diarrhea: Diarrhea may be an early symptom of incomplete intestinal obstruction, especially in patients with ileostomy or colostomy. Treatment of diarrhea with these drugs is inappropriate and possibly harmful.

Anticholinergic psychosis: Anticholinergic psychosis has been reported in sensitive individuals given anticholinergic drugs.

Gastric ulcer: Gastric ulcer may produce a delay in gastric emptying time and may complicate therapy (antral stasis).

Elderly: Elderly patients may react with excitement, agitation, drowsiness, and other untoward manifestations to even small doses of anticholinergic drugs.

Pregnancy: Category B (glycopyrrolate, parenteral); Category C (hyoscyamine, atropine, scopolamine, propantheline, methantheline).

Lactation: **Hyoscyamine** is excreted in breast milk; other anticholinergics (especially **atropine**) may be excreted in milk, causing infant toxicity, and may reduce milk production.

Children: Safety and efficacy are not established. **Hyoscyamine** has been used in infant colic. Safety and efficacy of **glycopyrrolate** in children < 12 years of age are not established for peptic ulcer. **Dicyclomine** is contraindicated in infants < 6 months of age.

Precautions

Use with caution in:

Ocular – Glaucoma; light irides. Use caution in the elderly because of increased incidence of glaucoma.

GI – Hepatic disease; early evidence of ileus, as in peritonitis; ulcerative colitis; hiatal hernia associated with reflux esophagitis.

GU – Renal disease; prostatic hypertrophy.

Cardiovascular – Coronary heart disease; CHF; cardiac arrhythmias; tachycardia; hypertension.

Pulmonary – Debilitated patients with chronic lung disease; reduction in bronchial secretions can lead to inspissation and formation of bronchial plugs.

Miscellaneous: Autonomic neuropathy; hyperthyroidism.

Special risk: Use cautiously in infants, small children, and people with Down's syndrome, brain damage, or spastic paralysis.

Hazardous tasks: May produce drowsiness, dizziness, or blurred vision; observe caution while driving or performing other tasks requiring alertness.

Drug Interactions

Drugs that may interact with GI anticholinergics include amantadine, atenolol, digoxin, phenothiazines, and tricyclic antidepressants.

Adverse Reactions

Xerostomia; altered taste perception; nausea; vomiting; dysphagia; heartburn; constipation; bloated feeling; paralytic ileus; urinary hesitancy and retention; impotence; blurred vision; mydriasis; photophobia; cycloplegia; increased intraocular pressure; dilated pupils; palpitations; tachycardia (after higher doses); headache; flushing; nervousness; drowsiness; weakness; dizziness; confusion; insomnia; fever (especially in children); mental confusion or excitement; CNS stimulation (restlessness, tremor with large doses); severe allergic reactions including anaphylaxis, urticaria and other dermal manifestations; nasal congestion; decreased sweating.

HISTAMINE H₂ ANTAGONISTS

CIMETIDINE
Tablets: 100 mg (*otc*)   *Tagamet HB* (GlaxoSmithKline)
Tablets: 200, 300, 400, and 800 mg (*Rx*)   Various, *Tagamet* (GlaxoSmithKline)
Liquid: 300 mg (as HCl)/5 mL (*Rx*)   *Cimetidine Oral Solution* (Barre-National),
     Tagamet (GlaxoSmithKline)
Injection: 300 mg (as HCl)/2 mL (*Rx*)   *Cimetidine* (Endo), *Tagamet* (GlaxoSmithKline)
Injection, premixed: 300 mg (as HCl) in 50 mL 0.9%   *Tagamet* (GlaxoSmithKline)
Sodium Chloride (*Rx*)

FAMOTIDINE
Tablets: 10 mg (*otc*)   *Pepcid AC Acid Controller* (J & J Merck)
Tablets: 20 and 40 mg (*Rx*)   *Pepcid* (J & J Merck)
Gelcaps: 10 mg (*otc*)   *Pepcid AC* (J & J Merck)
Tablets, chewable: 10 mg (*otc*)   *Pepcid AC* (J & J Merck)
Tablets, orally disintegrating: 20 and 40 mg (*Rx*)   *Pepcid RPD* (J & J Merck)
Powder for oral suspension: 40 mg/5 mL when reconstituted (*Rx*)
Injection: 10 mg/mL (*Rx*)
Injection, premixed: 20 mg/50 mL in 0.9% HCl (*Rx*)

NIZATIDINE
Tablets: 75 mg (*otc*)   *Axid AR* (Whitehall-Robins)
Capsules: 150 and 300 mg (*Rx*)   *Axid Pulvules* (Lilly)

RANITIDINE
Tablets: 75 mg (*otc*)   *Zantac 75* (GlaxoSmithKline)
Tablets: 150 and 300 mg (as HCl) (*Rx*)   *Zantac* (GlaxoSmithKline)
Tablets, effervescent: 150 mg (*Rx*)   *Zantac EFFERdose* (GlaxoSmithKline)
Capsules: 150 and 300 mg (*Rx*)   *Zantac GELdose* (GlaxoSmithKline)
Syrup: 15 mg (as HCl)/mL (*Rx*)   *Ranitidine HCl* (UDL), *Zantac* (GlaxoSmith-
     Kline)
Granules, effervescent: 150 mg (*Rx*)   *Zantac EFFERdose* (GlaxoSmithKline)
Injection: 0.5 and 25 mg (as HCl)/mL (*Rx*)   *Zantac* (GlaxoSmithKline)

HISTAMINE H₂ ANTAGONIST COMBINATIONS
Tablets, chewable: 10 mg famotidine, 800 mg calcium   *Pepcid Complete* (J & J Merck)
carbonate, 165 mg magnesium hydroxide (*otc*)

Indications

Histamine H₂ Antagonists: Summary of Indications					
✔ – Labeled x – Unlabeled	Cimetidine	Famotidine	Nizatidine	Ranitidine	Combinations
Duodenal ulcer					
Treatment	✔	✔	✔	✔	
Maintenance	✔	✔	✔	✔	
GERD (including erosive esophagitis)	✔	✔	✔	✔	
Gastric ulcer					
Treatment	✔	✔	✔	✔	
Maintenance				✔	
Pathological hypersecretory conditions	✔	✔		✔	
Heartburn/acid indigestion/ sour stomach	✔[1,2]	✔[1,3]			✔
Erosive esophagitis, maintenance				✔	
Prevent upper GI bleeding	✔	x		x	
Peptic ulcer [4]	x	x	x	x	
Prevent aspiration pneumonitis	x	x	x	x	
Prophylaxis of stress ulcers	x	x		x	
Prevent gastric NSAID damage				x	

Histamine H₂ Antagonists: Summary of Indications					
✔ – Labeled x – Unlabeled	Cimetidine	Famotidine	Nizatidine	Ranitidine	Combinations
Hyperparathyroidism	x				
Secondary hyperparathyroidism in hemodialysis	x				
Tinea capitis	x				
Herpes virus infection	x				
Hirsute women	x				
Chronic idiopathic urticaria	x				
Anaphylaxis (dermatological)	x				
Acetaminophen overdose	x				
Dyspepsia	x				
Warts	x				
Colorectal cancer	x				

[1] otc use only.
[2] Relief of symptoms only.
[3] Relief and prevention of symptoms.
[4] As part of a multi-drug regimen to eradicate *Helicobacter pylori*.

Administration and Dosage

CIMETIDINE:

Duodenal ulcer –

Short-term treatment of active duodenal ulcer: 800 mg at bedtime. Alternate regimens are 300 mg 4 times/day with meals and at bedtime, or 400 mg twice/day.

Maintenance therapy: 400 mg at bedtime.

Active benign gastric ulcer – For short-term treatment, 800 mg at bedtime or 300 mg 4 times/day with meals and at bedtime.

Erosive gastroesophageal reflux disease (GERD) –

Adults: 1600 mg daily in divided doses (800 mg twice daily or 400 mg 4 times/day) for 12 weeks. Use > 12 weeks has not been established.

Pathological hypersecretory conditions – 300 mg 4 times/day with meals and at bedtime. If necessary, give 300 mg doses more often. Do not exceed 2400 mg/day.

Prevention of upper GI bleeding – Continuous IV infusion of 50 mg/hour. Patients with Ccr < 30 mL/min should receive half the recommended dose. Treatment > 7 days has not been studied.

Severely impaired renal function – Accumulation may occur. Use the lowest dose; 300 mg every 12 hours orally or IV has been recommended. Dosage frequency may be increased to every 8 hours or even further with caution.

Parenteral – The usual dose is 300 mg IM or IV every 6 to 8 hours. If it is necessary to increase dosage, do so by more frequent administration of a 300 mg dose, not to exceed 2400 mg/day.

IM: Administer undiluted.

IV: Dilute to a total volume of 20 mL; inject over ≥ 2 minutes.

Intermittent IV infusion: Dilute 300 mg in at least 50 mL of compatible IV solution; infuse over 15 to 20 minutes.

Continuous IV infusion: 37.5 mg/hour (900 mg/day).

FAMOTIDINE:

Duodenal ulcer –

Acute therapy: 40 mg/day at bedtime. 20 mg twice/day is also effective.

Maintenance therapy: 20 mg once a day at bedtime.

Benign gastric ulcer –

Acute therapy: 40 mg orally once a day at bedtime.

Pathological hypersecretory conditions – The adult starting dose is 20 mg every 6 hours.

GERD – 20 mg twice daily for up to 6 weeks. For esophagitis including erosions and ulcerations and accompanying symptoms caused by GERD, 20 or 40 mg twice daily for up to 12 weeks.

Severe renal insufficiency –

Ccr < 10 mL/min: To avoid excess accumulation of the drug, the dose may be reduced to 20 mg at bedtime or the dosing interval may be prolonged to 36 to 48 hours, as indicated.

Parenteral –

IV: Give famotidine IV 20 mg every 12 hours.

Children – Studies suggest the following starting doses in pediatric patients 1 to 16 years of age.

Peptic ulcer: 0.5 mg/kg/day orally at bedtime or divided twice daily up to 40 mg/day.

GERD with or without esophagitis including erosions and ulcerations: 1 mg/kg/day orally divided twice daily up to 40 mg twice daily.

Heartburn, acid indigestion, and sour stomach (otc only) –

Acute therapy: 10 mg (1 tablet) with water.

Prevention: 10 mg 15 minutes before eating food or drinking a beverage that is expected to cause symptoms.

Use: Can be used up to twice daily (up to 2 tablets in 24 hours). Do not take maximum dose for > 2 weeks continuously unless otherwise directed by a physician.

Children: Do not give to children < 12 years of age unless otherwise directed.

Moderate (Ccr < 50 mL/min) or severe renal insufficiency (Ccr < 10 mL/min) – To avoid excess accumulation of the drug, the dose may be reduced to half the dose or the dosing interval may be prolonged to 36 to 48 hours, as indicated.

NIZATIDINE:

Active duodenal ulcer – 300 mg once daily at bedtime. An alternative dosage regimen is 150 mg twice daily.

Maintenance of healed duodenal ulcer – 150 mg once daily at bedtime.

GERD – 150 mg twice daily.

Benign gastric ulcer – 300 mg given either as 150 mg twice daily or 300 mg once daily at bedtime.

Heartburn, acid indigestion, and sour stomach (otc only) – Can be used up to twice daily (up to 2 tablets in 24 hours).

Relief: For relief of symptoms, take 1 tablet with a full glass of water.

Prevention: For prevention of symptoms, take 1 tablet with a full glass of water right before eating or up to 60 minutes before consuming food and beverages that cause heartburn.

Moderate to severe renal insufficiency –

Nizatidine Dosage in Renal Insufficiency		
	Dosage	
Ccr	Active duodenal ulcer	Maintenance therapy
20 to 50 mL/min	150 mg/day	150 mg every other day
< 20 mL/min	150 mg every other day	150 mg every 3 days

RANITIDINE:

Duodenal ulcer –

Short-term treatment of active duodenal ulcer: 150 mg orally twice daily. An alternate dosage of 300 mg once daily at bedtime can be used for patients in whom dosing convenience is important.

Maintenance therapy: 150 mg at bedtime.

Pathological hypersecretory conditions – 150 mg orally twice a day. More frequent doses may be necessary. Doses up to 6 g/day have been used.

Benign gastric ulcer (oral doseforms only) and GERD – 150 mg twice daily.

Gastric ulcer –

Treatment: 150 mg twice daily.

Maintenance: 150 mg at bedtime.

Erosive esophagitis –

Treatment: 150 mg 4 times daily.

Maintenance: 150 mg twice daily.

Heartburn (otc only) –

Treatment: For relief of symptoms, swallow 1 tablet with a glass of water.

Prevention: To prevent symptoms, swallow 1 tablet with a glass of water 30 to 60 minutes before eating food or drinking beverages that cause heartburn.

Maintenance: Can be used up to twice daily (up to 2 tablets in 24 hours).

Children – The safety and effectiveness of ranitidine have been established in children from 1 month to 16 years of age. There is insufficient information about the pharmacokinetics of ranitidine in neonatal patients < 1 month of age to make dosing recommendations. Do not give *otc* ranitidine to children < 12 years of age unless directed by physician.

Active duodenal and gastric ulcers:

Treatment – 2 to 4 mg/kg/day twice daily to a maximum of 300 mg/day.

Maintenance – 2 to 4 mg/kg once daily to a maximum of 150 mg/day.

GERD and erosive esophagitis: Although limited data exist for these conditions in pediatric patients, published literature supports a dosage of 5 to 10 mg/kg/day, usually given as 2 divided doses.

EFFERdose (tablets and granules) – Dissolve each dose in ≈ 6 to 8 oz. of water before drinking.

Renal impairment – (Ccr < 50 mL/min): 150 mg orally every 24 hours or 50 mg parenterally every 18 to 24 hours. The frequency of dosing may be increased to every 12 hours or further with caution.

Parenteral –

IM: 50 mg (2 mL) every 6 to 8 hours (no dilution necessary).

IV injection: 50 mg (2 mL) every 6 to 8 hours. Dilute 50 mg to a total volume of 20 mL; inject over ≥ 5 minutes.

Intermittent IV infusion: 50 mg (2 mL) every 6 to 8 hours. Dilute 50 mg and infuse over 15 to 20 minutes; do not exceed 400 mg/day.

Continuous IV infusion: Add ranitidine injection to 5% Dextrose Injection or other compatible IV solution. Deliver at a rate of 6.25 mg/hr (eg, 150 mg [6 mL] ranitidine injection in 250 mL of 5% Dextrose Injection at 10.7 mL/hr).

Children – The recommended dose in pediatric patients is for a total daily dose of 2 to 4 mg/kg, to be divided and administered every 6 to 8 hours up to a maximum of 50 mg given every 6 to 8 hours. Limited data in neonatal patients (< 1 month of age) receiving ECMO have shown that a dose of 2 mg/kg is usually sufficient to increase gastric pH to > 4 for at least 15 hours. Therefore, consider doses of 2 mg/kg given every 12 to 24 hours or as a continuous infusion.

COMBINATIONS:

≥ *12 years of age* – To relieve symptoms, chew 1 tablet before swallowing. Do not use > 2 tablets in 24 hours. Do not swallow tablet whole; chew completely.

Actions

Pharmacology: Histamine H₂ antagonists are reversible competitive blockers of histamine at the H₂ receptors, particularly those in the gastric parietal cells. They also inhibit fasting and nocturnal secretions, and secretions stimulated by food, insulin, caffeine, pentagastrin, and betazole. **Cimetidine**, **ranitidine**, and **famotidine** have no effect on gastric emptying, and cimetidine and famotidine have no effect on lower esophageal sphincter pressure. Ranitidine, **nizatidine**, and famotidine have little or no effect on fasting or postprandial serum gastrin.

Pharmacokinetics:

H₂ receptor antagonist	Bioavailability (%)	Time to peak plasma concentration (hr)	Peak plasma concentration[1] (mcg/mL)	Half-life (hr)	Protein binding (%)	Volume of distribution (L/kg)	Elimination (%) Urine, unchanged Oral	IV	Metabolized
Cimetidine	60-70	0.75-1.5	0.7-3.2 (300 mg dose) (3.5-7.5 IV)	≈ 2[2]	13-25	0.8-1.2	48	75	30-40
Famotidine	40-45	1-3	0.076-0.1 (40 mg dose)	2.5-3.5[3]	15-20	1.1-1.4	25-30	65-70	30-35
Nizatidine	> 90	0.5-3	0.7-1.8/ 1.4-3.6 (150/ 300 mg dose)	1-2[3]	≈ 35	0.8-1.5	60	na[4]	< 18
Ranitidine	50-60 (90-100 IM)	1-3 (0.25 IM)	0.44-0.55 (0.58 IM)	2-3[3]	15	1.2-1.9	30-35	68-79	< 10

[1] Dose-dependent.
[2] Increased in renal and hepatic impairment and in the elderly.
[3] Increased in renal impairment.
[4] na = not applicable.

Contraindications

Hypersensitivity to individual agents or to other H₂-receptor antagonists.

Warnings

Benzyl alcohol: Benzyl alcohol, contained in some of these products as a preservative, has been associated with a fatal "gasping syndrome" in premature infants.

Hypersensitivity reactions: Rare cases of anaphylaxis have occurred as well as rare episodes of hypersensitivity (eg, bronchospasm, laryngeal edema, rash, eosinophilia).

Renal function impairment: Because these agents are excreted primarily via the kidneys, decreased clearance may occur; reduced dosage may be necessary.

Hepatic function impairment: Observe caution. Decreased clearance may occur; these agents are partly metabolized in the liver.

Elderly: Safety and efficacy appear similar to those of younger age; however, the elderly may have reduced renal function. Decreased **cimetidine** clearance may be more common.

Pregnancy: (Category B - cimetidine, famotidine, nizatidine, ranitidine.). Cimetidine crosses the placenta.

Lactation: **Cimetidine** is excreted in breast milk with milk:plasma ratios of ≈ 5:1 to 12:1. Potential daily infant ingestion is ≈ 6 mg.
  Ranitidine is excreted in breast milk with milk:plasma ratios of 1:1 to 6.7:1.
  Nizatidine is excreted in breast milk in a concentration of 0.1% of the oral dose in proportion to plasma concentrations.
  Famotidine is excreted in the breast milk of rats. It is not known whether it is excreted in human breast milk.

Children: Safety and efficacy are not established. **Cimetidine** is not recommended for children < 16 years of age, unless anticipated benefits outweigh potential risks. In very limited experience, cimetidine 20 to 40 mg/kg/day has been used.

Precautions

Gastric malignancy: Symptomatic response to these agents does not preclude gastric malignancy.

CNS effects: Reversible CNS effects (eg, mental confusion, agitation, psychosis, depression, anxiety, hallucinations, disorientation) have occurred with **cimetidine,** predominantly in severely ill patients. Advancing age (≥ 50 years) and preexisting liver or renal disease appear to be contributing factors.

Hepatocellular injury: Hepatocellular injury may occur with **nizatidine** as evidenced by elevated liver enzymes (AST, ALT, or alkaline phosphatase).

Occasionally, reversible hepatitis, hepatocellular, or hepatocanalicular or mixed, with or without jaundice have occurred with oral **ranitidine.**

Monitoring – Laboratory test monitoring for liver abnormalities is appropriate.

Antiandrogenic effect: **Cimetidine** has a weak antiandrogenic effect in animals. Gynecomastia in patients treated for ≥ 1 month may occur.

Immunocompromised patients: Decreased gastric acidity, including that produced by acid-suppressing agents such as H$_2$ antagonists, may increase the possibility of strongyloidiasis.

Drug Interactions

Cimetidine reduces the hepatic metabolism of drugs metabolized via the cytochrome P-450 pathway, delaying elimination and increasing serum levels.

Cimetidine Drug Interactions (Decreased Hepatic Metabolism)	
Benzodiazepines[1]	Propafenone
Caffeine	Propranolol
Calcium channel blockers	Quinidine
Carbamazepine	Quinine
Chloroquine	Sulfonylureas
Labetalol	Tacrine
Lidocaine	Theophyllines[2]
Metoprolol	Triamterene
Metronidazole	Tricyclic antidepressants
Moricizine	Valproic acid
Pentoxifylline	Warfarin
Phenytoin	

[1] Does not include agents metabolized by glucuronidation (lorazepam, oxazepam, temazepam).
[2] Does not include dyphilline.

Ranitidine (which weakly binds to cytochrome P450 in vitro), **famotidine,** and **nizatidine** do not inhibit the cytochrome P450-linked oxygenase enzyme system in the liver. Drug interactions with these agents mediated by inhibition of hepatic metabolism are not expected.

Drugs that may affect histamine H$_2$ antagonists include antacids, anticholinergics, metoclopramide, and cigarette smoking. Drugs that may be affected by histamine H$_2$ antagonists include ferrous salts, indomethacin, ketoconazole, tetracyclines, carmustine, digoxin, flecainide, fluconazole, fluorouracil, narcotic analgesics, procainamide, succinylcholine, tocainide, salicylates, diazepam, sulfonylureas, theophyllines, warfarin, and ethanol.

Drug/Lab test interactions: False-positive tests for urobilinogen may occur during **nizatidine** therapy. False-positive tests for urine protein with *Multistix* may occur during **ranitidine** therapy; testing with sulfosalicylic acid is recommended.

Drug/Food interactions: Food may increase bioavailability of **famotidine** and **nizatidine;** this is of no clinical consequence. **Cimetidine** and **ranitidine** are not affected.

Adverse Reactions

Adverse reactions may include headache, somnolence/fatigue, dizziness, confusional states, hallucinations, insomnia, nausea, vomiting, abdominal discomfort, diarrhea, constipation, thrombocytopenia, alopecia, rash, gynecomastia, impotence, loss of libido, and arthralgia.

MISOPROSTOL

Tablets: 100 and 200 mcg (*Rx*)

Cytotec (Searle)

Warning:
Misoprostol is contraindicated in pregnant women because of its abortifacient property. Advise patients of the abortifacient property and warn them not to give the drug to others. Do not use in women of childbearing potential unless the patient requires nonsteroidal anti-inflammatory drugs (NSAIDs) and is at high risk of complications from gastric ulcers associated with use of NSAIDs, or is at high risk of developing gastric ulceration. In such patients, misoprostol may be prescribed if the patient:

- Is capable of complying with effective contraceptive measures;
- Has received oral and written warnings of the hazards of misoprostol, the risk of possible contraception failure, and the danger to other women of childbearing potential should the drug be taken by mistake;
- Has had a negative *serum* pregnancy test within 2 weeks prior to beginning therapy;
- Will begin therapy only on the second or third day of the next normal menstrual period.

Indications

Gastric ulcers: Prevention of NSAID- (including aspirin) induced gastric ulcers in patients at high risk of complications from a gastric ulcer, (eg, the elderly, patients with concomitant debilitating disease) as well as patients at high risk of developing gastric ulceration, such as patients with a history of ulcer. Take misoprostol for the duration of NSAID therapy.

Unlabeled uses: In doses of at least 400 mcg/day, misoprostol appears effective in treating duodenal ulcers, and may be useful in treating duodenal ulcers unresponsive to histamine H_2 antagonists; however, it does not prevent duodenal ulcers in patients on NSAIDs.

In one study, misoprostol 200 mcg 4 times daily for 12 weeks (concurrently with cyclosporine and prednisone) reduced the incidence of acute graft rejection in renal transplant recipients by improving renal function.

Administration and Dosage

Adults: 200 mcg 4 times daily with food. If this dose cannot be tolerated, 100 mcg can be used. Take misoprostol for the duration of NSAID therapy as prescribed. Take with meals, with the last dose of the day taken at bedtime.

Actions

Pharmacology: Misoprostol, a synthetic prostaglandin E_1 analog, has antisecretory (inhibiting gastric acid secretion). NSAIDs inhibit prostaglandin synthesis; a deficiency of prostaglandins within the gastric mucosa may lead to diminishing bicarbonate and mucous secretion and may contribute to the mucosal damage caused by these agents. Misoprostol can increase bicarbonate and mucus production.

Uterine effects – Misoprostol produces uterine contractions that may endanger pregnancy.

Pharmacokinetics: Misoprostol is extensively absorbed, and undergoes rapid de-esterification to its free acid, which is responsible for its clinical activity and, unlike the parent compound, is detectable in plasma. In healthy volunteers, misoprostol is rapidly absorbed after oral administration with a time-to-reach peak concentration of misoprostol acid of 12 minutes and a terminal half-life of 20 to 40 minutes.

Mean plasma levels after single doses show a linear relationship with doses over the range of 200 to 400 mcg. No accumulation was noted in multiple-dose studies; plasma steady-state was achieved within 2 days. After oral administration of radio-labeled misoprostol, $\approx$ 80% of detected radioactivity appears in urine.

Misoprostol does not affect the hepatic mixed function oxidase (cytochrome P450) enzyme system in animals. The serum protein binding of misoprostol acid is < 90% and is concentration-independent in the therapeutic range.

Contraindications
History of allergy to prostaglandins; pregnancy.

Warnings
Duodenal ulcers: Misoprostol does not prevent duodenal ulcers in patients on NSAIDs. Compared with placebo, it had no effect on GI pain or discomfort associated with NSAIDs.

Renal function impairment: Pharmacokinetic studies in patients with varying degrees of renal impairment showed an approximate doubling of half-life, maximum concentration and area under the curve (AUC), but no clear correlation between degree of impairment and AUC was shown. No routine dosage adjustment is recommended, but dosage may need to be reduced if usual dose is not tolerated.

Fertility impairment: Results of animal studies suggest the possibility of a general adverse effect on fertility in males and females.

Elderly: In subjects > 64 years of age, the AUC for misoprostol acid is increased; however, no routine dosage adjustment is recommended. Reduce the dose if the usual dose is not tolerated.

Pregnancy: Category X. Misoprostol may cause miscarriage. Uterine contractions, uterine bleeding, and expulsion of the products of conception occur. Miscarriages caused by misoprostol may be incomplete.

Lactation: It is not known if the active metabolite (misoprostol acid) is excreted in breast milk. Therefore, do not administer to nursing mothers because the potential excretion of misoprostol acid could cause significant diarrhea in nursing infants.

Children: Safety and efficacy in children < 18 years of age have not been established.

Precautions
Women of childbearing potential: Advise women of childbearing potential that they must not be pregnant when misoprostol therapy is initiated and that they must use an effective contraception method while taking misoprostol.

Diarrhea: Diarrhea (13% to 40%) is dose-related and usually develops early in the course of therapy (after 13 days), usually is self-limiting (often resolving after 8 days), but sometimes requires discontinuation of misoprostol (2% of the patients). The incidence of diarrhea can be minimized by administering after meals and at bedtime, and by avoiding coadministration of misoprostol with magnesium-containing antacids.

Drug Interactions
Antacids: Antacids reduce the total availability of misoprostol acid, but this does not appear clinically important.

Drug/Food interactions: Maximum plasma concentrations of misoprostol acid are diminished when taken with food.

Adverse Reactions
Adverse reactions associated with misoprostol may include diarrhea, abdominal pain, and nausea.

PROTON PUMP INHIBITORS

OMEPRAZOLE
Capsules, delayed release: 10 mg, 20 mg (Rx) — *Prilosec* (AstraZeneca)

LANSOPRAZOLE
Capsules, delayed release: 15 mg, 30 mg (Rx) — *Prevacid* (TAP Pharm.)

RABEPRAZOLE
Tablets, delayed release: 20 mg (Rx) — *Aciphex* (Eisai/Janssen)

PANTOPRAZOLE
Tablets, delayed release: 20 and 40 mg (Rx) — *Protonix* (Wyeth-Ayerst)
Powder for injection, freeze-dried: 40 mg/vial (Rx) — *Protonix I.V.* (Wyeth-Ayerst)

ESOMEPRAZOLE
Capsules, delayed release: 20 mg, 40 mg (Rx) — *Nexium* (AstraZeneca)

Indications

Gastric ulcers: For treatment or symptomatic relief of various gastric disorders including gastric and duodenal ulcers, gastroesophageal reflux disease (GERD), erosive esophagitis, or pathological hypersecretory conditions.

IV (pantoprazole): Short-term treatment (7 to 10 days) of GERD, as an alternative to oral therapy in patients who are unable to continue taking oral pantoprazole. Safety and efficacy of IV pantoprazole as initial treatment for GERD have not been established.

Unlabeled uses: Posterior laryngitis (**omeprazole** 40 mg at bedtime 6 to 24 weeks); enhanced efficacy of pancreatin (for treatment of steatorrhea in cystic fibrosis patients).

Administration and Dosage

OMEPRAZOLE: Take before eating. Do not open, crush, or chew the capsule; swallow whole. In clinical trials, antacids were used concomitantly with omeprazole.

Duodenal ulcer –

Treatment: 20 mg daily for 4 to 8 weeks; most patients heal within 4 weeks, although some may require an additional 4 weeks.

Associated with H. pylori:

Triple therapy (omeprazole/clarithromycin/amoxicillin) – Omeprazole 20 mg plus clarithromycin 500 mg plus amoxicillin 1000 mg each given twice daily for 10 days. If an ulcer is present at the initiation of therapy, continue omeprazole 20 mg for an additional 18 days.

Dual therapy (omeprazole/clarithromycin) – Omeprazole 40 mg once daily plus clarithromycin 500 mg 3 times daily for 14 days. If an ulcer is present at the initiation of therapy, continue omeprazole 20 mg for an additional 14 days.

Gastric ulcer, treatment – 40 mg once a day for 4 to 8 weeks.

Erosive esophagitis –

Treatment: 20 mg daily for 4 to 8 weeks.

Maintenance: 20 mg daily.

GERD –

GERD without esophageal lesions: 20 mg daily for 4 weeks.

GERD with erosive esophagitis: 20 mg daily for 4 to 8 weeks.

Pathological hypersecretory conditions – Individualize dosage. Initial adult dose is 60 mg/day. Doses up to 120 mg 3 times/day have been administered. Administer daily dosages > 80 mg in divided doses.

No dosage adjustment is necessary for patients with renal impairment, hepatic dysfunction, or for the elderly.

LANSOPRAZOLE: Take before meals. For patients who have difficulty swallowing capsules, lansoprazole can be opened and the intact granules contained within can be sprinkled on one tablespoon of applesauce, *Ensure* pudding, cottage cheese, yogurt, or strained pears and swallowed immediately. The delayed-release capsules may be emptied into a small volume of either orange juice or tomato juice (60 mL; ≈ 2 oz), mixed briefly, and swallowed immediately. To ensure complete delivery of the dose, rinse the glass with ≥ 2 volumes of juice (apple, cranberry, grape, orange, pineapple, prune, tomato, or V-8 vegetable juice). Do not chew or crush the granules.

Duodenal ulcer –

Treatment: 15 mg once daily for 4 weeks.

Maintenance: 15 mg once daily to maintain healing of duodenal ulcers.

Associated with H. pylori:

Triple therapy – 30 mg lansoprazole plus 500 mg clarithromycin and 1 g amoxicillin given twice daily for 10 to 14 days.

Dual therapy – 30 mg lansoprazole plus 1 g amoxicillin 3 times daily for 14 days for patients intolerant or resistant to clarithromycin.

Gastric ulcer –

Treatment: 30 mg once daily for ≤ 8 weeks.

Associated with NSAIDs:

Treatment – 30 mg once daily for 8 weeks.

Risk reduction – 15 mg once daily for ≤ 12 weeks.

GERD – 15 mg once daily for ≤ 8 weeks.

Erosive esophagitis –

Treatment: 30 mg/day for up to 8 weeks. For patients who do not heal within 8 weeks (5% to 10%) give an additional 8 weeks of treatment. If there is a recurrence of erosive esophagitis, consider an additional 8-week course.

Maintenance: 15 mg once daily to maintain healing of erosive esophagitis.

Hypersecretory conditions including Zollinger-Ellison syndrome – Individualize dosage. The recommended starting dose is 60 mg/day. Adjust doses to individual patient needs and continue for as long as clinically indicated. Dosages up to 90 mg twice daily have been administered. Administer daily dosages of > 120 mg in divided doses.

Hepatic function impairment – Consider dosage adjustment in patients with severe liver disease.

Nasogastric (NG) tube – For patients who have an NG tube in place, lansoprazole can be opened and the intact granules mixed in 40 mL of apple juice and injected through the NG tube into the stomach. After administering the granules, flush the NG tube with additional apple juice to clear the tube.

RABEPRAZOLE: Swallow tablets whole. Do not chew, crush, or split.

Duodenal ulcer – 20 mg once daily after the morning meal for a period of ≤ 4 weeks. Most patients with duodenal ulcers heal within 4 weeks.

Erosive or ulcerative GERD –

Treatment: 20 mg once daily for 4 to 8 weeks. For those patients not healed after 8 weeks of treatment, consider an additional 8-week course.

Maintenance: 20 mg once daily.

Hypersecretory conditions, including Zollinger-Ellison syndrome – Individualize dosage. Start dosing at 60 mg once daily. Adjust doses to individual patient needs and continue for as long as clinically indicated. Dosing may be divided. Doses ≤ 100 mg/day and 60 mg twice daily have been administered.

Hepatic impairment – Use caution in patients with mild to moderate hepatic impairment.

PANTOPRAZOLE: Swallow tablets whole. Do not chew, crush, or split.

Oral –

Erosive esophagitis associated with GERD:

Treatment – 40 mg once daily for ≤ 8 weeks. For those patients who have not healed after 8 weeks consider an additional 8-week course.

Maintenance – 40 mg once daily.

IV –

Treatment of erosive esophagitis: As an alternative to continued oral therapy, 40 mg pantoprazole once daily by infusion for 7 to 10 days.

Administration – Administer IV pantoprazole admixtures over a period of ≈ 15 minutes at a rate ≤ 3 mg/min (7 mL/min) through a dedicated line, using the in-line filter provided. Do not simultaneously administer IV pantoprazole through the same line with other IV solutions.

Discontinue treatment with IV pantoprazole as soon as the patient is able to resume treatment with pantoprazole delayed-release tablets. Safety and efficacy of IV pantoprazole as a treatment for GERD for > 10 days have not been demonstrated.

ESOMEPRAZOLE: Swallow capsules whole. Take ≥ 1 hour before eating.

Difficulty swallowing – For patients who have difficulty swallowing capsules, 1 tablespoon of applesauce can be added to an empty bowl and the esomeprazole capsule opened and the pellets inside carefully emptied onto the applesauce. The pellets should be mixed with the applesauce and swallowed immediately. The applesauce should not be hot and should be soft enough to swallow without chewing. Do not chew or crush the pellets. Do not store the pellet/applesauce mixture for future use.

In vitro, the pellets have been shown to remain intact when exposed to tap water, orange juice, apple juice, and yogurt.

Erosive esophagitis –

Treatment: 20 to 40 mg once daily for 4 to 8 weeks.

Maintenance: 20 mg once daily.

GERD – 20 mg once daily for 4 weeks.

Duodenal ulcer associated with H. pylori –

Esomeprazole: 40 mg once daily for 10 days.

Amoxicillin: 1000 mg twice daily for 10 days.

Clarithromycin: 500 mg twice daily for 10 days.

Actions

Pharmacology: Proton pump inhibitors do not exhibit anticholinergic or H_2 histamine antagonistic properties, but suppress gastric acid secretion by specific inhibition of the H^+/K^+ ATPase enzyme system at the secretory surface of the gastric parietal cell. Because this enzyme system is the "acid (proton) pump" within the gastric mucosa, these agents have been characterized as gastric acid pump inhibitors; they block the final step of acid production. This effect is dose-related and inhibits basal and stimulated acid secretion regardless of the stimulus.

Pharmacokinetics:

Absorption/Distribution – Proton pump inhibitors are acid-labile and are thus formulated as enteric-coated granules. Absorption is rapid and begins after the granules leave the stomach.

Metabolism/Excretion – These agents are extensively metabolized by the liver. The metabolites have very little or no antisecretory activity. The plasma elimination half-life is < 2 hours while the acid inhibitory effect lasts > 24 hours, apparently because of prolonged binding to the parietal H^+/K^+ ATPase enzyme. When the drug is discontinued, secretory activity returns over 3 to 5 days.

Little unchanged drug is excreted in urine. Approximately 33% of **lansoprazole**, 90% of **rabeprazole**, ≈ 71% of **pantoprazole**, and the majority of **omeprazole** (≈ 77%) is eliminated in urine. The remainder of the dose is excreted in feces. This implies a significant biliary excretion of the metabolites of omeprazole and lansoprazole.

	Select Pharmacokinetics of Proton Pump Inhibitors					
Drug	Absolute bioavailability (%)	T_{max} (hours)	t½ (hours)	Duration of action (hours)	Clearance (mL/min)	Protein binding (%)
Omeprazole	≈ 30 to 40[1]	0.5 to 3.5	0.5 to 1	≤ 72	500 to 600	≈ 95
Lansoprazole	> 80	≈ 1.7	1.5	> 24	—	97
Rabeprazole	52	2 to 5	1 to 2	> 24	301 to 588	96.3
Pantoprazole	≈ 77	2.4	≈ 1	> 24	127 to 233	≈ 98

[1] The bioavailability of omeprazole increases slightly upon repeat administration.

Races: An increase in AUC of **omeprazole** of ≈ 4-fold was noted in Asian subjects compared with Caucasians. Consider dose adjustment for Asian subjects, particularly where maintenance of healing of erosive esophagitis is indicated.

Contraindications

Hypersensitivity to any component of the formulation; substituted benzimidazoles (**rabeprazole**).

Warnings

Atrophic gastritis: Atrophic gastritis has been noted occasionally in gastric corpus biopsies from patients treated long-term with **omeprazole**.

Hepatic function impairment: In patients with various degrees of chronic hepatic disease, the mean plasma half-life of **lansoprazole**, **rabeprazole**, and **pantoprazole** was prolonged, and the mean AUC increased. Consider dose reduction in severe hepatic disease.

Elderly: Bioavailability of **omeprazole** may be increased. The clearance of **lansoprazole** is decreased in the elderly, with an increase of elimination half-life of ≈ 50% to 100%. Because the mean half-life in the elderly remains between 1.9 and 2.9 hours, repeated once-daily dosing does not result in accumulation of lansoprazole.

Pregnancy: Category C (**omeprazole**); Category B (**lansoprazole**, **rabeprazole**, **pantoprazole**).

Lactation: It is not known whether these agents are excreted in breast milk.

Children: Safety and efficacy in children have not been established.

Precautions

Gastric malignancy: Symptomatic response to therapy with proton pump inhibitors does not preclude gastric malignancy.

Drug Interactions

Drugs that may be affected by proton pump inhibitors include clarithromycin, cyclosporine, ketoconazole, digoxin, benzodiazepines, phenytoin, theophylline, and warfarin. Drugs that affect proton pump inhibitors include clarithromycin and sucralfate.

Proton pump inhibitors cause a profound and long-lasting inhibition of gastric acid secretion; therefore, it is theoretically possible that proton pump inhibitors may interfere with the absorption of drugs where gastric pH is an important determinant of bioavailability (eg, ketoconazole, ampicillin, iron salts, digoxin, cyanocobalamin).

P450 system: **Omeprazole** may interact with other drugs also metabolized via the cytochrome P450 (CYP450) system. There are clinical reports of interaction with other drugs metabolized via the cytochrome P450 system (eg, cyclosporine, disulfiram, benzodiazepines). **Lansoprazole** is metabolized through the cytochrome P450 system via CYP3A and CYP2C19 isoenzymes; however, lansoprazole does not have clinically significant interactions with other drugs metabolized by the cytochrome P450 system. **Rabeprazole** and **pantoprazole** are also metabolized by the cytochrome P450 system, but does not have clinically significant interactions with other drugs metabolized by CYP450. Pantoprazole is metabolized via cytochrome P450 system (CYPC19 and CYP3A4), but does not have clinically relevant interactions with other drugs metabolized by CYP450. In clinical trials, antacids were used concomitantly with these agents.

Drug/Food interactions: C_{max} and AUC are diminished by ≈ 50% if **lansoprazole** is given 30 minutes after food as opposed to in the fasting condition. There is no significant food effect if given before meals.

Adverse Reactions

The most common adverse effects (> 3%) of **omeprazole**, **lansoprazole**, and **rabeprazole** include headache and diarrhea.

ORLISTAT

Capsules: 120 mg	*Xenical* (Roche)

Indications

Obesity management: For management of obesity including weight loss and weight maintenance when used in conjunction with a reduced-calorie diet. Orlistat also is indicated to reduce the risk for weight regain after prior weight loss. Orlistat is indicated for obese patients with an initial body mass index (BMI) $\geq$ 30 kg/m^2, or $\geq$ 27 kg/m^2 in the presence of other risk factors (eg, hypertension, diabetes, dyslipidemia).

Administration and Dosage

The recommended dose of orlistat is one 120 mg capsule 3 times a day with each main meal containing fat (during or up to 1 hour after the meal).

Place the patient on a nutritionally balanced, reduced-calorie diet that contains $\approx$ 30% of calories from fat. Distribute the daily intake of fat, carbohydrate, and protein over 3 main meals. If a meal is occasionally missed or contains no fat, the dose of orlistat can be omitted.

Because orlistat reduces the absorption of some fat-soluble vitamins and beta-carotene, counsel patients to take a multivitamin containing fat-soluble vitamins to ensure adequate nutrition. Instruct the patient to take the supplement once a day, $\geq$ 2 hours before or after the administration of orlistat, such as at bedtime.

Doses > 120 mg 3 times a day have not been shown to provide additional benefit.

Based on fecal fat measurements, the effect of orlistat is seen as soon as 24 to 48 hours after dosing. Upon discontinuation of therapy, fecal fat content usually returns to pretreatment levels within 48 to 72 hours.

Safety and effectiveness beyond 2 years have not been determined at this time.

Actions

Pharmacology: Orlistat is a reversible lipase inhibitor for obesity management that acts by inhibiting the absorption of dietary fats. It exerts its therapeutic activity in the lumen of the stomach and small intestine.

Pharmacokinetics:

Absorption – Systemic exposure to orlistat is minimal. Peak plasma concentrations occurred at $\approx$ 8 hours following oral dosing with 360 mg orlistat; plasma concentrations of intact orlistat were near the limits of detection (< 5 ng/mL).

Distribution – In vitro orlistat was > 99% bound to plasma proteins (lipoproteins and albumin were major binding proteins). Orlistat minimally partitioned into erythrocytes.

Metabolism – It is likely that the metabolism of orlistat occurs mainly within the GI wall. In obese patients, 2 metabolites, M1 (4-member lactone ring hydrolyzed) and M3 (M1 with N-formyl leucine moiety cleaved), accounted for $\approx$ 42% in plasma.

Excretion – Fecal excretion was the major route of elimination following a single oral dose of 360 mg orlistat in healthy and obese subjects. Orlistat and its M1 and M3 metabolites also underwent biliary excretion. Approximately 97% was excreted in feces; 83% of that was found to be unchanged orlistat. The cumulative renal excretion was < 2%. Based on limited data, the half-life of the absorbed drug is in the range of 1 to 2 hours.

Contraindications

Chronic malabsorption syndrome or cholestasis; hypersensitivity to orlistat or to any component of this product.

Warnings

Causes of obesity: Exclude organic causes of obesity (eg, hypothyroidism) before prescribing orlistat.

Pregnancy: Category B.

Lactation: It is not known if orlistat is secreted in breast milk.

Children: Safety and efficacy in pediatric patients have not been established.

Precautions

Diet: Advise patients to adhere to dietary guidelines. GI events may increase when orlistat is taken with a diet high in fat (> 30% total daily calories from fat). The daily intake of fat should be distributed over 3 main meals. If orlistat is taken with any 1 meal that is very high in fat, the possibility of GI effects increases.

Vitamin supplement: Counsel patients to take a multivitamin supplement that contains fat-soluble vitamins to ensure adequate nutrition because orlistat reduces the absorption of some fat-soluble vitamins and beta-carotene. Instruct patients to take the supplement once a day ≥ 2 hours before or after the administration of orlistat, such as at bedtime.

Urinary oxalate: Some patients may develop increased levels of urinary oxalate following treatment. Exercise caution in patients with a history of hyperoxaluria or calcium oxalate nephrolithiasis.

Diabetic patients: Weight-loss induction by orlistat may be accompanied by improved metabolic control in diabetic patients, which might require a reduction in dose of oral hypoglycemic medication (eg, sulfonylureas, metformin) or insulin.

Misuse potential: As with any weight-loss agent, the potential exists for misuse of orlistat in inappropriate patient populations (eg, patients with anorexia nervosa or bulimia).

Drug Interactions

Drugs that may interact with orlistat include cyclosporine, fat-soluble vitamins, pravastatin, and warfarin.

Adverse Reactions

Adverse reactions occurringe in ≥ 3% of patients include the following:

GI: Oily spotting; flatus with discharge; fecal urgency; fatty/oily stool; oily evacuation; increased defecation; fecal incontinence.

Miscellaneous: Anxiety; depression; dizziness; headache; rash; abdominal pain/discomfort; gingival disorder; infectious diarrhea; nausea; rectal pain/discomfort; tooth disorder; vomiting; arthritis; back pain; myalgia; lower extremitiy pain; menstrual irregularity; vaginitis; influenza; upper/lower respiratory tract infection; fatigue; otitis; sleep disorder; urinary tract infection.

METOCLOPRAMIDE

Tablets: 5 and 10 mg (*Rx*)	Various, *Reglan* (Robins), *Maxolon* (GlaxoSmith-Kline)
Syrup: 5 mg/5 mL (*Rx*)	Various, *Reglan* (Robins)
Concentrated solution: 10 mg/mL (*Rx*)	*Metoclopramide Intensol* (Roxane)
Injection: 5 mg/mL (*Rx*)	Various, *Octamide PFS* (Adria), *Reglan* (Robins)

Indications

Diabetic gastroparesis: Relief of symptoms associated with acute and recurrent diabetic gastroparesis (diabetic gastric stasis). Usual manifestations of delayed gastric emptying (ie, nausea, vomiting, heartburn, persistent fullness after meals, anorexia) respond within different time intervals. Significant relief of nausea occurs early and improves over 3 weeks. Relief of vomiting and anorexia may precede the relief of abdominal fullness by ≥ 1 week.

Oral:

Symptomatic gastroesophageal reflux – Short-term (4 to 12 weeks) therapy for adults with symptomatic documented gastroesophageal reflux who fail to respond to conventional therapy.

Parenteral: For prevention of nausea and vomiting associated with emetogenic cancer chemotherapy.

Prophylaxis of postoperative nausea and vomiting when nasogastric suction is undesirable.

Single doses may facilitate small bowel intubation when the tube does not pass the pylorus with conventional maneuvers.

Stimulates gastric emptying and intestinal transit of barium in cases where delayed emptying interferes with radiological examination of the stomach or small intestine.

Unlabeled uses: Used to improve lactation. Doses of 30 to 45 mg/day have increased milk secretion, possibly by elevating serum prolactin levels (see Warnings). Also for treatment of postoperative gastric bezoars (10 mg 3 or 4 times daily).

Administration and Dosage

Diabetic gastroparesis: 10 mg 30 minutes before each meal and at bedtime for 2 to 8 weeks. Determine initial route of administration by the severity of symptoms. With only the earliest manifestations of diabetic gastric stasis, initiate oral administration. If symptoms are severe, begin with parenteral therapy. Administer 10 mg IV over 1 to 2 minutes. Parenteral administration up to 10 days may be required before symptoms subside, then oral administration may be instituted. Reinstitute therapy at the earliest manifestation.

Symptomatic gastroesophageal reflux: 10 to 15 mg orally up to 4 times daily 30 minutes before each meal and at bedtime. If symptoms occur only intermittently or at specific times of the day, single doses up to 20 mg prior to the provoking situation may be preferred rather than continuous treatment. Occasionally, patients who are more sensitive to the therapeutic or adverse effects of metoclopramide (eg, elderly) will require only 5 mg/dose. Guide therapy directed at esophageal lesions by endoscopy. Therapy > 12 weeks has not been evaluated and cannot be recommended.

Prevention of postoperative nausea and vomiting: Inject IM near the end of surgery. The usual adult dose is 10 mg; however, doses of 20 mg may be used.

Prevention of chemotherapy-induced emesis: Infuse slowly IV over not less than 15 minutes, 30 minutes before beginning cancer chemotherapy; repeat every 2 hours for 2 doses, then every 3 hours for 3 doses.

The initial 2 doses should be 2 mg/kg if highly emetogenic drugs such as cisplatin or dacarbazine are used alone or in combination. For less emetogenic regimens, 1 mg/kg/dose may be adequate.

If extrapyramidal symptoms occur, administer 50 mg diphenhydramine IM.

IV admixture: When diluted in a parenteral solution, administer IV slowly over a period of not less than 15 minutes.

Direct IV injection: Inject undiluted metoclopramide slowly IV allowing 1 to 2 minutes for 10 mg, because a transient but intense feeling of anxiety and restlessness followed by drowsiness may occur with rapid administration.

Facilitation of small bowel intubation – If the tube has not passed the pylorus with conventional maneuvers in 10 minutes, administer a single undiluted dose slowly IV over 1 to 2 minutes.

Recommended single dose –

Adults: 10 mg (2 mL).

Children (6 to 14 years of age): 2.5 to 5 mg (0.5 to 1 mL).

Children (< 6 years of age): 0.1 mg/kg.

Radiological examinations – In patients where delayed gastric emptying interferes with radiological examination of the stomach or small intestine, a single dose may be administered slowly IV over 1 to 2 minutes.

Rectal administration: For outpatient treatment when oral dosing is not possible, suppositories containing 25 mg metoclopramide have been extemporaneously compounded (5 pulverized oral tablets in polyethylene glycol). Administer 1 suppository 30 to 60 minutes before each meal and at bedtime.

Renal/Hepatic function impairment: Because metoclopramide is excreted principally through the kidneys, in those patients whose Ccr is < 40 mL/min, initiate therapy at ≈ ½ the recommended dosage. Depending on clinical efficacy and safety considerations, the dosage may be increased or decreased as appropriate.

Metoclopramide undergoes minimal hepatic metabolism, except for simple conjugation. Its safe use has been described in patients with advanced liver disease whose renal function was normal.

Admixture compatibilities/incompatibilities:

Physically and chemically compatible up to 48 hours – Cimetidine; mannitol; potassium acetate; potassium chloride; potassium phosphate.

Physically compatible up to 48 hours – Ascorbic acid; benztropine; cytarabine; dexamethasone sodium phosphate; diphenhydramine; doxorubicin; heparin sodium; hydrocortisone sodium phosphate; lidocaine; magnesium sulfate; multivitamin infusion (must be refrigerated) vitamin B complex with ascorbic acid.

Incompatible – Cephalothin; chloramphenicol; sodium bicarbonate.

Actions

Pharmacology: Metoclopramide stimulates motility of the upper GI tract without stimulating gastric, biliary, or pancreatic secretions. Its mode of action is unclear.

Pharmacokinetics:

Absorption/Distribution – Metoclopramide is rapidly and well absorbed. Onset of action is 1 to 3 minutes following an IV dose, 10 to 15 minutes following IM administration, and 30 to 60 minutes following an oral dose. Effects persist for 1 to 2 hours.

Relative to an IV dose of 20 mg, the absolute oral bioavailability of metoclopramide is ≈ 80%. Peak plasma concentrations occur at ≈ 1 to 2 hours after a single oral dose. Similar time to peak is observed after individual doses at steady-state. The area under the drug concentration-time curve increases linearly with doses from 20 to 100 mg; peak drug concentrations also increase linearly with dose. The whole body volume of distribution is high (≈ 3.5 L/kg), which suggests extensive distribution of drug to the tissues.

Metabolism/Excretion – Approximately 85% of an orally administered dose appears in the urine within 72 hours. Of the 85% eliminated in the urine, about one-half is present as free or conjugated metoclopramide. The average elimination half-life in individuals with normal renal function is 5 to 6 hours. The drug is not extensively bound to plasma proteins (about 30%).

Contraindications

When stimulation of GI motility might be dangerous (eg, in the presence of GI hemorrhage, mechanical obstruction, or perforation); pheochromocytoma (the drug may cause a hypertensive crisis, probably because of release of catecholamines from the tumor; control such crises with phentolamine); sensitivity or intolerance to metoclopramide; epileptics or patients receiving drugs likely to cause extrapyramidal reactions (the frequency and severity of seizures or extrapyramidal reactions may be increased).

Warnings

Depression: Depression has occurred in patients with and without a history of depression. Give metoclopramide to patients with a prior history of depression only if the expected benefits outweigh the potential risks.

Extrapyramidal symptoms: Extrapyramidal symptoms, manifested primarily as acute dystonic reactions, occur in ≈ 0.2% to 1% of patients treated with the usual adult dosages of 30 to 40 mg/day. These usually are seen during the first 24 to 48 hours of treatment, occur more frequently in children and young adults, and are even more frequent at the higher doses used in prophylaxis of vomiting caused by cancer chemotherapy. If symptoms occur, they usually subside following 50 mg diphenhydramine IM. Benztropine 1 to 2 mg IM may also be used to reverse these reactions.

Parkinson-like symptoms: Parkinson-like symptoms have occurred, more commonly within the first 6 months after beginning treatment with metoclopramide but occasionally after longer periods. These symptoms generally subside within 2 to 3 months following discontinuance of metoclopramide. Give metoclopramide cautiously, if at all, to patients with preexisting Parkinson's disease, because such patients may experience exacerbation of parkinsonian symptoms when taking metoclopramide.

Tardive dyskinesia: Tardive dyskinesia, a syndrome consisting of potentially irreversible, involuntary, dyskinetic movements, may develop in patients treated with metoclopramide. Metoclopramide itself, however, may suppress (or partially suppress) the signs of tardive dyskinesia, thereby masking the underlying disease process. Therefore, the use of metoclopramide for the symptomatic control of tardive dyskinesia is not recommended.

Hypertension: In one study of hypertensive patients, IV metoclopramide released catecholamines. Use caution in hypertensive patients.

Anastomosis or closure of the gut: Giving a promotility drug such as metoclopramide could theoretically put increased pressure on suture lines following a gut anastomosis or closure.

Carcinogenesis: Elevated prolactin levels persist during chronic administration. Approximately one-third of human breast cancers are prolactin-dependent in vitro; use caution if metoclopramide is contemplated in a patient with previously detected breast cancer. Although galactorrhea, amenorrhea, gynecomastia, and impotence have occurred with prolactin-elevating drugs, the clinical significance of elevated serum prolactin levels is unknown.

Pregnancy: Category B.

Lactation: Metoclopramide is excreted into breast milk and may concentrate at about twice the plasma level at 2 hours postdose. There appears to be no risk to the nursing infant with maternal doses ≤ 45 mg/day.

Children: Infants and children (21 days to 3.3 years of age) with symptomatic gastroesophageal reflux have been treated with metoclopramide at a dosage of 0.5 mg/kg/day; symptoms improved, the duration of the disease was shortened, and surgery was avoided.

Methemoglobinemia has occurred in premature and full-term neonates given metoclopramide orally, IV or IM, 1 to 4 mg/kg/day for 1 to ≥ 3 days; this did not occur at 0.5 mg/kg/day. Reverse methemoglobinemia by IV administration of methylene blue.

Precautions

Hypoglycemia: Gastroparesis (gastric stasis) may be responsible for poor diabetic control. Exogenously administered insulins may act before food has left the stomach, leading to hypoglycemia.

Hazardous tasks: May cause drowsiness; observe caution while driving or performing other tasks requiring alertness, coordination or physical dexterity.

Drug Interactions

Drugs that may affect metoclopramide include levodopa, anticholinergics, and narcotic analgesics. Drugs that may be affected by metoclopramide include alcohol, cimetidine, cyclosporine, digoxin, levodopa, MAO inhibitors, and succinylcholine.

Adverse Reactions

Adverse reactions occurring in ≥ 3% of patients include restlessness; drowsiness; fatigue; lassitude; akathisia; dizziness; anxiety; dystonia; insomnia; headache; myoclonus; confusion; convulsive seizures; hallucinations; nausea; bowel disturbances, primarily diarrhea.

LAXATIVES

BISACODYL

Tablets, enteric coated: 5 mg *(otc)* — Various, *Dulcolax* (Ciba Consumer), *Fleet Laxative* (Fleet), *Modane* (Savage), *Women's Gentle Laxative* (Goldline Consumer), *Bisac-Evac* (G & W), *Caroid* (Metholatum Co.), *Correctol* (Schering-Plough), *Feen-a-mint* (Schering-Plough)

Tablets, enteric coated, delayed-release: 5 mg — *Reliable Gentle Laxative* (Goldline Consumer)

Suppositories: 10 mg *(otc)* — Various, *Bisacodyl Uniserts* (Upsher-Smith), *Bisac-Evac* (G & W), *Dulcolax* (Novartis Consumer), *Reliable Gentle Laxative* (Goldline Consumer), *Fleet Laxative* (Fleet)

CASCARA SAGRADA

Tablets: 325 mg *(otc)* — Various

Liquid: *(otc)* — *Aromatic Cascara Fluidextract* (Various), *Cascara Aromatic* (Humco)

CASTOR OIL

Liquid: 95% castor oil *(otc)* — Various, *Purge* (Fleming)

Emulsion: 95% castor oil with emulsifying agents *(otc)* — *Emulsoil* (Paddock)

36.4% castor oil with 0.1% sodium benzoate, 0.2% potassium sorbate *(sf, otc)* — *Neoloid* (Kenwood)

CO$_2$ RELEASING SUPPOSITORIES

Suppositories: Sodium bicarbonate and potassium bitartrate in a water soluble polyethylene glycol base *(otc)* — *Ceo-Two* (Beutlich)

DOCUSATE CALCIUM (DIOCTYL CALCIUM SULFOSUCCINATE)

Capsules: 240 mg *(otc)* — Various, *DC Softgels* (Goldline), *Stool Softener* (Apothecary), *Stool Softener DC* (Rugby), *Surfak Liquigels* (Pharmacia)

DOCUSATE SODIUM (DIOCTYL SODIUM SULFOSUCCINATE; DSS)

Tablets: 100 mg *(otc)* — *ex-lax Stool Softener* (Novartis Consumer)

Capsules: 50 and 100 mg *(otc)* — Various, *Colace* (Roberts), *D-S-S* (Magno-Humphries), *Modane Soft* (Savage), *Non-Habit Forming Stool Softener*, *Stool Softener* (Rugby), *Regulax SS* (Republic)

Capsules: 250 mg *(otc)* — Various, *Stool Softener* (Rugby)

Capsules, soft gel: 50, 100, and 250 mg *(otc)* — Various, *D.O.S.*, *Genasoft* (Goldline Consumer), *Phillip's Liqui-Gels* (Bayer Consumer), *Stool Softener* (Rugby)

Syrup: 50, 60, 150 mg/15 mL, 20 mg/5 mL, 100 mg/30 mL *(otc)* — Various, *Colace* (Roberts), *Diocto* (Various), *Docu* (Hi-Tech Pharmacal), *Silace* (Silax)

GLYCERIN

Suppositories: Glycerin *(otc)* — Various, *Sani-Supp* (G & W), *Colace* (Roberts)

Liquid: 4 mL/applicator *(otc)* — *Fleet Babylax* (Fleet)

LACTULOSE

Syrup: 10 g lactulose/15 mL (< 1.6 g galactose, < 1.2 g lactose, and ≤ 1.2 g other sugars) *(Rx)* — Various, *Cephulac*, *Chronulac* (Aventis), *Cholac* (Alra), *Constilac* (Alra), *Constulose*, *Enulose* (Alpharma), *Duphalac* (Solvay Pharm.)

MINERAL OIL

Liquid: mineral oil *(otc)* — Various

Emulsion: Mineral oil with an emulsifier *(otc)* — *Kondremul Plain* (Heritage Consumer)

POLYCARBOPHIL

Tablets: 500 and 625 mg *(otc)* — *FiberNorm* (G & W), *Konsyl Fiber* (Konsyl)

Tablets, chewable: 625 mg (as calcium) *(otc)* — *Equalactin* (Numark), *Mitrolan* (Whitehall-Robins)

Tablets: 625 mg (as calcium) *(otc)* — *Bulk Forming Fiber Laxative* (Goldline Consumer), *Fiber-Lax* (Rugby), *FiberCon* (Lederle)

PSYLLIUM

Powder: Psyllium (*otc*)

Various, *Fiberall Tropical Fruit Flavor, Fiberall Orange Flavor* (Heritage Consumer), *Genfiber, Genfiber, Orange Flavor* (Goldline Consumer), *Hydrocil Instant* (Numark), *Konsyl, Konsyl-D, Konsyl-Orange, Konsyl Easy Mix Formula* (Konsyl Pharm.), *Metamucil, Metamucil Sugar Free, Metamucil Orange Flavor* (Procter & Gamble), *Modane Bulk* (Savage), *Natural Fiber Laxative* (Apothecary), *Reguloid, Reguloid, Orange, Reguloid, Sugar Free Orange* (Rugby), *Syllact* (Wallace)

Wafers: Psyllium (*otc*)

Metamucil (Procter & Gamble)

Granules: Psyllium (*otc*)

Serutan (Menley & James)

SALINE LAXATIVES

Granules: Magnesium sulfate (*otc*)

Epsom Salt (Various)

Suspension: Magnesium hydroxide (*otc*)

Milk of Magnesia, Milk of Magnesia, Concentrated (Various), *Phillips' Milk of Magnesia, Phillips' Milk of Magnesia, Concentrated* (Bayer)

Solution: Magnesium citrate (*otc*)

Magnesium Citrate Solution (Humco)

Solution: Sodium phosphates (*otc*)

Various, *Fleet Phospho-soda* (Fleet)

SENNOSIDES

Tablets: 6, 8.6, 15, 17, and 25 mg (*otc*)

ex•lax, ex•lax, chocolated, Maximum Relief ex•lax (Novartis Consumer), *Black-Draught* (Monticello), *Senokot* (Purdue Frederick), *Senna-Gen* (Zenith-Goldline), *SenokotXTRA* (Purdue Frederick)

Granules: 15 mg/5 mL and 20 mg/5 mL

Black-Draught (Monticello), *Senokot* (Purdue Frederick)

Liquid: 25 mg sennosides A and B/15 mL and 33.3 mg/mL senna concentrate (*otc*)

Agoral (Numark), *Fletcher's Castoria* (Mentholatum)

Syrup: 8.8 mg/5 mL sennosides (*otc*)

Senokot (Purdue Frederick)

ENEMAS

Disposable enemas

Fleet, Fleet Bisacodyl, Fleet Mineral Oil (Fleet), *Therevac-SB, Therevac-Plus* (Jones Medical)

LAXATIVE COMBINATIONS

Capsules and tablets: 50 mg docusate sodium, 8.6 mg senna concentrate (*otc*)

Senokot-S Tablets (Purdue Frederick)

100 mg docusate sodium, 30 mg casanthranol (*otc*)

Various, *Doxidan Capsules* (Pharmacia), *DSS 100 Plus* (Magno-Humphries), *Genasoft Plus Softgels, Peri-Dos Softgels* (Goldline), *Peri-Colace* (Roberts), *Nature's Remedy* (Block Drug)

150 mg cascara sagrada (*otc*)

Nature's Remedy Tablets (Block Drug)

Liquids, syrups, emulsions, suspensions: 60 mg docusate sodium and 30 mg casanthranol/15 mL (*otc*)

Diocto C (Various), *Peri-Colace* (Roberts), *DOK-Plus* (Major)

Mineral oil in emulsifying base (*otc*)

Liqui-Doss (Ferndale)

≈ 900 mg magnesium hydroxide and 3.75 mL mineral oil/15 mL (*otc*)

Haley's M-O (Bayer)

90 mg/15 mL casanthranol with senna extract, rhubarb, methyl salicylate, and menthol (*otc*)

Black-Draught (Monticello)

30 mg casanthranol, 60 mg docusate sodium/15 mL (*otc*)

Silace-C (Silarx)

15 mL equiv. to 30 mL milk of magnesia and 5 mL aromatic cascara fluid extract (*otc*)

Concentrated Milk of Magnesia-Cascara (Roxane)

Granules: 3.25 g psyllium, 0.74 g senna, 1.8 mg sodium, 35.5 mg potassium/rounded teaspoonful (*otc*)

Perdiem Overnight Relief (Novartis Consumer)

MISCELLANEOUS BOWEL EVACUANTS

Miscellaneous Bowel Evacuants (*otc*)

Evac-Q-Kwik (Savage), *Fleet Prep Kit 1, 2, and 3* (Fleet), *X-Prep Liquid, X-Prep Bowel Evacuant Kit-1, X-Prep Bowel Kit-2* (Gray), *Tridate Bowel Cleansing System* (Lafayette)

MISCELLANEOUS BULK-PRODUCING LAXATIVES

Powder: 2 mg methylcellulose per heaping tbsp (*otc*)

Citrucel, Citrucel Sugar Free (GlaxoSmithKline)

Powder: Powdered cellulose (*otc*)

Unifiber (Niche)

Tablets, coated: 750 mg malt soup extract (*otc*)

Maltsupex (Wallace)

Powder: 8 g malt soup extract/scoop (*otc*)

Maltsupex (Wallace)

Liquid: 16 g malt soup extract/tbsp (*otc*)	*Maltsupex* (Wallace)

Indications

Constipation: Treatment of constipation.

Rectal/Bowel examinations: Certain stimulant, lubricant, and saline laxatives are used to evacuate the colon for rectal and bowel examinations.

Prophylaxis: Laxatives, generally **fecal softeners** or **mineral oil**, are useful prophylactically in patients who should not strain during defecation (ie, following anorectal surgery, MI).

Lactulose (certain brands): Prevention and treatment of portal-systemic encephalopathy, including the stages of hepatic precoma and coma.

Psyllium: Useful in patients with irritable bowel syndrome and diverticular disease.

Polycarbophil: For constipation or diarrhea associated with conditions such as irritable bowel syndrome and diverticulosis; acute nonspecific diarrhea.

Mineral oil (enema): Relief of fecal impaction.

Docusate sodium: Prevention of dry, hard stools.

Unlabeled uses: **Psyllium** appears to be useful in the reduction of cholesterol levels as an adjunct to a dietary program.

Administration and Dosage

BISACODYL: Swallow whole; do not chew. Do not take within 1 hour of antacids or milk.

    Tablets –

        Adults and children ≥ 12 years of age: 10 to 15 mg (usually 10 mg) in a single dose once daily.

        Children (6 to < 12 years of age): 5 mg once daily.

    Suppositories –

        Adults: 10 mg once daily.

        Children (6 to < 12 years of age): 5 mg once daily.

CASCARA SAGRADA:

    Tablets – 1 tablet at bedtime.

    Liquid – 5 mL.

CASTOR OIL:

    Liquid –

        Adults: Daily dose range, 15 to 60 mL.

        Children (2 to 12 years of age): 5 to 15 mL.

        Infants: 2.5 to 7.5 mL.

    Emulsion –

        Adults: 67%, 15 to 60 mL; 95%, 45 mL (should be mixed with ½ to 1 glass liquid).

        Children (2 to 12 years of age): 67%, 15 mL; 95%, 5 to 10 mL (should be mixed with ½ to 1 glass liquid).

DOCUSATE CALCIUM (*Dioctyl Calcium Sulfosuccinate*):

    Adults and children ≥ 12 years of age – 240 mg daily until bowel movements are normal.

DOCUSATE SODIUM (*Dioctyl Sodium Sulfosuccinate; DSS*): Give in milk, fruit juice, or infant formula to mask taste. In enemas, add 50 to 100 mg (5 to 10 mL liquid) to a retention or flushing enema.

    Adults and older children – 50 to 500 mg.

    Children (6 to 12 years of age) – 40 to 120 mg.

    Children (3 to 6 years of age) – 20 to 60 mg.

    Children (< 3 years of age) – 10 to 40 mg.

GLYCERIN:

    Suppositories – Insert 1 suppository high in the rectum and retain 15 to 30 minutes; it need not melt to produce laxative action.

    Rectal liquid – With gentle, steady pressure, insert stem with tip pointing towards navel. Squeeze unit until nearly all the liquid is expelled, then remove. A small amount of liquid will remain in unit.

LACTULOSE:
> Chronulac, Constilac, Duphalac, Constulose –
>> Treatment of constipation: 15 to 30 mL (10 to 20 g lactulose) daily, increased to 60 mL/day, if necessary.
>
> Cephulac, Cholac, Enulose – Prevent and treat portal-systemic encephalopathy
>> Oral:
>>> Adults – 30 to 45 mL 3 or 4 times daily. Adjust dosage every day or two to produce 2 or 3 soft stools daily. Hourly doses of 30 to 45 mL may be used to induce rapid laxation in the initial phase of therapy. When the laxative effect has been achieved, reduce dosage to recommended daily dose. Improvement may occur within 24 hours, but may not begin before 48 hours or later. Continuous long-term therapy is indicated to lessen severity and prevent recurrence of portal-systemic encephalopathy.
>>> Children – Recommended initial daily oral dose in infants is 2.5 to 10 mL in divided doses. For older children and adolescents, the total daily dose is 40 to 90 mL. If the initial dose causes diarrhea, reduce immediately. If diarrhea persists, discontinue use.
>>>> May be more palatable when mixed with fruit juice, water, or milk.
>> Rectal: Administer to adults during impending coma or coma stage of portal-systemic encephalopathy when the danger of aspiration exists or when endoscopic or intubation procedures interfere with oral administration. The goal of treatment is reversal of the coma stage so the patient can take oral medication. Reversal of coma may occur within 2 hours of the first enema. Start recommended oral doses before enema is stopped entirely.
>>> Lactulose may be given as a retention enema via a rectal balloon catheter. Do not use cleansing enemas containing soap suds or other alkaline agents.
>>> Mix 300 mL lactulose with 700 mL water or physiologic saline and retain for 30 to 60 minutes. The enema may be repeated every 4 to 6 hours. If the enema is inadvertently evacuated too promptly, it may be repeated immediately.

MINERAL OIL:
> Dose –
>> Adults and children ≥ 12 years of age: 15 to 45 mL, take at bedtime; Kondremul, 30 to 75 mL.
>> Children 6 to < 12 years of age: 5 to 15 mL; Kondremul, 10 to 25 mL.

POLYCARBOPHIL:
> Adults and children ≥ 12 years of age – 1 g 1 to 4 times daily or as needed. Do not exceed 4 g in 24 hours.
>> Children 6 to < 12 years of age – 500 mg ≤ 4 times daily or as needed. Do not exceed 2 g/day.
>> Children < 6 years of age – Products vary. Consult product labeling for specific guidelines.
> For severe diarrhea, repeat dose every 30 min; do not exceed maximum daily dose.
> When using as a laxative, drink 8 oz water or other liquid with each dose.

PSYLLIUM: Refer to respective package inserts for particular dosing.

SALINE LAXATIVES:
> Magnesium sulfate –
>> Adults: 10 to 15 g in glass of water.
>> Children: 5 to 10 g in glass of water.
> Magnesium hydroxide –
>> Adults: Recommended dosage varies from product to product, ranging from 10 to 60 mL/day. See individual package labeling for specific dosing information.
>> Children (≥ 2 years of age): 5 to 30 mL, depending on age (must be at least 2 years of age).
> Magnesium citrate –
>> Adults: 1 glassful (≈ 240 mL) as needed.
>> Children: ½ the adult dose as needed; repeat if necessary.

Sodium phosphates –
> *Adults:* 20 to 30 mL mixed with ½ glass cool water.
> *Children:* 5 to 15 mL.

SENNOSIDES: The following dosages are for senna concentrate *only*. For other forms of senna, consult labeling. Dosages are different.

Tablets (6 and 8.6 mg) –
> *Adults:* 2 tablets, up to 8/day.
> *Children:* 1 tablet, up to 4/day.

Tablets (15 mg) –
> *Adults:* 1 tablet at bedtime, up to 4/day.

Granules –
> *Adults:* 1 tsp, up to 4 tsp/day.
> *Children:* ½ tsp, up 2 tsp/day.

Suppositories –
> *Adults:* 1 at bedtime; repeat in 2 hours if necessary.
> *Children:* ½ suppository at bedtime.

Liquid –
> *Adults:* 15 to 30 mL with or after meals or at bedtime.
> *Children (6 to 15 years of age):* 10 to 15 mL at bedtime.
> *Children (2 to 5 years of age):* 5 to 10 mL at bedtime.

Syrup –
> *Adults:* 10 to 15 mL at bedtime (up to 30 mL/day).
> *Children (5 to 15 years of age):* 5 to 10 mL at bedtime (up to 20 mL/day).
> *Children (1 to 5 years of age):* 2.5 to 5 mL at bedtime (up to 10 mL/day).
> *Children (1 month to 1 year of age):* 1.25 to 2.5 mL at bedtime (up to 5 mL/day).

MISCELLANEOUS BULK-PRODUCING LAXATIVES:

Citrucel –
> *Adults and children ≥ 12 years:* 1 heaping tbsp (19 g) in 8 oz cold water 1 to 3 times daily.
>
> *Children (6 to < 12 years of age):* ½ the adult dose in 8 oz cold water once daily.

Unifiber – Dose is 1 tbsp in 3 or 4 oz of fruit juice, milk, or water, or mix with soft foods such as applesauce, mashed potatoes, or pudding. Can be taken up to 3 times daily if needed or as recommended by a doctor.

Maltsupex –
> *Tablets:* Adults, 12 to 36 g/day. Initially, 4 tablets 4 times daily (meals and bedtime).
>
> *Powder:* 16 g = 1 heaping tablespoon.
>
> Adults, up to 32 g twice daily for 3 or 4 days, then 16 to 32 g at bedtime. Children 6 to 12 years, up to 16 g twice daily for 3 or 4 days; 2 to 6 years, 8 g twice daily for 3 or 4 days. For infants < 2 years, consult a doctor.
>
> *Liquid:* Adults, 2 tbsp twice daily for 3 or 4 days, then 1 to 2 tbsp at bedtime. Children 6 to 12 years, 1 tbsp twice daily for 3 or 4 days; 2 to 6 years, ½ tbsp twice daily for 3 or 4 days. For infants < 2 years, consult a doctor.

Actions

Pharmacology:

Pharmacologic Actions of Laxatives					
	Laxatives	Onset of action (hrs)	Site of action	Mechanism of action	Comments
Saline	Dibasic sodium phosphate[1,2] Magnesium citrate Magnesium hydroxide Magnesium sulfate Monobasic sodium phosphate[1,2] Sodium biphosphate[1]	0.5-3	Small & large intestine	Attract/Retain water in intestinal lumen increasing intraluminal pressure; cholecysto-kinin release	May alter fluid and electrolyte balance. Sulfate salts are considered the most potent.

Pharmacologic Actions of Laxatives					
	Laxatives	Onset of action (hrs)	Site of action	Mechanism of action	Comments
Stimulant/Irritant	Cascara	6-8	Colon	Direct action on intestinal mucosa or nerve plexus, alters water and electrolyte secretion	May prefer castor oil when more complete evacuation is required.
	Bisacodyl tablets Casanthranol Senna	6-10			
	Bisacodyl suppository	0.25-1			
Bulk-Producing	Methylcellulose Polycarbophil Psyllium	12-72	Small & large intestine	Holds water in stool to increase bulk-stimulating peristalsis; forms emollient gel	Safe; minimal side effects. Take with plenty of water (240 mL/dose).
Emollient	Mineral oil	6-8	Colon	Retards colonic absorption of fecal water; softens stool	May decrease absorption of fat-soluble vitamins.
Fecal Softeners/ Surfactants	Docusate[3]	12-72	Small & large intestine	Facilitates admixture of fat and water to soften stool	Beneficial in anorectal conditions where passage of a firm stool is painful.
Hyperosmotic	Glycerin suppository	0.25-1	Colon	Local irritation; hyperosmotic action	Sodium stearate in preparation causes the local irritation.
	Lactulose	24-48	Colon	Osmotic effect retains fluid in the colon, lowering the pH and increasing colonic peristalsis	Also indicated in portal-systemic encephalopathy.
Miscellaneous	Castor oil	2-6	Small intestine	Direct action on intestinal mucosa or nerve plexus, alters water and electrolyte secretion	Castor oil is converted to ricinoleic acid (active component) in the gut.

[1] Onset of action for rectal preparations is 2 to 15 min.
[2] Colon is site of action for rectal preparations.
[3] Site of action for potassium salt is in the colon.

Contraindications

Hypersensitivity to any ingredient; nausea, vomiting, or other symptoms of appendicitis; fecal impaction; intestinal obstruction; undiagnosed abdominal pain; patients who require a low galactose diet (**lactulose**).

Do not give **docusate sodium** if **mineral oil** is being given.

Warnings

Fluid and electrolyte balance: Excessive laxative use may lead to significant fluid and electrolyte imbalance. Monitor patients periodically.

Preparations containing sodium should be used cautiously by individuals on a sodium-restricted diet, and in the presence of edema, CHF, renal failure, or borderline hypertension.

Megacolon, bowel obstruction, imperforate anus, or CHF: Do not use sodium phosphate and sodium biphosphate in these patients; hypernatremic dehydration may occur.

Abuse/Dependency: Chronic use of laxatives, particularly stimulants, may lead to laxative dependency, which in turn may result in fluid and electrolyte imbalances, steatorrhea, osteomalacia, vitamin and mineral deficiencies, and a poorly functioning colon. Also known as laxative abuse syndrome (LAS), it is difficult to diagnose.

Cathartic colon: Cathartic colon, a poorly functioning colon, results from the chronic abuse of stimulant cathartics.

Melanosis coli: Melanosis coli is a darkened pigmentation of the colonic mucosa resulting from chronic use of anthraquinone derivatives (**casanthrol, cascara sagrada, senna**).

Lipid pneumonitis: Lipid pneumonitis may result from oral ingestion and aspiration of mineral oil, especially when the patient reclines. The young, elderly, debilitated, and dysphagic are at greatest risk.

Electrocautery procedures: A theoretical hazard may exist for patients being treated with **lactulose** who may undergo electrocautery procedures during proctoscopy or colonoscopy. Accumulation of H_2 gas in significant concentration in the presence of an electrical spark may result in an explosion. Although this complication has not been reported with lactulose, patients should have a thorough bowel cleansing with a nonfermentable solution.

Renal function impairment: Up to 20% of the magnesium in magnesium salts may be absorbed. Do not use products containing phosphate, sodium, magnesium, or potassium salts in the presence of renal dysfunction.

Pregnancy: Category B. (**Lactulose, magnesium sulfate**). Category C. (**Casanthranol, cascara sagrada, danthron, docusate sodium, docusate calcium, docusate potassium, mineral oil, senna**). Do not use **castor oil** during pregnancy; its irritant effect may induce premature labor. Mineral oil may decrease absorption of fat-soluble vitamins. Improper use of saline cathartics can lead to dangerous electrolyte imbalance. If needed, limit use to bulk-forming or surfactant laxatives.

Lactation: Anthraquinone derivatives (eg, **casanthranol, cascara sagrada, danthron**) are excreted in breast milk resulting in a potential increased incidence of diarrhea in the nursing infant. Sennosides A and B (eg, **senna**) are not excreted in breast milk. It is not known whether **docusate calcium, docusate potassium, docusate sodium, lactulose,** and **mineral oil** are excreted in breast milk.

Children: Physical manipulation of a glycerin suppository in infants often initiates defecation; hence, adverse effects are minimal. Do not administer enemas to children < 2 years of age.

Precautions

Monitoring: In the overall management of portal-systemic encephalopathy, there is serious underlying liver disease with complications such as electrolyte disturbance (eg, hypokalemia, hypernatremia), which may require other specific therapy. Elderly, debilitated patients who receive **lactulose** for > 6 months should have serum electrolytes (potassium, chloride) and carbon dioxide measured periodically.

Diabetic patients: **Lactulose** syrup contains galactose (< 1.6 g/15 mL) and lactose (< 1.2 g/ 15 mL). Use with caution in diabetic patients.

Concomitant laxative use: Do not use other laxatives, especially during the initial phase of therapy for portal-systemic encephalopathy; the resulting loose stools may falsely suggest adequate **lactulose** dosage.

Rectal bleeding or response failure: Rectal bleeding or failure to respond to therapy may indicate a serious condition that may require further medical attention.

Discoloration: Discoloration of acid urine to yellow-brown or black may occur with cascara sagrada or senna. Pink-red, red-violet, or red-brown discoloration of alkaline urine may occur with phenolphthalein, cascara sagrada, or senna.

Impaction or obstruction: Impaction or obstruction may be caused by bulk-forming agents if temporarily arrested in their passage through the alimentary canal (eg, patients with esophageal strictures). Administer bulk-forming agents with at least 240 mL fluid.

Drug Interactions

Drugs that may interact with laxatives include mineral oil, milk or antacids, H_2 antagonists, proton pump inhibitors, lipid soluble vitamins (A, D, E, and K), and tetracycline.

Adverse Reactions

Excessive bowel activity (griping, diarrhea, nausea, vomiting); perianal irritation; weakness; dizziness; fainting; palpitations; sweating; bloating; flatulence; abdominal cramps.

Esophageal, gastric, small intestinal, and rectal obstruction caused by the accumulation of mucilaginous components of bulk laxatives have occurred.

Large doses of mineral oil may cause anal seepage, resulting in itching (pruritus ani), irritation, hemorrhoids, and perianal discomfort.

Lactulose – Gaseous distention with flatulence, belching, abdominal discomfort such as cramping ($\approx 20\%$); nausea; vomiting. Excessive dosage can lead to diarrhea.

POLYETHYLENE GLYCOL-ELECTROLYTE SOLUTION (PEG-ES)

Oral solution: 146 mg NaCl, 168 mg sodium bicarb, 1.29 g sodium sulfate decahydrate, 75 mg KCl, 6 g PEG 3350, 30 mg polysorbate-80/100 mL (*Rx*)	*OCL* (Abbott)
Powder for oral solution: 1 gal: 227.1 g PEG 3350, 21.5 g sodium sulfate, 6.36 g sodium bicarb, 5.53 g NaCl, 2.82 g KCl (*Rx*)	*CoLyte* (Schwarz Pharma)
4 L: 240 g PEG 3350, 22.72 g sodium sulfate, 6.72 g sodium bicarb, 5.84 g NaCl, 2.98 g KCl. (*Rx*)	
Powder for oral solution: 236 g PEG 3350, 22.74 g sodium sulfate, 6.74 g sodium bicarb, 5.86 g NaCl, 2.97 g KCl; 227.1 g PEG 3350, 21.5 g sodium sulfate, 6.36 g sodium bicarb, 5.53 g NaCl, 2.82 g KCl (*Rx*)	*GoLYTELY* (Braintree Labs)
Powder for reconstitution: 420 g PEG 3350, 5.72 g sodium bicarb, 11.2 g NaCl, 1.48 g KCl (*Rx*)	*NuLytely* (Braintree)

Indications

For bowel cleansing prior to GI examination.

Unlabeled uses: PEG electrolyte solutions are useful in the management of acute iron overdose in children.

Administration and Dosage

The patient should fast ≈ 3 to 4 hours prior to ingestion of the solution; solid foods should never be given < 2 hours before solution is administered.

One method is to schedule patients for midmorning exam, allowing 3 hours for drinking and 1 hour to complete bowel evacuation. Another method is to give the solution the evening before the exam, particularly if the patient is to have a barium enema. No foods except clear liquids are permitted after solution administration.

Adult dosage: Adult dosage is 4 L orally of solution prior to GI exam. May be given via a nasogastric tube to patients unwilling or unable to drink the preparation. Drink 240 mL every 10 minutes until 4 L are consumed or until the rectal effluent is clear. Rapid drinking of each portion is preferred to drinking small amounts continuously. Nasogastric tube administration is at the rate of 20 to 30 mL/min (1.2 to 1.8 L/hour). The first bowel movement should occur in ≈ 1 hour.

Actions

Pharmacology: Oral solution induces diarrhea (onset, 30 to 60 minutes) that rapidly cleanses the bowel, usually within 4 hours. Polyethylene glycol 3350 (PEG 3350), a nonabsorbable solution, acts as an osmotic agent.

Contraindications

GI obstruction; gastric retention; bowel perforation; toxic colitis, megacolon, or ileus.

Warnings

Pregnancy: Category C.

Children: Safety and efficacy for use in children have not been established.

Several studies in infants and children ranging in age from 3 to 14 years of age showed that the use of PEG-electrolyte solutions are safe and effective in bowel evacuation.

Precautions

Regurgitation/Aspiration: Observe unconscious or semiconscious patients with impaired gag reflex and those who are otherwise prone to regurgitation or aspiration during use, especially if given via a nasogastric tube. If GI obstruction or perforation is suspected, rule out these contraindications before administration.

Severe bloating: If a patient experiences severe bloating, distention, or abdominal pain, slow or temporarily discontinue administration until symptoms abate.

Severe ulcerative colitis: Use with caution.

Drug Interactions

Oral medication given within 1 hour of start of therapy may be flushed from the GI tract and not absorbed.

Adverse Reactions

Nausea, abdominal fullness, bloating (≤ 50%); abdominal cramps, vomiting, anal irritation (less frequent).

POLYETHYLENE GLYCOL (PEG) SOLUTION

Powder for Oral Solution: 255 g PEG 3350, 527 g PEG 3350 *(Rx)*   *MiraLax* (Braintree Labs.)

For complete prescribing information, refer to the Laxatives group monograph.

Indications

For the treatment of occasional constipation. Do not use for > 2 weeks.

Administration and Dosage

The usual dose is 17 g of powder/day in 8 ounces of water. Each bottle is supplied with a measuring cap marked to contain 17 g of laxative powder when filled to the indicated line.

Two to 4 days (48 to 96 hours) may be required to produce a bowel movement.

DIFENOXIN HCl WITH ATROPINE SULFATE

Tablets: 1 mg difenoxin (as HCl) and 0.025 mg atropine sulfate (c-iv) *Motofen* (Carnrick)

Indications
Adjunctive therapy in management of acute nonspecific diarrhea and acute exacerbations of chronic functional diarrhea.

Administration and Dosage
Adults: Recommended starting dose: 2 tablets, then 1 tablet after each loose stool; 1 tablet every 3 to 4 hours as needed. The total dosage during any 24-hour treatment period should not exceed 8 tablets. For diarrhea in which clinical improvement is not observed in 48 hours, continued administration is not recommended. For acute diarrhea and acute exacerbations of functional diarrhea, treatment beyond 48 hours is usually not necessary.

Actions
Pharmacology: Difenoxin is an antidiarrheal agent chemically related to meperidine. Atropine sulfate is present to discourage deliberate overdosage.

Difenoxin manifests its antidiarrheal effect by slowing intestinal motility. The mechanism of action is by a local effect on the GI wall.

Difenoxin is the principal active metabolite of diphenoxylate and is effective at one-fifth the dosage of diphenoxylate.

Pharmacokinetics: Difenoxin is rapidly and extensively absorbed orally. Mean peak plasma levels occur within 40 to 60 minutes. Plasma levels decline to < 10% of their peak values within 24 hours and to < 1% of their peak values within 72 hours. This decline parallels the appearance of difenoxin and its metabolites in the urine. Difenoxin is metabolized to an inactive hydroxylated metabolite. The drug and its metabolites are excreted, mainly as conjugates, in urine and feces.

Contraindications
Diarrhea associated with organisms that penetrate the intestinal mucosa (eg, toxigenic *E. coli*, *Salmonella* sp., *Shigella*;) and pseudomembranous colitis associated with broad-spectrum antibiotics. Antiperistaltic agents may prolong or worsen diarrhea.

Children: Children < 2 years of age because of the decreased margin of safety of drugs in this class in younger age groups.

Hypersensitivity to difenoxin, atropine, or any of the inactive ingredients; jaundice.

Warnings
Difenoxin HCl with atropine sulfate is not innocuous; strictly adhere to dosage recommendations. Overdosage may result in severe respiratory depression and coma, possibly leading to permanent brain damage or death.

Fluid and electrolyte balance: The use of this drug does not preclude the administration of appropriate fluid and electrolyte therapy. Dehydration, particularly in children, may further influence the variability of response and may predispose to delayed difenoxin intoxication. Drug-induced inhibition of peristalsis may result in fluid retention in the colon, and this may further aggravate dehydration and electrolyte imbalance.

Ulcerative colitis: Agents that inhibit intestinal motility or delay intestinal transit time have induced toxic megacolon. Consequently, carefully observe patients with acute ulcerative colitis.

Liver and kidney disease: Use with extreme caution in patients with advanced hepatorenal disease and in all patients with abnormal liver function tests because hepatic coma may be precipitated.

Atropine: A subtherapeutic dose of atropine has been added to difenoxin to discourage deliberate overdosage. A recommended dose is not likely to cause prominent anticholinergic side effects, but avoid in patients in whom anticholinergic drugs are contraindicated. In children, signs of atropinism may occur even with recommended doses, particularly in patients with Down's Syndrome.

Pregnancy: Category C.

Lactation: Decide whether to discontinue nursing or to discontinue the drug, taking into account the importance of the drug to the mother.

Children: Contraindicated in children under 2 years of age. Safety and efficacy in children below the age of 12 have not been established.

Precautions

Drug abuse and dependence: Addiction to (dependence on) difenoxin is theoretically possible at high dosage. Therefore, do not exceed recommended dosage.

Drug Interactions

Drugs that may interact include MAO inhibitors, barbiturates, tranquilizers, narcotics, and alcohol.

Adverse Reactions

Adverse reactions may include nausea, dry mouth, dizziness, lightheadedness, and drowsiness.

DIPHENOXYLATE HCl WITH ATROPINE SULFATE

Tablets: 2.5 mg diphenoxylate HCl and 0.025 mg atropine sulfate (*c-v*)

Various, *Logen* (Goldline), *Lomotil* (Searle), *Lonox* (Geneva)

Liquid: 2.5 mg diphenoxylate HCl and 0.025 mg atropine sulfate per 5 mL (*c-v*)

Various, *Lomotil* (Searle)

Indications

Adjunctive therapy in the management of diarrhea.

Administration and Dosage

Adults: Individualize dosage. Initial dose is 5 mg 4 times/day.

Children: In children 2 to 12 years of age, use liquid form only. The recommended initial dosage is 0.3 to 0.4 mg/kg daily, in 4 divided doses.

Diphenoxylate w/Atropine Pediatric Dosage			
	Approximate weight		Dosage (mL)
Age (years)	kg	lb	(4 times daily)
2	11-14	24-31	1.5-3
3	12-16	26-35	2-3
4	14-20	31-44	2-4
5	16-23	35-51	2.5-4.5
6-8	17-32	38-71	2.5-5
9-12	23-55	51-121	3.5-5

Reduce dosage: Reduce dosage as soon as initial control of symptoms is achieved. Maintenance dosage may be as low as ¼ of the initial daily dosage. Do not exceed recommended dosage. Clinical improvement of acute diarrhea is usually observed within 48 hours. If clinical improvement of chronic diarrhea is not seen within 10 days after a maximum daily dose of 20 mg, symptoms are unlikely to be controlled by further use.

Actions

Pharmacology: Diphenoxylate, a constipating meperidine congener, lacks analgesic activity. High doses cause opioid activity.

Pharmacokinetics: Bioavailability of tablet vs liquid is ≈ 90%. Diphenoxylate is rapidly, extensively metabolized to diphenoxylic acid (difenoxine), the active major metabolite. Elimination half-life is ≈ 12 to 14 hours. An average of 14% of drug and metabolites are excreted over 4 days in urine, 49% in feces. Urinary excretion of unmetabolized drug is < 1%; difenoxine plus its glucuronide conjugate constitutes ≈ 6%.

Contraindications

Children < 2 years of age because of greater variability of response; hypersensitivity to diphenoxylate or atropine; obstructive jaundice; diarrhea associated with pseudomembranous enterocolitis or enterotoxin-producing bacteria.

Warnings

Diarrhea: Diphenoxylate may prolong or aggravate diarrhea associated with organisms that penetrate intestinal mucosa (ie, toxigenic *Escherichia coli*, *Salmonella*, *Shigella*) or in pseudomembranous enterocolitis associated with broad-spectrum antibiotics. Do not use diphenoxylate in these conditions. In some patients with acute ulcerative colitis, diphenoxylate may induce toxic megacolon.

Fluid/Electrolyte balance: Dehydration, particularly in younger children, may influence variability of response and may predispose to delayed diphenoxylate intoxication. Inhibition of peristalsis may result in fluid retention in the intestine, which may further aggravate dehydration and electrolyte imbalance.

Hepatic function impairment: Use with extreme caution in patients with advanced hepatorenal disease or abnormal liver function; hepatic coma may be precipitated.

Pregnancy: Category C.

Lactation: Diphenoxylic acid may be excreted in breast milk and atropine is excreted in breast milk.

Children: Use with caution; signs of atropinism may occur with recommended doses, particularly in Down's syndrome patients. Use with caution in young children because of variable response. Not recommended in children < 2 years of age.

Precautions

Drug abuse and dependence: In recommended doses, diphenoxylate has not produced addiction and is devoid of morphine-like subjective effects. At high doses, it exhibits codeine-like subjective effects; therefore, addiction to diphenoxylate is possible. A subtherapeutic dose of atropine may discourage deliberate abuse.

Drug Interactions

Drugs that may interact include MAO inhibitors, barbiturates, tranquilizers, and alcohol.

Adverse Reactions

Adverse reactions may include dry skin and mucous membranes, flushing, hyperthermia, tachycardia, urinary retention (especially in children), pruritus, gum swelling, angioneurotic edema, urticaria, anaphylaxis, dizziness, drowsiness, sedation, headache, malaise, lethargy, restlessness, euphoria, depression, numbness of extremities, confusion, anorexia, nausea, vomiting, abdominal discomfort, toxic megacolon, and pancreatitis.

LOPERAMIDE HCl

Tablets: 2 mg *(otc)*	*Imodium A-D Caplets* (McNeil-CPC), *Kaopectate II Caplets* (Upjohn), *Maalox Anti-Diarrheal Caplets* (Aventis)
Capsules: 2 mg *(Rx)*	Various, *Imodium* (Janssen)
Liquid: 1 mg/5 mL *(otc)*	Various, *Imodium A-D* (McNeil-CPC)
Liquid: 1 mg/mL *(otc)*	*Pepto Diarrhea Control* (Procter & Gamble)

Indications

Rx: Control and symptomatic relief of acute nonspecific diarrhea and of chronic diarrhea associated with inflammatory bowel disease.

For reducing the volume of discharge from ileostomies.

OTC: Control of symptoms of diarrhea, including traveler's diarrhea.

Administration and Dosage

Rx:

   Acute diarrhea –

      Adults: 4 mg followed by 2 mg after each unformed stool. Do not exceed 16 mg/day. Clinical improvement is usually observed within 48 hours.

     Children:

Loperamide Pediatric Dosage (First Day Schedule)			
Age (years)	Weight (kg)	Doseform	Amount
2-5	13-20	liquid	1 mg tid
6-8	20-30	liquid or capsule	2 mg bid
8-12	> 30	liquid or capsule	2 mg tid

   Subsequent doses: Administer 1 mg/10 kg only after a loose stool. Total daily dosage should not exceed recommended dosages for the first day.

   Chronic diarrhea –

      Adults: 4 mg followed by 2 mg after each unformed stool until diarrhea is controlled. When optimal daily dosage (average, 4 to 8 mg) has been established, administer as a single dose or in divided doses.

       If clinical improvement is not observed after treatment with 16 mg/day for at least 10 days, symptoms are unlikely to be controlled by further use.

     Children – Dose has not been established.

OTC:

   Acute diarrhea, including traveler's diarrhea –

      Adults: 4 mg after first loose bowel movement followed by 2 mg after each subsequent loose bowel movement but no more than 8 mg/day for no more than 2 days.

     Children:

        9 to 11 years of age (60 to 95 lbs) – 2 mg after first loose bowel movement followed by 1 mg after each subsequent loose bowel movement but no more than 6 mg/day for no more than 2 days.

        6 to 8 years of age (48 to 59 lbs) – 1 mg after first loose bowel movement followed by 1 mg after each subsequent loose bowel movement but no more than 4 mg/day for no more than 2 days.

        < 6 years of age (up to 47 lbs) – Consult physician (not for use in children < 6).

Actions

Pharmacology: Loperamide slows intestinal motility and affects water and electrolyte movement through the bowel. It inhibits peristalsis by a direct effect on the circular and longitudinal muscles of the intestinal wall. It reduces daily fecal volume, increases viscosity and bulk density and diminishes the loss of fluid and electrolytes.

Pharmacokinetics:

   Absorption/Distribution – Loperamide is 40% absorbed after oral administration and does not penetrate well into the brain. Peak plasma levels occur ≈ 5 hours after capsule administration, 2.5 hours after liquid administration and are similar for both formulations.

   Metabolism/Excretion – The apparent elimination half-life is 10.8 hours (range, 9.1 to 14.4 hrs). Of a 4 mg oral dose, 25% is excreted unchanged in the feces, and 1.3% is excreted in the urine as free drug and glucuronic acid conjugate within 3 days.

Contraindications

Hypersensitivity to the drug and in patients who must avoid constipation.

OTC use: Bloody diarrhea; body temperature > 101°F.

Warnings

Diarrhea: Do not use loperamide in acute diarrhea associated with organisms that penetrate the intestinal mucosa (enteroinvasive *Escherichia coli*, *Salmonella*, and *Shigella*) or in pseudomembranous colitis associated with broad-spectrum antibiotics.

Acute ulcerative colitis: In some patients with acute ulcerative colitis, agents that inhibit intestinal motility or delay intestinal transit time may induce toxic megacolon.

Fluid/electrolyte depletion: Fluid/electrolyte depletion may occur in patients who have diarrhea. Loperamide use does not preclude administration of appropriate fluid and electrolyte therapy.

Pregnancy: Category B.

Lactation: It is not known whether loperamide is excreted in breast milk.

Children: Not recommended for use in children < 2 years of age. Use special caution in young children because of the greater variability of response in this age group. Dehydration may further influence variability of response. Dosage has not been established for children in treatment of chronic diarrhea.

Precautions

Acute diarrhea: If clinical improvement is not observed in 48 hours, discontinue use.

Hepatic dysfunction: Monitor patients with hepatic dysfunction closely for signs of CNS toxicity because of the apparent large first-pass biotransformation.

Adverse Reactions

Adverse reactions may include abdominal pain, distention, or discomfort; constipation; dry mouth; nausea; vomiting; tiredness, drowsiness, or dizziness; hypersensitivity reactions (including skin rash).

BISMUTH SUBSALICYLATE (BSS)

Tablets, chewable: 262 mg (*otc*)	Various, *Pepto-Bismol* (Procter & Gamble)
Caplets: 262 mg (*otc*)	*Pepto-Bismol* (Procter & Gamble)
Liquid: 130 mg/15 mL (*otc*), 262 mg/15 mL (*otc*), 524 mg/15 mL (*otc*)	Various, *Pepto-Bismol* (Procter & Gamble)

Indications

For indigestion without causing constipation; nausea; control of diarrhea, including traveler's diarrhea, within 24 hours. Also relieves abdominal cramps.

Administration and Dosage

Adults: 2 tablets or 30 mL.

Children: 9 to 12 years of age – 1 tablet or 15 mL.
6 to 9 years of age – ⅔ tablet or 10 mL.
3 to 6 years of age – ⅓ tablet or 5 mL.
< 3 years of age – Consult physician.

Repeat dosage every 30 minutes to 1 hour, as needed, up to 8 doses in 24 hours.

Actions

Pharmacology: BSS appears to have antisecretory and antimicrobial effects in vitro and may have some anti-inflammatory effects. The salicylate moiety provides the antisecretory effect, while the bismuth moiety may exert direct antimicrobial effects against bacterial and viral enteropathogens.

Pharmacokinetics: BSS undergoes chemical dissociation in the GI tract. Two BSS tablets yield 204 mg salicylate. Following ingestion, salicylate is absorbed, with > 90% recovered in the urine; plasma levels are similar to levels achieved after a comparable dose of aspirin. Absorption of bismuth is negligible.

Precautions

Impaction: Impaction may occur in infants and debilitated patients.

Radiologic examinations: May interfere with radiologic examinations of GI tract. Bismuth is radiopaque.

Drug Interactions

Drugs that may be affected by bismuth include aspirin and tetracyclines.

MESALAMINE (5-aminosalicylic acid, 5-ASA)

Tablets, delayed release: 400 mg (*Rx*)	*Asacol* (Procter & Gamble)
Capsules, controlled release: 250 mg (*Rx*)	*Pentasa* (Aventis)
Suppositories: 500 mg (*Rx*)	*Rowasa* (Solvay)
Rectal suspension: 4 g/60 mL (*Rx*)	*Rowasa* (Solvay)

Indications
Chronic inflammatory bowel disease:
> *Oral* – Remission and treatment of mildly to moderately active ulcerative colitis.
> *Rectal* – Treatment of active mild to moderate distal ulcerative colitis, proctosigmoiditis, or proctitis.

Administration and Dosage
Oral:
> *Tablets* – 800 mg 3 times daily for a total dose of 2.4 g/day for 6 weeks.
> *Capsules* – 1 g 4 times daily for a total dose of 4 g for up to 8 weeks.

Suppository: One suppository (500 mg) 2 times daily. Retain the suppository in the rectum for 1 to 3 hours or more if possible to achieve maximum benefit. While the effect may be seen within 3 to 21 days, the usual course of therapy is 3 to 6 weeks depending on symptoms and sigmoidoscopic findings.

Suspension: The usual dosage of mesalamine suspension enema in 60 mL units is 1 rectal instillation (4 g) once a day, preferably at bedtime, and retained for ≈ 8 hours. While the effect may be seen within 3 to 21 days, the usual course of therapy is 3 to 6 weeks depending on symptoms and sigmoidoscopic findings.

Actions
Pharmacology: Sulfasalazine is split by bacterial action in the colon into sulfapyridine and mesalamine (5-ASA).

The mechanism of action of mesalamine (and sulfasalazine) is unknown, but appears to be topical rather than systemic, and it is possible that mesalamine diminishes inflammation by blocking cyclooxygenase and inhibiting prostaglandin production in the colon.

Pharmacokinetics:
> *Absorption/Distribution* –
> *Rectal:* Mesalamine administered rectally as a suspension enema is poorly absorbed from the colon and is excreted principally in the feces during subsequent bowel movements. At steady state, ≈ 10% to 30% of the daily 4 g dose can be recovered in cumulative 24 hour urine collections.
> *Oral:*
>> *Tablets* – Mesalamine tablets are coated with an acrylic-based resin that delays release of mesalamine until it reaches the terminal ileum and beyond. Approximately 28% is absorbed after oral ingestion, leaving the remainder available for topical action and excretion in the feces. Mesalamine from oral mesalamine tablets appears to be more extensively absorbed than that released from sulfasalazine.
>> *Capsules* – Mesalamine capsules are designed to release therapeutic quantities of the drug throughout the GI tract; 20% to 30% of mesalamine is absorbed. Plasma mesalamine concentration peaked at ≈ 1 mcg/mL 3 hours after administration of a 1 g dose and declined in a biphasic manner. Mean terminal half-life was 42 minutes after IV administration.
> *Metabolism/Excretion* –
> *Rectal:* Whatever the metabolic site, most absorbed mesalamine is excreted in urine as the N-acetyl-5-ASA metabolite. While the elimination half-life of mesalamine is short (0.5 to 1.5 hours), the acetylated metabolite exhibits a half-life of 5 to 10 hours.
> *Oral:*
>> *Tablets* – Following oral administration, the absorbed mesalamine is rapidly acetylated in the gut mucosal wall and by the liver. It is excreted mainly by the kid-

neys as N-acetyl-5-ASA. The half-lives of elimination for mesalamine and the metabolite are usually ≈ 12 hours, but are variable ranging from 2 to 15 hours.

Capsules – Elimination of free mesalamine and salicylates in feces increased proportionately with the dose. N-acetyl-5-ASA was the primary compound excreted in the urine (19% to 30%).

Contraindications
Hypersensitivity to mesalamine, salicylates, or any component of the formulation.

Warnings
Intolerance/Colitis exacerbation: Mesalamine has been implicated in the production of an acute intolerance syndrome or exacerbation of colitis characterized by cramping, acute abdominal pain and bloody diarrhea, and occasionally fever, headache, malaise, pruritus, conjunctivitis, and rash. Symptoms usually abate when mesalamine is discontinued.

Pancolitis: While using mesalamine, some patients have developed pancolitis.

Hypersensitivity reactions: Most patients who were hypersensitive to sulfasalazine were able to take mesalamine enemas without evidence of any allergic reaction. Nevertheless, exercise caution when mesalamine is initially used in patients known to be allergic to sulfasalazine.

Renal function impairment: Renal impairment, including minimal change nephropathy, and acute and chronic interstitial nephritis, has occurred.

Pregnancy: Category B. Mesalamine is known to cross the placental barrier.

Lactation: Low concentrations of mesalamine and higher concentrations of N-acetyl-5-ASA have been detected in breast milk.

Children: Safety and efficacy for use in children have not been established.

Precautions
Pericarditis: Pericarditis has occurred rarely with mesalamine-containing products including sulfasalazine.

Adverse Reactions
Adverse reactions may include abdominal pain/cramps/discomfort; colitis exacerbation; constipation; diarrhea; dyspepesia; eructation; flatulence/gas; nausea; vomiting; asthenia; chills; dizziness; fever; headache; malaise/fatigue/weakness; sweating; pharyngitis; rhinitis; pruritus; rash/spots; arthralgia; back pain; hypertonia; myalgia; chest pain; dysmenorrhea; edema; flu syndrome; pain.

OLSALAZINE SODIUM

Capsules: 250 mg *(Rx)*

Dipentum (Pharmacia)

Indications

Maintenance of remission of ulcerative colitis in patients intolerant of sulfasalazine.

Administration and Dosage

1 g/day in 2 divided doses.

Actions

Pharmacology: Olsalazine sodium is a sodium salt of a salicylate compound that is effectively bioconverted to 5-aminosalicylic acid (mesalamine; 5-ASA), which has anti-inflammatory activity in ulcerative colitis. Approximately 98% to 99% of an oral dose will reach the colon, where each molecule is rapidly converted into 2 molecules of 5-ASA by colonic bacteria. The liberated 5-ASA is absorbed slowly, resulting in very high local concentrations in the colon.

Mechanism of action of mesalamine is unknown, but appears topical rather than systemic. It may diminish colonic inflammation by blocking cyclooxygenase and inhibiting colon prostaglandin production in bowel mucosa.

Pharmacokinetics: After oral administration ≈ 2.4% of a single 1 g oral dose is absorbed. Maximum serum concentrations appear after ≈ 1 hour, and are low even after a single 1 g dose. Olsalazine has a very short serum half-life of ≈ 0.9 hours and is > 99% bound to plasma proteins. Urinary recovery is < 1%. Total oral olsalazine recovery ranges from 90% to 97%.

Serum concentrations of 5-ASA are detected after 4 to 8 hours. Of the total urinary 5-ASA, > 90% is in the form of N-acetyl-5-ASA (Ac-5-ASA).

Contraindications

Hypersensitivity to salicylates.

Warnings

Pregnancy: Category C.

Lactation: It is not known whether this drug is excreted in breast milk.

Children: Safety and efficacy in children have not been established.

Precautions

Diarrhea: About 17%, resulting in drug withdrawal in 6%; appears dose-related, but may be difficult to distinguish from underlying disease symptoms.

Colitis symptoms: Exacerbation of the symptoms of colitis thought to have been caused by mesalamine or sulfasalazine has been noted.

Renal abnormalities: Renal abnormalities were not reported in clinical trials with olsalazine; however, the possibility of renal tubular damage caused by absorbed mesalamine or its n-acetylated metabolite must be kept in mind, particularly in pre-existing renal disease.

Adverse Reactions

Adverse reactions may include headache; diarrhea; pain/cramps; nausea; dyspepsia; arthralgia.

BALSALAZIDE DISODIUM

Capsules: 750 mg (*Rx*)	*Colazal* (Salix)

Indications
Active ulcerative colitis: Treatment of mildly to moderately active ulcerative colitis.

Administration and Dosage
Ulcerative colitis: Take three 750 mg capsules 3 times a day for a total daily dose of 6.75 g for a duration of 8 weeks. Some patients in clinical trials required treatment for ≤ 12 weeks. Safety and efficacy of balsalazide disodium beyond 12 weeks have not been established.

Actions
Pharmacology: Balsalazide is delivered intact to the colon where it is cleaved by bacterial azoreduction to release equimolar quantities of mesalamine, which is the therapeutically active portion of the molecule and 4-aminobenzoyl-β-alanine. The recommended dose of 6.75 g/day for the treatment of active disease provides 2.4 g of free 5-aminosalicylic acid (5-ASA) to the colon.

Pharmacokinetics:

    Absorption – In healthy individuals, the systemic absorption of intact balsalazide was very low and variable. The mean C_{max} occurs ≈ 1 to 2 hours after single oral doses of 1.5 or 2.25 g. There was a large intersubject variability in the plasma concentration of balsalazide vs time profiles in all studies, thus its half-life could not be determined.

    Distribution – The binding of balsalazide to human plasma proteins was ≥ 99%.

    Metabolism – The products of the azoreduction of this compound, 5-ASA and 4-aminobenzoyl-β-alanine, and their N-acetylated metabolites have been identified in plasma, urine, and feces.

    Excretion – Less than 1% of an oral dose was recovered as parent compound, 5-ASA, or 4-aminobenzoyl-β-alanine in the urine of healthy subjects.

Contraindications
Hypersensitivity to salicylates or any of the components of balsalazide capsules or balsalazide metabolites.

Warnings
Renal function impairment: There have been no reported incidents of renal impairment in patients taking balsalazide. Renal toxicity has been observed in patients given other mesalamine products. Therefore, exercise caution when administering balsalazide to patients with known renal dysfunction or a history of renal disease.

Pregnancy: Category B.

Lactation: It is not known whether balsalazide is excreted in breast milk. Exercise caution when administering to a nursing woman.

Children: Safety and efficacy of balsalazide in pediatric patients have not been established.

Precautions
Exacerbation of symptoms: Exacerbation of the symptoms of colitis, possibly related to drug use, has been reported.

Pyloric stenosis: Patients with pyloric stenosis may have prolonged gastric retention of balsalazide capsules.

Adverse Reactions
Adverse reactions occurring in ≥ 3% of patients include the following: Headache; abdominal pain; diarrhea and nausea; vomiting; respiratory infection; arthralgia.

SULFASALAZINE

Tablets: 500 mg (*Rx*)	Various, *Azulfidine* (Pharmacia)
Tablets, delayed-release: 500 mg (*Rx*)	*Azulfidine EN-tabs* (Pharmacia)

Sulfasalazine also is indicated for use in rheumatoid arthritis and juvenile rheumatoid arthritis. Refer to the monograph in the CNS chapter.

Indications

Ulcerative colitis: In the treatment of mild to moderate ulcerative colitis and as adjunctive therapy in severe ulcerative colitis; for the prolongation of the remission period between acute attacks of ulcerative colitis.

Rheumatoid arthritis (RA; enteric-coated tablets): In the treatment of patients with RA who have responded inadequately to salicylates or other nonsteroidal anti-inflammatory drugs (NSAIDs).

Juvenile rheumatoid arthritis (JRA; enteric-coated tablets): In the treatment of pediatric patients ≥ 6 years of age with polyarticular-course JRA who have responded inadequately to salicylates or other NSAIDs.

Unlabeled uses: Psoriatic arthritis (2 g/day).

Administration and Dosage

Give the drug in evenly divided doses over each 24-hour period; intervals between nighttime doses should not exceed 8 hours, with administration after meals recommended when feasible. Swallow tablets whole; do not crush or chew. Experience suggests that with daily dosages of ≥ 4 g, the incidence of adverse effects tends to increase.

Some patients may be sensitive to treatment with sulfasalazine. Various desensitization-like regimens have been reported to be effective. These regimens suggest starting with a total daily dose of 50 to 250 mg initially, and doubling it every 4 to 7 days until the desired therapeutic level has been achieved. If the symptoms of sensitivity recur, discontinue sulfasalazine. Do not attempt desensitization in patients who have a history of agranulocytosis, or who have experienced an anaphylactoid reaction while previously receiving sulfasalazine.

Ulcerative colitis:

Initial therapy –

Adults: 3 to 4 g daily in evenly divided doses. It may be advisable to initiate therapy with a lower dosage (eg, 1 to 2 g daily), to reduce possible GI intolerance.

Children ≥ 2 years of age: 40 to 60 mg/kg in each 24-hour period, divided into 3 to 6 doses.

Maintenance therapy –

Adults: 2 g daily.

Children ≥ 2 years of age: 30 mg/kg in each 24-hour period, divided into 4 doses.

It is often necessary to continue medication even when clinical symptoms, including diarrhea, have been controlled. When endoscopic examination confirms satisfactory improvement, reduce dosage to a maintenance level. If diarrhea recurs, increase dosage to previously effective levels.

Actions

Pharmacology: The mode of action of sulfasalazine or its metabolites, 5-aminosalicylic acid (5-ASA) and sulfapyridine (SP), is still under investigation but may be related to the anti-inflammatory or immunomodulatory properties that have been observed in animals and in vitro, to its affinity for connective tissue, or to the relatively high concentration it reaches in serous fluids, the liver, and intestinal walls. In ulcerative colitis, the major therapeutic action may reside in the 5-ASA moiety.

Pharmacokinetics:

Absorption – The absolute bioavailability of oral sulfasalazine is < 15% for parent drug. In the intestine, sulfasalazine is metabolized by intestinal bacteria to SP and 5-ASA. Of the two, SP is relatively well absorbed from the colon and highly metabolized with an estimated bioavailability of 60%. 5-ASA is much less well absorbed with an estimated bioavailability of 10% to 30%. Peak plasma levels of both occur ≈ 10 hours after dosing.

Distribution – Following IV injection, the calculated volume of distribution (Vd_{ss}) for sulfasalazine was ≈ 7.5 L. Sulfasalazine is highly bound to albumin (> 99.3%), while SP is only ≈ 70% bound to albumin.

Metabolism – The observed plasma half-life for IV sulfasalazine is 7.6 hours. The primary route of metabolism of SP is via acetylation to form AcSP. The rate of metabolism of SP to AcSP is dependent on acetylator phenotype. In fast acetylators, the mean plasma half-life of SP is 10.4 hours, while in slow acetylators it is 14.8 hours.

Excretion – Absorbed SP and 5-ASA and their metabolites are primarily eliminated in the urine either as free metabolites or as glucuronide conjugates. The majority of 5-ASA stays within the colonic lumen and is excreted as 5-ASA and acetyl-5-ASA with the feces.

Contraindications

Pediatric patients < 2 years of age; intestinal or urinary obstruction; porphyria, hypersensitivity to sulfasalazine, its metabolites, salicylates, or sulfonamides.

Warnings

Porphyria: Patients with porphyria should not receive sulfonamides as these drugs have been reported to precipitate an acute attack.

GI intolerance: Sulfasalazine enteric-coated tablets are particularly indicated in patients with ulcerative colitis who cannot take uncoated sulfasalazine tablets because of GI intolerance, and in whom there is evidence that this intolerance is not primarily the result of high blood levels of sulfapyridine and its metabolites (eg, patients experiencing nausea and vomiting with the first few doses of the drug, or patients in whom a reduction in dosage does not alleviate the adverse GI effects).

Special risk patients: The presence of clinical signs such as sore throat, fever, pallor, purpura, or jaundice may be indications of serious blood disorders. Use with caution in patients with severe allergy or bronchial asthma.

Deaths: Deaths associated with the administration of sulfasalazine have been reported from hypersensitivity reactions, agranulocytosis, aplastic anemia, other blood dyscrasias, renal and liver damage, irreversible neuromuscular and CNS changes, and fibrosing alveolitis. If toxic or hypersensitivity reactions occur, discontinue sulfasalazine immediately.

Renal/Hepatic function impairment: Only after critical appraisal should sulfasalazine be given to patients with hepatic or renal damage or blood dyscrasias.

Fertility impairment: Oligospermia and infertility have been observed in men treated with sulfasalazine. Withdrawal of the drug appears to reverse these effects.

Elderly: Elderly patients with rheumatoid arthritis showed a prolonged plasma half-life for sulfasalazine, SP, and their metabolites.

Pregnancy: Category B.

Lactation: Sulfonamides are excreted in breast milk. In newborns, they compete with bilirubin for binding sites on the plasma proteins and may cause kernicterus.

Children: The safety and efficacy of sulfasalazine in pediatric patients < 2 years of age with ulcerative colitis have not been established.

Precautions

Monitoring: Perform complete blood counts, including differential white cell count and liver function tests before starting sulfasalazine and every second week during the first 3 months of therapy. During the second 3 months, perform the same tests once monthly and, thereafter, once every 3 months and as clinically indicated. Also perform urinalysis and assess renal function periodically during treatment.

The determination of serum sulfapyridine levels may be useful because concentrations > 50 mcg/mL appear to be associated with an increased incidence of adverse reactions.

Ulcerative colitis: Inform patients with this condition that ulcerative colitis rarely remits completely, and that the risk of relapse can be substantially reduced by continued administration of sulfasalazine at a maintenance dosage.

Glucose-6-phosphate dehydrogenase deficiency: Observe patients with glucose-6-phosphate dehydrogenase deficiency closely for signs of hemolytic anemia. This reaction is frequently dose-related.

Undisintegrated tablets: Isolated instances have occurred where sulfasalazine enteric-coated tablets have passed undisintegrated. If this is observed, discontinue the administration of the drug immediately.

Fluid intake: Adequate fluid intake must be maintained in order to prevent crystalluria and stone formation.

Drug Interactions

Drugs that may interact with sulfasalazine include digoxin, sulfonylureas, and folic acid.

Adverse Reactions

Adverse events occurring in ≥ 3% of patients with ulcerative colitis include the following: Anorexia; headache; nausea; vomiting; gastric distress; reversible oligospermia.

HELICOBACTER PYLORI AGENTS

Helicobacter pylori: H. pylori is found in ≈ 100% of chronic active antral gastritis cases, 90% to 95% of duodenal ulcer patients, and 50% to 80% of gastric ulcer patients. The treatment of documented H. pylori infection in patients with confirmed peptic ulcer on first presentation or recurrence has been recommended by the National Institutes for Health in a 1994 Consensus Conference. Once H. pylori eradication has been achieved, reinfection rates are < 0.5% per year, and ulcer recurrence rates are dramatically reduced.

Numerous clinical trials have been done to determine the optimal regimen for H. pylori eradication, but there remains no gold standard of therapy to date. When selecting a regimen, take into account efficacy, tolerability, compliance, and cost. H. pylori is easily suppressed but, to ensure successful eradication, requires the use of 2 antimicrobial agents with either a bismuth compound, an antisecretory agent, or both. These combinations have been shown to enhance H. pylori cure, shorten the duration of treatment and decrease treatment failure caused by antimicrobial resistance.

Double antimicrobial therapy plus an antisecretory drug:

Regimens Used in the Eradication of *H. pylori* [1]			
Regimen	Dosing	Duration	Eradication
Metronidazole	500 mg twice daily with meals	1 week	87% to 91%
Omeprazole	20 mg twice daily with meals		
Clarithromycin	500 mg twice daily with meals		
Amoxicillin	1 g twice daily with meals	1 to 2 weeks	77% to 83%
Omeprazole	20 mg twice daily before meals		
Clarithromycin	500 mg twice daily with meals		
Metronidazole	500 mg twice daily with meals	1 to 2 weeks	77% to 83%
Omeprazole	20 mg twice daily before meals		
Amoxicillin	1 g twice daily with meals		

[1] Extending therapy to 10 to 14 days in the above regimens may provide additional benefit. H_2 blockers may be used with 2 antibiotics, but a longer treatment course (10 to 14 days), higher antibiotic doses, and 3 times daily administration are required.

Triple-therapy regimens: These regimens have proven to be very effective in eradicating H. pylori. The primary disadvantage of these regimens is compliance because of the variety and number of medications used. Likewise, adverse effects are more common in patients taking these regimens compared with alternatives.

Regimens Used in the Eradication of *H. pylori* [1]			
Regimen	Dosing	Duration	Eradication
Bismuth subsalicylate	525 mg 4 times daily with meals and at bedtime	2 weeks	88% to 90%
Metronidazole	250 mg 4 times daily with meals and at bedtime	1 week	86% to 90%
Tetracycline	500 mg 4 times daily		
Bismuth subsalicylate	525 mg 4 times daily with meals and at bedtime	1 week	94% to 98%
Metronidazole	250 mg 4 times daily with meals and at bedtime		
Tetracycline	500 mg 4 times daily		
Omeprazole	20 mg 2 times daily before meals		
Bismuth subsalicylate	525 mg 4 times daily with meals and at bedtime	2 weeks	80% to 86%
Metronidazole	250 mg 4 times daily with meals and at bedtime	1 week	75% to 81%
Amoxicillin	500 mg 4 times daily with meals and at bedtime		

[1] One week of 4 times daily therapy may be sufficient in the absence of antibiotic resistance. Adding a proton pump inhibitor facilitates shorter treatment periods. Until more data is available, the use of H_2 antagonists or proton pump inhibitors with the above regimens is appropriate to enhance ulcer healing and provide symptomatic relief.

Quadruple therapy regimens (2 antibiotics, bismuth, antisecretory agent): Like triple therapy regimens, these have proven to be effective in H. pylori eradication. The primary disadvantage of these regimens is compliance. In addition, because of the variety and number of medications used, adverse effects are more common in patients taking these regimens compared with alternatives.

FDA-Approved Regimens for the Eradication of *H. pylori*			
Regimen	Dosing	Eradication	Comments
Omeprazole	40 mg once daily followed by a 2-week course of 20 mg once daily	64% to 74%	The American College of Gastroenterology recommends that either tetracycline or amoxicillin be added to this regimen.
Clarithromycin	500 mg 3 times daily for 2 weeks		
Ranitidine bismuth citrate	400 mg twice daily for 4 weeks	82%	The American College of Gastroenterology recommends that either tetracycline or amoxicillin be added to this regimen.
Clarithromycin	500 mg 3 times daily for 2 weeks		
Metronidazole	250 mg 4 times daily at meals and bedtime	82%	*Helidac* therapy combines bismuth subsalicylate, metronidazole, and tetracycline in a consumer-tested, patient-friendly kit.
Tetracycline HCl	500 mg 4 times daily at meals and bedtime		
Bismuth subsalicylate	525 mg 4 times daily at meals and bedtime		

Practice Guidelines from the American College of Gastroenterology: In the 1996 Consensus Statement on Medical Treatment of Peptic Ulcer Disease, the American College of Gastroenterology does not recommend single-antibiotic combinations of either clarithromycin or amoxicillin with proton pump inhibitors because efficacy is < 70% (cure), and a high-dose, 2-week treatment period is required. The Consensus Statement recommends a 2-antibiotic combination of clarithromycin, metronidazole, or amoxicillin in regimens that do not employ a bismuth compound. In addition, the American College of Gastroenterology suggests adding either tetracycline or amoxicillin to the recently approved ranitidine-bismuth citrate-clarithromycin combination to enhance successful *H. pylori* eradication. Combining a proton pump inhibitor, either omeprazole or lansoprazole, with 2 antibiotics is thought to enhance effectiveness and allow for a shorter duration of treatment.

There are a number of factors that limit the effectiveness of regimens designed to eradicate *H. pylori*. The first, antibiotic resistance, is seen with metronidazole and clarithromycin but has not been reported with bismuth, amoxicillin, or tetracycline.

Second, mild adverse effects (eg, diarrhea, metallic taste, black stools) do occur in ≈ 30% to 50% of patients. Therefore, shorter treatment periods in this group of patients may be better tolerated.

Finally, patient compliance is often a problem because of cumbersome regimens and adverse effects.

Maintenance therapy with antisecretory agents: Currently, it is advisable to continue maintenance until *H. pylori* cure has been confirmed in patients with a history of complications, frequent or troublesome recurrences or refractory ulcers.

Successful eradication: Confirming successful eradication is important in patients with a history of complicated or refractory ulcers but is controversial in those with uncomplicated ulcers who remain asymptomatic after therapy.

Refractory ulcers: Refractory ulcers in patients receiving antibiotic therapy for *H. pylori* eradication is often due to failure to successfully eradicate *H. pylori* infection. Resistance patterns, as well as noncompliance, and concurrent NSAID use may play a role in refractory cases.

PILOCARPINE HCl

Tablets: 5 mg (*Rx*)	*Salagen* (MGI Pharma)

Indications
Xerostomia: Treatment of symptoms of xerostomia from salivary gland hypofunction caused by radiotherapy for cancer of the head and neck.

Administration and Dosage
The recommended dose for the initiation of treatment is 5 mg 3 times/day. Titration up to 10 mg 3 times/day may be considered for patients who have not responded adequately and who can tolerate lower doses. The incidence of the most common adverse events increases with dose. Use the lowest dose that is tolerated and effective for maintenance.

Actions
Pharmacology: Pilocarpine is a cholinergic parasympathomimetic agent exerting a broad spectrum of pharmacologic effects with predominant muscarinic action. Pilocarpine can increase secretion by the exocrine glands, can stimulate intestinal tract smooth muscle (dose-related), and may increase bronchial smooth muscle tone. The tone and motility of urinary tract, gallbladder, and biliary duct smooth muscle may be enhanced. Pilocarpine may have paradoxical effects on the cardiovascular system. The expected effect of a muscarinic agonist is vasodepression, but administration of pilocarpine may produce hypertension after a brief episode of hypotension. Bradycardia and tachycardia have been reported with use of pilocarpine.

Pharmacokinetics: Following single 5 and 10 mg oral doses, unstimulated salivary flow was time-related with an onset at 20 minutes and a peak at 1 hour with a duration of 3 to 5 hours.

Following 2 days of 5 or 10 mg oral pilocarpine given at 8 am, noon, and 6 pm, the mean elimination half-life was 0.76 and 1.35 hours for the 5 and 10 mg doses, respectively. T_{max} was 1.25 and 0.85 hours and C_{max} was 15 and 41 ng/mL, respectively. The AUC was 33 and 108 hr•ng/mL, respectively, following the last 6 hour dose.

Inactivation of pilocarpine is thought to occur at neuronal synapses and probably in plasma. Pilocarpine and its minimally active or inactive degradation products, including pilocarpic acid, are excreted in the urine.

Contraindications
Uncontrolled asthma; hypersensitivity to pilocarpine; when miosis is undesirable.

Warnings
Cardiovascular disease: Patients with significant cardiovascular disease may be unable to compensate for transient changes in hemodynamics or rhythm induced by pilocarpine. Pulmonary edema has been reported as a complication of pilocarpine toxicity from high ocular doses given for acute angle-closure glaucoma. Administer pilocarpine with caution and under close medical supervision in patients with cardiovascular disease.

The dose-related cardiovascular effects of pilocarpine include hypotension, hypertension, bradycardia, and tachycardia.

Ocular effects: Carefully examine the fundus prior to initiating therapy with pilocarpine. An association of ocular pilocarpine use and retinal detachment in patients with preexisting retinal disease has been reported. The systemic blood level that is associated with this finding is not known.

Ocular formulations of pilocarpine have caused visual blurring that may result in decreased visual acuity, especially at night and in patients with central lens changes, and impairment of depth perception. Advise caution while driving at night or performing hazardous activities in reduced lighting.

Pulmonary disease: Pilocarpine has been reported to increase airway resistance, bronchial smooth muscle tone, and bronchial secretions. Administer with caution and under close medical supervision in patients with controlled asthma, chronic bronchitis, or chronic obstructive pulmonary disease.

Elderly: Adverse events reported by those > 65 and those ≤ 65 years of age were comparable. Elderly women volunteers had a higher C_{max} and AUC than elderly men.

Pregnancy: Category C.

Lactation: It is not known whether this drug is excreted in breast milk.

Children: Safety and efficacy in children have not been established.

Precautions

Toxicity: Toxicity is characterized by an exaggeration of parasympathomimetic effects which may include the following: Headache; visual disturbance; lacrimation; sweating; respiratory distress; GI spasm; nausea; vomiting; diarrhea; AV block; tachycardia; bradycardia; hypotension; hypertension; shock; mental confusion; cardiac arrhythmia; tremors.

Biliary tract: Administer with caution to patients with known or suspected cholelithiasis or biliary tract disease. Contractions of the gallbladder or biliary smooth muscle could precipitate complications including cholecystitis, cholangitis, and biliary obstruction.

Renal colic: Pilocarpine may increase ureteral smooth muscle tone and could theoretically precipitate renal colic (or "ureteral reflux"), particularly in patients with nephrolithiasis.

Psychiatric disorder: Cholinergic agonists may have dose-related CNS effects. Consider this when treating patients with underlying cognitive or psychiatric disturbances.

Drug Interactions

Drugs that may interact with pilocarpine include beta blockers and anticholinergics.

Drug/Food interactions: The rate of absorption of pilocarpine is decreased when taken with a high-fat meal. Maximum concentration is decreased and time to reach maximum concentration is increased.

Adverse Reactions

The most frequent adverse experiences associated with pilocarpine were a consequence of the expected pharmacologic effects. Adverse reactions occurring in ≥ 3% of patients include the following: Sweating, nausea, rhinitis, chills, flushing, urinary frequency, dizziness, asthenia, headache, dyspepsia, lacrimation, diarrhea, edema, abdominal pain, amblyopia, vomiting, pharyngitis, and hypertension.

Chapter 9
SYSTEMIC ANTI-INFECTIVE AGENTS

Penicillins, 719
Cephalosporins, 740
Carbapenem, 766
   Meropenem, 766
   Imipenem-Cilastatin, 768
   Ertapenem, 772
Monobactams, 775
   Aztreonam, 775
Chloramphenicol, 778
Fluoroquinolones, 781
Tetracyclines, 804
Macrolides, 811
Vancomycin, 822
Oxalodinones, 825
   Linezolid, 825
Lincosamides, 828
Aminoglycosides, Parenteral, 832
Aminoglycosides, Oral, 840
Metronidazole, 842
Antifungal Agents, 845
   Nystatin, 845
   Miconazole, 845
   Ketoconazole, 846
   Amphotericin B, 848
   Griseofulvin, 853
   Fluconazole, 854
   Itraconazole, 857
   Terbinafine, 862
Sulfonamides, 864
Antituberculosis Drugs, 867
   Isoniazid, 869
   Rifampin, 871
   Rifabutin, 873
   Ethambutol HCl, 875
   Pyrazinamide, 876
   Aminosalicylate Sodium, 878
   Ethionamide, 879
   Cycloserine, 880
   Streptomycin Sulfate, 882
   Capreomycin, 884
   Rifapentine, 886

Antiviral Agents, 888
   Foscarnet, 888
   Ganciclovir, 891
   Valganciclovir, 895
   Acyclovir, 898
   Famciclovir, 901
   Valacyclovir, 903
   Amantadine, 905
   Ribavirin, 908
   Rimantadine HCl, 913
   Zanamivir, 915
   Oseltamivir, 916
Antiretroviral Agents, 919
   Saquinavir, 919
   Ritonavir, 921
   Indinavir, 924
   Nelfinavir, 926
   Amprenavir, 928
   Lopinavir/Ritonavir, 930
   Tenofovir Disoproxil Fumarate, 933
   Didanosine, 935
   Lamivudine, 940
   Stavudine, 944
   Zalcitabine, 947
   Zidovudine, 951
   Abacavir, 954
   Lamivudine/Zidovudine, 957
   Abacavir Sulfate/Lamivudine/Zidovudine, 958
   Nevirapine, 962
   Delavirdine, 964
   Efavirenz, 966
Miscellaneous Anti-Infectives, 970
   Trimethoprim/Sulfamethoxazole, 970
   Erythromycin/Sulfisoxazole, 973
   Pentamidine Isethionate, 973
   Atovaquone, 975
   Trimetrexate, 977
Anthelmintics, 979

PENICILLINS

AMOXICILLIN
Tablets, chewable: 125 and 250 mg (as trihydrate) (*Rx*)
Capsules: 250 and 500 mg (as trihydrate) (*Rx*)

Various, *Amoxil* (GlaxoSmithKline)
Various, *Amoxil* (GlaxoSmithKline), *Trimox* (Apothecon), *Wymox* (Wyeth-Ayerst)

Powder for oral suspension: 50 mg/mL, 125 and 250 mg/5 mL (as trihydrate) when reconstituted (*Rx*)

Various, *Amoxil* (GlaxoSmithKline), *Amoxil Pediatric Drops* (GlaxoSmithKline), *Trimox* (Apothecon), *Trimox Pediatric Drops* (Apothecon), *Wymox* (Wyeth-Ayerst)

AMOXICILLIN AND POTASSIUM CLAVULANATE
Tablets: 250, 500, or 875 mg amoxicillin (as trihydrate) and 125 mg clavulanic acid (*Rx*)

Augmentin (GlaxoSmithKline)

Tablets, chewable: 125 mg amoxicillin (as trihydrate) and 31.25 mg clavulanic acid; 200 mg amoxicillin (as trihydrate) and 28.5 mg clavulanic acid; 250 mg amoxicillin (as trihydrate) and 62.5 mg clavulanic acid; 400 mg amoxicillin (as trihydrate) and 57 mg clavulanic acid (*Rx*)

Powder for oral suspension: 125 mg amoxicillin and 31.25 mg clavulanic acid/5 mL; 200 mg amoxicillin and 28.5 mg clavulanic acid/5 mL; 250 mg amoxicillin and 62.5 mg clavulanic acid/5 mL; 400 mg amoxicillin and 57 mg clavulanic acid/5 mL (*Rx*)

AMPICILLIN
Capsules: 250 and 500 mg (as trihydrate or anhydrous) (*Rx*)

Various, *Principen* (Apothecon), *Totacillin* (GlaxoSmithKline), *Omnipen* (Wyeth-Ayerst), *Marcillin* (Marnel)

Powder for oral suspension: 125 and 250 mg/5 mL (as trihydrate) when reconstituted (*Rx*)

Various, *Omnipen* (Wyeth-Ayerst), *Totacillin* (GlaxoSmithKline), *Principen* (Apothecon)

AMPICILLIN SODIUM, PARENTERAL
Powder for injection: 125, 250, and 500 mg and 1, 2, and 10 g (*Rx*)

Various, *Omnipen-N* (Wyeth-Ayerst)

AMPICILLIN SODIUM AND SULBACTAM SODIUM
Powder for injection: 1.5 g (1 g ampicillin sodium/0.5 g sulbactam sodium), 3 g (2 g ampicillin sodium/1 g sulbactam sodium), 10 g (10 g ampicillin sodium/5 g sulbactam sodium) (*Rx*)

Unasyn (Roerig)

BACAMPICILLIN HCl
Tablets: 400 mg (chemically equivalent to 280 mg ampicillin) (*Rx*)

Spectrobid (Roerig)

CARBENICILLIN INDANYL SODIUM
Tablets, film-coated: 382 mg carbenicillin (118 mg indanyl sodium ester) (*Rx*)

Geocillin (Roerig)

CLOXACILLIN SODIUM
Capsules: 250 and 500 mg (*Rx*)
Powder for oral suspension: 125 mg/5 mL when reconstituted (*Rx*)

Various, *Cloxapen* (GlaxoSmithKline)
Various

DICLOXACILLIN SODIUM
Capsules: 125, 250, and 500 mg (*Rx*)

Various, *Dycill* (GlaxoSmithKline), *Pathocil* (Wyeth-Ayerst), *Dynapen* (Apothecon)

Powder for oral suspension: 62.5 mg/5 mL reconstituted (*Rx*)

Dynapen (Apothecon), *Pathocil* (Wyeth-Ayerst)

MEZLOCILLIN SODIUM
Powder for injection: 1, 2, 3, 4, and 20 g (*Rx*)

Mezlin (Bayer)

NAFCILLIN SODIUM
Capsules: 250 mg (*Rx*)
Powder for injection: 500 mg, 1, 2, and 10 g (*Rx*)

Unipen (Wyeth-Ayerst)
Nallpen (GlaxoSmithKline)

OXACILLIN SODIUM
Capsules: 250 and 500 mg (*Rx*)
Powder for oral solution: 250 mg/5 mL when reconstituted (*Rx*)

Various
Various

OXACILLIN SODIUM, PARENTERAL
Powder for injection: 250 and 500 mg, 1, 2, 4, and 10 g (*Rx*)

Various, *Bactocill* (GlaxoSmithKline)

PENICILLIN G (AQUEOUS)	
Injection, premixed, frozen: 1, 2, and 3 million units (*Rx*)	*Penicillin G Potassium* (Baxter)
Powder for injection: 1, 5, 10, and 20 million units/vial (*Rx*)	*Pfizerpen* (Roerig), *Penicillin G Potassium*, *Penicillin G Sodium* (Marsam)
PENICILLIN G BENZATHINE, IM	
Injection: 300,000 units/mL; 600,000 units, 1,200,000, and 2,400,000 units/dose (*Rx*)	*Bicillin L-A* (Wyeth-Ayerst), *Permapen* (Roerig)
PENICILLIN G PROCAINE, IM	
Injection: 600,000, 1,200,000, and 2,400,000 units/unit dose (*Rx*)	*Wycillin* (Wyeth-Ayerst)
PENICILLIN G BENZATHINE AND PROCAINE COMBINED, IM	
Injection: 300,000 units/mL; 600,000, 1,200,000, and 2,400,000 units/dose; 900,000 units penicillin G benzathine and 300,000 units penicillin G procaine/dose (*Rx*)	*Bicillin C-R*, *Bicillin C-R 900/300* (Wyeth-Ayerst)
PENICILLIN V (PHENOXYMETHYL PENICILLIN)	
Tablets: 250 and 500 mg (*Rx*)	*Various*, *Beepen-VK* (GlaxoSmithKline), *Pen•Vee K* (Wyeth-Ayerst), *Veetids* (Apothecon)
Powder for oral solution: 125 or 250 mg/5 mL when reconstituted (*Rx*)	*Various*, *Beepen-VK* (GlaxoSmithKline), *Pen•Vee K* (Wyeth-Ayerst), *Veetids* (Apothecon), *Veetids '250'* (Apothecon)
PIPERACILLIN SODIUM	
Powder for injection: 2, 3, 4, and 40 g (*Rx*)	*Pipracil* (Lederle)
PIPERACILLIN SODIUM AND TAZOBACTAM SODIUM	
Powder for injection: 2 g piperacillin/0.25 g tazobactam; 3 g piperacillin/0.375 g tazobactam; 4 g piperacillin/0.5 g tazobactam; 36 g piperacillin/4.5 g tazobactam (*Rx*)	*Zosyn* (Wyeth-Ayerst)
TICARCILLIN DISODIUM	
Powder for injection: 1, 3, 6, 20, and 30 g (as disodium) (*Rx*)	*Ticar* (GlaxoSmithKline)
TICARCILLIN AND CLAVULANATE POTASSIUM	
Powder for injection: 3 g ticarcillin (as disodium) and 0.1 g clavulanic acid (as potassium) (*Rx*)	*Timentin* (GlaxoSmithKline)
Injection solution: 3 g ticarcillin (as disodium) and 0.1 g clavulanic acid (as potassium)/100 mL (*Rx*)	

Indications

Oral: Penicillins are generally indicated in the treatment of mild to moderately severe infections caused by penicillin-sensitive microorganisms.

Penicillinase-resistant penicillins: The percentage of staphylococcal isolates resistant to **penicillin G** outside the hospital is increasing, approximating the high percentage found in the hospital. Therefore, use a penicillinase-resistant penicillin as initial therapy for any suspected staphylococcal infection until culture and sensitivity results are known.

When treatment is initiated before definitive culture and sensitivity results are known, consider that these agents are only effective in the treatment of infections caused by pneumococci, group A beta-hemolytic streptococci, and penicillin G-resistant and penicillin G-sensitive staphylococci.

Parenteral: In patients with severe infection, or when there is nausea, vomiting, gastric dilatation, cardiospasm, or intestinal hypermotility.

Administration and Dosage

Therapy may be initiated prior to obtaining results of bacteriologic studies when there is reason to believe the causative organisms may be susceptible. Once results are known, adjust therapy.

Continue treatment of all infections for a minimum of 48 to 72 hours beyond the time that the patient becomes asymptomatic or evidence of bacterial eradication has been obtained, unless single-dose therapy is employed.

AMOXICILLIN: Larger doses may be required for persistent or severe infections. The children's dose is intended for individuals whose weight will not cause the calculated dosage to be greater than that recommended for adults; the children's dose should not exceed the maximum adult dose.

Amoxicillin Uses and Dosages	
Organisms/Infections	Dosage
Infections of the ear, nose, and throat caused by strepto-cocci, pneumococci, nonpenicillinase-producing staphylo-cocci, and *Haemophilus influenzae* *Infections of the GU tract* caused by *Escherichia coli*, *Proteus mirabilis*, and *Streptococcus faecalis* *Infections of the skin and soft tissues* caused by streptococci, susceptible staphylococci, and *E. coli*	*Adults and children (> 20 kg)* – 250 to 500 mg every 8 hrs *Children* – 20 to 40 mg/kg/day in divided doses every 8 hrs
Infections of the lower respiratory tract caused by strepto-cocci, pneumococci, nonpenicillinase-producing staphylo-cocci, and *H. influenzae*	*Adults and children (> 20 kg)* – 500 mg every 8 hrs *Children* – 40 mg/kg/day in divided doses every 8 hrs
Gonorrheal infections: Uncomplicated urethral, endocervical, or rectal infection	*Adults:* 3 g as a single oral dose *Prepubertal children (> 2 years):* 50 mg/kg amoxicillin combined with 25 mg/kg probenecid as a single dose
Prevention of bacterial endocarditis: For dental, oral, or upper respiratory tract procedures in patients at risk Standard regimen:	2 g (50 mg/kg for children) orally 1 hr prior to procedure
For GU or GI procedures Standard regimen:	2 g ampicillin (50 mg/kg for children) plus 1.5 mg/kg genta-micin (2 mg/kg for children) not to exceed 80 mg, both IM or IV ½ hr prior to procedure, followed by 1.5 g amoxicillin (25 mg/kg for children)
Moderate-risk patients:	2 g (50 mg/kg for children) orally 1 hr prior to procedure
Alternate low-risk patient regimen:	3 g 1 hr before procedure, then 1.5 g 6 hrs after initial dose
Unlabeled use: *Chlamydia trachomatis* in pregnancy	As an alternative to erythromycin; 500 mg orally 3 times/day for 7 days.

Children –

Administration and Dosage of Pediatric Amoxicillin Drops
Usual dosage for all indications except infections of the lower respiratory tract:
< 6 kg (13 lbs): 0.75 mL every 8 hrs
6 to 7 kg (13 to 15 lbs): 1 mL every 8 hrs
8 kg (16 to 18 lbs): 1.25 mL every 8 hrs
Infections of the lower respiratory tract:
< 6 kg (13 lbs): 1.25 mL every 8 hrs
6 to 7 kg (13 to 15 lbs): 1.75 mL every 8 hrs
8 kg (16 to 18 lbs): 2.25 mL every 8 hrs
Children weighing > 8 kg (18 lbs) should receive the appropriate dose of the oral suspension, 125 mg or 250 mg/5 mL.

AMOXICILLIN AND POTASSIUM CLAVULANATE: May be administered without regard to meals.

Because the 250 and 500 mg tablets contain the same amount of clavulanic acid (125 mg as potassium salt), two 250 mg tablets are not equivalent to one 500 mg tablet.

The 875 mg tablet also contains 125 mg potassium clavulanate. In addition, the 250 mg tablet and 250 mg chewable tablet do not contain the same amount of potassium clavulanate and should not be substituted for each other, as they are not interchangeable.

Usual dose – Children's dose is based on amoxicillin content.

Adults: One 250 mg tablet every 8 hours or one 500 mg tablet every 12 hours.

Suspension – Adults who have difficulty swallowing may be given the 125 mg/5 mL or 250 mg/5 mL suspension in place of the 500 mg tablet or give 200 mg/5 mL or 400 mg/5 mL suspension in place of the 875 mg tablet.

Children:

< 3 months old – 30 mg/kg/day divided every 12 hours, based on the amoxi-cillin component. Use of the 125 mg/5 mL oral suspension is recommended.

≥ 3 months old – Children's dose is based on amoxicillin content. Refer to the following table. Because of the different amoxicillin to clavulanic acid ratios

in the 250 mg tablets (250/125) vs the 250 mg chewable tablets (250/62.5), do not use the 250 mg tablet until the child weighs ≥ 40 kg.

≥ 40 kg – Dose according to adult recommendations.

Amoxicillin/Potassium Clavulanate Dosing in Children ≥ 3 Months of Age		
Infections	Dosing regimen	
	200 mg/5 mL or 400 mg/5 mL (q 12 hr)[1,2]	125 mg/5 mL or 250 mg/5 mL (q 8 hr)[2]
Otitis media,[3] sinusitis, lower respiratory tract infections, severe infections	45 mg/kg/day	40 mg/kg/day
Less severe infections	25 mg/kg/day	20 mg/kg/day

[1] The every-12-hour regimen is associated with significantly less diarrhea; however, the 200 and 400 mg formulations (suspension and chewable tablets) contain aspartame and should not be used by phenylketonurics.
[2] Each strength of the suspension is available as a chewable tablet for use by older children.
[3] Recommended duration is 10 days.

Severe infections and respiratory tract infections –

Adults: One 500 mg tablet every 8 hours or one 875 mg tablet every 12 hours.

Renal function impairment – Renal function impairment does not generally require a dose reduction unless impairment is severe. Severely impaired patients with a glomerular filtration rate (GFR) of < 30 mL/min should not receive the 875 mg tablet. Give patients with a GFR of 10 to 30 mL/min 500 or 250 mg every 12 hours, depending on the severity of infection. Give patients with a GFR < 10 mL/min 500 or 250 mg every 24 hours, depending on severity of infection. Give hemodialysis patients 500 or 250 mg every 24 hours, and an additional dose during and at the end of dialysis.

Hepatic function impairment – Dose with caution and monitor hepatic function.

AMPICILLIN:

Ampicillin Uses and Dosages	
Organisms/Infections	Dosage
Labeled uses:	
Respiratory tract and soft tissue infections:	*Parenteral:* Patients ≥ 40 kg – 250 to 500 mg every 6 hrs; < 40 kg – 25 to 50 mg/kg/day in divided doses at 6- to 8-hr intervals *Oral:* Patients ≥ 20 kg – 250 mg every 6 hrs; < 20 kg – 50 mg/kg/day in divided doses at 6- to 8-hr intervals
Bacterial meningitis: Haemophilus influenzae, Streptococcus pneumoniae, or *Neisseria meningitidis*	150 to 200 mg/kg/day in divided doses every 3 to 4 hrs. Initial treatment is usually by IV drip, followed by frequent (every 3 to 4 hrs) IM injections.
Septicemia:	*Adults and children:* 150 to 200 mg/kg/day. Give IV at least 3 days; continue IM every 3 to 4 hrs.
GI and GU infections: Other than *Neisseria gonorrhea*	*Oral:* Adults/children > 20 kg: 500 mg orally every 6 hrs. Use larger doses for severe or chronic infections, if needed. Children ≤ 20 kg: 100 mg/kg/day every 6 hrs
N. gonorrhea	*Oral:* Single dose of 3.5 g administered simultaneously with 1 g probenecid *Parenteral:* Adults/Children ≥ 40 kg: 500 mg IV or IM every 6 hrs Children < 40 kg: 50 mg/kg/day IV or IM in equally divided doses 6- to 8-hr intervals
Urethritis caused by *N. gonorrhea* in males	*Parenteral:* Males ≥ 40 kg: Two 500 mg doses, IV or IM, at an interval of 8 to 12 hrs. Treatment may be repeated if necessary or extended if required. In complicated gonorrheal urethritis (eg, prostatitis, epididymitis), prolonged and intensive therapy is recommended.

| Ampicillin Uses and Dosages ||
Organisms/Infections	Dosage
Prevention of bacterial endocarditis: For dental, oral or upper respiratory tract procedures in patients at moderate risk or patients unable to take oral medications	2 g (50 mg/kg for children), both IM or IV 30 min prior to procedure
High-risk	*Adults:* 2 g ampicillin IM/IV plus 1.5 mg/kg gentamicin 30 min prior to procedure; 6 hrs later, ampicillin 1 g IM/IV or amoxicillin 1 g orally *Children:* Ampicillin 50 mg/kg IM/IV plus gentamicin 1.5 mg/kg 30 min prior to procedure; 6 hrs later, ampicillin 25 mg/kg IM/IV or amoxicillin 25 mg/kg orally
Unlabeled use:	
Prophylaxis in cesarean section in certain high-risk patients	Single IV dose, administered immediately after cord clamping

Renal impairment – Increase dosing interval to 12 hours in severe renal impairment (Ccr ≤ 10 mL/min).

Adults – 1 to 12 g daily in divided doses every 4 to 6 hours.

Children – 50 to 400 mg/kg/day in divided doses every 4 to 6 hours.

Infants > 7 days: 25 mg/kg/day in divided doses every 8 hours (meningitis: 50 mg/kg every 6 hours).

Infants < 7 days: 25 mg/kg/day in divided doses every 12 hours (meningitis: 50 mg/kg every 12 hours).

AMPICILLIN SODIUM AND SULBACTAM SODIUM: Give IV or IM. The recommended adult dosage is 1.5 g (1 g ampicillin plus 0.5 g sulbactam) to 3 g (2 g ampicillin plus 1 g sulbactam) every 6 hours. Do not exceed 4 g/day sulbactam.

Renal function impairment – The elimination kinetics of ampicillin and sulbactam are similarly affected; hence, the ratio of one to the other will remain constant whatever the renal function. In patients with renal impairment, give as follows:

| Ampicillin/Sulbactam Dosage Guide For Patients With Renal Impairment |||
Ccr (mL/min/1.72 m^2)	Half-life (hours)	Recommended dosage
≥ 30	1	1.5 to 3 g q 6 to 8 h
15 to 29	5	1.5 to 3 q 12 h
5 to 14	9	1.5 to 3 g q 24 h

Children – Do not routinely exceed 14 days of IV therapy. Safety and efficacy of IM administration have not been established.

Children ≥ 1 year of age (< 40 kg): 300 mg/kg/day IV (200 mg ampicillin/100 mg sulbactam) in divided doses every 6 hours.

Children ≥ 40 kg: Dose according to adult recommendations; total sulbactam dose should not exceed 4 g/day.

The safety and efficacy of ampicillin/sulbacatam sodium have been established for pediatric patients ≥ 1 year of age for skin and skin structure infections as approved in adults but have not been established for pediatric patients for intra-abdominal infections.

BACAMPICILLIN HCl: Tablets may be given without regard to meals; administer suspension to fasting patients.

Upper respiratory tract infections – Upper respiratory tract infections (including otitis media) caused by streptococci, pneumococci, nonpenicillinase-producing staphylococci, and *H. influenzae*; urinary tract infections caused by *E. coli*, *P. mirabilis*, and *S. faecalis*; skin and skin structure infections caused by streptococci and susceptible staphylococci:

Adults: 400 mg every 12 hours.

Children (≥ 25 kg): 25 mg/kg/day in equally divided doses at 12-hour intervals.

Severe infections or those caused by less-susceptible organisms –
 Adults: 800 mg every 12 hours.
 Children (≥ 25 kg): 50 mg/kg/day in equally divided doses at 12-hour intervals.
Lower respiratory tract infections – Lower respiratory tract infections caused by streptococci, pneumococci, nonpenicillinase-producing staphylococci, and *H. influenzae:*
 Adults: 800 mg every 12 hours.
 Children (≥ 25 kg): 50 mg/kg/day in equally divided doses at 12-hour intervals.
Gonorrhea, uncomplicated – The usual adult dosage (males and females) is 1.6 g bacampicillin plus 1 g probenecid as a single oral dose. No pediatric dosage has been established.

CARBENICILLIN INDANYL SODIUM:
 Urinary tract infections –
  E. coli, Proteus species, and Enterobacter: 382 to 764 mg 4 times daily.
  Pseudomonas and enterococci: 764 mg 4 times daily.
  Prostatitis caused by E. coli, P. mirabilis, Enterobacter, and enterococcus (S. faecalis) – 764 mg 4 times daily.

CLOXACILLIN SODIUM:
 Mild to moderate upper respiratory and localized skin and soft tissue infections –
  Adults and children (≥ 20 kg): 250 mg every 6 hours.
  Children (< 20 kg): 50 mg/kg/day in equally divided doses every 6 hours.
 Severe infections (lower respiratory tract or disseminated infections) –
  Adults and children (≥ 20 kg): ≥ 500 mg every 6 hours.
  Children (< 20 kg): ≥ 100 mg/kg/day in equal doses every 6 hours.
  Another suggested dosage for infants and children is 50 to 100 mg/kg/day, up to a maximum of 4 g/day, divided every 6 hours.

DICLOXACILLIN SODIUM:
 For mild to moderate upper respiratory and localized skin and soft tissue infections –
  Adults and children (≥ 40 kg): 125 mg every 6 hours.
  Children (< 40 kg): 12.5 mg/kg/day in equal doses every 6 hours.
 For more severe infections, such as lower respiratory tract or disseminated infections –
  Adults and children (≥ 40 kg): 250 mg every 6 hours.
  Children (< 40 kg): 25 mg/kg/day in equally divided doses every 6 hours.
  Use in the newborn is not recommended.

MEZLOCILLIN SODIUM: Administer IV for serious infections. IM doses should not exceed 2 g/injection.
 Adults – The recommended adult dosage for serious infections is 200 to 300 mg/kg/day given in 4 to 6 divided doses. The usual dose is 3 g given every 4 hours (18 g/day) or 4 g given every 6 hours (16 g/day).
 Infants and children – Limited data are available on the safety and effectiveness in the treatment of infants and children with serious infection.

Mezlocillin Dosage Guidelines for Neonates		
Body weight (g)	Age	
	≤ 7 Days	> 7 Days
≤ 2000	75 mg/kg every 12 hours (150 mg/kg/day)	75 mg/kg every 8 hours (225 mg/kg/day)
> 2000	75 mg/kg every 12 hours (150 mg/kg/day)	75 mg/kg every 6 hours (300 mg/kg/day)

 For infants > 1 month of age and children < 12 years, administer 50 mg/kg every 4 hours (300 mg/kg/day); infuse IV over 30 minutes or administer by IM injection.
 Renal function impairment – After an IV dose of 3 g, the serum half-life is ≈ 1 hour in patients with Ccr > 60 mL/min, 1.3 hours in those with Ccr of 30 to 59 mL/min, 1.6 hours in those with Ccr of 10 to 29 mL/min, and ≈ 3.6 hours in patients with Ccr of < 10 mL/min.

Mezlocillin Uses and Dosages	
Organisms/Infections	Dosage
Urinary infection: Uncomplicated with normal renal function (Ccr ≥ 30 mL/min)	100 to 125 mg/kg/day (6 to 8 g/day); 1.5 to 2 g every 6 hrs IV or IM
Uncomplicated with renal impairment	1.5 g every 8 hrs
Complicated with normal renal function	150 to 200 mg/kg/day (12 g/day); 3 g every 6 hrs IV
Complicated with renal impairment – Ccr	
10 to 30 mL/min	1.5 g every 6 hrs
< 10 mL/min	1.5 g every 8 hrs
Lower respiratory tract infection, intra-abdominal infection, gynecological infection, skin and skin structure infections, septicemia:	225 to 300 mg/kg/day (16 to 18 g/day); 4 g every 6 hrs or 3 g every 4 hrs IV
Serious systemic infection with renal impairment – Ccr	
10 to 30 mL/min	3 g every 8 hrs
< 10 mL/min	2 g every 8 hrs
Serious systemic infection undergoing hemodialysis for renal failure peritoneal dialysis	3 to 4 g after each dialysis; then every 12 hrs. 3 g every 12 hrs
Life-threatening infections:	Up to 350 mg/kg/day; 4 g every 4 hrs (24 g/day maximum)
In patients with renal impairment- Ccr	
10 to 30 mL/min	3 g every 8 hrs
< 10 mL/min	2 g every 8 hrs
Acute, uncomplicated gonococcal urethritis:	1 to 2 g IV or IM; plus 1 g probenecid at time of dosing or up to ½ hour before
Prophylaxis: To prevent postoperative infection in contaminated or potentially contaminated surgery	4 g IV, ½ to 1½ hr prior to start of surgery; 4 g IV, 6 and 12 hrs later
Caesarean section patients –	First dose: 4 g IV when umbilical cord is clamped; second dose: 4 g IV, 4 hrs after first dose; third dose: 4 g IV, 8 hrs after first dose

NAFCILLIN SODIUM:
> Parenteral –
>> IV: 3 to 6 g per 24 hours. Use this route for short-term therapy (24 to 48 hours) because of occasional occurrence of thrombophlebitis, particularly in the elderly.
>> IM:
>>> Adults – 500 mg every 4 to 6 hours.
>>> Infants and children (< 40 kg) – 25 mg/kg twice daily. Other suggested dosing is 100 to 200 mg/kg/day IM or IV, given in 4 or 6 divided doses.
>>> Neonates – 10 mg/kg twice daily. Other suggested doses include: Weight < 2000 g – 50 mg/kg/day divided every 12 hours (age < 7 days) or 75 mg/kg/day divided every 8 hours (age > 7 days).
>>> Weight > 2000 g – 50 mg/kg/day divided every 8 hours (age < 7 days) or 75 mg/kg/day divided every 6 hours (age > 7 days).
> Oral – Serum levels of oral nafcillin are low and unpredictable.
>> Adults: 250 to 500 mg every 4 to 6 hours for mild to moderate infections. In severe infections – 1 g every 4 to 6 hours.
>> Children:
>>> Staphylococcal infections – 50 mg/kg/day in 4 divided doses. For neonates, 10 mg/kg 3 to 4 times daily. If inadequate, change to parenteral nafcillin sodium.
>>> Scarlet fever and pneumonia – 25 mg/kg/day in 4 divided doses.
>>> Streptococcal pharyngitis – 250 mg 3 times daily for 10 days. (Penicillin V is the drug of choice for streptococcal infections.)
>> Neonates: 10 mg/kg 3 to 4 times daily. If inadequate, change to parenteral nafcillin sodium.

OXACILLIN SODIUM:

Oxacillin Dosage		
Indication	Adults	Children (< 40 kg)
Oral		
Mild to moderate infection	500 mg every 4 to 6 hours	50 mg/kg/day in equally divided doses every 6 hours
Severe infection	1 g every 4 to 6 hours	100 mg/kg/day in equally divided doses every 4 to 6 hours
Parenteral (IM or IV)		
Mild to moderate infection	250 to 500 mg IM or IV every 4 to 6 hours	50 mg/kg/day IM or IV in equally divided doses every 6 hours
Severe infection	1 g IM or IV every 4 to 6 hours	100 mg/kg/day IM or IV in equally divided doses every 4 to 6 hours. **Premature/neonates**: 25 mg/kg/day IM or IV

Other suggested doses for children and neonates include –
Children: 50 to 100 mg/kg/day divided every 6 hours.
Neonates: Weight < 2000 g – 50 mg/kg/day divided every 12 hours (age < 7 days) or 100 mg/kg/day divided every 8 hours (age > 7 days).
Weight > 2000 g – 75 mg/kg/day divided every 8 hours (age < 7 days) or 150 mg/kg/day divided every 6 hours (age > 7 days).

PENICILLIN G (AQUEOUS): Give recommended daily dosage IM or by continuous IV infusion.

IM – Keep total volume of injection small. The IM route is the preferred route of administration. Solutions containing ≤ 100,000 units/mL may be used with a minimum of discomfort. Use greater concentrations as required.

Continuous IV infusion – When larger doses are required, administer aqueous solutions by means of continuous IV infusion. Determine volume and rate of fluid administration required by the patient in a 24-hour period. Add appropriate daily dosage to this fluid.

Intrapleural or other local infusion – If fluid is aspirated, give infusion in a volume equal to ¼ or ½ the amount of fluid aspirated; otherwise, prepare as for the IM injection.

Intrathecal use – Must be highly individualized. Use only with full consideration of the possible irritating effects of penicillin when used by this route. The preferred route of therapy in bacterial meningitis is IV, supplemented by IM injection. It has been suggested that intrathecal use has no place in therapy.

Infants – Preferably administered IV as 15- to 30-minute infusions.
Over 7 days old: 75,000 units/kg/day in divided doses every 8 hours (meningitis – 200,000 to 300,000 units/kg/day every 6 hours).
Under 7 days old: 50,000 units/kg/day in divided doses every 12 hours (group B streptococcus – 100,000 units/kg/day; meningitis – 100,000 to 150,000 units/kg/day).

Parenteral Penicillin G Use and Dosages in Adults	
Indications	Adult dosage
Labeled uses:	
Meningococcal meningitis/septicemia:	24 million units/day; 1 to 2 million units IM every 2 hours; or 20 to 30 million units/day continuous IV drip for 14 days or until afebrile for 7 days; or 200,000 to 300,000 units/kg/day every 2 to 4 hours in divided doses for a total of 24 doses
Actinomycosis	
For cervicofacial cases	1 to 6 million units/day
For thoracic and abdominal disease	10 to 20 million units/day IV every 4 to 6 hours for 6 weeks. May be followed by oral penicillin V, 500 mg 4 times daily for 2 to 3 months

Parenteral Penicillin G Use and Dosages in Adults	
Indications	Adult dosage
Clostridial infections: Botulism (adjunctive therapy to antitoxin), gas gangrene and tetanus (adjunctive therapy to human tetanus immune globulin)	20 million units/day every 4 to 6 hours as adjunct to antitoxin
Fusospirochetal infections: Severe infections of oropharynx, lower respiratory tract and genital area	5 to 10 million units/day every 4 to 6 hours
Rat-bite fever (Spirillum minus, Streptobacillus moniliformis), Haverhill fever	12 to 20 million units/day every 4 to 6 hours for 3 to 4 weeks
Listeria infections (Listeria monocytogenes): Meningitis (adults)	15 to 20 million units/day every 4 to 6 hours for 2 weeks
Endocarditis (adults)	15 to 20 million units/day every 4 to 6 hours for 4 weeks
Pasteurella infections (Pasteurella multocida): Bacteremia and meningitis	4 to 6 million units/day every 4 to 6 hours for 2 weeks
Erysipeloid (Erysipelothrix rhusiopathiae): Endocarditis	12 to 20 million units/day every 4 to 6 hours for 4 to 6 weeks
Diphtheria: Adjunct to antitoxin to prevent carrier state	2 to 3 million units/day in divided doses every 4 to 6 hours for 10 to 12 days
Anthrax: (Bacillus anthracis is often resistant)	Minimum 5 million units/day; 12 to 20 million units/day have been used
Serious streptococcal infections (S. pneumoniae): Empyema, pneumonia, pericarditis, endocarditis, meningitis	5 to 24 million units/day in divided doses every 4 to 6 hours
Syphilis: Neurosyphilis	18 to 24 million units/day IV (3 to 4 million units every 4 hours) for 10 to 14 days. Many recommend benzathine penicillin G 2.4 million units IM weekly for 3 weeks following the completion of this regimen
Disseminated gonococcal infections: (eg, meningitis, endocarditis, arthritis)	10 million units/day every 4 to 6 hours, with the exception of meningococcal meningitis/septicemia (ie, every 2 hours)
Unlabeled uses: Lyme disease (Borrelia burgdorferi): Erythema chronicum migrans	Use oral penicillin V
Neurologic complications (eg, meningitis, encephalitis)	200,000 to 300,000 units/kg/day (up to 20 million units) IV for 10 to 14 days
Carditis	200,000 to 300,000 units/kg/day (up to 20 million units) IV for 10 days with cardiac monitoring and a temporary pacemaker for complete heart block
Arthritis	200,000 to 300,000 units/kg/day (up to 20 million units) IV for 10 to 20 days

Children –

Parenteral Penicillin G Use and Dosages in Children

Indications	Pediatric dosage
Serious streptococcal infections, such as pneumonia and endocarditis (*S. pneumoniae*) and meningococcus	150,000 units/kg/day divided in equal doses every 4 to 6 hours; duration depends on infecting organism and type of infection
Meningitis caused by susceptible strains of pneumococcus and meningococcus	250,000 units/kg/day divided in equal doses every 4 hours for 7 to 14 days depending on the infecting organism (maximum dose of 12 to 20 million units/day)
Disseminated gonococcal infections (penicillin-susceptible strains):	*Weight < 45 kg:*
Arthritis	100,000 units/kg/day in 4 equally divided doses for 7 to 10 days
Meningitis	250,000 units/kg/day in equal doses every 4 hours for 10 to 14 days
Endocarditis	250,000 units/kg/day in equal doses every 4 hours for 4 weeks
	Weight ≥ 45 kg:
Arthritis, meningitis, endocarditis	10 million units/day in 4 equally divided doses with the duration of therapy depending on the type of infection
Syphilis (congenital and neurosyphilis) after the newborn period:	200,000 to 300,000 units/kg/day (administered as 50,000 units/kg every 4 to 6 hours) for 10 to 14 days
Congenital syphilis: Symptomatic or asymptomatic infants	*Infants:* 50,000 units/kg/dose IV every 12 hours the first 7 days, thereafter every 8 hours for total of 10 days. *Children:* 50,000 units/kg every 4 to 6 hours for 10 days.
Diphtheria (adjunctive therapy to antitoxin and for prevention of carrier state)	150,000 to 250,000 units/kg/day in equal doses every 6 hours for 7 to 10 days
Rat-bite fever; Haverhill fever (with endocarditis caused by S. moniliformis)	150,000 to 250,000 units/kg/day in equal doses every 4 hours for 4 weeks

PENICILLIN G BENZATHINE, IM: Administer by deep IM injection in the upper outer quadrant of the buttock. In infants and small children, the midlateral aspect of the thigh may be preferable. Do not inject benzathine penicillin into the gluteal region of children < 2 years of age. When doses are repeated, rotate the injection site. Do not administer IV.

Penicillin G Benzathine Uses and Dosages

Organisms/Infections	Dosage
Streptococcal (group A): Upper respiratory tract infections	*Adults:* 1.2 million units IM as a single injection *Older children:* 900,000 units IM as a single injection *Infants and children (< 60 lbs; 27 kg):* 300,000 to 600,000 units
Syphilis: Early syphilis - Primary, secondary or latent syphilis	*Adults:* 2.4 million units IM in single dose *Children:* 50,000 units/kg IM, up to adult dosage
Gummas and cardiovascular syphilis - Latent	*Adults:* 2.4 million units IM once weekly for 3 weeks *Children:* 50,000 units/kg IM, up to adult dosage

| Penicillin G Benzathine Uses and Dosages ||
Organisms/Infections	Dosage
Neurosyphilis	Aqueous penicillin G, 18 to 24 million units/day IV (3 to 4 million units every 4 hours) for 10 to 14 days. Many recommend benzathine penicillin G, 2.4 million IM units following completion of this regimen.
	or
	Procaine penicillin G, 2.4 million units/day IM *plus* probenecid 500 mg orally 4 times daily, both for 10 to 14 days. Many recommend benzathine penicillin G, 2.4 million units IM following completion of this regimen.
Syphilis in pregnancy	Dosage schedule appropriate for stage of syphilis recommended for nonpregnant patients.
Yaws, bejel and pinta	1.2 million units IM in a single dose
Prophylaxis for rheumatic fever and glomerulo-nephritis	Following an acute attack, may be given IM in doses of 1.2 million units once a month or 600,000 units every 2 weeks

PENICILLIN G PROCAINE, IM: Administer by deep IM injection only into the upper outer quadrant of the buttock. In infants and small children, the midlateral aspect of the thigh may be preferable. When doses are repeated, rotate the injection site. Do not inject into or near an artery or nerve. Penicillin G procaine must never be used IV.

Adults and children – 600,000 to 1.2 million units/day IM in 1 or 2 doses (up to a maximum of 4.8 million units/day) for 10 days to 2 weeks.

Newborns – 50,000 units/kg IM once daily. Avoid use in these patients because sterile abscesses and procaine toxicity are of much greater concern than in older children.

| Penicillin G Procaine Uses and Dosages ||
Organisms/Infections	Dosage
Pneumococcal infections: Moderately severe upper respiratory tract infections	*Adults:* 600,000 to 1 million units/day IM *Children (< 60 lbs):* 300,000 units/day IM
Streptococcal infections (group A): Moderately severe to severe tonsillitis, erysipelas, scarlet fever, upper respiratory tract, and skin and skin structure infections	*Adults:* 600,000 to 1 million units/day IM for a minimum of 10 days *Children (< 60 lbs):* 300,000 units daily IM
Bacterial endocarditis – Only in extremely sensitive infections (*S. viridans, S. bovis*)	600,000 to 1 million units/day IM
Staphylococcal infections: Moderately severe infections of the skin and skin structure	*Adults:* 600,000 to 1 million units/day IM *Children (< 60 lbs):* 300,000 units daily
Diphtheria: Adjunctive therapy with antitoxin	300,000 to 600,000 units/day IM
Carrier state	300,000 units/day IM for 10 days
Anthrax: Cutaneous	600,000 to 1 million units/day IM
Vincent's gingivitis and pharyngitis (fusospirochetosis)	600,000 to 1 million units/day IM. Obtain necessary dental care in infections involving gum tissue.
Erysipeloid	600,000 to 1 million units/day IM
Rat-bite fever (*S. moniliformis and S. minus*)	600,000 to 1 million units/day IM

Penicillin G Procaine Uses and Dosages

Organisms/Infections	Dosage
Gonorrheal infections (uncomplicated)	4.8 million units divided into at least 2 doses at one visit; 1 g oral probenecid is given just before the injections. Obtain follow-up cultures from the original site(s) of infection 7 to 14 days after therapy. In women, it is also desirable to obtain culture test-of-cure from both the endocervical and anal canals. Note: Treat gonorrheal endocarditis intensively with aqueous penicillin G. Test all gonorrhea patients for syphilis and treat appropriately.
Syphilis: Primary, secondary, and latent with a negative spinal fluid (adults and children > 12 years of age)	600,000 units IM daily for 8 days; total 4.8 million units
Late (tertiary, neurosyphilis, and latent syphilis with positive spinal-fluid examination or no spinal-fluid examination):	600,000 units IM daily for 10 to 15 days; total 6 to 9 million units
Neurosyphilis (as an alternative to the recommended regimen of penicillin G aqueous)	2.4 million units/day IM plus probenecid 500 mg orally 4 times daily, both for 10 to 14 days; many recommend benzathine penicillin G 2.4 million/units IM following the completion of this regimen
Congenital syphilis: Symptomatic and asymptomatic infants	50,000 units/kg/day (administered once IM) for 10 days
Yaws, bejel and pinta:	Treat same as syphilis in corresponding stage of disease

PENICILLIN G BENZATHINE AND PROCAINE COMBINED, IM: Administer by deep IM injection in the upper outer quadrant of the buttock. In infants and small children, the midlateral aspect of the thigh may be preferable. when doses are repeated, rotate the injection site.

Streptococcal infections – Treatment with the recommended dosage is usually given in a single session using multiple IM sites when indicated. An alternative dosage schedule may be used, giving half the total dose on day 1 and half on day 3. This will also ensure adequate serum levels over a 10-day period; however, use only when the patient's cooperation can be ensured.

Adults and children (> 60 lbs; 27 kg): 2.4 million units.

Children (30 to 60 lbs; 14 to 27 kg): 900,000 to 1.2 million units.

Infants and children (< 30 lbs; 14 kg): 600,000 units.

Pneumococcal infections (except pneumococcal meningitis) –

Children: 600,000 units.

Adults: 1.2 million units. Repeat every 2 or 3 days until the patient has been afebrile for 48 hours.

PENICILLIN V (PHENOXYMETHYL PENICILLIN): 250 mg = 400,000 units.

Adults – 125 to 500 mg 4 times/day; in renal impairment (Ccr ≤ 10 mL/min) - Do not exceed 250 mg every 6 hours.

Children – 25 to 50 mg/kg/day in divided doses every 6 to 8 hours.

Penicillin V Uses and Dosages for Adults and Children > 12 Years of Age

Organisms/Infections	Dosage
Labeled uses:	
Streptococcal infections: Infections of the upper respiratory tract, including scarlet fever and mild erysipelas	125 to 250 mg orally every 6 to 8 hours for 10 days
Pharyngitis in children	500 mg orally every 6 hours
Pneumococcal infections: Mild to moderately severe respiratory tract infections including otitis media	250 mg orally every 6 hours until afebrile at least 2 days

Penicillin V Uses and Dosages for Adults and Children > 12 Years of Age	
Organisms/Infections	Dosage
Staphylococcal infections: Mild infections of skin and soft tissue	250 mg orally every 6 to 8 hours
Fusospirochetosis (Vincent's infection) of the oropharynx: Mild-to-moderately severe infections	250 mg orally every 6 to 8 hours
For prevention of recurrence following rheumatic fever or chorea	125 mg orally 2 times daily on a continuing basis
Unlabeled uses:	
Prophylactic treatment of children with sickle cell anemia (to reduce the incidence of S. pneumoniae septicemia)	125 mg orally 2 times daily
Anaerobic infections: Mild to moderate infections	250 mg orally 4 times daily
Lyme disease (Borrelia burgdorferi):	
Erythema chronicum migrans:	
Pregnant or lactating women, tetracycline treatment failures	250 to 500 mg orally 4 times a day for 10 to 20 days
Children < 2 years of age	50 mg/kg/day (up to 2 g/day) orally in 4 divided doses for 10 to 20 days

PIPERACILLIN SODIUM: Administer IM or IV. For serious infections, give 3 to 4 g every 4 to 6 hours as a 20 to 30 minute IV infusion. Maximum daily dose is 24 g/day, although higher doses have been used. Limit IM injections to 2 g/site.

Hemodialysis – Maximum dose is 6 g/day (2 g every 8 hours). Hemodialysis removes 30% to 50% of piperacillin in 4 hours; administer an additional 1 g after dialysis.

Renal failure and hepatic insufficiency – Measure serum levels to provide additional guidance for adjusting dosage; however, this may not be practical.

Infants and children < 12 years of age – Dosages have not been established; however, the following doses have been suggested:

> *Neonates:*
> *Less than 36 weeks of age –* 75 mg/kg IV every 12 hours in the first week of life, then every 8 hours in the second week.
> *Full-term –* 75 mg/kg IV every 8 hours the first week of life, then every 6 hours thereafter.

Other conditions, 200 to 300 mg/kg/day, up to a maximum of 24 g/day divided every 4 to 6 hours.

Piperacillin Uses and Dosages	
Organisms/Infections	Dosage
Serious infections: Septicemia, nosocomial pneumonia, intra-abdominal infections, aerobic and anaerobic gynecologic infections, and skin and soft tissue infections:	12 to 18 g/day IV (200 to 300 mg/kg/day) in divided doses every 4 to 6 hrs
Renal impairment – Ccr	
20 to 40 mL/min	12 g/day; 4 g every 8 hrs
< 20 mL/min	8 g/day; 4 g every 12 hrs
Urinary tract infections: Complicated (normal renal function)	8 to 16 g/day (125 to 200 mg/kg/day) in divided doses every 6 to 8 hrs
Renal impairment – Ccr	
20 to 40 mL/min	9 g/day; 3 g every 8 hrs
< 20 mL/min	6 g/day; 3 g every 12 hrs
Uncomplicated UTI and most community-acquired pneumonia (normal renal function)	6 to 8 g/day IM or IV (100 to 125 mg/kg/day) in divided doses every 6 to 12 hrs
Uncomplicated UTI with renal impairment – Ccr	
< 20 mL/min	6 g/day; 3 g every 12 hrs
Uncomplicated gonorrhea infections:	2 g IM in a single dose with 1 g probenecid ½ hr prior to injection

Piperacillin Uses and Dosages	
Organisms/Infections	Dosage
Prophylaxis: Intra-abdominal surgery	2 g IV just prior to anesthesia; 2 g during surgery; 2 g every 6 hrs post-op for no more than 24 hrs
Vaginal hysterectomy	2 g IV just prior to anesthesia; 2 g 6 hrs after initial dose; 2 g 12 hrs after first dose
Cesarean section	2 g IV after cord is clamped; 2 g 4 hrs after initial dose; 2 g 8 hrs after first dose
Abdominal hysterectomy	2 g IV just prior to anesthesia; 2 g on return to recovery room; 2 g after 6 hrs

PIPERACILLIN SODIUM AND TAZOBACTAM SODIUM: Administer by IV infusion over 30 minutes. The usual total daily dose for adults is 12 g/1.5 g, given as 3.375 g every 6 hours.

Nosocomial pneumonia – Start with 3.375 g every 4 hours plus an aminoglycoside. Continue the aminoglycoside in patients from whom *Pseudomonas aeruginosa* is isolated. If it is not isolated, the aminoglycoside may be discontinued at the discretion of the treating physician as guided by the severity of the infection and the patient's clinical and bacteriological progress.

Renal function impairment – In patients with renal insufficiency (Ccr < 40 mL/min), adjust the IV dose to the degree of actual renal function impairment. Measurement of serum levels of piperacillin and tazobactam will provide additional guidance for adjusting dosage.

Piperacillin Sodium and Tazobactam Sodium Dosage Recommendations	
Creatinine clearance (mL/min)	Recommended dosage regimen
> 40	12 g/1.5 g/day in divided doses of 3.375 g every 6 hours
20 to 40	8 g/1 g/day in divided doses of 2.25 g every 6 hours
< 20	6 g/0.75 g/day in divided doses of 2.25 g every 8 hours

Hemodialysis – The maximum dose is 2.25 g every 8 hours. In addition, because hemodialysis removes 30% to 40% of a dose in 4 hours, give one additional dose of 0.75 g following each dialysis period.

TICARCILLIN DISODIUM: Use IV therapy in higher doses in serious urinary tract and systemic infections. IM injections should not exceed 2 g/injection.

Ticarcillin Uses and Dosages	
Organisms/Infections	Dosage
Bacterial septicemia, respiratory tract infections, skin and soft tissue infections, intra-abdominal infections and infections of the female pelvis and genital tract	*Adults:* 200 to 300 mg/kg/day by IV infusion in divided doses every 4 or 6 hrs (3 g every 4 hrs or 4 g every 6 hrs), depending on weight of patient and severity of infection *Children (< 40 kg):* 200 to 300 mg/kg/day by IV infusion in divided doses every 4 or 6 hr.[1]
Urinary tract infections: Complicated infections	*Adults and children:* 150 to 200 mg/kg/day IV infusion in divided doses every 4 or 6 hrs. Usual dose for average adult (70 kg) is 3 g 4 times daily.
Uncomplicated infections	*Adults:* 1 g IM or direct IV every 6 hours. *Children (< 40 kg):* 50 to 100 mg/kg/day IM or direct IV in divided doses every 6 or 8 hours.
Neonates: Severe infections (sepsis) caused by susceptible strains of *Pseudomonas* sp., *Proteus* sp., and *E. coli*	Give IM or by 10- to 20-min IV infusions.
< 2 kg	*< 7 days* – 75 mg/kg/12 hr (150 mg/kg/day) *> 7 days* – 75 mg/kg/8 hr (225 mg/kg/day)
> 2 kg	*< 7 days* – 75 mg/kg/8 hr (225 mg/kg/day) *> 7 days* – 100 mg/kg/8 hr (300 mg/kg/day)

[1] Daily dose for children should not exceed adult dosage.

Admixture incompatibilities – Do not mix ticarcillin together with gentamicin, amikacin, or tobramycin in the same IV solution because of the gradual inactivation of gentamicin, amikacin, or tobramycin under these circumstances. The therapeutic effect of these drugs remains unimpaired when administered separately.

TICARCILLIN AND CLAVULANATE POTASSIUM: Administer by IV infusion over 30 minutes.

Adults –

Ticarcillin/Clavulanate Potassium Administration in Adults			
	Systemic and urinary tract infections	Gynecological infections	
		Moderate	Severe
Adults ≥ 60 kg	3.1 g every 4 to 6 hours	200 mg/kg/day every 6 hours	300 mg/kg/day every 4 hours
Adults < 60 kg	200 to 300 mg/kg/day every 4 to 6 hours		

Children –

Dosage Guidelines for Ticarcillin/Clavulanate Potassium in Children ≥ 3 months of age		
	Mild to moderate infections	Severe infections
Children ≥ 60 kg	3.1 g every 6 hours	3.1 g every 4 hours
Children < 60 kg (dosed at 50 mg/kg/dose)	200 mg/kg/day every 6 hours	300 mg/kg/day every 4 hours

Renal function impairment –

Dosage of Ticarcillin/Clavulanate Potassium in Renal Insufficiency[1]	
Ccr (mL/min)	Dosage
> 60	3.1 g[2] every 4 hrs
30 to 60	2 g every 4 hrs
10 to 30	2 g every 8 hrs
< 10	2 g every 12 hrs
< 10 with hepatic dysfunction	2 g every 24 hrs
Patients on peritoneal dialysis	3.1 g[2] every 12 hrs
Patients on hemodialysis	2 g every 12 hrs supplemented with 3.1 g[2] after each dialysis

[1] Half-life of ticarcillin in patients with renal failure is ≈ 13 hours. Initial loading dose is 3.1 g. Follow with doses based on Ccr and type of dialysis.
[2] 3 g ticarcillin plus 100 mg clavulanic acid.

Admixture incompatibility – Incompatible with sodium bicarbonate.

Actions

Pharmacology: Penicillins inhibit the biosynthesis of cell wall mucopeptide. They are bactericidal against sensitive organisms when adequate concentrations are reached, and they are most effective during the stage of active multiplication. Inadequate concentrations may produce only bacteriostatic effects.

Penicillins					
	Routes of administration	Penicillinase-resistant	Acid stable	% Protein bound	May be taken with meals
Natural penicillins					
Penicillin G	IM-IV	no	†[1]	60	†[1]
Penicillin V	Oral	no	yes	80	yes
Penicillinase-resistant					
Cloxacillin	Oral	yes	yes	95	no
Dicloxacillin	Oral	yes	yes	98	no
Nafcillin	IM-IV-Oral	yes	yes	87 to 90	no
Oxacillin	IM-IV-Oral	yes	yes	94	no

Penicillins					
	Routes of administration	Penicillinase-resistant	Acid stable	% Protein bound	May be taken with meals
Aminopenicillins					
Amoxicillin	Oral	no	yes	20	yes
Amoxicillin/ potassium clavulanate	Oral	yes	yes	18/25	yes
Ampicillin	IM-IV-Oral	no	yes	20	no
Ampicillin/ sulbactam	IM-IV	yes	†[1]	28/38	†[1]
Bacampi-cillin	Oral	no	yes	20	yes
Extended-spectrum					
Carbeni-cillin	Oral	no	yes	50	no
Mezlocillin	IM-IV	no	†[1]	16 to 42	†[1]
Piperacillin	IM-IV	no	†[1]	16	†[1]
Piperacillin/ Tazobactam sodium	IV	yes	†[1]	30/30	†[1]
Ticarcillin	IM-IV	no	†[1]	45	†[1]
Ticarcillin/ Potassium clavulanate	IV	yes	†[1]	45/9	†[1]

[1] Available only for IM or IV use.

Pharmacokinetics:

Absorption – Peak serum levels occur ≈ 1 hour after oral use. Parenteral **penicillin G** (sodium and potassium) gives rapid and high but transient blood levels; derivatives provide prolonged penicillin blood levels with IM use.

Distribution – Penicillins are bound to plasma proteins, primarily albumin, in varying degrees. They diffuse readily into most body tissues and fluids.

Excretion – Penicillins are excreted largely unchanged in the urine by glomerular filtration and active tubular secretion. Nonrenal elimination includes hepatic inactivation and excretion in bile; this is only a minor route for all penicillins except **nafcillin** and **oxacillin**. Excretion by renal tubular secretion can be delayed by coadministration of probenecid. Elimination half-life of most penicillins is short (≤ 1.5 hours). Impaired renal function prolongs the serum half-life of penicillins eliminated primarily by renal excretion.

Microbiology: The following table indicates the organisms that are generally susceptible to the penicillins in vitro:

Organisms Generally Susceptible to Penicillins

Organisms (✓ = generally susceptible)	Penicillin G	Penicillin V	Cloxacillin	Dicloxacillin	Nafcillin	Oxacillin	Amoxicillin	Ampicillin	Bacampicillin	Amoxicillin/Potassium clavulanate	Ampicillin/Sulbactam	Carbenicillin	Mezlocillin	Piperacillin	Ticarcillin	Ticarcillin/Potassium clavulanate	Piperacillin/Tazobactam sodium
Gram-positive																	
Staphylococci	✓[1]	✓[1]	✓	✓	✓	✓	✓[1]	✓[1]	✓[1]	✓	✓	✓[1]		✓[1]	✓[1]	✓	
Staphylococcus aureus	✓[1]	✓[1]	✓	✓	✓	✓				✓	✓	✓[1]	✓[1]	✓[1]	✓[1]	✓	✓
Staphyloccus epidermidis																	✓[5]
Streptococci	✓	✓						✓			✓						
Streptococcus pneumoniae	✓	✓	✓	✓	✓	✓	✓	✓	✓	✓	✓	✓	✓	✓	✓	✓	✓[2]
Beta-hemolytic streptococci	✓	✓			✓		✓	✓	✓	✓	✓	✓	✓	✓	✓	✓	
Enterococcus (Streptococcus) faecalis	✓[4]	✓					✓	✓	✓	✓	✓	✓	✓	✓	✓	✓	✓
Streptococcus viridans	✓	✓			✓		✓	✓		✓	✓			✓		✓	
Corynebacterium diphtheriae	✓	✓															
Bacillus anthracis	✓	✓						✓			✓						
Streptococcus agalactiae																✓	
Streptococcus pyogenes																✓	
Erysipelothrix rhusiopathiae	✓																
Listeria monocytogenes	✓	✓					✓	✓			✓						
Gram-negative																	
Escherichia coli	✓						✓	✓	✓	✓	✓	✓	✓	✓	✓	✓	✓
Haemophilus influenzae							✓	✓	✓	✓	✓	✓	✓	✓[2]	✓	✓	✓
Haemophilus parainfluenzae														✓			
Eikenella corrodens											✓						
Bacteroides melaninogenicus																	✓
Pseudomonas sp.																✓	✓
Klebsiella sp.										✓	✓		✓	✓		✓	✓
Neisseria gonorrhoeae	✓[1]	✓					✓	✓	✓	✓	✓	✓	✓	✓	✓	✓	✓
Neisseria meningitidis	✓							✓		✓	✓			✓	✓	✓	✓[2]
Proteus mirabilis	✓						✓	✓	✓	✓	✓	✓	✓	✓	✓	✓	✓
Salmonella sp.	✓							✓			✓	✓	✓	✓	✓	✓	
Shigella sp.	✓							✓			✓		✓	✓			
Morganella morganii											✓	✓	✓	✓	✓	✓	✓
Proteus vulgaris											✓	✓	✓	✓	✓	✓	✓
Providencia rettgeri											✓	✓	✓	✓	✓	✓	
Providencia stuartii											✓		✓			✓	
Enterobacter sp.		✓								✓	✓	✓	✓	✓	✓	✓	
Citrobacter sp.												✓	✓	✓	✓	✓	
Pseudomonas aeruginosa												✓	✓	✓	✓	✓	✓
Serratia sp.													✓	✓	✓	✓	✓
Acinetobacter sp.											✓		✓	✓		✓	
Streptobacillus moniliformis	✓	✓															
Moraxella (Branhamella) catarrhalis										✓	✓			✓		✓	✓

Organisms Generally Susceptible to Penicillins															
Organisms	Natural penicillins		Penicillinase-resistant				Aminopenicillins					Extended spectrum					
✔ = generally susceptible	Penicillin G	Penicillin V	Cloxacillin	Dicloxacillin	Nafcillin	Oxacillin	Amoxicillin	Ampicillin	Bacampicillin	Amoxicillin/Potassium clavulanate	Ampicillin/Sulbactam	Carbenicillin	Mezlocillin	Piperacillin	Ticarcillin	Ticarcillin/Potassium clavulanate	Piperacillin/Tazobactam sodium
Anaerobic Clostridium sp.	✔	✔					✔	✔		✔	✔	✔	✔	✔	✔	✔	✔
Peptococcus sp.	✔	✔					✔	✔		✔	✔	✔	✔	✔	✔	✔	
Peptostreptococcus sp.	✔	✔					✔			✔	✔	✔	✔	✔	✔	✔	
Bacteroides sp.	✔[3]									✔	✔	✔	✔	✔	✔	✔	✔
Fusobacterium sp.	✔									✔	✔	✔	✔	✔	✔	✔	✔
Eubacterium sp.	✔											✔	✔	✔	✔		
Treponema pallidum	✔	✔															
Actinomyces bovis	✔	✔											✔				
Veillonella sp.												✔	✔	✔	✔		

[1] Non–penicillinase-producing.
[2] Non–beta-lactamase-producing.
[3] Many strains of B. fragilis are resistant.
[4] Bacteriostatic effect.
[5] Nonmethicillin/oxacillin-resistant strains.

Contraindications

History of hypersensitivity to penicillins, cephalosporins, or imipenem.

Do not treat severe pneumonia, empyema, bacteremia, pericarditis, meningitis, or purulent or septic arthritis with an oral penicillin during the acute stage.

Warnings

Bleeding abnormalities: **Ticarcillin**, **mezlocillin**, or **piperacillin** may induce hemorrhagic manifestations associated with abnormalities of coagulation tests.

Cystic fibrosis: Cystic fibrosis patients have a higher incidence of side effects (eg, fever, rash) when treated with extended-spectrum penicillins (eg, **piperacillin**, **carbenicillin**).

Hypersensitivity reactions: Serious and occasionally fatal immediate-hypersensitivity reactions have occurred. The incidence of anaphylactic shock is between 0.015% and 0.04%. Anaphylactic shock resulting in death has occurred in ≈ 0.002% of the patients treated. These reactions are likely to be immediate and severe in penicillin-sensitive individuals with a history of atopic conditions.

Hypersensitivity myocarditis – Hypersensitivity myocarditis is not dose-dependent and may occur at any time during treatment.

An urticarial rash, not representing a true penicillin allergy, occasionally occurs with **ampicillin** (9%). Typically, the rash appears 7 to 10 days after the start of oral ampicillin therapy and remains for a few days to a week after drug discontinuance. In most cases, the rash is maculopapular, pruritic, and generalized.

Desensitization: Patients with a positive skin test to one of the penicillin determinants can be desensitized, a relatively safe procedure. This is recommended in instances when penicillin must be given where no proven alternatives exist.

Cross-allergenicity with cephalosporins: Individuals with a history of penicillin hypersensitivity have experienced severe reactions when treated with a cephalosporin. The incidence of cross-allergenicity between penicillins and cephalosporins is estimated to range from 5% to 16%; however, it is possible the incidence is much lower, possibly 3% to 7%.

Renal function impairment: Because **carbenicillin** is primarily excreted by the kidney, patients with severe renal impairment (Ccr < 10 mL/min) will not achieve the therapeutic urine levels of carbenecillin.

In patients with Ccr 10 to 20 mL/min, it may be necessary to adjust dosage to prevent accumulation of the drug.

Pregnancy: Category B. Penicillins cross the placenta.

Lactation: Penicillins are excreted in breast milk in low concentrations; use may cause diarrhea, candidiasis, or allergic response in the nursing infant.

Children: Safety and efficacy of **carbenicillin**, **piperacillin**, and the β-lactamase inhibitor/penicillin combinations have not been established in infants and children < 12 years of age. Use caution in administering to newborns and evaluate organ system function frequently.

Precautions

Monitoring: Obtain blood cultures, white blood cell, and differential cell counts prior to initiation of therapy and at least weekly during therapy with penicillinase-resistant penicillins. Measure AST and ALT during therapy to monitor for liver function abnormalities.

Perform periodic urinalysis, BUN, and creatinine determinations during therapy with penicillinase-resistant penicillins, and consider dosage alterations if these values become elevated.

Monitoring is particularly important in newborns and infants and when high dosages are used.

Streptococcal infections: Therapy must be sufficient to eliminate the organism (a minimum of 10 days); otherwise, sequelae (eg, endocarditis, rheumatic fever) may occur.

Sexually transmitted diseases: When treating gonococcal infections in which primary and secondary syphilis are suspected, perform proper diagnostic procedures, including darkfield examinations and monthly serological tests for at least 4 months.

Resistance: The number of strains of staphylococci resistant to penicillinase-resistant penicillins has been increasing; widespread use of penicillinase-resistant penicillins may result in an increasing number of resistant staphylococcal strains.

Pseudomembranous colitis: Pseudomembranous colitis has occurred with the use of broad-spectrum antibiotics caused by overgrowth of clostridia; therefore, it is important to consider its diagnosis in patients who develop diarrhea in association with antibiotic use.

Procaine sensitivity: If sensitivity to the procaine in **penicillin G procaine** is suspected, inject 0.1 mL of a 1% to 2% procaine solution intradermally. Development of erythema, wheal, flare, or eruption indicates procaine sensitivity; treat by the usual methods.

Parenteral administration: Inadvertent intravascular administration, including direct intra-arterial injection or injection immediately adjacent to arteries, has resulted in severe neurovascular damage, including transverse myelitis with permanent paralysis, gangrene requiring amputation of digits and more proximal portions of extremities, and necrosis and sloughing at and surrounding the injection site.

Electrolyte imbalance: Patients given continuous IV therapy with **potassium penicillin G** in high dosage (> 10 million units daily) may suffer severe or even fatal potassium poisoning particularly if renal insufficiency is present. High dosage of **sodium salts of penicillins** may result in or aggravate CHF caused by high sodium intake. Individuals with liver disease or those receiving cytotoxic therapy or diuretics rarely demonstrated a decrease in serum potassium concentrations with high doses of **piperacillin**. **Sodium penicillin G** contains 2 mEq sodium per million units,

potassium penicillin G contains 1.7 mEq potassium and 0.3 mEq sodium per million units. The sodium content of other IV penicillin derivatives is listed below:

Sodium Content of IV Penicillins			
Penicillin	Maximum recommended daily dose (g)	Sodium content (mEq/g)[1]	Sodium (mEq/day)[1,2]
Ampicillin sodium	14	2.9 to 3.1	40.6 to 43.4
Mezlocillin sodium	24	1.85	44.4
Nafcillin sodium	6	2.9	17.4
Oxacillin sodium	6	2.5 to 3.1	15 to 18.6
Piperacillin sodium	24	1.85	44.4
Piperacillin/Tazobactam sodium	12	2.35	28.2
Ticarcillin disodium	18	5.2 to 6.5	93.6 to 117

[1] 1 mEq sodium equals 23 mg.
[2] Based on maximum daily dose.

Hypokalemia – Hypokalemia has occurred in a few patients receiving **mezlocillin**, **ticarcillin**, and **piperacillin**.

Drug Interactions

Drugs that may affect penicillins include allopurinol, aminoglycosides (parenteral), aspirin, beta blockers, chloramphenicol, erythromycin, ethacrynic acid, furosemide, indomethacin, phenylbutazone, probenecid, sulfonamides, tetracycline, and thiazide diuretics. Drugs that may be affected by penicillins include aminoglycosides (parenteral), anticoagulants, beta blockers, chloramphenicol, cyclosporine, oral contraceptives, erythromycin, heparin, and vecuronium.

Drug/Lab test interactions: False-positive **urine glucose** reactions may occur with penicillin therapy if *Clinitest*, *Benedict's Solution*, or *Fehling's Solution* are used. It is recommended that enzymatic glucose oxidase tests (such as *Clinistix* or *Tes-Tape*) be used. Positive Coombs' tests have occurred. High urine concentrations of some penicillins may produce false-positive protein reactions (pseudoproteinuria) with the following methods: Sulfosalicylic acid and boiling test, acetic acid test, biuret reaction and nitric acid test. The bromphenol blue (*Multi-Stix*) reagent strip test has been reported to be reliable.

Drug/Food interactions: Absorption of most penicillins is affected by food; these medications are best taken on an empty stomach, 1 hour before or 2 hours after meals. **Penicillin V** may be given with meals; however, blood levels may be slightly higher when taken on an empty stomach. **Amoxicillin, amoxicillin/potassium clavulanate,** and **bacampicillin** tablets may be given without regard to meals; absorption of bacampicillin suspension is affected by food.

Adverse Reactions

CNS: Penicillins have caused neurotoxicity (manifested as lethargy, neuromuscular irritability, hallucinations, convulsions, and seizures) when given in large IV doses, especially in patients with renal failure.

GI: Glossitis; stomatitis; gastritis; sore mouth or tongue; dry mouth; furry tongue; black "hairy" tongue; abnormal taste sensation; nausea; vomiting; abdominal pain or cramp; epigastric distress; diarrhea or bloody diarrhea; rectal bleeding; flatulence; enterocolitis; pseudomembranous colitis.

Hematologic/Lymphatic: Anemia; hemolytic anemia; thrombocytopenia; thrombocytopenic purpura; eosinophilia; leukopenia; granulocytopenia; neutropenia; bone marrow depression; agranulocytosis; reduction of hemoglobin or hematocrit; prolongation of bleeding and prothrombin time; decrease in WBC and lymphocyte counts; increase in lymphocytes, monocytes, basophils, and platelets.

Hypersensitivity: Adverse reactions (estimated incidence, 1% to 10%) are more likely to occur in individuals with previously demonstrated hypersensitivity. In penicillin-sensitive individuals with a history of allergy, asthma, or hay fever, the reactions may be immediate and severe.

Allergic symptoms include urticaria; angioneurotic edema; laryngospasm; bronchospasm; hypotension; vascular collapse; death; maculopapular to exfoliative dermatitis; vesicular eruptions; erythema multiforme; reactions resembling serum sickness (eg, chills, fever, edema, arthralgia, arthritis, malaise); laryngeal edema; skin rashes; prostration.

Lab test abnormalities: Elevations of AST, ALT, bilirubin, and LDH have been noted in patients receiving semisynthetic penicillins (particularly **oxacillin** and **cloxacillin**); such reactions are more common in infants. Elevations of serum alkaline phosphatase and hypernatremia and reduction in serum potassium, albumin, total proteins, and uric acid may occur.

Local: Pain (accompanied by induration) at the site of injection; ecchymosis; deep vein thrombosis; hematomas.

Miscellaneous: Vaginitis and anorexia.

CEPHALOSPORINS AND RELATED ANTIBIOTICS

CEFACLOR
Tablets, extended release: 375 and 500 mg (*Rx*)
Capsules: 250 and 500 mg (*Rx*)
Powder for oral suspension: 125, 187, 250, and 375 mg/5 mL (*Rx*)

Ceclor CD (Eli Lilly)
Various, *Ceclor Pulvules* (Eli Lilly)
Various, *Ceclor* (Eli Lilly)

CEFADROXIL
Capsules: 500 mg (as monohydrate) (*Rx*)
Tablets: 1 g (as monohydrate) (*Rx*)
Powder for oral suspension: 125, 250, and 500 mg/5 mL (*Rx*)

Various, *Duricef* (Bristol-Myers Squibb)
Various, *Duricef* (Bristol-Myers Squibb)
Various, *Duricef* (Bristol-Myers Squibb)

CEFAMANDOLE NAFATE
Powder for injection: 1 g/10 mL and 2 g/20 mL (*Rx*)

Mandol (Lilly)

CEFAZOLIN SODIUM
Powder for injection: 250 and 500 mg, 1, 5, 10, and 20 g (*Rx*)
Injection: 500 mg or 1 g (*Rx*)

Various, *Ancef* (GlaxoSmithKline), *Zolicef* (Apothecon), *Kefzol* (Eli Lilly)
Ancef (GlaxoSmithKline), *Kefzol* (Eli Lilly)

CEFDINIR
Capsules: 300 mg (*Rx*)
Oral suspension: 125 mg/5 mL (*Rx*)

Omnicef (Parke-Davis)
Omnicef (Parke-Davis)

CEFDITOREN PIVOXIL
Tablets: 200 mg (*Rx*)

Spectracef (TAP Pharm.)

CEFEPIME HCl
Powder for injection: 500 mg, 1 and 2 g (*Rx*)

Maxipime (Dura)

CEFIXIME
Tablets: 200 and 400 mg (*Rx*)
Powder for oral suspension: 100 mg/5 mL (*Rx*)

Suprax (Lederle)
Suprax (Lederle)

CEFMETAZOLE SODIUM
Powder for injection: 1 and 2 g (*Rx*)
Injection: 1 and 2 g/50 mL (*Rx*)

Zefazone (Pharmacia)
Zefazone (Pharmacia)

CEFONICID SODIUM
Powder for injection: 1 and 10 g (*Rx*)

Monocid (GlaxoSmithKline)

CEFOPERAZONE SODIUM
Powder for injection: 1 and 2 g (*Rx*)
Injection: 1, 2, and 10 g (*Rx*)

Cefobid (Roerig)
Cefobid (Roerig)

CEFOTAXIME SODIUM
Powder for injection: 500 mg, 1, 2, and 10 g (*Rx*)
Injection: 1 and 2 g (*Rx*)

Claforan (Aventis)
Claforan (Aventis)

CEFOTETAN DISODIUM
Powder for injection: 1, 2, and 10 g (*Rx*)
Injection: 1 and 2 g/50 mL (*Rx*)

Cefotan (AstraZeneca)
Cefotan (AstraZeneca)

CEFOXITIN SODIUM
Powder for injection: 1, 2, and 10 g (*Rx*)
Injection: 1 and 2 g (*Rx*)

Mefoxin (Merck)
Mefoxin (Merck)

CEFPODOXIME PROXETIL
Tablets: 100 and 200 mg (*Rx*)
Granules for suspension: 50 and 100 mg/5 mL (*Rx*)

Vantin (Pharmacia)
Vantin (Pharmacia)

CEFPROZIL
Tablets: 250 and 500 mg (as anhydrous) (*Rx*)
Powder for oral suspension: 125 and 250 mg (as anhydrous)/5 mL (*Rx*)

Cefzil (Bristol-Myers Squibb)
Cefzil (Bristol-Myers Squibb)

CEFTAZIDIME
Powder for injection: 500 mg, 1, 2, 6, and 10 g (*Rx*)

Injection: 1 and 2 g (*Rx*)

Fortaz (GlaxoSmithKline), *Tazidime* (Eli Lilly), *Ceptaz* (GlaxoSmithKline), *Tazicef* (GlaxoSmithKline/Bristol-Myers Squibb)
Fortaz (GlaxoSmithKline), *Tazicef* (GlaxoSmithKline/Bristol-Myers Squibb)

CEFTIBUTEN

Capsules: 400 mg (*Rx*)	*Cedax* (Schering-Plough)
Powder for oral suspension: 90 and 180 mg/5 mL (*Rx*)	*Cedax* (Schering-Plough)

CEFTIZOXIME SODIUM

Powder for injection: 500 mg, 1, 2, and 10 g (as sodium) (*Rx*)	*Cefizox* (Fujisawa)
Injection: 1 and 2 g (as sodium) (*Rx*)	*Cefizox* (Fujisawa)

CEFTRIAXONE SODIUM

Powder for injection: 250 and 500 mg, 1, 2, and 10 g (*Rx*)	*Rocephin* (Roche)
Injection: 1 and 2 g (*Rx*)	*Rocephin* (Roche)

CEFUROXIME

Tablets: 125, 250, and 500 mg (*Rx*)	*Ceftin* (GlaxoSmithKline)
Suspension: 125 and 250 mg (as axetil)/5 mL (when reconstituted) (*Rx*)	*Ceftin* (GlaxoSmithKline)
Powder for injection: 750 mg, 1.5 and 7.5 g (as sodium)/vial (*Rx*)	Various, *Zinacef* (GlaxoSmithKline), *Kefurox* (Lilly)
Injection: 750 mg and 1.5 g (as sodium) (*Rx*)	*Zinacef* (GlaxoSmithKline)

CEPHALEXIN

Capsules: 250 and 500 mg (*Rx*)	Various, *Keflex* (Dista), *Biocef* (Inter Ethical Labs)
Tablets: 250 and 500 mg and 1 g (*Rx*)	Various
Powder for oral suspension: 125 and 250 mg/5 mL (*Rx*)	Various, *Biocef* (Inter. Ethical Labs), *Keflex* (Dista)

CEPHALEXIN HCl MONOHYDRATE

Tablets: 500 mg (*Rx*)	*Keftab* (Dista)

CEPHAPIRIN SODIUM

Powder for injection: 1 g (*Rx*)	*Cefadyl* (Apothecon)

CEPHRADINE

Capsules: 250 and 500 mg (*Rx*)	Various, *Velosef* (Bristol-Myers Squibb)
Powder for oral suspension: 125 and 250 mg/5 mL (when reconstituted) (*Rx*)	Various, *Velosef* (Bristol-Myers Squibb)
Powder for injection: 250 and 500 mg, 1 and 2 g (*Rx*)	*Velosef* (Bristol-Myers Squibb)

LORACARBEF

Pulvules (capsules): 200 and 400 mg (*Rx*)	*Lorabid* (Eli Lilly)
Powder for oral suspension: 100 and 200 mg/5 mL (*Rx*)	*Lorabid* (Eli Lilly)

Indications

For approved indications, refer to the Administration and Dosage section.

Administration and Dosage

Duration of therapy: Continue administration for a minimum of 48 to 72 hours after fever abates or after evidence of bacterial eradication has been obtained.

Perioperative prophylaxis: Discontinue prophylactic use within 24 hours after the surgical procedure. In surgery where infection may be particularly devastating, prophylactic use may be continued for 3 to 5 days following surgery completion.

CEFACLOR:

Adults – Usual dosage is 250 mg every 8 hours. In severe infections or those caused by less susceptible organisms, dosage may be doubled.

Capsules: Food does not affect the extent of absorption.

Tablets, extended release: Administer with food to enhance absorption. Do not cut, crush, or chew.

Acute bacterial exacerbations of chronic bronchitis – 500 mg/12 hours for 7 days.
Secondary bacterial infection of acute bronchitis – 500 mg/12 hours for 7 days.
Pharyngitis or tonsillitis – 375 mg/12 hours for 10 days.
Uncomplicated skin and skin structure infections – 375 mg/12 hours for 7 to 10 days.

Children – Give 20 mg/kg/day in divided doses, every 8 hours. In more serious infections, otitis media, and infections caused by less susceptible organisms, administer 40 mg/kg/day, with a maximum dosage of 1 g/day.

Twice-daily treatment option: For otitis media and pharyngitis, the total daily dosage may be divided and administered every 12 hours.

CEFADROXIL: Can be given without regard to meals.

Urinary tract infections – For uncomplicated lower urinary tract infection (eg, cystitis), the usual dosage is 1 or 2 g/day in single or 2 divided doses. For all other urinary tract infections, the usual dosage is 2 g/day in 2 divided doses.

Skin and skin structure infections – 1 g/day in single or 2 divided doses.

Pharyngitis and tonsillitis –

Group A β-hemolytic streptococci: 1 g/day in single or 2 divided doses for 10 days.

Children –

Urinary tract infections, skin and skin structure infections: 30 mg/kg/day in divided doses every 12 hours.

Pharyngitis, tonsillitis: 30 mg/kg/day in single or 2 divided doses. For β-hemolytic streptococcal infections, continue treatment for at least 10 days.

Renal impairment – Adjust dosage according to Ccr rates to prevent drug accumulation.

Initial adult dose: 1 g: The maintenance dose (based on Ccr rate, mL/min/1.73 m^2) is 500 mg at the intervals below:

Cefadroxil Dosage in Renal Impairment	
Ccr (mL/min)	Dosage interval (hours)
0 to 10	36
10 to 25	24
25 to 50	12
> 50	No adjustment

CEFAMANDOLE NAFTATE:

Adults – Usual dosage range is 500 mg to 1 g every 4 to 8 hours; 500 mg every 6 hours is adequate in uncomplicated skin and skin structure infections. In uncomplicated urinary tract infections, 500 mg every 8 hours; in more serious urinary tract infections, the dose may be increased to 1 g every 8 hours. In severe infections, administer 1 g at 4- to 6-hour intervals. In life-threatening infections or infections caused by less susceptible organisms, up to 2 g every 4 hours may be needed.

Infants and children – 50 to 100 mg/kg/day in equally divided doses every 4 to 8 hours is effective for most infections susceptible to cefamandole. This may be increased to 150 mg/kg/day (not to exceed the maximum adult dose) for severe infections.

Perioperative prophylaxis –

Adults: 1 or 2 g IM or IV, ½ to 1 hour prior to the surgical incision, followed by 1 or 2 g every 6 hours for 24 to 48 hours.

Children (3 months of age and older): 50 to 100 mg/kg/day in equally divided doses by the routes and schedule designated above.

Renal function impairment – Reduce dosages and monitor the serum levels. After an initial dose of 1 to 2 g (depending on the severity of infection), follow maintenance dosage in table.

Maintenance Cefamandole Dosage Guide for Patients with Renal Impairment			
Renal function impairment	Ccr (mL/min/ 1.73 m^2)	Life-threatening infections (Maximum dosage)	Less severe infections
Normal	> 80	2 g q 4 h	1 to 2 g q 6 h
Mild	50 to 80	1.5 g q 4 h or 2 g q 6 h	0.75 to 1.5 g q 6 h
Moderate	25 to 50	1.5 g q 6 h or 2 g q 8 h	0.75 to 1.5 g q 8 h
Severe	10 to 25	1 g q 6 h or 1.25 g q 8 h	0.5 to 1 g q 8 h
Marked	2 to 10	0.67 g q 8 h or 1 g q 12 h	0.5 to 0.75 g q 12 h
None	< 2	0.5 g q 8 h or 0.75 g q 12 h	0.25 to 0.5 g q 12 h

CEFAZOLIN SODIUM: Total daily dosages are the same for IM and IV administration.

Mild infections caused by susceptible gram-positive cocci – 250 to 500 mg every 8 hours.

Moderate-to-severe infections – 500 mg to 1 g every 6 to 8 hours.

Pneumococcal pneumonia – 500 mg every 12 hours.

Severe, life-threatening infections (eg, endocarditis, septicemia) – 1 to 1.5 g every 6 hours. Rarely, 12 g/day have been used.

Acute uncomplicated urinary tract infections – 1 g every 12 hours.

Perioperative prophylaxis –

   Preoperative: 1 g IV or IM, ½ to 1 hour prior to surgery.

   Intraoperative (≥ 2 hrs): 0.5 to 1 g IV or IM during surgery at appropriate intervals.

   Postoperative: 0.5 to 1 g IV or IM every 6 to 8 hours for 24 hours after surgery.

Renal function impairment – All reduced dosage recommendations apply after an initial loading dose appropriate to the severity of the infection.

Cefazolin Dosage in Renal Impairment				
Serum Creatinine (mg %)	Ccr (mL/min)	Dose		Dosage interval (hrs)
		≤ 1.5	≥ 55	
≤ 1.5	≥ 55	250 to 500	500 to 1000	6 to 8
1.6 to 3	35 to 54	250 to 500	500 to 1000	≥ 8
3.1 to 4.5	11 to 34	125 to 250	250 to 500	12
≥ 4.6	≤ 10	125 to 250	250 to 500	18 to 24

Children –

   Mild to moderately severe infections: A total daily dosage of 25 to 50 mg/kg (≈ 10 to 20 mg/lb) in 3 or 4 equal doses.

   Severe infections: Total daily dosage may be increased to 100 mg/kg (45 mg/lb).

CEFDINIR:

Adults/Adolescents – Capsules may be taken without regard to meals.

Cefdinir Dosage in Adults and Adolescents (≥ 13 years of age)		
Type of infection	Dosage	Duration
Community-acquired pneumonia	300 mg q 12 hrs	10 days
Acute exacerbations of chronic bronchitis	300 mg q 12 hrs or 600 mg q 24 hrs	10 days 10 days
Acute maxillary sinusitis	300 mg q 12 hrs or 600 mg q 24 hrs	10 days 10 days
Pharyngitis/Tonsillitis	300 mg q 12 hrs or 600 mg q 24 hrs	5 to 10 days 10 days
Uncomplicated skin and skin structure infections	300 mg q 12 hrs	10 days

Children –

   Powder for oral suspension: The recommended dosage in pediatric patients is 14 mg/kg, up to a maximum dose of 600 mg/day. Oral suspension may be administered without regard to meals.

Cefdinir Dosage in Pediatric Patients (6 Months Through 12 Years of Age)		
Type of infection	Dosage	Duration
Acute bacterial otitis media	7 mg/kg q 12 h or 14 mg/kg q 24 h	10 days 10 days
Acute maxillary sinusitis	7 mg/kg q 12 h or 14 mg/kg q 24 h	10 days 10 days

Cefdinir Dosage in Pediatric Patients (6 Months Through 12 Years of Age)		
Type of infection	Dosage	Duration
Pharyngitis/Tonsillitis	7 mg/kg q 12 h or 14 mg/kg q 24 h	5 to 10 days 10 days
Uncomplicated skin and skin structure infections	7 mg/kg q 12 h	10 days

Cefdinir for Oral Suspension Pediatric Dosage Chart		
Weight		
kg	lb	125 mg/5 mL
9	20	2.5 mL (½ tsp) q 12 h or 5 mL (1 tsp) q 24 h
18	40	5 mL (1 tsp) q 12 h or 10 mL (2 tsp) q 24 h
27	60	7.5 mL (1½ tsp) q 12 h or 15 mL (3 tsp) q 24 h
36	80	10 mL (2 tsp) q 12 h or 20 mL (4 tsp) q 24 h
≥ 43[1]	95	12 mL (2½ tsp) q 12 h or 24 mL (5 tsp) q 24 h

[1] Pediatric patients who weigh ≥ 43 kg should receive the maximum daily dose of 600 mg.

Renal function impairment – For adult patients with Ccr < 30 mL/min, the dose of cefdinir should be 300 mg given once daily.

For pediatric patients with a Ccr of < 30 mL/min/1.73 m^2, the dose of cefdinir should be 7 mg/kg (≤ 300 mg) given once daily.

Hemodialysis – Hemodialysis removes cefdinir from the body. In patients maintained on chronic hemodialysis, the recommended initial dosage regimen is a 300 mg or 7 mg/kg dose every other day. At the conclusion of each hemodialysis session, give 300 mg (or 7 mg/kg). Subsequent doses (300 mg or 7 mg/kg) are then administered every other day.

CEFDITOREN PIVOXIL:

Cefditoren Dosage and Administration in Adults and Adolescents ≥ 12 Years of Age[1]		
Type of infection	Dosage	Duration (days)
Acute bacterial exacerbation of chronic bronchitis	400 mg BID	
Pharyngitis/Tonsillitis	200 mg BID	10
Uncomplicated skin and skin structure infections		

[1] Take with meals.

Renal impairment – It is recommended that ≤ 200 mg twice daily be administered to patients with moderate renal impairment (Ccr 30 to 49 mL/min/1.73 m^2) and 200 mg every day be administered to patients with severe renal impairment (Ccr < 30 mL/min/1.73 m^2).

CEFEPIME:

Recommended Dosage Schedule for Cefepime			
Site and type of infection	Dose	Frequency	Duration (days)
Mild to moderate uncomplicated or complicated urinary tract infections, including pyelonephritis, caused by *Escherichia coli*, *Klebsiella pneumoniae*, or *Proteus mirabilis*.[1]	0.5 to 1 g IV/IM[2]	q 12 hrs	7 to 10
Severe uncomplicated or complicated urinary tract infections, including pyelonephritis, caused by *E. coli* or *K. pneumoniae*.[1]	2 g IV	q 12 hrs	10

Recommended Dosage Schedule for Cefepime			
Site and type of infection	Dose	Frequency	Duration (days)
Moderate to severe pneumonia caused by *Streptococcus pneumoniae*,[1] *Pseudomonas aeruginosa*, *K. pneumoniae*, or *Enterobacter* sp.	1 to 2 g IV	q 12 hrs	10
Moderate to severe uncomplicated skin and skin structure infections caused by *Staphylococcus aureus* or *Streptococcus pyogenes*.	2 g IV	q 12 hrs	10
Empiric therapy for febrile neutropenic patients.	2 g IV	q 8 hrs	7[3]
Complicated intra-abdominal infections (used in combination with metronidazole) caused by *E. coli*, viridans group streptococci, *P. aeruginosa*, *K. pneumoniae*, *Enterobacter* species, or *Bacteroides fragilis*.	2 g IV	q 12 hrs	7 to 10

[1] Including cases associated with concurrent bacteremia.
[2] IM route of administration is indicated only for mild to moderate, uncomplicated, or complicated UTIs caused by *E. coli* when the IM route is a more appropriate route of drug administration.
[3] Or until resolution of neutropenia. In patients whose fever resolves but who remain neutropenic for > 7 days, frequently re-evaluate the need for continued antimicrobial therapy.

Empiric therapy for febrile neutropenic patients – As monotherapy for empiric treatment of febrile neutropenic patients. In patients at high risk for severe infection (including patients with a history of recent bone marrow transplantation, with hypotension at presentation, with an underlying hematologic malignancy, or with severe or prolonged neutropenia), antimicrobial monotherapy may not be appropriate. Insufficient data exist to support the efficacy of cefepime monotherapy in such patients.

Complicated intra-abdominal infections – In combination with metronidazole for complicated intra-abdominal infections caused by *E. coli*, viridans group streptococci, *P. aeruginosa*, *K. pneumoniae*, *Enterobacter* sp., or *B. fragilis*.

Pediatric patients (2 months to 16 years of age) – Treatment of uncomplicated and complicated urinary tract infections (including pyelonephritis), uncomplicated skin and skin structure infections, pneumonia, and as empiric therapy for febrile neutropenic patients.

Renal function impairment – In patients with impaired renal function (Ccr < 60 mL/min), adjust the dose of cefepime to compensate for the slower rate of renal elimination. The recommended initial dose should be the same as in patients with normal renal function.

In patients undergoing hemodialysis, ≈ 68% of the total amount of cefepime present in the body at the start of dialysis will be removed during a 3-hour dialysis period. Give a repeat dose, equivalent to the initial dose, at the completion of each dialysis session.

In elderly patients with renal insufficiency, adjust dosage and administration.

In patients undergoing continuous ambulatory peritoneal dialysis, administer cefepime at normal recommended doses at a dosage interval of every 48 hours.

Recommended Cefepime Maintenance Schedule in Patients with Renal Impairment				
Ccr (mL/min)	Recommended maintenance schedule			
> 60	500 mg q 12 h [1]	1 g q 12 h	2 g q 12 h	2 g q 8 h
30 to 60	500 mg q 24 h	1 g q 24 h	2 g q 24 h	2 g q 12 h
11 to 29		500 mg q 24 h	1 g q 24 h	2 g q 24 h
≤ 11	250 mg q 24 h	250 mg q 24 h	500 mg q 24 h	1 g q 24 h

[1] Normal recommended dosing schedule.

IV administration – Administer over ≈ 30 minutes. Reconstitute with 50 or 100 mL of a compatible IV fluid. Cefepime is compatible at concentrations of 1 to 40 mg/

mL with 0.9% Sodium Chloride Injection, 5% and 10% Dextrose Injection, M/6 Sodium Lactate Injection, 5% Dextrose and 0.9% Sodium Chloride Injection, Lactated Ringers and 5% Dextrose Injection, *Normosol-R* or *Normosol-M* in 5% Dextrose injection.

Cefepime Admixture Stability				
Cefepime concentration (mg/mL)	Admixture and concentration	IV Infusion solutions	Stability time for RT/L[1] (20° to 25°C) (hours)	Stability time for refrigeration (2° to 8°C)
40	Amikacin 6 mg/mL	NS[2] or D5W[3]	24	7 days
40	Ampicillin 1 mg/mL	D5W[3]	8	8 hrs
40	Ampicillin 10 mg/mL	D5W[3]	2	8 hrs
40	Ampicillin 1 mg/mL	NS[2]	24	48 hrs
40	Ampicillin 10 mg/mL	NS[2]	8	48 hrs
4	Ampicillin 40 mg/mL	NS[2]	8	8 hrs
4 to 40	Clindamycin phosphate 0.25 to 6 mg/mL	NS[2] or D5W[3]	24	7 days
4	Heparin 10 to 50 units/mL	NS[2] or D5W[3]	24	7 days
4	Potassium chloride 10 to 40 mEq/L	NS[2] or D5W[3]	24	7 days
4	Theophylline 0.8 mg/mL	D5W[3]	24	7 days
1 to 4	na	*Aminosyn II 4.25%* with electrolytes and calcium	8	3 days
0.125 to 0.25	na	*Inpersol* with 4.25% dextrose	24	7 days

[1] Ambient room temperature and light.
[2] 0.9% sodium chloride injection.
[3] 5% dextrose injection.

Admixture compatibility/incompatibility: Intermittent IV infusion with a Y-type administration set can be accomplished with compatible solutions; however, during infusion of a solution containing cefepime, it is desirable to discontinue the other solution.

Solutions of cefepime, like those of most β-lactam antibiotics, should not be added to solutions of ampicillin at a concentration > 40 mg/mL, and should not be added to metronidazole, vancomycin, gentamicin, tobramycin, netilmicin sulfate, or aminophylline because of potential interaction. However, if concurrent therapy with cefepime is indicated, each of these antibiotics can be administered separately.

IM administration: Reconstitute cefepime with the following diluents: Sterile Water for Injection, 0.9% Sodium Chloride, 5% Dextrose Injection, 0.5% or 1% lidocaine HCl, or Sterile Bacteriostatic Water for Injection with parabens or benzyl alcohol.

Pediatric dosing: The usual recommended daily dosage in pediatric patients up to 40 kg in weight is 50 mg/kg/dose administered every 12 hours (every 8 hours for febrile neutropenic patients), for 7 to 10 days, depending on the indication and severity of infection. The maximum dose for pediatric patients (2 months to 16 years of age) should not exceed the recommended adult dose.

Renal impairment – Data in pediatric patients with impaired renal function are not available; however, because cefepime pharmacokinetics are similar in adult and pediatric patients, changes in dosing regimen similar to those in adults are recommended for pediatric patients.

CEFIXIME:

Adults – 400 mg/day as a single 400 mg tablet (recommended for gonococcal infections) or as 200 mg every 12 hours.

Children – 8 mg/kg/day suspension as a single daily dose or as 4 mg/kg every 12 hours. Treat children > 50 kg or > 12 years of age with the recommended adult dose.

Treat otitis media with the suspension.

For *S. pyogenes* infections, administer cefixime for ≥ 10 days.

Renal function impairment –

| Cefixime Dosing in Renal Impairment ||
Ccr (mL/min)	Dosage
> 60	Standard
21 to 60 or renal hemodialysis	75% of standard
≤ 20 or continuous ambulatory peritoneal dialysis	50% of standard

CEFMETAZOLE SODIUM:

Adults –

General guidelines: 2 g IV every 6 to 12 hours for 5 to 14 days.

Prophylaxis –

| Cefmetazole Dosing Regimen for Prophylaxis ||
Surgery	Dosing Regimen
Vaginal hysterectomy	2 g single dose 30 to 90 min before surgery or 1 g doses 30 to 90 min before surgery and repeated 8 and 16 hrs later.
Abdominal hysterectomy	1 g dose 30 to 90 min before surgery and repeated 8 and 16 hrs later.
Cesarean section	2 g single dose after clamping cord or 1 g doses after clamping cord; repeated at 8 and 16 hrs.
Colorectal surgery	2 g single dose 30 to 90 min before surgery or 2 g doses 30 to 90 min before surgery and repeated 8 to 16 hrs later.
Cholecystectomy (high risk)	1 g doses 30 to 90 min before surgery and repeated 8 and 16 hrs later.

Renal function impairment –

| Cefmetazole Dosage Guidelines in Renal Function Impairment ||||
Renal function	Ccr (mL/min/1.73 m^2)	Dose (g)	Frequency (hrs)
Mild impairment	50 to 90	1 to 2	q 12
Moderate impairment	30 to 49	1 to 2	q 16
Severe impairment	10 to 29	1 to 2	q 24
Essentially no function	< 10	1 to 2	q 48[1]

[1] Administered after hemodialysis.

CEFONICID SODIUM:

Adults – Usual dose is 1 g/24 hours, IV or by deep IM injection. Doses > 1 g/day are rarely necessary; however, up to 2 g/day have been well tolerated.

| General Cefonicid Dosage Guidelines (IM or IV) |||
Type of infection	Daily dosage (g)	Frequency
Uncomplicated urinary tract	0.5	once every 24 hrs
Mild to moderate	1	once every 24 hrs
Severe or life-threatening	2[1]	once every 24 hrs
Surgical prophylaxis	1	1 hr preoperatively

[1] When administering 2 g IM doses once daily, divide dose in half and give each half in a different large muscle mass.

Preoperative prophylaxis – Administer 1 g 1 hour prior to appropriate surgical procedures to provide protection from most infections caused by susceptible organisms for ≈ 24 hours after administration.

Renal function impairment – Renal function impairment requires modification of dosage. Following an initial loading dosage of 7.5 mg/kg, IM or IV, follow maintenance schedule below. It is not necessary to administer additional dosage following dialysis.

Cefonicid Dosage in Adults with Reduced Renal Function		
Ccr (mL/min/ 1.73²)	Mild to moderate infections	Severe infections
60 to 79	10 mg/kg q 24 hr	25 mg/kg q 24 hr
40 to 59	8 mg/kg q 24 hr	20 mg/kg q 24 hr
20 to 39	4 mg/kg q 24 hr	15 mg/kg q 24 hr
10 to 19	4 mg/kg q 48 hr	15 mg/kg q 48 hr
5 to 9	4 mg/kg q 3 to 5 days	15 mg/kg q 3 to 5 days
< 5	3 mg/kg q 3 to 5 days	4 mg/kg q 3 to 5 days

CEFOPERAZONE SODIUM: Administer IM or IV.

Usual adult dose is 2 to 4 g/day administered in equally divided doses every 12 hours.

In severe infections or infections caused by less sensitive organisms, the total daily dose or frequency may be increased. Patients have been successfully treated with a total daily dosage of 6 to 12 g divided into 2, 3, or 4 administrations ranging from 1.5 to 4 g/dose. A total daily dose of 16 g by constant infusion has been given without complications.

Hepatic disease or biliary obstruction – In general, total daily dosage > 4 g should not be necessary.

Renal function impairment –

Hemodialysis: The half-life is reduced slightly during hemodialysis. Thus, schedule dosing to follow a dialysis period.

CEFOTAXIME SODIUM:

Adults – Administer IV or IM. Maximum daily dosage should not exceed 12 g.

Cefotaxime Dosage Guidelines for Adults		
Type of infection	Daily dosage (g)	Frequency and route
Gonococcal urethritis/cervicitis in males and females	0.5	0.5 g IM (single dose)
Rectal gonorrhea in females	0.5	0.5 g IM (single dose)
Rectal gonorrhea in males	1	1 g IM (single dose)
Uncomplicated infections	2	1 g every 12 hrs IM or IV
Moderate to severe infections	3 to 6	1 to 2 g every 8 hrs IM or IV
Infections commonly needing higher dosage (eg, septicemia)	6 to 8	2 g every 6 to 8 hrs IV
Life-threatening infections	≤ 12	2 g every 4 hrs IV

Perioperative prophylaxis: 1 g IV or IM, 30 to 90 minutes prior to surgery.

Cesarean section: Administer the first 1 g dose IV as soon as the umbilical cord is clamped. Administer the second and third doses as 1 g IV or IM at 6- and 12-hour intervals after the first dose.

Children –

Cefotaxime Dosage Guidelines in Pediatrics			
Age	Weight (kg)	Dosage schedule	Route
0 to 1 week	-	50 mg/kg every 12 hrs	IV
1 to 4 weeks	-	50 mg/kg every 8 hrs	IV
1 month to 12 years	< 50[1]	50 to 180 mg/kg/day in 4 to 6 divided doses[2]	IV or IM

[1] For children ≥ 50 kg, use adult dosage.
[2] Use higher doses for more severe or serious infections including meningitis.

Renal function impairment – In patients with estimated Ccr < 20 mL/min/1.73 m², reduce dosage by ½.

When only serum creatinine is available, the following formula may be used to convert this value into Ccr. The serum creatinine should represent steady-state renal function.

CDC-recommended treatment schedules for gonorrhea –

Disseminated gonococcal infection: Give 1 g IV every 8 hours.

Gonococcal ophthalmia in adults: For penicillinase-producing *Neisseria gonorrhoeae* (PPNG), give 500 mg IV 4 times/day.

CEFOTETAN DISODIUM:

Adults – The usual dosage is 1 or 2 g IV or IM every 12 hours for 5 to 10 days. Determine proper dosage and route of administration by the condition of the patient, severity of the infection and susceptibility of the causitive organism.

General Cefotetan Dosage Guidelines		
Type of Infection	Daily Dose	Frequency and Route
Urinary tract	1 to 4 g	500 mg every 12 hrs IV or IM
		1 or 2 g every 24 hrs IV or IM
		1 or 2 g every 12 hrs IV or IM
Skin/Skin structure Mild to moderate[2]	2 g	2 g q 24 hrs IV
		1 g q 12 hrs IV or IM
Severe	4 g	2 g q 12 hrs IV
Other sites	2 to 4 g	1 or 2 g every 12 hrs IV or IM
Severe	4 g	2 g every 12 hrs IV
Life-threatening	6 g[1]	3 g every 12 hrs IV

[1] Maximum daily dosage should not exceed 6 g.
[2] Treat *K. pneumoniae* skin and skin structure infections with 1 or 2 g every 12 hours IV or IM.

Prophylaxis – To prevent postoperative infection in clean contaminated or potentially contaminated surgery in adults, give a single 1 or 2 g IV dose 30 to 60 minutes prior to surgery. In patients undergoing cesarean section, give the dose as soon as the umbilical cord is clamped.

Renal function impairment – Reduce the dosage schedule using the following guidelines:

Cefotetan Dosage in Renal Impairment		
Ccr (mL/min)	Dose	Frequency
> 30	Usual recommended dose[1]	Every 12 hrs
10 to 30	Usual recommended dose[1]	Every 24 hrs
< 10	Usual recommended dose[1]	Every 48 hrs

[1] Dose determined by the type and severity of infection and susceptibility of the causitive organism.

Alternatively, the dosing interval may remain constant at 12-hour intervals, but reduce dose by ½ for patients with a Ccr of 10 to 30 mL/min, and by ¼ for patients with a Ccr < 10 mL/min.

Dialysis – Cefotetan is dialyzable; for patients undergoing intermittent hemodialysis, give ¼ of the usual recommended dose every 24 hours on days between dialysis and ½ of the usual recommended dose on the day of dialysis.

CEFOXITIN SODIUM:

Adult – Adult dosage range is 1 to 2 g every 6 to 8 hours.

Cefoxitin Dosage Guidelines		
Type of infection	Daily dosage	Frequency and route
Uncomplicated (pneumonia, urinary tract, cutaneous)[1]	3 to 4 g	1 g every 6 to 8 hrs IV or IM
Moderately severe or severe	6 to 8 g	1 g every 4 hrs or 2 g every 6 to 8 hrs IV
Infections commonly requiring higher dosage (eg, gas gangrene)	12 g	2 g every 4 hrs or 3 g every 6 hrs IV

[1] Including patients in whom bacteremia is absent or unlikely.

Uncomplicated gonorrhea – 2 g IM with 1 g oral probenecid given concurrently or up to 30 minutes before cefoxitin.

Prophylactic use, surgery – Administer 2 g IV or IM 30 to 60 minutes prior to surgery followed by 2 g every 6 hours after the first dose for no more than 24 hours.

Prophylactic use, cesarean section – Administer 2 g IV as soon as the umbilical cord is clamped. If a 3-dose regimen is used, give the second and third 2 g dose IV, 4 and 8 hours after the first dose.

Prophylactic use, transurethral prostatectomy – Administer 1 g prior to surgery; 1 g every 8 hours for up to 5 days.

Renal function impairment –

Adults: Initial loading dose is 1 to 2 g. Mantenance doses:

Maintenance Cefoxitin Dosage in Renal Impairment			
Renal function	Ccr (mL/min/1.73 m^2)	Dose (g)	Frequency (hrs)
Mild impairment	30 to 50	1 to 2	8 to 12
Moderate impairment	10 to 29	1 to 2	12 to 24
Severe impairment	5 to 9	0.5 to 1	12 to 24
Essentially no function	< 5	0.5 to 1	24 to 48

Hemodialysis – Administer a loading dose of 1 to 2 g after each hemodialysis. Give the maintenance dose as indicated in the table above.

Infants and children ≥ 3 months: 80 to 160 mg/kg/day divided every 4 to 6 hours. Use higher dosages for more severe or serious infections. Do not exceed 12 g/day.

Prophylactic use (≥ 3 months) – 30 to 40 mg/kg/dose every 6 hours

Renal function impairment – Modify consistent with recommendation for adults.

CDC recommended treatment schedules for acute pelvic inflammatory disease (PID) – 2 g IV every 6 hours plus 100 mg doxycycline IV or orally every 12 hours.

CEFPODOXIME PROXETIL: Administer with food to enhance absorption.

Dosage/Duration of Cefpodoxime			
Type of infection	Total daily dose	Dose frequency	Duration
Adults ≥ 13 years of age			
Acute community-acquired pneumonia	400 mg	200 mg every 12 hrs	14 days
Acute bacterial exacerbations of chronic bronchitis (tablets)	400 mg	200 mg every 12 hrs	10 days
Uncomplicated gonorrhea (men and women) and rectal gonococcal infections (women)	200 mg	single dose	
Skin and skin structure	800 mg	400 mg every 12 hrs	7 to 14 days
Pharyngitis/Tonsillitis	200 mg	100 mg every 12 hrs	5 to 10 days

Dosage/Duration of Cefpodoxime			
Type of infection	Total daily dose	Dose frequency	Duration
Uncomplicated urinary tract infection	200 mg	100 mg every 12 hrs	7 days
Children (5 months through 12 years of age):[1] Acute otitis media	10 mg/kg/day (max 400 mg/day)	10 mg/kg every 24 hrs (max 400 mg/dose) or 5 mg/kg every 12 hrs (max 200 mg/dose)	10 days
Pharyngitis/Tonsillitis	10 mg/kg/day (max 200 mg/day)	5 mg/kg every 12 hrs (max 100 mg/dose)	5 to 10 days

[1] Do not exceed adult recommended doses.

Renal dysfunction – For patients with severe renal impairment (Ccr < 30 mL/min), increase the dosing intervals to every 24 hours. In patients maintained on hemodialysis, use a frequency of 3 times/week after hemodialysis.

CEFPROZIL:

Cefprozil Dosage and Duration		
Population/Infection	Dosage (mg)	Duration (days)
Adults (≥ 13 years of age) Pharyngitis/Tonsillitis	500 q 24 hrs	10[1]
Acute sinusitis (use higher dose for moderate to severe infections)	250 q 12 hrs or 500 q 12 hrs	10
Secondary bacterial infection of acute bronchitis and acute bacterial exacerbation of chronic bronchitis	500 q 12 hrs	10
Uncomplicated skin and skin structure infections	250 q 12 hrs, 500 q 24 hrs, or 500 q 12 hrs	10
Children (2 to 12 years of age)[2] Pharyngitis/Tonsillitis	7.5 mg/kg q 12 hrs	10[1]
Uncomplicated skin and skin structure infections	20 mg/kg q 24 hrs	10
Infants and children (6 months to 12 years of age)[2] Otitis media	15 mg/kg q 12 hrs	10
Acute sinusitis (use higher dose for moderate to severe infections)	7.5 mg/kg q 12 hrs or 15 mg/kg q 12 hrs	10

[1] For infections caused by S. *pyogenes*, administer for ≥ 10 days.
[2] Not to exceed adult recommended doses.

Renal function impairment – For Ccr of 30 to 120 mL/min, use standard dosage and dosing interval. For Ccr < 30 mL/min, use a dosage 50% of standard at the standard dosing interval.

Cefprozil is in part removed by hemodialysis; therefore, administer after the completion of hemodialysis.

CEFTAZIDIME:

Ceftazidime Dosage Guidelines		
Patient/Infection site	Dose	Frequency
Adults Usual recommended dose	1 g IV or IM	q 8 to 12 h
Uncomplicated urinary tract infections	250 mg IV or IM	q 12 h
Complicated urinary tract infections	500 mg IV or IM	q 8 to 12 h
Uncomplicated pneumonia; mild skin and skin structure infections	500 mg to 1 g IV or IM	q 8 h

Ceftazidime Dosage Guidelines		
Patient/Infection site	Dose	Frequency
Bone and joint infections	2 g IV	q 12 h
Serious gynecological and intra-abdominal infections	2 g IV	q 8 h
Meningitis		
Very severe life-threatening infections, especially in immunocompromised patients		
Pseudomonal lung infections in cystic fibrosis patients w/normal renal function[1]	30 to 50 mg/kg IV up to 6 g/day	q 8 h
Neonates (0 to 4 weeks)	30 mg/kg IV	q 12 h
Infants and children (1 month to 12 years of age)	30 to 50 mg/kg IV up to 6 g/day[2]	q 8 h

[1] Although clinical improvement has been shown, bacteriological cures cannot be expected in patients with chronic respiratory disease and cystic fibrosis.
[2] Reserve the higher dose for immunocompromised children or children with cystic fibrosis or meningitis.

Renal function impairment – Ceftazidime is excreted by the kidneys, almost exclusively by glomerular filtration. In patients with impaired renal function (glomerular filtration rate (GFR) < 50 mL/min), reduce dosage to compensate for slower excretion. In patients with suspected renal insufficiency, give an initial loading dose of 1 g. Estimate GFR to determine the appropriate maintenance dose.

Ceftazidime Dosage in Renal Impairment		
Ccr (mL/min)	Recommended unit dose of ceftazidime	Frequency of dosing
31 to 50	1 g	q 12 h
16 to 30	1 g	q 24 h
6 to 15	500 mg	q 24 h
≤ 5	500 mg	q 48 h

In patients with severe infections who normally receive 6 g ceftazidime daily were it not for renal insufficiency, the unit dose given in the table above may be increased by 50% or the dosing frequency increased appropriately.

Dialysis – Give a 1 g loading dose, followed by 1 g after each hemodialysis period.

Ceftazidime also can be used in patients undergoing intraperitoneal dialysis (IPD) and continuous ambulatory peritoneal dialysis (CAPD). Give a loading dose of 1 g, followed by 500 mg every 24 hours. In addition to IV use, ceftazidime can be incorporated in the dialysis fluid at a concentration of 250 mg per 2 L of dialysis fluid.

CEFTIBUTEN: Ceftibuten suspension must be administered ≥ 2 hours before or 1 hour after a meal.

Ceftibutin Dosage and Duration			
Type of infection	Daily maximum dose	Dose and frequency	Duration
Adults ≥ 12 years of age			
Acute bacterial exacerbations of chronic bronchitis caused by *H. influenzae*, *M. catarrhalis*, or *Streptococcus pneumoniae*	400 mg	400 mg/day	10 days
Pharyngitis and tonsillitis caused by *S. pyogenes*			
Acute bacterial otitis media caused by *H. influenzae*, *M. catarrhalis*, or *S. pyogenes*			

Ceftibutin Dosage and Duration			
Type of infection	Daily maximum dose	Dose and frequency	Duration
Children Pharyngitis and tonsillitis caused by S. pyogenes Acute bacterial otitis media caused by H. influenzae, M. catarrhalis, or S. pyogenes	400 mg	9 mg/kg/day	10 days

Ceftibuten Oral Suspension Pediatric Dosage Chart[1]			
Weight		90 mg/5 mL	180 mg/5 mL
kg	lb		
10	22	5 mL (1 tsp)/day	2.5 mL (½ tsp)/day
20	44	10 mL (2 tsp)/day	5 mL (1 tsp)/day
40	88	20 mL (4 tsp)/day	10 mL (2 tsp)/day

[1] Children > 45 kg should receive the maximum daily dose of 400 mg.

Renal function impairment – Ceftibuten may be given at normal doses in impaired renal function with creatinine clearance of ≥ 50 mL/min. Dosing recommendations for patients with varying degrees of renal insufficiency are presented in the following table.

Ceftibuten Dosage in Renal Impairment	
Ccr (mL/min)	Recommended dosing schedules
> 50	9 mg/kg or 400 mg q 24 h (normal dosing schedule)
30 to 49	4.5 mg/kg or 200 mg q 24 h
5 to 29	2.25 mg/kg or 100 mg q 24 h

Hemodialysis patients – In patients undergoing hemodialysis 2 or 3 times weekly, a single 400 mg dose of ceftibuten capsules or a single dose of 9 mg/kg (maximum of 400 mg) oral suspension may be given at the end of each hemodialysis session.

CEFTIZOXIME SODIUM:
Adults – Usual dosage is 1 or 2 g every 8 to 12 hours.

Ceftizoxime Dosage Guidelines in Adults		
Type of infection	Daily dose (g)	Frequency and route
Uncomplicated urinary tract	1	500 mg every 12 hrs IM or IV
Pelvic inflammatory disease (PID)[1]	6	2 g every 8 hrs IV
Other sites	2 to 3	1 g every 8 to 12 hrs IV or IM
Severe or refractory	3 to 6	1 g every 8 hours IM or IV 2 g every 8 to 12 hrs IM [1] or IV
Life-threatening[2]	9 to 12	3 to 4 g every 8 hrs IV

[1] Dosages up to 2 g every 4 hours have been given.
[2] Divide 2 g IM doses and give in different large muscle masses.

Urinary tract infections – Higher dosage is recommended.

Gonorrhea, uncomplicated – A single 1 g IM injection is the usual dose.

Life-threatening infections – The IV route may be preferable for patients with bacterial septicemia, localized parenchymal abscesses (such as intra-abdominal abscess), peritonitis or other severe or life-threatening infections.

In those patients with normal renal function, the IV dosage is 2 to 12 g daily. In conditions such as bacterial septicemia, 6 to 12 g/day IV may be given initially for several days, and the dosage gradually reduced according to clinical response and laboratory findings.

Pediatric –

Children (≥ 6 months): 50 mg/kg every 6 to 8 hours. Dosage may be increased to 200 mg/kg/day. Do not exceed the maximum adult dose for serious infection.

Renal function impairment: Renal function impairment requires modification of dosage. Following an initial loading dose of 500 mg to 1 g IM or IV, use the maintenance dosing schedule in the following table.

Hemodialysis – No additional supplemental dosing is required following hemodialysis; give the dose (according to the table below) at the end of dialysis.

Ceftizoxime Dosage in Adults with Renal Impairment			
Renal function	Ccr (mL/min)	Less severe infections	Life-threatening infections
Mild impairment	50 to 79	500 mg q 8 h	750 mg to 1.5 g q 8 h
Moderate to severe impairment	5 to 49	250 to 500 mg q 12 h	500 mg to 1 g q 12 h
Dialysis patients	0 to 4	500 mg q 48 h or 250 mg q 24 h	500 mg to 1 g q 48 h or 500 mg q 24 h

CEFTRIAXONE SODIUM: Administer IV or IM.

Adults – Usual daily dosage is 1 to 2 g once a day (or in equally divided doses twice a day) depending on type and severity of infection. Do not exceed a total daily dose of 4 g.

Uncomplicated gonococcal infections: Give a single IM dose of 250 mg.

Surgical prophylaxis: Give a single 1 g dose ½ to 2 hours before surgery.

Children – To treat serious infections other than meningitis, administer 50 to 75 mg/kg/day (not to exceed 2 g) in divided doses every 12 hours.

Meningitis: 100 mg/kg/day (not to exceed 4 g). Thereafter, a total daily dose of 100 mg/kg/day (not to exceed 4 g/day) is recommended. May give daily dose once per day or in equally divided doses every 12 hours. Usual duration is 7 to 14 days.

Skin and skin structure infections: Give 50 to 75 mg/kg once daily (or in equally divided doses twice daily), not to exceed 2 g.

CDC-recommended treatment schedules for chancroid, gonorrhea, and acute PID –

Chancroid (Haemophilus ducreyi infection): 250 mg IM as a single dose.

Gonococcal infections:

Uncomplicated – 125 mg IM in a single dose plus 1 g azithromycin in single oral dose or 100 mg doxycycline twice a day for 7 days.

Conjunctivitis – 1 g IM single dose.

Disseminated – 1 g IM or IV every 24 hours.

Meningitis/Endocarditis – 1 to 2 g IV every 12 hours for 10 to 14 days (meningitis) or for ≥ 4 weeks (endocarditis).

Children (< 45 kg) – With bacteremia or arthritis, use 50 mg/kg (maximum, 1 g) IM or IV in a single dose for 7 days. For meningitis, increase duration to 10 to 14 days and maximum dose to 2 g.

Infants – 25 to 50 mg/kg/day IV or IM in a single daily dose, not to exceed 125 mg. For disseminated infection, continue for 7 days, with a duration of 7 to 14 days with documented meningitis.

Acute PID (ambulatory): 250 mg IM plus doxycycline.

CEFUROXIME:

Oral – Tablets and suspension are not bioequivalent and not substitutable on a mg/mg basis.

Tablets: The tablets may be given without regard to meals.

Suspension: Administer with food.

Dosage for Cefuroxime Axetil Tablets		
Population/Infection	Dosage	Duration (days)
Adults (≥ 13 years of age)		
Pharyngitis/Tonsillitis	250 mg bid	10
Acute bacterial exacerbations of chronic bronchitis[1]	250 or 500 mg bid	10
Secondary bacterial infections of acute bronchitis		5 to 10
Uncomplicated skin and skin structure infections	250 or 500 mg bid	10
Uncomplicated urinary tract infections	125 or 250 mg bid	7 to 10
Uncomplicated gonorrhea	1000 mg once	single dose
Early Lyme disease	500 mg bid	20
Children who can swallow tablets whole[2]		
Pharyngitis/Tonsillitis	125 mg bid	10
Acute otitis media	250 mg bid	10

[1] Safety and efficacy of drug administered < 10 days in patients with acute exacerbations of chronic bronchitis have not been established.
[2] Do not exceed adult recommended doses.

Dosage for Cefuroxime Axetil Suspension			
Population/Infection	Dosage	Daily maximum dose	Duration (days)
Infants and children (3 months to 12 years of age)			
Pharyngitis/Tonsillitis	20 mg/kg/day divided bid	500 mg	10
Acute otitis media	30 mg/kg/day divided bid	1000 mg	10
Impetigo	30 mg/kg/day divided bid	1000 mg	10

Renal failure: Because cefuroxime is renally eliminated, its half-life will be prolonged in patients with renal failure.

Parenteral –

Dosage:

Adults – 750 mg to 1.5 g IM or IV every 8 hours, usually for 5 to 10 days.

Cefuroxime Dosage Guidelines		
Type of infection	Daily dosage (g)	Frequency
Uncomplicated urinary tract, skin and skin structure, disseminated gonococcal, uncomplicated pneumonia	2.25	750 mg every 8 hrs
Severe or complicated	4.5	1.5 g every 8 hrs
Bone and joint	4.5	1.5 g every 8 hrs
Life-threatening or caused by less susceptible organisms	6	1.5 g every 6 hrs
Bacterial meningitis	9	≤ 3 g every 8 hrs
Uncomplicated gonococcal	1.5 g IM[1]	single dose

[1] Administered at 2 different sites together with 1 g oral probenecid.

Preoperative prophylaxis: For clean-contaminated or potentially contaminated surgical procedures, administer 1.5 g IV prior to surgery (≈ ½ to 1 hour before). Thereafter, give 750 mg IV or IM every 8 hours when the procedure is prolonged.

For preventative use during open heart surgery, give 1.5 g IV at the induction of anesthesia and every 12 hours thereafter for a total of 6 g.

Renal function impairment: Reduce dosage.

Parenteral Cefuroxime Dosage in Renal Impairment (Adults)	
Ccr (mL/min)	Dose and frequency
> 20	750 mg to 1.5 g every 8 hrs
10 to 20	750 mg every 12 hrs
< 10	750 mg every 24 hrs [1]

[1] Because cefuroxime is dialyzable, give patients on hemodialysis a further dose at the end of the dialysis.

Infants and children (> 3 months) – 50 to 100 mg/kg/day in equally divided doses every 6 to 8 hours. Use 100 mg/kg/day (not to exceed maximum adult dose) for more severe or serious infections.

Bone and joint infections: 150 mg/kg/day (not to exceed maximum adult dose) in equally divided doses every 8 hours.

Bacterial meningitis: Initially, 200 to 240 mg/kg/day IV in divided doses every 6 to 8 hours.

In renal insufficiency, modify dosage frequency per adult guidelines.

CEPHALEXIN:

Adults – 1 to 4 g/day in divided doses.

Usual dose: 250 mg every 6 hours.

Streptococcal pharyngitis, skin and skin structure infections, uncomplicated cystitis in patients > 15 years: 500 mg every 12 hours.

May need larger doses for more severe infections or less susceptible organisms. If dose is > 4 g/day, use parenteral drugs.

Children – Do not exceed adult recommended doses.

Monohydrate: 25 to 50 mg/kg/day in divided doses. For streptococcal pharyngitis in patients > 1 year of age and for skin and skin structure infections, divide total daily dose and give every 12 hours. In severe infections, double the dose.

Otitis media – 75 to 100 mg/kg/day in 4 divided doses.

β-*hemolytic streptococcal infections* – Continue treatment for ≥ 10 days.

HCl monohydrate – Safety and efficacy not established for use in children.

CEPHAPIRIN SODIUM:

Adults – 500 mg to 1 g every 4 to 6 hours IM or IV. The lower dose is adequate for certain infections, such as skin and skin structure and most urinary tract infections; the higher dose is recommended for more serious infections.

Serious or life-threatening infections – Up to 12 g daily. Use the IV route when high doses are indicated.

Renal function impairment: Patients with reduced renal function (moderately severe oliguria or serum creatinine > 5 mg/100 mL) may be treated adequately with a lower dose, 7.5 to 15 mg/kg every 12 hours. Patients who are to be dialyzed should receive the same dose just prior to dialysis and every 12 hours thereafter.

Perioperative prophylaxis: 1 to 2 g IM or IV administered ½ to 1 hour prior to the start of surgery; 1 to 2 g during surgery (administration modified depending on duration of operation); 1 to 2 g IV or IM every 6 hours for 24 hours postoperatively.

Children – Recommended total daily dose is 40 to 80 mg/kg (20 to 40 mg/lb) administered in 4 equally divided doses.

Infants – Cephapirin has not been extensively studied in infants; therefore, in the treatment of children < 3 months of age, consider the relative benefit to risk.

CEPHRADINE:

Oral – May be given without regard to meals.

Adults:

Skin, skin structure, and respiratory tract infections (other than lobar pneumonia) – Usual dose is 250 mg every 6 hours or 500 mg every 12 hours.

Lobar pneumonia – 500 mg every 6 hours or 1 g every 12 hours.

Uncomplicated urinary tract infections – The usual dose is 500 mg every 12 hours. In more serious infections and prostatitis, 500 mg every 6 hours or 1 g every 12 hours. Severe or chronic infections may require larger doses (up to 1 g every 6 hours).

Children: No adequate information is available on the efficacy of twice a day regimens in children < 9 months of age. For children > 9 months, the usual dose is 25 to 50 mg/kg/day, in equally divided doses every 6 or 12 hours. For otitis media caused by *H. influenzae*, 75 to 100 mg/kg/day in equally divided doses every 6 or 12 hours is recommended; do not exceed 4 g/day.

All patients regardless of age and weight: Larger doses (up to 1 g 4 times/day) may be given for severe or chronic infections.

Parenteral – Parenteral therapy may be followed by oral. To minimize pain and induration, inject IM deep into a large muscle mass.

Adults: Daily dose is 2 to 4 g in equally divided doses 4 times/day, IM or IV. In bone infections, the usual dosage is 1 g IV 4 times/day. A dose of 500 mg 4 times/day is adequate in uncomplicated pneumonia, skin and skin structure infections, and most urinary tract infections. In severe infections, dose may be increased by giving every 4 hours or by increasing dose up to a maximum of 8 g/day.

Perioperative prophylaxis – Recommended doses are 1 g IV or IM administered 30 to 90 minutes prior to the start of surgery, followed by 1 g every 4 to 6 hours after the first dose for 1 or 2 doses, or for up to 24 hours postoperatively.

Cesarean section – Give 1 g IV as soon as the umbilical cord is clamped. Give the second and third doses as 1 g IM or IV at 6 to 12 hours after the first dose.

Infants and children – 50 to 100 mg/kg/day in 4 equally divided doses; determine by age, weight, and infection severity.

Renal impairment dosage –

Patients not on dialysis:

Cephradine Dosage in Renal Impairment		
Ccr (mL/min)	Dose (mg)	Time interval (hours)
> 20	500	6
5 to 20	250	6
< 5	250	12

Patients on chronic, intermittent dialysis: 250 mg initially; repeat at 12 hours and after 36 to 48 hours.

LORACARBEF: Administer ≥ 1 hour before or 2 hours after a meal.

Dosage/Duration of Loracarbef		
Population/Infection	Dosage (mg)	Duration (days)
Adults ≥ 13 years of age		
Lower respiratory tract		
Secondary bacterial infection of acute bronchitis	200 to 400 q 12 hrs	7
Acute bacterial exacerbation of chronic bronchitis	400 q 12 hrs	7
Pneumonia	400 q 12 hrs	14
Upper respiratory tract		
Pharyngitis/Tonsillitis	200 q 12 hrs	10[1]
Sinusitis	400 q 12 hrs	10
Skin and skin structure		
Uncomplicated	200 q 12 hrs	7
Urinary tract		
Uncomplicated cystitis	200 q 24 hrs	7
Uncomplicated pyelonephritis	400 q 12 hrs	14
Infants and children (6 months to 12 years)[2]		
Upper respiratory tract		
Acute otitis media[3]	30 mg/kg/day in divided doses q 12 hrs	10
Acute maxillary sinusitis		
Pharyngitis/Tonsillitis	15 mg/kg/day in divided doses q 12 hrs	10[1]

Dosage/Duration of Loracarbef		
Population/Infection	Dosage (mg)	Duration (days)
Skin and skin structure Impetigo	15 mg/kg/day in divided doses q 12 hrs	7

[1] In treatment of infections caused by *S. pyogenes*, administer for ≥ 10 days.
[2] Do not exceed adult recommended doses.
[3] Use suspension; it is more rapidly absorbed than capsules, resulting in higher peak plasma concentrations when given at the same dose.

Renal function impairment – Use usual dose and schedule in patients with Ccr levels ≥ 50 mL/min. Patients with Ccr between 10 and 49 mL/min may be given half the recommended dose at the usual dosage interval. Patients with Ccr levels < 10 mL/min may receive recommended dose given every 3 to 5 days; patients on hemodialysis should receive another dose following dialysis.

Actions

Pharmacology: Cephalosporins are structurally and pharmacologically related to penicillins. **Cefoxitin** and **cefotetan** (cephamycins) and **loracarbef** (a carbacephem) are included because of their similarity.

Cephalosporins inhibit mucopeptide synthesis in the bacterial cell wall, making it defective and osmotically unstable. The drugs are usually bactericidal, depending on organism susceptibility, dose, tissue concentrations, and the rate at which organisms are multiplying. They are more effective against rapidly growing organisms forming cell walls.

Pharmacokinetics:

Pharmacokinetic Parameters of Cephalosporins								
		Half-Life						
	Drug	Routes	Normal renal function (minutes)	ESRD[1] (hours)	Hemodialysis (hours)	Protein bound (%)	Recovered unchanged in urine (%)	Peak serum level 1 g IV dose (mcg/mL)	Sodium (mEq/g)
First	Cefadroxil	Oral	78-96	20-25	3-4	20	> 90	—	—
	Cefazolin	IM-IV	90–120	3-7	9-14	80-86	60-80	185	2-2.1
	Cephalexin	Oral	50-80	19-22	4-6	10	> 90	—	—
	Cephapirin	IM-IV	36	1.8-4	1.8	44-50	70	73	2.4
	Cephradine	Oral/IM-IV	48-80	8-15	—	8-17	> 90	86	6[2]
Second	Cefaclor	Oral	35-54	2-3	1.6-2.1	25	60-85	—	—
	Cefamandole	IM-IV	30-60	8-11	7	70	65-85	139	3.3
	Cefmetazole	IM-IV	72-90	—	—	65	85	—	2
	Cefonicid	IM-IV	270	11	—	90	99	221.3	3.7
	Cefotetan	IM-IV	180-276	13-35	5	88-90	51-81	158	3.5
	Cefoxitin	IV	40-60	20	4	73	85	110	2.3
	Cefprozil	Oral	78	5.2-5.9	decreased	36	60	—	—
	Cefuroxime	Oral/IM-IV	80	16-22[3]	3.5	50	66-100	100[4]	2.4[3]
	Loracarbef	Oral	60	32	4	25	> 90	—	—

Pharmacokinetic Parameters of Cephalosporins								
		Half-Life						
Drug	Routes	Normal renal function (minutes)	ESRD[1] (hours)	Hemodialysis (hours)	Protein bound (%)	Recovered unchanged in urine (%)	Peak serum level 1 g IV dose (mcg/mL)	Sodium (mEq/g)
Cefdinir	Oral	100	16	3.2	60-70	12-18	—	—
Cefepime	IM-IV	102-138	17-21	11-16	20	85	79	—
Cefixime	Oral	180-240	11.5	—	65	50	—	—
Cefopera-zone	IM-IV	120	1.3-2.9	2	82-93	20-30	73-153	1.5
Cefotaxime	IM-IV	60	3-11	2.5	30-40	60	42-102	2.2
Cefpodox-ime[2]	Oral	120-180	9.8	—	21-29	29-33	—	—
Ceftazidime	IM-IV	114-120	14-30	—	< 10	80-90	69-90	2.3
Ceftibuten	Oral	144	13.4-22.3	2-4	65	56	—	—
Ceftizoxime	IM-IV	102	25-30	6	30	80	60-87	2.6
Ceftriaxone	IM-IV	348-522	15.7	14.7	85-95	33-67	151	3.6

(Third)

[1] ESRD = End stage renal disease (Ccr < 10 mL/min/1.73 m^2).
[2] Also available in sodium-free form.
[3] Injection only.
[4] Following 1.5 g IV dose.
[5] Extended spectrum agent.

Cephalexin, cephradine, cefaclor, cefixime, cefprozil, cefadroxil, ceftibuten, and **loracarbef** are well absorbed from the GI tract. Cephalosporins are widely distributed to most tissues and fluids. First and second generation agents do not readily enter cerebrospinal fluid (CSF), except **cefuroxime**, even when meninges are inflamed. Third generation compounds (little data for cefixime) readily diffuse into the CSF of patients with inflamed meninges. However, CSF levels of **cefoperazone** are relatively low. Most cephalosporins and metabolites are primarily excreted renally.

Microbiology:

Organisms Generally Susceptible to Cephalosporins

✓ = generally susceptible
++ = demonstrated in vitro activity

Organisms (Gram-positive)	First Generation					Second Generation									Third Generation									
	Cefadroxil	Cefazolin	Cephalexin	Cephapirin	Cephradine	Cefaclor	Cefamandole	Cefonicid	Cefoxitin	Cefuroxime	Cefmetazole	Cefotetan	Cefprozil	Loracarbef	Cefdinir	Cefepime[1]	Cefixime	Cefoperazone	Cefotaxime	Cefpodoxime[2]	Ceftazidime	Ceftibuten	Ceftizoxime	Ceftriaxone
Staphylococci[3]	✓	✓	✓[4]	✓	✓	✓[4]		✓[4]	✓	✓	✓	✓	✓	✓	✓[5]	✓[6]		✓	✓[5]	✓[4]	✓		✓	✓
Staphylococcus aureus							✓																	
Staphylococcus epidermidis						++	✓			++				++	++[6]									
Staphylococcus saprophyticus	✓									++				✓										
Streptococci, beta-hemolytic	✓	✓	✓	✓	✓	✓	✓	✓	✓	++	✓	✓	✓	++	++	++	✓	✓	✓	✓	✓		✓	✓
Streptococcus agalactiae														++										
Streptococcus bovis														++										
Streptococcus pneumoniae	✓	✓	✓	✓	✓	✓	✓	✓		✓	✓	✓	✓	✓	✓[7]	✓[8]	✓	✓	✓	✓	✓	✓[7]	✓	✓
Streptococcus pyogenes		✓	✓	✓	✓	✓	✓	✓	✓	✓	✓	✓	✓	✓	✓	✓	✓	✓	✓	✓	✓	✓	✓	✓
Streptococcus viridans														++	++									

Organisms Generally Susceptible to Cephalosporins

Legend: ✓ = generally susceptible; + = demonstrated in vitro activity

Gram-negative

Organisms	First Generation					Second Generation									Third Generation									
	Cefadroxil	Cefazolin	Cephapirin	Cephalexin	Cephradine	Cefaclor	Cefamandole	Cefonicid	Cefoxitin	Cefuroxime	Cefmetazole	Cefotetan	Cefprozil	Loracarbef	Cefdinir	Cefepime[1]	Cefixime	Cefoperazone	Cefotaxime	Cefpodoxime[2]	Ceftazidime	Ceftibuten	Ceftizoxime	Ceftriaxone
Acinetobacter sp.		✓														+	+	✓[4]	✓		+		✓	+
Citrobacter sp.								+		✓[4]	+	+	+	+	+	+	+	✓	✓	+	✓		+	+
Enterobacter sp.		✓[4]					✓	+		✓[4]	+	✓				✓	✓	✓	✓		✓		✓	✓
Escherichia coli	✓	✓	✓	✓	✓	✓	✓	✓[5]	✓	✓[5]	✓[5]	✓[5]	+	✓	+	✓	✓	✓	✓	✓	✓		✓	✓
Haemophilus influenzae		✓	✓			✓[5]	✓[4]		✓[5]	+			✓[5]	✓[5]	✓[5]	+[5]	✓[5]	✓[5]	✓[5]	✓[5]	✓[5]	✓[5]	✓[5]	✓[5]
Haemophilus parainfluenzae						+								+	✓[5]		+[5]	✓	✓	+	+			✓
Hafnia alvei													+	+	+	+	+				✓			
Klebsiella sp.		✓	✓	✓	✓	✓	✓	✓	✓		✓	✓	+	+	+	✓	+	✓	✓	✓	✓		✓	✓
Klebsiella pneumoniae				+		+		+																
Moraxella (Branhamella) catarrhalis	+					✓[5]				✓[4]	+	+	✓[5]	✓[5]	✓[5]	+[5]	✓[5]	✓[5]	✓	✓	✓	✓[5]	+	
Morganella (Proteus) morganii	✓						✓	✓	✓		✓	✓				+		✓	✓	✓	+		✓	✓

Organisms Generally Susceptible to Cephalosporins

Legend: ✔ = generally susceptible; + = demonstrated in vitro activity

Organisms (Gram-negative cont'd)	First Generation						Second Generation									Third Generation								
	Cefadroxil	Cefazolin	Cephalexin	Cephapirin	Cephradine	Cefaclor	Cefamandole	Cefonicid	Cefoxitin	Cefuroxime	Cefmetazole	Cefotetan	Cefprozil	Loracarbef	Cefdinir	Cefepime[1]	Cefixime	Cefoperazone	Cefotaxime	Cefpodoxime[2]	Ceftazidime	Cefibuten	Ceftizoxime	Ceftriaxone
Neisseria catarrhalis	✔		✔																					
Neisseria gonorrhoeae						++		++	✔	✔	++	++	++	+[3]			++	✔[5]	✔	✔[4]	++		✔	✔
Neisseria meningitidis										✔								++	✔		✔		++	✔
Pasteurella multocida											++			++										
Proteus inconstans															++									
Proteus mirabilis	✔	✔	✔	✔	✔	✔	✔	✔	✔	✔	✔	✔	++	++		✔	✔	✔	✔	✔	✔		✔	✔
Proteus vulgaris								✔	✔		✔	✔				++	++	✔	++	++	++		++	++
Providencia sp.							✔[4]	✔	✔	✔	++					++	++	✔	✔	++	++		✔	++
Providencia rettgeri																++	++	✔	✔[4]	++	++		✔	++
Pseudomonas aeruginosa																✔		++	✔[4]		✔		✔[4]	✔[4]
Salmonella sp.									✔		++	++	++	++			++	++	++	++	++		++	++
Salmonella typhi												++				++	++		++				++	++
Serratia sp.												++				++	++	✔	✔		✔		✔	✔
Shigella sp.										✔	++	++	++	++		++	++	++	++	++	++		++	++
Yersinia enterocolitica												✔		++										+

Organisms Generally Susceptible to Cephalosporins

Legend: ✓ = generally susceptible; ‡ = demonstrated in vitro activity

Organisms	First Generation					Second Generation									Third Generation									
	Cefadroxil	Cefazolin	Cephalexin	Cephapirin	Cephradine	Cefaclor	Cefamandole	Cefonicid	Cefoxitin	Cefuroxime	Cefmetazole	Cefotetan	Cefprozil	Loracarbef	Cefdinir	Cefepime[1]	Cefixime	Cefoperazone	Cefotaxime	Cefpodoxime[2]	Ceftazidime	Ceftibuten	Ceftizoxime	Ceftriaxone
Anaerobes																								
Bacteroides sp.						✓	✓		✓	✓	✓	✓[4]	‡					✓	✓		✓[4]		‡	✓
Bacteroides fragilis								‡	✓		✓	✓						✓	✓				✓	‡
Clostridium sp.							✓		✓	✓	✓	✓	‡	‡				✓	✓		‡		‡	‡
Clostridium difficile												‡	‡					‡						
Eubacterium sp.																		‡						‡
Fusobacterium sp.							✓	‡	✓	✓	✓	✓	‡	‡				‡	✓				‡	‡
Peptococcus sp.						‡	✓	‡	✓	✓	‡	✓	‡	‡				✓	✓	‡	‡		✓	‡
Peptococcus niger						‡	✓	‡						‡										
Peptostreptococcus sp.							✓	‡	✓	✓	‡	✓	‡	‡				✓	✓	‡	‡		✓	‡
Porphyromonas asaccharolytica																								
Prevotella bivia												✓												
Prevotella disiens												✓												
Prevotella melaninogenica												‡												
Prevotella oralis												‡												
Propionibacterium acnes						‡								‡										
Propionibacterium sp.												‡												
Veillonella sp.												‡												
Other																								
Borrelia burgdorferi										✓														

[1] Extended spectrum agent.
[2] Some other references consider this fourth generation.
[3] Coagulase-positive, coagulase-negative and penicillinase-producing.
[4] Some strains are resistant.
[5] Including some β-lactamase-producing strains.
[6] Methicillin-susceptible strains only.
[7] Penicillin-susceptible strains only.
[8] Lancefield's Group A streptococci.

Contraindications

Hypersensitivity to cephalosporins or related antibiotics.

Cefditoren: Cefditoren is contraindicated in patients with carnitine deficiency or inborn errors of metabolism that may result in clinically significant carnitine deficiency because use of cefditoren causes renal excretion of carnitine.

Cefditoren contains sodium caseinate, a milk protein. Do not administer cefditoren to patients with milk protein hypersensitivity (not lactose intolerance).

Warnings

Hypersensitivity: Reactions range from mild to life-threatening. Before therapy is instituted, inquire about previous hypersensitivity reactions to cephalosporins and penicillins.

Cross-allergenicity with penicillin: Administer cautiously to penicillin-sensitive patients. There is evidence of partial cross-allergenicity; cephalosporins cannot be assumed to be an absolutely safe alternative to penicillin in the penicillin-allergic patient. The estimated incidence of cross-sensitivity is 5% to 16%; however, it is possibly as low as 3% to 7%.

Serum sickness-like reactions: (erythema multiforme or skin rashes accompanied by polyarthritis, arthralgia and, frequently, fever) have been reported; these reactions usually occurred following a second course of therapy. Signs and symptoms occur after a few days of therapy and resolve a few days after drug discontinuation with no serious sequelae.

Seizures: Several cephalosporins have been implicated in triggering seizures, particularly in patients with renal impairment when the dosage was not reduced.

Coagulation abnormalities: **Cefamandole, cefmetazole, cefoperazone, cefotetan,** and **ceftriaxone** may be associated with a fall in prothrombin activity. Those at risk include patients with renal impairment, cancer, impaired vitamin K synthesis, or low vitamin K stores (eg, chronic hepatic disease or malnutrition), as well as patients receiving a protracted course of antimicrobial therapy. Monitor prothrombin time for patients at risk and administer exogenous vitamin K as indicated. Vitamin K administration may be necessary if the prothrombin time is prolonged before therapy.

Predisposing factors – Predisposing factors to cephalosporin bleeding abnormalities include hepatic and renal dysfunction, thrombocytopenia and the concomitant use of "high dose" heparin (> 20,000 units/day), oral anticoagulants, or other drugs that affect hemostasis (eg, aspirin). Elderly, malnourished or debilitated patients are more likely to experience bleeding abnormalities than other patients.

Pseudomembranous colitis: Pseudomembranous colitis occurs with the use of cephalosporins (and other broad spectrum antibiotics); therefore, consider its diagnosis in patients who develop diarrhea with antibiotic use.

Immune hemolytic anemia: Immune hemolytic anemia has been observed in patients receiving cephalosporin class antibiotics.

Renal function impairment: Cephalosporins may be nephrotoxic; use with caution in the presence of markedly impaired renal function (Ccr < 50 mL/min/1.73 m^2).

Hepatic function impairment: Cefoperazone is extensively excreted in bile. Serum half-life increases 2-fold to 4-fold in patients with hepatic disease or biliary obstruction.

Pregnancy: Category B. These agents cross the placenta.

Lactation: Most of these agents are excreted in breast milk in small quantities.

Children: When using cephalosporins in infants, consider the relative benefit to risk. In neonates, accumulation of cephalosporin antibiotics (with resulting prolongation of drug half-life) has occurred.

Safety and efficacy in children < 1 month (**cefazolin** and **cefaclor** capsule and suspension), < 3 months (**cefuroxime, cephapirin,** and **cefoxitin),** < 5 months (**cefpodoxime**), < 6 months (**cefdinir, loracarbef, cefixime, ceftozoxime,** and **cefprozil**), < 9 months (**oral cephradine**) and < 1 year of age (**cefepime** and **parenteral cephradine**) have not been established.

Safety and efficacy of **cefaclor** extended-release tablets in children < 16 years of age have not been established.

Safety and efficacy of **cefonicid, cefmetazole, cefoperazone, cephalexin,** and **cefotetan** in children have not been established.

Precautions

Parenteral use: Inject IM preparations deep into musculature; properly dilute IV preparations and administer over an appropriate time interval.

Gonorrhea: In the treatment of gonorrhea, all patients should have a serologic test for syphilis. Patients with incubating syphilis (seronegative without clinical signs of syphilis) are likely to be cured by the regimens used for gonorrhea.

Superinfection: Use of antibiotics (especially prolonged or repeated therapy) may result in bacterial or fungal overgrowth of nonsusceptible organisms.

Drug Interactions

Agents that may interact with cephalosporins include ethanol, aminoglycosides, anticoagulants, polypeptide antibiotics, probenecid, antacids, H_2 antagonists, iron supplements, and loop diuretics.

Drug/Lab test interactions: A false-positive reaction for **urine glucose** may occur with *Benedict's* solution, *Fehling's* solution, or with *Clinitest* tablets, but not with enzyme-based tests such as *Clinistix* and *Tes-Tape.*

Cephradine may cause false-positive reactions in urinary protein tests that use sulfosalicylic acid.

Cefuroxime may cause a false-negative reaction in the ferricyanide test for blood glucose.

Cefdinir may cause a false-positive reaction for ketones in urine when measured using nitroprusside but not nitroferricynide.

A false-positive direct *Coombs' test* has occurred in some patients receiving cephalosporins.

Cephalosporins may falsely elevate *urinary 17-ketosteroid* values.

High concentrations of **cefoxitin** (> 100 mcg/mL) may interfere with measurement of *creatinine levels* by the Jaffe reaction and produce false results. **Cefotetan** may also affect these measurements.

Drug/Food interactions: Food increases absorption of **cefpodoxime** and oral **cefuroxime**.

Adverse Reactions

Most common – GI disturbances (nausea, vomiting, diarrhea); hypersensitivity phenomena (most common); hypotension; fever; dyspnea; candidal overgrowth consisting of oral candidiasis, vaginitis, genital moniliasis, vaginal discharge and genitoanal pruritus; nervousness; insomnia; confusion; hypertonia; dizziness; somnolence.

CNS: Headache; dizziness; lethargy; fatigue; paresthesia; confusion; diaphoresis; flushing.

Hematologic: Eosinophilia; transient neutropenia; leukocytosis; leukopenia; thrombocythemia; thrombocytopenia; agranulocytosis; granulocytopenia; hemolytic anemia; bone marrow depression; pancytopenia; decreased platelet function; anemia; aplastic anemia; hemorrhage.

Hepatic: Elevated AST, ALT, GGTP, total bilirubin, alkaline phosphatase, LDH; hepatitis.

Local: IM administration commonly results in pain, induration, temperature elevation, and tenderness.

Renal: Transitory elevations in BUN with and without elevated serum creatinine (frequency increases in patients > 50 years of age and in children < 3 years of age).

MEROPENEM

Powder for injection: 500 mg and 1 g (*Rx*)   *Merrem IV* (AstraZeneca)

Indications

For the treatment of the following infections when caused by susceptible strains of the designated microorganisms:

Intra-abdominal infections: Complicated appendicitis and peritonitis caused by viridans group streptococci, *Escherichia coli*, *Klebsiella pneumoniae*, *Pseudomonas aeruginosa*, *Bacterioides fragilis*, *Bacterioides thetaiotaomicron*, and *Peptostreptococcus* sp.

Bacterial meningitis (pediatric patients ≥ 3 months only): Bacterial meningitis caused by *Streptococcus pneumoniae*, *Haemophilus influenzae* (β-lactamase and non-β-lactamase-producing strains), and *Neisseria meningitidis*.

Administration and Dosage

Adults: 1 g IV every 8 hours. Give over ≈ 15 to 30 minutes or as an IV bolus injection (5 to 20 mL) over ≈ 3 to 5 minutes.

Renal function impairment: Reduce dosage in patients with Ccr < 50 mL/min.

Recommended Meropenem IV Dosage Schedule for Adults with Impaired Renal Function		
Ccr (mL/min)	Dose (dependent on type of infection)	Dosing interval
26 to 50	recommended dose (100 mg)	every 12 hours
10 to 25	½ recommended dose	every 12 hours
< 10	½ recommended dose	every 24 hours

Use in pediatric patients: For pediatric patients from ≥ 3 months of age, the meropenem dose is 20 or 40 mg/kg every 8 hours (maximum dose, 2 g every 8 hours), depending on the type of infection (intra-abdominal or meningitis). Administer pediatric patients weighing > 50 kg 1 g every 8 hours for intra-abdominal infections and 2 g every 8 hours for meningitis. Give over ≈ 15 to 30 minutes or as an IV bolus injection (5 to 20 mL) over ≈ 3 to 5 minutes.

Recommended Meropenem IV Dosage Schedule for Pediatric Patients with Normal Renal Function		
Type of infection	Dose (mg/kg)	Dosing interval
Intra-abdominal	20	every 8 hours
Meningitis	40	every 8 hours

Actions

Pharmacology: Meropenem is a broad-spectrum carbapenem antibiotic. The bactericidal activity of meropenem results from the inhibition of cell-wall synthesis. Meropenem readily penetrates the cell wall of most gram-positive and gram-negative bacteria to reach penicillin-binding-protein (PBP) targets.

Pharmacokinetics: Meropenem has dose-dependent kinetics.

In subjects with normal renal function, the elimination half-life of meropenem is ≈ 1 hour. Meropenem is excreted by the kidney with a half-life of 0.8 to 1.24 hours; 65% to 83% of the dose is recovered in the urine as meropenem and 20% to 28% as the inactive open β-lactam metabolite.

Plasma protein binding of meropenem is ≈ 2%. The volume of meropenem distribution is 15.7 to 26.68 L. Meropenem penetrates well into most body fluids and tissues, including cerebrospinal fluid, achieving concentrations matching or exceeding those required to inhibit most susceptible bacteria.

The pharmacokinetics of meropenem in pediatric patients ≥ 2 years of age are essentially similar to those in adults. In infants and children 2 months to 12 years of age, no age- or dose-dependent effects on pharmacokinetic parameters were observed. Mean half-life was 1.13 hours, mean volume of distribution at steady state was 0.43 L/kg, mean residence time was 1.57 hours, clearance was 5.63 mL/min/kg and renal clearance was 2.53 mL/min/kg. The elimination half-life is slightly prolonged (1.5 hours) in pediatric patients 3 months to 2 years of age.

Microbiology: Meropenem has significant stability to hydrolysis by β-lactamases of most categories, both penicillinases and cephalosporinases produced by gram-positive and gram-negative bacteria, with the exception of matallo-β-lactamases. Do not use to treat methicillin-resistant staphylococci. Cross-resistance is sometimes observed with strains resistant to other carbapenems. In vitro tests show meropenem to act synergistically with aminoglycoside antibiotics against some isolates of *P. aeruginosa*.

Contraindications

Hypersensitivity to any component of this product or to other drugs in the same class or in patients who have demonstrated anaphylactic reactions to β-lactams.

Warnings

Pseudomembranous colitis: Pseudomembranous colitis has been reported with nearly all antibacterial agents, including meropenem and may range in severity from mild to life-threatening. Therefore, it is important to consider this diagnosis in patients who develop diarrhea subsequent to the administration of antibacterial agents.

Hypersensitivity reactions: Serious and occasionally fatal hypersensitivity (anaphylactic) reactions have been reported in patients receiving therapy with β-lactams. These reactions are more likely to occur with a history of sensitivity to multiple allergens.

There have been reports of individuals with a history of penicillin hypersensitivity who have experienced severe hypersensitivity reactions when treated with other β-lactams.

Renal function impairment: Plasma clearance of meropenem correlates with Ccr. In moderate renal dysfunction (Ccr 30 to 80 mL/min), mean half-life has been prolonged to 1.93 to 3.36 hours. In patients with greater dysfunction (Ccr 2 to 30 mg/min), mean half-life has been further prolonged to 3.82 to 5.73 hours. Patients undergoing hemodialysis (patients with end-stage renal disease) had mean predialysis half-lives of 7 to 10 hours. Hemodialysis shortened elimination half-life to 1.4 to 2.9 hours during the dialysis period.

Elderly: Elderly patients with renal insufficiency have shown a reduction in plasma clearance of meropenem that correlates with age-associated reduction in creatinine clearance. The mean terminal half-life is prolonged slightly to 1.27 hours.

Pregnancy: Category B.

Lactation: It is not known whether this drug is excreted in breast milk.

Children: The safety and efficacy of meropenem have not been established for children < 3 months of age (see Administration and Dosage).

Precautions

Monitoring: Periodic assessment of organ system functions, including renal, hepatic, and hematopoietic is advisable during prolonged therapy.

Seizures: Seizures and other CNS adverse experiences have been reported during treatment with meropenem. These adverse experiences have occurred most commonly in patients with CNS disorders (eg, brain lesions or history of seizures) or with bacterial meningitis or compromised renal function.

Superinfection: As with other broad-spectrum antibiotics, prolonged use of meropenem may result in overgrowth of nonsusceptible organisms.

Drug Interactions

Probenecid: Probenecid may interact with meropenem.

Adverse Reactions

Adverse reactions occurring in ≥ 3% of patients include inflammation at the injection site, diarrhea, nausea, and vomiting.

Adverse reactions occuring in ≥ 3% of pediatric patients include diarrhea, vomiting, and rash (mostly diaper-area moniliasis).

IMIPENEM-CILASTATIN

Powder for injection: 250, 500, and 750 mg imipenem equivalent and cilastatin equivalent (*Rx*)

Primaxin I.V. (Merck), *Primaxin I.M.* (Merck)

Indications

IV: Treatment of serious infections caused by susceptible strains of the designated microorganisms in the conditions listed below:

Lower respiratory tract infections – Staphylococcus aureus (penicillinase-producing), Escherichia coli, Klebsiella sp., Enterobacter sp., Haemophilus influenzae, Haemophilus parainfluenzae, Acinetobacter sp., Serratia marcescens.

Urinary tract infections (complicated and uncomplicated) – Enterococcus faecalis, S. aureus (penicillinase-producing), E. coli, Klebsiella sp., Enterobacter sp., Proteus vulgaris, Providencia rettgeri, Morganella morganii, Pseudomonas aeruginosa.

Intra-abdominal infections – Enterococcus faecalis, S. aureus (penicillinase-producing), Staphylococcus epidermidis, E. coli, Klebsiella sp., Enterobacter sp., Proteus sp., M. morganii, P. aeruginosa, Citrobacter sp., Clostridium sp., Bacteroides sp. including Bacteroides fragilis, Fusobacterium sp.; Peptococcus sp., Peptostreptococcus sp., Eubacterium sp., Propionibacterium sp., Bifidobacterium sp.

Gynecologic infections – E. faecalis; S. aureus (penicillinase-producing), S. epidermidis, Streptococcus agalactiae (group B streptococcus), E. coli, Klebsiella sp., Proteus sp., Enterobacter sp., Bifidobacterium sp., Bacteroides sp. including B. fragilis, Gardnerella vaginalis; Peptococcus sp., Peptostreptococcus sp., Propionibacterium sp.

Bacterial septicemia – E. faecalis, S. aureus (penicillinase-producing), E. coli, Klebsiella sp., P. aeruginosa, Serratia sp., Enterobacter sp., Bacteroides sp.

Bone and joint infections – E. faecalis; S. aureus (penicillinase-producing), S. epidermidis, Enterobacter sp., P. aeruginosa.

Skin and skin structure infections – E. faecalis, S. aureus (penicillinase-producing), S. epidermidis, E. coli, Klebsiella sp., Enterobacter sp., P. vulgaris, P. rettgeri, M. morganii, P. aeruginosa, Serratia sp., Citrobacter sp., Acinetobacter sp., Bacteroides sp., Fusobacterium sp.; Peptococcus sp., Peptostreptococcus sp.

Endocarditis – S. aureus (penicillinase-producing).

Polymicrobic infections – Polymicrobic infections, including those in which S. pneumoniae (pneumonia, septicemia), S. pyogenes (skin and skin structure) or nonpenicillinase-producing S. aureus is one of the causative organisms. However, these monobacterial infections usually are treated with narrower spectrum antibiotics (eg, penicillin G). Although clinical improvement has been observed in patients with cystic fibrosis, chronic pulmonary disease, and lower respiratory tract infections caused by P. aeruginosa, bacterial eradication may not be achieved.

IM: Treatment of serious infections of mild to moderate severity where IM therapy is appropriate. Not intended for severe or life-threatening infections, including bacterial sepsis or endocarditis, or in major physiological impairments (eg, shock).

Lower respiratory tract infections – Lower respiratory tract infections, including pneumonia and bronchitis as an exacerbation of COPD, caused by S. pneumoniae and H. influenzae.

Intra-abdominal infections – Intra-abdominal infections, including acute gangrenous or perforated appendicitis and appendicitis with peritonitis, caused by group D streptococcus including E. faecalis; Streptococcus (viridans group); E. coli; Klebsiella pneumoniae; P. aeruginosa; Bacteroides sp. including B. fragilis, B. distasonis, B. intermedius, and B. thetaiotaomicron; Fusobacterium sp.; Peptostreptococcus sp.

Skin and skin structure infections – Skin and skin structure infections, including abscesses, cellulitis, infected skin ulcers, and wound infections caused by S. aureus (including penicillinase-producing strains); Streptococcus pyogenes; group D streptococcus including E. faecalis; Acinetobacter sp. including A. calcoaceticus; Citrobacter sp.; E. coli; Enterobacter cloacae; K. pneumoniae; P. aeruginosa; Bacteroides sp. including B. fragilis.

Gynecologic infections – Gynecologic infections, including postpartum endomyometritis, caused by group D streptococcus such as *E. faecalis*; *E. coli*; *K. pneumoniae*; *B. intermedius*; *Peptostreptococcus* sp.

Infections resistant to other antibiotics (eg, cephalosporins, penicillins, aminoglycosides) have responded to treatment with imipenem.

Administration and Dosage

Dosage recommendations represent the quantity of imipenem to be administered. An equivalent amount of cilastatin is also present in the solution.

IV:

  Adults – Give a 125, 250, or 500 mg dose by IV infusion over 20 to 30 minutes. Infuse a 750 or 1 g dose over 40 to 60 minutes. In patients who develop nausea, slow the infusion rate.

    Because of high antimicrobial activity, do not exceed 50 mg/kg/day or 4 g/day, whichever is lower.

Imipenem-Cilastatin IV Dosing Schedule for Adults with Normal Renal Function				
Type or severity of infection	Fully susceptible organisms[1]	Total daily dose	Moderately susceptible organisms, primarily some strains of *P. aeruginosa*	Total daily dose
Mild	250 mg q 6 hr	1 g	500 mg q 6 hr	2 g
Moderate	500 mg q 8 hr or 500 mg q 6 hr	1.5 or 2 g	500 mg q 6 hr or 1 g q 8 hr	2 or 3 g
Severe, life-threatening	500 mg q 6 hr	2 g	1 g q 8 hr or 1 g q 6 hr	3 or 4 g
Uncomplicated UTI	250 mg q 6 hr	1 g	250 mg q 6 hr	1 g
Complicated UTI	500 mg q 6 hr	2 g	500 mg q 6 hr	2 g

[1] Including gram-positive and -negative aerobes and anaerobes

  Children –

Pediatric Dosing Guidelines (≥ 3 months old)
≥ 3 months old (non-CNS infections)
15 to 25 mg/kg/dose every 6 hours
Maximum daily dose for fully susceptible organisms is 2 g/day, and for infections with moderately susceptible organisms (primarily some strains of *P. aeruginosa*) is 4 g/day (based on adults studies).
Higher doses (≤ 90 mg/kg/day in older children) have been used in cystic fibrosis patients.

Pediatric Dosing Guidelines (≤ 3 months old)
≤ 3 months old (weighing ≥ 1500 g; non-CNS infections)
< 1 week old: 25 mg/kg every 12 hours
1 to 4 weeks old: 25 mg/kg every 8 hours
4 weeks to 3 months old: 25 mg/kg every 6 hours

    Give doses ≤ 500 mg by IV infusion over 15 to 30 minutes. Give doses > 500 mg by IV infusion over 40 to 60 minutes.

    Imipenem-cilastatin IV is not recommended in pediatric patients with CNS infections because of the risk of seizures and in pediatric patients < 30 kg with impaired renal function, as no data are available.

Renal function impairment –

Reduced IV Dosage in Adult Patients with Impaired Renal Function or Body Weight < 70 kg					
Body weight	≥ 70 kg	60 kg	50 kg	40 kg	30 kg
Ccr (mL/min/1.73 m²)	If total daily dose for normal renal function is 1 g/day, use:				
≥ 71	250 q 6 hr	250 q 8 hr	125 q 6 hr	125 q 6 hr	125 q 8 hr
41 to 70	250 q 8 hr	125 q 6 hr	125 q 6 hr	125 q 8 hr	125 q 8 hr
21 to 40	250 q 12 hr	250 q 12 hr	125 q 8 hr	125 q 12 hr	125 q 12 hr
6 to 20	250 q 12 hr	125 q 12 hr	125 q 12 hr	125 q 12 hr	125 q 12 hr
	If total daily dose for normal renal function is 1.5 g/day, use:				
≥ 71	500 q 8 hr	250 q 6 hr	250 q 6 hr	250 q 8 hr	125 q 6 hr
41 to 70	250 q 6 hr	250 q 8 hr	250 q 8 hr	125 q 6 hr	125 q 8 hr
21 to 40	250 q 8 hr	250 q 8 hr	250 q 12 hr	125 q 8 hr	125 q 8 hr
6 to 20	250 q 12 hr	250 q 12 hr	250 q 12 hr	125 q 12 hr	125 q 12 hr
	If total daily dose for normal renal function is 2 g/day, use:				
≥ 71	500 q 6 hr	500 q 8 hr	250 q 6 hr	250 q 6 hr	250 q 8 hr
41 to 70	500 q 8 hr	250 q 6 hr	250 q 6 hr	250 q 8 hr	125 q 6 hr
21 to 40	250 q 6 hr	250 q 8 hr	250 q 8 hr	250 q 12 hr	125 q 8 hr
6 to 20	250 q 12 hr	250 q 12 hr	250 q 12 hr	250 q 12 hr	125 q 12 hr
	If total daily dose for normal renal function is 3 g/day, use:				
≥ 71	1000 q 8 hr	750 q 8 hr	500 q 6 hr	500 q 8 hr	250 q 6 hr
41 to 70	500 q 6 hr	500 q 8 hr	500 q 8 hr	250 q 6 hr	250 q 8 hr
21 to 40	500 q 8 hr	500 q 8 hr	250 q 6 hr	250 q 8 hr	250 q 8 hr
6 to 20	500 q 12 hr	500 q 12 hr	250 q 12 hr	250 q 12 hr	250 q 12 hr
	If total daily dose for normal renal function is 4 g/day, use:				
≥ 71	1000 q 6 hr	1000 q 8 hr	750 q 8 hr	500 q 6 hr	500 q 8 hr
41 to 70	750 q 8 hr	750 q 8 hr	500 q 6 hr	500 q 8 hr	250 q 6 hr
21 to 40	500 q 6 hr	500 q 8 hr	500 q 8 hr	250 q 6 hr	250 q 8 hr
6 to 20	500 q 12 hr	500 q 12 hr	500 q 12 hr	250 q 12 hr	250 q 12 hr

IM: Total daily IM dosages > 1500 mg/day are not recommended.

Administer by deep IM injection into a large muscle mass (such as the gluteal muscles or lateral part of the thigh) with a 21-gauge 2" needle.

Imipenem-Cilastatin IM Dosage Guidelines		
Type/Location of infection	Severity	Dosage regimen
Lower respiratory tract Skin and skin structure Gynecologic	Mild/Moderate	500 or 750 mg q 12 h depending on the severity of infection
Intra-abdominal	Mild/Moderate	750 mg q 12 h

Hemodialysis – Imipenem-cilastatin is cleared by hemodialysis. The patient should receive imipenem-cilastatin after hemodialysis and at 12-hour intervals timed from the end of that dialysis session.

Actions

Pharmacology: This product is a formulation of imipenem, a thienamycin antibiotic, and cilastatin sodium, the inhibitor of the renal dipeptidase, dehydropeptidase-1, which is responsible for the extensive metabolism of imipenem when it is administered alone. Cilastatin prevents the metabolism of imipenem, increasing urinary recovery and decreasing possible renal toxicity. The bactericidal activity of imipenem results from the inhibition of cell-wall synthesis, related to binding to penicillin-binding proteins (PBP).

Pharmacokinetics:
Absorption/Distribution –
    IV: IV infusion over 20 minutes results in peak plasma levels of imipenem antimicrobial activity that range from 14 to 83 mcg/mL, depending on the dose. Plasma levels declined to ≤ 1 mcg/mL in 4 to 6 hours. Peak plasma levels of cilastatin following a 20-minute IV infusion range from 15 to 88 mcg/mL, depending on the dose. The plasma half-life of each component is ≈ 1 hour. Protein binding is 20% for imipenem and 40% for cilastatin.
    IM: Following IM administration of 500 or 750 mg doses, peak plasma levels of imipenem antimicrobial activity occur within 2 hours and average 10 and 12 mcg/mL, respectively. When compared with IV administration, imipenem is ≈ 75% bioavailable following IM administration, while cilastatin is ≈ 95% bioavailable. The prolonged absorption of imipenem following IM use results in an effective plasma half-life of ≈ 2 to 3 hours and plasma levels that remain > 2 mcg/mL for ≥ 6 or 8 hours following a 500 or 750 mg dose, respectively. This plasma profile for imipenem permits IM administration every 12 hours with no accumulation of cilastatin and only slight accumulation of imipenem.
    Imipenem urine levels remain above 10 mcg/mL for the 12-hour dosing interval following IM administration of 500 or 750 mg doses. Total urinary excretion of imipenem and cilastatin averages 50% and 75%, respectively, following either dose.
    Metabolism/Excretion – Cilastatin prevents renal metabolism of imipenem. The protein binding of imipenem and cilastatin is ≈ 20% and 40%, respectively. Approximately 70% of imipenem and cilastatin is recovered in urine within 10 hours of administration.
Microbiology: Imipenem-cilastatin has a high degree of stability in the presence of β-lactamases, including penicillinases and cephalosporinases produced by gram-negative and gram-positive bacteria.

Contraindications
Hypersensitivity to any component of this product.

IM: Hypersensitivity to local anesthetics of the amide type and in patients with severe shock or heart block due to the use of lidocaine HCl diluent.

IV: Patients with meningitis (safety and efficacy have not been established).

Warnings
Resistance: As with other β-lactam antibiotics, some strains of *P. aeruginosa* may develop resistance fairly rapidly during treatment with imipenem-cilastatin.

Pseudomembranous colitis: Pseudomembranous colitis has occurred with virtually all antibiotics.

Hypersensitivity reactions: Serious and occasionally fatal hypersensitivity reactions have occurred in patients receiving therapy with β-lactams. They are more apt to occur in people with a history of sensitivity to multiple allergens. Patients with a history of penicillin hypersensitivity have experienced severe reactions when treated with another β-lactam.

Renal function impairment: Do not give imipenem-cilastatin IV to patients with Ccr ≤ 5 mL/min/1.73 m^2, unless hemodialysis is instituted within 48 hours. For patients on hemodialysis, imipenem-cilastatin IV is recommended only when the benefit outweighs the potential risk of seizures.

Pregnancy: Category C.

Lactation: It is not known whether this drug is excreted in breast milk.

Children:
    IM – Safety and efficacy for use in children < 12 years of age are not established for IM use.
    IV – Use of IV in neonates to 16 years of age (with non-CNS infections) is supported by evidence from adequate and well-controlled studies. IV use is not recom-

mended in pediatric patients with CNS infections because of the risk of seizures, or in pediatric patients < 30 kg with impaired renal function as no data are available.

Precautions

Monitoring: Periodically assess organ system function during prolonged therapy.

CNS adverse experiences: CNS adverse experiences have occurred with the IV formulation, especially when recommended dosages were exceeded. They are most common in patients with CNS disorders who also have compromised renal function and are rare when no underlying CNS disorder exists. (Continue anticonvulsants in patients with a known seizure disorder.) If focal tremors, myoclonus, or seizures occur, neurologically evaluate the patient, institute anticonvulsants, re-examine the dose, and determine whether to decrease dosage or discontinue the drug. If these effects occur with the IM formulation, discontinue the drug.

Drug Interactions

Drugs that may interact with imipenem-cilastatin include ganciclovir, probenecid, and cyclosporine.

Adverse Reactions

Adverse reactions occurring in ≥ 3% of patients include phlebitis and thrombophlebitis; in newborn patients to ≥ 3 months of age, diarrhea and convusions have occurred.

ERTAPENEM

Powder, lyophilized: 1.046 g ertapenem sodium (equivalent to 1 g ertapenem) (*Rx*)	*Invanz* (Merck)	

Indications

For the treatment of adult patients with the following moderate to severe infections caused by susceptible strains of the designated microorganisms.

Complicated intra-abdominal infections: Caused by *Escherichia coli, Clostridium clostridioforme, Eubacterium lentum, Peptostreptococcus* sp., *Bacteroides fragilis, B. distasonis, B. ovatus, B. thetaiotaomicron,* or *B. uniformis.*

Complicated skin and skin structure infections: Caused by *Staphylococcus aureus* (methicillin-susceptible strains only), *Streptococcus pyogenes, E. coli,* or *Peptostreptococcus* sp.

Community-acquired pneumonia: Caused by *Streptococcus pneumoniae* (penicillin-susceptible strains only), including cases with concurrent bacteremia, *Haemophilus influenzae* (beta-lactamase-negative strains only), or *Moraxella catarrhalis.*

Complicated urinary tract infections, including pyelonephritis: Caused by *E. coli,* including cases with concurrent bacteremia, or *Klebsiella pneumoniae.*

Acute pelvic infections, including postpartum endomyometritis, septic abortion, and postsurgical gynecologic infections: Caused by *Streptococcus agalactiae, E. coli, B. fragilis, Porphyromonas asaccharolytica, Peptostreptococcus* sp., or *Prevotella bivia.*

Administration and Dosage

1 g given once a day.

Ertapenem may be administered by IV infusion for up to 14 days or IM injection for up to 7 days. When administered IV, infuse ertapenem over a period of 30 minutes.

IM administration of ertapenem may be used as an alternative to IV administration in the treatment of those infections for which IM therapy is appropriate.

Do not mix or co-infuse ertapenem with other medications. Do not use diluents containing dextrose (α-D-glucose).

Ertapenem Dosage Guidelines for Adults with Normal Renal Function[1] and Body Weight		
Infection[2]	Daily dose (IV or IM)	Recommended duration of total antimicrobial treatment
Complicated intra-abdominal infections	1 g	5 to 14 days
Complicated skin and skin-structure infections	1 g	7 to 14 days
Community-acquired pneumonia	1 g	10 to 14 days[3]
Complicated urinary tract infections, including pyelo-nephritis	1 g	10 to 14 days[3]
Acute pelvic infections, including postpartum endomyo-metritis, septic abortion, and postsurgical gynecologic infections	1 g	3 to 10 days

[1] Defined as Ccr > 90 mL/min/1.73 m².
[2] Caused by the designated pathogens (see Indications).
[3] Duration includes a possible switch to an appropriate oral therapy after ≥ 3 days of parenteral therapy once clinical improvement has been demonstrated.

Renal insufficiency: Patients with advanced renal insufficiency (Ccr ≤ 30 mL/min/1.73 m²) and end-stage renal insufficiency (Ccr ≤ 10 mL/min/1.73 m²) should receive 500 mg daily.

Hemodialysis: When patients on hemodialysis are given the recommended daily dose of 500 mg of ertapenem within 6 hours prior to hemodialysis, a supplementary dose of 150 mg is recommended following the hemodialysis session. If ertapenem is given ≥ 6 hours prior to hemodialysis, no supplementary dose is needed. There are no data in patients undergoing peritoneal dialysis or hemofiltration.

Actions

Pharmacokinetics:

Absorption – The mean bioavailability is ≈ 90%. Following 1 g daily IM administration, mean peak plasma concentrations (C_{max}) are achieved in ≈ 2.3 hours (T_{max}).

Distribution – Ertapenem is highly bound to human plasma proteins, primarily albumin.

The apparent volume of distribution at steady state of ertapenem is ≈ 8.2 L.

Metabolism – In vitro studies in human liver microsomes indicate that ertapenem does not inhibit metabolism mediated by any of the following cytochrome P450 (CYP) isoforms: 1A2, 2C9, 2C19, 2D6, 2E1, and 3A4.

Excretion – Ertapenem is eliminated primarily by the kidneys. The mean plasma half-life in healthy young adults is ≈ 4 hours, and the plasma clearance is ≈ 1.8 L/hour.

Following the administration of 1 g IV radiolabeled ertapenem to healthy young adults, ≈ 80% is recovered in urine and 10% in feces. Of the 80% recovered in urine, ≈ 38% is excreted as unchanged drug and ≈ 37% as the ring-opened metabolite.

Contraindications

Ertapenem is contraindicated in patients with known hypersensitivity to any component of this product or to other drugs in the same class or in patients who have demonstrated anaphylactic reactions to beta-lactams.

Warnings

Seizures: Seizures and other CNS adverse experiences have been reported during treatment with ertapenem.

Pseudomembranous colitis: Pseudomembranous colitis has been reported and may range in severity from mild to life-threatening.

Hypersensitivity reactions: Serious and occasionally fatal hypersensitivity (anaphylactic) reactions have been reported in patients receiving therapy with beta-lactams. These reactions are more likely to occur in individuals with a history of sensitivity to multiple allergens. There have been reports of individuals with a history of penicillin hypersensitivity who have experienced severe hypersensitivity reactions when treated with another beta-lactam.

Elderly: This drug is known to be substantially excreted by the kidney, and the risk of toxic reactions to this drug may be greater in patients with impaired renal function. Because elderly patients are more likely to have decreased renal function, take care in dose selection; it may be useful to monitor renal function.

Pregnancy: Category B.

Lactation: Ertapenem is excreted in breast milk. Exercise caution when ertapenem is administered to a nursing woman. Administer ertapenem to nursing mothers only when the expected benefit outweighs the risk.

Children: Safety and effectiveness in pediatric patients have not been established.

Precautions

Monitoring: As with other antibiotics, prolonged use of ertapenem may result in overgrowth of nonsusceptible organisms.

While ertapenem possesses toxicity similar to the beta-lactam group of antibiotics, periodic assessment of organ system function, including renal, hepatic, and hematopoietic, is advisable during prolonged therapy.

Special risk: Seizures, irrespective of drug relationship, occurred in 0.5% of patients during study therapy plus 14-day follow-up period. These experiences have occurred most commonly in patients with CNS disorders (eg, brain lesions or history of seizures) or compromised renal function.

Drug Interactions

Ertapenem interacts with probenecid.

Adverse Reactions

The most common drug-related adverse experiences in patients treated with ertapenem, including those who were switched to therapy with an oral antimicrobial, were diarrhea, infused vein complication, nausea, headache, vaginitis, phlebitis/thrombophlebitis, and vomiting.

Adverse reactions occurring in ≥ 3% of patients included the following: Altered mental status, headache, insomnia, infused vein complication, abdominal pain, constipation, diarrhea, nausea, vomiting, edema/swelling, fever, and vaginitis.

Drug-related laboratory adverse experiences that were reported during therapy in ≥ 1% of patients treated with ertapenem in clinical studies were ALT increased, AST increased, serum alkaline phosphatase increased, platelet count increased, and eosinophils increased.

AZTREONAM

Powder for injection (lyophilized cake): 500 mg, 1 g, and *Azactam* (Squibb)
2 g (*Rx*)

Indications

Urinary tract infections: Urinary tract infections (complicated and uncomplicated), including pyelonephritis and cystitis (initial and recurrent) caused by *Escherichia coli, Klebsiella pneumoniae, Proteus mirabilis, Pseudomonas aeruginosa, Enterobacter cloacae, Klebsiella oxytoca, Citrobacter* sp., and *Serratia marcescens.*

Lower respiratory tract infections: Lower respiratory tract infections, including pneumonia and bronchitis caused by *E. coli, K. pneumoniae, P. aeruginosa, Haemophilus influenzae, P. mirabilis, Enterobacter* sp. and *S. marcescens.*

Septicemia: Septicemia caused by *E. coli, K. pneumoniae, P. aeruginosa, P. mirabilis, S. marcescens,* and *Enterobacter* sp.

Skin and skin structure infections: Skin and skin structure infections, including those associated with postoperative wounds, ulcers, and burns caused by *E. coli, P. mirabilis, S. marcescens, Enterobacter* sp., *P. aeruginosa, K. pneumoniae,* and *Citrobacter* sp.

Intra-abdominal infections: Intra-abdominal infections, including peritonitis caused by *E. coli, Klebsiella* sp. including *K. pneumoniae, Enterobacter* sp. including *E. cloacae, P. aeruginosa, Citrobacter* sp. including *C. freundii* and *Serratia* sp. including *S. marcescens.*

Gynecologic infections: Gynecologic infections, including endometritis and pelvic cellulitis caused by *E. coli, K. pneumoniae, Enterobacter* sp. including *E. cloacae,* and *P. mirabilis.*

Surgery: For adjunctive therapy to surgery to manage infections caused by susceptible organisms.

Concurrent initial therapy: Concurrent initial therapy with other antimicrobials and aztreonam is recommended before the causative organism(s) is known in seriously ill patients who also are at risk of having an infection caused by gram-positive aerobic pathogens. If anaerobic organisms are also suspected, initiate therapy concurrently with aztreonam.

Unlabeled uses: 1 g IM may be beneficial for acute uncomplicated gonorrhea in patients with penicillin-resistant gonococci, as an alternative to spectinomycin.

Administration and Dosage

Give IM or IV.

Aztreonam Dosage Guide (Adults)		
Type of infection	Dose[1]	Frequency (hours)
Urinary tract infection	500 mg or 1 g	8 or 12
Moderately severe systemic infections	1 or 2 g	8 or 12
Severe systemic or life-threatening infections	2 g	6 or 8

[1] Maximum recommended dose is 8 g/day.

Aztreonam Dosage Guide (Children)		
Type of infection	Dose[1]	Frequency (hours)
Mild to moderate infections	30 mg/kg	8
Moderate to severe infections	30 mg/kg	6 or 8

[1] Maximum recommended dose is 120 mg/kg/day.

IV route: IV route is recommended for patients requiring single doses > 1 g or those with bacterial septicemia, localized parenchymal abscess (eg, intra-abdominal abscess), peritonitis, or other severe systemic or life-threatening infections. For infections due to *P. aeruginosa,* a dosage of 2 g every 6 or 8 hours is recommended, at least upon initiation of therapy.

Duration: Duration of therapy depends on the severity of infection. Generally, continue aztreonam for at least 48 hours after the patient becomes asymptomatic or evidence of bacterial eradication has been obtained. Persistent infections may require treatment for several weeks.

Children: Administer aztreonam IV to pediatric patients with normal renal function. There are insufficient data regarding IM administration to pediatric patients or dosing in pediatric patients with renal impairment.

Renal function impairment: Reduce dosage by 50% in patients with estimated Ccr between 10 and 30 mL/min/1.73 m² after an initial loading dose of 1 or 2 g.

In patients with severe renal failure, give 500 mg, 1 or 2 g initially. The maintenance dose should be 25% of the usual initial dose given at the usual fixed interval of 6, 8, or 12 hours. For serious or life-threatening infections, in addition to the maintenance doses, give 12.5% of the initial dose after each hemodialysis session.

Elderly: Obtain estimates of Ccr and make appropriate dosage modifications.

IV: Bolus injection may be used to initiate therapy. Slowly inject directly into a vein, or into the tubing of a suitable administration set, over 3 to 5 minutes.

IM: Inject deeply in large muscle mass.

Actions

Pharmacology: Aztreonam, a synthetic bactericidal antibiotic, is the first of a class identified as monobactams. The monobactams have a monocyclic β-lactam nucleus. Aztreonam's bactericidal action results from the inhibition of bacterial cell wall synthesis because of a high affinity of aztreonam for penicillin-binding protein 3 (PBP3).

Pharmacokinetics:

Absorption/Distribution – Following single IM injections of 500 mg and 1 g, maximum serum concentrations occur at about 1 hour.

The serum half-life averaged 1.7 hours in subjects with normal renal function. In healthy subjects, the serum clearance was 91 mL/min and renal clearance was 56 mL/min; the apparent mean volume of distribution at steady state averaged 12.6 L.

Metabolism/Excretion – In healthy subjects, aztreonam is excreted in the urine about equally by active tubular secretion and glomerular filtration. Approximately 60% to 70% of an IV or IM dose was recovered in the urine by 8 hours; recovery was complete by 12 hours.

Administration IV or IM of a single 500 mg or 1 g dose every 8 hours for 7 days to healthy subjects produced no apparent accumulation; serum protein binding averaged 56% and was independent of dose.

Contraindications

Hypersensitivity to aztreonam or any other component in the formulation.

Warnings

Pseudomembranous colitis: Pseudomembranous colitis has been reported with nearly all antibacterial agents, including aztreonam, and may range in severity from mild to life-threatening.

Epidermal necrolysis: Epidermal necrolysis rarely has been reported in association with aztreonam in patients undergoing bone marrow transplant with multiple risk factors.

Hypersensitivity reactions: Make careful inquiry for a history of hypersensitivity reactions. Monitor patients who have had immediate hypersensitivity reactions to penicillins or cephalosporins. If an allergic reaction occurs, discontinue the drug and institute supportive treatment. Cross-sensitivity with other penicillins or β-lactam antibiotics is rare.

Renal/Hepatic function impairment: Appropriate monitoring is recommended.

In patients with impaired renal function, the serum half-life is prolonged.

Pregnancy: Category B. Aztreonam crosses the placenta and enters fetal circulation.

Lactation: Aztreonam is excreted in breast milk in concentrations that are < 1% of maternal serum. Consider temporary discontinuation of nursing.

Children: Safety and efficacy of IV aztreonam have been established children 9 months to 16 years of age. Sufficient data are not available for pediatric patients < 9 months of age or for treatment of the following indications/pathogens: Septicemia and skin and skin-structure infections (where the skin infection is caused by *H. influenzae* type b). In pediatric patients with cystic fibrosis, higher doses of aztreonam may be warranted.

Drug Interactions

Drugs that may interact with aztreonam include other β-lactamase-inducing antibiotics and aminoglycosides.

Adverse Reactions

Adults: No adverse reactions have been reported in ≥ 3% of adult patients.

Children: Of patients < 2 years of age receiving 30 mg/kg every 6 hours, 11.6% experienced neutropenia; of patients > 2 years of age receiving 50 mg/kg every 6 hours, 15% to 20% had elevations of AST and ALT > 3 times the upper limit of normal. The increased frequency of these reported laboratory adverse events may be caused by increased severity of illness treated or higher doses of aztreonam administered.

CHLORAMPHENICOL

Capsules: 250 mg (Rx)
Powder for injection: 100 mg/mL (as sodium succinate) when reconstituted (Rx)

Various, *Chloromycetin Kapseals* (Parke-Davis)
Various, *Chloromycetin Sodium Succinate* (Parke-Davis)

Warning:
Serious and fatal blood dyscrasias occur after short-term and prolonged therapy with chloramphenicol. Aplastic anemia, which later terminated in leukemia, has been reported. Chloramphenicol must not be used when less potentially dangerous agents are effective. It must not be used to treat trivial infections or infections other than indicated, or as prophylaxis for bacterial infections.

Indications

Serious infections: Serious infections for which less potentially dangerous drugs are ineffective or contraindicated caused by susceptible strains of *Salmonella* sp.; *Haemophilus influenzae*, specifically, meningeal infections; rickettsiae; lymphogranuloma-psittacosis group; various gram-negative bacteria causing bacteremia, meningitis or other serious gram-negative infections; infections involving anaerobic organisms, when *Bacteroides fragilis* is suspected; or other susceptible organisms that have been demonstrated to be resistant to all other appropriate antimicrobial agents.

If presumptive therapy is initiated, perform in vitro sensitivity tests concurrently, so that the drug may be discontinued if less potentially dangerous agents are indicated.

Acute infections: In acute infections caused by *Salmonella typhi*, chloramphenicol is a drug of choice.

Cystic fibrosis regimens: In cystic fibrosis regimens.

Administration and Dosage

Therapeutic concentrations: Therapeutic concentrations generally should be maintained as follows: Peak 10 to 20 mcg/mL; trough 5 to 10 mcg/mL.

Monitoring: Monitoring serum levels is important because of the variability of chloramphenicol's pharmacokinetics. Monitor serum concentrations weekly; monitor more often in patients with hepatic dysfunction, in therapy > 2 weeks, or with potentially interacting drugs.

Adults: 50 mg/kg/day in divided doses every 6 hours for typhoid fever and rickettsial infections. Exceptional infections (ie, meningitis, brain abscess) caused by moderately resistant organisms may require dosage up to 100 mg/kg/day to achieve blood levels inhibiting the pathogen; decrease high doses as soon as possible.

Renal/Hepatic function impairment – An initial loading dose of 1 g followed by 500 mg every 6 hours has been recommended in impaired hepatic function.

Children: 50 to 75 mg/kg/day in divided doses every 6 hours has been recommended for most indications. For meningitis, 50 to 100 mg/kg/day in divided doses every 6 hours has been recommended.

Newborns: 25 mg/kg/day in 4 doses every 6 hours usually produces and maintains adequate concentrations in blood and tissues. Give increased dosage demanded by severe infections only to maintain the blood concentration within an effective range. After the first 2 weeks of life, full-term infants ordinarily may receive up to 50 mg/kg/day in 4 doses every 6 hours.

Neonates (< 2 kg) – 25 mg/kg once daily.
Neonates from birth to 7 days (> 2 kg) – 25 mg/kg once daily.
Neonates over 7 days (> 2 kg) – 50 mg/kg/day in divided doses every 12 hours.

These dosage recommendations are extremely important because blood concentration in all premature and full-term infants < 2 weeks of age differs from that of other infants because of variations in the maturity of the metabolic functions of the liver and kidneys.

Infants and children with immature metabolic processes: 25 mg/kg/day usually produces therapeutic concentrations. In this group particularly, carefully monitor the concentration of drug in the blood.

IV administration: Chloramphenicol sodium succinate is intended for IV use only; it is ineffective when given IM. Administer IV as a 10% solution injected over ≥ 1 minute. Substitute oral dosage as soon as feasible.

Actions

Pharmacology: Chloramphenicol binds to 50 S ribosomal subunits of bacteria and interferes with or inhibits protein synthesis.

Pharmacokinetics:

    Absorption – Chloramphenicol base is absorbed rapidly from the intestinal tract and is 75% to 90% bioavailable. The inactive prodrug, chloramphenicol palmitate, is rapidly hydrolyzed to active chloramphenicol base. Bioavailability is ≈ 80% for the palmitate ester. The bioavailability of the IV succinate is ≈ 70%. Approximately 30% is eliminated in the urine as unhydrolyzed ester.

    Distribution – The therapeutic range for total serum chloramphenicol concentration is: Peak, 10 to 20 mcg/mL; trough, 5 to 10 mcg/mL. The drug is ≈ 60% bound to plasma proteins. Chloramphenicol enters the cerebrospinal fluid (CSF), even in the absence of meningeal inflammation.

    Metabolism/Excretion – Total urinary excretion of chloramphenicol ranges from 68% to 99% over 3 days. Most chloramphenicol detected in the blood is in the active free form. The elimination half-life of chloramphenicol is ≈ 4 hours.

Contraindications

History of hypersensitivity to, or toxicity from, chloramphenicol.

Chloramphenicol must not be used to treat trivial infections or infections other than those indicated, or as prophylaxis for bacterial infections.

Warnings

Blood dyscrasias: An irreversible type of marrow depression leading to aplastic anemia with a high rate of mortality is characterized by appearance of bone marrow aplasia or hypoplasia weeks or months after therapy. Peripherally, pancytopenia is most often observed, but only 1 or 2 of the 3 major cell types may be depressed.

    A dose-related reversible type of bone marrow depression may occur and is associated with sustained serum levels at peak ≥ 25 mcg/mL, trough ≥ 10 mcg/mL.

Renal/Hepatic function impairment: Excessive blood levels may result in patients with impaired liver or kidney function, including that caused by immature metabolic processes in the infant.

Pregnancy: Chloramphenicol readily crosses the placental barrier; cautious use is particularly important during pregnancy at term or during labor because of potential toxic effects on the fetus.

Lactation: Chloramphenicol appears in breast milk with a milk:plasma ratio of 0.5. Use with caution, if at all, during lactation.

Children: Use with caution and in reduced dosages in premature and full-term infants to avoid gray syndrome toxicity. Monitor drug serum levels carefully during therapy of the newborn.

Precautions

Hematology: Evaluate baseline and periodic blood studies approximately every 2 days during therapy. Discontinue the drug upon appearance of reticulocytopenia, leukopenia, thrombocytopenia, anemia, or any other findings attributable to chloramphenicol. Avoid concurrent therapy with other drugs that may cause bone marrow depression.

    Avoid repeated courses if at all possible. Do not continue treatment longer than required to produce a cure.

Acute intermittent porphyria or glucose-6-phosphate dehydrogenase deficiency: Use with caution in patients with acute intermittent porphyria or glucose-6-phosphate dehydrogenase deficiency.

Drug Interactions

Drugs that may affect chloramphenicol include barbiturates, rifampin, and hydantoins. Drugs that may be affected by chloramphenicol include barbiturates, anticoagulants, cyclophosphamide, hydantoins, iron salts, penicillins, sulfonylureas, and vitamin B_{12}.

Adverse Reactions

Adverse reactions may include nausea; vomiting; glossitis; stomatitis; diarrhea; headache; mild depression; mental confusion; fever; macular/vesicular rashes; angioedema; urticaria; anaphylaxis; optic and peripheral neuritis.

Toxic reactions including fatalities ($\approx 40\%$) have occurred in the premature infant and newborn; the signs and symptoms associated with these reactions have been referred to as the "gray syndrome."

FLUOROQUINOLONES

CIPROFLOXACIN
Tablets: 250, 500, and 750 mg (*Rx*) — *Cipro* (Bayer)
Suspension, oral: 5 g/100 mL (5%) and 10 g/100 mL (10%) — *Cipro* (Bayer)
Injection: 200 and 400 mg (*Rx*) — *Cipro IV* (Bayer)

ENOXACIN
Tablets: 200 and 400 mg (*Rx*) — *Penetrex* (Aventis)

GATIFLOXACIN
Tablets: 200 and 400 mg (*Rx*) — *Tequin* (Bristol-Myers Squibb)
Solution for Injection (single-use vials): 200 and 400 mg (*Rx*) — *Tequin* (Bristol-Myers Squibb)
Solution for Injection (premix): 200 and 400 mg (*Rx*) — *Tequin* (Bristol-Myers Squibb)

LEVOFLOXACIN
Tablets: 250, 500, and 750 mg (*Rx*) — *Levaquin* (Ortho-McNeil)
Injection (single-use vials): 500 mg (25 mg/mL) and 750 mg (25 mg/mL) (*Rx*) — *Levaquin* (Ortho-McNeil)
Injection (premix): 250 (5 mg/mL), 500 mg (5 mg/mL), and 750 mg (5 mg/mL) (*Rx*) — *Levaquin* (Ortho-McNeil)

LOMEFLOXACIN HCl
Tablets: 400 mg (*Rx*) — *Maxaquin* (Unimed)

MOXIFLOXACIN HCl
Tablets: 400 mg (*Rx*) — *Avelox* (Bayer)
Injection (premix): 400 mg (*Rx*) — *Avelox* (Bayer)

NORFLOXACIN
Tablets: 400 mg (*Rx*) — *Noroxin* (Merck)

OFLOXACIN
Tablets: 200, 300, and 400 mg (*Rx*) — *Floxin* (Ortho-McNeil)
Injection: 200 and 400 mg (*Rx*) — *Floxin* (Ortho-McNeil)

SPARFLOXACIN
Tablets: 200 mg (*Rx*) — *Zagam* (Bertek)

TROVAFLOXACIN MESYLATE/ALATROFLOXACIN MESYLATE
Tablets: 100 and 200 mg trovafloxacin mesylate (*Rx*) — *Trovan* (Pfizer)
Solution for injection: 5 mg/mL alatrofloxacin mesylate (*Rx*) — *Trovan* (Pfizer)

Warning:
Trovafloxacin: Trovafloxacin has been associated with serious liver injury leading to liver transplantation or death. Trovafloxacin-associated liver injury has been reported with short-term and long-term drug exposure. Trovafloxacin use exceeding 2 weeks in duration is associated with a significantly increased risk of serious liver injury. Liver injury also has been reported following trovafloxacin re-exposure. Reserve trovafloxacin for use in patients with serious, life- or limb-threatening infections who receive their initial therapy in an inpatient health care facility (eg, hospital, long-term nursing care facility). Do not use trovafloxacin when safer, alternative antimicrobial therapy will be effective.

Indications
For specific approved indications, refer to the Administration and Dosage section.

Administration and Dosage
CIPROFLOXACIN:

Ciprofloxacin Dosage Guidelines

Location of infection	Type or severity	Unit dose	Frequency	Daily dose	Usual durations[1] (oral doseforms only)
Urinary tract	acute uncomplicated	100 or 250 mg	q 12 h	200 or 500 mg	3 days
	mild/moderate	250 mg (200 mg IV)	q 12 h	500 mg (400 mg IV)	7 to 14 days
	severe/complicated[2]	500 mg (400 mg IV)	q 12 h	1000 mg (800 mg IV)	7 to 14 days
Lower respiratory tract Bone and joint Skin and skin structure	mild/moderate	500 mg (400 mg IV)	q 12 h	1000 mg (800 mg IV)	7 to 14 days ≥ 4 to 6 weeks (bone and joint only)
	severe/complicated	750 mg (400 mg IV)	q 12 h (q 8 h)	1500 mg (1200 mg)	7 to 14 days ≥ 4 to 6 weeks (bone and joint only)
Nosocomial pneumonia	mild/moderate/severe	400 mg IV	q 8 h	1200 mg IV	
Intra-abdominal[3]	complicated	500 mg (400 mg IV)	q 12 h	1000 mg (800 mg IV)	7 to 14 days
Acute sinusitis	mild/moderate	500 mg (400 mg IV)	q 12 h	1000 mg (800 mg IV)	10 days
Chronic bacterial prostatitis	mild/moderate	500 mg (400 mg IV)	q 12 h	1000 mg (800 mg IV)	28 days
Empirical therapy in febrile neutropenic patients	severe: ciprofloxacin	400 mg IV	q 8 h	1200 mg IV	
	+ piperacillin	50 mg/kg IV	q 4 h	not to exceed 24 g/day	
Infectious diarrhea	mild/moderate/severe	500 mg	q 12 h	1000 mg	5 to 7 days
Typhoid fever	mild/moderate	500 mg	q 12 h	1000 mg	10 days
Urethral/Cervical gonococcal infections	uncomplicated	250 mg	single dose	250 mg	single dose

Ciprofloxacin Dosage Guidelines

Location of infection	Type or severity	Unit dose	Frequency	Daily dose	Usual durations[1] (oral doseforms only)
Inhalational anthrax (postexposure)[4]	adult	500 mg (400 mg IV)	q 12 h	1000 mg (800 mg IV)	60 days
	pediatric	15 mg/kg/dose, not to exceed 500 mg/dose (10 mg/kg/IV dose, not to exceed 400 mg/IV dose)	q 12 h	not to exceed 1000 mg (not to exceed 800 mg IV)	60 days

[1] Generally, ciprofloxacin should be continued for ≥ 2 days after the signs and symptoms of infection have disappeared, except for inhalational anthrax (postexposure).

[2] Including secondary bacteremia from *Escherichia coli* (IV only).

[3] Used in conjunction with metronidazole.

[4] Begin drug administration as soon as possible after suspected or confirmed exposure. This indication is based on a surrogate endpoint, ciprofloxacin serum concentrations achieved in humans, reasonably likely to predict clinical benefit. Total duration of ciprofloxacin administration (IV or oral) for inhalational anthrax (postexposure) is 60 days.

The duration of treatment depends upon the severity of infection. Generally, continue ciprofloxacin for ≥ 2 days after the signs and symptoms of infection have disappeared. The usual duration is 7 to 14 days; however, for severe and complicated infections, more prolonged therapy may be required. Bone and joint infections may require treatment for 4 to 6 weeks or longer. Infectious diarrhea may be treated for 5 to 7 days. Typhoid fever should be treated for 10 days. Treat chronic prostatitis for 28 days.

Administer sucralfate or divalent and trivalent cations such as antacids or iron containing magnesium, aluminum, or calcium 6 hours before or 2 hours after ciprofloxacin dosing.

Renal function impairment –

Ciprofloxacin Dosage in Impaired Renal Function	
Ccr (mL/min)	Dose
> 50 (oral); > 30 (IV)	See usual dosage
30 to 50	250 to 500 mg q 12 h
5 to 29	250 to 500 mg q 18 h (oral); 200 to 400 mg q 18 to 24 h (IV)
Hemodialysis or peritoneal dialysis	250 to 500 mg q 24 h (after dialysis)

In patients with severe infections and severe renal impairment, 750 mg may be administered orally at the intervals noted in the table.

CDC-recommended treatment schedules for chancroid and gonorrhea –

Chancroid (H. ducreyi infection): 500 mg orally 2 times/day for 3 days.

Gonococcal infections:

Disseminated (alternative initial regimen) – 500 mg IV every 12 hours for 24 to 48 hours after improvement begins, then 500 mg orally twice daily for 7 days.

Uncomplicated – 500 mg orally in a single dose plus azithromycin 1 g orally in a single dose or doxycycline 100 mg orally twice a day for 7 days.

IV: Administer by IV infusion over 60 minutes. Slow infusion of a dilute solution into a large vein will minimize patient discomfort and reduce the risk of venous irritation.

IV admixture compatibility/stability – Stable for ≤ 14 days at refrigerated or room temperature when diluted with 0.9% NaCl Injection, 5% Dextrose Injection, Sterile Water for Injection, 10% Dextrose for Injection, 5% Dextrose and 0.225% NaCl for Injection, 5% Dextrose and 0.45% NaCl for Injection, or Lactated Ringer's for Injection. Protect from light and freezing. If a Y-type IV infusion set or a piggyback method is used, temporarily discontinue the administration of any other solutions during the ciprofloxacin infusion.

NORFLOXACIN: Take 1 hour before or 2 hours after meals or dairy products and with a glass of water. Patients should be well hydrated.

Recommended Norfloxacin Dosage					
Infection	Description	Dose	Frequency	Duration	Daily dose
Urinary tract infections (UTI)	Uncomplicated (cystitis) caused by E. coli, Klebsiella pneumoniae, or Proteus mirabilis	400 mg	q 12 h	3 days	800 mg
	Uncomplicated caused by other organisms	400 mg	q 12 h	7 to 10 days	800 mg
	Complicated	400 mg	q 12 h	10 to 21 days	800 mg
Sexually transmitted diseases	Uncomplicated gonorrhea	800 mg	single dose	1 day	800 mg
Prostatitis	Acute or chronic	400 mg	q 12 h	28 days	800 mg

Renal function impairment – In patients with Ccr ≤ 30 mL/min/1.73 m^2, administer 400 mg once daily for the duration given above.

Elderly – Dose based on normal or impaired renal function.

CDC-recommended treatment schedules for gonorrhea –

Gonococcal infections, uncomplicated: 800 mg as a single dose (alternative regimen to **ciprofloxacin** or **ofloxacin**).

OFLOXACIN: Usual daily dose is 200 to 400 mg every 12 hours as described in the following table:

Ofloxacin Dosage Guidelines (Oral and IV)[1]					
Infection	Description	Dose	Frequency	Duration	Daily dose
Lower respiratory tract	Exacerbation of chronic bronchitis	400 mg	q 12 h	10 days	800 mg
	Community acquired pneumonia	400 mg	q 12 h	10 days	800 mg
Sexually transmitted diseases	Acute, uncomplicated urethral and cervical gonorrhea	400 mg	single dose	1 day	400 mg
	Cervicitis/Urethritis caused by *Chlamydia trachomatis*	300 mg	q 12 h	7 days	600 mg
	Cervicitis/Urethritis caused by *C. trachomatis* and *Neisseria gonorrhoeae*	300 mg	q 12 h	7 days	600 mg
	Acute pelvic inflammatory disease	400 mg	q 12 h	10 to 14 days	800 mg
Skin and skin structure	Uncomplicated	400 mg	q 12 h	10 days	800 mg
Urinary tract	Uncomplicated cystitis caused by *E. coli* or *K. pneumoniae*	200 mg	q 12 h	3 days	400 mg
	Uncomplicated cystitis caused by other organisms	200 mg	q 12 h	7 days	400 mg
	Complicated UTIs	200 mg	q 12 h	10 days	400 mg
Prostatitis	Caused by *E. coli*	300 mg	q 12 h	6 weeks[2]	600 mg

[1] Caused by the designated pathogens (see Indications).
[2] Because there are no safety data presently available to support the use of the IV formulation for > 10 days, switch to oral or other appropriate therapy after 10 days.

Do not take antacids containing calcium, magnesium, or aluminum; sucralfate; divalent or trivalent cations such as iron; multivitamins containing zinc; or didanosine (chewable/buffered tablets or pediatric powder for oral solution) 2 hours before or 2 hours after taking ofloxacin.

Renal function impairment – Adjust dosage in patients with Ccr ≤ 50 mL/min. After a normal initial dose, adjust the dosing interval as follows:

Ofloxacin Dosage in Impaired Renal Function		
Ccr (mL/min)	Maintenance dose	Frequency
20 to 50	usual recommended unit dose	q 24 hr
< 20	½ usual recommended unit dose	q 24 hr

Chronic hepatic impairment (cirrhosis) – The excretion of ofloxacin may be reduced in patients with severe liver function disorders (eg, cirrhosis with or without ascites). Do not exceed a maximum dose of 400 mg/day.

CDC-recommended treatment schedules for chlamydia, epididymitis, pelvic inflammatory disease (PID), and gonorrhea – †

Chlamydia: 300 mg orally 2 times/day for 7 days (alternative regimen).

Epididymitis: 300 mg orally 2 times/day for 10 days.

PID, outpatient: 400 mg orally 2 times/day for 14 days plus metronidazole.

Gonococcal infections, uncomplicated: 400 mg orally in a single dose plus doxycycline or azithromycin.

IV – Administer by IV infusion only. Do not give IM, intrathecally, intraperitoneally, or SC. Avoid rapid or bolus IV infusion; administer slowly over a period of ≥ 60 minutes.

Compatible IV solutions: 0.9% Sodium Chloride; 5% Dextrose; 5% Dextrose/0.9% Sodium Chloride; 5% Dextrose in Lactated Ringer's; 5% Sodium Bicarbonate; *Plasma-Lyte* 56 in 5% Dextrose; 5% Dextrose, 0.45% Sodium Chloride and 0.15% Potassium Chloride; Sodium Lactate (M/6); Water for Injection.

† CDC 1998 Sexually Transmitted Diseases Treatment Guidelines. *MMWR.* 1998 ;47(RR-1): 1-118.

ENOXACIN: Take ≥ 1 hour before or 2 hours after a meal.

Enoxacin Dosage Guidelines					
Infection	Description	Dose	Frequency	Duration	Daily dose
Urinary tract infections	Uncomplicated (cystitis)	200 mg	q 12 h	7 days	400 mg
	Complicated	400 mg	q 12 h	14 days	800 mg
Sexually transmitted diseases	Uncomplicated urethral or cervical gonorrhea	400 mg	single dose	1 day	400 mg

Renal function impairment – Adjust dosage in patients with Ccr ≤ 30 mL/min/1.73 m². After a normal initial dose, use a 12-hour interval and ½ the recommended dose.

Elderly – Dosage adjustment is not necessary with normal renal function.

CDC recommended treatment schedules for gonorrhea –

Gonococcal infections, uncomplicated: 400 mg as a single dose (alternative regimen to ciprofloxacin or ofloxacin).

LOMEFLOXACIN HCl: Risk of reaction to solar UVA light may be reduced by taking lomefloxacin ≥ 12 hours before exposure to the sun (eg, in the evening). Lomefloxacin may be taken without regard to meals (see Actions).

Recommended Daily Dose of Lomefloxacin					
Body system	Infection	Dose	Frequency	Duration	Daily dose
Lower respiratory tract	Acute bacterial exacerbation of chronic bronchitis	400 mg	once daily	10 days	400 mg
Urinary tract	Uncomplicated cystitis caused by *K. pneumoniae, P. mirabilis,* or *Staphylococcus saprophyticus*	400 mg	once daily	10 days	400 mg
	Uncomplicated cystitis in females caused by *E. coli*	400 mg	once daily	3 days	400 mg
	Complicated UTI	400 mg	once daily	14 days	400 mg

Elderly – No dosage adjustment needed for elderly patients with normal renal function (Ccr ≥ 40 mL/min/1.73 m²).

Renal function impairment – Lomefloxacin primarily is eliminated by renal excretion. Modification of dosage is recommended in patients with renal dysfunction. In patients with a Ccr > 10 but < 40 mL/min/1.73 m², the recommended dosage is an initial loading dose of 400 mg followed by daily maintenance doses of 200 mg once daily for the duration of the treatment.

Dialysis patients – Hemodialysis removes only a negligable amount of lomefloxacin (3% in 4 hours). Give hemodialysis patients an initial loading dose of 400 mg followed by maintenance dose of 200 mg once daily for duration of treatment.

Preoperative prevention –

Transrectal prostate biopsy: The recommended dose for transrectal prostate biopsy is a single 400 mg dose 1 to 6 hours prior to the procedure.

Transurethral surgical procedures: A single 400 mg dose 2 to 6 hours prior to surgery when oral preoperative prophylaxis for transurethral surgical procedures is considered appropriate.

CDC-recommended treatment schedules for gonorrhea –

Gonococcal infections, uncomplicated: 400 mg as a single dose (alternative regimen to ciprofloxacin or ofloxacin).

SPARFLOXACIN: Sparfloxacin may be taken with or without food.

Community-acquired pneumonia; acute bacterial exacerbations of chronic bronchitis – The recommended daily dose of sparfloxacin in patients with normal renal function is two 200 mg tablets taken on the first day as a loading dose. Thereafter, take one 200 mg tablet every 24 hours for a total of 10 days of therapy (11 tablets).

Renal function impairment – The recommended daily dose of sparfloxacin in patients with renal impairment (Ccr < 50 mL/min) is two 200 mg tablets taken on the first

† CDC 1998 Guidelines for the Treatment of Sexually Transmitted Diseases. *MMWR.* 1998;47(RR-1):1-118.

day as a loading dose. Thereafter, take one 200 mg tablet every 48 hours for a total of 9 days of therapy (6 tablets).

LEVOFLOXACIN: The usual dose of levofloxacin tablets/injection is 250 or 500 mg administered orally or by slow infusion over 60 minutes every 24 hours or 750 mg administered by slow infusion over 90 minutes every 24 hours, as indicated by infection and described in the following dosing chart. These recommendations apply to patients with normal renal function (ie, Ccr > 80 mL/min). For patients with altered renal function, see Levofloxacin Dosing with Renal Function Impairment table. Administer oral doses ≥ 2 hours before or 2 hours after antacids containing magnesium or aluminum, as well as sucralfate, metal cations such as iron and multivitamin preparations with zinc, or didanosine (chewable/buffered tablets or pediatric powder for oral solution).

Levofloxacin Dosing with Normal Renal Function				
Infection[1]	Unit dose	Frequency	Duration[2]	Daily dose
Acute bacterial exacerbation of chronic bronchitis	500 mg	q 24 hr	7 days	500 mg
Community-acquired pneumonia	500 mg	q 24 hr	7 to 14 days	500 mg
Acute maxillary sinusitis	500 mg	q 24 hr	10 to 14 days	500 mg
Complicated SSSI[3]	750 mg	q 24 hr	7 to 14 days	750 mg
Uncomplicated SSSI[3]	500 mg	q 24 hr	7 to 10 days	500 mg
Complicated UTI	250 mg	q 24 hr	10 days	250 mg
Uncomplicated UTI	250 mg	q 24 hr	3 days	250 mg
Acute pyelonephritis	250 mg	q 24 hr	10 days	250 mg

[1] Caused by the designated pathogens (see Indications).
[2] Sequential therapy (IV to oral) may be instituted at the discretion of the physician.
[3] Skin and skin structure infection.

Levofloxacin Dosing with Renal Function Impairment		
Renal status	Initial dose	Subsequent dose
Acute bacterial exacerbation of chronic bronchitis/community-acquired pneumonia/acute maxillary sinusitis/uncomplicated SSSI		
Ccr from 50 to 80 mL/min	No dosage adjustment required	
Ccr from 20 to 49 mL/min	500 mg	250 mg q 24 hr
Ccr from 10 to 19 mL/min	500 mg	250 mg q 48 hr
Hemodialysis	500 mg	250 mg q 48 hr
CAPD[1]	500 mg	250 mg q 48 hr
Complicated SSSI		
Ccr from 50 to 80 mL/min	No dosage adjustment required	
Ccr from 20 to 49 mL/min	750 mg	750 mg q 48 hr
Ccr from 10 to 19 mL/min	750 mg	500 mg q 48 hr
Hemodialysis	750 mg	500 mg q 48 hr
CAPD[1]	750 mg	500 mg q 48 hr
Complicated UTI/acute pyelonephritis		
Ccr ≥ 20 mL/min	No dosage adjustment required	
Ccr from 10 to 19 mL/min	250 mg	250 mg q 48 hr
Uncomplicated UTI	No dosage adjustment required	

[1] CAPD = chronic ambulatory peritoneal dialysis.

IV administration – Administer by IV infusion only, slowly over a period of ≥ 60 minutes. Avoid rapid or bolus IV infusion. Do not administer by IM, intrathecal, intraperitoneal, or SC routes.

TROVAFLOXACIN MESYLATE/ALATROFLOXACIN MESYLATE: Administer oral doses ≥ 2 hours before or 2 hours after antacids containing magnesium or aluminum, as well as sucralfate, citric acid buffered with sodium citrate, metal cations (eg, ferrous sulfate), and didanosine (chewable/buffered tablets or pediatric powder for oral solution).

If trovafloxacin is taken on an empty stomach, administer IV morphine ≥ 2 hours later. If trovafloxacin is taken with food, administer IV morphine ≥ 4 hours later.

Administer alatrofloxacin only by IV infusion. Do not administer by IM, intrathecal, intraperitoneal, or SC routes.

Single-use vials require dilution prior to administration.

Trovafloxacin/Alatrofloxacin Dosage Guidelines			
Infection[1]/ Location and type	Daily unit dose and route of administration	Frequency	Total duration
Nosocomial pneumonia[2]	300 mg IV[3] followed by 200 mg oral	q 24 hr	10 to 14 days
Community-acquired pneumonia	200 mg oral or 200 mg IV followed by 200 mg oral	q 24 hr	7 to 14 days
Complicated intra- abdominal infections, including post- surgical infections	300 mg IV[3] followed by 200 mg oral	q 24 hr	7 to 14 days
Gynecologic and pelvic infections	300 mg IV[3] followed by 200 mg oral	q 24 hr	7 to 14 days
Skin and skin structure infections, complicated, including diabetic foot infections	200 mg oral or 200 mg IV followed by 200 mg oral	q 24 hr	10 to 14 days

[1] Caused by the designated pathogens (see Indications).
[2] As with other antimicrobials, where *Pseudomonas aeruginosa* is a documented or presumptive pathogen, combination therapy with either an aminoglycoside or aztreonam may be clinically indicated.
[3] Where the 300 mg IV dose is indicated, decrease therapy to 200 mg as soon as clinically indicated.

Do not administer trovafloxacin for > 2 weeks unless the treating physician believes the benefits to the individual patient clearly outweigh the risks of longer-term treatment.

Renal function impairment – No dosage adjustment is necessary in patients with impaired renal function.

Chronic hepatic disease (cirrhosis) – The following table provides dosing guidelines for patients with mild or moderate cirrhosis (Child-Pugh Class A and B). There are no data in patients with severe cirrhosis (Child-Pugh Class C).

Trovafloxacin/Alatrofloxacin Dosage in Chronic Hepatic Disease	
Indicated dose (normal hepatic function)	Chronic hepatic disease dose
300 mg IV	200 mg IV
200 mg IV or oral	100 mg IV or oral

IV administration – After dilution with an appropriate diluent, administer by IV infusion over a period of 60 minutes.

Admixture incompatibility – Do not dilute alatrofloxacin with 0.9% Sodium Chloride Injection (normal saline), alone or in combination with other diluents. A precipitate may form under these conditions. In addition, do not dilute alatrofloxacin with Lactated Ringer's.

Compatible IV solutions: 5% Dextrose Injection; 0.45% Sodium Chloride Injection; 5% Dextrose and 0.45% Sodium Chloride Injection; 5% Dextrose and 0.2% Sodium Chloride Injection; Lactated Ringer's and 5% Dextrose Injection.

Normal saline, 0.9% Sodium Chloride Injection, can be used for flushing IV lines prior to or after administration of alatrofloxacin.

MOXIFLOXACIN HCl: The dose of moxifloxacin is 400 mg (orally or as an IV infusion) once every 24 hours.

Administer IV moxifloxacin by IV infusion only. It is not intended for IM, intrathecal, intraperitoneal, or SC administration.

Administer by IV infusion over a period of 60 minutes by direct infusion or through a Y-type IV infusion set that may already be in place. Caution: Rapid or bolus IV infusion must be avoided.

Moxifloxacin Dosage Guidelines (IV and Oral)			
Infection[1]	Daily dose (mg)	Frequency	Duration (days)
Acute bacterial sinusitis	400	q 24 hr	10
Acute bacterial exacerbation of chronic bronchitis	400	q 24 hr	5
Community-acquired pneumonia	400	q 24 hr	10
Uncomplicated skin and skin structure infections	400	q 24 hr	7

[1] Caused by the designated pathogens (see Indications).

Impaired renal function: No dosage adjustment is required in renally impaired patients. Moxifloxacin has not been studied in patients on hemodialysis or continuous ambulatory peritoneal dialysis (CAPD).

Impaired hepatic function: No dosage adjustment is required in patients with mild hepatic insufficiency. The use of moxifloxacin is not recommended in patients with moderate and severe hepatic insufficiency.

Switching from IV to oral dosing: When switching from IV to oral dosage administration, no dosage adjustment is necessary.

GATIFLOXACIN: Gatifloxacin may be administered without regard to food, including milk and dietary supplements containing calcium, and without regard to age (≥ 18 years) or gender.

Oral: Administer oral gatifloxacin ≥ 4 hours before the administration of ferrous sulfate; dietary supplements containing zinc, magnesium, or iron (such as multivitamins); aluminum/magnesium-containing antacids; or didanosine (buffered tablets, buffered solution, or buffered powder for oral suspension).

When switching from IV to oral dosage administration, no dosage adjustment is necessary. Patients whose therapy is started with the injection may be switched to tablets when clinically indicated at the discretion of the physician.

IV: Administer injection by IV infusion only. It is not intended for IM, intrathecal, intraperitoneal, or SC administration.

Gatifloxacin Dosage Guidelines			
Infection[1]	Daily dose (mg)[2]	Frequency	Duration
Acute bacterial exacerbation of chronic bronchitis	400	q 24 hr	5 days
Acute sinusitis	400	q 24 hr	10 days
Community-acquired pneumonia	400	q 24 hr	7 to 14 days
Uncomplicated UTIs (cystitis)	400	q 24 hr	Single dose
	or 200		3 days
Complicated UTIs	400	q 24 hr	7 to 10 days
Acute pyelonephritis	400	q 24 hr	7 to 10 days
Uncomplicated urethal gonorrhea in men; endocervical and rectal gonorrhea in women	400	q 24 hr	Single dose

[1] Caused by the designated pathogens (see Indications).
[2] For either the oral and IV routes of administration.

Renal function impairment: Because gatifloxacin is eliminated primarily by renal excretion, a dosage modification of gatifloxacin is recommended for patients with Ccr < 40 mL/min, including patients on hemodialysis and on continuous ambulatory peritoneal dialysis (CAPD). The recommended dosage of gatifloxacin follows:

Recommended Dosage of Gatifloxacin in Adult Patients with Renal Impairment		
Ccr	Initial dose (mg)	Subsequent dose[1]
≥ 40 mL/min	400	400 mg daily
< 40 mL/min	400	200 mg daily
Hemodialysis	400	200 mg daily
Continuous peritoneal dialysis	400	200 mg daily

[1] Start of subsequent dose on day 2 of dosing.

Administer gatifloxacin after a dialysis session for patients on hemodialysis.

Uncomplicated UTIs and gonorrhea – Single 400 mg dose regimen (for the treatment of uncomplicated UTIs and gonorrhea) and 200 mg once daily for 3 days regimen (for the treatment of uncomplicated UTIs) require no dosage adjustment in patients with impaired renal function.

Actions

Pharmacology: The fluoroquinolones are synthetic, broad-spectrum antibacterial agents that inhibit DNA gyrase and topoisomerase IV. DNA gyrase is an essential enzyme that is involved in the replication, transcription, and repair of bacterial DNA. Topoisomerase IV is an enzyme known to play a key role in the partitioning of the chromosomal DNA during bacterial cell division.

Pharmacokinetics:

Pharmacokinetics of Fluoroquinolones

Fluoroquinolone	Bioavailability (%)	Max urine concentration (mcg/mL) (dose)	Mean peak plasma concentration (mcg/mL) (dose)	Area under curve (AUC) (mcg • hr/mL) (dose)	Protein binding (%)	t½ (hr)	Urine recovery unchanged (%)
Ciprofloxacin Oral	≈ 70-80	> 200 (250 mg)	1.2 (250 mg) 2.4 (500 mg) 4.3 (750 mg) 5.4 (1000 mg)	4.8 (250 mg) 11.6 (500 mg) 20.2 (750 mg) 30.8 (1000 mg)	20 to 40	≈ 4	≈ 40 to 50
IV		> 200 (200 mg) > 400 (400 mg)	4.4 (400 mg)	4.8 (200 mg) 11.6 (400 mg)		≈ 5 to 6	≈ 50 to 70
Enoxacin	≈ 90	nd[1]	0.93 (200 mg) 2 (400 mg)		≈ 40	3 to 6	> 40
Gatifloxacin[2] Oral	≈ 96		≈ 2 (200 mg single dose) ≈ 3.8 (400 mg single dose) ≈ 4.2 (400 mg multiple dose)	≈ 14.2 (200 mg single dose) ≈ 33 (400 mg single dose) ≈ 34.4 (400 mg multiple dose)	≈ 20	≈ 7.8 (400 mg single dose) ≈ 7.1 (400 mg multiple dose)	≈ 73.8 (200 mg single dose) ≈ 72.4 (400 mg single dose) ≈ 80.2 (400 mg multiple dose)
IV			≈ 2.2 (200 mg single dose) ≈ 2.4 (200 mg multiple dose) ≈ 5.5 (400 mg single dose) ≈ 4.6 (400 mg multiple dose)	≈ 15.9 (200 mg single dose) ≈ 16.8 (200 mg multiple dose) ≈ 35.1 (400 mg single dose) ≈ 35.4 (400 mg multiple dose)		≈ 11.1 (200 mg single dose) ≈ 12.3 (200 mg multiple dose) ≈ 7.4 (400 mg single dose) ≈ 13.9 (400 mg multiple dose)	≈ 71.7 (200 mg single dose) ≈ 72.4 (200 mg multiple dose) ≈ 62.3 (400 mg single dose) ≈ 83.5 (400 mg multiple dose)
Levofloxacin	≈ 99		≈ 2.8 to 11.5 (single dose oral or IV) ≈ 5.7 to 12.1 (multiple dose oral or IV)	27.2 to 110 (single dose oral or IV) ≈ 47.5 to 108 (multiple dose oral or IV)	≈ 24-38	≈ 6.3 to 7.5 (single dose oral or IV) ≈ 7 to 8.8 (multiple dose oral or IV)	≈ 87 (oral)
Lomefloxacin	≈ 95-98	> 300 (400 mg)	0.8 (100 mg) 1.4 (200 mg) 3.2 (400 mg)	5.6 (100 mg) 10.9 (200 mg) 26.1 (400 mg)	≈ 10	≈ 8	≈ 65
Moxifloxacin	≈ 90		4.5 (400 mg)	≈ 48 (400 mg)	≈ 50	≈ 12	≈ 20
Norfloxacin	30 to 40	≥ 200 (400 mg)	0.8 (200 mg) 1.5 (400 mg) 2.4 (800 mg)		10 to 15	3 to 4	26 to 32

Pharmacokinetics of Fluoroquinolones

Fluoroquinolone	Bioavailability (%)	Max urine concentration (mcg/mL) (dose)	Mean peak plasma concentration (mcg/mL) (dose)	Area under curve (AUC) (mcg • hr/mL) (dose)	Protein binding (%)	$t\frac{1}{2}$ (hr)	Urine recovery unchanged (%)
Ofloxacin Oral	≈ 98	≈ 220 (200 mg)	1.5 (200 mg) 2.4 (300 mg) 2.9 (400 mg) 4.6 (400 mg steady-state)	14.1 (200 mg) 21.2 (300 mg) 31.4 (400 mg) 61 (400 mg steady-state)	≈ 32	≈ 9	65 to 80
IV		nd[1]	2.7 (200 mg) 4 (400 mg)	43.5 (400 mg)	≈ 32	5 to 10	≈ 65
Sparfloxacin	92	> 12 (400 mg)[3]	≈ 1.3 (400 mg)	≈ 34 (400 mg)	≈ 45	≈ 20	≈ 10
Trovafloxacin/ Alatrofloxacin[2] Trovafloxacin Single-dose	≈ 88 (oral)		≈ 1 (100 mg) ≈ 2.1 (200 mg)	≈ 11.2 (100 mg) ≈ 26.7 (200 mg)	≈ 76	9.1 (100 mg) 9.6 (200 mg)	≈ 6 (oral)
Multiple dose		≈ 12.1 (200 mg)	≈ 1.1 (100 mg) ≈ 3.1 (200 mg)	≈ 11.8 (100 mg) 34.4 (200 mg)		10.5 (100 mg) 12.2 (200 mg)	
Alatrofloxacin[4] Single-dose			2.7 (200 mg) ≈ 3.6 (300 mg)	28.1 (200 mg) 46.1 (300 mg)		9.4 (200 mg) 11.2 (300 mg)	
Multiple dose			3.1 (200 mg) 4.4 (300 mg)	32.2 (200 mg) 46.3 (300 mg)		11.7 (200 mg) 12.7 (300 mg)	

[1] nd = no data.
[2] Single dose: AUC (0-∞); Multiple dose: AUC (0-24).
[3] Following a 400 mg loading dose of sparfloxacin, the mean urine concentration 4 hours postdose was in excess of 12 mcg/mL.
[4] Trovafloxacin equivalents.

Microbiology:

Organisms Generally Susceptible to Fluoroquinolones In Vitro

Organism	Ciprofloxacin	Enoxacin	Gatifloxacin	Levofloxacin	Lomefloxacin	Moxifloxacin	Norfloxacin	Ofloxacin	Sparfloxacin	Trovafloxacin/Alatrofloxacin
Acinetobacter anitratus	✓[1]								✓[1]	✓[1]
Acinetobacter iwoffi	✓[1]			✓[1]					✓[1]	
Acinetobacter calcoaceticus								✓[1]		
Aeromonas hydrophilia	✓[1]	✓[1]			✓[1]					
Bacteroides distasonis										✓[1]
Bacteroides ovatus										✓[1]
Bordetella pertussis				✓[1]				✓[1]		
Campylobacter jejuni	✓[2]									
Chlamydia trachomatis								✓[1]		
Citrobacter diversus	✓	✓[1]	✓[1]	✓[1]	✓		✓[1]	✓[1]	✓[1]	✓
Citrobacter freundii	✓	✓[1]	✓[1]		✓[1]	✓[1]	✓	✓[1]		✓[1]
Citrobacter koseri		✓[1]	✓[1]							
Enterobacter cloacae	✓	✓	✓[1]	✓	✓	✓[1]	✓	✓[1]	✓	✓[1]
Enterobacter aerogenes	✓[1]	✓[1]	✓[1]	✓[1]	✓[1]		✓	✓	✓[1]	
Enterobacter agglomerans				✓[1]	✓[1]		✓[1]		✓	
Enterobacter sakazakii				✓[1]						
Escherichia coli	✓	✓	✓	✓	✓	✓[1]	✓	✓	✓	✓
Edwardsiella tarda	✓[1]						✓[1]			
Fusobacterium sp.						✓[1]				
Gardenella vaginalis		✓[1]								
Haemophilus ducreyi								✓	✓	✓
Haemophilus influenzae	✓		✓	✓[1]	✓[1]	✓	✓[1]	✓[1]	✓	✓
Haemophilus parainfluenzae	✓		✓	✓[1]	✓[1]	✓		✓	✓	✓
Hafnia alvei									✓	
Klebsiella pneumoniae	✓	✓	✓	✓	✓	✓	✓	✓	✓	✓

Gram-negative

Organisms Generally Susceptible to Fluoroquinolones In Vitro

Organism	Ciprofloxacin	Enoxacin	Gatifloxacin	Levofloxacin	Lomefloxacin	Moxifloxacin	Norfloxacin	Ofloxacin	Sparfloxacin	Trovafloxacin/Alatrofloxacin
Klebsiella oxytoca	✓[1]	✓[1]	✓[1]	✓[1]		✓[1]	✓[1]	✓[1]	✓[1]	
Klebsiella ozaenae		✓[1]			✓[1]					
Moraxella catarrhalis	✓[2]		✓	✓	✓[1]			✓[1]	✓	✓
Morganella morganii	✓	✓[1]	✓[1]	✓[1]	✓	✓	✓[1]	✓[1]	✓[1]	✓[1]
Mycoplasma hominis					✓[1]	✓		✓[1]		✓[1]
Neisseria gonorrhoeae	✓[2]	✓	✓					✓		
Pasteurella multocida	✓[1]						✓			
Prevotella sp.						✓[1]				
Proteus mirabilis	✓	✓	✓	✓	✓	✓[1]	✓	✓	✓[1]	✓
Proteus vulgaris	✓	✓[1]	✓[1]	✓[1]	✓[1]	✓	✓	✓[1]	✓[1]	✓[1]
Providencia alcalifaciens	✓	✓[1]			✓[1]		✓[1]		✓[1]	✓[1]
Providencia rettgeri	✓	✓[1]		✓[1]	✓[1]		✓[1]	✓[1]		
Providencia stuartii	✓	✓		✓[3]			✓[1]	✓[1]		
Pseudomonas aeruginosa	✓	✓		✓[3]	✓[4]		✓	✓[3]		✓
Pseudomonas fluorescens				✓[1]			✓[1]			
Pseudomonas stutzeri							✓[1]			
Salmonella sp.	✓[5]		✓	✓		✓		✓	✓	✓
Salmonella typhi	✓									
Salmonella enteritidis	✓[1]									
Serratia marcescens	✓	✓[1]		✓[1]	✓[1]		✓	✓[1]		
Serratia proteomaculans		✓[1]			✓[1]					
Shigella sp.	✓[5]		✓	✓		✓		✓	✓	✓
Shigella boydii	✓[2]									
Shigella dysenteriae	✓[2]									
Shigella flexneri	✓[2]									
Shigella sonnei	✓[2]									

Gram-negative (cont'd.)

Organisms Generally Susceptible to Fluoroquinolones In Vitro

	Organism	Ciprofloxacin	Enoxacin	Gatifloxacin	Levofloxacin	Lomefloxacin	Moxifloxacin	Norfloxacin	Ofloxacin	Sparfloxacin	Trovafloxacin/ Alatrofloxacin
Gram-negative (cont'd.)	Ureoplasma urealyticum							✓[1]	✓[1]		✓[1]
	Vibrio parahemolyticus	✓[1]									
	Vibrio vulnificus	✓[1]									
	Vibrio cholerae	✓[1]									
	Yersinia enterocolitica	✓[1]									
Gram-positive	Staphylococcus aureus methicillin susceptible	✓		✓	✓	✓[1]	✓	✓[6]	✓	✓[6]	✓
	Staphylococcus aureus methicillin resistant					✓[1]					
	Staphylococcus epidermidis methicillin susceptible	✓[6]	✓[6]	✓	✓[1]	✓[1]	✓	✓[6]	✓[1]	✓	✓
	Staphylococcus epidermidis methicillin resistant			✓		✓[1]	✓				
	Staphylococcus hemolyticus	✓									
	Staphylococcus hominis	✓									
	Staphylococcus saprophyticus	✓	✓	✓[1]	✓	✓		✓	✓[1]		
	Streptococci pyogenes	✓		✓[1]	✓		✓[1]		✓	✓[1]	✓
	Streptococcus viridans				✓[1]					✓[1]	✓
	Streptococcus group c/f, g				✓[1]						
	Streptococcus milleri				✓[1]						✓[7]
	Streptococcus agalactiae				✓[1]		✓	✓[1]		✓[1]	✓[1]
	Enterococcus faecalis	✓[7]			✓[7]			✓[1]			✓[1]
	Penicillin susceptible			✓	✓		✓		✓	✓	✓
	Penicillin resistant			✓[1]	✓		✓[1]		✓[1]	✓[1]	✓[1]

Organisms Generally Susceptible to Fluoroquinolones In Vitro

	Organism	Ciprofloxacin	Enoxacin	Gatifloxacin	Levofloxacin	Lomefloxacin	Moxifloxacin	Norfloxacin	Ofloxacin	Sparfloxacin	Trovafloxacin/Alatrofloxacin
Atypical bacteria	Legionella pneumophilia	✓[1]		✓	✓	✓[1]	✓[1]		✓[1]	✓[1]	✓
	Mycoplasma pneumoniae			✓	✓		✓		✓[1]	✓	✓
	Chlamydia pneumoniae			✓	✓	✓	✓		✓[1]	✓	✓
Anaerobe bacteria	Bacteroides fragilis										✓
	Peptostreptococcus sp.			✓[1]	✓[1]		✓[1]				✓
	Clostridium perfringes				✓[1]			✓	✓[1]		✓[1]

1 Exhibits in vitro MIC of ≤ 1 mcg/mL (ciprofloxacin, sparfloxacin); ≤ 2 mcg/mL (enoxacin, gatifloxacin, levofloxacin, lomefloxacin, moxifloxacin, ofloxacin, and trovafloxacin); ≤ 4 mcg/mL norfloxacin against most (≥ 90%) strains of microorganisms; however, the safety and effectiveness in treating clinical infections caused by these microorganisms have not been established in adequate and well-controlled clinical trials.

2 Oral ciprofloxacin.

3 As with other drugs in this class, some strains of *P. aeruginosa* may develop resistance fairly rapidly during treatment.

4 Urinary tract only.

5 See following text for individual microorganisms.

6 Does not specify susceptible or resistant.

7 Many strains are moderately susceptible.

Contraindications

Hypersensitivity to fluoroquinolones or the quinolone group; tendinitis or tendon rupture associated with quinolone use; patients receiving disopyramide and amiodarone as well as other QT_c-prolonging antiarrhythmic drugs reported to cause torsade de pointes, such as class IA antiarrhythmic agents (eg, quinidine, procainamide), class III antiarrhythmic agents (eg, sotalol), and bepridil (**sparfloxacin**); patients with known QT_c prolongation or in patients being treated concomitantly with medications known to produce an increase in the QT_c interval or torsades de pointes (**sparfloxacin**); patients whose lifestyle or employment will not permit compliance with required safety precautions concerning phototoxicity (**sparfloxacin**).

Warnings

Phototoxicity: Moderate-to-severe phototoxic reactions have occurred in patients exposed to direct or indirect sunlight or to artificial ultraviolet light (eg, sunlamps) during or following treatment with **lomefloxacin**, **sparfloxacin**, **ofloxacin**, or **trovafloxacin/alatrofloxacin**.

Avoid direct exposure to direct or indirect sunlight (even when using sunscreens or sunblocks) while taking lomefloxacin and other fluoroquinolones for several days following therapy. Discontinue therapy at first signs or symptoms of phototoxicity.

Hepatic failure: **Trovafloxacin/alatrofloxacin**-associated liver enzyme abnormalities, symptomatic hepatitis, jaundice, and liver failure (including rare reports of acute hepatic necrosis with eosinophilic infiltration, liver transplantation, or death) have been reported with short- and long-term drug exposure in men and women. Use exceeding 2 weeks in duration is associated with a significantly increased risk of serious liver injury. Liver injury also has been reported following trovafloxacin/alatrofloxacin re-exposure. Monitor liver function tests (eg, AST, ALT, bilirubin) in recipients who develop signs or symptoms consistent with hepatitis. Consider discontinuing the drug in those patients who develop liver function test abnormalities (see Warning Box).

Cardiac toxicity: **Moxifloxacin** and **gatifloxacin** have been shown to prolong the QT interval of the electrocardiogram in some patients. Avoid in patients with known prolongation of the QT interval, patients with uncorrected hypokalemia, and patients receiving class IA (eg, quinidine, procainamide) or class III (eg, amiodarone, sotalol) antiarrhythmic agents, because of the lack of clinical experience with these drugs in these patient populations.

Increases in the QT_c interval have been observed in healthy volunteers treated with **sparfloxacin**.

Avoid the concomitant prescription of medications known to prolong the QT_c interval (eg, erythromycin, terfenadine, astemizole, cisapride, pentamidine, tricyclic antidepressants, some antipsychotics including phenothiazines). **Sparfloxacin** is not recommended for use in patients with proarrhythmic conditions (eg, hypokalemia, significant bradycardia, CHF, myocardial ischemia, atrial fibrillation).

Hypotension: Life-threatening hypotension has been reported with **alatrofloxacin** administration. This has occurred in patients receiving alatrofloxacin either at the recommended rate of infusion or if given more rapidly. Hypotension may be potentiated with the concomitant administration of anesthetic agents. Alatrofloxacin should be only administered by slow IV infusion over a period of 60 minutes. Monitor blood pressure closely during infusion.

Tendon rupture/Tendinitis: Ruptures of the shoulder, hand, and Achilles tendons that required surgical repair or resulted in prolonged disability have been reported with fluoroquinolone antimicrobials. Discontinue therapy if the patient experiences pain, inflammation, or rupture of a tendon. Patients should rest and refrain from exercise until the diagnosis of tendinitis or tendon rupture has been confidently excluded. Tendon rupture can occur at any time during or after therapy.

Convulsions: Increased intracranial pressure, convulsions, and toxic psychosis have occurred. CNS stimulation also may occur and may lead to tremor, restlessness, lightheadedness, confusion, dizziness, depression, hallucinations, and rarely, suicidal thoughts or acts. Use with caution in patients with known or suspected CNS disorders (eg, severe cerebral arteriosclerosis, epilepsy) or other factors that predispose to seizures or lower the seizure threshold, or in the presence of other risk factors that may predispose to seizures or lower the seizure threshold (eg, certain drug therapy, renal dysfunction). If these reactions occur, stop the drug, and institute appropriate measures.

Syphilis: **Ciprofloxacin, enoxacin, gatifloxacin, norfloxacin, ofloxacin,** and **trovafloxacin** are not effective for syphilis. High doses of antimicrobial agents for short periods of time to treat gonorrhea may mask or delay symptoms of incubating syphilis. All patients should have a serologic test for syphilis at the time of gonorrhea diagnosis. Patients treated with ciprofloxacin, enoxacin, gatifloxacin, norfloxacin, ofloxacin, and trovafloxacin should have a follow-up serologic test after 3 months.

Chronic bronchitis due to Streptococcus pneumoniae: **Lomefloxacin** is not indicated for the empiric treatment of acute bacterial exacerbation of chronic bronchitis when it is probable that *S. pneumoniae* is a causative pathogen because it exhibits in vitro resistance to lomefloxacin.

P. aeruginosa: In clinical trials of complicated UTIs due to *P. aeruginosa*, 12 of 16 patients had the microorganism eradicated from the urine after therapy with **lomefloxacin.** No patients had concomitant bacteremia. Serum levels of lomefloxacin do not reliably exceed the MIC of *Pseudomonas* isolates. The safety and efficacy of lomefloxacin in treating patients with *Pseudomonas* bacteremia have not been established.

Hypersensitivity reactions: Hypersensitivity reactions, serious and occasionally fatal, have occurred in patients receiving quinolone therapy, some following the first dose. Refer to Management of Acute Hypersensitivity Reactions.

Pseudomembranous colitis: Pseudomembranous colitis has been reported with nearly all antibacterial agents, including fluoroquinolones, and may range from mild to life-threatening in severity.

Renal function impairment: Alteration in dosage regimen is necessary. See Administration and Dosage.

Hepatic function impairment: The oral clearance of **trovafloxacin** in mild and moderate cirrhosis is reduced ≈ 30%, which corresponds to prolongation of half-life by 2 to 2.5 hours (25% to 30%) increase. There are no data in patients with severe cirrhosis. Dosage adjustment is recommended in patients with mild-to-moderate cirrhosis.

Elderly: **Norfloxacin** is eliminated more slowly because of decreased renal function; absorption appears unaffected. The apparent half-life of **ofloxacin** is 6 to 8 hours, compared to ≈ 5 hours in younger adults; absorption is unaffected. **Lomefloxacin** plasma clearance was reduced by ≈ 25% and the AUC was increased by ≈ 33% in the elderly, which may be caused by decreased renal function in this population. **Enoxacin** plasma concentrations are 50% higher in the elderly than in young adults.

Pregnancy: Category C.

Lactation: **Norfloxacin** was not detected in breast milk following the administration of 200 mg to nursing mothers; however, this was a low dose. **Ciprofloxacin** is excreted in breast milk. **Ofloxacin,** as a single 200 mg dose, resulted in breast milk concentrations in nursing females that were similar to those found in plasma. **Levofloxacin** has not been measured in breast milk. Based upon data from ofloxacin, it can be presumed that levofloxacin will be excreted in breast milk. **Sparfloxacin** is excreted in breast milk. **Gatifloxacin** and **moxifloxacin** are excreted in the breast milk of rats. **Trovafloxacin** is excreted in breast milk and was found in measurable concentrations in the breast milk of lactating subjects. It is not known whether lomefloxacin, gatifloxacin, or enoxacin are excreted in breast milk. Because of the potential for serious adverse reactions in nursing infants, decide whether to discontinue nursing or to discontinue the drug, taking into account the importance of the drug to the mother.

Children: Safety and efficacy of enoxacin, gatifloxacin, levofloxacin, lomefloxacin, moxifloxacin, norfloxacin, ofloxacin, sparfloxacin, and trovafloxacin in children < 18 years of age have not been established. Ciprofloxacin, enoxacin, gatifloxacin, levofloxacin, lomefloxacin, moxifloxacin, ofloxacin, sparfloxacin, and trovafloxacin cause arthropathy and osteochondrosis in immature animals. Administration of ciprofloxacin, moxifloxacin, and norfloxacin caused lameness in immature dogs because of permanent cartilage lesions.

Precautions

Monitoring: Periodic assessment of organ system functions, including renal, hepatic, and hematopoietic, is advisable during prolonged therapy.

Symptomatic pancreatitis has been reported with trovafloxacin/alatrofloxacin therapy. Monitor pancreatic tests in patients who develop symptoms consistent with pancreatitis.

Crystalluria: Needle-shaped crystals were found in the urine of some volunteers who received either placebo or 800 or 1600 mg norfloxacin. While crystalluria is not expected to occur under usual conditions with 400 mg twice daily, do not exceed the daily recommended dosage. Crystalluria related to ciprofloxacin has occurred only rarely in humans because human urine is usually acidic. The patient should drink sufficient fluids to ensure proper hydration and adequate urinary output.

Hemolytic reactions: Rarely, hemolytic reactions have been reported in patients with latent or actual defects in glucose-6-phosphate dehydrogenase activity who take quinolone antibacterial agents, including norfloxacin.

Myasthenia gravis: Quinolones may exacerbate the signs of myasthenia gravis and lead to life-threatening weakness of the respiratory muscles. Exercise caution when using quinolones in patients with myasthenia gravis.

Blood glucose abnormalities: As with other quinolones, disturbances of blood glucose, including symptomatic hyper- and hypoglycemia, have been reported, usually in diabetic patients receiving concomitant treatment with an oral hypoglycemic agent (eg, glyburide/glibenclamide) or with insulin. In these patients, careful monitoring of blood glucose is recommended. If a hypoglycemic reaction occurs, initiate appropriate therapy immediately.

Drug Interactions

Drugs that may affect fluoroquinolones include antacids, didanosine, iron salts, sucralfate, azlocillin, bismuth subsalicylate, cimetidine, nitrofurantoin, cisapride, nonsteroidal anti-inflammatory drugs (NSAIDs), morphine, and probenecid.

Drugs that may be affected by fluoroquinolones include caffeine, cyclosporine, digoxin, antiarrhythmic agents, bepridil, erythromycin, phenothiazine, tricyclic antidepressants, procainamide, anticoagulants, cyclosporine, and theophylline.

Drug/Food interactions: Food may decrease the absorption of norfloxacin. Food delays the absorption of ciprofloxacin, resulting in peak concentrations that are closer to 2 hours after dosing rather than 1 hour; however, overall absorption is not substantially affected. Dairy products such as milk and yogurt reduce the absorption of ciprofloxacin; avoid concurrent use. The bioavailability of ciprofloxacin may also be decreased by enteral feedings. Food delays the rate of absorption of lomefloxacin and decreases the extent of absorption (AUC) by 12%.

Adverse Reactions

	Adverse reaction	Ciprofloxacin[1]	Enoxacin[2]	Gatifloxacin	Levofloxacin	Lomefloxacin	Moxifloxacin	Norfloxacin[2]	Ofloxacin[1]	Sparfloxacin	Trovafloxacin/Alatrofloxacin[1]
Fluoroquinolone Adverse Reactions (%)											
CNS	Headache	1.2	≤ 2	3	0.1-6.4	3.6	2	2-2.8	1-9	4.2-8.1	1-5
	Dizziness	< 1	≤ 3	3	0.3-2.7	2.1	3	1.7-2.6	1-5	2-3.8	2-11
	Fatigue/Lethargy/Malaise	< 1	< 1		< 1-1.2	< 1	> 0.05-< 1	0.3-1	1-3	< 1	< 1
	Somnolence/Drowsiness	< 1	< 1	< 0.1	< 1	< 1	> 0.05-< 1	0.3-1	1-3	< 1-1.5	< 1
	Depression	< 1	< 1	< 0.1	< 1	< 1		0.1-0.2	< 1	< 1	< 1
	Insomnia	< 1	1	≥ 0.1-< 3	0.5-4.6	< 1	> 0.05-< 1	0.3-1	3-7	1.9	< 1
	Seizures/Convulsions[3]	< 1	< 1	< 0.1	< 1	< 1		✓[4]	< 1		< 1
	Confusion	≤ 1	< 1	< 0.1	< 1	< 1	> 0.05-< 1	✓[4]	< 1	< 1	< 1
	Psychotic reactions	< 1	< 0.1					✓[4]			
	Paresthesia	< 1	< 1	≥ 0.1-< 3	< 1	< 1			< 1	< 1	
	Hallucinations	< 1	< 0.1	< 0.1	< 1		> 0.05-< 1	✓[4]	< 1	< 1	< 1
Dermatologic	Photosensitivity[3]	< 1	< 1			2.3			✓[4]		
	Rash	1.1	≤ 1	≥ 0.1-< 3	0.3-1.2	< 1	> 0.05-< 1	0.3-1	1-3	1.1	< 1-2
	Pruritus	< 1	1	< 0.1	0.4-1.3	< 1	> 0.05-< 1	0.3-1	1-3	1.8-3.3	< 1-2
	Toxic epidermal necrolysis	< 1	< 1					✓[4]			
	Stevens-Johnson syndrome	< 1	< 1					✓[4]			
	Exfoliative dermatitis	< 1						✓[4]			
	Hypersensitivity[3]	< 1				< 1		✓[4]	✓[3]		

Fluoroquinolone Adverse Reactions (%)

Adverse reaction	Ciprofloxacin[1]	Enoxacin[2]	Gatifloxacin	Levofloxacin	Lomefloxacin	Moxifloxacin	Norfloxacin[2]	Ofloxacin[1]	Sparfloxacin	Trovafloxacin/ Alatrofloxacin[1]
GI										
Nausea	5.2	2-8	8	1.3-7.2	3.5	8	2.6-4.2	3-10	4.3-7.6	4-8
Abdominal pain/discomfort/cramping	≤1-1.7	≤2	≥0.1-<3	0.4-2.5	1.2	>0.05≤2	0.3-1.6	1-3	1.8-2.4	1
Diarrhea	2.3	1-2	4	1-5.6	1.4	6	0.3-1	1-4	3.2-4.6	2
Vomiting	≤1-2	2-9	≥0.1-<3	0.2-2.3	<1	2	0.3-1	1-4	<1-1.3	1-3
Dry/Painful mouth	<1	<1		<1	<1	>0.05-<1	0.3-1	1-3	<1-1.4	
Dyspepsia/Heartburn	<1	1	≥0.1-<3	0.3-2.4	<1	1	0.3-1	<1	1.6-2.3	
Constipation	<1	<1	≥0.1-<3	0.1-3.2	<1	>0.05-<1	0.3-1	1-3	<1	
Flatulence	<1	<1	<0.1	0.4-1.5	<1		0.3-1	1-3	<1-1.1	<1
Pseudomembranous colitis[3]	<1	<0.1	<0.1	<1	✓[4]		✓[4]	✓[3]		<1
Miscellaneous										
Visual disturbances	<1	<1			<1		0.1-0.2	1-3		<1
Hearing loss	<1						✓[4]	<1		
Vaginitis	<1	<1	6	0.7-1.8	<1	>0.05-<1		1-5	<1	<1-2
Hypertension	<1		<0.1	<1	<1	>0.05-<1		<1	<1	<1
Palpitations	<1	<1	≥0.1-<3	<1		>0.05-<1		<1	<1	
Syncope	<1	<1		<1	<1			<1		<1
Chills	<1	<1	≥0.1-<3	<1	<1	>0.05-<1	0.1-0.2	<1	<1	
Edema	<1	<1	<0.1	<1	<1		0.1-0.2	<1		<1
Fever	<1	<1	≥0.1-<3	<1			0.3-1	1-3	<1	<1

Fluoroquinolone Adverse Reactions (%)

Adverse reaction	Ciprofloxacin[1]	Enoxacin[2]	Gatifloxacin	Levofloxacin	Lomefloxacin	Moxifloxacin	Norfloxacin[2]	Ofloxacin[1]	Sparfloxacin	Trovafloxacin/Alatrofloxacin[1]
↑ ALT/↑ AST	1.9/1.7	≥1	<1		≤0.4		1.4/1.4-1.6	≥1	2-2.3	≥1
↑ Alkaline phosphatase	0.8	<1	<1		0.1		1.1	≥1	<1	≥1
↑ LDH	0.4			<1			✓			
↑ or ↓ Bilirubin	0.3	<1	<1		0.1	≥2			<1	
Eosinophilia	0.6	<1			0.1	>0.05-<1	0.6-1.5	≥1		≥1
Leukopenia	0.4	<1		<1	0.1	>0.05-<1	1.4	≥1		
↑ or ↓ Platelets	0.1	<1			<1		1		<1	≥1
Pancytopenia	0.1									
↑ ESR/Lymphocytopenia					<0.1			≥1		
Neutropenia			<1				1.4	≥1		
↑ Serum creatinine	1.1				0.1		✓	≥1		
↑ BUN	0.9				0.1		✓	≥1		
Crystalluria/Cylinduria/Candiduria	✓						✓			
Hematuria	✓							≥1		
Glucosuria/Pyuria								≥1		
Proteinuria/Albuminuria		<1			<0.1		1	≥1		

Abnormal laboratory values

Fluoroquinolone Adverse Reactions (%)

Adverse reaction	Ciprofloxacin[1]	Enoxacin[2]	Gatifloxacin	Levofloxacin	Lomefloxacin	Moxifloxacin	Norfloxacin[2]	Ofloxacin[1]	Sparfloxacin	Trovafloxacin/Alatrofloxacin[1]
↑ γ-glutamyltransferase	< 0.1				< 0.1					
↑ Serum amylase	< 0.1		< 1						< 1	
↑ Uric acid	< 0.1									
↑ or ↓ Blood glucose	< 0.1			2.2	< 0.1			≥ 1	< 1	
↑ or ↓ Hemoglobin/Hematocrit	< 0.1	< 1			< 0.1	≥ 2	0.6			≥ 1
↑ or ↓ Potassium	✔[4]	< 1			0.1				< 1	
Anemia	< 0.1				< 0.1			≥ 1		
Bleeding/↑ PT	< 0.1				< 0.1					
↑ Monocytes	< 0.1				0.2				< 1	
Leukocytosis	< 0.1	< 1		< 1	0.1			≥ 1		
↑ Triglycerides/Cholesterol	✔[4]									

Abnormal laboratory values con't

[1] Includes data for oral and IV formulations.
[2] From single- and multiple-dose studies.
[3] See Warnings or Precautions.
[4] ✔ = Adverse reaction observed; incidence not reported.

TETRACYCLINES

TETRACYCLINE HCl	
Tablets: 250 and 500 mg (*Rx*)	*Sumycin 250 and 500* (Apothecon)
Capsules: 100, 250 and 500 mg (*Rx*)	Various, *Achromycin V* (Lederle)
Oral suspension: 125 mg/5 mL (*Rx*)	Various, *Achromycin V* (Lederle)
DEMECLOCYCLINE HCl	
Tablets: 150 and 300 mg (*Rx*)	*Declomycin* (Lederle)
Capsules: 50 and 100 mg (*Rx*)	*Declomycin* (Lederle)
DOXYCYCLINE	
Tablets: 50 and 100 mg (as hyclate) (*Rx*)	Various, *Vibra-Tabs* (Pfizer), *Bio-Tab* (Inter. Ethical Labs)
Capsules: 50 and 100 mg (*Rx*)	Various, *Monodox* (Oclassen), *Vibramycin* (Pfizer)
Capsules, coated pellets: 100 mg (as hyclate) (*Rx*)	*Doryx* (Parke-Davis)
Capsules: 50 and 100 mg (as monohydrate) (*Rx*)	*Monodox* (Oclassen)
Powder for oral suspension: 25 mg/5 mL (as monohydrate when reconstituted) (*Rx*)	*Vibramycin* (Pfizer)
Syrup: 50 mg/5 mL (as calcium) (*Rx*)	*Vibramycin* (Pfizer)
Powder for injection: 100 and 200 mg (as hyclate) (*Rx*)	Various, *Vibramycin IV* (Pfizer)
MINOCYCLINE	
Capsules: 50 and 100 mg (*Rx*)	Various, *Dynacin* (Medicis Dermatologics)
Capsules, pellet filled: 50 and 100 mg (*Rx*)	*Minocin* (Lederle)
Oral suspension: 50 mg/5 mL (*Rx*)	*Minocin* (Lederle)
Powder for injection: 100 mg (*Rx*)	*Minocin IV* (Lederle)
OXYTETRACYCLINE	
Capsules: 250 mg (*Rx*)	Various, *Terramycin* (Pfizer)
Injection: 50 and 125 mg/mL (*Rx*)	*Terramycin IM* (Roerig)

Indications

Infections caused by the following microorganisms: Rickettsiae (Rocky Mountain spotted fever, typhus fever and the typhus group, Q fever, rickettsialpox, and tick fevers); *Mycoplasma pneumoniae* (PPLO, Eaton agent); agents of psittacosis and ornithosis; agents of lymphogranuloma venereum and granuloma inguinale; the spirochetal agent of relapsing fever (*Borrelia recurrentis*).

Infections caused by the following gram-negative microorganisms: *Haemophilus ducreyi* (chancroid); *Yersinia pestis* and *Francisella tularensis* (formerly *Pasteurella pestis* and *Pasturella tularensis*); *Bartonella bacilliformis*; *Bacteroides* sp.; *Campylobacter fetus* (formerly *Vibrio fetus*); *Vibrio cholerae* (formerly *Vibrio comma*); *Brucella* sp. (in conjunction with streptomycin).

Infections caused by the following microorganisms, when bacteriologic testing indicates appropriate susceptibility to the drug:
Gram-negative – *Escherichia coli*; *Enterobacter aerogenes* (formerly *Aerobacter aerogenes*); *Shigella* sp.; *Acinetobacter calcoaceticus* (formerly *Mima* and *Herellea* sp.); *Haemophilus influenzae* (respiratory infections); *Klebsiella* sp. (respiratory and urinary infections).

Gram-positive – *Streptococcus* sp. including *S. pneumoniae*. Up to 44% of strains of *S. pyogenes* and 74% of *S. faecalis* are resistant to tetracyclines.

Staphylococcus aureus: *S. aureus*, skin and soft tissue infections. Tetracyclines are not the drugs of choice in the treatment of any type of staphylococcal infection.

Treatment of trachoma: Treatment of trachoma, although the infectious agent is not always eliminated, as judged by immunofluorescence.

When penicillin is contraindicated: When penicillin is contraindicated, tetracyclines are alternatives for treatment of infections caused by: *Neisseria gonorrhoeae*; *Treponema pallidum and T. pertenue* (syphilis and yaws); *Listeria monocytogenes*; *Clostridium* sp.; *Bacillus anthracis*; *Fusobacterium fusiforme* (Vincent's infection); *Actinomyces* sp.; *Neisseria meningitidis* (IV only).

Acute intestinal amebiasis: Tetracyclines may be a useful adjunct to amebicides.

Oral tetracyclines:

Adults – Treatment of uncomplicated urethral, endocervical, or rectal infections caused by *Chlamydia trachomatis*.

Severe acne – Severe acne (where it may be useful as adjunctive therapy).

Inclusion conjunctivitis – Inclusion conjunctivitis (which may be treated with oral tetracyclines or with a combination of oral and topical agents).

Doxycycline, oral – Treatment of uncomplicated gonococcal infections in adults (except for anorectal infections in men); gonococcal arthritis-dermatitis syndrome; acute epididymo-orchitis caused by *N. gonorrhoeae* and *C. trachomatis*; nongonococcal urethritis caused by *C. trachomatis* and *Ureaplasma urealyticum*.

Minocycline, oral – Treatment of asymptomatic carriers of *N. meningitidis* to eliminate meningococci from the nasopharynx. Not indicated for the treatment of meningococcal infection.

Oral minocycline has been successful in *Mycobacterium marinum* infections.

Minocycline also is indicated for the treatment of uncomplicated urethral, endocervical, or rectal infections in adults caused by *U. urealyticum*; uncomplicated gonococcal urethritis in men caused by *N. gonorrhoeae*.

Unlabeled uses: Tetracycline suspension has been used as a mouthwash in the treatment of nonspecific mouth ulcerations, aphthous ulcers, and canker sores. Dosages have ranged from 5 to 10 mL of 125 mg/mL 3 times/day for 5 to 7 days.

Doxycycline has been used to prevent "traveler's diarrhea" commonly caused by enterotoxigenic *Escherichia coli*. In limited trials, this prophylactic (100 mg/day) therapy appears to be superior to placebo.

Lyme disease – Lyme disease (the etiologic agent is a spirochete, *Borrelia burgdorferi*): Oral **tetracycline** 250 mg daily for 10 days is the drug of choice for stage I disease in adults; **doxycycline** has also been recommended for early disease. Both agents have been recommended for stage II disease, and they are being evaluated for treatment of stage III disease. However, the efficacy of tetracycline at the recommended dose for early Lyme disease has been questioned.

Administration and Dosage

Avoid rapid IV administration. Thrombophlebitis may result from prolonged IV therapy.

Continue therapy at least 24 to 48 hours after symptoms and fever subside. Treat all infections caused by group A β-hemolytic streptococci for at least 10 days.

TETRACYLINE HCl:

Adults –

Usual dose: 1 to 2 g/day in 2 or 4 equal doses.

Children (> 8 years of age) – Daily dose is 10 to 20 mg/lb (25 to 50 mg/kg in 4 equal doses.

Brucellosis – 500 mg 4 times/day for 3 weeks, accompanied by 1 g streptomycin IM twice/day the first week, and once daily the second week.

Syphilis – 30 to 40 g in equally divided doses over 10 to 15 days. Perform close follow-up and laboratory tests.

Gonorrhea – 1.5 g initially, then 500 mg every 6 hours, to a total of 9 g.

Gonorrhea in patients sensitive to penicillin – Initially, 1.5 g; follow with 500 mg every 6 hours for 4 days to a total of 9 g.

Uncomplicated urethral, endocervical, or rectal infections caused by Chlamydia trachomatis – 500 mg 4 times/day for at least 7 days.

Severe acne (long-term therapy) – Initially, 1 g/day in divided doses. For maintenance, give 125 to 500 mg/day.

CDC-recommended treatment schedules for sexually transmitted diseases –

Chlamydia trachomatis – *Uncomplicated urethral, endocervical, or rectal infections in adults:* 500 mg 4 times/day for 7 days.

Gonococcal infections – *Uncomplicated urethral, endocervical, or rectal infections in adults:* 3 g amoxicillin, 3.5 g oral ampicillin, 4.8 million units IM aqueous procaine penicillin G or 250 mg IM ceftriaxone. Each (except ceftriaxone) should be accompanied by 1 g oral probenecid. Follow with 500 mg tetracycline 4 times/day for 7 days.

In adults allergic to penicillins, cephalosporins, or probenecid – 500 mg 4 times/day for 7 days.

Penicillinase-producing Neisseria gonorrheae (PPNG): 2 g IM spectinomycin or 250 mg IM ceftriaxone. Follow with 500 mg tetracycline 4 times/day for 7 days.

Children – 40 mg/kg/day in 4 divided doses for 5 days.

In PPNG-endemic and -hyperendemic areas: 250 mg IM ceftriaxone plus 100 mg oral doxycycline twice daily for 7 days or 500 mg oral tetracycline 4 times/day for 7 days. If tetracyclines are contraindicated or not tolerated, follow the single-dose regimen with erythromycin.

Disseminated gonococcal infections in patients allergic to penicillins or cephalosporins: 500 mg 4 times/day for ≥ 7 days.

Lymphogranuloma venereum – Genital, inguinal, or anorectal: 500 mg 4 times/day for ≥ 2 weeks.

Nongonococcal urethritis: 500 mg 4 times/day for 7 days.

Acute pelvic inflammatory disease – Ambulatory treatment: 2 g IM cefoxitin, 3 g amoxicillin, 3.5 g oral ampicillin, 4.8 million units IM aqueous procaine penicillin G at 2 sites or 250 mg IM ceftriaxone. Each (except for ceftriaxone) should be accompanied by 1 g oral probenecid. Follow with 500 mg tetracycline 4 times/day. (However, doxycycline is preferred.)

Children > 7 years of age – 150 mg/kg/day IV cefuroxime or 100 mg/kg/day IV ceftriaxone followed by 30 mg/kg/day IV tetracycline in 3 doses, continued for ≥ 4 days. Thereafter, continue tetracycline orally to complete ≥ 14 days of therapy.

Syphilis (penicillin-allergic patients):

Early – 500 mg 4 times/day for 15 days.

More than 1 year's duration – 500 mg 4 times/day for 30 days.

Sexually transmitted epididymo-orchitis: 3 g oral amoxicillin, 3.5 g oral ampicillin, 4.8 million units IM aqueous procaine penicillin G at 2 sites (each with 1 g oral probenecid), 2 g IM spectinomycin or 250 mg ceftriaxone followed by 500 mg tetracycline 4 times/day for 10 days.

Urethral syndrome in women: 500 mg 4 times/day for 7 days.

Rape victims – Prophylaxis: 500 mg 4 times/day for 7 days.

DEMECLOCYCLINE HCl:

Adults –

Daily dose: 4 divided doses of 150 mg each or 2 divided doses of 300 mg each.

Children (over 8 years of age) –

Usual daily dose: 3 to 6 mg/lb (6 to 12 mg/kg), depending upon the severity of the disease, divided into 3 or 4 doses.

Gonorrhea patients sensitive to penicillin – Initially, 600 mg; follow with 300 mg every 12 hours for 4 days to a total of 3 g.

DOXYCYCLINE:

Oral –

Adults:

Usual dose – 200 mg on the first day of treatment (100 mg every 12 hours); follow with a maintenance dose of 100 mg/day. The maintenance dose may be administered as a single dose or as 50 mg every 12 hours.

More severe infections (particularly chronic urinary tract infections) – 100 mg every 12 hours.

Children (> 8 years of age):

≤ 100 lbs (< 45 kg) – 2 mg/lb (4.4 mg/kg) divided into 2 doses on the first day of treatment; follow with 1 mg/lb (2.2 mg/kg) given as a single daily dose or divided into 2 doses on subsequent days.

More severe infections – Up to 2 mg/lb (4.4 mg/kg) may be used. For children > 100 lbs (45 kg), use the usual adult dose.

Acute gonococcal infection: 200 mg immediately, then 100 mg at bedtime on the first day. Follow by 100 mg 2 times/day for 3 days.

Single visit dose – Immediately give 300 mg; follow with 300 mg in 1 hour, which may be administered with food, milk, or carbonated beverage.

Primary and secondary syphilis: 300 mg/day in divided doses for ≥ 10 days.

Uncomplicated urethral, endocervical, or rectal infections in adults caused by Chlamydia trachomatis: 100 mg twice daily for ≥ 7 days.

Endometritis, salpingitis, parametritis, or peritonitis: Give 100 mg doxycycline IV, twice/day and 2 g cefoxitin IV 4 times/day. Continue IV administration for ≥ 4 days and for ≥ 48 hours after patient improves. Then continue oral doxycycline (100 mg) twice daily to complete 10 to 14 days total therapy.

Parenteral – Do not inject IM or SC. The duration of IV infusion may vary with the dose (100 to 200 mg/day), but is usually 1 to 4 hours. A recommended minimum infusion time for 100 mg of a 0.5 mg/mL solution is 1 hour.

Adults: The usual dosage is 200 mg IV on the first day of treatment, administered in 1- or 2-hour infusions. Subsequent daily dosage is 100 to 200 mg, depending upon the severity of infection, with 200 mg administered in 1 or 2 infusions.

Primary and secondary syphilis – 300 mg daily for ≥ 10 days.

Children (> 8 years): ≤ 100 lbs (45 kg), give 2 mg/lb (4.4 mg/kg) on the first day of treatment, in 1 or 2 infusions. Subsequent daily dosage is 1 to 2 mg/lb (2.2 to 4.4 mg/kg) given as 1 or 2 infusions, depending on the severity of the infection. For children > 100 lbs (45 kg), use the usual adult dose.

Children (< 8 years): Safety of IV use has not been established.

CDC-recommended treatment schedules for sexually transmitted diseases –

Chlamydia trachomatis – Uncomplicated urethral, endocervical, or rectal infections in adults: 100 mg 2 times/day for 7 days.

Gonococcal infections:

Uncomplicated urethral, endocervical, or rectal infections in adults – 3 g oral amoxicillin, 3.5 g oral ampicillin, 4.8 million units IM aqueous procaine penicillin G or 250 mg IM ceftriaxone. Each (except for ceftriaxone) should be accompanied by 1 g oral probenecid. Follow with 100 mg doxycycline twice daily for 7 days.

In adults allergic to penicillins, cephalosporins, or probenecid: 100 mg twice daily for 7 days.

In PPNG-endemic and -hyperendemic areas: 250 mg IM ceftriaxone plus 100 mg oral doxycycline twice daily for 7 days. If tetracyclines are contraindicated or not tolerated, follow the single-dose regimen with erythromycin.

PPNG: 2 g IM spectinomycin or 250 mg IM ceftriaxone. Follow with 100 mg doxycycline, twice daily for 7 days.

Disseminated gonococcal infections in patients allergic to penicillins or cephalosporins: 100 mg, twice daily for ≥ 7 days.

Lymphogranuloma venereum:

Genital, inguinal, or anorectal – 100 mg twice daily for ≥ 2 weeks.

Nongonococcal urethritis: 100 mg twice daily for 7 days.

Acute pelvic inflammatory disease:

Ambulatory treatment – 250 mg single IM dose of ceftriaxone plus 100 mg oral doxycycline twice daily for 10 to 14 days. Other effective third-generation cephalosporins may be substituted in the appropriate doses for ceftriaxone.

Inpatient treatment – 100 mg IV doxycycline twice daily, plus 2 g IV cefoxitin 4 times/day. Continue drugs IV for ≥ 4 days and ≥ 48 hours after patient improves. Then continue doxycycline 100 mg orally twice daily to complete 10 to 14 days of total therapy.

Sexually transmitted epididymo-orchitis: 3 g oral amoxicillin, 3.5 g oral ampicillin, 4.8 million units IM aqueous procaine penicillin G at 2 sites (each with 1 g oral probenecid), 2 g IM spectinomycin or 250 mg IM ceftriaxone followed by 100 mg doxycycline twice daily for 7 days.

Rape victims prophylaxis: 100 mg twice daily for 7 days.

MINOCYCLINE:

Oral –

Usual dosage:

Adults – 200 mg initially, followed by 100 mg every 12 hours. If more frequent doses are preferred, give 100 or 200 mg initially; follow with 50 mg 4 times/day.

Children (over 8 years of age) – Initially, 4 mg/kg; follow with 2 mg/kg every 12 hours.

Syphilis: Administer usual dose over a period of 10 to 15 days. Close follow-up, including laboratory tests, is recommended.

Uncomplicated urethral, endocervical, or rectal infections in adults caused by Chlamydia trachomatis: 100 mg 2 times/day for ≥ 7 days.

Uncomplicated gonococcal urethritis in men: 100 mg 2 times/day for 5 days.

Mycobacterium marinum infections: Although optimal doses are not established, 100 mg twice daily for 6 to 8 weeks has been successful in a limited number of cases.

Parenteral –

Adults: 200 mg followed by 100 mg every 12 hours; do not exceed 400 mg in 24 hours.

Children (over 8 years of age): Usual pediatric dose is 4 mg/kg, followed by 2 mg/kg every 12 hours.

OXYTETRACYCLINE:

Oral – See Tetracycline HCl.

Parenteral –

Adults: The usual daily dose is 250 mg administered once every 24 hours or 300 mg given in divided doses at 8- to 12-hour intervals.

Children (> 8 years of age): 15 to 25 mg/kg, up to a maximum of 250 mg/single daily injection. Dosage may be divided and given at 8 to 12 hour intervals.

Actions

Pharmacology: The tetracyclines are bacteriostatic. They exert their antimicrobial effect by inhibition of protein synthesis.

Pharmacokinetics:

Tetracycline Pharmacokinetic Variables and Dosage Regimens					
Tetracyclines	Serum protein binding (%)	Normal serum half-life (hrs)	% excreted unchanged in urine	Usual oral adult maintenance dosage	Lipid solubility
Tetracycline	65	16 to 12	60	250 mg q 6 h or 500 mg q 6 to 12 h	Intermediate
Demeclocycline	65 to 91	12 to 16	39	150 mg q 6 h or 300 mg q 12 h	Intermediate
Doxycycline	80 to 95	15 to 25	30 to 42	150 mg q 12 h or 100 mg q 24 h	High
Minocycline	70 to 80	11 to 18	16 to 12	100 mg q 12 h	High
Oxytetracycline	20 to 40	16 to 12	70	250 to 500 mg q 6 h	Low

Contraindications

Hypersensitivity to any of the tetracyclines.

Warnings

Photosensitivity: Photosensitivity manifested by an exaggerated sunburn reaction has been observed in some individuals taking tetracyclines. Advise patients who are apt to be exposed to direct sunlight or ultraviolet light that this reaction can occur with tetracycline drugs, and discontinue treatment at the first evidence of skin erythema.

Phototoxic reactions are most frequent with demeclocycline, and occur less frequently with the other tetracyclines; minocycline is least likely to cause phototoxic reactions.

Parenteral therapy: Reserve for situations in which oral therapy is not indicated. Institute oral therapy as soon as possible. If given IV over prolonged periods, thrombophlebitis may result. IM use produces lower blood levels than recommended oral dosages.

Nephrogenic diabetes insipidus: Administration of **demeclocycline** has resulted in appearance of the diabetes insipidus syndrome (polyuria, polydipsia, and weakness) in some patients on long-term therapy.

Hazardous tasks: Lightheadedness, dizziness or vertigo may occur with **minocycline.** Patients should observe caution while driving or performing other tasks requiring alertness.

Renal function impairment: If renal impairment exists, even usual doses may lead to excessive systemic accumulation of the tetracyclines (with the exception of doxycycline and minocycline) and possible liver toxicity. Use lower than usual doses.

Hepatic function impairment: Doses > 2 g/day IV can be extremely dangerous. In the presence of renal dysfunction, and particularly in pregnancy, IV tetracycline > 2 g/day has been associated with death secondary to liver failure.

Pregnancy: Category D (**doxycycline**). Do not use during pregnancy. They readily cross the placenta; concentrations of oxytetracycline in cord blood are ≈ 50% of those of the mother. Tetracyclines are found in fetal tissues and can have toxic effects on the developing fetus (retardation of skeletal development).

Lactation: Tetracyclines are excreted in breast milk. A dosage of 2 g/day for 3 days has achieved a milk:plasma ratio of 0.6 to 0.8.

Children: Tetracyclines generally should not be used in children < 8 years of age unless other drugs are not likely to be effective or are contraindicated.

    Teeth – The use of tetracyclines during the period of tooth development (from the last half of pregnancy through the eighth year of life) may cause permanent discoloration (yellow-gray-brown) of deciduous and permanent teeth. Doxycycline and oxytetracycline may be less likely to affect teeth.

    Bone – Tetracycline forms a stable calcium complex in any bone-forming tissue. Decreased fibula growth rate occurred in premature infants given 25 mg/kg oral tetracycline every 6 hours.

Precautions

Pseudotumor cerebri: Pseudotumor cerebri (benign intracranial hypertension) in adults has been associated with tetracycline use.

Outdated products: Under no circumstances should outdated tetracyclines be administered; the degradation products of tetracyclines are highly nephrotoxic and have, on occasion, produced a Fanconi-like syndrome.

Drug Interactions

Drugs that may affect tetracyclines include antacids containing aluminum, calcium, zinc, magnesium, bismuth salts, divalent and trivalent cations; barbiturates; carbamazepine; hydantoins; cimetidine; oral iron salts; methoxyflurane; and sodium bicarbonate.

Drugs that may be affected by tetracyclines include oral anticoagulants, digoxin, insulin, lithium, methoxyflurane, oral contraceptives, and penicillins.

Drug/Food interactions: Food and some dairy products interfere with absorption of tetracyclines. Administer oral tetracycline 1 hour before or 2 hours after meals. Doxycycline has a low affinity for calcium binding. GI absorption of minocycline and doxycycline is not significantly affected by food or dairy products.

Adverse Reactions

CNS: Lightheadedness, dizziness, or vertigo has been reported with **minocycline.**

Dermatologic: Maculopapular and erythematous rashes.

GI:

    Oral and parenteral – Anorexia; nausea; vomiting; diarrhea; epigastric distress; bulky loose stools; stomatitis; sore throat; glossitis; hoarseness.

    Oral – Esophageal ulcers, most commonly in patients with an esophageal obstructive element or hiatal hernia.

Hematologic: Hemolytic anemia; thrombocytopenia; thrombocytopenic purpura; neutropenia; eosinophilia.

Hepatic: Fatty liver; increases in liver enzymes.

Hypersensitivity: Urticaria; angioneurotic edema; anaphylaxis; anaphylactoid purpura; pericarditis; exacerbated systemic lupus erythematosus; polyarthralgia; serum sickness-like reactions (eg, fever, rash, arthralgia).

Miscellaneous: Pseudotumor cerebri (adults); bulging fontanels (infants). Nephrogenic diabetes insipidus has been reported with **demeclocycline**.

MACROLIDES

AZITHROMYCIN
Tablets: 250 mg (as dihydrate) and 600 mg (*Rx*) — Zithromax (Pfizer)
Powder for oral suspension: 100 mg and 200 mg/5 mL, 1 g/packet (*Rx*)
Powder for injection: 500 mg (*Rx*)

CLARITHROMYCIN
Tablets: 250 and 500 mg (*Rx*) — Biaxin (Abbott)
Tablets, extended release: 500 mg (*Rx*) — Biaxin XL (Abbott)
Granules for oral suspension: 125 and 250 mg/5 mL (*Rx*) — Biaxin (Abbott)

DIRITHROMYCIN
Tablets, enteric coated: 250 mg (*Rx*) — Dynabac (Sanofi)

ERYTHROMYCIN BASE
Tablets, enteric coated: 250, 333, and 500 mg (*Rx*) — E-Mycin (Knoll), Ery-Tab (Abbott), E-Base (Barr)
Tablets with polymer-coated particles: 333 and 500 mg (*Rx*) — PCE Dispertab (Abbott)
Tablets, film coated: 250 and 500 mg (*Rx*) — Erythromycin Filmtabs (Abbott)
Capsules, delayed release: 250 mg (*Rx*) — Various, Eryc (Warner Chilcott)

ERYTHROMYCIN ESTOLATE
Tablets: 500 mg (as estolate) — Ilosone (Lilly)
Capsules: 250 mg (as estolate) — Various, Ilosone Pulvules (Lilly)
Suspension: 235 and 250 mg (as estolate)/5 mL — Various, Ilosone (Lilly)

ERYTHROMYCIN LACTOBIONATE
Powder for injection: 500 mg and 1 g (as lactobionate) (*Rx*) — Various, Erythrocin (Abbott)

ERYTHROMYCIN GLUCEPTATE
Injection: 1 g (as gluceptate) (*Rx*) — Ilotycin Gluceptate (Lilly)

ERYTHROMYCIN ETHYLSUCCINATE
Tablets, chewable: 200 mg (as ethylsuccinate) (*Rx*) — EryPed (Abbott)
Tablets: 400 mg (as ethylsuccinate) (*Rx*) — Various, E.E.S. 400 (Abbott)
Suspension: 200 and 400 mg (as ethylsuccinate)/5 mL (*Rx*) — Various, E.E.S. 200 (Abbott), E.E.S. 400 (Abbott), EryPed 200 (Abbott), EryPed 400 (Abbott)
Drops, suspension: 100 mg (as ethylsuccinate)/2.5 mL (*Rx*) — EryPed Drops (Abbott)
Powder for oral suspension: 200 mg (as ethylsuccinate)/5 mL when reconstituted (*Rx*) — E.E.S. Granules (Abbott)

ERYTHROMYCIN STEARATE
Tablets, film coated: 250 and 500 mg (*Rx*) — Various, Erythrocin Stearate (Abbott)

TROLEANDOMYCIN
Capsules: 250 mg (*Rx*) — Tao (Pfizer)

Indications
For specific approved indications, refer to the Administration and Dosage sections.

Administration and Dosage
AZITHROMYCIN: Administer at least 1 hour before or 2 hours after a meal. Do not give with food. Azithromycin *tablets* can be taken with or without food.

Adults –

Mild-to-moderate acute bacterial exacerbations of chronic obstructive pulmonary disease, community-acquired pneumonia of mild severity, pharyngitis/tonsillitis (as second-line therapy), and uncomplicated skin and skin structure infections: 500 mg as a single dose on the first day followed by 250 mg once daily on days 2 through 5.

Genital ulcer disease caused by Haemophilus ducreyi (chancroid): Single 1 g dose.
Nongonococcal urethritis and cervicitis due to Chlamydia trachomatis: Single 1 g dose.
Gonococcal urethritis/cervitis caused by C. trachomatis: Single 2 g dose.
Uncomplicated gonococcal infections of the cervix, urethra, and rectum caused by Neisseria gonorrhoeae: Single 1 g dose (plus a single dose of 400 mg oral cefixime, 125 mg IM ceftriaxone, 500 mg oral ciprofloxacin, or 400 mg oral ofloxacin).

Gonococcal pharyngitis: Single 1 g dose (plus a single dose of 125 mg IM ceftriaxone, 500 mg ciprofloxacin, or 400 mg ofloxacin).

Chlamydial infections caused by C. trachomatis: Single 1 g dose.

Children –

Acute otitis media/community-acquired pneumonia: The recommended dose for oral suspension is 10 mg/kg as a single dose on the first day (not to exceed 500 mg/day, followed by 5 mg/kg on days 2 through 5 (not to exceed 250 mg/day). See the following table.

Pediatric Dosage Guidelines for Otitis Media (≥ 6 months of age)					
Dosing calculated on 10 mg/kg on day 1 dose, followed by 5 mg/kg on days 2 to 5					
Weight		Amount of 100 mg/5 mL suspension		Amount of 200 mg/5 mL suspension		Total mL per treatment course
kg	lbs	Day 1	Days 2 to 5	Day 1	Days 2 to 5	
10	22	5 mL	2.5 mL			15 mL
20	44			5 mL	2.5 mL	15 mL
30	66			7.5 mL	3.75 mL	22.5 mL
40	88			10 mL	5 mL	30 mL

Chlamydial infections caused by C. trachomatis (≥ 45 kg and < 8 years of age or ≥ 8 years of age): 1 g orally in single dose.

Pharyngitis/tonsillitis: The recommended dose for children with pharyngitis/tonsillitis is 12 mg/kg qd for 5 days (not to exceed 500 mg/day). See the following.

Pediatric Dosage Guidelines for Pharyngitis/Tonsillitis (≥ 2 years of age)			
Dosing calculated on 12 mg/kg once daily on days 1 through 5			
Weight		Amount of 200 mg/5 mL suspension	
kg	lbs	Days 1 to 5	Total mL per treatment course
8	18	2.5 mL	12.5 mL
17	37	5 mL	25 mL
25	55	7.5 mL	37.5 mL
33	73	10 mL	50 mL
40	88	12.5	62.5 mL

Parenteral – Infuse injections over a period of > 60 minutes. Do not administer azithromycin for injection as a bolus or IM injection.

Community-acquired pneumonia: 500 mg as a single daily dose IV for ≥ 2 days. Follow IV therapy by the oral route at a single daily dose of 500 mg to complete a 7- to 10-day course of therapy.

Pelvic inflammatory disease (PID): 500 mg as a single daily dose for 1 or 2 days. Follow IV therapy by the oral route at a single daily dose of 250 mg to complete a 7-day course of therapy. If anaerobic microorganisms are suspected of contributing to the infection, administer an antimicrobial agent with anaerobic activity in combination with azithromycin.

The infusate concentration and rate of infusion for azithromycin for injection should be either 1 mg/mL over 3 hours or 2 mg/mL over 1 hour.

CLARITHROMYCIN: Clarithromycin may be given with or without meals.

Helicobacter pylori –

Clarithromycin and Omeprazole Dosage Regimens for Active Duodenal Ulcer Associated with *H. pylori* Infection (28-Day Therapy)	
Days 1 to 14	Days 15 to 28
500 mg clarithromycin tablet 3 times daily plus omeprazole 2 × 20 mg every morning	Omeprazole 20 mg every morning

Clarithromycin and Ranitidine Bismuth Citrate Dosage Regimens for Active Duodenal Ulcer Associated with *H. pylori* Infection (28-Day Therapy)	
Days 1 to 14	Days 15 to 28
500 mg clarithromycin tablet 3 times daily plus ranitidine bismuth citrate 400 mg tablet twice daily	Ranitidine bismuth citrate 400 mg tablet twice daily

H. pylori eradication to reduce the risk of duodenal ulcer recurrence triple therapy:
Clarithromycin/Lansoprazole/Amoxicillin – 500 mg clarithromycin, 30 mg lansoprazole, and 1 g amoxicillin every 12 hours for 14 days.

Clarithromycin/Omeprazole/Amoxicillin – 500 mg clarithromycin, 20 mg omeprazole, and 1 g amoxicillin every 12 hours for 10 days. In patients with an ulcer present at the time of initiation of therapy, an additional 18 days of omeprazole 20 mg once daily is recommended for ulcer healing and symptom relief.

Adults –

Clarithromycin Dosage Guidelines				
	Tablets		Extended-release tablets	
Infection	Dosage (q 12 hr)	Duration (days)	Dosage (q 24 hr)	Duration (days)
Pharyngitis/Tonsillitis	250 mg	10	-	-
Acute maxillary sinusitis	500 mg	14	2 × 500 mg	14
Acute exacerbation of chronic bronchitis caused by:				
Haemophilus parainfluenzae	500 mg	7	2 × 500 mg	7
Streptococcus pneumoniae	250 mg	7 to 14	2 × 500 mg	7
Moraxella catarrhalis	250 mg	7 to 14	2 × 500 mg	7
Haemophilus influenzae	500 mg	7 to 14	2 × 500 mg	7
Community-acquired pneumonia caused by:				
S. pneumoniae	250 mg	7 to 14	2 × 500 mg	7
Mycoplasma pneumoniae	250 mg	7 to 14	2 × 500 mg	7
H. influenzae	250 mg	7	2 × 500 mg	7
H. parainfluenzae	-	-	2 × 500 mg	7
M. catarrhalis	-	-	2 × 500 mg	7
Chlamydia pneumoniae	250 mg	7 to 14	2 × 500 mg	7
Uncomplicated skin and skin structure infection	250 mg	7 to 14	-	-

Mycobacterial infections – Recommended as the primary agent for the treatment of disseminated *Mycobacterium avium* complex (MAC). Use in combination with other antimycobacterial drugs that have shown an in vitro activity against MAC. Continue therapy for life if clinical and mycobacterial improvements are observed.

Dosage for mycobacterial infection:
Adults – 500 mg twice daily.

Children – 7.5 mg/kg twice daily up to 500 mg twice daily. Refer to the Pediatric Dosing table.

Children – Usual recommended daily dosage is 15 mg/kg/day divided every 12 hours for 10 days.

Pediatric Dosage Guidelines (based on body weight)			
Dosing calculated on 7.5 mg/kg q 12 h			
Weight	Dose (q 12 h)	125 mg/5 mL (q 12 h)	250 mg/5 mL (q 12 h)
kg | lb			
9 | 20	62.5 mg	2.5 mL	1.25 mL
17 | 37	125 mg	5 mL	2.5 mL
25 | 55	187.5 mg	7.5 mL	3.75 mL
33 | 73	250 mg	10 mL	5 mL

Renal/Hepatic function impairment – In the presence of severe renal impairment (Ccr < 30 mL/min) with or without co-existing hepatic impairment, halved doses or prolongation of dosing intervals may be needed.

DIRITHROMYCIN: Administer with food or within 1 hour of eating. Do not cut, crush, or chew the tablets.

Recommended Dosage Schedule for Dirithromycin (≥ 12 years of age)			
Infection (mild-to-moderate severity)	Dose	Frequency	Duration (days)
Acute bacterial exacerbations of chronic bronchitis caused by *H. influenzae*, *M. catarrhalis*, or *S. pneumoniae*.	500 mg	once a day	5 to 7
Secondary bacterial infection of acute bronchitis caused by *M. catarrhalis* or *S. pneumoniae*.	500 mg	once a day	7
Community-acquired pnemonia caused by *Legionella pneumophila*, *M. pneumoniae*, or *S. pneumoniae*.	500 mg	once a day	14
Pharyngitis/Tonsillitis caused by *Streptococcus pyogenes*.	500 mg	once a day	10
Uncomplicated skin and skin structure infections caused by *Staphylococcus aureus* (methicillin-susceptible) or *S. pyogenes*.	500 mg	once a day	5 to 7

ERYTHROMYCIN, IV:

Erythromycin IV – Erythromycin IV is indicated when oral use is impossible, or when severity of the infection requires immediate high serum levels. Replace IV therapy with oral as soon as possible.

Continuous infusion: Continuous infusion is preferable, but intermittent infusion in 20- to 60-minute periods at intervals of ≤ 6 hours is also effective. Because of irritative properties of erythromycin, IV push is unacceptable.

Severe infections – 15 to 20 mg/kg/day. Up to 4 g/day in very severe infections.

ERYTHROMYCIN, ORAL: Dosages and product strengths are expressed as erythromycin base equivalents. Because of differences in absorption and biotransformation, varying quantities of each salt form are required to produce the same free erythromycin serum levels.

Optimal serum levels of erythromycin are reached when erythromycin base or stearate is taken in the fasting state or immediately before meals. Erythromycin ethylsuccinate, estolate, and enteric-coated erythromycin may be administered without regard to meals.

Usual dosage –

Adults: 250 mg (or 400 mg ethylsuccinate) every 6 hours, or 500 mg every 12 hours, or 333 mg every 8 hours. May increase up to ≥ 4 g/day, according to severity of infection. If twice-daily dosage is desired, the recommended dose is 500 mg every 12 hours. Twice-daily dosing is not recommended when doses > 1 g daily are administered.

Children: 30 to 50 mg/kg/day in divided doses.

Erythromycin Uses and Dosages	
Indication (Organism)	Dosage (Stated as erythromycin base)
Labeled uses:	
Upper respiratory tract infections of mild-to-moderate severity	
S. pyogenes (group A beta-hemolytic streptococcus)	250 to 500 mg 4 times/day or 20 to 50 mg/kg/day for children (not to exceed the adult dose) in divided doses for 10 days.
S. pneumoniae	250 to 500 mg every 6 hours.
H. influenzae (used concomitantly with a sulfonamide)	Erythromycin ethylsuccinate: 50 mg/kg/day for children (not to exceed 6 g/day). Sulfisoxazole: 150 mg/kg/day. Combination given for 10 days.
Lower respiratory tract infections of mild to moderate severity	
S. pyogenes (group A beta-hemolytic streptococcus)	250 to 500 mg 4 times/day or 20 to 50 mg/kg/day for children (not to exceed the adult dose) in divided doses for 10 days.
S. pneumoniae	250 to 500 mg every 6 hours.

Erythromycin Uses and Dosages	
Indication (Organism)	Dosage (Stated as erythromycin base)
Respiratory tract infections M. pneumoniae (Eaton agent, PPLO)	500 mg every 6 hours for 5 to 10 days. Treat severe infections for up to 3 weeks.
Skin and skin structure infections of mild to moderate severity S. pyogenes	250 to 500 mg 4 times/day or 20 to 50 mg/kg/day for children (not to exceed the adult dose) in divided doses for 10 days.
S. aureus (resistant organisms may emerge)	250 mg every 6 hours or 500 mg every 12 hours, maximum 4 g/day.
Pertussis (whooping cough) Bordetella pertussis: Effective in eliminating the organism from the nasopharynx of infected patients. May be helpful in prophylaxis of pertussis in exposed individuals.	40 to 50 mg/kg/day for children (not to exceed the adult dose) in divided doses for 5 to 14 days, or 500 mg 4 times/day for 10 days.
Diphtheria Corynebacterium diphtheriae: Adjunct to antitoxin to prevent establishment of carriers and to eradicate organism in carriers.	500 mg every 6 hours for 10 days.
Erythrasma Corynebacterium minutissiumum	250 mg 3 times daily for 21 days.
Intestinal amebiasis Entamoeba histolyticia: Oral erythromycin only.	*Adults:* 250 mg 4 times daily for 10 to 14 days. *Children:* 30 to 50 mg/kg/day in divided doses for 10 to 14 days.
Pelvic inflammatory disease (PID), acute N. gonorrhoeae: Erythromycin lactobionate IV followed by oral erythromycin.[1]	500 mg IV every 6 hours for 3 days, then 250 mg orally every 6 hours for 7 days.
Conjunctivitis of the newborn, pneumonia of infancy, urogenital infections during pregnancy	50 mg/kg/day for children (not to exceed the adult dose) in 4 divided doses for 10 to ≥ 14 days (conjunctivitis) or ≥ 21 days (pneumonia)
C. trachomatis	500 mg 4 times daily for 7 days or 250 mg 4 times daily on an empty stomach for ≥ 14 days (urogenital infections).
Urethral, endocervical, or rectal infections, uncomplicated C. trachomatis[1]	500 mg ≥ 4 times daily for 7 days or 250 mg 4 times daily for 14 days if patient cannot tolerate high-dose erythromycin.[2]
Nongonococcal urethritis Ureaplasma urealyticum[1]	500 mg 4 times daily for at least 7 days or 250 mg orally 4 times daily for 14 days if patient cannot tolerate high-dose erythromycin.[2]
Primary syphilis Treponema pallidum: Oral erythromycin only[1]	20 to 40 g in divided doses over 10 to 15 days.
Legionnaire's disease Legionella pneumophila: No controlled clinical efficacy studies have been conducted, but data suggest effectiveness	1 to 4 g daily in divided doses for 10 to 14 days.
Rheumatic fever S. pyogenes (group A beta-hemolytic streptococci): Prevention of initial or recurrent attacks.[1]	250 mg 2 times daily.
Bacterial endocarditis (in penicillin-allergic patients with valvular heart disease who are to undergo dental procedures or surgical procedures of the upper respiratory tract).	

| Erythromycin Uses and Dosages ||
Indication (Organism)	Dosage (Stated as erythromycin base)
Alpha-hemolytic streptococcus (viridans)[1]	Adults: 1 g 1 to 2 hours prior to procedure, then 500 mg 6 hours after initial dose.[3] Children: 20 mg/kg 2 hours prior to procedure, then 10 mg/kg 6 hours after initial dose.[3]
Listeria monocytogenes	Adults: 250 mg every 6 hours or 500 mg every 12 hours, maximum 4 g/day.
Unlabeled uses:	
Campylobacter jejuni: Has been successful in severe or prolonged diarrhea associated with *Campylobacter enteritis* or enterocolitis.[2]	500 mg 4 times a day for 7 days.
Lymphogranuloma venereum: Genital, inguinal, or anorectal.[2]	500 mg 4 times a day for 21 days.
Haemophilus ducreyi (chancroid): Treat until ulcers or lymph nodes are healed.[2]	500 mg 4 times a day for 7 days.
T. pallidum: Early syphilis (primary or secondary)	500 mg 4 times a day for 14 days.
Prior to elective colorectal surgery, to reduce wound complications	Combination of erythromycin base and neomycin is a popular preoperative preparation.
Clostridium tetani: Tetanus[1]	500 mg every 6 hours for 10 days.
Granuloma inguinale *Calymmatobacterium granulomatis*[2,4]	500 mg orally 4 times daily for ≥ 21 days.

[1] Use as alternative drug in penicillin or tetracycline hypersensitivity or when penicillin or tetracycline are contraindicated or not tolerated.
[2] CDC 1998 Guidelines for Sexually Transmitted Diseases Treatment. *MMWR.* 1998;47:1-117.
[3] American Heart Association statement. *JAMA.* 1990;264:2919-2922.
[4] Use as alternate therapy to trimethoprim-sulfamethoxazole or doxycycline.

ERYTHROMYCIN ETHYLSUCCINATE: Expressed in base equivalents, 400 mg erythromycin ethylsuccinate produces the same free erythromycin serum levels as 250 mg of erythromycin base, stearate, or estolate.

TROLEANDOMYCIN: Continue therapy for 10 days when used for streptococcal infection.

Adults – 250 to 500 mg 4 times a day.

Children – 125 to 250 mg (6.6 to 11 mg/kg) every 6 hours.

Actions

Pharmacology: Macrolide antibiotics reversibly bind to the P site of the 50S ribosomal subunit of susceptible organisms and inhibit RNA-dependent protein synthesis by stimulating the dissociation of peptidyl t-RNA from ribosomes. They may be bacteriostatic or bactericidal, depending on such factors as drug concentration.

Macrolides are weak bases; their activity increases in alkaline pH. Macrolides enter pleural fluid, ascitic fluid, middle-ear exudates, and sputum. When meninges are inflamed, macrolides may enter the CSF. They are used for respiratory, genital, GI tract, and skin and soft tissue infections, especially when beta-lactam antibiotics or tetracyclines are contraindicated.

Despite differing structures, macrolides have similar antibacterial spectrum, mechanisms of action and resistance, but relatively different pharmacokinetics (see table).

Pharmacokinetics:

Various Pharmacokinetic Parameters of Macrolides								
Macrolide	Route of administration	Protein binding (%)	Bioavailability (%)	Effect of food	C_{max}^* (mcg/mL)	T_{max}^* (hr)	Half-life (hr)	Metabolism	Elimination
Azithromycin	Oral IV	51 (0.02 mcg/L) 7 (2 mcg/L)	≈ 40	Food increases absorption, C_{max} by 23% and suspension by 56%; take on empty stomach.	0.5 1.14^3 3.63^4	2.2	68^1	Some hepatic but mainly excreted unchanged	6% excreted unchanged in urine; primarily excreted unchanged in bile
Clarithromycin	Oral	40-70	≈ 50	Food delays onset of absorption and formation of metabolite; does not affect extent of bioavailability. Take without regard to meals.	1-3	2-3	3-7	Metabolized to active metabolite (14-OH clarithromycin)	Primarily renal; rate approximates normal GFR
Dirithromycin	Oral	$15-30^2$	≈ 10	Take with food or within an hour of eating.	$0.3 - 0.4^2$	$3.9 - 4.1^2$	2-36	Nonenzymatic conversion to erythromycylamine	81%-97% fecal/hepatic²
Erythromycin	Oral IV	70-80 (96 estolate)	> 35	Base or stearate: Take on an empty stomach. Estolate, ethylsuccinate, delayed release base: Take without regard to meals.	0.3-2	1.6	1.6	Hepatic; demethylation	< 5% (oral) and 12% to 15% (IV) excreted unchanged in urine; significant quantity excreted in bile
Troleandomycin	Oral				2	2			20% excreted in urine; significant quantity excreted in bile

* C_{max} = Maximum concentration; T_{max} = Time to reach maximum concentration.
[1] Average terminal half-life.
[2] Value listed for erythromycylamine, the active moiety.
[3] At a concentration of 1 mg/mL.
[4] At a concentration of 2 mg/mL.

Microbiology:

	Organisms (✔ = generally susceptible)	Azithromycin	Clarithromycin	Dirithromycin	Erythromycin	Troleandomycin[1]
Gram-positive aerobes	Staphylococcus aureus	✔	✔	✔	✔	
	Streptococcus pyogenes	✔	✔	✔	✔	✔
	Streptococcus pneumoniae	✔	✔	✔	✔	✔
	Streptococcus agalactiae	✔	✔	✔	✔	
	Streptococcus sp.	✔	✔	✔		
	Streptococcus viridans	✔	✔	✔	✔	
	Listeria monocytogenes			✔	✔	
	Corynebacterium diphtheriae				✔	
	Corynebacterium minutissimum				✔	

Organisms Generally Susceptible to Macrolides In Vitro

Organisms Generally Susceptible to Macrolides In Vitro					
Organisms (🖛 = generally susceptible)	Azithromycin	Clarithromycin	Dirithromycin	Erythromycin	Troleandomycin[1]
Gram-negative aerobes					
Haemophilus influenzae	🖛	🖛	🖛	†[2]	
Haemophilus ducreyi	🖛				
Moraxella catarrhalis	🖛	🖛	🖛	🖛	
Bordetella pertussis	🖛	🖛	🖛	🖛	
Legionella pneumophila	🖛	🖛	🖛	🖛	
Neisseria gonorrhoeae	🖛	🖛		🖛	
Pasteurella multocida		🖛			
Anaerobes					
Prevotella (formerly Bacteroides) bivius	🖛				
Prevotella (formerly Bacteroides) melaninogenicus		🖛			
Clostridium perfringens		🖛			
Propionibacterium acnes		🖛	🖛		
Peptococcus niger		🖛			
Peptostreptococcus sp.	🖛				
Other					
Borrelia burgdorferi	🖛				
Chlamydia trachomatis	🖛	🖛		🖛	
Mycobacterium kansasii		🖛			
Mycoplasma pneumoniae	🖛	🖛	🖛	🖛	
Treponema pallidum	🖛			🖛	
Ureaplasma urealyticum	🖛			🖛	
Entamoeba histolytica				🖛	
Chlamydia pneumoniae (TWAR strain)	🖛	🖛			
Mycoplasma hominis	🖛				
Mycobacterium avium		🖛			
Mycobacterium intracellulare		🖛			
Helicobacter pylori		🖛			
Clostridium tetani				🖛	

[1] Data is limited for troleandomycin.
[2] Many strains resistant to erythromycin alone; may be susceptible to erythromycin plus a sulfonamide.

The in vitro spectrum of erythromycin covers primarily gram-positive microorganisms and gram-negative cocci.

Azithromycin is less active than **erythromycin** against most *Staphylococcus* and *Streptococcus* sp, but it is more potent against other organisms, including many gram-negative bacteria considered resistant to erythromycin. Azithromycin may expand the therapeutic range traditionally assigned to macrolides.

Clarithromycin exhibits the same spectrum of in vitro activity as erythromycin, but appears to have significantly increased potency against those organisms.

Troleandomycin, an acetylated ester of oleandomycin, is less active than erythromycin and offers no advantage. It also can cause hepatotoxicity.

Contraindications

Hypersensitivity to any of the macrolide antibiotics; patients receiving astemizole, cisapride, or pimozide; known, suspected, or potential bacteremias (**dirithromycin**); pre-existing liver disease (**erythromycin estolate**).

Warnings

Pseudomembranous colitis: Pseudomembranous colitis has occurred with nearly all antibacterial agents and may range in severity from mild to life-threatening. Consider this diagnosis in patients who present with diarrhea subsequent to the administration of antibacterial agents.

Cardiac effects: Ventricular arrhythmias in individuals with prolonged QT intervals have occurred with macrolide products.

Acute porphyria: Do not use **clarithromycin** in combination with ranitidine bismuth citrate in patients with a history of acute porphyria.

Azithromycin:

Pneumonia – Do not use oral **azithromycin** in patients with pneumonia who are judged to be inappropriate for oral therapy because of moderate-to-severe illness or risk factors such as any of the following: Nosocomially acquired infections; known or suspected bacteremia; conditions requiring hospitalization; cystic fibrosis; significant underlying health problems that may compromise patients' ability to respond to their illness (including immunodeficiency or functional asplenia); elderly or debilitated patients.

Hypersensitivity – Rare serious allergic reactions, including angioedema, anaphylaxis, and dermatologic reactions including Stevens-Johnson syndrome and toxic epidermal necrolysis have occurred in patients on **azithromycin** therapy.

Dirithromycin:

Bacteremias – Dirithromycin should not be used in patients with known, suspected or potential bacteremias as serum levels are inadequate to provide antibacterial coverage of the blood stream.

Erythromycin:

Hepatotoxicity – Erythromycin administration has been associated with the infrequent occurrence of cholestatic hepatitis. This effect is most common with erythromycin estolate; however, it has also occurred with other erythromycin salts.

Although initial symptoms have developed after a few days of treatment, they generally have followed 1 or 2 weeks of continuous therapy. Symptoms reappear promptly, usually within 48 hours after the drug is readministered to sensitive patients. The syndrome seems to result from a form of sensitization, occurs chiefly in adults, and is reversible when medication is discontinued.

Myasthenia gravis – **Erythromycin** may aggravate the weakness of patients with myasthenia gravis.

Troleandomycin:

Hepatic effects – Troleandomycin has been associated with allergic cholestatic hepatitis. Some patients receiving troleandomycin for > 2 weeks or in repeated courses have developed jaundice accompanied by right upper quadrant pain, fever, nausea, vomiting, eosinophilia, and leukocytosis. These have reversed on drug discontinuance. Readministration reproduces hepatotoxicity, often within 24 to 48 hours.

Renal/Hepatic function impairment:

Clarithromycin – In the presence of severe renal impairment (creatinine < 30 mL/min) with or without coexisting hepatic impairment, decreased dosage or prolonged dosing intervals may be appropriate.

Azithromycin and troleandomycin – Exercise caution when administering to patients with impaired renal or hepatic function.

Erythromycin – Erythromycin is principally excreted by the liver. Exercise caution in administering to patients with impaired hepatic function.

Dirithromycin – No dosage adjustment should be necessary in patients with impaired renal function, including dialysis patients. In patients with mild hepatic impairment, mean peak serum concentration, AUC and volume of distribution increased somewhat with multiple-dose administration; however, based on the magnitude of these changes, no dosage adjustment should be necessary in patients with mildly impaired hepatic function.

Elderly:

Clarithromycin – Studies show age-related decreases in renal function. Consider dosage adjustment in elderly patients with severe renal impairment.

Azithromycin – Dosage adjustment does not appear to be necessary for older patients with normal renal and hepatic function.

Dirithromycin – No dosage adjustment should be necessary in elderly patients.

Pregnancy: Category B (azithromycin, erythromycin); *Category* C (clarithromycin, dirithromycin, troleandomycin).

Lactation:

Clarithromycin, dirithromycin, and azithromycin – It is not known whether these agents are excreted in breast milk.

Erythromycin – Erythromycin is excreted in breast milk, and may concentrate (observed milk:plasma ratio of 0.5 to 3). Erythromycin is considered compatible with breastfeeding by the American Academy of Pediatrics.

Children:

Dirithromycin – Safety and efficacy in children < 12 years of age have not been established.

Clarithromycin – Safety and efficacy in children < 6 months of age have not been established.

Azithromycin – Safety and efficacy in children < 6 months of age (acute otitis media, community-acquired pneumonia) or < 2 years of age (pharyngitis/tonsillitis) have not been established.

IV use: Safety and efficacy of azithromycin for IV injection in children or adolescents < 16 years of age have not been established.

Precautions

Azithromycin:

Local IV site reactions – Local IV site reactions have been reported with the IV administration of azithromycin. The incidence and severity of these reactions were the same when 500 mg was given over 1 hour (2 mg/mL as 250 mL infusion) or over 3 hours (1 mg/mL as 500 mL infusion). All volunteers who received infusate concentrations > 2 mg/mL experienced local IV site reactions; therefore, avoid higher concentrations.

Drug Interactions

Clarithromycin: Drugs that may be affected by clarithromycin include anticoagulants, astemizole, benzodiazepines, buspirone, carbamazepine, cisapride, cyclosporine, digoxin, disopyramide, ergot alkaloids, HMG-CoA reductase inhibitors, omeprazole, ranitidine bismuth citrate, tacrolimus, theophylline, and zidovudine. Also consider all drug interactions with erythromycin. Drugs that may affect clarithromycin include fluconazole, ranitidine bismuth citrate, pimozide, rifamycins, and omeprazole.

Azithromycin: Drugs that may interact with azithromycin include antacids, cyclosporine, HMG-CoA reductase inhibitors, pimozide, tacrolimus, theophyllines, and warfarin. Also consider all drug interactions with erythromycin.

Dirithromycin: Drugs that may be affected by dirithromycin include antacids. Drugs that may affect dirithromycin include antacids, pimozide, and H_2 antagonists. Also consider all drug interactions with erythromycin.

Erythromycin: Drugs that may be affected by erythromycin include alfentanil, anticoagulants, astemizole, benzodiazepines, buspirone, carbamazepine, cisapride, cyclosporine, digoxin, disopyramide, ergot alkaloids, felodipine, fluoroquinolones, HMG-CoA reductase inhibitors, lincosamides, methylprednisolone, penicillins, and theophyllines. Drugs that may affect erythromycin include antacids, pimozide, rifamycins, and theophyllines.

Troleandomycin: Drugs that may be affected by troleandomycin include astemizole, benzodiazepines, buspirone, carbamazepine, cisapride, oral contraceptives, cyclosporine, ergot alkaloids, methylprednisolone, tacrolimus, and theophyllines. Drugs that may affect troleandomycin include rifamycins.

Drug/Food interactions:

Clarithromycin – Following tablet administration, food delays both the onset of clarithromycin absorption and the formulation of 14 OH clarithromycin, but does not affect bioavailability. Following the suspension, food decreases mean peak clarithromycin levels and extent of absorption.

Azithromycin – When azithromycin suspension was administered with food, the rate of absorption (C_{max}) was increased by 56% while the extent of absorption (AUC) was unchanged. Take 1 hour before or 2 hours after a meal. Do not take with food.

Dirithromycin – Dirithromycin should be administered with food or within an hour of eating. After administration of two 250 mg tablets 1 or 4 hours before food and immediately after a standard breakfast indicated an increase in absorption of erythromycylamine when dirithromycin was administered after food, while a significant decrease in C_{max} (33%) and AUC (31%) occurred when administered 1 hour before food.

Erythromycin – Antimicrobial effectiveness of erythromycin stearate and certain formulations of erythromycin base may be reduced. Take at least 2 hours before or after a meal. Erythromycin estolate and ethylsuccinate and the base in a delayed release form may be administered without regard to meals.

Adverse Reactions

Clarithromycin – Adverse reactions occurring in ≥ 3% of patients include diarrhea, nausea, abdominal pain, rash, increased BUN, and abnormal taste.

Azithromycin – Adverse reactions occurring in ≥ 3% of patients include diarrhea/loose stools, vomiting, nausea, abdominal pain, increased ALT and AST, increased serum creatinine, and increased bilirubin.

Dirithromycin – Adverse reactions occurring in ≥ 3% of patients include abdominal pain/discomfort, diarrhea/loose stools, nausea, vomiting, increased platelet count, and headache.

Erythromycin – Adverse reactions occurring in ≥ 3% of patients include abdominal pain/discomfort, diarrhea/loose stools, nausea, increased platelet count, and headache.

Hepatic – Hepatotoxicity is most commonly associated with erythromycin estolate.

Local – Venous irritation and phlebitis have occurred with parenteral administration, but the risk of such reactions may be reduced if the infusion is given slowly, in dilute solution, by continuous IV infusion or intermittent infusion over 20 to 60 minutes.

VANCOMYCIN

Pulvules: 125 mg and 250 mg (Rx)	*Vancocin* (Lilly)
Powder for oral solution: 1 and 10 g (Rx)	*Vancomycin HCl* (ESI Lederle), *Vancocin* (Lilly)
Powder for injection: 500 mg, 1, 5, and 10 g (Rx)	Various, *Vancocin* (Lilly), *Vancoled* (Lederle)

Indications

Parenteral: Serious or severe infections not treatable with other antimicrobials, including the penicillins and cephalosporins.

Severe staphylococcal infections – Severe staphylococcal infections (including methicillin-resistant staphylococci) in patients who cannot receive or who have failed to respond to penicillins and cephalosporins, or who have infections with resistant staphylococci. Infections may include endocarditis, bone infections, lower respiratory tract infections, septicemia, and skin and skin structure infections.

Endocarditis –

Staphylococcal: Vancomycin is effective alone.

Streptococcal: Vancomycin is effective alone or in combination with an aminoglycoside for endocarditis caused by *S. viridans* or *S. bovis*. It is only effective in combination with an aminoglycoside for endocarditis caused by enterococci (eg, *S. faecalis*).

Diphtheroid: Vancomycin is effective for diphtheroid endocarditis, and has been used successfully with rifampin, an aminoglycoside, or both in early onset prosthetic valve endocarditis caused by *Staphylococcus epidermidis* or diphtheroids.

Prophylactic: Although no controlled clinical efficacy studies have been conducted, IV vancomycin has been suggested for prophylaxis against bacterial endocarditis in penicillin-allergic patients who have congenital heart disease or rheumatic or other acquired or valvular heart disease when these patients undergo dental procedures or surgical procedures of the upper respiratory tract.

Pseudomembranous colitis/staphylococcal enterocolitis caused by Clostridium difficile – The parenteral form may be administered orally; parenteral use alone is unproven. The oral use of parenteral vancomycin is not effective for other infections.

Oral: Staphylococcal enterocolitis and antibiotic-associated pseudomembranous colitis produced by *C. difficile*. The parenteral product may also be given orally for these infections. Oral vancomycin is not effective for other types of infection.

Administration and Dosage

Complete full course of therapy; do not discontinue therapy without notifying physician.

Oral:

Adults – 500 mg to 2 g/day given in 3 or 4 divided doses for 7 to 10 days.

Alternatively, dosages of 125 mg 3 or 4 times daily for *C. difficile* colitis may be as effective as the 500 mg dose regimen.

Children – 40 mg/kg/day in 3 or 4 divided doses for 7 to 10 days. Do not exceed 2 g/day.

Neonates – 10 mg/kg/day in divided doses.

Parenteral: Administer each dose over at least 60 minutes. Intermittent infusion is the preferred administration method.

Adults – 500 mg IV every 6 hours or 1 g every 12 hours.

Children – 10 mg/kg/dose given every 6 hours.

Infants and neonates – Initial dose of 15 mg/kg, followed by 10 mg/kg every 12 hours for neonates in the first week of life and every 8 hours thereafter up to the age of 1 month.

Prevention of bacterial endocarditis:

GU/GI procedures (high-risk, penicillin-allergic patients) – 1 g IV over 1 to 2 hours (children, 20 mg/kg) plus gentamicin 1.5 mg/kg IV or IM for both adult (not to exceed 120 mg) and children. Complete injection or infusion within 30 minutes of starting procedure.

(Moderate-risk, penicillin-allergic patients) – 1 g IV over 1 to 2 hours (children 20 mg/kg). Complete infusion within 30 minutes of starting procedure.

Renal function impairment: Adjust dosage; check serum levels regularly. In premature infants and the elderly, dosage reduction may be necessary caused by decreasing renal function.

For most patients, if Ccr can be measured or estimated accurately, the dosage may be calculated by using the following table.

Vancomycin Dosage in Impaired Renal Function	
Ccr (mL/min)	Dose (mg/24 hr)
100	1545
90	1390
80	1235
70	1080
60	925
50	770
40	620
30	465
20	310
10	155

The table is not valid for functionally anephric patients on dialysis. For such patients, give a loading dose of 15 mg/kg to achieve therapeutic serum levels promptly and a maintenance dose of 1.9 mg/kg/24 hr. In patients with marked renal impairment, it may be more convenient to give maintenance doses of 250 to 1000 mg once every several days rather than administering the drug on a daily basis. In anuria a dose of 1000 mg every 7 to 10 days has been recommended.

Actions
Pharmacology: Vancomycin is a tricyclic glycopeptide antibiotic that inhibits cell-wall biosynthesis. It also alters bacterial-cell-membrane permeability and RNA synthesis.

Pharmacokinetics:
    Absorption/Distribution – Systemic absorption of oral vancomycin is generally poor.
    Metabolism/Excretion – In the first 24 hours, ≈ 75% of a dose is excreted in urine by glomerular filtration. Elimination half-life is 4 to 6 hours in adults and 2 to 3 hours in children. About 60% of an intraperitoneal dose administered during peritoneal dialysis is absorbed systemically in 6 hours. Accumulation occurs in renal failure. Serum half-life in anephric patients is ≈ 7.5 days. Vancomycin is not significantly removed by hemodialysis or continuous ambulatory peritoneal dialysis, although there have been reports of increased clearance with hemoperfusion and hemofiltration.

Contraindications
Hypersensitivity to vancomycin.

Warnings
Ototoxicity: Ototoxicity has occurred in patients receiving vancomycin. It may be transient or permanent. It has occurred mostly in patients who have been given excessive doses, who have an underlying hearing loss, or who are receiving concomitant therapy with another ototoxic agent.

Hypotension: Rapid bolus administration may be associated with exaggerated hypotension, including shock, and rarely, cardiac arrest. To avoid hypotension, administer in a dilute solution over ≥ 60 minutes. Stopping the infusion usually results in prompt cessation of these reactions. Frequently monitor blood pressure and heart rate.

Pseudomembranous colitis: In rare instances, pseudomembranous colitis has occurred because of C. *difficile* developing in patients who received IV vancomycin.

Reversible neutropenia: Reversible neutropenia has occurred in patients receiving vancomycin.

Tissue irritation: Vancomycin is irritating to tissue and must be given by a secure IV route of administration. Pain, tenderness, and necrosis occur with IM injection or inadvertent extravasation.

Reports have revealed that administration of sterile vancomycin by the intraperitoneal route during continuous ambulatory peritoneal dialysis (CAPD) has resulted in a syndrome of chemical peritonitis. This syndrome has ranged from a cloudy dialysate alone to a cloudy dialysate accompanied by variable degrees of abdominal pain and fever. This syndrome appears to be short-lived after discontinuation of intraperitoneal vancomycin.

Nephrotoxicity: The risk of toxicity may be appreciably increased by high serum concentrations or prolonged therapy. Factors that may increase the risk of nephrotoxicity include use in elderly and neonatal patients and concomitant use with other nephrotoxic drugs.

Renal function impairment: Because of its nephrotoxicity, use carefully in renal insufficiency.

Pregnancy: Category C; Category B (pulvules only).

Lactation: Vancomycin is excreted in breast milk.

Children: In premature and full-term neonates it may be appropriate to confirm desired vancomycin serum concentrations.

Precautions

Monitoring: Perform auditory function serial tests and monitor serum levels. When monitoring vancomycin serum levels, draw a peak concentration 1.5 to 2.5 hours after the completion of a 1-hour infusion and a trough concentration within 1 hour of the next scheduled dose. Peak levels are generally expected to be in the 30 to 40 mg/mL range and trough levels in the 10 to 15 mg/mL range.

Systemic absorption: Clinically significant serum concentrations may occur in some patients who have taken multiple oral doses for active *C. difficile*-induced pseudomembranous colitis or who have inflammatory disorders of the intestinal mucosa; the risk is greater with the presence of renal impairment.

Red Man (or Redneck) syndrome: Red Man (or Redneck) syndrome is usually stimulated by a too-rapid IV infusion (dose given over a few minutes), but it has been reported rarely when given as recommended and following oral or intraperitoneal administration. The onset may occur anytime within a few minutes of starting an IV infusion to a short time after infusion completion. The rash generally resolves several hours after termination of administration.

Drug Interactions

Drugs that may interact with vancomycin include aminoglycosides, anesthetics, neurotoxic/nephrotoxic agents, and nondepolarizing muscle relaxants.

Adverse Reactions

Adverse reactions may include renal impairment; hearing loss; neutropenia; vertigo; dizziness; anaphylaxis; drug fever; nausea; chills; eosinophilia; rashes; hypotension; wheezing; dyspnea; urticaria; inflammation at injection site; Red Man (or Redneck) syndrome; chemical peritonitis has been reported following intraperitoneal administration of vancomycin.

LINEZOLID

Tablets: 400[1] and 600 mg[2] (Rx)
Powder for reconstitution:[3] 100 mg/5 mL (Rx)
Injection:[4] 2 mg/mL (Rx)

Zyvox (Pharmacia)

[1] Sodium content is 1.95 mg/400 mg tablet (0.1 mEq/tablet).
[2] Sodium content is 2.92 mg/600 mg tablet (0.1 mEq/tablet).
[3] Sodium content is 8.52 mg/5 mL (0.4 mEq/5 mL).
[4] Sodium content 0.38 mg/mL (5 mEq/300 mL bag, 3.3 mEq/200 mL bag, 1.7 mEq/100 mL bag).

Indications

Vancomycin-resistant Enterococcus faecium infections: For the treatment of vancomycin-resistant *E. faecium* infections including cases with concurrent bacteremia.

Nosocomial pneumonia: For the treatment of nosocomial pneumonia caused by *Staphylococcus aureus* (methicillin-susceptible and -resistant strains), or *Streptococcus pneumoniae* (penicillin-susceptible strains only). Combination therapy may be indicated if the documented or presumptive pathogens include gram-negative organisms.

Complicated skin and skin structure infections: For the treatment of complicated skin and skin structure infections caused by *S. aureus* (methicillin-susceptible and -resistant strains), *Streptococcus pyogenes*, or *Streptococcus agalactiae*. It has not been studied in the treatment of diabetic foot and decubitus ulcers. Combination therapy may be clinically indicated if the documented or presumptive pathogens include gram-negative organisms.

Uncomplicated skin and skin structure infections: For the treatment of uncomplicated skin and skin structure infections caused by *S. aureus* (methicillin-susceptible strains only) or *S. pyogenes.*

Community-acquired pneumonia: For the treatment of community-acquired pneumonia caused by *S. pneumoniae* (penicillin-susceptible strains only), including cases with concurrent bacteremia, or *S. aureus* (methicillin-susceptible strains only).

Because of concerns about inappropriate use of antibiotics leading to increase in resistant organisms, carefully consider alternatives before initiating treatment with linezolid in the outpatient setting.

Administration and Dosage

Administer without regard to meals.

Linezolid Dosage Guidelines		
Infection[1]	Dosage and route of administration	Recommended duration of treatment (consecutive days)
Vancomycin-resistant *E. faecium* infections, including concurrent bacteremia	600 mg IV or oral[2] q12hr	14 to 28
Nosocomial pneumonia Complicated skin and skin structure infections Community-acquired pneumonia, including concurrent bacteremia	600 mg IV or oral[2] q12hr	10 to 14
Uncomplicated skin and skin structure infections	400 mg oral[2] q12hr	10 to 14

[1] Because of the designated pathogens (see Indications).
[2] Oral dosing using either linezolid tablets or oral suspension.

Treat patients with methicillin-resistant *S. aureus* (MRSA) infection with linezolid 600 mg/12 hours.

No dose adjustment is necessary when switching from IV to oral administration. Patients who are started on IV therapy may be switched to tablets or oral suspension when clinically indicated.

IV administration: Administer over a period of 30 to 120 minutes. Do not use IV infusion bag in series connections. Do not introduce additives into this solution. Do not administer concomitantly with another drug; administer each drug separately.

Compatible IV solutions: 5% Dextrose Injection, 0.9% NaCl Injection; Lactated Ringer's Injection.

Admixture incompatibilities: Physical incompatibilities resulted when linezolid IV injection was combined with the following drugs during simulated Y-site administration: Amphotericin B, chlorpromazine HCl, diazepam, pentamidine isothionate, erythromycin lactobionate, phenytoin sodium, and trimethoprim-sulfamethoxazole. Additionally, chemical incompatibility resulted when linezolid IV injection was combined with ceftriaxone sodium.

If the same IV line is used for sequential infusion of several drugs, the line should be flushed before and after infusion of IV injection with an infusion solution compatible with linezolid IV injection and with any other drug(s) administered via this common line.

Actions

Pharmacology: Linezolid binds to a site on the bacterial 23S ribosomal RNA of the 50S subunit and prevents the formation of a functional 70S initiation complex, which is an essential component of the bacterial translation process. The results of time-kill studies have shown linezolid to be bacteriostatic against *Enterococci* and *Staphylococci*. For *Streptococci*, linezolid was found to be bactericidal for the majority of strains.

Pharmacokinetics:

Absorption – Linezolid is rapidly and extensively absorbed after oral dosing with an absolute bioavailability of ≈ 100%.

Distribution – The plasma protein binding of linezolid is ≈ 31% and is concentration-independent. The volume of distribution of linezolid at steady-state averaged 40 to 50 L in healthy adult volunteers.

Metabolism – Linezolid is primarily metabolized by oxidation of the morpholine ring, which results in 2 inactive ring-opened carboxylic acid metabolites.

Excretion – Nonrenal clearance accounts for ≈ 65% of the total clearance of linezolid. Under steady-state conditions, ≈ 30% of the dose appears in the urine as linezolid, 40% as metabolite B, and 10% as metabolite A. The renal clearance of linezolid is low (average, 40 mL/min) and suggests net tubular reabsorption. Virtually, no linezolid appears in the feces, while ≈ 6% of the dose appears in the feces as metabolite B and 3% as metabolite A.

Special populations –

Children: Currently, there are limited data on the pharmacokinetics of linezolid during multiple dosing in pediatric patients of all ages. No data have been collected in infants < 3 months of age.

Pharmacokinetic information indicates that pediatric patients dosed with 10 mg/kg IV have a similar C_{max} but a higher average clearance when corrected by body weight and shorter apparent elimination half-life than adults receiving 625 mg of linezolid.

Gender: Females have a slightly lower volume of distribution of linezolid than males. Plasma concentrations are higher in females than in males, which is partly due to body weight differences. After a 600 mg dose, mean oral clearance is ≈ 38% lower in females than in males. However, there are no significant gender differences in mean apparent elimination-rate constant or half-life. Thus, drug exposure in females is not expected to substantially increase beyond levels known to be well tolerated. Therefore, dose adjustment by gender does not appear to be necessary.

Renal function impairment: The pharmacokinetics of the parent drug, linezolid, are not altered in patients with any degree of renal insufficiency; however, the 2 primary metabolites of linezolid may accumulate in patients with renal insufficiency, with the amount of accumulation increasing with the severity of renal dysfunction. The clinical significance of accumulation of these 2 metabolites has not been determined in patients with severe renal insufficiency. Given the absence of information on the clinical significance of accumulation of the primary metabolites, weigh the use of linezolid in patients with renal insufficiency against the potential risks of accumulation of these metabolites. Linezolid and the 2 metabolites are eliminated by dialysis. No information is available on the effect of peritoneal dialysis on the pharmacokientics of linezolid. Approximately 30% of a dose was eliminated in a 3-hour dialysis session beginning 3 hours after the dose of linezolid was administered; therefore, give linezolid after hemodialysis.

Contraindications
Hypersensitivity to linezolid or any of the other product components.

Warnings
Myelosuppression: Myelosuppression (including anemia, leukopenia, pancytopenia, and thrombocytopenia) has been reported in patients receiving linezolid. In cases where the outcome is known, when linezolid was discontinued, the affected hematologic parameters rose toward pretreatment levels. Monitor complete blood counts weekly in patients who receive linezolid, particularly in those who receive linezolid for > 2 weeks, those with preexisting myelosuppression, those receiving concomitant drugs that produce bone marrow suppression, or those with a chronic infection who have received previous or concomitant antibiotic therapy. Consider discontinuation of therapy with linezolid in patients who develop or have worsening myelosuppression.

Pseudomembranous colitis: Pseudomembranous colitis has been reported with nearly all antibacterial agents, including linezolid, and may range in severity from mild to life-threatening.

Pregnancy: Category C.

Lactation: Linezolid and its metabolites are excreted in the milk of lactating rats. Concentrations in milk were similar to those in maternal plasma. It is not known whether linezolid is excreted in human breast milk.

Children: Drug clearance of linezolid is increased in pediatric patients compared with adults, resulting in a shorter half-life. Pediatric dosing regimens that provide a pharmacokinetic profile similar to adults have not been determined.

Precautions
Duration of therapy: The safety and efficacy of linezolid formulations given for > 28 days have not been evaluated in controlled clinical trials.

Phenylketonurics: Each 5 mL of the 100 mg/5 mL oral suspension contains 20 mg phenylalanine. The other linezolid formulations do not contain phenylalanine. Advise patients to contact their physician or pharmacist.

Drug Interactions
Drugs that may interact with linezolid include monoamine oxidase inhibitors, SSRIs, and adrenergic agents.

Drug/Food interactions: Large quantities of foods or beverages with high tyramine content should be avoided while taking linezolid.

Adverse Reactions
Thrombocytopenia – Linezolid has been associated with thrombocytopenia when used in doses ≤ 600 mg every 12 hours for ≤ 28 days. Thrombocytopenia associated with the use of linezolid appears to be dependent on duration of therapy (generally > 2 weeks of treatment). The platelet counts for most patients returned to the normal range/baseline during the follow-up period.

During clinical trials, 2% to 3% of linezolid patients discontinued therapy because of adverse effects. Adverse reactions occurring in ≥ 3% of patients include diarrhea, nausea, and lab test abnormalities (hemoglobin, ALT, alkaline phosphatase, and lipase).

LINCOSAMIDES

LINCOMYCIN

Capsules: 500 mg (as HCl) (*Rx*)
Injection: 300 mg/mL (as HCl) (*Rx*)

Lincocin (Pharmacia)
Lincomycin HCl (Steris), *Lincocin* (Pharmacia),
Lincorex (Hyrex)

CLINDAMYCIN

Capsules: 75, 150, and 300 mg (as HCl) (*Rx*)
Granules for oral solution: 75 mg (as palmitate)/5 mL (*Rx*)
Injection: 150 mg (as phosphate)/mL (*Rx*)

Various, *Cleocin* (Pharmacia)
Cleocin Pediatric (Pharmacia)

Various, *Cleocin Phosphate* (Pharmacia)

Warning:

These agents can cause severe and possibly fatal colitis, characterized by severe persistent diarrhea, severe abdominal cramps, and possibly, the passage of blood and mucus.

Reserve for serious infections where less toxic antimicrobial agents are inappropriate. Do not use in patients with nonbacterial infections (ie, most upper respiratory tract infections).

Indications

Anaerobes: Serious respiratory tract infections such as empyema, anaerobic pneumonitis, and lung abscess; serious skin and soft tissue infections; septicemia, intra-abdominal infections such as peritonitis and intra-abdominal abscess (typically resulting from anaerobic organisms resident in the normal GI tract); infections of the female pelvis and genital tract such as endometritis, nongonococcal tubo-ovarian abscess, pelvic cellulitis, and postsurgical vaginal cuff infection.

Streptococci and staphylococci: Serious respiratory tract infections; serious skin and soft tissue infections; septicemia (parenteral only); acute staphylococcal hematogenous osteomyelitis (parenteral only).

Pneumococci: Serious respiratory tract infections.

Administration and Dosage

LINCOMYCIN:

Oral – Take ≥ 1 to 2 hours before or after eating to ensure optimum absorption.

    Adults:

        Serious infections – 500 mg every 8 hours.

        More severe infections – ≥ 500 mg every 6 hours.

    Children > 1 month of age:

        Serious infections – 30 mg/kg/day (15 mg/lb/day) divided into 3 or 4 equal doses.

        More severe infections – 60 mg/kg/day (30 mg/lb/day) divided into 3 or 4 equal doses.

IM –

    Adults:

        Serious infections – 600 mg every 24 hours.

        More severe infections – 600 mg every 12 hours or more often.

    Children > 1 month of age:

        Serious infections – 10 mg/kg (5 mg/lb) every 24 hours.

        More severe infections – 10 mg/kg (5 mg/lb) every 12 hours or more often.

IV – Dilute to 1 g/100 mL (minimum) and infuse over 1 hour/1 g dose. Severe cardiopulmonary reactions have occurred when given at greater than the recommended concentration and rate.

    Adults:

        Serious infections – 600 mg to 1 g every 8 to 12 hours.

        Severe to life-threatening situations – Doses of 8 g/day have been given.

        Maximum recommended dose – 8 g/day.

Children > 1 month of age: Infuse 10 to 20 mg/kg/day (5 to 10 mg/lb/day), depending on severity of infection, in divided doses as described above for adults.

Subconjunctival injection – 75 mg/0.25 mL injected subconjunctivally results in ocular fluid levels of antibiotic (lasting for ≥ 5 hours) with MICs sufficient for most susceptible pathogens.

Renal function impairment – When required, an appropriate dose is 25% to 30% of that recommended for patients with normal renal function.

CLINDAMYCIN:

Oral – Take with a full glass of water or with food to avoid esophageal irritation. Clindamycin absorption is not affected by food.

   Adults:

      Serious infections – 150 to 300 mg every 6 hours.

      More severe infections – 300 to 450 mg every 6 hours.

   Children:

      Clindamycin HCl –

         Serious infections: 8 to 16 mg/kg/day divided into 3 or 4 equal doses.

         More severe infections: 16 to 20 mg/kg/day divided into 3 or 4 equal doses.

      Clindamycin palmitate HCl –

         Serious infections: 8 to 12 mg/kg/day divided into 3 or 4 equal doses.

         Severe infections: 13 to 25 mg/kg/day divided into 3 or 4 equal doses. In children weighing ≤ 10 kg, administer 37.5 mg 3 times daily as the minimum dose.

   Parenteral –

      Adults:

         Serious infections – Serious infections due to aerobic gram-positive cocci and the more sensitive anaerobes: 600 to 1200 mg/day in 2 to 4 equal doses.

         More severe infections – More severe infections, particularly those caused by *Bacteroides fragilis, Peptococcus* sp. or *Clostridium* sp. other than *C. perfringens:* 1.2 to 2.7 g/day in 2 to 4 equal doses.

         In life-threatening situations – In life-threatening situations caused by aerobes or anaerobes, doses of 4.8 g/day have been given IV to adults. Single IM injections > 600 mg are not recommended.

      Children (> 1 month of age): 20 to 40 mg/kg/day in 3 or 4 equal doses, depending on the severity of infection.

      Alternatively, children may be dosed based on body surface area:

         Serious infections – 350 mg/m^2/day; *more serious infections –* 450 mg/m^2/day.

      Neonates (< 1 month of age): 15 to 20 mg/kg/day in 3 or 4 equal doses.

   CDC recommendation for acute pelvic inflammatory disease – 900 mg IV every 8 hours plus gentamicin loading dose 2 mg/kg IV or IM, followed by 1.5 mg/kg every 8 hours.

      After discharge from hospital, continue with oral doxycycline 100 mg 2 times/day for 10 to 14 days total. Alternatively, continue with oral clindamycin 450 mg 4 times daily for 10 to 14 days.

Actions

Pharmacology: **Lincomycin** and **clindamycin**, known collectively as lincosamides, bind exclusively to the 50 S subunit of bacterial ribosomes and suppress protein synthesis. Cross-resistance has been demonstrated between these 2 agents. Clindamycin is preferred because it is better absorbed and more potent.

Pharmacokinetics: Administration with food markedly impairs **lincomycin** (but not **clindamycin**) oral absorption.

Dialysis –

Select Pharmacokinetic Parameters of Lincosamides									
							Elimination (%)		
Lincosamides	Bioavailability (%)	Mean peak serum level (mcg/mL)	Time to peak serum level (hours)	Protein binding (%)	Half-life (hours)	Hepatic	Unchanged in urine (range)	Feces
Clindamycin[1]								
Oral	90	2.5	0.75	≈ 90	2.4 to 3[3]	> 90	10	3.6
IM		6 to 9	1 to 3					
IV		7 to 14	0[2]					
Lincomycin								
Oral	20 to 30	1.8 to 5.3	2 to 4	57 to 72	4.4 to 6.4	> 90	4 (1 to 31)	40
IM		9.3 to 18.5	0.5				17.3 (2 to 25)	
IV		15.9 to 20.9	0				13.8 (5 to 30)	

[1] Clindamycin palmitate and phosphate are rapidly hydrolyzed to the base.
[2] By end of infusion, peak levels are reached.
[3] Increased slightly in patients with markedly reduced renal or hepatic function.

Microbiology:

Organisms Generally Susceptible to Lincosamides			
✔ = generally susceptible		Lincosamides	
	Microorganism	Lincomycin	Clindamycin
Gram-positive	Staphylococcus aureus	✔	✔
	Staphylococcus epidermidis[1]	✔	✔
	Staphylococcus albus	✔	
	Streptococcus pneumoniae	✔	✔
	Streptococcus pyogenes	✔	✔
	β-hemolytic streptococci	✔	
	Streptococcus viridans	✔	✔
	Pneumococci		✔
	Corynebacterium diphtheriae	✔	✔
	Diplococcus pneumoniae	✔	
	Corynebacterium acnes	✔	
	Nocardia asteroides	✔	✔
Anaerobes	Bacteroides sp.	✔	✔[2]
	Fusobacterium sp.		✔
	Propionibacterium (same as C. acnes)	✔	✔
	Eubacterium sp.	✔	✔
	Actinomyces sp.	✔	✔
	Peptococcus sp.	✔	✔
	Peptostreptococcus	✔	✔
	Microaerophilic streptococci		✔
	Clostridium perfringens	✔	✔
	Clostridium tetani	✔	✔
	Veillonella sp.		✔

[1] Penicillinase and nonpenicillinase.
[2] Including B. fragilis and B. melaninogenicus.

Contraindications
Hypersensitivity to lincosamides; treatment of minor bacterial or viral infections.

Warnings
Meningitis: **Clindamycin** does not diffuse adequately into CSF; do not use for meningitis.

Diarrhea: If significant diarrhea occurs during therapy with **lincomycin** or **clindamycin**, discontinue therapy.

Hypersensitivity reactions: Use with caution in patients with a history of asthma or significant allergies. Refer to Management of Acute Hypersensitivity Reactions.

Renal function impairment: Cautiously give **clindamycin** to patients with severe renal or hepatic disease accompanied by severe metabolic aberrations. Use of **lincomycin** in pre-existing liver disease is not recommended unless special clinical circumstances so indicate.

Elderly: Older patients with associated severe illness may not tolerate diarrhea well.

Pregnancy: Category B (**clindamycin**).

Lactation: **Clindamycin** and **lincomycin** appear in breast milk. The American Academy of Pediatrics considers clindamycin to be compatible with breastfeeding.

Children: **Lincomycin** is not indicated for use in the newborn. When **clindamycin** is administered to newborns and infants, monitor organ system functions.

Precautions
Monitoring: In prolonged therapy, perform liver/kidney function tests and blood counts.

Drug Interactions
Drugs that may interact with lincosamides include erythromycin, kaolin-pectin, and neuromuscular blockers (nondepolarizing).

Drug/Food interactions: Food impairs the absorption of **lincomycin**; do not take anything by mouth (except water) for 1 to 2 hours before and after lincomycin. **Clindamycin** absorption is not affected by food.

Adverse Reactions
Nausea; vomiting; diarrhea (**clindamycin** 3.4% to 30%); pseudomembranous colitis (clindamycin 0.01% to 10%; 3 to 4 times more frequent with oral administration); neutropenia (sometimes transient); leukopenia; agranulocytosis; thrombocytopenic purpura; skin rashes, urticaria, erythema multiforme; anaphylaxis; jaundice; liver function test abnormalities (serum transaminase elevations).

AMINOGLYCOSIDES, PARENTERAL

STREPTOMYCIN SULFATE	
Injection: 400 mg/mL (*Rx*)	*Streptomycin Sulfate* (Pfizer)
KANAMYCIN SULFATE	
Injection: 500 mg and 1 g (*Rx*)	Various, *Kantrex* (Apothecon)
Pediatric injection: 75 mg (*Rx*)	Various, *Kantrex* (Apothecon)
GENTAMICIN	
Injection: 2, 10, and 40 mg/mL (*Rx*)	Various, *Garamycin* (Schering)
TOBRAMYCIN SULFATE	
Injection: 10 and 40 mg/mL (*Rx*)	Various, *Nebcin* (Lilly), *Nebcin Pediatric* (Lilly)
Pediatric injection: 10 mg/mL (*Rx*)	Various, *Nebcin Pediatric* (Lilly)
Powder for injection: 1.2 g (after reconstitution) (*Rx*)	*Nebcin* (Lilly)
Nebulizer solution: 300 mg/5 mL (*Rx*)	*TOBI* (PathoGenesis)
AMIKACIN SULFATE	
Injection: 250 mg/mL (*Rx*)	Various, *Amikin* (Apothecon)
Pediatric injection: 50 mg/mL (*Rx*)	Various, *Amikin* (Apothecon)
NETILMICIN SULFATE	
Injection: 100 mg/mL (*Rx*)	*Netromycin* (Schering)

Indications

Reserve these drugs for treatment of infections caused by organisms not sensitive to less toxic agents. Safety for treatment periods > 14 days has not been established.

For approved indications, refer to the Administration and Dosage section.

Unlabeled uses:

Gentamicin – An alternative regimen for pelvic inflammatory disease is gentamicin plus clindamycin. Continue for at least 4 days and at least 48 hours after patient improves; then continue clindamycin 450 mg orally 4 times daily for 10 to 14 days total therapy.

Amikacin sulfate – Intrathecal/intraventricular administration has been suggested at 8 mg/24 hours.

Administration and Dosage

Synergism: In vitro studies indicate that aminoglycosides combined with penicillins or cephalosporins act synergistically against some strains of gram-negative organisms and enterococci (*Streptococcus faecalis*). Aminoglycosides may exhibit a synergistic effect when combined with carbenicillin or ticarcillin for *Pseudomonas* infections.

STREPTOMYCIN SULFATE: Administer IM only.

Tuberculosis (TB) – The standard regimen for the treatment of drug-susceptible TB has been 2 months of INH, rifampin, and pyrazinamide followed by 4 months of INH and rifampin. When streptomycin is added to this regimen because of suspected or proven drug resistence, the recommended dosing for streptomycin is as follows:

Streptomycin Dosing for TB			
	Daily	Twice weekly	Three times weekly
Children	20 to 40 mg/kg max 1 g	25 to 30 mg/kg max 1.5 g	25 to 30 mg/kg max 1.5 g
Adults	15 mg/kg max 1 g	25 to 30 mg/kg max 1.5 g	25 to 30 mg/kg max 1.5 g

Streptomycin usually is administered daily as a single IM injection. Give a total dose of < 120 g over the course of therapy unless there are no other therapeutic options. In patients > 60 years of age, use a reduced dosage. The total period of drug treatment for TB is a minimum of 1 year.

Tularemia – 1 to 2 g/day in divided doses for 7 to 14 days, or until afebrile 5 to 7 days.

Plague – 2 g daily in 2 divided doses for a minimum of 10 days.

Bacterial endocarditis –

Streptococcal: In penicillin-sensitive alpha and nonhemolytic streptococci, use streptomycin for 2 weeks with penicillin: 1 g twice daily for 1 week, 0.5 g twice daily for the second week. If patient is > 60 years of age, give 0.5 g twice daily for the entire 2-week period.

Enterococcal: 1 g twice daily for 2 weeks and 0.5 g twice daily for 4 weeks in combination with penicillin.

Adults – 1 to 2 g in divided doses every 6 to 12 hours for moderate-to-severe infections. Doses should generally not exceed 2 g/day.

Children – 20 to 40 mg/kg/day in divided doses every 6 to 12 hours.

KANAMYCIN SULFATE: Do not exceed total 1.5 g/day by any route.

IM – For adults or children, 7.5 mg/kg every 12 hours (15 mg/kg/day). If continuously high blood levels are desired, give daily dose of 15 mg/kg in equally divided doses every 6 or 8 hours. Usual treatment duration is 7 to 10 days. Doses of 7.5 mg/kg give mean peak levels of 22 mcg/mL. At 8 hours after a 7.5 mg/kg dose, mean serum levels are 3.2 mcg/mL.

IV –

Adults: Do not exceed 15 mg/kg/day. Give slowly over 30 to 60 minutes. Divide daily doses into 2 to 3 equal doses.

Children: Use sufficient diluent to infuse drug over 30 to 60 minutes.

Renal failure – Calculate the dosage interval with the following formula: Serum creatinine (mg/dL) × 9 = dosage interval (in hours).

Intraperitoneal (following exploration for peritonitis or after peritoneal contamination caused by fecal spill during surgery) – 500 mg in 20 mL sterile distilled water instilled through a polyethylene catheter into wound.

Aerosol treatment – 250 mg 2 to 4 times/day.

Other routes – Concentrations of 0.25% have been used as irrigating solutions in abscess cavities, pleural space, peritoneal and ventricular cavities.

GENTAMICIN:

Dosage – May be given IM or IV. For patients with serious infections and normal renal function, give 3 mg/kg/day in 3 equal doses every 8 hours. For patients with life-threatening infections, administer up to 5 mg/kg/day in 3 or 4 equal doses. Reduce dosage to 3 mg/kg/day as soon as clinically indicated.

Obese patients: Base dosage on an estimate of lean body mass.

Children: 6 to 7.5 mg/kg/day (2 to 2.5 mg/kg every 8 hours).

Infants and neonates: 7.5 mg/kg/day (2.5 mg/kg every 8 hours).

Premature or full term neonates (≤ 1 week of age): 5 mg/kg/day (2.5 mg every 12 hours). A regimen of either 2.5 mg/kg every 18 hours or 3 mg/kg every 24 hours may also provide satisfactory peak and trough levels in preterm infants < 32 weeks gestational age.

Prevention of bacterial endocarditis –

In dental, oral, or upper respiratory tract procedures (alternate regimen): 1 to 2 g (50 mg/kg for children) ampicillin plus 1.5 mg/kg (2 mg/kg for children) gentamicin not to exceed 80 mg, both IM or IV ½ hour prior to procedure, followed by 1.5 g (25 mg/kg for children) amoxicillin 6 hours after initial dose or repeat parenteral dose 8 hours after initial dose.

GU or GI procedures (standard regimen): 2 g (50 mg/kg for children) ampicillin plus 1.5 mg/kg (2 mg/kg for children) gentamicin not to exceed 80 mg, both IM or IV ½ hour prior to procedure followed by 1.5 mg (25 mg/kg for children) amoxicillin.

Renal function impairment –

Rule of eights: Approximate the interval between doses (in hours) by multiplying the serum creatinine level (mg/dL) by 8. For example, a patient weighing 60 kg with a serum creatinine level of 2 mg/dL could be given 60 mg (1 mg/kg) every 16 hours (2 × 8).

IV – A 1 to 2 mg/kg loading dose may be used, followed by a maintenance dose.

Intrathecal – In general, the recommended dose for infants and children ≥ 3 months of age is 1 to 2 mg once a day. For adults, administer 4 to 8 mg once a day.

TOBRAMYCIN SULFATE:

Dosage – Use the patient's ideal body weight for dosage calculation. Peak and trough serum concentrations should be measured. Avoid prolonged peak concentrations > 12 mcg/mL or troughs > 2 mcg/mL.

Adults with serious infections – Administer 3 mg/kg/day in 3 equal doses every 8 hours.

Life-threatening infections: Administer up to 5 mg/kg/day in 3 or 4 equal doses. Reduce dosage to 3 mg/kg/day as soon as clinically indicated.

Children – Administer 6 to 7.5 mg/kg/day in 3 or 4 equally divided doses (2 to 2.5 mg/kg every 8 hours or 1.5 to 1.9 mg/kg every 6 hours).

Premature or full-term infants (≤ 1 year of age) – Administer up to 4 mg/kg/day in 2 equal doses every 12 hours. Preliminary data suggest that 2.5 mg/kg every 18 hours or 3 mg/kg every 24 hours may achieve safe and effective peak and trough serum concentrations in newborn infants weighing < 1 kg at birth.

Renal function impairment – Following a loading dose of 1 mg/kg, adjust subsequent dosage, either with reduced doses administered at 8-hour intervals or with normal doses given at prolonged levels.

An alternative guide for determining reduced dosage at 8-hour intervals (for patients whose steady-state serum creatinine values are known) is to divide the normally recommended dose by the patient's serum creatinine.

Hemodialysis – Hemodialysis removes ≈ 50% of a dose in 6 hours. In patients maintained by regular dialysis, the usual dose of 1.5 to 2 mg/kg given after every dialysis usually maintains therapeutic, nontoxic serum levels. In patients receiving intermittent peritoneal dialysis, patients dialyzed twice weekly should receive a 1.5 to 2 mg/kg loading dose followed by 1 mg/kg every 3 days. Where dialysis occurs every 2 days, a 1.5 mg/kg loading dose is given after the first dialysis and 0.75 mg/kg after each subsequent dialysis.

IV administration – The IV dose is the same as the IM dose. Infuse the diluted solution over a period of 20 to 60 minutes. Infusion periods of < 20 minutes are not recommended because peak serum levels may exceed < 20 mcg/mL.

Cystic fibrosis (nebulizer solution) – Recommended dosage for adults and children ≥ 6 years of age is 300 mg twice a day in repeating cycles of 28 days on drug/ 28 days off drug. Do not adjust dosage by age or weight. Take as close to 12 hours apart as possible; do not take < 6 hours apart. Administer by inhalation over a 10- to 15-minute period, using a hand-held *PARI LC PLUS* reusable nebulizer with a *DeVilbiss Pulmo-Aide* compressor. Do not dilute or mix with dornase alfa in the nebulizer. Instruct patients on multiple therapies to take them first, followed by tobramycin. Bronchospasm, which can occur with inhalation of tobramycin, may be reduced if inhalation of tobramycin nebulization solution follows bronchodilator therapy.

Monitoring: In patients with normal renal function, serum tobramycin concentrations are ≈ 1 mcg/mL 1 hour after dose administration. Monitoring of serum concentrations in patients with renal dysfunction or patients treated with concomitant parenteral tobramycin may reduce the risk of toxicity.

AMIKACIN SULFATE:

Adults and children – Use the patient's ideal body weight for dosage calculation. Administer IM or IV. Administer 15 mg/kg/day divided into 2 or 3 equal doses at equally divided intervals. Treatment of heavier patients should not exceed 1.5 g/ day. In uncomplicated UTIs, use 250 mg twice daily.

Neonates: A loading dose of 10 mg/kg is recommended, followed by 7.5 mg/kg every 12 hours. Lower dosages may be safer during the first 2 weeks of life.

Renal function impairment – Adjust doses in patients with impaired renal function by administering normal doses at prolonged intervals or by administering reduced doses at a fixed interval.

Normal dosage at prolonged intervals: If the Ccr is not available and the patient's condition is stable, calculate a dosage interval (in hours) for the normal dose by multiplying the patient's serum creatinine by 9.

Reduced dosage at fixed time intervals: Measure serum concentration to ensure accurate administration and to avoid concentrations > 35 mcg/mL. Initiate therapy by administering a normal dose, 7.5 mg/kg, as a loading dose.

To determine maintenance doses administered every 12 hours, reduce the loading dose in proportion to the reduction in the patient's Ccr:

$$\frac{\text{Maintenance dose}}{\text{every 12 hours}} = \frac{\text{observed Ccr (mL/min)}}{\text{normal Ccr (mL/min)}} \times \frac{\text{calculated loading}}{\text{dose (mg)}}$$

Dialysis: Approximately half the normal mg/kg dose can be given after hemodialysis; in peritoneal dialysis, a parenteral dose of 7.5 mg/kg is given, and then amikacin is instilled in peritoneal dialysate at a concentration desired in serum.

NETILMICIN SULFATE:

Dosage – Administer IM or IV. The recommended dosage for both methods is identical.

Obtain the patient's pretreatment body weight for calculation of correct dosage. Base the dosage in obese patients on an estimate of the lean body mass.

Patients with normal renal function –

Adults: Complicated UTIs: 1.5 to 2 mg/kg every 12 hours (3 to 4 mg/kg/day).

Serious systemic infections – 1.3 to 2.2 mg/kg every 8 hours or 2 to 3.25 mg/kg every 12 hours (4 to 6.5 mg/kg/day).

Infants and children (6 weeks through 12 years of age): Administer 1.8 to 2.7 mg/kg every 8 hours or 2.7 to 4 mg/kg every 12 hours (5.5 to 8 mg/kg/day).

Neonates (< 6 weeks of age): Administer 2 to 3.25 mg/kg every 12 hours (4 to 6.5 mg/kg/day).

Renal function impairment – If netilmicin serum concentrations are not available and renal function is stable, serum creatinine and Ccr values are the most reliable, readily available indicators of the degree of renal impairment to guide dosage adjustment. The BUN level is much less reliable for this purpose. Periodically reassess renal function during therapy.

Hemodialysis – In adults with renal failure who are undergoing hemodialysis, the amount of netilmicin removed from the blood may vary, depending upon the dialysis equipment and methods used. In adults, a dose of 2 mg/kg at the end of each dialysis period is recommended until the results of tests measuring serum levels become available.

Actions

Pharmacology: The aminoglycosides are bactericidal antibiotics used primarily in the treatment of gram-negative infections.

Pharmacokinetics:

Absorption/Distribution – Absorption from IM injection is rapid, with peak blood levels achieved within 1 hour.

Excretion is by glomerular filtration, largely as unchanged drug; thus, high urine levels are attained. Aminoglycosides are removed by hemodialysis (4 to 6 hours removes ≈ 50%) and peritoneal dialysis (range, removal of 23% in 8 hours to only 4% in 22 hours).

Serum levels – Because of the narrow range between therapeutic and toxic serum levels, careful attention to dosage calculations is essential, especially in patients with renal impairment, geriatric and female patients, those requiring high peak serum levels, patients on prolonged therapy (> 10 days), patients with unstable renal function or those undergoing dialysis, those with abnormal extracellular fluid volume, or with prior exposure to ototoxic or nephrotoxic drugs. Age markedly affects peak concentration in children; it is generally lower in young children and infants. Monitor drug serum levels. Peak levels indicate therapeutic levels. Trough serum level determinations (just before next dose) best indicate drug accumulation. Obtain serum levels within 48 hours of start of therapy and every 3 to 4 days assuming stable renal function; also, levels are indicated when dose is changed or in changing renal function. Generally, to measure peak levels, draw a serum sample about 30 minutes after IV infusion or 1 hour after an IM dose. For trough levels, obtain serum samples at 8 hours or just prior to the next dose.

Various Pharmacokinetic Parameters of the Aminoglycosides						
	Half-life (hrs)		Therapeutic serum levels (peak) (mcg/mL)	Toxic serum levels (mcg/mL)		Dose (mg/kg/day) (normal Ccr)
Aminoglycoside	Normal	ESRD		Peak[1]	Trough[2]	
Amikacin	2 to 3	24 to 60	16 to 32	> 35	> 10	15
Gentamicin	2	24 to 60	4 to 8	> 12	> 2	3 to 5
Kanamycin	2 to 3	24 to 60	15 to 40	> 35	> 10	15
Netilmicin	2 to 2.7	40	6 to 10	> 16	> 4	3 to 6.5
Streptomycin	2.5	100	20 to 30	> 50	—	15
Tobramycin	2 to 2.5	24 to 60	4 to 8	> 12	> 2	3 to 5

[1] Measured 1 hour after IM administration.
[2] Measured immediately prior to next dose.

Microbiology:

Organisms Generally Susceptible to Aminoglycosides		Amikacin	Gentamicin	Kanamycin	Netilmicin	Streptomycin	Tobramycin
Gram-positive	*Mycobacterium tuberculosis*	✔[1]				✔[2]	
	Staphylococci	✔[3]	✔[3]		✔[3]		✔
	Staphylococcus aureus	✔	✔	✔[3]	✔[3]		✔
	Staphylococcus epidermidis	✔		✔	✔		
	Streptococci					✔[2]	
	Streptococcus faecalis		✔[2]		✔[2]	✔[2]	✔[2]
Gram-negative	*Acinetobacter* sp.	✔		✔	✔		
	Brucella sp.					✔	
	Citrobacter sp.	✔	✔	✔	✔	✔	✔
	Enterobacter sp.	✔	✔	✔	✔	✔	✔
	Escherichia coli	✔	✔	✔	✔	✔	✔
	Haemophilus influenzae	✔		✔		✔[2]	
	Haemophilus ducreyi					✔	
	Klebsiella sp.	✔	✔	✔	✔	✔[2]	✔
	Morganella morganii						✔
	Neisseria sp.	✔		✔	✔	✔	
	Proteus sp.	✔[4]	✔[4]	✔[4]	✔	✔	✔[4]
	Providencia sp.	✔	✔	✔	✔	✔	✔
	Pseudomonas sp.	✔			✔		
	P. aeruginosa	✔	✔[2]		✔	✔	✔
	Salmonella sp.	✔	✔	✔	✔	✔	✔
	Serratia sp.	✔	✔	✔	✔	✔	✔
	Shigella sp.	✔	✔	✔	✔	✔	✔
	Yersinia (Pasteurella) pestis	✔	✔	✔	✔	✔	✔

[1] ✔ = generally susceptible
[2] Usually used concomitantly with other anti-infectives.
[3] Penicillinase-producing and nonpenicillinase-producing.
[4] Indole-positive and indole-negative.

Contraindications

Previous reactions to these agents. With the exception of the use of streptomycin in tuberculosis, these agents generally are not indicated in long-term therapy because of the ototoxic and nephrotoxic hazards of extended administration.

Warnings

Toxicity: Aminoglycosides are associated with significant nephrotoxicity or ototoxicity. These agents are excreted primarily by glomerular filtration; thus, the serum half-life will be prolonged and significant accumulation will occur in patients with impaired renal function. Toxicity may develop even with conventional doses, particularly in prerenal azotemia or impaired renal function.

Ototoxicity – Neurotoxicity, manifested as auditory (cochlear) and vestibular ototoxicity, can occur with any of these agents. Auditory changes are irreversible, usually bilateral, and may be partial or total. Risk of hearing loss increases with degree of exposure to either high peak or high trough serum concentrations and continues to progress after drug withdrawal. Risk is greater with renal impairment and with pre-existing hearing loss. High frequency deafness usually occurs first and can be detected by audiometric testing. Relative ototoxicity is: **Streptomycin = Kanamycin > Amikacin = Gentamicin = Tobramycin > Netilmicin.**

Renal toxicity – Renal toxicity may be characterized by decreased creatinine clearance, cells or casts in the urine, decreased urine specific gravity, oliguria, proteinuria, or evidence of nitrogen retention. Renal damage is usually reversible. The relative nephrotoxicity of these agents is estimated to be: **Kanamycin = Amikacin = Gentamicin = Netilmicin > Tobramycin > Streptomycin.**

Monitoring – Closely observe all patients treated with aminoglycosides. Monitoring renal and eighth cranial nerve function at onset of therapy is essential for patients with known or suspected renal impairment and also in those whose renal function is initially normal but who develop signs of renal dysfunction.

Burn patients: In patients with extensive burns, altered pharmacokinetics may result in reduced serum concentrations of aminoglycosides.

Hypomagnesemia: Hypomagnesemia may occur in > ⅓ of patients whose oral diet is restricted or who are eating poorly.

Neuromuscular blockade: Neurotoxicity can occur. Aminoglycosides may aggravate muscle weakness because of a potential curare-like effect on the neuromuscular junction.

Neuromuscular blockade resulting in respiratory paralysis has occurred with these agents, especially if given with or soon after anesthesia or muscle relaxants.

Nephrotoxicity: Nephrotoxicity may occur. Risk factors include the elderly, patients with a history of renal impairment who are treated for longer periods or with higher doses than those recommended, a recent course of aminoglycosides (within 6 weeks), concurrent use of other nephrotoxic agents, frequent dosing, potassium depletion, and decreased intravascular volume. Adverse renal effects can occur in patients with initially normal renal function. Of patients receiving an aminoglycoside for several days or more, ≈ 8% to 26% will develop mild renal impairment that is generally reversible.

Hydration – These drugs reach high concentrations in the renal system; keep patients well hydrated to minimize chemical irritation of tubules.

Dosing interval: Preliminary evidence indicates that aminoglycosides may be administered on a once-daily basis without compromising efficacy and without increasing the potential for nephrotoxicity and ototoxicity. It is possible that the incidence of nephrotoxicity may even be decreased.

Elderly: Elderly patients may have reduced renal function that is not evident in the results of routine screening tests, such as BUN or serum creatinine. A Ccr determination may be more useful.

Pregnancy: Category D (amikacin, gentamicin, kanamycin, netilmicin, tobramycin).

Lactation: Small amounts of **streptomycin, kanamycin,** and **netilmicin** are excreted in breast milk.

Children: Use with caution in premature infants and neonates because of their renal immaturity and the resulting prolongation of serum half-life of these drugs.

Precautions

Intrathecal gentamicin: Use of excessive (40 to 160 mg) doses of intrathecal **gentamicin** has produced neuromuscular disturbances (eg, ataxia, paresis, incontinence).

Cross-allergenicity: Cross-allergenicity among the aminoglycosides has been demonstrated.

Monitoring: Monitor peak and trough serum concentrations periodically to ensure adequate levels and to avoid potentially toxic levels. Also monitor serum calcium, magnesium and sodium (see Adverse Reactions).

Eighth cranial nerve function testing – Serial audiometric tests are suggested, particularly when renal function is impaired or prolonged aminoglycoside therapy is required; also repeat such tests periodically after treatment if there is evidence of a hearing deficit or vestibular abnormality before or during therapy, or when consecutive or concomitant use of other potentially ototoxic drugs is unavoidable.

Syphilis: In the treatment of sexually transmitted disease, if concomitant syphilis is suspected, perform a darkfield examination before treatment is started. Perform monthly serologic tests for ≥ 4 months.

Topical use: Aminoglycosides are quickly and almost totally absorbed when applied topically in association with surgical procedures, except to the urinary bladder.

Drug Interactions

Drugs that may affect aminoglycosides include cephalosporins, enflurane, methoxyflurane, vancomycin, indomethacin IV, loop diuretics, and penicillins.

Drugs that may be affected by aminoglycosides include depolarizing and nondepolarizing neuromuscular blockers and polypeptide antibiotics.

Adverse Reactions

Aminoglycoside Adverse Reactions (%)						
Adverse Reaction	Amikacin	Gentamicin	Kanamycin	Netimicin	Streptomycin	Tobramycin
Central/Peripheral nervous system						
Headache	rare	✔[1]	rare	< 0.1		✔
Confusion		✔				✔
Fever		✔		0.1	✔	✔
Lethargy		✔				✔
Disorientation				< 0.1		✔
Neuromuscular blockade[2]	✔		✔	✔	✔	
Paresthesia	rare		rare	< 0.1		
GI						
Vomiting	rare	✔	rare	< 0.1	✔	✔
Nausea	rare	✔	rare		✔	✔
Diarrhea			rare	< 0.1		✔
Hematologic						
Anemia	rare	✔		< 0.1		✔
Eosinophilia	rare	✔		0.4	✔	✔
Leukopenia		✔		< 0.1	✔	✔
Thrombocytopenia		✔		< 0.1	✔	✔
Hypersensitivity						
Rash	rare	✔	rare	≤ 0.5	✔	✔
Urticaria		✔			✔	✔
Itching		✔		≤ 0.5		✔
Special senses						
Dizziness		✔		✔		✔
Tinnitus		✔		✔		✔
Vertigo		✔		✔	✔	✔
Hearing loss/deafness	✔	✔	✔[3]		✔	✔

Aminoglycoside Adverse Reactions (%)							
	Adverse Reaction	Amikacin	Gentamicin	Kanamycin	Netilmicin	Streptomycin	Tobramycin
Renal[1]	Oliguria	✔	✔	✔	✔		✔
	Proteinuria	✔	✔	✔	✔		✔
	Rising serum creatinine[2]	✔	✔	✔	✔		✔
	Casts	✔	✔		✔		
	Rising BUN[2]		✔	✔	✔		✔
	Red and white cells in urine	✔		✔	✔		
	Azotemia	✔				✔	
Lab test abnormalities	Increased AST/ALT		✔		1.5		✔
	Increased bilirubin		✔		1.5		✔
Other	Apnea	✔	✔	✔	✔	✔	✔
	Pain/Irritation at injection site		✔	✔	≈ 0.4		✔
	Hypotension	rare	✔		< 0.1		

[1] ✔ = Reported; no incidence given
[2] See Warnings
[3] Partially reversible to irreversible bilateral hearing loss.

AMINOGLYCOSIDES, ORAL

KANAMYCIN SULFATE
Capsules: 500 mg (*Rx*)
Kantrex (Apothecon)

NEOMYCIN SULFATE
Tablets: 500 mg (*Rx*)
Oral solution: 125 mg/5 mL (*Rx*)
Various, *Neo-Tabs* (Pharma-Tek)
Mycifradin (Pharmacia), *Neo-Fradin* (Pharma-Tek)

PAROMOMYCIN SULFATE
Capsules: 250 mg (*Rx*)
Humatin (Parke-Davis)

For complete information on the aminoglycosides, refer to the Aminoglycosides, Parenteral monograph.

Indications

Suppression of intestinal bacteria.

Hepatic coma.

Neomycin sulfate: Many studies have documented lipid-lowering efficacy of neomycin. Alone, it reduced LDL cholesterol levels by 24%. Combined with niacin, it reduced LDL cholesterol levels to below the 90th percentile in 92% of patients.

Administration and Dosage

KANAMYCIN SULFATE:

Suppression of intestinal bacteria – As an adjunct to mechanical cleansing of the large bowel in short-term therapy — 1 g for every hour for 4 hours, followed by 1 g every 6 hours for 36 to 72 hours.

Hepatic coma – 8 to 12 g/day in divided doses.

NEOMYCIN SULFATE:

Preoperative prophylaxis for elective colorectal surgery –

Recommended Bowel Preparation Regimen (Proposed Surgery Time 8 am)[1]			
Therapy	Day 3 before surgery	Day 2 before surgery	Day 1 before surgery
Diet	Minimum residue or clear liquid	Minimum residue or clear liquid	Clear liquid
Bisacodyl, 1 oral cap	6 pm (-62 hrs)		
Magnesium sulfate, 30 mL of a 50% solution orally		10 am (-46 hrs). Repeat at 2 pm (-42 hrs) and 6 pm (-38 hrs)	10 am (-22 hrs). Repeat at 2 pm (-18 hrs).
Enema		7 pm (-37 hrs) & 8 pm (-36 hrs). Repeat hourly until no solid feces return with last enema	None
Supplemental IV fluids			As needed
Neomycin and erythromycin tablets, 1 g each, orally			1 pm (-19 hrs). Repeat at 2 pm (-18 hrs) and 11 pm (-9 hrs)

[1] On day of surgery, patient should evacuate rectum at 6:30 am (-1½ hrs) for 8 am procedure.

Hepatic coma (as adjunct) –

Adults: 4 to 12 g/day in divided doses.

Children: 50 to 100 mg/kg/day in divided doses. Continue treatment over a period of 5 to 6 days; during this time, return protein to the diet incrementally. Chronic hepatic insufficiency may require up to 4 g/day over an indefinite period.

PAROMOMYCIN SULFATE:

Intestinal amebiasis –

Adults and children: Usual dose is 25 to 35 mg/kg/day, in 3 doses with meals for 5 to 10 days.

Management of hepatic coma –

Adults: Usual dose: 4 g/day in divided doses at regular intervals for 5 to 6 days. Paromomycin sulfate has been recommended for other parasitic infections — *Dientamoeba fragilis* (25 to 30 mg/kg/day in 3 doses for 7 days); *Diphyllobothrium latum, Taenia saginata, Taenia solium, Dipylidium caninum* (*adults:* 1 g every 15 minutes for 4 doses; *pediatric:* 11 mg/kg every 15 minutes for 4 doses); *Hymenolepis nana* (45 mg/kg/day for 5 to 7 days).

Actions

Pharmacokinetics: Oral aminoglycosides are poorly absorbed; therefore, use only for suppression of GI bacterial flora.

Contraindications

Presence of intestinal obstruction; hypersensitivity to aminoglycosides.

Warnings

Increased absorption: Although negligible amounts are absorbed through intact mucosa, consider the possibility of increased absorption from ulcerated or denuded areas.

Nephrotoxicity/Ototoxicity: Because of reported cases of deafness and potential nephrotoxic effects, closely observe patients. Refer to the Warning Box in the Aminoglycosides, Parenteral monograph concerning aminoglycoside toxicity.

Pregnancy:
Neomycin – *Category D.*

Lactation: It is not known whether **neomycin** is excreted in breast milk. Other aminoglycosides are excreted in breast milk.

Children: The safety and efficacy of oral **neomycin** in patients < 18 years of age have not been established. If treatment is necessary, use with caution; do not exceed a treatment period of 3 weeks because of absorption from the GI tract.

Precautions

Muscular disorders: Use with caution in patients with muscular disorders such as myasthenia gravis or parkinsonism.

GI effects:
Neomycin – Orally administered neomycin increases fecal bile acid excretion and reduces intestinal lactase activity.
Paromomycin – Use with caution in individuals with ulcerative lesions of the bowel to avoid renal toxicity through inadvertent absorption.

Drug Interactions

Drugs that may be affected by aminoglycosides include anticoagulants, digoxin, methotrexate, neuromuscular blockers (depolarizing and nondepolarizing).

Adverse Reactions

Nausea, vomiting, diarrhea (most common); "malabsorption syndrome" characterized by increased fecal fat, decreased serum carotene, and fall in xylose absorption. *Clostridium difficile*-associated colitis (following **neomycin** therapy); nephrotoxicity and ototoxicity (following prolonged and high-dosage therapy in hepatic coma).

METRONIDAZOLE

Tablets: 250 mg and 500 mg (*Rx*)	Various, *Flagyl* (Searle)
Capsules: 375 mg (*Rx*)	*Flagyl 375* (Searle)
Powder for injection, lyophilized: 500 mg (as HCl) (*Rx*)	*Flagyl I.V.* (Schiapparelli Searle)
Injection, ready-to-use: 500 mg/100 mL (*Rx*)	Various, *Metronidazole* (Abbott), *Flagyl I.V. RTU* (Schiapparelli Searle)

Metronidazole also is available for topical and intravaginal use and also is used orally as an amebicide.

> **Warning:**
> Metronidazole is carcinogenic in rodents. Avoid unnecessary use.

Indications

Anaerobic infections: Treatment of serious infections caused by susceptible anaerobic bacteria. Effective in *Bacteroides fragilis* infections resistant to clindamycin, chloramphenicol, and penicillin.

Intra-abdominal infections – Intra-abdominal infections (peritonitis, intra-abdominal abscess, and liver abscess) caused by *Bacteroides* sp. (*B. fragilis*, *B. distasonis*, *B. ovatus*, *B. thetaiotaomicron*, *B. vulgatus*), *Clostridium* sp., *Eubacterium* sp., *Peptostreptococcus* sp., and *Peptococcus* sp.

Skin and skin structure infections – Skin and skin structure infections, caused by *Bacteroides* sp. including the *B. fragilis* group, *Clostridium* sp., *Peptococcus* sp., *Peptostreptococcus* sp., and *Fusobacterium* sp.

Gynecologic infections – Gynecologic infections (endometritis, endomyometritis, tubo-ovarian abscess, and postsurgical vaginal cuff infection), caused by *Bacteroides* sp. including the *B. fragilis* group, *Clostridium* sp., *Peptococcus* sp., and *Peptostreptococcus* sp.

Bacterial septicemia – Bacterial septicemia caused by *Bacteroides* sp. including the *B. fragilis* group and *Clostridium* sp.

Bone and joint infections – Bone and joint infections caused by *Bacteroides* sp. including the *B. fragilis* group, as adjunctive therapy.

CNS infections – CNS infections (meningitis and brain abscess), caused by *Bacteroides* sp. including the *B. fragilis* group.

Lower respiratory tract infections – Lower respiratory tract infections (pneumonia, empyema, and lung abscess) caused by *Bacteroides* sp. including the *B. fragilis* group.

Endocarditis – Endocarditis caused by *Bacteroides* sp. including the *B. fragilis* group.

Prophylaxis: Preoperative, intraoperative, and postoperative IV metronidazole may reduce the incidence of postoperative infection in patients undergoing elective colorectal surgery which is classified as contaminated or potentially contaminated.

Metronidazole also is indicated for amebiasis and trichomoniasis, intravaginally for bacterial vaginosis, and topically for acne rosacea.

Unlabeled uses: The CDC has recommended the use of oral metronidazole for bacterial vaginosis (500 mg twice daily for 7 days). Single-dose therapy for bacterial vaginosis (2 g) also appears to be as effective as multiple-dose therapy.

Administration and Dosage

May cause GI upset; take with food. Avoid alcoholic beverages.

Anaerobic bacterial infections: In the treatment of most serious anaerobic infections, metronidazole is usually administered IV initially.

Loading dose – 15 mg/kg infused over 1 hour ($\approx$ 1 g for a 70 kg adult).

Maintenance dose – 7.5 mg/kg infused over 1 hour every 6 hours ($\approx$ 500 mg for a 70 kg adult). Administer the first maintenance dose 6 hours following the initiation of loading dose. Do not exceed a maximum of 4 g in 24 hours.

The usual duration of therapy is 7 to 10 days; however, infections of the bone and joints, lower respiratory tract, and endocardium may require longer treatment.

Administer by slow IV, continuous or intermittent drip infusion only. Do not give by direct IV bolus injection because of the low pH (0.5 to 2) of the reconstituted product. The drug must be further diluted and neutralized for infusion.

Oral – Following IV therapy, use oral metronidazole when conditions warrant. The usual adult oral dosage is 7.5 mg/kg every 6 hours. Do not exceed a maximum of 4 g in 24 hours.

Prophylaxis: To prevent postoperative infection in contaminated or potentially contaminated colorectal surgery, the recommended adult dosage is 15 mg/kg infused over 30 to 60 minutes and completed ≈ 1 hour before surgery, followed by 7.5 mg/kg infused over 30 to 60 minutes at 6 and 12 hours after the initial dose.

It also has been suggested that a dose of 1500 mg infused at the beginning of surgery achieves significantly higher concentrations against B. *fragilis* than the 500 mg infusion and may be beneficial in ensuring adequate metronidazole levels.

Hepatic disease: Hepatic disease patients metabolize metronidazole slowly; accumulation of metronidazole and its metabolites occurs. Therefore, reduce doses below those usually recommended.

Renal disease: Do not specifically reduce the dose in anuric patients because accumulated metabolites may be rapidly removed by dialysis.

Actions
Pharmacology: Metronidazole, a nitroimidazole, is active against various anaerobic bacteria and protozoa.

Pharmacokinetics:
Absorption – Metronidazole is well absorbed after oral administration. Peak serum levels occur at about 1 to 2 hours. Food delays peak serum levels up to 2 hours.

Distribution – Metronidazole has a large apparent volume of distribution. It diffuses well into all tissues.

Excretion – The major route of elimination of metronidazole and its metabolites is via the urine (60% to 80% of the dose); fecal excretion accounts for 6% to 15% of the dose. Renal clearance is ≈ 10 mL/min/1.73 m^2. Metronidazole has an average elimination half-life in healthy subjects of 8 hours. Patients with Ccr < 10 mL/min (not receiving dialysis) will accumulate both metabolites. Metronidazole and its 2 major metabolites are removed by hemodialysis. Metronidazole is also removed by peritoneal dialysis.

Contraindications
Hypersensitivity to metronidazole or other nitroimidazole derivatives; pregnancy (first trimester in patients with trichomoniasis).

Warnings
Neurologic effects: Seizures (associated with high cumulative doses) and peripheral neuropathy (characterized by numbness or paresthesia of an extremity) have occurred. In some cases, neuropathy is not reversible.

Hepatic function impairment: Patients with severe hepatic disease metabolize metronidazole slowly. Accumulation of the drug and its metabolites may occur.

Elderly: Because the pharmacokinetics of metronidazole may be altered in the elderly, monitoring of serum levels may be necessary to adjust the dosage accordingly.

Pregnancy: Category B. Restrict metronidazole for trichomoniasis in the second and third trimesters to those in whom local palliative treatment has been inadequate to control symptoms.

Lactation: Safety for use in nursing mothers has not been established. A nursing mother should express and discard any breast milk produced while on the drug and resume nursing 24 to 48 hours after the drug is discontinued.

Children: Safety and efficacy in children have not been established, except for the treatment of amebiasis. Newborns demonstrate a diminished capacity to eliminate metronidazole; half-life may be as high as 22 hours.

Precautions

Crohn's disease: Crohn's disease patients are known to have an increased incidence of GI and certain extraintestinal cancers.

Candidiasis: Candidiasis may present more prominent symptoms during therapy and requires treatment with a candicidal agent.

Hematologic effects: Metronidazole is a nitroimidazole; use with care in patients with evidence or history of blood dyscrasia. Perform total and differential leukocyte counts before and after therapy.

Amebic liver abscess: Metronidazole does not obviate the need for aspiration of pus.

Drug Interactions

Drugs that may affect metronidazole include barbiturates and cimetidine. Drugs that may be affected by metronidazole include anticoagulants, disulfiram, ethanol, hydantoins, and lithium.

Drug/Lab test interactions: The drug may interfere with chemical analyses for AST, ALT, LDH, triglycerides, and hexokinase glucose.

Adverse Reactions

Adverse reactions may include dysuria; cystitis; polyuria; incontinence; proliferation of *Candida* in the vagina; dyspareunia; darkened urine; seizures and peripheral neuropathy; dizziness; vertigo; incoordination; ataxia; confusion; irritability; depression; weakness; insomnia; headache; syncope; nausea; diarrhea; epigastric distress; constipation; proctitis; glossitis; stomatitis; unpleasant metallic taste; urticaria; erythematous rash; flushing; nasal congestion.

NYSTATIN, ORAL

| Tablets: 500,000 units (*Rx*) | Various, Nystatin (Major), Mycostatin (Apothecon) |

Indications
Nonesophageal membrane GI candidiasis: Treatment of nonesophageal membrane GI candidiasis

Administration and Dosage
500,000 to 1,000,000 units 3 times daily. Continue treatment for at least 48 hours after clinical cure to prevent relapse.

Actions
Pharmacology: A polyene antibiotic with antifungal activity. Nystatin probably acts by binding to sterols in the cell membrane of the fungus, with a resultant change in membrane permeability allowing leakage of intracellular components.

Pharmacokinetics: Sparingly absorbed after oral use.

Contraindications
Hypersensitivity to nystatin.

Adverse Reactions
Nystatin is virtually nontoxic and nonsensitizing and is well tolerated by all age groups including debilitated infants, even on prolonged administration.

MICONAZOLE

| Injection: 10 mg/mL (*Rx*) | Monistat i.v. (Janssen) |

Indications
Use only to treat severe systemic fungal disease: Coccidioidomycosis, candidiasis, cryptococcosis, pseudoallescheriosis (petriellidiosis, allescheriosis), paracoccidioidomycosis, and for the treatment of chronic mucocutaneous candidiasis.

In the treatment of fungal meningitis or *Candida* urinary bladder infections, IV infusion alone is inadequate. It must be supplemented with intrathecal administration or bladder irrigation.

Administration and Dosage
Adults: The following daily doses are recommended:

Recommended Miconazole Daily Doses		
Organism	Total daily dosage range[1] (mg)	Duration of therapy (weeks)
Coccidioidomycosis	1800 to 3600	3 to > 20
Cryptococcosis	1200 to 2400	3 to > 12
Pseudoallescheriosis	1600 to 3000	5 to> 20
Candidiasis	1600 to 1800	1 to > 20
Paracoccidioidomycosis	1200 to 1200	2 to > 16

[1] May be divided over 3 infusions.

Repeated courses may be necessitated by relapse or reinfection.

Children:
    < 1 year of age – 15 to 30 mg/kg/day.
    1 to 12 years of age – 20 to 40 mg/kg/day. Do not exceed 15 mg/kg/dose.

IV: For doses ≤ 2400 mg/day, infuse at a rate of ≈ 2 hours/amp. For doses > 2400 mg/day, adjust infusion rate and diluent according to patient tolerability.

Intrathecal: Administer undiluted solution by various intrathecal routes (20 mg/dose) as an adjunct to IV treatment in fungal meningitis. Succeeding intrathecal injections may be alternated between lumbar, cervical, and cisternal punctures every 3 to 7 days.

Bladder instillation: 200 mg diluted solution for *Candida* of the urinary bladder.

Actions

Pharmacology: Miconazole, an imidazole derivative, exerts a fungicidal effect by altering the permeability of the fungal cell membrane.

Pharmacokinetics:

Absorption/Distribution – CSF levels following IV administration are undetectable. Penetration of the drug into inflamed joints, the vitreous body of the eye, and the peritoneal cavity is good. Greater than 90% is bound to serum protein.

Metabolism/Excretion – Miconazole is rapidly metabolized in the liver. About 14% to 22% of the administered dose is excreted in the urine, mainly as inactive metabolites. The terminal elimination half-life is 20 to 25 hours.

Contraindications

Hypersensitivity to miconazole.

Warnings

Cardiac effects: Cardiorespiratory arrest or anaphylaxis has occurred, possibly because of excessively rapid administration in some cases. Rapid injection of undiluted miconazole may produce transient tachycardia or arrhythmia.

Pregnancy: Category C.

Children: Safety for use in children < 1 year of age has not been extensively studied.

Precautions

Give by IV infusion. Start treatment under stringent conditions of hospitalization. Subsequently, it may be given to suitable patients under ambulatory conditions with close clinical monitoring. Monitor hemoglobin, hematocrit, electrolytes, and lipids.

Systemic fungal mycoses: Systemic fungal mycoses may be complications of chronic underlying conditions which, in themselves, may require appropriate measures.

Drug Interactions

Drugs that may interact with miconazole include amphotericin B, astemizole, cisapride, oral anticoagulants, phenytoin, and terfenadine.

Adverse Reactions

Adverse reactions occurring in ≥ 3% of patients include phlebitis at infusion site, pruritus/rash (if severe, discontinuation may be necessary), nausea, vomiting, fever, and chills.

KETOCONAZOLE

Tablets: 200 mg *(Rx)* Various, *Nizoral* (Janssen)

> **Warning:**
> Ketoconazole has been associated with hepatic toxicity, including some fatalities. Closely monitor patients and inform them of the risk.

Indications

Treatment of the following systemic fungal infections: Candidiasis, chronic mucocutaneous candidiasis, oral thrush, candiduria, blastomycosis, coccidioidomycosis, histoplasmosis, chromomycosis, and paracoccidioidomycosis.

Treatment of severe recalcitrant cutaneous dermatophyte infections not responding to topical therapy or oral griseofulvin or in patients unable to take griseofulvin.

Do not use ketoconazole for fungal meningitis because it penetrates poorly into the CSF.

Administration and Dosage

If antacids, anticholinergics, or H_2 blockers are needed, give at least 2 hours after administration. Take with food to alleviate GI disturbance.

Adults: Initially, 200 mg once daily. In very serious infections, or if clinical response is insufficient, increase dose to 400 mg once daily.

Children:
>   (> *2 years of age*) – 3.3 to 6.6 mg/kg/day as a single daily dose.
>   (< *2 years of age*) – Daily dosage has not been established.

Minimum treatment is 1 or 2 weeks for candidiasis and 6 months for the other indicated systemic mycoses. Chronic mucocutaneous candidiasis usually requires maintenance therapy.

Minimum treatment of recalcitrant dermatophyte infections is 4 weeks in cases involving glabrous skin. Palmar and plantar infections may respond more slowly.

Actions

Pharmacology: Ketoconazole, an imidazole broad-spectrum antifungal agent, impairs the synthesis of ergosterol, the main sterol of fungal cell membranes, allowing increased permeability and leakage of cellular components.

Pharmacokinetics:

   Absorption/Distribution – Bioavailability depends on an acidic pH for dissolution and absorption. In vitro, plasma protein binding is ≈ 95% to 99%, mainly to albumin.

   Metabolism/Excretion – The drug undergoes extensive hepatic metabolism to inactive metabolites. Plasma elimination is biphasic; half-life is 2 hours during the first 10 hours, 8 hours thereafter. The major excretory route is enterohepatic. From 85% to 90% is excreted in bile and feces, 13% in urine.

Contraindications

Hypersensitivity to ketoconazole. Do not use ketoconazole for the treatment of fungal meningitis because it penetrates poorly into the CSF. Concomitant administration of ketoconazole with oral triazolam is contraindicated.

Warnings

Hepatotoxicity: Hepatotoxicity, primarily of the hepatocellular type, has been associated with ketoconazole, including rare fatalities. Measure liver function before starting treatment and frequently during treatment. Monitor patients receiving ketoconazole concurrently with other potentially hepatotoxic drugs, particularly those patients requiring prolonged therapy or those with a history of liver disease. Transient minor elevations in liver enzymes have occurred.

Prostatic cancer: In clinical trials involving 350 patients with metastatic prostatic cancer, 11 deaths were reported within 2 weeks of starting high-dose ketoconazole (1200 mg/day). It is not known whether death was related to therapy. High ketoconazole doses are known to suppress adrenal corticosteroid secretion.

Hypersensitivity reactions: Anaphylaxis occurs rarely after the first dose. Hypersensitivity reactions, including urticaria, have been reported.

Pregnancy: Category C.

Lactation: Ketoconazole is excreted in breast milk. Administer to nursing mothers only if the potential benefits outweigh the potential risks to the infant.

Children: Safety for use in children < 2 years of age has not been established.

Precautions

Hormone levels: Testosterone levels are impaired with doses of 800 mg/day and abolished by 1600 mg/day. It also decreases ACTH-induced corticosteroid serum levels at similar high doses.

Gastric acidity: Ketoconazole requires acidity for dissolution and absorption. In achlorhydria, dissolve each tablet in 4 mL aqueous solution of 0.2 N HCl. Use a glass or plastic straw to avoid contact with teeth. Follow with a glass of water.

Drug Interactions

Ketoconazole is a potent inhibitor of the cytochrome P450 3A4 enzyme system. Coadministration of ketoconazole with other drugs metabolized by the same enzyme system may result in increased plasma concentrations of the drugs that could increase or prolong both therapeutic and adverse effects. Unless otherwise specified, dosage adjustment may be necessary.

Drugs that may affect ketoconazole include antacids, didanosine, histamine H_2 antagonists, isoniazid, sucralfate, proton pump inhibitors, and rifampin. Drugs that may be affected by ketoconazole include oral anticoagulants, corticosteroids, cyclosporine, protease inhibitors, tricyclic antidepressants, carbamazepine, quinidine, sulfonylureas, benzodiazepines, buspirone, oral contraceptives, donepezil, nisoldipine, tacrolimus, vinca alkaloids, zolpidem, and theophylline.

Adverse Reactions

Adverse reactions occurring in ≥ 3% of patients include nausea and vomiting.

AMPHOTERICIN B

Powder for injection: 50 mg (as deoxycholate) (Rx)	Amphotericin B (PharmaTek), Fungizone Intravenous (Apothecon), Amphocin (Pharmacia)
Suspension for injection: 100 mg/20 mL (as lipid complex) (Rx)	Abelcet (Liposome Co.)
Powder for injection: 50 mg and 100 mg (as cholesteryl) (Rx)	Amphotec (Sequus Pharmaceuticals)
Powder for injection: 50 mg (as liposomal) (Rx)	AmBisome (Fujisawa)

Warning:
Use primarily for treatment of patients with progressive and potentially fatal fungal infections. Do not use to treat noninvasive forms of fungal disease such as oral thrush, vaginal candidiasis, and esophageal candidiasis in patients with normal neutrophil counts.

Indications

Fungal infections, systemic:

Amphotericin B deoxycholate – Intended to treat the following potentially life-threatening invasive fungal infections: Aspergillosis; cryptococcosis (torulosis); North American blastomycosis; candidiasis; coccidioidomycosis; histoplasmosis; zygomycosis including mucormycosis caused by *Mucor*, *Rhizopus*, and *Absidia* sp.; infections caused by related susceptible species of *Conidiobolus* and *Basidiobolus*; sporotrichosis.

Lipid-based formulations – For use in patients refractory to conventional amphotericin B deoxycholate therapy or where renal impairment or unacceptable toxicity precludes the use of the deoxycholate formulation for the treatment of invasive fungal infections (lipid complex); for the treatment of invasive aspergillosis (cholesteryl); for the treatment of infections caused by *Aspergillus*, *Candida*, or *Cryptococcus* sp. (liposomal).

Fungal infections, empirical: For empirical treatment in febrile, neutropenic patients with presumed fungal infection (liposomal only).

Cryptococcal meningitis in HIV: Treatment of cryptococcal meningitis in HIV-infected patients (*AmBisome* only).

Leishmaniasis: For treatment of visceral leishmaniasis (liposomal only); treatment of American mucocutaneous leishmaniasis but not as primary therapy (deoxycholate).

Unlabeled uses: Prophylaxis for fungal infection in patients with bone marrow transplantation (0.1 mg/kg/day).

Administration and Dosage

Fungal infection, empirical: Administer 3 mg/kg/day of liposomal amphotericin B using a controlled infusion device over ≈ 120 minutes; infusion time may be reduced to 60 minutes if well tolerated or increased if patient experiences discomfort.

Fungal infection, systemic:
  Amphotericin B deoxycholate (eg, Fungizone) –

Suggested Indication-Specific Dosage Regimens for Amphotericin B Deoxycholate		
Fungal infection, systemic	Treatment regimen	Dose[1] (mg/kg/day)
Aspergillosis	up to 3.6 g total dose	1 to 1.5
Blastomyces	4 to 12 weeks	0.5 to 0.6
Candidiasis	4 to 12 weeks	0.5 to 1
Coccidioidomycosis	4 to 12 weeks	0.5 to 1
Cryptococcus	4 to 12 weeks	0.5 to 0.7
Histoplasmosis	4 to 12 weeks	0.5 to 0.6
Mucormycosis	4 to 12 weeks	1 to 1.5
Rhinocerebral phycomycosis	3 to 4 g total dose	0.25 to 0.3 up to 1 to 1.5
Sporotrichosis	up to 2.5 g total dose	0.5

[1] Some of these dosages are not FDA-approved.

Because patient tolerance varies greatly, a test dose may be preferred; 1 mg in 20 mL of 5% Dextrose delivered IV over 20 to 30 minutes. Record patient's temperature, pulse, respiration, and blood pressure every 30 minutes for 2 to 4 hours.

The recommended initial dose is 0.25 to 0.3 mg/kg/day prepared as 0.1 mg/mL infusion and delivered slowly over 2 to 6 hours. Depending on the patient's cardio-renal status, dosage may be gradually increased by 5 to 10 mg/day up to a total dose of 0.5 to 0.7 mg/kg/day. Some mycoses may require total doses up to 1 to 1.5 mg/kg/day. Do not exceed a total daily dose of 1.5 mg/kg; overdoses can result in cardio-respiratory arrest. Alternate daily dosing is recommended for total daily doses of 1.5 mg/kg.

In patients with impaired cardio-renal function or a severe reaction to the test dose, initiate therapy with smaller daily doses (eg, 5 to 10 mg).

An in-line membrane filter of ≥ 1 micron mean pore diameter may be used.

Amphotericin B cholesteryl (Amphotec) – A test dose is advisable (eg, 10 mL of final preparation containing between 1.6 to 8.3 mg infused over 15 to 30 min). The recommended dose is 3 to 4 mg/kg/day prepared as a 0.6 mg/mL (range, 0.16 to 0.83 mg/mL) infusion delivered at a rate of 1 mg/kg/hr. Do not use an in-line filter.

Amphotericin B lipid complex (Abelcet) – The recommended dose is 5 mg/kg/day prepared as a 1 mg/mL infusion and delivered at a rate of 2.5 mg/kg/hr. For pediatric patients and patients with cardiovascular disease, the drug may be diluted to a final concentration of 2 mg/mL. If the infusion exceeds 2 hours, mix the contents by shaking the infusion bag every 2 hours. Do not use an in-line filter.

Liposomal amphotericin B (AmBisome) – The recommended dose is 3 to 5 mg/kg/day prepared as a 1 to 2 mg/mL infusion delivered initially over 120 minutes; infusion time may be reduced to 60 minutes if well tolerated or increased if patient experiences discomfort. Lower infusion concentrations of 0.2 to 0.5 mg/mL may be appropriate for infants and small children to provide sufficient volume for infusion. An in-line membrane filter of ≥ 1 micron mean pore diameter may be used.

Cryptococcal meningitis in HIV:
  AmBisome – Administer 6 mg/kg/day using a controlled infusion device over ≈ 120 minutes; infusion time may be reduced to 60 minutes if well tolerated or increased if patient experiences discomfort.

Leishmaniasis:
  Liposomal amphotericin B (AmBisome) – Administer 3 mg/kg/day on days 1 through 5, 14 and 21 to immunocompetent patients; a repeat course of therapy may be useful if parasitic clearance is not achieved. Administer 4 mg/kg/day on days 1 through 5, 10, 17, 24, 31, and 38 to immunosuppressed patients; seek expert advice regarding further therapy if parasitic clearance is not achieved.

Amphotericin B deoxycholate (eg, Fungizone) – 0.5 mg/kg/day administered on alternate days for 14 doses has been effective but is not recommended as primary therapy.

Rhinocerebral phycomycosis: A cumulative dose of ≥ 3 g amphotericin B is recommended. Although a total dose of 3 to 4 g will infrequently cause lasting renal impairment, it is a reasonable minimum where there is clinical evidence of deep tissue invasion. Rhinocerebral phycomycosis usually follows a rapidly fatal course; therapy must be more aggressive than that for more indolent mycoses.

Unlabeled:

Cystitis, candidal – Irrigate bladder with a 50 mcg/mL solution, instilled periodically or continuously for 5 to 10 days.

Meningitis, coccidioidal or cryptococcal – Adminsiter amphotericin B deoxycholate intrathecally at initial doses of 0.025 mg, gradually increased to the maximum tolerable dose. The usual dose is 0.25 to 1 mg every 48 to 72 hours. A maximum total dose of 15 mg has been suggested.

Paracoccidioidomycosis – Administer 0.4 to 0.5 mg/kg/day slow IV infusion, treat for 4 to 12 weeks.

Actions

Pharmacology: Amphotericin B is fungistatic or fungicidal, depending on the concentration obtained in body fluids and on the susceptibility of the fungus. It acts by binding to sterols in the fungal cell membrane with a resultant change in membrane permeability, allowing leakage of a variety of intracellular components.

Liposomal encapsulation or incorporation in a lipid complex can substantially affect a drug's functional properties relative to those of the unencapsulated or non-lipid-associated drug. Lipid-based formulations increase the circulation time and alter the biodistribution of associated amphotericin. Increasing drug levels at site of action and reducing levels in normal tissues offers 2 distinct clinical advantages: An increased therapeutic index and altered toxicity profile relative to free drug.

Different lipid-based formulations with a common active ingredient may vary from one another in the chemical composition (eg, phospholipid and cholesterol content) and physical form of the lipid component (eg, sphere, disc, or ribbon). Such differences may affect functional properties of these drug products.

Pharmacokinetics:

Absorption/Distribution – Amphotericin B is highly protein bound (> 90%) and is poorly dialyzable.

Metabolism/Excretion – Amphotericin B has a relatively short initial serum half-life of 24 hours, followed by a second elimination phase with a half-life of ≈ 15 days. The drug is slowly excreted by the kidneys with 2% to 5% as the biologically active form. The following table presents pharmacokinetic parameters at steady-state for lipid-based formulations of amphotericin B; the assay used to measure serum levels did not distinguish between free and complex amphotericin B.

Pharmacokinetic Parameters of Lipid-Based Amphotericin B Formulations[1]						
Parameter	AmBisome 1 mg/kg/day (n = 7)	AmBisome 2.5 mg/kg/day (n = 7)	AmBisome 5 mg/kg/day (n = 9)	Amphotec 3 mg/kg/day (predicted)[2]	Amphotec 4 mg/kg/day (predicted)[2]	Abelcet 5 mg/kg/day (n = varied)[3]
Cmax (mcg/mL)	≈ 12.2	≈ 31.4	≈ 83	2.6	2.9	≈ 1.7
AUC (mcg/mL•hr)	≈ 60	≈ 197	≈ 555	29	36	≈ 14
t½ (hrs)	≈ 7	≈ 6.3	≈ 6.8	27.5 (100 to 153)[4]	28.2 (100 to 153)[4]	≈ 173.4
Vss (L/kg)	≈ 0.14	≈ 0.16	≈ 0.1	3.8	4.1	≈ 131
CL (mL/hr/kg)	≈ 17	≈ 22	≈ 11	105	112	≈ 436

[1] Data are pooled from separate studies and are not necessarily comparable.
[2] Values based on the population model developed from 51 bone marrow transplant patients with systemic fungal infections given *Amphotec* 0.5 to 8 mg/kg/day.
[3] Data obtained from various studies in patients with mucocutaneous leishmaniasis or cancer with presumed or proven fungal infections.
[4] Based on total amphotericin B levels measured within a 24-hour dosing interval (or up to 49 days after dosing).

Contraindications

Hypersensitivity to amphotericin B, unless the condition requiring treatment is life-threatening and amenable only to amphotericin B therapy.

Warnings

Fatal fungal diseases: Amphotericin B is frequently the only effective treatment for potentially fatal fungal diseases. Balance its possible lifesaving effect against its dangerous side effects.

Nephrotoxicity: Renal damage is a limiting factor for the use of amphotericin B. Renal dysfunction usually improves upon interruption of therapy, dose reduction or increased dosing interval; however, some permanent impairment often occurs, especially in patients receiving large doses (> 5 g) or receiving other nephrotoxic agents. Decreased glomerular filtration rate and renal blood flow, increased serum creatinine and renal tubular dysfunction are prominent. In some patients, hydration and sodium repletion prior to amphotericin B administration may reduce the risk of developing nephrotoxicity.

Lipid formulations of amphotericin B have been shown to reduce the severe kidney toxicity of amphotericin B and are indicated in patients with renal impairment or when unacceptable toxicity precludes the use of amphotericin B deoxycholate in effective doses.

Infusion reactions: Acute reactions including fever, shaking chills, hypotension, anorexia, vomiting, nausea, headache, and tachypnea are common 1 to 3 hours after starting an IV infusion. These reactions usually are more severe with the first few doses of amphotericin B and usually diminish with subsequent doses. Avoid rapid IV infusion because it has been associated with hypotension, hypokalemia, arrhythmias, bronchospasm, and shock.

Leukoencephalopathy: This has been reported following use of amphotericin B. The literature has suggested that total body irradiation may be a predisposition.

Rhinocerebral phycomycosis: A fulminating disease, this generally occurs in association with diabetic ketoacidosis. Diabetic control must be instituted before successful treatment with amphotericin B can be accomplished. Pulmonary phycomycosis, which is more common in association with hematologic malignancies, is often an incidental finding at autopsy.

Hypersensitivity reactions: Anaphylaxis has been reported with amphotericin B. If severe respiratory distress occurs, discontinue the infusion immediately. Do not give further infusions. Have cardiopulmonary resuscitation facilities available during administration.

Renal function impairment: Use amphotericin B desoxycholate with care in patients with reduced renal function; frequent monitoring is recommended (see Precautions). Lipid formulations have been reported to overcome most problems of chronic nephrotoxicity, even in patients with impaired renal function following previous treatment with amphotericin B desoxycholate.

Pregnancy: Category B.

Lactation: It is not known whether amphotericin B is excreted in breast milk; however, consider discontinuing nursing.

Children: Safety and efficacy of amphotericin B desoxycholate in children have not been established. Systemic fungal infections have been successfully treated in children without reports of unusual side effects. Limit administration to the least amount compatible with an effective therapeutic regimen.

Pediatric patients < 16 years of age (n = 97) with systemic fungal infections have been treated with amphotericin B cholesteryl at daily mg/kg doses similar to those given in adults and had significantly less renal toxicity than the desoxycholate formulation (12% vs 52%); 273 pediatric patients age 1 month to 16 years with presumed fungal infections, confirmed systemic fungal infections or with visceral leishmaniasis have been successfully treated with liposomal amphotericin B (*AmBisome*); 111 children < 16 years of age, including 11 patients < 1 year of age, have been treated with amphotericin B lipid complex (*Abelcet*) at 5 mg/kg/day and 5 children with hepatosplenic candidiasis were effectively treated with 2.5 mg/kg/day. Safety and efficacy in patients < 1 month of age have not been established.

Precautions

Monitoring: Monitor renal function frequently during amphotericin B therapy. It is also advisable to monitor liver function, serum electrolytes (particularly magnesium and potassium), blood counts, and hemoglobin concentrations on a regular basis. Use laboratory test results as a guide to subsequent dose adjustments. Monitor complete blood count and prothrombin time as medically indicated.

Record the patient's temperature, pulse, respiration, and blood pressure every 30 minutes for 2 to 4 hours after administration.

Resistance: Variants with reduced susceptibility to amphotericin B have been isolated from several fungal species after serial passage in cell culture media containing the drug and from some patients receiving prolonged therapy with amphotericin B desoxycholate. The relevance of drug resistance to clinical outcome has not been established.

Therapy interruption: Whenever medication is interrupted for > 7 days, resume therapy with the lowest dosage level; increase gradually.

Pulmonary reactions: Pulmonary reactions characterized by acute dyspnea, hypoxemia, and interstitial infiltrates have been observed in neutropenic patients receiving amphotericin B and leukocyte transfusions. Separate the infusion as far as possible from the time of a leukocyte transfusion.

Lab test abnormalities:

Serum electrolyte abnormalities – Hypomagnesemia, hyperkalemia, hypokalemia, hypercalcemia, hypocalcemia, hypophosphatemia.

Liver function test abnormalities – Increased AST, ALT, GGT, bilirubin, alkaline phosphatase, and LDH.

Renal function impairment – Increased BUN and serum creatinine.

Other test abnormalities – Acidosis, hyperamylasemia, hypoglycemia, hyperglycemia, hyperuricemia.

Drug Interactions

Drugs that may interact with amphotericin B include antineoplastic agents, corticosteroids, zidovudine, other nephrotoxic agents, digitalis glycosides, flucytocine, skeletal muscle relaxants, cyclosporine, azole antifungal agents, and thiazides.

Adverse Reactions

Prevention of adverse reactions – Most patients will exhibit some intolerance, often at less than full therapeutic dosage. Severe reactions may be lessened by giving aspirin, antipyretics (eg, acetaminophen), antihistamines, and antiemetics before the infusion and by maintaining sodium balance. Administration on alternate days may decrease anorexia and phlebitis. Small doses of IV adrenal corticosteroids given prior to or during the infusion may decrease febrile reactions. Meperidine (25 to 50 mg IV) has been shown in some patients to decrease the duration of shaking chills and fever that may accompany infusion of amphotericin B.

Adverse reactions may include abdominal pain; acidosis; anemia; anorexia; anxiety; apnea; asthenia; asthma; arrhthmias; azotemia; bilirubinemia; blood product transfusion reaction; chest/back pain; coagulation disorder; confusion; cough increased; cramping; decreased prothrombin time; depression; diarrhea; dizziness; dry mouth; dyspepsia; dyspnea; edema; epigastric pain; epistaxis; eye hemorrhage; face edema; fever (sometimes with shaking chills); generalized pain, including muscle and joint pains; GI hemorrhage; headache; heart arrest; hematemesis; hematuria; hemoptysis; hemorrhage; hypernatremia; hypertension; hyperventilation; hypokalemia; hypovolemia; hyposthenuria; hypotension; hypoxia; increased serum creatinine; infection; insomnia; jaundice; leukopenia; lung disorder; maculopapular rash; malaise; mucous membrane disorder; multiple organ failure; nausea; normochromic, normycytic anemia; pain; peripheral edema; pleural effusion; pneumonia; pruritus; rash; renal tubular acidosis and nephrocalcinosis; respiratory disorder;

respiratory failure; rhinitis; sepsis; somnolence; stomatitis; sweating; tachycardia; tachypnea; thinking abnormal; thrombocytopenia; tremor; vomiting; venous pain at the injection site with phlebitis and thrombophlebitis; weight loss/gain.

GRISEOFULVIN

GRISEOFULVIN MICROSIZE

Tablets: 250 and 500 mg (*Rx*)   *Fulvicin U/F* (Schering), *Grifulvin V* (Ortho Derm), *Grisactin 500* (Wyeth-Ayerst)

Capsules: 250 mg (*Rx*)   *Grisactin 250* (Wyeth-Ayerst)

Oral suspension: 125 mg/5 mL (*Rx*)   *Grifulvin V* (Ortho Derm)

GRISEOFULVIN ULTRAMICROSIZE

Tablets: 125, 165, 250, and 330 mg (*Rx*)   Various, *Fulvicin P/G* (Schering), *Grisactin Ultra* (Westwood Squibb), *Gris-PEG* (Allergan Herbert)

Indications

Treatment of ringworm infections of the skin, hair, and nails, namely: Tinea corporis, tinea pedis, tinea cruris, tinea barbae, tinea capitis, tinea unguium (onychomycosis) when caused by one or more of the following genera of fungi: *Trichophyton rubrum*; *Trichophyton tonsurans*; *Trichophyton mentagrophytes*; *Trichophyton interdigitalis*; *Trichophyton verrucosum*; *Trichophyton megnini*; *Trichophyton gallinae*; *Trichophyton crateriform*; *Trichophyton sulphureum*; *Trichophyton schoenleini*; *Microsporum audouini*; *Microsporum canis*; *Microsporum gypseum*; *Epidermophyton floccosum*.

Note: Prior to therapy, identify the types of fungi responsible for the infection. Use of this drug is not justified in minor or trivial infections that will respond to topical agents alone.

Griseofulvin is not effective in bacterial infections; candidiasis (moniliasis); histoplasmosis; actinomycosis; sporotrichosis; chromoblastomycosis; coccidioidomycosis; North American blastomycosis; cryptococcosis (torulosis); tinea versicolor; nocardiosis.

Administration and Dosage

Duration of therapy: Representative treatment periods are: Tinea capitis, 4 to 6 weeks; tinea corporis, 2 to 4 weeks; tinea pedis, 4 to 8 weeks; tinea unguium (depending on rate of growth) – fingernails, at least 4 months, toenails, at least 6 months.

Adults:

Tinea corporis, tinea cruris, tinea capitis – A single or divided daily dose of 500 mg microsize (330 to 375 mg ultramicrosize) will give a satisfactory response in most patients.

Tinea pedis, tinea unguium – 0.75 to 1 g microsize (660 to 750 mg ultramicrosize) per day in divided doses.

Children: Approximately 11 mg microsize/kg/day (5 mg/lb/day) or 7.3 mg ultramicrosize/kg/day (3.3 mg/lb/day) is an effective dose for most children.

Griseofulvin Dosage for Children Based on Weight			
Weight		Daily dose (mg)	
lb	kg	microsize	ultramicrosize
30 to 50	13.6 to 23	125 to 250	82.5 to 165
> 50	> 22.6	250 to 500	165 to 330

Clinical experience indicates that a single daily dose is effective in children with tinea capitis.

Children (≤ 2 years of age) – Dosage not established.

Actions

Pharmacology: Griseofulvin, an antibiotic derived from a species of *Penicillium*, is deposited in the keratin precursor cells, which are gradually exfoliated and replaced by noninfected tissue; it has a greater affinity for diseased tissue.

Pharmacokinetics: The peak serum level found in fasting adults given 0.5 g griseofulvin microsize occurs at ≈ 4 hours and ranges between 0.5 to 2 mcg/mL. Some individuals are consistently "poor absorbers" and tend to attain lower blood levels at all times. The serum level may be increased by giving the drug with a meal with a high fat content.

Contraindications
Hypersensitivity to griseofulvin; porphyria; hepatocellular failure.

Warnings
Hypersensitivity reactions: Hypersensitivity reactions (eg, skin rashes, urticaria, angioneurotic edema, erythema multiforme-like reactions) may occur and necessitate withdrawal of therapy. Institute appropriate counter measures.

Fertility impairment: Because griseofulvin has demonstrated harmful effects in vitro on the genotype bacteria, plants, and fungi, males should wait ≥ 6 months after completing therapy before fathering a child. Females should avoid risk of pregnancy while receiving griseofulvin.

Pregnancy: Category C.

Precautions
Prolonged therapy: Closely observe patients on prolonged therapy. Periodically monitor renal, hepatic, and hematopoietic function.

Penicillin cross-sensitivity: Penicillin cross-sensitivity is possible because griseofulvin is derived from species of *Penicillium*.

Lupus erythematosus,: Lupus erythematosus, lupus-like syndromes or exacerbation of lupus erythematosus have occurred in patients receiving griseofulvin.

Photosensitivity: Photosensitivity may occur. Photosensitivity reactions may aggravate lupus erythematosus.

Drug Interactions
Drugs that may interact with griseofulvin include anticoagulants, oral contraceptives, cyclosporine, salicylates, and barbiturates.

Adverse Reactions
Adverse reactions may include hypersensitivity reactions such as skin rashes and urticaria; oral thrush; nausea; vomiting; epigastric distress; diarrhea; headache; fatigue; dizziness; insomnia; mental confusion; impairment of performance of routine activities.

FLUCONAZOLE

Tablets: 50, 100, 150, and 200 mg (*Rx*)
Powder for oral suspension: 10 and 40 mg/mL when reconstituted (*Rx*)
Injection: 2 mg/mL (*Rx*)

Diflucan (Roerig)

Indications
Candidiasis:
> *Treatment* – Oropharyngeal and esophageal candidiasis.
>> Candidal urinary tract infections, peritonitis, and systemic candidal infections including candidemia, disseminated candidiasis and pneumonia.
>> Vaginal candidiasis (vaginal yeast infections caused by *Candida*).
> *Prophylaxis* – To decrease the incidence of candidiasis in patients undergoing bone marrow transplantation who receive cytotoxic chemotherapy or radiation therapy.

Cryptococcal meningitis: Treatment of cryptococcal meningitis.

Administration and Dosage
Single dose:
> *Vaginal candidiasis* – 150 mg as a single oral dose.

Multiple dose: The daily dose of fluconazole is the same for oral and IV administration. In general, a loading dose of twice the daily dose is recommended on the first day of therapy to result in plasma levels close to steady state by the second day of therapy.

Patients with AIDS and cryptococcal meningitis or recurrent oropharyngeal candidiasis usually require maintenance therapy to prevent relapse.

Adults –

Oropharyngeal candidiasis: 200 mg on the first day, followed by 100 mg once daily. Continue treatment for at least 2 weeks to decrease the likelihood of relapse.

Esophageal candidiasis: 200 mg on the first day, followed by 100 mg once daily. Doses up to 400 mg/day may be used, based on the patient's response. Treat patients with esophageal candidiasis for a minimum of 3 weeks and for at least 2 weeks following resolution of symptoms.

Candidiasis, other: For candidal UTIs and peritonitis, 50 to 200 mg/day has been used. For systemic candidal infections (including candidemia, disseminated candidiasis, and pneumonia), optimal dosage and duration have not been determined, although doses up to 400 mg/day have been used.

Prevention of candidiasis in bone marrow transplant: 400 mg once daily. In patients who are anticipated to have severe granulocytopenia (< 500 neutrophils/mm^3), start fluconazole prophylaxis several days before the anticipated onset of neutropenia, and continue for 7 days after the neutrophil count rises above 1000 cells/mm^3.

Cryptococcal meningitis: 400 mg on the first day, followed by 200 mg once daily. A dosage of 400 mg once daily may be used, based on the patient's response to therapy. The duration of treatment for initial therapy of cryptococcal meningitis is 10 to 12 weeks after the cerebrospinal fluid becomes culture negative. The dosage of fluconazole for suppression of relapse of cryptococcal meningitis in patients with AIDS is 200 mg once daily.

Children –

Fluconazole Dosage in Children	
Pediatric Patients	Adults
3 mg/kg	100 mg
6 mg/kg	200 mg
12 mg/kg[1]	400 mg

[1] Some older children may have clearances similar to that of adults. Absolute doses > 600 mg/day are not recommended.

Based on the prolonged half-life seen in premature newborns (gestational age 26 to 29 weeks), these children, in the first 2 weeks of life, should receive the same dosage (mg/kg) as older children, but administered every 72 hours. After the first 2 weeks, dose these children once daily.

Oropharyngeal candidiasis: The recommended dosage is 6 mg/kg on the first day, followed by 3 mg/kg once daily. Administer treatment for at least 2 weeks.

Esophageal candidiasis: The recommended dosage is 6 mg/kg on the first day followed by 3 mg/kg once daily. Doses up to 12 mg/kg/day may be used based on medical judgment of the patient's response to therapy. Treat patients with esophageal candidiasis for a minimum of 3 weeks and for at least 2 weeks following the resolution of symptoms.

Systemic Candida infections: For the treatment of candidemia and disseminated *Candida* infections, daily doses of 6 to 12 mg/kg/day have been used.

Cryptococcal meningitis: The recommended dosage is 12 mg/kg on the first day, followed by 6 mg/kg once daily. A dosage of 12 mg/kg once daily may be used. The recommended duration of treatment for initial therapy of cryptococcal meningitis is 10 to 12 weeks after the CSF becomes culture negative. For suppression of relapse of cryptococcal meningitis in children with AIDS, the recommended dose is 6 mg/kg once daily.

Renal function impairment: There is no need to adjust single dose therapy for vaginal candidiasis in patients with impaired renal function. In patients with impaired renal function who will receive multiple doses, give an initial loading dose of 50 to 400 mg. After the loading dose, base the daily dose on the following table:

| Fluconazole Dose in Impaired Renal Function ||
Ccr (mL/min)	Percent of recommended dose
> 50	100%
≤ 50	50%
Patients receiving regular hemodialysis	One recommended dose after each dialysis

Injection: Fluconazole injection has been used safely for up to 14 days of IV therapy. Administer the IV infusion of fluconazole at a maximum rate of ≈ 200 mg/hr, given as a continuous infusion. Fluconazole injections are intended only for IV administration.

Actions

Pharmacology: Fluconazole, a synthetic broad spectrum bis-triazole antifungal agent, is a highly selective inhibitor of fungal cytochrome P450 and sterol C-14 alpha-demethylation.

Pharmacokinetics:

Absorption/Distribution – The pharmacokinetic properties of fluconazole are similar following administration by the IV or oral routes. In healthy volunteers, the bio-availability of oral fluconazole is > 90% compared with IV administration.

Peak plasma concentrations (C_{max}) in fasted healthy volunteers occur between 1 and 2 hours with a terminal plasma elimination half-life of ≈ 30 hours (range, 20 to 50 hours) after oral administration.

Steady-state concentrations are reached within 5 to 10 days following oral doses of 50 to 400 mg given once daily. The apparent volume of distribution approximates that of total body water. Plasma protein binding is low (11% to 12%).

Metabolism/Excretion – Fluconazole is cleared primarily by renal excretion, with ≈ 80% of the dose appearing in the urine unchanged, ≈ 11% as metabolites. The dose may need to be reduced in patients with impaired renal function. A 3-hour hemodialysis session decreases plasma concentrations by ≈ 50%.

Contraindications

Hypersensitivity to fluconazole or to any excipients in the product. There is no information regarding cross-hypersensitivity between fluconazole and other azole antifungal agents; use with caution in patients with hypersensitivity to other azoles.

Warnings

Hepatic injury: Fluconazole has been associated with rare cases of serious hepatic toxicity. Instances of fatal hepatic reactions occurred primarily in patients with serious underlying medical conditions (predominantly AIDS or malignancy) and often while taking multiple concomitant medications.

Anaphylaxis: In rare cases, anaphylaxis has occurred.

Dermatologic changes: Patients have rarely developed exfoliative skin disorders during treatment with fluconazole.

Pregnancy: Category C.

Lactation: The use of fluconazole in nursing mothers is not recommended.

Children: Efficacy has not been established in children < 6 months of age.

Precautions

Single-dose use: Weigh the convenience and efficacy of the single dose regimen for treatment of vaginal yeast infections against the acceptability of a higher incidence of adverse reactions with fluconazole (26%) vs intravaginal agents (16%).

Drug Interactions

Fluconazole is a potent inhibitor of the cytochrome P450 3A4 enzyme system. Coadministration of fluconazole with other drugs metabolized by the same enzyme system may result in increased plasma concentrations of the drugs, which could increase or prolong therapeutic and adverse effects. Unless otherwise specified, dosage adjustment may be necessary.

Drugs that may affect fluconazole include cimetidine, hydrochlorothiazide, and rifampin. Drugs that may be affected by fluconazole include oral contraceptives, cyclosporine, phenytoin, theophylline, sulfonylureas, warfarin, alfentanil, zolpidem, vinca alkaloids, tacrolimus, nisoldipine, benzodiazepines, corticosteroids, buspirone, tricyclic antidepressants, losartan, and zidovudine.

Adverse Reactions

Adverse reactions occurring in ≥ 3% of patients include headache, nausea, abdominal pain, and diarrhea.

ITRACONAZOLE

Capsules: 100 mg (Rx)	*Sporanox* (Janssen-Ortho)
Oral solution: 10 mg/mL (Rx)	*Sporanox* (Janssen-Ortho)
Injection: 10 mg/mL (Rx)	*Sporanox* (Ortho Biotech)

Warning:

CHF: Do not administer itraconazole for the treatment of onychomycosis or dermatomycoses in patients with evidence of cardiac dysfunction, such as CHF or a history of CHF. Discontinue if signs and symptoms of CHF occur during treatment of onychomycosis or dermatomycoses. If signs and symptoms of CHF occur during treatment for more serious fungal infections involving other parts of the body, reassess continued use of itraconazole.

Drug interactions: Coadministration of pimozide, dofetilide, or quinidine with itraconazole is contraindicated. Itraconazole is a potent inhibitor of the cytochrome P450 3A4 isoenzyme system and may raise plasma concentrations of drugs metabolized by this pathway. Serious cardiovascular events, including QT prolongation, torsades de pointes, ventricular tachycardia, cardiac arrest, or sudden death have occurred in patients taking itraconazole concomitantly with cisapride, pimozide, or quinidine, which are inhibitors of the cytochrome P450 3A4 system.

Indications

Capsules: For treatment of the following fungal infections in normal, predisposed, or immunocompromised patients:

- Dermatomycoses caused by tinea corporis, tinea cruris, tinea pedis, and pityriasis versicolor when oral therapy is considered appropriate
- Onychomycosis
- Invasive and noninvasive pulmonary aspergillosis
- Oral and oral/esophageal candidiasis
- Chronic pulmonary histoplasmosis
- Cutaneous and lymphatic sporotrichosis
- Paracoccidioidomycosis
- Chromomycosis
- Blastomycosis

Oral solution:

Candidiasis – Treatment of oral or esophageal candidiasis in adult HIV-positive or other immunocompromised patients.

Injection: For empiric therapy of febrile neutropenic patients with suspected fungal infections.

For treatment of the following fungal infections in immunocompromised and nonimmunocompromised patients:

- Blastomycosis, pulmonary and extrapulmonary
- Histoplasmosis, including chronic cavitary pulmonary disease and disseminated, nonmeningeal histoplasmosis
- Aspergillosis, pulmonary and extrapulmonary, in patients who are intolerant

of or refractory to amphotericin B therapy.

Unlabeled uses: Itraconazole appears to be beneficial in the treatment of the following conditions. Dosage is generally 50 to 400 mg/day; duration of therapy varies from 1 day to ≥ 6 months depending on the condition and mycological response.

Itraconazole Unlabeled Uses		
Superficial mycoses	Systemic mycoses	Miscellaneous
Dermatophytoses Tinea capitis Tinea manuum Tinea pedis Sebopsoriasis	Cryptococcal infections Disseminated Meningitis Dimorphic infections Coccidioidomycosis	Alternariosis Fungal keratitis Leishmaniasis, cutaneous Zygomycosis

Administration and Dosage

Do not use capsules and oral solution interchangeably.

Capsules: Taking immediately after a full meal is essential to ensure maximal absorption. Capsules must be swallowed whole.

Blastomycosis/Chronic pulmonary histoplasmosis – The recommended dose is 200 mg once daily. If there is no obvious improvement or there is evidence of progressive fungal disease, increase the dose in 100 mg increments to a maximum of 400 mg daily. Give doses > 200 mg/day in 2 divided doses.

Continue treatment for a minimum of 3 months and until clinical parameters and laboratory tests indicate that the active fungal infection has subsided. An inadequate period of treatment may lead to recurrence of active infection.

Oral and oral/esophageal candidiasis – The recommended dose is 100 mg daily for 2 weeks. Increase the dose to 200 mg/day in patients with AIDS and neutropenic patients. In patients with oral/esophageal candidiasis, treatment should last 4 weeks.

Other systemic mycoses –

Other Systemic Mycoses Dose and Duration of Therapy		
Indication	Dose	Median duration (months)
Aspergillosis		
Pulmonary	200 mg QD	3 to 4
Invasive pulmonary	200 mg BID	3 to 4
Sporotrichosis	100 mg QD	3
Paracoccidioidomycosis	100 mg QD	6
Chromomycosis		
Caused by *Fonsecaea pedrosoi*	200 mg QD	6
Caused by *Cladosporium carrionii*	100 mg QD	3

Dermatomycoses –

  Standard dosages:

    Tinea corporis/tinea cruris – Recommended dose is 100 mg once daily for 14 consecutive days.

    Tinea pedis – Recommended dose is 100 mg once daily for 28 consecutive days.

    Pityriasis versicolor – Recommended dose is 200 mg once daily for 7 consecutive days.

  Alternative dosages: Shorter dosing schedules have also been found to be effective in the treatment of tinea corporis/tinea cruris and tinea pedis. The shorter dosages are:

    Tinea corporis/tinea cruris – 200 mg once daily for 7 consecutive days.

    Tinea pedis – 200 mg BID for 7 consecutive days.

    Equivalency between standard and alternative dosages was not established. Patients with chronic recalcitrant tinea pedis may benefit from the standard dosage of a lower daily dose (100 mg) for a longer period of time (4 weeks).

  Onychomycosis – A 1-week treatment course consists of 200 mg twice daily for 7 days. Treatment with 2 one-week courses is recommended for fingernail infections and 3 one-week courses for toenail infections. The one-week courses are always separated by a 3-week drug-free interval. Clinical response will become evident as the nail regrows, following discontinuation of the treatment.

Itraconazole Onychomycosis Dosing Schedule									
	Pulse 1[1]				Pulse 2[1]				Pulse 3[1]
Site of onychomycosis	Week 1	Week 2	Week 3	Week 4	Week 5	Week 6	Week 7	Week 8	Week 9
Toenails with/ without fingernail involvement	200 mg BID for 7 days	Itraconazole-free weeks			200 mg BID for 7 days	Itraconazole-free weeks			200 mg BID for 7 days
Fingernails only	200 mg BID for 7 days	Itraconazole-free weeks			200 mg BID for 7 days				

[1] A pulse = 1 week course of treatment.

Oral solution: For optimal absorption, do not take with food. Swish in oral cavity and swallow. Do not rinse after swallowing. Discard unused product 3 months after opening.

Oropharyngeal candidiasis – The recommended dosage for oropharyngeal candidiasis is 200 mg (20 mL) daily in single or divided doses for 1 to 2 weeks to decrease likelihood of relapse.

Esophageal candidiasis – The recommended dosage for esophageal candidiasis is 100 mg (10 mL) daily for a minimum of 3 weeks. Continue treatment for 2 weeks following resolution of symptoms. Doses ≤ 200 mg (20 mL) per day may be used based on medical judgement of the patient's response to therapy.

Injection: Use only the components provided in the kit. Do not substitute.

Admixture incompatibility – The compatibility of itraconazole injection with diluents other than 0.9% Sodium Chloride Injection (Normal Saline) is not known. Do not dilute with 5% Dextrose Injection or with Lactated Ringer's Injection alone or in combination with any other diluent. Not for IV bolus injection.

Preparation/Administration – Use only a dedicated infusion line for administration of itraconazole injection. Do not introduce concomitant medication in the same bag or through the same line used for itraconazole injection. Other medications may be administered after flushing the line/catheter with 0.9% Sodium Chloride Injection.

Empiric therapy in febrile, neutropenic patients with suspected fungal infections (ETFN) – The recommended dose of itraconazole injection is 200 mg twice daily for 4 doses, followed by 200 mg once daily for up to 14 days. Infuse each IV dose over 1 hour. Continue treatment with itraconazole oral solution 200 mg (20 mL) twice daily until resolution of clinically significant neutropenia. The safety and efficacy of itraconazole use exceeding 28 days in ETFN is not known.

Blastomycosis, histoplasmosis, and aspergillosis – 200 mg IV twice daily for 4 doses, followed by 200 mg/day. Infuse each IV dose over 1 hour.

For the treatment of blastomycosis, histoplasmosis, and aspergillosis, itraconazole can be given as oral capsules or IV. The safety and efficacy of the injection administered for > 14 days are not known.

Continue total itraconazole therapy (injection followed by capsules) for a minimum of 3 months and until clinical parameters and laboratory tests indicate that the active fungal infection has subsided. An inadequate period of treatment may lead to recurrence of active infection.

Renal function impairment: Do not use in patients with Ccr < 30 mL/min.

Actions

Pharmacology: Itraconazole is a synthetic triazole antifungal agent. In vitro, itraconazole inhibits the cytochrome P450-dependent synthesis of ergosterol, which is a vital component of fungal cell membranes.

Pharmacokinetics:

Absorption/Distribution –

Oral solution/injection: The oral bioavailability is maximal when itraconazole oral solution is taken without food. Steady state is reached after 1 to 2 weeks during chronic administration. Peak plasma levels are observed 2 hours (fasting) to 5 hours (with food) following oral administration. Steady-state plasma concentrations are ≈ 25% lower when the oral solution is taken with food.

Plasma protein binding is 99.8%. It is extensively distributed into tissues that are prone to fungal invasion. Concentrations in the lung, kidney, liver, bone, stomach, spleen, and muscle were found to be 2 to 3 times higher than the corresponding plasma concentration. Following IV administration, the volume of distribution averaged 796 ± 185 L.

Metabolism/Excretion – Itraconazole is extensively metabolized by the cytochrome P450 3A4 to several metabolites including the major metabolite hydroxyitraconazole. Fecal excretion of the parent drug varies between 3% and 18% of the dose. Renal excretion of the parent drug is < 0.03% of the dose. Itraconazole is not removed by hemodialysis.

The estimated mean half-life at steady-state of itraconazole after IV infusion was 35.4 hours.

Contraindications

CHF: Do not administer itraconazole capsules for the treatment of onychomycosis or dermatomycoses in patients with evidence of ventricular dysfunction such as CHF or a history of CHF.

Coadministration of pimozide, quinidine, dofetilide, cisapride, triazolam, or oral midazolam (see Warning Box and Drug Interactions); hypersensitivity to the drug or its excipients (there is no information regarding cross-hypersensitivity between itraconazole and other azole antifungal agents; use caution in prescribing to patients with hypersensitivity to other azoles); HMG-CoA reductase inhibitors metabolized by the CYP3A4 enzyme system (eg, lovastatin, simvastatin) during itraconazole therapy (see Drug Interactions); treatment of onychomycosis in pregnant women or in women contemplating pregnancy.

Warnings

Cardiac dysrhythmias: Life-threatening cardiac dysrhythmias or sudden death have occurred in patients using pimozide or quinidine concomitantly with itraconazole or other CYP3A4 inhibitors. Concomitant administration of these drugs with itraconazole is contraindicated.

CHF: Do not administer itraconazole for the treatment of onychomycosis or dermatomycoses in patients with evidence of ventricular dysfunction such as CHF or a history of CHF. Do not use itraconazole capsules for other indications in patients with evidence of ventricular dysfunction unless the benefit clearly outweighs the risk.

Itraconazole has been shown to have a negative inotropic effect, and has been associated with reports of CHF. Do not use itraconazole in patients with CHF or with a history of CHF unless the benefit clearly outweighs the risk. This individual benefit/risk assessment should take into consideration factors such as the severity of the indication, the dosing regimen, and the individual risk factors for CHF.

Hepatotoxicity: Itraconazole has been associated with rare cases of serious hepatotoxicity, including liver failure and death. Some of these cases had neither pre-existing liver disease, nor a serious underlying medical condition. If liver function tests are abnormal, discontinue treatment. In patients with raised liver enzymes or an active liver disease or who have experienced liver toxicity with other drugs, do not start treatment unless the expected benefit exceeds the risk of hepatic injury. In such cases, liver enzyme monitoring is necessary.

Bioequivalency: Do not use itraconazole capsules and oral solution interchangeably. Drug exposure is greater with the oral solution than with the capsules when the same dose of drug is given. Additionally, the topical effects of mucosal exposure may be different between the 2 formulations.

AIDS and neutropenic patients: Studies with itraconazole capsules in neutropenic and AIDS patients have indicated that itraconazole plasma concentrations are lower than those in healthy subjects (particularly in those patients who are achlorhydric). However, the bioavailability of itraconazole oral solution, when tested in AIDS patients, was found satisfactory and not altered by the stage of HIV infection.

Renal function impairment: Do not use itraconazole injection in patients with severe renal dysfunction (Ccr < 30 mL/min) because of prolonged elimination of hydroxypropyl-β-cyclodextrin.

Hepatic function impairment: Itraconazole is predominantly metabolized in the liver. The terminal half-life of itraconazole in cirrhotic patients is somewhat prolonged. A decrease in the oral bioavailability of itraconazole from itraconazole capsules was observed in cirrhotic patients; this can also be expected with the oral solution. It is advisable to monitor itraconazole plasma concentrations and to adapt the dose when necessary. In patients with raised liver enzymes or an active liver disease or who have experienced liver toxicity with other drugs, do not start treatment unless the expected benefit exceeds the risk of hepatic injury. In such cases, liver enzyme monitoring is necessary.

Elderly:
 Oral solution – Since clinical data on the use of itraconazole oral solution in elderly patients is limited, it is advised to use the oral solution in these patients only if the potential benefit outweighs the potential risks.

Pregnancy: Category C.

Lactation: Itraconazole is excreted in breast milk.

Children: Safety and efficacy have not been established. A small number of patients from 3 to 16 years of age have been treated with 100 mg/day for systemic fungal infections and no serious adverse effects have been reported.

Precautions
Monitoring: Monitor plasma levels 3 to 4 hours after dosing in patients requiring treatment for > 1 month, in patients with systemic mycoses who have factors predisposing to poor absorption (eg, achlorhydria, renal insufficiency, neutropenia, AIDS) or in those who are taking drugs that may alter itraconazole absorption or metabolism (eg, rifampicin, phenytoin).

 Monitor hepatic function periodically in all patients receiving continuous treatment for > 1 month or when a patient develops signs or symptoms suggestive of hepatitis (eg, anorexia, nausea, vomiting, fatigue, abdominal pain, dark urine). If tests are abnormal, terminate treatment.

 Monitor serum potassium in patients at risk during high-dose itraconazole therapy.

Neuropathy: Discontinue if neuropathy occurs that may be attributable to itraconazole capsules or oral solution.

Decreased gastric acidity: Absorption of itraconazole from the capsules is impaired when gastric acidity is decreased. In patients also receiving acid-neutralizing medicines (eg, aluminum hydroxide), these should be given at least 2 hours after the intake of itraconazole capsules. In patients with achlorhydria, such as certain AIDS patients on acid secretion suppressors (eg, H_2 antagonists, proton pump inhibitors), it is advisable to give itraconazole capsules with a cola beverage.

Drug Interactions
Both itraconazole and its major metabolite, hydroxyitraconazole, are inhibitors of the cytochrome P450 3A4 enzyme system. Coadministration of itraconazole and drugs primarily metabolized by the cytochrome P450 3A4 enzyme system may result in increased plasma concentrations of the drugs that could increase or prolong both therapeutic and adverse effects.

Drugs that may affect itraconazole include antacids, didanosine, H_2 antagonists, macrolide antibiotics, phenytoin, protease inhibitors, proton pump inhibitors, and rifamycins.

Drugs that may be affected by itraconazole include benzodiazepines, buspirone, calcium blockers, cyclosporine, digoxin, tacrolimus, warfarin, alfentanil, zolpidem, vinca alkaloids, corticosteroids, protease inhibitors, HMG-CoA reductase inhibitors, triazolam, oral midazolam, alprazolam, carbamazepine, dofetilide, haloperidol, hydantoins (phenytoin), pimozide, polyenes, amphotericin B, quinidine, toltero-dine, hypoglycemic agents, and rifamycins.

Adverse Reactions

Adverse reactions occurring in ≥ 3% of patients include the following: Nausea, vom-iting, diarrhea, rash, hypokalemia, bilirubinemia, increased ALT.

TERBINAFINE HCl

Tablets: 250 mg (*Rx*)   *Lamisil* (Novartis)

> **Warning:**
> Rare cases of hepatic failure, some leading to death or liver transplant, have
> occurred with the use of terbinafine for the treatment of onychomycosis in indi-
> viduals with and without pre-existing liver disease. In the majority of liver cases
> reported in association with terbinafine use, the patients had serious underlying
> systemic conditions and an uncertain causal relationship with terbinafine. Ter-
> binafine is not recommended for patients with chronic or active liver disease.
> Before prescribing terbinafine, assess pre-existing liver disease. Hepatotoxicity
> may occur in patients with and without preexisting liver disease. Pretreatment
> serum transaminase (ALT and AST) tests are advised for all patients before tak-
> ing terbinafine.

Indications

Onychomycosis: Treatment of onychomycosis of the toenail or fingernail caused by der-matopytes.

Administration and Dosage

Onychomycosis:

    Fingernail – 250 mg/day for 6 weeks.

    Toenail – 250 mg/day for 12 weeks.

The optimal clinical effect is seen some months after mycological cure and ces-sation of treatment. This is related to the period required for outgrowth of healthy nail.

Actions

Pharmacology: Terbinafine is a synthetic allylamine derivative that exerts its antifungal effect by inhibiting squalene epoxidase, a key enzyme in sterol biosynthesis in fungi. This action results in a deficiency in ergosterol and a corresponding accumula-tion of squalene within the fungal cell and causes fungal cell death.

Pharmacokinetics: Terbinafine is well absorbed (> 70%). Bioavailability is ≈ 40%. Peak plasma concentrations of 1 mcg/mL appear ≤ 2 hours after a single 250 mg dose, the AUC is ≈ 4.56 mcg•hr/mL.

Prior to excretion, terbinafine is extensively metabolized. No metabolites have been identified that have antifungal activity similar to terbinafine. Approximately 70% of the administered dose is eliminated in the urine.

Contraindications

Hypersensitivity to terbinafine or any component of the product.

Warnings

Hepatic failure: Rare cases of liver failure, some leading to death or liver transplant, have occurred with the use of terbinafine for the treatment of onychomycosis in individu-als with and without pre-existing liver disease.

The severity of hepatic events or their outcome may be worse in patients with active or chronic liver disease. Discontinue treatment with terbinafine if biochemi-cal or clinical evidence of liver injury develops.

Ophthalmic: Changes in the ocular lens and retina have been reported following the use of terbinafine.

Neutropenia: Isolated cases of severe neutropenia have been reported but were reversible with discontinuation of treatment with or without supportive therapy. If the neutrophil count is ≤ 1000 cells/mm³, discontinue treatment and start supportive management.

Dermatologic: There have been isolated reports of serious skin reactions (eg, Stevens-Johnson syndrome, toxic epidermal necrolysis).

Renal/Hepatic function impairment: In patients with renal impairment (Ccr ≤ 50 mL/min) or chronic or active liver disease, the use of terbinafine is not recommended

Pregnancy: Category B.

Lactation: After oral administration, terbinafine is present in the breast milk of nursing mothers. Use of terbinafine tablets is not recommended in nursing mothers.

Children: Safety and efficacy in children have not been established.

Precautions

Monitoring:

Immunodeficiency – Monitor CBC in patients receiving treatment for > 6 weeks.

Hepatic – Pretreatment serum transaminase (ALT and AST) tests are advised for all patients before taking terbinafine. Warn patients to immediately report to their physician any symptoms of persistent nausea, anorexia, fatigue, vomiting, right upper abdominal pain or jaundice, dark urine, or pale stools. Patients with these symptoms should discontinue taking oral terbinafine, and the patient's liver function should be immediately evaluated.

Drug Interactions

Drugs that may interact with terbinafine include the following: Cimetidine, rifampin, terfenadine, caffeine, dextromethorphan, cyclosporine.

Adverse Reactions

Adverse reactions occurring in ≥ 3% of patients include the following: Diarrhea, dyspepsia, rash, liver enzyme abnormalities, headache.

SULFONAMIDES

SULFADIAZINE
Tablets: 500 mg (*Rx*)　　　　　　　　　Various, *Sulfadiazine* (Stanley)

SULFISOXAZOLE
Tablets: 500 mg (*Rx*)　　　　　　　　　Various, *Gantrisin* (Roche)

SULFAMETHOXAZOLE
Tablets: 500 mg (*Rx*)　　　　　　　　　Various, *Gantanol* (Roche), *Urobak* (Shionogi)
Oral suspension: 500 mg/5 mL (*Rx*)　　　*Gantanol* (Roche)

SULFAMETHIZOLE
Tablets: 500 mg (*Rx*)　　　　　　　　　*Thiosulfil Forte* (Wyeth-Ayerst)

Indications

Sulfonamide Indications					
✔ – Labeled Indications	Multiple sulfas	Sulfadiazine	Sulfamethizole	Sulfamethoxazole	Sulfisoxazole
Chancroid	✔	✔		✔	✔
Inclusion conjunctivitis	✔	✔		✔	✔
Malaria[1]	✔	✔		✔	✔
Meningitis, *Haemophilus influenzae*[2]	✔	✔			✔
Meningitis, meningococcal[3]	✔	✔		✔	✔
Nocardiosis	✔	✔		✔	✔
Otitis media, acute[4]	✔	✔		✔	✔
Rheumatic fever		✔			
Rheumatoid arthritis					
Toxoplasmosis[5]	✔	✔		✔	✔
Trachoma	✔	✔		✔	✔
Urinary tract infections[6] (pyelonephritis, cystitis)	✔	✔	✔	✔	✔

[1] As adjunctive therapy because of chloroquine-resistant strains of *Plasmodium falciparum*.
[2] As adjunctive therapy with parenteral streptomycin.
[3] When the organism is susceptible and for prophylaxis when sulfonamide-sensitive group A strains prevail.
[4] Caused by *H. influenzae* when used with penicillin or erythromycin.
[5] As adjunctive therapy with pyrimethamine.
[6] In the absence of obstructive uropathy or foreign bodies, when caused by *Escherichia coli*, *Klebsiella-Enterobacter*, *Staphylococcus aureus*, *Proteus mirabilis*, and *Proteus vulgaris*.

Administration and Dosage

CDC-recommended treatment schedules for sexually transmitted diseases:

Lymphogranuloma venereum – As an alternative regimen to doxycycline, sulfisoxazole 500 mg 4 times/day for 21 days or equivalent sulfonamide course.

Treatment of uncomplicated urethral, endocervical, or rectal Chlamydia trachomatic infections – As an alternative regimen to doxycycline or tetracycline (or if erythromycin is not tolerated), sulfisoxazole 500 mg 4 times/day for 10 days or equivalent sulfonamide course.

SULFADIAZINE:

Adults – Loading dose - 2 to 4 g. Maintenance dose - 4 to 8 g/day in 4 to 6 divided doses.

Children (> 2 months of age) –
Loading dose: 75 mg/kg (or 2 g/m^2).
Maintenance dose: 120 to 150 mg/kg/day (4 g/m^2/day) in 4 to 6 divided doses.
Maximum dose: 6 g/day.

Infants (< 2 months of age) – Contraindicated, except as adjunctive therapy with pyrimethamine in the treatment of congenital toxoplasmosis.

Loading dose – 75 to 100 mg/kg.

Maintenance dose – 100 to 150 mg/kg/day in 4 divided doses.

Other recommended doses for toxoplasmosis (for 3 to 4 weeks) include –

Infants (< 2 months of age): 25 mg/kg/dose 4 times daily.

Children (> 2 months of age): 25 to 50 mg/kg/dose 4 times daily.

Prevention of recurrent attacks of rheumatic fever – Prevention of recurrent attacks of rheumatic fever (not for initial treatment of streptococcal infections): Patients > 30 kg (> 66 lbs) - 1 g/day; < 30 kg (< 66 lbs) - 0.5 g/day.

SULFISOXAZOLE:

Loading dose – 2 to 4 g.

Maintenance dose: 4 to 8 g/day in 4 to 6 divided doses. Although recommended, a loading dose is unnecessary because sulfisoxazole is rapidly absorbed and appears in high concentrations in the urine.

Children and infants (> 2 months of age) –

Initial dose: 75 mg/kg.

Maintenance dose: 120 to 150 mg/kg/day (4 g/m^2/day) in 4 to 6 divided doses (max, 6 g/day).

SULFAMETHOXAZOLE:

Adults –

Mild to moderate infections: 2 g initially; maintenance dose is 1 g morning and evening therafter.

Severe infections: 2 g initially, then 1 g 3 times daily.

Children and infants (> 2 months of age) – Initially, 50 to 60 mg/kg; maintenance dose is 25 to 30 mg/kg morning and evening. Do not exceed 75 mg/kg/day.

Another recommended dose is 50 to 60 mg/kg/day divided every 12 hours, not to exceed 3 g/24 hours.

SULFAMETHIZOLE:

Adults – 0.5 to 1 g 3 or 4 times daily.

Children and infants (> 2 months of age) – 30 to 45 mg/kg/day in 4 divided doses.

Actions

Pharmacology: Sulfonamides exert their bacteriostatic action by competitive antagonism of para-aminobenzoic acid (PABA), an essential component in folic acid synthesis.

Pharmacokinetics:

Absorption/Distribution – The oral sulfonamides are readily absorbed from the GI tract. Approximately 70% to 100% of an oral dose is absorbed. Sulfonamides are bound to plasma proteins in varying degrees.

Metabolism – Metabolism occurs in the liver by conjugation, acetylation, and other metabolic pathways to inactive metabolites.

Excretion – Renal excretion is mainly by glomerular filtration; tubular reabsorption occurs in varying degrees.

Microbiology: Sulfonamides have a broad antibacterial spectrum that includes grampositive and gram-negative organisms.

Contraindications

Hypersensitivity to sulfonamides or chemically related drugs (eg, sulfonylureas, thiazide and loop diuretics, carbonic anhydrase inhibitors, sunscreens with PABA, local anesthetics); pregnancy at term; lactation; infants < 2 months of age (except in congenital toxoplasmosis as adjunct with pyrimethamine); porphyria; salicylate hypersensitivity.

Warnings

Group A beta-hemolytic streptococcal infections: Do not use for treatment of these infections.

Severe reactions: Severe reactions including deaths caused by sulfonamides have been associated with hypersensitivity reactions, agranulocytosis, aplastic anemia, other blood dyscrasias, and renal and hepatic damage. Irreversible neuromuscular and CNS changes and fibrosing alveolitis may occur.

Porphyria: In patients with porphyria, these drugs have precipitated an acute attack.

Photosensitivity: Photosensitization (photoallergy or phototoxicity) may occur.

Renal/Hepatic function impairment: Use with caution. The frequency of renal complications is considerably lower in patients receiving the more soluble sulfonamides (sulfisoxazole and sulfamethizole).

Pregnancy: Category B; Category D near term. Significant levels may persist in the neonate if these drugs are given near term; jaundice, hemolytic anemia, and kernicterus may occur. Do not use at term.

Lactation: According to the American Academy of Pediatrics, breastfeeding and sulfonamide use are compatible. However, do not nurse premature infants or those with hyperbilirubinemia or G-6-PD deficiency.

Children: Do not use in infants < 2 months of age (except for congenital toxoplasmosis as adjunctive therapy with pyrimethamine).

Precautions

Allergy or asthma: Give with caution to patients with severe allergy or bronchial asthma.

Hemolytic anemia: Hemolytic anemia, frequently dose-related, may occur in G-6-PD deficient individuals.

Drug Interactions

Drugs that may interact with sulfonamides include oral anticoagulants, cyclosporine, hydantoins, methotrexate, and sulfonylureas.

Drugs that may interact with sulfisoxazole include barbiturate anesthetics.

Drug/Lab test interactions: Sulfonamides may produce false-positive **urinary glucose tests** when performed by Benedict's method. Sulfisoxazole may interfere with the **Urobilistix test** and may produce false-positive results with sulfosalicylic acid tests for urinary protein.

Adverse Reactions

Agranulocytosis; aplastic anemia; thrombocytopenia; leukopenia; hemolytic anemia; purpura; hypoprothrombinemia; cyanosis; methemoglobinemia; megaloblastic (macrocytic) anemia; Stevens-Johnson type erythema multiforme; generalized skin eruptions; epidermal necrolysis; urticaria; serum sickness; pruritus; exfoliative dermatitis; anaphylactoid reactions; periorbital edema; nausea; emesis; abdominal pains; diarrhea; bloody diarrhea; anorexia; pancreatitis; stomatitis; hepatitis; pseudomembranous enterocolitis; glossitis; headache; peripheral neuropathy; mental depression; convulsions; ataxia; hallucinations; tinnitus; vertigo; insomnia; hearing loss; drowsiness; apathy; crystalluria; hematuria; proteinuria; elevated creatinine; drug fever; chills; pyrexia; alopecia; arthralgia; myalgia.

ANTITUBERCULOSIS DRUGS

Antituberculosis drugs have been described in terms of the following 3 areas of activity: Bactericidal activity, sterilizing activity, and drug resistance prevention.

Standard treatment regimens are divided into the following 2 phases: An initial phase, during which agents are used to kill rapidly multiplying populations of Mycobacterium tuberculosis and to prevent the emergence of drug resistance, followed by a continuation phase, during which sterilizing drugs kill the intermittently dividing populations.

The initial phase of the regimen must contain ≥ 3 of the following drugs: Isoniazid, rifampin, and pyrazinamide, along with either ethambutol or streptomycin if the local resistance pattern to isoniazid is not documented or is > 4%.

Directly observed therapy (DOT): Adherence to the treatment regimen can be achieved by DOT, the "gold standard." The health care provider watches the patient swallow each dose of medication. This allows for monitoring of the number of doses that an individual has taken.

Recommended Drugs for the Treatment of Tuberculosis in Children and Adults[1]					
	Daily dose[2]		Maximum daily dose in children and adults	Twice weekly dose	
Drug	Children	Adults		Children	Adults
Initial treatment					
Isoniazid	10 to 20 mg/kg PO or IM	5 mg/kg PO or IM	300 mg	20 to 40 mg/kg max. 900 mg	15 mg/kg max. 900 mg
Rifampin	10 to 20 mg/kg PO	10 mg/kg PO	600 mg	10 to 20 mg/kg max. 600 mg	10 mg/kg max. 600 mg
Pyrazinamide	15 to 30 mg/kg PO	15 to 30 mg/kg PO	2 g	50 to 70 mg/kg	50 to 70 mg/kg
Streptomycin	20 to 40 mg/kg IM	15 mg/kg IM	1 g[3]	25 to 30 mg/kg IM	25 to 30 mg/kg IM
Ethambutol	15 to 25 mg/kg PO	15 to 25 mg/kg PO	2.5 g	50 mg/kg	50 mg/kg
Second-line treatment					
Cycloserine	10 to 20 mg/kg PO	15 to 20 mg/kg PO	1 g	—	—
Ethionamide	15 to 20 mg/kg PO	15 to 20 mg/kg PO	1 g	—	—
Capreomycin	15 to 30 mg/kg IM	15 to 30 mg/kg IM	1 g	—	—
Kanamycin	15 to 20 mg/kg IM or IV	15 to 30 mg/kg IM or IV	1 g	—	—
Ciprofloxacin	—	500 to 750 mg PO BID	750 mg	—	—
Ofloxacin	—	600 to 800 mg/day PO	800 mg	—	—
Levofloxacin	—	500 to 750 mg/day PO	750 mg	—	—
Sparfloxacin	—	200 mg/day PO	200 mg	—	—
P-amino-salicylic acid	150 to 360 mg/kg PO	150 mg/kg to 12 g PO	12 g	—	—
Rifabutin	—	300 mg/day PO	300 mg	—	—

[1] For detailed dosing information and frequency, see individual monographs.
[2] Doses based on weight. Adjust as weight changes.
[3] In people > 60 years of age, limit the daily dose of streptomycin to 10 mg/kg with a maximum dose of 750 mg.

Treatment regimens: The CDC recommends at least a 3-drug regimen with rifampin, isoniazid, and pyrazinamide for a minimum of 2 months, followed by rifampin and isoniazid for 4 months in areas with a low incidence of tuberculosis. Administer streptomycin or ethambutol for the first 2 months in areas with a high incidence of tuberculosis.

Retreatment: Retreatment is necessary when treatment fails because of noncompliance or inadequate drug treatment. Retreatment regimens include ≥ 4 drugs; however, depending on disease progression and the bacteriostatic or bactericidal activity of the drug, ≤ 7 drugs can be used. Retreatment drug regimens most commonly include the second-line agents of ethionamide, aminosalicylic acid, cycloserine, and capreomycin, as well as ofloxacin and ciprofloxacin.

Individualize treatment on the basis of the susceptibility pattern of the infecting organism when retreating patients known to be infected with drug-resistant isolates. Include in this regimen ≥ 3 new drugs to which the organism is susceptible. Continue therapy until sputum cultures convert to negative, and then continue therapy for an additional 12 months with 2 drugs. Treatment may be continued for 24 months after sputum culture conversion.

HIV: The initial phase of a 6-month tuberculosis regimen consists of isoniazid, rifabutin, pyrazinamide, and ethambutol for patients receiving therapy with protease inhibitors or nonnucleoside reverse transcriptase inhibitors. These drugs are administered a) daily for at least the first 2 weeks, followed by twice weekly dosing for 6 weeks or b) daily for 8 weeks to complete the 2-month induction phase. The second phase of treatment consists of rifabutin and isoniazid administered twice weekly or daily for 4 months.

Do not use tuberculosis regimens consisting of isoniazid, ethambutol, and pyrazinamide (ie, 3-drug regimens that do not contain a rifamycin, an aminoglycoside [eg, streptomycin, amikacin, kanamycin], or capreomycin) for the treatment of patients with HIV-related tuberculosis. The minimum duration of therapy is 18 months (or 12 months after documented culture conversion) if these regimens are used for the treatment of tuberculosis.

Administer pyridoxine (vitamin B_6) 25 to 50 mg daily or 50 to 100 mg twice weekly to all HIV-infected patients who are undergoing tuberculosis treatment with isoniazid to reduce the occurrence of isoniazid-induced side effects in the central and peripheral nervous system.

Because the *MMWR*'s most recent recommendations for the use of antiretroviral therapy strongly advise against interruptions of therapy, and because alternative tuberculosis treatments that do not contain rifampin are available, previous antituberculosis therapy options that involved stopping protease inhibitor therapy to allow the use of rifampin are no longer recommended.

Pregnancy: Do not delay treatment for suspected or confirmed tuberculosis during pregnancy. The best therapeutic choices with the least danger to the fetus appear to be combinations of isoniazid, ethambutol, and rifampin. Pyrazinamide and streptomycin are not recommended during pregnancy because of possible teratogenic effects. Administer pyridoxine to all pregnant women receiving tuberculosis treatment to prevent peripheral neuropathy as a result of taking isoniazid. In pregnant women, delay prophylaxis until after delivery.

Multidrug resistance: The most recent cultures should undergo susceptibility testing to all antituberculosis drugs if cultures remain positive after 3 to 4 months of treatment.

Chemoprophylaxis: Administer isoniazid to adults in a daily dose of 300 mg for 1 year. Administer 10 mg/kg to a maximum daily dose of 300 mg for 1 year to children.

ISONIAZID (Isonicotinic acid hydrazide; INH)

Tablets: 100 and 300 mg (*Rx*)
Syrup: 50 mg/5 mL (*Rx*)
Injection: 100 mg/mL (*Rx*)

Various, *Isoniazid* (Barr)
Isoniazid (Carolina Medical)
Nydrazid (Apothecon)

Warning:
Severe and sometimes fatal hepatitis associated with isoniazid therapy may occur or develop even after many months of treatment. The risk of developing hepatitis is age-related. Risk of hepatitis increases with daily alcohol consumption.

Carefully monitor and interview patients at monthly intervals. For people > 35 years of age, in addition to a monthly symptom review, measure hepatic enzymes (specifically AST and ALT) prior to starting isoniazid therapy and periodically throughout treatment. Isoniazid-associated hepatitis usually occurs during the first 3 months of treatment. Enzyme levels generally return to normal despite continuance of the drug, but in some cases, progressive liver dysfunction occurs. Other factors associated with an increased risk of hepatitis include daily use of alcohol, chronic liver disease, and injection drug use. A report suggests an increased risk of fatal hepatitis associated with isoniazid among women, particularly black and Hispanic women. The risk also may be increased during the postpartum period. Consider more careful monitoring in these groups, possibly including more frequent laboratory monitoring. If abnormalities of liver function exceed 3 to 5 times the upper limit of normal, consider discontinuation of isoniazid. Liver function tests are not a substitute for a clinical evaluation at monthly intervals or for the prompt assessment of signs or symptoms of adverse reactions occurring between regularly scheduled evaluations. Instruct patients to report immediately signs or symptoms consistent with liver damage or other adverse effects. If these symptoms appear, or if signs suggestive of hepatic damage are detected, discontinue isoniazid promptly because continued use of the drug in such cases may cause a more severe form of liver damage.

Treat patients with tuberculosis who have hepatitis attributed to isoniazid with appropriate alternative drugs. Reinstitute isoniazid after symptoms and laboratory abnormalities have become normal. Restart the drug in very small doses; gradually increase doses and withdraw immediately if there is any indication of recurrent liver involvement.

Defer preventive treatment in people with acute hepatic diseases.

Indications
Used for all forms of tuberculosis in which organisms are susceptible.

Also recommended as preventive therapy (chemoprophylaxis) for specific situations.

IM administration is intended for use whenever oral is not possible.

Administration and Dosage
Treatment of tuberculosis: Use in conjunction with other effective antituberculosis agents.
    Adults – 5 mg/kg/day (up to 300 mg total) in a single dose, or 15 mg/kg (≤ 900 mg daily) 2 to 3 times weekly.
    Children – 10 to 15 mg/kg (≤ 300 mg daily) in a single dose, or 20 to 40 mg/kg (≤ 900 mg/day) 2 to 3 times weekly.

Preventive treatment:
    Adults (> 30 kg) – 300 mg/day in a single dose.
    Infants and children – 10 mg/kg/day (up to 300 mg total) in a single dose.

Actions
Pharmacology: Isoniazid inhibits the synthesis of mycoloic acids, an essential component of the bacterial cell wall. At therapeutic levels, isoniazid is bacteriocidal against actively growing intracellular and extracellular *Mycobacterium tuberculosis* organisms.

Pyridoxine (vitamin B_6) deficiency sometimes is observed in adults taking high doses of INH and is probably caused by the drug's competition with pyridoxal phosphate for the enzyme apotryptophanase.

Pharmacokinetics:

Absorption – INH is rapidly and completely absorbed orally and parenterally and produces peak blood levels within 1 to 2 hours. However, the rate and extent of absorption is decreased by food.

Distribution – INH readily diffuses into all body fluids (including cerebrospinal, pleural, and ascitic), tissues, organs, and excreta (saliva, sputum, feces). It also passes through the placental barrier and into breast milk in concentrations comparable to those in plasma.

Metabolism – The half-life of INH is widely variable and dependent on acetylator status. Isoniazid is primarily acetylated by the liver; this process is genetically controlled. Fast acetylators metabolize the drug about 5 to 6 times faster than slow acetylators. Several minor metabolites have been identified, one or more of which may be "reactive" (monoacetylhydrazine is suspected), and responsible for liver damage. The rate of acetylation does not significantly alter the effectiveness of INH. However, slow acetylation may lead to higher blood levels of the drug, and thus to an increase in toxic reactions.

Excretion – Approximately 50% to 70% of a dose of isoniazid is excreted as unchanged drug and metabolites by the kidneys in 24 hours.

Contraindications

Previous isoniazid-associated hepatic injury or other severe adverse reactions.

Warnings

Hypersensitivity reactions: Stop all drugs and evaluate at the first sign of a hypersensitivity reaction. If isoniazid must be reinstituted, give only after symptoms have cleared. Restart the drug in very small and gradually increasing doses and withdraw immediately if there is any indication of recurrent hypersensitivity reaction.

Renal/Hepatic function impairment: Monitor patients with active chronic liver disease or severe renal dysfunction.

Carcinogenesis: Isoniazid induces pulmonary tumors in a number of strains of mice.

Pregnancy: Category C.

Lactation: The small concentrations of isoniazid in breast milk do not produce toxicity in the nursing newborn; therefore, do not discourage breastfeeding. However, because levels of isoniazid are so low in breast milk, they cannot be relied upon for prophylaxis or therapy in nursing infants.

Precautions

Laboratory tests: Because there is a higher frequency of isoniazid-associated hepatitis among certain patient groups, obtain transaminase measurements prior to starting and monthly during preventative therapy, or more frequently as needed. If any of the values exceed 3 to 5 times the upper limit of normal, temporarily discontinue isoniazid and consider restarting therapy.

Periodic ophthalmologic examinations: Periodic ophthalmologic examinations during isoniazid therapy are recommended even when visual symptoms do not occur.

Pyridoxine administration: Pyridoxine administration is recommended in individuals likely to develop peripheral neuropathies secondary to INH therapy. Prophylactic doses of 10 to 25 mg of pyridoxine daily have been recommended.

Drug Interactions

Drugs that may interact with isoniazid include acetaminophen, carbamazepine, chlorzoxazone, disulfiram, enflurane, hydantoins, ketoconazole, rifampin, and theophylline.

Drug/Food interactions: Rate and extent of INH absorption is decreased by food.

Adverse Reactions

Toxic effects are usually encountered with higher doses of isoniazid; the most frequent are those affecting the nervous system and the liver.

Adverse reactions include pyridoxine deficiency; hyperglycemia; gynecomastia; peripheral neuropathy; convulsions; optic neuritis and atrophy; memory impairment; toxic psychosis; nausea; vomiting; epigastric distress; elevated AST, ALT; bilirubinemia; jaundice; anorexia; fatigue; malaise; weakness; agranulocytosis; hemolytic, sideroblastic, or aplastic anemia; thrombocytopenia; eosinophilia; fever; skin eruptions; lymphadenopathy; vasculitis.

RIFAMPIN

Capsules: 150 and 300 mg (*Rx*)
Powder for injection: 600 mg (*Rx*)

Various, *Rifadin* (Aventis), *Rimactane* (Novartis)
Rifadin (Aventis)

Indications
Tuberculosis:
> *Oral* – Oral treatment is for all forms of tuberculosis. A 3-drug regimen consisting of rifampin, isoniazid, and pyrazinamide is recommended in the initial phase of short-course therapy that is usually continued for 2 months.

> *IV* – Initial treatment and retreatment of tuberculosis when the drug cannot be taken by mouth.

Neisseria meningitidis carriers: Treatment of asymptomatic carriers of *N. meningitidis* to eliminate meningococci from the nasopharynx. Not indicated for treatment of meningococcal infection.

Administration and Dosage
Oral: Administer once daily, either 1 hour before or 2 hours after meals.
> Data is not available to determine dosage for children < 5 years of age.

Oral and IV:
> *Tuberculosis: Adults* – 10 mg/kg in a single daily administration not to exceed 600 mg once daily.

> *Children* – 10 to 20 mg/kg, not to exceed 600 mg/day.

The 2-month regimen: According to the MMWR, the 2-month daily regimen of rifampin and pyrazinamide is recommended in HIV-infected people. However, the drug toxicities may be increased.

The 4-month regimen: According to the MMWR, rifampin given daily for 3 months has resulted in better protection than placebo in treatment of LTBI in non-HIV patients with silicosis in a randomized prospective trial. However, because the patients receiving rifampin had a high rate of active tuberculosis (4%), experts have concluded that a 4-month regimen would be more prudent when using rifampin alone. This option may be useful for patients who cannot tolerate isoniazid or pyrazinamide.

The 6-month regimen: Ordinarily this consists of an initial 2-month phase of rifampin, isoniazid, and pyrazinamide and, if clinically indicated, streptomycin or ethambutol, followed by 4 months of rifampin and isoniazid. Reassess the need for a fourth drug when the results of susceptibility testing are known. If community rates of INH resistance are currently < 4%, an initial treatment regimen with < 4 drugs may be considered. Continue treatment for > 6 months if the patient is still sputum- or culture-positive, if resistant organisms are present, or if the patient is HIV positive.

Meningococcal carriers: Once daily for 4 consecutive days in the following doses:
> *Adults* – 600 mg.
> *Children* – 10 to 20 mg/kg, not to exceed 600 mg/day.
> *The following dosage has also been recommended* –
>> *Adults:* 600 mg every 12 hours for 2 days.
>> *Children (≥ 1 month of age):* 10 mg/kg every 12 hours for 2 days.
>> *Children (< 1 month of age):* 5 mg/kg every 12 hours for 2 days.

Actions

Pharmacology: Rifampin inhibits DNA-dependent RNA polymerase activity in susceptible cells. Specifically, it interacts with bacterial RNA polymerase, but does not inhibit the mammalian enzyme. Cross-resistance has only been shown with other rifamycins. Rifampin at therapeutic levels has demonstrated bactericidal activity against intracellular and extracellular *Mycobacterium tuberculosis* organisms.

Pharmacokinetics:

Oral –

Absorption/Distribution: Rifampin is almost completely absorbed and achieves mean peak plasma levels within 1 to 4 hours. Absorption of rifampin is reduced by ≈ 30% when the drug is ingested with food.

Metabolism: Rifampin is metabolized in the liver by deacetylation; the metabolite is still active against *Mycobacterium tuberculosis.* About 40% is excreted in bile and undergoes enterohepatic circulation; however, the deacetylated metabolite is poorly absorbed. The half-life is ≈ 3 hours after a 600 mg oral dose, up to 5.1 after a 900 mg oral dose. With repeated administration, the half-life decreases and averages ≈ 2 to 3 hours.

Excretion: Elimination occurs mainly through the bile and, to a much lesser extent, the urine. Dosage adjustment is not necessary in renal failure, but is with hepatic dysfunction. Rifampin is not significantly removed by hemodialysis.

Contraindications

Hypersensitivity to any rifamycin.

Warnings

Hepatotoxicity: There have been fatalities associated with jaundice in patients with liver disease or patients receiving rifampin concomitantly with other hepatotoxic agents. Carefully monitor liver function, especially AST and ALT, prior to therapy and then every 2 to 4 weeks during therapy.

Hyperbilirubinemia: Hyperbilirubinemia, resulting from competition between rifampin and bilirubin for excretory pathways of the liver at the cell level, can occur in early days of treatment.

Porphyria: Isolated reports have associated porphyria exacerbation with rifampin administration.

Meningococci resistance: The possibility of rapid emergence of resistant meningococci restricts use to short-term treatment of asymptomatic carrier state. Not for treatment of meningococcal disease.

Hypersensitivity reactions: Hypersensitivity reactions have occurred during intermittent therapy or when treatment was resumed following accidental or intentional interruption and were reversible with rifampin discontinuation and appropriate therapy.

Hepatic function impairment: Dosage adjustment is necessary.

Pregnancy: Category C.

Lactation: Rifampin is excreted in breast milk.

Precautions

Monitoring: Perform baseline measurements of hepatic enzymes, bilirubin, serum creatinine, CBC, and platelet count (or estimate) in adults treated for tuberculosis with rifampin. Baseline tests are unnecessary in pediatric patients unless a complicating condition is known or clinically suspected.

Intermittent therapy: Intermittent therapy may be used if the patient cannot or will not self-administer drugs on a daily basis. Closely monitor patients on intermittent therapy for compliance, and caution against intentional or accidental interruption of prescribed therapy because of increased risk of serious adverse reactions.

Urine, feces, saliva, sputum, sweat, and tears may be colored red-orange. Soft contact lenses may be permanently stained. Advise patients of these possibilities.

IV: For IV infusion only. Must not be administered by IM or SC route.

Thrombocytopenia: Thrombocytopenia has occurred, primarily with high dose intermittent therapy, but has also been noted after resumption of interrupted treatment.

Cerebral hemorrhage and fatalities have occurred when rifampin administration has continued or resumed after appearance of purpura.

Drug Interactions

Rifampin is known to induce the hepatic microsomal enzymes that metabolize various drugs such as acetaminophen, oral anticoagulants, barbiturates, benzodiazepines, beta blockers, chloramphenicol, clofibrate, oral contraceptives, corticosteroids, cyclosporine, disopyramide, estrogens, hydantoins, mexiletine, quinidine, sulfones, sulfonylureas, theophyllines, tocainide, verapamil, digoxin, enalapril, morphine, nifedipine, ondansetron, progestins, protease inhibitors, buspirone, delavirdine, doxycycline, fluoroquinolones, losartan, macrolides, sulfonylureas, tacrolimus, thyroid hormones, TCAs, zolpidem, zidovudine, and ketoconazole. The therapeutic effects of these drugs may be decreased.

Enzyme induction properties: Rifampin has enzyme induction properties that can enhance the metabolism of endogenous substrates including adrenal hormones, thyroid hormones, and vitamin D. Rifampin and isoniazid have been reported to alter vitamin D metabolism. In some cases, reduced levels of circulating 25-hydroxy vitamin D and 1,25-dihydroxy vitamin D have been accompanied by reduced serum calcium and phosphate, and elevated parathyroid hormone.

Drug/Lab test interactions: Therapeutic levels of rifampin inhibit standard assays for serum folate and vitamin B_{12}.

Transient abnormalities in liver function tests (eg, elevation in serum bilirubin, alkaline phosphatase, serum transaminases), and reduced biliary excretion of contrast media used for visualization of the gallbladder have also been observed.

Drug/Food interactions: Food interferes with the absorption of rifampin, possibly resulting in decreased peak plasma concentrations. Take on an empty stomach with a full glass of water.

Adverse Reactions

High doses of rifampin (> 600 mg) given once or twice weekly have resulted in a high incidence of adverse reactions including the following: "Flu-like" syndrome; hematopoietic reactions; cutaneous, GI, and hepatic reactions; shortness of breath; shock; renal failure; asymptomatic elevations of liver enzymes; rash.

RIFABUTIN

Capsules: 150 mg (*Rx*)	*Mycobutin* (Pharmacia)

Indications

Prevention of disseminated *Mycobacterium avium* complex (MAC) disease in patients with advanced HIV infection.

Administration and Dosage

Usual dose: 300 mg once daily. For those patients with propensity to nausea, vomiting, or other GI upset, administration of rifabutin at doses of 150 mg twice daily taken with food may be useful.

Actions

Pharmacology: Rifabutin, an antimycobacterial agent, is a semisynthetic ansamycin antibiotic derived from rifamycin S. It is not known whether rifabutin inhibits DNA-dependent RNA polymerase in *Mycobacterium avium* or in *Mycobacterium intracellulare* that comprise MAC.

Pharmacokinetics: Following a single oral dose of 300 mg to healthy adult volunteers, rifabutin was readily absorbed from the GI tract with mean peak plasma levels attained in 3.3 hours. Plasma concentrations post-C_{max} declined in an apparent biphasic manner. Rifabutin was slowly eliminated from plasma in healthy adult volunteers, presumably because of distribution-limited elimination, with a mean terminal half-life of 45 hours. Although the systemic levels of rifabutin following multiple dosing decreased by 38%, its terminal half-life remained unchanged. Estimates of apparent steady-state distribution volume (9.3 L/kg) in HIV-positive patients, following IV dosing, exceed total body water by ≈ 15-fold. About 85% of the drug is bound in a concentration-independent manner to plasma proteins over a concentration range of 0.05 to 1 mcg/mL.

Mean systemic clearance in healthy adult volunteers following a single oral dose was 0.69 L/hr/kg; renal and biliary clearance of unchanged drug each contribute ≈ 5%. About 30% of the dose is excreted in the feces; 53% of the oral dose is excreted in the urine, primarily as metabolites. Of the five metabolites that have been identified, 25-O-desacetyl and 31-hydroxy are the most predominant, and show a plasma metabolite:parent AUC ratio of 0.1 and 0.07, respectively. The 25-O-desacetyl metabolite has an activity equal to the parent drug and contributes ≤ 10% to the total antimicrobial activity.

Absolute bioavailability assessed in HIV-positive patients averaged 20%. Somewhat reduced drug distribution and faster drug elimination in compromised renal function may result in decreased drug concentrations.

Contraindications

Hypersensitivity to this drug or to any other rifamycins.

Warnings

Active tuberculosis: Rifabutin prophylaxis must not be administered to patients with active tuberculosis. HIV-positive patients are likely to have a nonreactive purified protein derivative (PPD) despite active disease. Chest X-ray, sputum culture, blood culture, urine culture, or biopsy of a suspicious lymph node may be useful in the diagnosis of tuberculosis in the HIV-positive patient.

There is no evidence that rifabutin is effective prophylaxis against M. *tuberculosis*. Patients requiring prophylaxis against both M. *tuberculosis* and M. *avium* complex may be given isoniazid and rifabutin concurrently.

Pregnancy: Category B.

Lactation: It is not known whether rifabutin is excreted in breast milk. Because of the potential for serious adverse reactions in nursing infants, decide whether to discontinue nursing or discontinue the drug, taking into account the importance of the drug to the mother.

Children: Safety and efficacy in children have not been established. Limited safety data are available from treatment use in 22 HIV-positive children with MAC who received rifabutin in combination with ≥ 2 other antimycobacterials for periods from 1 to 183 weeks. Mean doses (mg/kg) for these children were: 18.5 for infants 1 year of age; 8.6 for children 2 to 10 years of age; and 4 for adolescents 14 to 16 years of age. There is no evidence that doses > 5 mg/kg/day are useful.

Precautions

Monitoring: Because rifabutin may be associated with neutropenia, and, more rarely, thrombocytopenia, consider obtaining hematologic studies periodically in patients receiving prophylaxis.

Drug Interactions

CYP450: Rifabutin has liver enzyme-inducing properties. The related drug, rifampin, is known to reduce the activity of a number of other drugs. Because of the structural similarity of rifabutin and rifampin, rifabutin may be expected to have similar interactions. However, unlike rifampin, rifabutin appears not to affect the acetylation of isoniazid. Rifabutin appears to be a less potent enzyme inducer than rifampin. The significance of this finding for clinical drug interactions is not known.

Drugs that may interact with rifabutin include the following: Anticoagulants, azole antifungal agents, benzodiazepines, beta blockers, buspirone, corticosteroids, cyclosporine, delavirdine, doxycycline, hydantoins, indinavir, rifamycins, losartan, macrolide antibiotics, methadone, morphine, nelfinavir, quinine, quinidine, theophylline, aminophylline, tricyclic antidepressants, and zolpidem.

Drug/Food interactions: High-fat meals slow the rate of absorption without influencing the extent.

Adverse Reactions

Rifabutin is generally well tolerated. Discontinuation of therapy because of an adverse event was required in 16% of patients receiving rifabutin vs 8% with placebo.

Adverse reactions occurring in ≥ 3% of patients include the following: Abdominal pain, headache, diarrhea, dyspepsia, eructation, nausea, vomiting, rash, taste perversion, discolored urine, increased AST and ALT, anemia, leukopenia, neutropenia, and thrombocytopenia.

ETHAMBUTOL HCl

Tablets: 100 and 400 mg (*Rx*)	*Myambutol* (Dura)

Indications

Pulmonary tuberculosis: Use in conjunction with ≥ 1 other antituberculosis drug(s).

In patients who have received previous therapy, mycobacterial resistance to other drugs used in initial therapy is frequent. In retreatment patients, combine ethambutol with ≥ 1 of the second-line drug(s) not previously administered to the patient, and to which bacterial susceptibility has been indicated.

Administration and Dosage

Do not use ethambutol alone. Administer once every 24 hours only. Absorption is not significantly altered by administration with food. Continue therapy until bacteriological conversion has become permanent and maximal clinical improvement has occurred.

Initial treatment: In patients who have not received previous antituberculosis therapy, administer 15 mg/kg (7 mg/lb) as a single oral dose once every 24 hours. Isoniazid has been administered concurrently in a single, daily oral dose.

Retreatment: In patients who have received previous antituberculosis therapy, administer 25 mg/kg (11 mg/lb) as a single oral dose once every 24 hours. Concurrently administer ≥ 1 other antituberculosis drug(s) to which the organisms have been demonstrated to be susceptible by in vitro tests. Suitable drugs usually include those not previously used in the treatment of the patient. After 60 days of administration, decrease the dose to 15 mg/kg and administer as a single oral dose once every 24 hours.

Children: Not recommended for use in children < 13 years of age.

Actions

Pharmacology: Ethambutol diffuses into actively growing mycobacterium cells such as tubercle bacilli. It inhibits the synthesis of ≥ 1 metabolite, thus causing impairment of cell metabolism, arrest of multiplication, and cell death. No cross-resistance with other agents has been demonstrated.

Pharmacokinetics:

Absorption/Distribution – Ethambutol absorption is not influenced by food. Following a single oral dose of 15 to 25 mg/kg, ethambutol attains a peak of 2 to 5 mcg/mL in serum 2 to 4 hours after administration. Serum levels are similar after prolonged dosing. The serum level is undetectable 24 hours after the last dose except in some patients with abnormal renal function.

Metabolism – During the 24 hours following oral administration, ≈ 20% of ethambutol is metabolized by the liver.

Excretion – Unchanged drug is excreted (≈ 50%) in the urine, 8% to 15% as metabolites and 20% to 22% unchanged in the feces. Marked accumulation may occur with renal insufficiency. Ethambutol is not significantly removed by hemodialysis.

Contraindications

Hypersensitivity to ethambutol; known optic neuritis, unless clinical judgment determines that it may be used.

Warnings

Renal function impairment: Patients with decreased renal function require reduced dosage (as determined by serum levels) because this drug is excreted by the kidneys.

Pregnancy: Category B.

Children: Not recommended for use in children < 13 years of age.

Precautions

Monitoring: Perform periodic assessment of renal, hepatic, and hematopoietic systems during long-term therapy.

Visual effects: This drug may have adverse effects on vision. The effects are generally reversible when the drug is discontinued promptly. Perform testing before beginning therapy and periodically during drug administration (monthly when a patient is receiving > 15 mg/kg/day).

Advise patients to report promptly any change in visual acuity. If evaluation confirms visual change and fails to reveal other causes, discontinue drug and reevaluate patient at frequent intervals.

Drug Interactions

Aluminum salts: Aluminum salts may delay and reduce the absorption of ethambutol. Separate their administration by several hours.

Adverse Reactions

Adverse reactons may include anaphylactoid reactions, dermatitis, pruritus, decreases in visual acuity, anorexia, nausea, vomiting, GI upset, abdominal pain, fever, malaise, headache, dizziness, mental confusion, disorientation, possible hallucinations, peripheral neuritis, elevated serum uric acid levels, precipitation of acute gout, transient impairment of liver function, and joint pain.

PYRAZINAMIDE

Tablets: 500 mg (*Rx*) *Pyrazinamide (UDL, ESI)*

Indications

Tuberculosis: Initial treatment of active tuberculosis in adults and children when combined with other antituberculosis agents.

The current CDC recommendation for drug-susceptible initial treatment of active tuberculosis disease is a 6-month regimen consisting of isoniazid, rifampin, and pyrazinamide given for 2 months, followed by isoniazid and rifampin for 4 months.

Treatment failure: After treatment failure with other primary drugs in any form of active tuberculosis.

Administration and Dosage

Administer pyrazinamide with other effective antituberculosis drugs. It is administered for the initial 2 months of a 6-month or longer treatment regimen for drug susceptible patients. Treat patients who are known or suspected to have drug-resistant disease with regimens individualized to their situation. Pyrazinamide frequently will be an important component of such therapy.

HIV infection: Patients with concomitant HIV infection may require longer courses of therapy. Be alert to any revised recommendations from CDC for this group of patients.

Usual dose: 15 to 30 mg/kg once daily. Do not exceed 2 g/day.

Alternative dosing: Alternatively, a twice weekly dosing regimen (50 to 70 mg/kg twice weekly based on lean body weight) has been developed to promote patient compliance on an outpatient basis. In studies evaluating the twice weekly regimen, doses of pyrazinamide in excess of 3 g twice weekly have been administered without an increased incidence of adverse reactions.

Actions
Pharmacology: Pyrazinamide, the pyrazine analog of nicotinamide, may be bacteriostatic or bactericidal against *Mycobacterium tuberculosis* depending on the concentration of the drug attained at the site of infection. The mechanism of action is unknown.

Pharmacokinetics:

Absorption/Distribution – Pyrazinamide is well absorbed from the GI tract and attains peak plasma concentrations within 2 hours. It is widely distributed in body tissues and fluids including the liver, lungs, and cerebrospinal fluid. Pyrizinamide is ≈ 10% bound to plasma proteins.

Metabolism/Excretion – The half-life is 9 to 10 hours; it may be prolonged in patients with impaired renal or hepatic function.

Approximately 70% of an oral dose is excreted in urine, mainly by glomerular filtration, within 24 hours. Pyrazinamide is significantly dialyzed and should be dosed after hemodialysis.

Contraindications
Severe hepatic damage; hypersensitivity; acute gout.

Warnings
Combination therapy: Use only in conjunction with other effective antituberculosis agents.

Hyperuricemia: Pyrazinamide inhibits renal excretion of urates, frequently resulting in hyperuricemia that is usually asymptomatic. Patients started on pyrazinamide should have baseline serum uric acid determinations. Discontinue the drug and do not resume if signs of hyperuricemia accompanied by acute gouty arthritis appear.

Renal function impairment: It does not appear that patients with impaired renal function require a reduction in dose. It may be prudent to select doses at the low end of the dosing range, however.

Hepatic function impairment: Patients started on pyrazinamide should have baseline liver function determinations. Closely follow those patients with pre-existing liver disease or those at increased risk for drug-related hepatitis. Discontinue pyrazinamide and do not resume if signs of hepatocellular damage appear.

Elderly: In general, dose selection for an elderly patient should be cautious, usually starting at the low end of the dosing range, reflecting the greater frequency of decreased hepatic or renal function, and of concomitant disease or other drug therapy.

Pregnancy: Category C.

Lactation: Pyrazinamide has been found in small amounts in breast milk. Therefore, it is advised that pyrazinamide be used with caution in nursing mothers, taking into account the risk-benefit of this therapy.

Children: Pyrazinamide appears to be well tolerated in children.

Precautions
Monitoring: Determine baseline liver function studies and uric acid levels prior to therapy. Perform appropriate laboratory testing at periodic intervals and if any clinical signs or symptoms occur during therapy.

HIV infection: In patients with concomitant HIV infection, be aware of current recommendations of CDC. It is possible these patients may require a longer course of treatment.

Diabetes mellitus: Use with caution in patients with a history of diabetes mellitus, as management may be more difficult.

Primary resistance of M. tuberculosis: Primary resistance of M. *tuberculosis* to pyrazinamide is uncommon. In cases with known or suspected drug resistance, perform in vitro susceptibility tests with recent cultures of M. *tuberculosis* against pyrazinamide and the usual primary drugs.

Drug Interactions
Drug/Lab test interactions: Pyrazinamide has been reported to interfere with *Acetest* and *Ketostix* urine tests to produce a pink-brown color.

Adverse Reactions

Adverse reactions may include the following: Fever; porphyria; dysuria; gout; hepatic reaction; nausea; vomiting; anorexia; thrombocytopenia and sideroblastic anemia with erythroid hyperplasia; vacuolation of erythrocytes; increased serum iron concentration; adverse effects on blood clotting mechanisms; mild arthralgia and myalgia; hypersensitivity reactions including rashes, urticaria, pruritus; fever; acne; photosensitivity; porphyria; dysuria; interstitial nephritis.

AMINOSALICYLATE SODIUM (Para-Aminosalicylate Sodium)

Granules, delayed-release: 4 g (*Rx*)   *Paser* (Jacobus Pharm.)

Refer to the general discussion in the Antituberculosal Agents introduction.

Indications

Tuberculosis: Treatment of tuberculosis in combination with other active agents. It is most commonly used in patients with multi-drug resistant tuberculosis (MDR-TB) or in situations when therapy with isoniazid and rifampin is not possible because of a combination of resistance and intolerance.

Administration and Dosage

Tuberculosis: The adult dosage of 4 g (1 packet) 3 times/day, or correspondingly smaller doses in children, is to be taken without chewing by sprinkling on applesauce or yogurt or by swirling in the glass to suspend the granules in an acidic drink such as tomato or orange juice or food such as applesauce or yogurt. The coating will last ≥ 2 hours.

Do not use if packet is swollen or the granules have lost their tan color, turning dark brown or purple.

Actions

Pharmacology: Aminosalicylic acid is bacteriostatic against *Mycobacterium tuberculosis.* It inhibits the onset of bacterial resistance to streptomycin and isoniazid. The mechanism of action has been postulated to be inhibition of folic acid synthesis (but without potentiation with antifolic compounds) or inhibition of synthesis of the cell wall component, mycobactin, thus reducing iron uptake by M. *tuberculosis.*

Pharmacokinetics:

Absorption/Distribution – In a single 4 g pharmacokinetic study with food in normal volunteers, the initial time to a 2 mcg/mL serum level of aminosalicylic acid was 2 hours; the median time to peak was 6 hours; the mean peak level was 20 mcg/mL; a level of 2 mcg/mL was maintained for an average of 7.9 hours; a level of 1 mcg/mL was maintined for an average of 6.8 hours. Approximately 50% to 60% of aminosalicylic acid is protein-bound; binding is reported to be reduced 50% in kwashiorkor.

Excretion – 80% of aminosalicylic acid is excreted in the urine by glomerular filtration, with ≥ 50% of the dosage excreted in acetylated form.

Contraindications

Hypersensitivity to any component of this medication; severe renal disease.

Warnings

Hepatitis: In 1 retrospective study of 7492 patients on rapidly absorbed aminosalicylic acid preparations, drug-induced hepatitis occurred in 38 patients (0.5%); in these 38, the first symptom usually appeared within 3 months of the start of therapy with a rash as the most common event followed by fever and much less frequently by GI disturbances of anorexia, nausea, or diarrhea.

Hypersensitivity reactions: Stop all drugs at the first sign suggesting a hypersensitivity reaction. They may be restarted one at a time in very small but gradually increasing doses to determine whether the manifestations are drug-induced and, if so, which drug is responsible.

Desensitization has been accomplished successfully.

Renal function impairment: Patients with severe renal disease will accumulate amino-salicylic acid and its acetyl metabolite but will continue to acetylate, thus leading exclusively to the inactive acetylated form; deacetylation, if any, is not significant. Patients with end-stage renal disease should not receive aminosalicylic acid.

Hepatic function impairment: Use with caution.

Pregnancy: Category C.

Lactation: Aminosalicylic acid is excreted in breast milk.

Precautions
Malabsorption syndrome: A malabsorption syndrome can develop in patients on amino-salicylic acid but usually is not complete.

Lab test abnormalities: Aminosalicylic acid has been reported to interfere technically with the serum determinations of albumin by dye-binding AST by the azoene dye method and with qualitative urine tests for ketones, bilirubin, urobilinogen, or porphobilinogen.

Crystalluria may develop and can be prevented by the maintenance of urine at a neutral or alkaline pH.

Drug Interactions
Aminosalicylic acid may affect isoniazid, digoxin, and vitamin B_{12}.

Adverse Reactions
GI: The most common side effect is GI intolerance manifested by nausea, vomiting, diarrhea, and abdominal pain.

Hypersensitivity: Fever, skin eruptions of various types, including exfoliative dermatitis, infectious mononucleosis-like, or lymphoma-like syndrome, leukopenia, agranulocytosis, thrombocytopenia, Coombs' positive hemolytic anemia, jaundice, hepatitis, pericarditis, hypoglycemia, optic neuritis, encephalopathy, Leoffler's syndrome, vasculitis, and a reduction in prothrombin.

ETHIONAMIDE

Tablets: 250 mg (*Rx*)	*Trecator-SC* (Wyeth-Ayerst)

Indications
Recommended for any form of active tuberculosis when treatment with first-line drugs (isoniazid, rifampin) has failed. Use only with other effective antituberculosis agents.

Administration and Dosage
Administer with ≥ 1 other effective antituberculosis drug(s).

Average adult dose: 15 to 20 mg/kg/day taken once daily up to a maximum of 1 g/day.

Children: A dose of 10 to 20 mg/kg/day in 2 to 3 divided doses given after meals or 15 mg/kg/24 hours as a single daily dose has been recommended.

Concomitant administration of pyridoxine is recommended.

Actions
Pharmacology: Ethionamide may be bacteriostatic or bactericidal in action, depending on the concentration of the drug attained at the site of infection and the susceptibility of the infecting organism. The exact mechanism of action of ethionamide has not been fully elucidated, but the drug appears to inhibit peptide synthesis in susceptible organisms.

Pharmacokinetics:
Absorption/Distribution – Ethionamide is essentially completely absorbed following oral administration and is not subjected to any appreciable first pass metabolism.

The drug is ≈ 30% bound to plasma proteins. Ethionamide is rapidly and widely distributed into body tissues and fluids, with concentrations in plasma and various organs being approximately equal. Significant concentrations also are present in cerebrospinal fluid.

Metabolism/Excretion – Ethionamide is extensively metabolized to active and inactive metabolites with < 1% excreted as the free form in urine. Ethionamide has a plasma elimination half-life of ≈ 2 hours after oral dosing.

Monitoring – Normal serum concentrations of 1 to 5 mcg/mL are usually seen 2 hours following doses of 250 to 500 mg and approximate the therapeutic range for this drug.

Contraindications
Severe hypersensitivity to ethionamide; severe hepatic damage.

Warnings
Resistance: The use of ethionamide alone in the treatment of tuberculosis results in rapid development of resistance.

Compliance: It is recommended that directly observed therapy be practiced when patients are receiving antituberculosis medication.

Pregnancy: Category C.

Lactation: Because no information is available on the excretion of ethionamide in breast milk, administer to nursing mothers only if the benefits outweigh the risks.

Children: Investigations have been limited; do not use in pediatric patients < 12 years of age except when the organisms are definitely resistant to primary therapy and systemic dissemination of the disease, or other life-threatening complications of tuberculosis, is judged to be imminent.

Precautions
Monitoring: Make determinations of serum transaminase (AST, ALT) prior to and monthly during therapy. Monitor blood glucose and thyroid function tests periodically.

Drug Interactions
Ethionamide may interact with isoniazid and cycloserine.

Adverse Reactions
Adverse reactions may include the following: Depression; drowsiness and asthenia; convulsions; peripheral neuritis and neuropathy; olfactory disturbances; blurred vision; diplopia; optic neuritis; dizziness; headache; restlessness; tremors; psychosis; anorexia; nausea and vomiting; diarrhea; metallic taste; hepatitis; jaundice; stomatitis; postural hypotension; skin rash; acne; alopecia; thrombocytopenia; pellagra-like syndrome; gynecomastia; impotence; menorrhagia; and increased difficulty managing diabetes mellitus.

CYCLOSERINE

Capsules: 250 mg (*Rx*)   *Seromycin Pulvules* (Dura)

Indications
Treatment of active pulmonary and extrapulmonary tuberculosis (including renal disease) when organisms are susceptible, after failure of adequate treatment with the primary medications. Use in conjunction with other effective chemotherapy.

May be effective in the treatment of acute urinary tract infections caused by susceptible strains of gram-positive and gram-negative bacteria, especially *Enterobacter* sp. and *Escherichia coli.* It usually is less effective than other antimicrobial agents in the treatment of urinary tract infections caused by bacteria other than mycobacteria. Consider using only when the more conventional therapy has failed and when the organism has demonstrated sensitivity.

Administration and Dosage
Administer 500 mg to 1 g daily in divided doses monitored by blood levels. The usual initial dosage is 250 mg twice daily at 12-hour intervals for the first 2 weeks. Do not exceed 1 g/day.

Pyridoxine 200 to 300 mg/day may prevent the neurotoxic effects.

Actions

Pharmacology: Inhibits cell-wall synthesis in susceptible strains of gram-positive and gram-negative bacteria and in *Mycobacterium tuberculosis.*

Pharmacokinetics:

Absorption/Distribution – When given orally, cycloserine is rapidly absorbed, reaching peak plasma concentrations in 4 to 8 hours. It is widely distributed throughout body fluids and tissues; cerebrospinal fluid levels are similar to plasma.

Metabolism/Excretion – Approximately 35% of the drug is metabolized; 50% of a parenteral dose is excreted unchanged in the urine in the first 12 hours. About 65% of the drug is recoverable in 72 hours.

Contraindications

Hypersensitivity to cycloserine; epilepsy; depression; severe anxiety; psychosis; severe renal insufficiency; excessive concurrent use of alcohol.

Warnings

CNS toxicity: Discontinue or reduce dosage if patient develops symptoms of CNS toxicity, such as convulsions, psychosis, somnolence, depression, confusion, hyperreflexia, headache, tremor, vertigo, paresis, or dysarthria. The risk of convulsions is increased in chronic alcoholics.

Allergic dermatitis: Discontinue the drug or reduce dosage if patient develops allergic dermatitis.

Toxicity: Toxicity is closely related to excessive blood levels (> 30 mcg/mL) that are caused by high dosage or inadequate renal clearance. The therapeutic index in tuberculosis is small.

Renal function impairment: Patients will accumulate cycloserine and may develop toxicity if the dosage regimen is not modified. Patients with severe impairment should not receive the drug.

Pregnancy: Category C.

Lactation: Because of the potential for serious adverse reactions in nursing infants, decide whether to discontinue nursing or to discontinue the drug.

Children: Safety and dosage not established for pediatric use.

Precautions

Monitoring: Monitor patients by hematologic, renal excretion, blood level, and liver function studies.

Obtain cultures: Obtain cultures and determine susceptibility before treatment.

Determine blood levels: Determine blood levels weekly for patients having reduced renal function, for individuals receiving > 500 mg/day, and for those with symptoms of toxicity. Adjust dosage to maintain blood level < 30 mcg/mL.

Anticonvulsant drugs or sedatives: Anticonvulsant drugs or sedatives may be effective in controlling symptoms of CNS toxicity, such as convulsions, anxiety, and tremor. Closely observe patients receiving > 500 mg/day for such symptoms. Pyridoxine may prevent CNS toxicity, but its efficacy has not been proven.

Anemia: Administration has been associated in a few cases with vitamin B_{12} or folic acid deficiency, megaloblastic anemia, and sideroblastic anemia. If evidence of anemia develops, institute appropriate studies and therapy.

Drug Interactions

Drugs that may interact with cycloserine include alcohol, ethionamide, and isoniazid.

Adverse Reactions

Adverse reactions related to > 500 mg/day may include the following: Convulsions; drowsiness and somnolence; headache; tremor; dysarthria; vertigo; confusion and disorientation with loss of memory; psychoses, possibly with suicidal tendencies, character changes, hyperirritability, aggression; paresis; hyperreflexia; paresthesias; major and minor (localized) clonic seizures; coma; sudden development of CHF; skin rash; and elevated transaminase.

STREPTOMYCIN SULFATE

Powder, lyophilized: 1 g　　　　　　　　*Streptomycin Sulfate* (Pharma-Tek)

Also refer to the streptomycin sulfate monograph in the Aminoglycosides, Parenteral section.

Warning:

The risk of severe neurotoxic reactions is sharply increased in patients with impaired renal function or prerenal azotemia. These include disturbances of vestibular and cochlear function, optic nerve dysfunction, peripheral neuritis, arachnoiditis, and encephalopathy. The incidence of clinically detectable, irreversible vestibular damage is particularly high in patients treated with streptomycin.

Monitor renal function carefully; patients with renal impairment and/or nitrogen retention should receive reduced doses. Do not exceed peak serum concentrations of 20 to 25 mcg/mL in individuals with kidney damage.

Avoid concurrent or sequential use of other neurotoxic and/or nephrotoxic drugs with streptomycin sulfate, including neomycin, kanamycin, gentamicin, cephaloridine, paromomycin, viomycin, polymyxin B, colistin, tobramycin, and cyclosporine.

The neurotoxicity of streptomycin can result in respiratory paralysis from neuromuscular blockage, especially when the drug is given soon after the use of anesthesia or muscle relaxants. Reserve the administration of streptomycin in parenteral form for patients where adequate laboratory and audiometric testing facilities are available during therapy.

Indications

Add either streptomycin or ethambutol as a fourth drug in a regimen containing isoniazid (INH), rifampin, and pyrazinamide for initial treatment of tuberculosis unless the likelihood of INH or rifampin resistance is very low.

For more indications, see individual monograph in Aminoglycosides, Parenteral section.

Administration and Dosage

Administer by the IM route only.

Tuberculosis: The standard regimen for the treatment of drug-susceptible tuberculosis has been 2 months of INH, rifampin, and pyrazinamide followed by 4 months of INH and rifampin (patients with concomitant infection with tuberculosis and HIV may require treatment for a longer period). When streptomycin is added to this regimen because of suspected or proven drug resistance, the recommended dosing for streptomycin is as follows:

Streptomycin Recommended Dosing			
Patient	Daily	Twice daily	3 times/week
Children	20 to 40 mg/kg; max: 1 g	25 to 30 mg/kg; max: 1.5 g	25 to 30 mg/kg; max: 1.5g
Adults	15 mg/kg; max: 1 g	25 to 30 mg/kg; max: 1.5 g	25 to 30 mg/kg; max: 1.5 g

Streptomycin usually is administered daily as a single IM injection. Do not give a total dose ≥ 120 g over the course of therapy unless there are no other therapeutic options. In patients > 60 years of age, reduce dosage because of the risk of increased toxicity (see Warning Box).

As with other aminoglycosides, reduce dosage in impaired renal function.

Actions

Pharmacology: Streptomycin sulfate is a bactericidal antibiotic. It acts by interfering with normal protein synthesis.

Pharmacokinetics: Following IM injection of 1 g of streptomycin as the sulfate, a peak serum level of 25 to 50 mcg/mL is reached within 1 hour, diminishing slowly to ≈ 50% after 5 to 6 hours.

Appreciable concentrations are found in all organ tissues except the brain.

Streptomycin is excreted by glomerular filtration. Any reduction of glomerular function results in decreased excretion of the drug and a concurrent rise in serum and tissue levels.

Contraindications
Hypersensitivity to streptomycin sulfate or any other aminoglycoside.

Warnings
Ototoxicity: Both vestibular and auditory dysfunction can follow the administration of streptomycin. The degree of impairment is directly proportional to the dose and duration of streptomycin administration, the age of the patient, the level of renal function, and the amount of underlying existing auditory dysfunction.

Renal function impairment: Exercise extreme caution in selecting a dosage regimen in the presence of pre-existing renal insufficiency.

Pregnancy: Category D.

Lactation: Because of the potential for serious adverse reactions in nursing infants from streptomycin, decide whether to discontinue nursing or to discontinue the drug, taking into account the importance of the drug to the mother.

Children:
    Infants – A syndrome of apparent CNS depression, characterized by stupor and flaccidity, occasionally coma and deep respiratory depression, has been reported in young infants in whom streptomycin dosage had exceed the recommended limits. Thus, do not give infants streptomycin in excess of the recommended dosage.

Precautions
Monitoring: Baseline and periodic caloric stimulation tests and audiometric tests are advisable with extended streptomycin therapy. Tinnitus, roaring noises, or a sense of fullness in the ears indicates need for audiometric examination, termination of streptomycin therapy, or both.

Drug Interactions
The ototoxic effects of the aminoglycosides, including streptomycin, are potentiated by the coadministration of ethacrynic acid, furosemide, mannitol, and possibly other diuretics.

Adverse Reactions
The following reactions are common: Vestibular ototoxicity (eg, nausea, vomiting, vertigo); paresthesia of face; rash; fever; urticaria; angioneurotic edema; eosinophilia.

The following reactions are less frequent: Cochlear ototoxicity (deafness); exfoliative dermatitis; anaphylaxis; azotemia; leukopenia; thrombocytopenia; pancytopenia; hemolytic anemia; muscular weakness; amblyopia.

    Vestibular dysfunction – Vestibular dysfunction resulting from the parenteral administration of streptomycin is cumulatively related to the total daily dose. When 1.8 to 2 g/day are given, symptoms are likely to develop in a large percentage of patients (especially in the elderly or patients with impaired renal function) within 4 weeks. Therefore, it is recommended that caloric and audiometric tests be done prior to, during, and following intensive therapy with streptomycin in order to facilitate detection of any vestibular dysfunction or impairment of hearing that may occur.

    Vestibular symptoms generally appear early and usually are reversible with early detection and cessation of streptomycin administration. Two to 3 months after stopping the drug, gross vestibular symptoms usually disappear, except from the relative inability to walk in total darkness or on very rough terrain.

    Nephrotoxicity – Although streptomycin is the least nephrotoxic of the aminoglycosides, nephrotoxicity does occur rarely.

CAPREOMYCIN

Powder for injection: 1 g (as sulfate)/10 mL vial (*Rx*)   *Capastat Sulfate* (Dura)

Warning:
Undertake the use of capreomycin in patients with renal insufficiency or pre-existing auditory impairment with great caution. Weigh the risk of additional eighth nerve impairment or renal injury against benefits to be derived from therapy.

Because other parenteral antituberculosis agents (eg, streptomycin, viomycin) also have similar and sometimes irreversible toxic effects, particularly on eighth cranial nerve and renal function, simultaneous administration of these agents with capreomycin is not recommended. Use concurrent nonantituberculosis drugs (eg, polymyxin A sulfate, colistin sulfate, amikacin, gentamicin, tobramycin, vancomycin, kanamycin, neomycin) having ototoxic or nephrotoxic potential only with great caution.

Indications
Intended for use concomitantly with other antituberculosis agents in pulmonary infections caused by capreomycin-susceptible strains of *Mycobacterium tuberculosis*, when the primary agents (eg, isoniazid, rifampin) have been ineffective or cannot be used because of toxicity or the presence of resistant tubercle bacilli.

Administration and Dosage
May be administered IM or IV following reconstitution.

IV: For IV infusion, further dilute reconstituted capreomycin solution in 100 mL of 0.9% Sodium Chloride Injection and administer over 60 minutes.

IM: Give reconstituted capreomycin by deep IM injection into a large muscle mass; superficial injections may be associated with increased pain and sterile abscesses.

Usual dose: 1 g daily (not to exceed 20 mg/kg/day) given IM or IV for 60 to 120 days, followed by 1 g by either route 2 or 3 times weekly.

Renal function impairment: Reduce the dosage based on Ccr using the guidelines in the table. These dosages are designed to achieve a mean steady-state capreomycin level of 10 mcg/L.

| Capreomycin Dosage in Renal Function Impairment |||||
| Ccr (mL/min) | Capreomycin clearance (L/kg/hr×10⁻²) | Half-life (hours) | Dose[1] (mg/kg) for the following dosing intervals |||
			24 hr	48 hr	72 hr
0	0.54	55.5	1.29	2.58	3.87
10	1.01	29.4	2.43	4.87	7.30
20	1.49	20.0	3.58	7.16	10.7
30	1.97	15.1	4.72	9.45	14.2
40	2.45	12.2	5.87	11.7	
50	2.92	10.2	7.01	14	
60	3.40	8.8	8.16		
80	4.35	6.8	10.4[2]		
100	5.31	5.6	12.7[2]		
110	5.78	5.2	13.9[2]		

[1] Initial maintenance dose estimates are given for optional dosing intervals; longer dosing intervals are expected to provide greater peak and lower trough serum capreomycin levels than shorter dosing intervals.
[2] The usual dosage for patients with normal renal function is 1 g daily, not to exceed 20 mg/kg/day, for 60 to 120 days, then 1 g 2 to 3 times weekly.

Actions
Pharmacology: A polypeptide antibiotic isolated from *Streptomyces capreolus.*

Pharmacokinetics:

Absorption – Capreomycin sulfate is not absorbed in significant quantities from the GI tract and must be administered parenterally. The AUC is similar for single-dose capreomycin (1 g) administered IM and by IV (over 1 hour) routes of administration. Capreomycin peak concentrations after IV infusion were ≈ 30% higher than after IM administration.

Distribution – Peak serum concentrations following IM administration of 1 g are achieved in 1 to 2 hours. Low serum concentrations are present at 24 hours. Doses of 1 g daily for ≥ 30 days produce no significant accumulation in subjects with normal renal function.

Excretion – Capreomycin is excreted essentially unaltered; 52% is excreted in the urine within 12 hours.

Contraindications
Hypersensitivity to capreomycin.

Warnings
Hypersensitivity reactions: Has occurred when capreomycin and other antituberculosis drugs were given concomitantly.

Renal function impairment: Dosage reduction is necessary. See Administration and Dosage.

Pregnancy: Category C.

Lactation: It is not known whether this drug is excreted in breast milk.

Children: Safety for use in infants and children has not been established.

Precautions
Neuromuscular blockade: A partial neuromuscular blockade was demonstrated after large IV doses of capreomycin. This action was enhanced by ether anesthesia (as has been reported for neomycin) and was antagonized by neostigmine.

Ototoxicity: Perform audiometric measurements and assessment of vestibular function prior to initiation of therapy and at regular intervals during treatment.

Nephrotoxicity: Perform regular tests of renal function throughout treatment, and reduce dose in patients with renal impairment. Renal injury with tubular necrosis, elevation of BUN or serum creatinine, and abnormal sediment have been noted. Reduce the dosage or withdraw the drug.

Hypokalemia: Hypokalemia may occur during therapy; therefore, determine serum potassium levels frequently.

Drug Interactions
Drugs that may interact with capreomycin include aminoglycosides and nondepolarizing neuromuscular blocking agents.

Adverse Reactions
Adverse reactions may include the following: Ototoxicity; tinnitus; vertigo; pain, induration, and excessive bleeding at the injection sites; sterile abscesses; leukocytosis; leukopenia; eosinophilia; abnormal results in liver function tests; urticaria; and maculopapular skin rashes.

RIFAPENTINE

Tablets: 150 mg (*Rx*)	*Priftin* (Aventis)

Indications
Tuberculosis: For the treatment of pulmonary tuberculosis (TB). Rifapentine must always be used in conjunction with ≥ 1 other antituberculosis drug(s) to which the isolate is susceptible.

Administration and Dosage
Do not use rifapentine alone. Concomitant administration of pyridoxine (vitamin B_6) is recommended in the malnourished, in those predisposed to neuropathy (eg, alcoholics, diabetics), and in adolescents.

Tuberculosis:

Intensive phase – 600 mg (four 150 mg tablets twice weekly) with an interval of ≥ 3 days (72 hours) between doses continued for 2 months. May be given with food if stomach upset, nausea, or vomiting occurs.

Continuation phase – Continue treatment with rifapentine once weekly for 4 months in combination with isoniazid or an appropriate agent for susceptible organisms. If the patient is still sputum-smear- or culture-positive, if resistant organisms are present, or if the patient is HIV-positive, follow ATS/CDC treatment guidelines.

Actions
Pharmacology: Rifapentine is a rifamycin-derivative antibiotic and has a similar profile of microbiological activity to rifampin.

Pharmacokinetics:

Absorption/Distribution – The absolute bioavailability of rifapentine has not been determined. C_{max} is 15.05 mcg/mL and half-life is 13.19 hours. The estimated apparent volume of distribution is ≈ 70 L. In healthy volunteers, rifapentine and 25-desacetyl rifapentine (active metabolite) were 97.7% and 93.2% bound to plasma proteins, respectively, mainly to albumin.

Metabolism/Excretion – Rifapentine is hydrolyzed by an esterase enzyme to form a microbiologically active 25-desacetyl rifapentine. Rifapentine and 25-desacetyl rifapentine account for 99% of total drug in plasma. Plasma AUC and C_{max} values of the 25-desacetyl rifapentine metabolite are 50% and 33% those of rifapentine, respectively. Eighty-seven percent of the total dose was recovered in the urine (17%) and feces (70%); > 80% was excreted within 7 days.

Special populations –

Gender: The estimated apparent oral clearance of rifapentine for males and females was ≈ 2.51 and ≈ 1.69 L/hr, respectively. The clinical significance of the difference in the estimated apparent oral clearance is not known.

Contraindications
Hypersensitivity to any of the rifamycins (rifampin and rifabutin).

Warnings
Compliance: Poor compliance with the dosage regimen, particularly daily administered nonrifamycin drugs in the intensive phase, was associated with late sputum conversion and a high relapse rate.

Hyperbilirubinemia: An isolated report showing a moderate rise in bilirubin or transaminase level is not an indication to interrupt treatment; rather, repeat tests, noting trends in the levels, and consider them in conjunction with the patient's clinical condition.

Pseudomembranous colitis: If suspected, stop rifapentine immediately and treat the patient with supportive and specific treatment without delay (eg, oral vancomycin). Products inhibiting peristalsis are contraindicated in this clinical situation.

HIV-infected patients: As with other antituberculosis treatments, when rifapentine is used in HIV-infected patients, employ a more aggressive regimen (eg, more frequent dosing). Once-weekly dosing during the continuation phase of treatment is not recommended at this time.

Hepatic function impairment: Only give patients with abnormal liver tests or liver disease rifapentine in cases of necessity and then with caution and under strict medical supervision. In these patients, carefully monitor liver tests (especially serum transaminases) prior to therapy and then every 2 to 4 weeks during therapy. If signs of liver disease occur or worsen, discontinue rifapentine.

Pregnancy: Category C.

Lactation: Because of the potential for serious adverse reactions in nursing infants, decide whether to discontinue nursing or discontinue the drug, taking into account the importance of the drug to the mother.

Children: Safety and efficacy in children < 12 years of age have not been established.

Precautions

Monitoring: Obtain baseline measurements of hepatic enzymes, bilirubin, a CBC, and a platelet count (or estimate). Assess patients at least monthly during therapy. Routine laboratory monitoring for toxicity in people with normal baseline measurements is generally not necessary.

Resistance: M. tuberculosis organisms resistant to other rifamycins are likely to be resistant to rifapentine. Cross-resistance does not appear between rifapentine and non-rifamycin antimycobacterial agents such as isoniazid and streptomycin.

Red discoloration of body fluids: Rifapentine may produce a predominately red-orange discoloration of body tissues or fluids (eg, skin, teeth, tongue, urine, feces, saliva, sputum, tears, sweat, cerebrospinal fluid). Contact lenses may become permanently stained.

Drug Interactions

Use rifapentine with extreme caution, if at all, in patients who are also taking protease inhibitors (eg, indinavir).

Cytochrome P450: Rifapentine is an inducer of cytochromes P450 3A4 and P450 2C8/9 and may increase the metabolism of other coadministered drugs that are metabolized by these enzymes.

Note: Advise patients using oral or other systemic hormonal contraceptives to change to nonhormonal methods of birth control.

Amitriptyline	Doxycycline	Phenytoin
Barbiturates	Fluconazole	Progestins
Beta blockers	Fluoroquinolones	Quinidine
Buspirone	Haloperidol	Quinine
Cardiac glycosides	Indinavir	Ritonavir
Chloramphenicol	Itraconazole	Saquinavir
Clarithromycin	Ketoconazole	Sildenafil
Clofibrate	Levothyroxine	Sulfonylureas
Corticosteroids	Methadone	Tacrolimus
Cyclosporine	Mexiletine	Theophylline
Dapsone	Morphine	Tocainide
Delavirdine	Nelfinavir	Verapamil
Diazepam	Nifedipine	Warfarin
Diltiazem	Nortriptyline	Zidovudine
Disopyramide	Oral contraceptives	Zolpidem

Drug/Lab test interactions: Therapeutic concentrations of rifampin have been shown to inhibit standard microbiological assays for serum folate and vitamin B_{12}.

Drug/Food interactions: Food (850 total calories: 33 g protein, 55 g fat, and 58 g carbohydrate) increased AUC and C_{max} in healthy volunteers by 43% and 44%, respectively, and in asymptomatic HIV-infected volunteers by 51% and 53%, respectively.

Adverse Reactions

Adverse reactions occurring in ≥ 3% of patients receiving rifapentine combination therapy include the following: Rash; pyuria; proteinuria; hematuria; urinary casts; neutropenia; lymphopenia; hyperuricemia; and an increase in ALT and AST.

FOSCARNET SODIUM (Phosphonoformic acid)

Injection: 24 mg/mL (*Rx*)   *Foscavir* (Astra)

Warning:

Renal impairment, the major toxicity, occurs to some degree in most patients. Continual assessment of a patient's risk and frequent monitoring of serum creatinine with dose adjustment for changes in renal function are imperative.

Seizures related to alterations in plasma minerals and electrolytes have been associated with foscarnet treatment. Therefore, patients must be carefully monitored for such changes and their potential sequelae. Mineral and electrolyte supplementation may be required.

Foscarnet causes alterations in plasma minerals and electrolytes that have led to seizures. Monitor patients frequently for such changes and their potential sequelae.

Indications

Cytomegalovirus (CMV) retinitis: Treatment of CMV retinitis in patients with AIDS.

Combination: Combination therapy with ganciclovir for patients who have relapsed after monotherapy with either drug.

Herpes simplex virus (HSV) infections: Treatment of acyclovir-resistant mucocutaneous HSV infections in immunocompromised patients.

Administration and Dosage

HSV infections: Foscarnet is not a cure for HSV infections. While complete healing may occur, relapse occurs in most patients.

Caution: Do not administer by rapid or bolus IV injection. Toxicity may be increased as a result of excessive plasma levels. An infusion pump must be used.

It is recommended that 750 to 1000 mL of normal saline or 5% dextrose solution be given prior to the first infusion of foscarnet to establish diuresis. With subsequent infusions, 750 to 1000 mL of hydration fluid should be given with 90 to 120 mg/kg of foscarnet, and 500 mL with 40 to 60 mg/kg of foscarnet. Hydration fluid may need to be decreased if clinically warranted. After the first dose, administer the hydration fluid concurrently with each infusion of foscarnet.

Induction treatment: The recommended initial dose for patients with normal renal function is 60 mg/kg, adjusted for individual patients' renal function, given IV at a constant rate over a minimum of 1 hour every 8 hours for 2 to 3 weeks, depending on clinical response.

Maintenance treatment: 90 to 120 mg/kg/day (individualized for renal function) as an IV infusion over 2 hours. It is recommended that most patients be started on maintenance treatment with 90 mg/kg/day. Escalation to 120 mg/kg/day may be considered should early reinduction be required because of retinitis progression.

Patients who experience progression of retinitis while receiving maintenance therapy may be retreated with the induction and maintenance regimens above.

Dose adjustment in renal impairment:

Foscarnet Dosing Guide Based on Ccr for Induction			
	HSV: Equivalent to		CMV: Equivalent to
Ccr (mL/min/kg)	80 mg/kg/day	120 mg/kg/day	180 mg/kg/day
> 1.4	40 q 12 hr	40 q 8 hr	60 q 8 hr
> 1 to 1.4	30 q 12 hr	30 q 8 hr	45 q 8 hr
> 0.8 to 1	20 q 12 hr	35 q 12 hr	50 q 12 hr
> 0.6 to 0.8	35 q 24 hr	25 q 12 hr	40 q 12 hr
> 0.5 to 0.6	25 q 24 hr	40 q 24 hr	60 q 24 hr
≥ 0.4 to 0.5	20 q 24 hr	35 q 24 hr	50 q 24 hr
< 0.4	Not recommended	Not recommended	Not recommended

Foscarnet Dosing Guide Based on Ccr for Maintenance		
Ccr (mL/min/kg)	CMV: Equivalent to	
	90 mg/kg/day	120 mg/kg/day
> 1.4	90 q 24 hr	120 q 24 hr
> 1 to 2.4	70 q 24 hr	90 q 24 hr
> 0.8 to 1	50 q 24 hr	65 q 24 hr
> 0.6 to 0.8	80 q 48 hr	105 q 48 hr
> 0.5 to 0.6	60 q 48 hr	30 q 48 hr
≥ 0.4 to 0.5	50 q 48 hr	65 q 48 hr
< 0.4	Not recommended	Not recommended

Actions

Pharmacology: Foscarnet exerts its antiviral activity by a selective inhibition at the pyrophosphate binding site on virus-specific DNA polymerases and reverse transcriptases at concentrations that do not affect cellular DNA polymerases. CMV strains resistant to ganciclovir may be sensitive to foscarnet. Acyclovir- or ganciclovir-resistant mutants may be resistant to foscarnet.

Pharmacokinetics: Foscarnet is 14% to 17% bound to plasma protein at plasma drug concentrations of 1 to 1000 mcM.

Approximately 80% to 90% of IV foscarnet is excreted unchanged in the urine of patients with normal renal function. Both tubular secretion and glomerular filtration account for urinary elimination of foscarnet.

Plasma half-life increases with the severity of renal impairment. Half-lives of 2 to 8 hours occurred in patients having estimated or measured 24-hour Ccr of 44 to 90 mL/min.

The foscarnet terminal half-life determined by urinary excretion was 87.5 ± 41.8 hours, possibly because of release of foscarnet from bone. Postmortem data provide evidence that foscarnet does accumulate in bone in humans.

Variable penetration into cerebrospinal fluid (CSF) has been observed. Disease-related defects in the blood-brain barrier may be responsible for the variations seen.

Contraindications

Hypersensitivity to foscarnet.

Warnings

Mineral and electrolyte imbalances: Foscarnet has been associated with changes in serum electrolytes including hypocalcemia (15%), hypophosphatemia (8%) and hyperphosphatemia (6%), hypomagnesemia (15%), and hypokalemia (16%). Foscarnet is associated with a transient, dose-related decrease in ionized serum calcium, which may not be reflected in total serum calcium.

Accidental exposure: Accidental skin and eye contact with foscarnet sodium solution may cause local irritation and burning sensation. Flush the exposed area with water.

Other CMV infections: Safety and efficacy have not been established for the treatment of other CMV infections (eg, pneumonitis, gastroenteritis); congenital or neonatal CMV disease; nonimmunocompromised individuals.

Neurotoxicity and seizures: Foscarnet was associated with seizures in AIDS patients.

Statistically significant risk factors associated with seizures were low baseline absolute neutrophil count (ANC), impaired baseline renal function, and low total serum calcium. Several cases of seizures were associated with death.

Renal function impairment: The major toxicity of foscarnet is renal impairment, which occurs to some degree in most patients. Approximately 33% of 189 patients with AIDS and CMV retinitis who received IV foscarnet in clinical studies developed significant impairment of renal function, manifested by a rise in serum creatinine concentration to ≥ 2 mg/dL.

Elderly: Because these individuals frequently have reduced glomerular filtration, pay particular attention to assessing renal function before and during administration.

Pregnancy: Category C.

Lactation: It is not known whether foscarnet is excreted in breast milk.

Children: The safety and efficacy of foscarnet in children have not been studied.

Precautions

Monitoring: The majority of patients will experience some decrease in renal function due to foscarnet administration. Therefore, it is recommended that Ccr be determined at baseline, 2 to 3 times/week during induction therapy, and at least once every 1 to 2 weeks during maintenance therapy, with foscarnet dose adjusted accordingly. More frequent monitoring may be required for some patients. It also is recommended that a 24-hour Ccr be determined at baseline and periodically thereafter to ensure correct dosing. Discontinue if Ccr drops to < 0.4 mL/min/kg.

Because of foscarnet's propensity to chelate divalent metal ions and alter levels of serum electrolytes, closely monitor patients for such changes. It is recommended that a schedule similar to that recommended for serum creatinine be used to monitor serum calcium, magnesium, potassium, and phosphorus.

Careful monitoring and appropriate management of creatinine are of particular importance in patients with conditions that may predispose them to seizures.

Diagnosis of CMV retinitis: Diagnosis of CMV retinitis should be established by an ophthalmologist familiar with the retinal presentation of these conditions.

Toxicity/Local irritation: The maximum single-dose administered was 120 mg/kg by IV infusion over 2 hours. It is likely that larger doses, or more rapid infusions, would result in increased toxicity. Infuse solutions containing foscarnet only into veins with adequate blood flow to permit rapid dilution and distribution, and avoid local irritation. Local irritation and ulcerations of penile epithelium have occurred in patients receiving foscarnet, possibly because of drug in urine. Adequate hydration with close attention to personal hygiene may minimize the occurrence of such events.

Anemia: Anemia occurred in 33% of patients. Granulocytopenia occurred in 17% of patients.

Drug Interactions

Drugs that may interact with foscarnet include nephrotoxic drugs (eg, aminoglycosides, amphotericin B, IV pentamidine), pentamidine, and zidovudine.

Foscarnet decreases serum levels of ionized calcium. Exercise particular caution when other drugs known to influence serum calcium levels are used concurrently.

Adverse Reactions

Adverse reactions occurring in ≥ 3% of patients include fever; nausea; anemia; diarrhea; abnormal renal function including acute renal failure, decreased Ccr and increased serum creatinine; vomiting; headache; seizure; death; marrow suppression; injection site pain or inflammation; paresthesia; dizziness; involuntary muscle contractions; hypoesthesia; neuropathy; sensory disturbances; influenza-like symptoms; bacterial/fungal infections; rectal hemorrhage; dry mouth; melena; flatulence; ulcerative stomatitis; pancreatitis; granulocytopenia; leukopenia; thrombocytopenia; platelet abnormalities; thrombosis; WBC abnormalities; lymphadenopathy; electrolyte abnormalities; neurotoxicity; renal impairment; decreased weight; increased alkaline phosphatase, LDH and BUN; acidosis; cachexia; thirst; depression; confusion; anxiety; aggressive reaction; hallucination; coughing; dyspnea; pneumonia; sinusitis; pharyngitis; rhinitis; respiratory disorders or insufficiency; pulmonary infiltration; stridor; pneumothorax; hemoptysis; bronchospasm; rash; increased sweating; pruritus; skin ulceration; seborrhea; erythematous rash; maculopapular rash; vision abnormalities; taste perversions; eye abnormalities; eye pain; conjunctivitis; hypertension; palpitations; ECG abnormalities.

GANCICLOVIR (DHPG)

Capsules: 250 and 500 mg (*Rx*)
Powder for injection, lyophilized: 500 mg/vial ganciclovir
(*Rx*)

Cytovene (Roche)

Warning:
> The clinical toxicity of ganciclovir includes granulocytopenia, anemia, and thrombocytopenia. In animal studies, ganciclovir was carcinogenic, teratogenic, and caused aspermatogenesis.
>
> Ganciclovir IV is indicated for use only in the treatment of cytomegalovirus (CMV) retinitis in immunocompromised patients and for the prevention of CMV disease in transplant patients at risk for CMV disease.
>
> Ganciclovir capsules are indicated only for prevention of CMV disease in patients with advanced HIV infection at risk for CMV disease and for maintenance treatment of CMV retinitis in immunocompromised patients.
>
> Because oral ganciclovir is associated with a risk of more rapid rate of CMV retinitis progression, use only in those patients for whom this risk is balanced by the benefit associated with avoiding daily IV infusions.

Indications

IV:
> CMV *retinitis* – Treatment of CMV retinitis in immunocompromised patients, including patients with AIDS.
>
> CMV *disease* – Prevention of CMV disease in transplant recipients at risk for CMV disease.

Oral:
> CMV *retinitis* – Alternative to the IV formulation for maintenance treatment of CMV retinitis in immunocompromised patients, including patients with AIDS, in whom retinitis is stable following appropriate induction therapy and for whom the risk of more rapid progression is balanced by the benefit associated with avoiding daily IV infusions.
>
> CMV *disease* – Prevention of CMV disease in individuals with advanced HIV infection at risk for developing CMV disease.

Administration and Dosage

IV: Do not administer by rapid or bolus IV injection. The toxicity may be increased as a result of excessive plasma levels. Do not exceed the recommended infusion rate. IM or SC injection of reconstituted ganciclovir may result in severe tissue irritation because of high pH.

CMV *retinitis treatment (normal renal function):*
> *Induction* – Recommended initial dose is 5 mg/kg (given IV at a constant rate of 1 hour) every 12 hours for 14 to 21 days. Do not use oral ganciclovir for induction.

> *Maintenance* –
>> IV: Following induction, the recommended maintenance dose is 5 mg/kg given as a constant rate IV infusion over 1 hour once per day 7 days per week, or 6 mg/kg once per day 5 days/week.
>>
>> Oral: Following induction, the recommended maintenance dose of oral ganciclovir is 1000 mg 3 times daily with food. Alternatively, the dosing regimen of 500 mg 6 times daily every 3 hours with food during waking hours may be used.
>>
>> For patients who experience progression of CMV retinitis while receiving maintenance treatment with either formulation of ganciclovir, reinduction treatment is recommended.

Prevention of CMV disease in transplant recipients with normal renal function:
   IV – The recommended initial dose of IV ganciclovir for patients with normal renal function is 5 mg/kg (given IV at a constant rate over 1 hour) every 12 hours for 7 to 14 days, followed by 5 mg/kg once daily 7 days/week or 6 mg/kg once daily 5 days/week.
   Oral – The recommended prophylactic dosage is 1000 mg 3 times daily with food. The duration of treatment with ganciclovir in transplant recipients is dependent on the duration and degree of immunosuppression. In controlled clinical trials in bone marrow allograft recipients, IV ganciclovir treatment was continued until day 100 to 120 posttransplantation. CMV disease occurred in several patients who discontinued treatment with IV ganciclovir prematurely. In heart allograft recipients, the onset of newly diagnosed CMV disease occurred after treatment with IV ganciclovir was stopped at day 28 post-transplant, suggesting that continued dosing may be necessary to prevent late occurrence of CMV disease in this patient population.

Prevention of CMV disease in patients with advanced HIV infection and normal renal function: The recommended dose of ganciclovir capsules is 1000 mg 3 times daily with food.

Renal function impairment:
   IV – Refer to the table for recommended doses and adjust the dosing interval as indicated.

IV Ganciclovir Dose in Renal Impairment				
Ccr (mL/min)	Ganciclovir induction dose (mg/kg)	Dosing interval (hours)	Ganciclovir maintenance dose (mg/kg)	Dosing interval (hours)
≥ 70	5	12	5	24
50 to 69	2.5	12	2.5	24
25 to 49	2.5	24	1.25	24
10 to 24	1.25	24	0.625	24
< 10	1.25	3 times/week following hemodialysis	0.625	3 times/week following hemodialysis

Hemodialysis: Dosing for patients undergoing hemodialysis should not exceed 1.25 mg/kg 3 times/week, following each hemodialysis session. Give shortly after completion of the hemodialysis session, since hemodialysis reduces plasma levels by ≈ 50%.

Oral: In renal impairment, modify the dose of oral ganciclovir as follows:

Oral Ganciclovir Dose in Renal Impairment	
Ccr (mL/min)	Ganciclovir doses
≥ 70	1000 mg TID or 500 mg q3h, 6 times/day
50 to 69	1500 mg QD or 500 mg TID
25 to 49	1000 mg QD or 500 mg BID
10 to 24	500 mg QD
< 10	500 mg 3 times/week, following hemodialysis

Patient monitoring: Because of the frequency of granulocytopenia, anemia, and thrombocytopenia, it is recommended that CBCs and platelet counts be performed frequently, especially in patients in whom ganciclovir or other nucleoside analogs have previously resulted in cytopenia, or in whom neutrophil counts are < 1000/mcL at the beginning of treatment. Patients should have serum creatinine or Ccr values followed carefully to allow for dosage adjustment in renally impaired patients.

Reduction of dose: Dose reductions are required with IV therapy and should be considered with oral therapy for patients with renal impairment and for those with neutropenia, anemia, or thrombocytopenia. Do not administer in severe neutropenia (ANC < 500/mcL) or severe thrombocytopenia (platelets < 25,000/mcL).

Actions

Pharmacology: Ganciclovir, a synthetic guanine derivative active against CMV, is an acyclic nucleoside analog of 2'-deoxyguanosine that inhibits replication of herpes viruses both in vitro and in vivo. Sensitive human viruses include CMV, herpes simplex virus (HSV)-1 and -2, herpes virus type 6, Epstein-Barr virus, varicella-zoster virus, and hepatitis B virus.

Pharmacokinetics:

Absorption – Absolute bioavailability of oral ganciclovir under fasting conditions was ≈ 5%; following food it was 6% to 9%. When given with a high-fat meal, steady-state AUC increased and there was a significant prolongation of time to peak serum concentrations.

At the end of a 1-hour IV infusion of 5 mg/kg, total AUC and C_{max} ranged between 22.1 and 26.8 mcg•hr/mL and 8.27 and 9 mcg/mL, respectively.

Distribution – The steady-state volume of distribution after IV administration was 0.74 L/kg. Cerebrospinal fluid concentrations obtained 0.25 and 5.67 hours post-dose in 3 patients who received 2.5 mg/kg ganciclovir IV every 8 or 12 hours ranged from 0.31 to 0.68 mcg/mL, representing 24% to 70% of the respective plasma concentrations. Binding to plasma proteins was 1% to 2% over ganciclovir concentrations of 0.5 and 51 mcg/mL.

Metabolism – Following oral administration of a single 1000 mg dose, 86% of the administered dose was recovered in the feces and 5% was recovered in the urine.

Excretion – When administered IV, ganciclovir exhibits linear pharmacokinetics over the range of 1.6 to 5 mg/kg and when administered orally, it exhibits linear kinetics up to a total daily dose of 4 g/day. Renal excretion of unchanged drug by glomerular filtration and active tubular secretion is the major route of elimination. In patients with normal renal function, 91.3% of IV ganciclovir was recovered unmetabolized in the urine. After oral administration, steady state is achieved within 24 hours. Renal clearance following oral administration was 3.1 mL/min/kg. Half-life was 3.5 hours following IV administration and 4.8 following oral use.

Children: At an IV dose of 4 or 6 mg/kg in 27 neonates (2 to 49 days of age), the pharmacokinetic parameters were, respectively, C_{max} of 5.5 and 7 mcg/mL, systemic clearance of 3.14 and 3.56 mL/min/kg and half-life of 2.4 hours for both.

Contraindications

Hypersensitivity to ganciclovir or acyclovir.

Warnings

CMV disease: Safety and efficacy have not been established for congenital or neonatal CMV disease, nor for the treatment of established CMV disease other than retinitis, nor for use in nonimmunocompromised individuals. The safety and efficacy of oral ganciclovir have not been established for treating any manifestation of CMV disease other than maintenance treatment of CMV retinitis.

Diagnosis of CMV retinitis: The diagnosis should be made by indirect ophthalmoscopy. Other conditions in the differential diagnosis of CMV retinitis include candidiasis, toxoplasmosis, histoplasmosis, retinal scars, and cotton wool spots, any of which may produce a retinal appearance similar to CMV. The diagnosis may be supported by a culture of CMV from urine, blood, or throat, but a negative CMV culture does not rule out CMV retinitis.

Retinal detachment: Retinal detachment has been observed in subjects with CMV retinitis both before and after initiation of therapy with ganciclovir. Its relationship to therapy is unknown. Patients with CMV retinitis should have frequent ophthalmologic evaluations to monitor the status of their retinitis and to detect any other retinal pathology.

Hematologic: Do not administer if the absolute neutrophil count is < 500/mm³ or the platelet count is < 25,000/mm³. Granulocytopenia (neutropenia), anemia, and thrombocytopenia have been observed in patients treated with ganciclovir. The frequency and severity of these events vary widely in different patient populations. Therefore, use with caution in patients with pre-existing cytopenias or with a history of cytopenic reactions to other drugs, chemicals, or irradiation. Granulocytopenia usually occurs during the first or second week of treatment, but may occur at any time during treatment. Cell counts usually begin to recover within 3 to

7 days of discontinuing the drug. Colony-stimulating factors have increased neutrophil and WBC counts in patients receiving IV ganciclovir for CMV retinitis.

Renal function impairment: Use ganciclovir with caution. Half-life and plasma/serum concentrations of ganciclovir will be increased because of reduced renal clearance (see Administration and Dosage).

If renal function is impaired, dosage adjustments are required for ganciclovir IV and should be considered for oral ganciclovir. Base such adjustments on measured or estimated Ccr values.

Hemodialysis reduces plasma levels of ganciclovir by $\approx$ 50%.

Carcinogenesis: Consider ganciclovir a potential carcinogen.

Mutagenesis: Because of the mutagenic and teratogenic potential of ganciclovir, advise women of childbearing potential to use effective contraception during treatment. Similarly, advise men to practice barrier contraception during and for at least 90 days following treatment with ganciclovir.

Fertility impairment: Although data in humans have not been obtained regarding this effect, it is considered probable that ganciclovir, at recommended doses, causes temporary or permanent inhibition of spermatogenesis.

Elderly: Pharmacokinetic profile in elderly patients is not established. Because elderly individuals frequently have a reduced glomerular filtration rate, pay particular attention to assessing renal function before and during ganciclovir therapy.

Pregnancy: Category C.

Lactation: It is not known whether ganciclovir is excreted in breast milk. The possibility of serious adverse reactions from ganciclovir in nursing infants is considered likely. Instruct mothers to discontinue nursing if they are receiving ganciclovir. The minimum interval before nursing can safely be resumed after the last dose of ganciclovir is unknown.

Children: Safety and efficacy in children have not been established. The use of ganciclovir in children warrants extreme caution to the probability of long-term carcinogenicity and reproductive toxicity. Administer to children only after careful evaluation and only if the potential benefits of treatment outweigh the risks. Oral ganciclovir has not been studied in children < 13 years of age.

There has been very limited clinical experience using ganciclovir for the treatment of CMV retinitis in patients < 12 years of age.

The spectrum of adverse reactions reported in 120 immunocompromised pediatric clinical trial participants with serious CMV infections receiving IV ganciclovir were similar to those reported in adults. Granulocytopenia (17%) and thrombocytopenia (10%) were most commonly reported.

Precautions

Monitoring: Because of the frequency of neutropenia, anemia, and thrombocytopenia in patients receiving ganciclovir, it is recommended that CBCs and platelet counts be performed frequently, especially in patients in whom ganciclovir or other nucleoside analogs have previously resulted in leukopenia, or in whom neutrophil counts are < 1000/mm^3 at the beginning of treatment. Patients should also have serum creatinine or Ccr values followed carefully.

Large doses/rapid infusion: The maximum single dose administered was 6 mg/kg by IV infusion over 1 hour. Larger doses have resulted in increased toxicity. It is likely that more rapid infusions would also result in increased toxicity.

Phlebitis/Pain at injection site: Initially, reconstituted ganciclovir solutions have a high pH (pH 11). Despite further dilution in IV fluids, phlebitis or pain may occur at the site of IV infusion. Take care to infuse solutions containing ganciclovir only into veins with adequate blood flow to permit rapid dilution and distribution.

Hydration: Because ganciclovir is excreted by the kidneys and normal clearance depends on adequate renal function, administration of ganciclovir should be accompanied by adequate hydration.

Drug Interactions

Drugs that may affect ganciclovir include imipenem-cilastatin, nephrotoxic drugs, probenecid, didanosine, and zidovudine. Drugs that may be affected by ganciclovir include cytotoxic drugs, didanosine, and zidovudine.

Adverse Reactions

Adverse reactions occurring in ≥ 3% of AIDS patients include fever; infection; chills; sepsis; diarrhea; anorexia; vomiting; leukopenia; anemia; thrombocytopenia; neuropathy; sweating; pruritus.

VALGANCICLOVIR

Tablets: 450 mg (Rx)	Valcyte (Roche)

Warning:
The clinical toxicity of valganciclovir, which is metabolized to ganciclovir, includes granulocytopenia, anemia, and thrombocytopenia. In animal studies, ganciclovir was carcinogenic, teratogenic, and caused aspermatogenesis.

Indications

Cytomegalovirus (CMV) retinitis: For the treatment of CMV retinitis in patients with acquired immunodeficiency syndrome (AIDS).

Administration and Dosage

Strict adherence to dosage recommendations is essential to avoid overdose. Valganciclovir tablets cannot be substituted for ganciclovir capsules on a one-to-one basis.

CMV retinitis (normal renal function):
  Induction – 900 mg (two 450 mg tablets) twice daily for 21 days with food.
  Maintenance – Following induction treatment, or in patients with inactive CMV retinitis, the recommended dosage is 900 mg (two 450 mg tablets) once daily with food.

Renal impairment: Monitor serum creatinine or Ccr levels carefully. Dosage adjustment is required according to Ccr, as shown in the table below. Increased monitoring for cytopenias may be warranted in patients with renal impairment.

Oral Valganciclovir in Renal Impairment		
Ccr (mL/min)	Induction dose	Maintenance dose
≥ 60	900 mg twice daily	900 mg once daily
40 to 59	450 mg twice daily	450 mg once daily
25 to 39	450 mg once daily	450 mg every 2 days
10 to 24	450 mg every 2 days	450 mg twice weekly

[1] An estimated creatinine clearance can be related to serum creatinine

by the following formulas: Males: $\dfrac{\text{Weight (kg)} \times (140 - \text{age})}{72 \times \text{serum creatinine (mg/dL)}} = \text{Ccr}$

Females: 0.85 × above value

Hemodialysis patients: Do not prescribe valganciclovir to patients receiving hemodialysis.

Handling and disposal: Exercise caution in the handling of valganciclovir tablets. Do not break or crush tablets. Because valganciclovir is considered a potential teratogen and carcinogen in humans, observe caution in handling broken tablets. Avoid direct contact of broken or crushed tablets with skin or mucous membranes. If such contact occurs, wash thoroughly with soap and water, and rinse eyes thoroughly with plain water.

Because ganciclovir shares some of the properties of antitumor agents (ie, carcinogenicity and mutagenicity), consider handling and disposing according to guidelines issued for antineoplastic drugs.

Actions

Pharmacology: Valganciclovir is an L-valyl ester (prodrug) of ganciclovir that exists as a mixture of 2 diastereomers. After oral administration, both diastereomers are rapidly converted to ganciclovir by intestinal and hepatic esterases.

Drug resistance – Viruses resistant to ganciclovir can arise after prolonged treatment with valganciclovir.

Pharmacokinetics:

Absorption – Valganciclovir is well absorbed from the GI tract and rapidly metabolized in the intestinal wall and liver to ganciclovir. The absolute bioavailability of ganciclovir from valganciclovir tablets following administration with food was $\approx$ 60%. Ganciclovir median T_{max} following administration of 450 to 2625 mg valganciclovir tablets ranged from 1 to 3 hours. Systemic exposure to the prodrug, valganciclovir, is transient and low, and the AUC_{24} and C_{max} values are $\approx$ 1% and 3% of those of ganciclovir, respectively.

Distribution – Plasma protein binding of ganciclovir is 1% to 2%. When ganciclovir was administered IV, the steady-state volume of distribution of ganciclovir was $\approx$ 0.703 L/kg (n = 69).

Metabolism – Valganciclovir is rapidly hydrolyzed to ganciclovir; no other metabolites have been detected.

Excretion – The major route of elimination of valganciclovir is by renal excretion as ganciclovir through glomerular filtration and active tubular secretion. Systemic clearance of IV administered ganciclovir was $\approx$ 3.07 mL/min (n = 68) while renal clearance was $\approx$ 2.99 mL/min/kg (n = 16).

The terminal half-life of ganciclovir following oral administration of valganciclovir tablets to either healthy or HIV-positive/CMV-positive subjects was $\approx$ 4.08 hours (n = 73), and that following administration of IV ganciclovir was $\approx$ 3.81 hours (n = 69).

Special populations –

Renal function impairment: Because the major elimination pathway for ganciclovir is renal, dosage reductions according to creatinine clearance are required for valganciclovir tablets.

Decreased renal function results in decreased clearance of ganciclovir from valganciclovir, and a corresponding increase in terminal half-life. Therefore, dosage adjustment is required for patients with impaired renal function.

Hemodialysis – Hemodialysis reduces plasma concentrations of ganciclovir by $\approx$ 50% following valganciclovir administration. Patients receiving hemodialysis (Ccr < 10 mL/min) cannot use valganciclovir tablets because the daily dose of valganciclovir tablets required for these patients is < 450 mg (see Administration and Dosage).

Liver transplant patients – In liver transplant patients, the ganciclovir $AUC_{0-24\ hr}$ achieved with 900 mg valganciclovir was $\approx$ 41.7 mcg•hr/mL (n = 28) and the $AUC_{0-24\ hr}$ achieved with the approved dosage of 5 mg/kg IV ganciclovir was $\approx$ 48.2 mcg•hr/mL (n = 27).

Contraindications

Hypersensitivity to valganciclovir or ganciclovir.

Warnings

Toxicity: The clinical toxicity of valganciclovir, which is metabolized to ganciclovir, includes granulocytopenia, anemia, and thrombocytopenia. In animal studies, ganciclovir was carcinogenic, teratogenic, and caused aspermatogenesis.

Hematologic: Valganciclovir tablets should not be administered if the absolute neutrophil count is < 500 cells/mm^3, the platelet count is < 25,000/mm^3, or the hemoglobin is < 8 g/dL.

Severe leukopenia, neutropenia, anemia, thrombocytopenia, pancytopenia, bone marrow depression, and aplastic anemia have been observed in patients treated with valganciclovir tablets (and ganciclovir) (see Precautions and Adverse Reactions).

Cytopenia may occur at any time during treatment and may increase with continued dosing. Cell counts usually begin to recover within 3 to 7 days of discontinuing drug.

Renal function impairment: If renal function is impaired, dosage adjustments are required for valganciclovir.

Carcinogenesis: Like ganciclovir, valganciclovir is a potential carcinogen.

Mutagenesis: Valganciclovir increases mutations in mouse lymphoma cells.

Fertility impairment: It is considered probable that in humans, valganciclovir at the recommended doses may cause temporary or permanent inhibition of spermatogenesis. Animal data also indicate that suppression of fertility in females may occur.

Because of the mutagenic and teratogenic potential of ganciclovir, advise women of childbearing potential to use effective contraception during treatment. Similarly, advise men to practice barrier contraception during and for at least 90 days following treatment with valganciclovir.

Elderly: The pharmacokinetic characteristics of valganciclovir in elderly patients have not been established. Since elderly individuals frequently have a reduced glomerular filtration rate, pay particular attention to assessing renal function before and during administration of valganciclovir.

Pregnancy: Category C.

Lactation: It is not known whether ganciclovir or valganciclovir is excreted in human milk. Because of potential for serious adverse events in nursing infants, mothers should be instructed not to breastfeed if they are receiving valganciclovir tablets. In addition, the Centers for Disease Control and Prevention recommend that HIV-infected mothers not breastfeed their infants to avoid risking postnatal transmission of HIV.

Children: Safety and efficacy of valganciclovir in pediatric patients have not been established.

Precautions

Monitoring: Because of the frequency of neutropenia, anemia, and thrombocytopenia in patients receiving valganciclovir tablets, it is recommended that complete blood counts and platelet counts be performed frequently, especially in patients in whom ganciclovir or other nucleoside analogs have previously resulted in leukopenia, or in whom neutrophil counts are < 1000 cell/mm³ at the beginning of treatment. Increased monitoring for cytopenias may be warranted if therapy with oral ganciclovir is changed to oral valganciclovir, because of increased plasma concentrations of ganciclovir after valganciclovir administration.

Increased serum creatinine levels have been observed in trials evaluating valganciclovir tablets. Patients should have serum creatinine or Ccr values monitored carefully to allow for dosage adjustments in renally impaired patients. The mechanism of impairment of renal function is not known.

Drug Interactions

No in vivo drug interaction studies were conducted with valganciclovir. However, because valganciclovir is rapidly and extensively converted to ganciclovir, interactions associated with ganciclovir will be expected for valganciclovir tablets (see Ganciclovir monograph).

Drugs that may affect valganciclovir include imipenem-cilastin, nephrotoxic drugs, probenecid, didanosine, and zidovudine. Drugs that may be affected by valganciclovir include cytotoxic drugs, didanosine, and zidovudine.

Drug/Food interactions: When valganciclovir tablets were administered with a high-fat meal containing ≈ 600 total calories (31.1 g fat, 51.6 g carbohydrates, and 22.2 g protein) at a dose of 875 mg once daily to 16 HIV-positive subjects, the steady-state ganciclovir AUC increased by 30% (95% CI 12% to 51%), and the C_{max} increased by 14% (95% CI −5% to 36%), without any prolongation in time to peak plasma concentrations (T_{max}). Administer valganciclovir tablets with food.

Adverse Reactions

Adverse reactions occurring in ≥ 3% of patients include the following: Headache, insomnia, peripheral neuropathy, paresthesia, diarrhea, nausea, vomiting, abdominal pain, neutropenia, anemia, thrombocytopenia, pyrexia, retinal detachment.

ACYCLOVIR (Acycloguanosine)

Tablets: 400 and 800 mg (*Rx*)
Capsules: 200 mg (*Rx*)
Suspension: 200 mg/5 mL (*Rx*)
Powder for injection: 500 and 1000 mg/vial (as sodium) (*Rx*)

Zovirax (GlaxoWellcome)

Indications

Parenteral: Treatment of initial and recurrent mucosal and cutaneous herpes simplex virus (HSV)-1 and -2 and varicella-zoster (shingles) infections in immunocompromised patients.

Herpes simplex encephalitis in patients > 6 months of age.

Severe initial clinical episodes of genital herpes in patients who are not immunocompromised.

Oral: Treatment of initial episodes and management of recurrent episodes of genital herpes in certain patients. Severity of the disease depends upon the immune status of the patient, frequency and duration of episodes, and degree of cutaneous or systemic involvement.

Acute treatment of herpes zoster (shingles) and chickenpox (varicella).

Administration and Dosage

Parenteral: For IV infusion only. Avoid rapid or bolus IV, IM, or SC injection. Administer over at least 1 hour to prevent renal tubular damage. Initiate therapy as soon as possible following onset of signs and symptoms.

IV Acyclovir Dosage/Management Guidelines		
	Dosage	
Indication	Adults	Children (< 12 years)
Mucosal and cutaneous HSV infections in immuno-compromised patients	5 mg/kg infused at a constant rate over 1 hour every 8 hours (15 mg/kg/day) for 7 days[1]	250 mg/m² infused at a constant rate over 1 hour every 8 hours (750 mg/m²/day) for 7 days[1]
Varicella-zoster infections (shingles) in immuno-compromised patients[2]	10 mg/kg infused at a constant rate over 1 hour every 8 hours for 7 days[3]	500 mg/m² infused at a constant rate over at least 1 hour every 8 hours for 7 days[3]
Herpes simplex encephalitis	10 mg/kg infused at a constant rate over at least 1 hour every 8 hours for 10 days	500 mg/m² infused at a constant rate over at least 1 hour every 8 hours for 10 days[4]

[1] For severe initial clinical episodes of herpes genitalis, use the same dose for 5 days.
[2] Base dosage for obese patients on ideal body weight (10 mg/kg).
[3] Do not exceed 500 mg/m² every 8 hours.
[4] > 6 months of age.

Renal function impairment, acute or chronic – Adjust the dosing interval as indicated below:

Parenteral Acyclovir Dosage in Renal Function Impairment		
Ccr (mL/min/1.73 m²)	Percent of recommended dose	Dosing interval (hours)
> 50	100%	8
25 to 50	100%	12
10 to 25	100%	24
0 to 10	50%	24

Hemodialysis – The mean plasma half-life of acyclovir during hemodialysis is ≈ 5 hours; a 60% decrease in plasma concentrations follows a 6-hour dialysis period. Therefore, administer a dose after each dialysis.

Oral:

Herpes simplex –

Initial genital herpes: 200 mg every 4 hours 5 times daily for 10 days. In patients with extremely severe episodes in which prostration, CNS involvement, urinary retention, or inability to take oral medication requires hospitalization and more aggressive management, initiate therapy with IV acyclovir (see above).

Chronic suppressive therapy for recurrent disease: 400 mg 2 times daily for up to 12 months, followed by reevaluation. Reevaluate the frequency and severity of the patient's HSV after 1 year of therapy to assess the need for continuation of therapy; frequency and severity of episodes of untreated genital herpes may change over time. Reevaluation usually requires a trial off acyclovir to assess the need for reinstitution of suppressive therapy. Some patients, such as those with very frequent or severe episodes before treatment, may warrant uninterrupted suppression for > 1 year.

Alternative regimens have included doses ranging from 200 mg 3 times daily to 200 mg 5 times daily.

Intermittent therapy: 200 mg every 4 hours 5 times daily for 5 days. Initiate therapy at the earliest sign or symptom (prodrome) of recurrence.

Herpes zoster, acute treatment – 800 mg every 4 hours 5 times daily for 7 to 10 days.

Chickenpox – 20 mg/kg (not to exceed 800 mg) 4 times daily for 5 days. Initiate at earliest sign or symptom.

Renal impairment, acute or chronic –

Oral Acyclovir Dosage in Renal Function Impairment			
Normal dosage regimen (5× daily)	Ccr (mL/min/1.73 m²)	Adjusted dosage regimen	
		Dose (mg)	Dosing interval
200 mg every 4 hours	> 10	200	Every 4 hours, 5× daily
	0 to 10	200	Every 12 hours
400 mg every 12 hours	> 10	400	Every 12 hours
	0 to 10	200	Every 12 hours
800 mg every 4 hours	> 25	800	Every 4 hours, 5× daily
	10 to 25	800	Every 8 hours
	0 to 10	800	Every 12 hours

Hemodialysis – For patients that require hemodialysis, adjust dosing schedule so that a dose is administered after each dialysis. No supplemental dose is necessary after peritoneal dialysis.

Actions

Pharmacology: A synthetic acyclic purine nucleoside analog, acyclovir has in vitro inhibitory activity against HSV-1 and HSV-2, varicella zoster, Epstein-Barr, and cytomegalovirus. Acyclovir is preferentially taken up and selectively converted to the active triphosphate form by HSV-infected cells. Acyclovir triphosphate interferes with HSV DNA polymerase and inhibits viral DNA replication. In vitro, acyclovir triphosphate can be incorporated into growing chains of DNA by viral DNA polymerase and, to a much smaller extent, by cellular DNA polymerase. When incorporation occurs, the DNA chain is terminated.

Pharmacokinetics:

Absorption/Distribution – When acyclovir was administered to adults at 5 mg/kg (≈ 250 mg/m²) by 1 hour infusions every 8 hours, mean steady-state peak and trough concentrations were 9.8 mcg/mL (5.5 to 13.8 mcg/mL) and 0.7 mcg/mL (0.2 to 1 mcg/mL), respectively. Similar concentrations are achieved in children > 1 year of age when doses of 250 mg/m² are given every 8 hours. Oral acyclovir is slowly and incompletely absorbed from the GI tract. Peak concentrations are reached in 1.5 to 2 hours; absorption is unaffected by food. Bioavailability is between 15% and 30% and decreases with increasing doses. Concentrations achieved in CSF are

≈ 50% of plasma values. Plasma protein binding is 9% to 33%. Acyclovir is widely distributed in tissues and body fluids, including brain, kidney, lung, liver, muscle, spleen, uterus, vaginal mucosa, vaginal secretions, CSF, and herpetic vesicular fluid.

Metabolism/Excretion – Renal excretion of unchanged drug by glomerular filtration and tubular secretion following IV use accounts for 62% to 91% of the dose. Mean renal excretion of unchanged drug following oral use is 14.4% (8.6% to 19.8%). The only major urinary metabolite may account for up to 14% of the dose in patients with normal renal function. An insignificant amount is recovered in feces and expired CO_2; there is no evidence of tissue retention.

Half-life and total body clearance depend on renal function:

Acyclovir Half-Life and Total Body Clearance Based on Renal Function		
Ccr (mL/min/1.73 m²)	Half-life (hr)	Total body clearance (mL/min/1.73 m²)
> 80	2.5	327
50 to 80	3	248
15 to 50	3.5	190
0 (Anuric)	19.5	29

The half-life and total body clearance of acyclovir in pediatric patients > 1 year of age is similar to those in adults with normal renal function.

Contraindications

Hypersensitivity to acyclovir or any component of the formulation.

Warnings

Pregnancy: Category C.

Lactation: Acyclovir concentrations in breast milk in women following oral administration have ranged from 0.6 to 4.1 times corresponding plasma levels. These concentrations would potentially expose the nursing infant to a dose of acyclovir up to 0.3 mg/kg/day.

Children: Safety and efficacy of oral acyclovir in children < 2 years of age have not been established.

Precautions

Diagnosis: Proof of HSV infection rests on viral isolation and identification in tissue culture. Although the cutaneous vesicular lesions associated with HSV are often characteristic, other etiologic agents can cause similar lesions.

Genital herpes: Avoid sexual intercourse when visible lesions are present.

Herpes zoster infections: Adults ≥ 50 years of age tend to have more severe shingles, and acyclovir treatment showed more significant benefit for older patients. Treatment was more useful if started within the first 48 hours of rash onset.

Chickenpox: Although chickenpox in otherwise healthy children is usually a self-limited disease of mild to moderate severity, adolescents and adults tend to have more severe disease. Treatment was initiated within 24 hours of the typical chickenpox rash in the controlled studies, and there is no information regarding the effects of treatment begun later in the disease course. It is unknown whether the treatment of chickenpox in childhood has any effect on long-term immunity. However, there is no evidence to indicate that acyclovir treatment of chickenpox would have any effect on either decreasing or increasing the incidence or severity of subsequent recurrences of herpes zoster (shingles) later in life.

Do not exceed: Do not exceed the recommended dosage, frequency, or length of treatment. Base dosage adjustments on estimated Ccr.

Renal effects: Precipitation of acyclovir crystals in renal tubules can occur if the maximum solubility of free acyclovir is exceeded or if the drug is administered by bolus injection. Serum creatinine and BUN rise and Ccr decreases.

Bolus administration of the drug leads to a 10% incidence of renal dysfunction, while infusion of 5 mg/kg (250 mg/m²) over an hour was associated with a lower frequency (4.6%). Concomitant use of other nephrotoxic drugs, pre-existing renal disease and dehydration make further renal impairment with acyclovir more likely. In most instances, alterations of renal function were transient and resolved spontaneously or with improvement of water and electrolyte balance, with drug dosage adjustments, or with drug discontinuation. However, these changes may progress to acute renal failure.

Hydration: Accompany IV infusion by adequate hydration. Because maximum urine concentration occurs within the first 2 hours following infusion, establish sufficient urine flow during that period to prevent precipitation in renal tubules.

Encephalopathic changes: Patients (1%) receiving acyclovir IV have manifested encephalopathic changes characterized by either lethargy, obtundation, tremors, confusion, hallucinations, agitation, seizures, or coma. Use with caution in those patients who have underlying neurologic abnormalities; those with serious renal, hepatic, or electrolyte abnormalities or significant hypoxia; and those who have manifested prior neurologic reactions to cytotoxic drugs.

Resistance: Exposure of HSV isolates to acyclovir in vitro can lead to the emergence of less sensitive viruses. In severely immunocompromised patients, prolonged or repeated courses of acyclovir may result in resistant viruses that may not fully respond to continued acyclovir therapy.

Drug Interactions

Drugs that may affect acyclovir include probenecid and zidovudine.

Adverse Reactions

Adverse reactions (parenteral) occurring in ≥ 3% of patients include inflammation or phlebitis at injection site, transient elevations of serum creatinine or BUN, and nausea or vomiting.

Adverse reactions (oral) occurring in ≥ 3% of patients include malaise, nausea, and headache.

FAMCICLOVIR

Tablets: 125, 250, and 500 mg (*Rx*)   *Famvir* (GlaxoSmithKline)

Indications

Acute herpes zoster: Management of acute herpes zoster (shingles).

Genital herpes: Treatment of recurrent episodes of genital herpes.

Administration and Dosage

Herpes zoster: The recommended dosage is 500 mg every 8 hours for 7 days. Initiate therapy promptly as soon as herpes zoster is diagnosed.

Genital herpes (recurrent episodes): The recommended dosage is 125 mg twice daily for 5 days. Initiate therapy at the first sign or symptom if medical management of a genital herpes recurrence is indicated.

Famciclovir Dosage in Renal Function Impairment	
Ccr (mL/min)	Dose regimen
Herpes zoster	
≥ 60	500 mg q 8 h
40 to 59	500 mg q 12 h
20 to 39	500 mg q 24 h
< 20	250 mg q 48 h
Recurrent genital herpes	
≥ 40	125 mg q 12 h
20 to 39	125 mg q 24 h
< 20	125 mg q 48 h

Hemodialysis patients: The recommended dose of famciclovir is 250 mg (herpes zoster) or 125 mg (genital herpes) administered following each dialysis treatment.

Actions

Pharmacology: Famciclovir undergoes rapid biotransformation to the active antiviral compound penciclovir, which has inhibitory activity against herpes simplex virus types 1 (HSV-1) and 2 (HSV-2), and varicella-zoster virus (VZV). In HSV-1-, HSV-2-, and VZV-infected cells, viral thymidine kinase phosphorylates penciclovir to a monophosphate form that, in turn, is converted to penciclovir triphosphate by cellular kinases. In vitro, penciclovir triphosphate inhibits HSV-2 polymerase competitively with deoxyguanosine triphosphate. Consequently, herpes viral DNA synthesis and, therefore, replication are selectively inhibited.

Pharmacokinetics:

Absorption – The absolute bioavailability of famciclovir is 77%. The area under the plasma concentration-time curve (AUC) was 8.6 mcg•hr/mL. The maximum concentration (C_{max}) was 3.3 mcg/mL and the time to C_{max} (T_{max}) was 0.9 hours.

After a 1-hour IV infusion of penciclovir at doses of 5 to 20 mg/kg, the volume of distribution (Vd_b) of penciclovir was 83.1 and 125 L, respectively. Penciclovir is < 20% bound to plasma proteins over the concentration range of 0.1 to 20 mcg/mL. The blood/plasma ratio of penciclovir is ≈ 1.

Metabolism – Famciclovir given orally is deacetylated and oxidized to form penciclovir. Inactive metabolites include 6-deoxy penciclovir, monoacetylated penciclovir, and 6-deoxy monoacetylated penciclovir (each < 0.5% of the dose). Cytochrome P450 does not play an important role in famciclovir metabolism.

Excretion – Following a single 500 mg oral dose of radio-labeled famciclovir, 73% and 27% of administered radioactivity were recovered in urine and feces over 72 hours, respectively. Penciclovir accounted for 82% and 6-deoxy penciclovir accounted for 7% of the radioactivity excreted in the urine. Approximately 60% of the administered radiolabeled dose was collected in urine in the first 6 hours.

Renal clearance of penciclovir following the oral administration of a single 500 mg dose of famciclovir was 27.7 L/hr.

The plasma elimination half-life of penciclovir was 2 hours after IV penciclovir and 2.3 hours after 500 mg oral famciclovir. The half-life in 7 herpes zoster patients was 3 hours.

Contraindications

Hypersensitivity to famciclovir.

Warnings

Renal function impairment: Apparent plasma clearance, renal clearance, and the plasma-elimination rate constant of penciclovir decreased linearly with reductions in renal function. After a single 500 mg oral famciclovir dose to healthy volunteers and to volunteers with varying degrees of renal insufficiency, the following results were obtained.

Pharmacokinetics of Famciclovir in Patients with Renal Function Impairment				
Parameter (mean)	Ccr ≥ 60 (mL/min; n = 15)	Ccr 40 to 59 (mL/min; n = 5)	Ccr 20 to 39 (mL/min; n = 4)	Ccr < 20 (mL/min; n = 3)
Ccr (mL/min)	88.1	49.3	26.5	12.7
CL_R (L/hr)	30.1	13[1]	4.2	1.6
CL/F^2 (L/hr)	66.9	27.3	12.8	5.8
Half-life (hr)	2.3	3.4	6.2	13.4

[1] n = 4
[2] CL/F consists of bioavailability factor and famciclovir to penciclovir conversion factor.

Dosage adjustment is recommended in renal insufficiency (see Administration and Dosage).

Hepatic function impairment: Well-compensated chronic liver disease (chronic hepatitis, chronic ethanol abuse, or primary biliary cirrhosis) had no effect on extent of availability (AUC) of penciclovir following a single dose of 500 mg famciclovir. However, there was a 44% decrease in penciclovir mean maximum plasma level and the time to maximum plasma concentration was increased by 0.75 hours in patients with hepatic insufficiency compared with normal volunteers. No dosage adjustment is recommended in well-compensated hepatic impairment. Penciclovir pharmacokinetics have not been evaluated in severe uncompensated hepatic impairment.

Elderly: Mean penciclovir AUC was 40% larger and penciclovir renal clearance was 22% lower after the oral administration of famciclovir in elderly volunteers (65 to 79 years of age) compared with younger volunteers.

Pregnancy: Category B.

Lactation: It is not known whether famciclovir is excreted in breast milk. Because of the potential for tumorigenicity shown for famciclovir in rats, discontinue nursing or the drug, taking into account the importance of the drug to the mother.

Children: Safety and efficacy in children < 18 years of age have not been established.

Drug Interactions
The conversion of 6-deoxy penciclovir to penciclovir is catalyzed by aldehyde oxidase. Interactions with other drugs metabolized by this enzyme could occur.

Drugs that may affect famciclovir include cimetidine, probenecid, and theophylline.

Drugs that may be affected by famciclovir include digoxin.

Drug/Food interactions: When famciclovir was administered with food, penciclovir C_{max} decreased $\approx$ 50%. Because the systemic availability of penciclovir (AUC) was not altered, it appears that famciclovir may be taken without regard to meals.

Adverse Reactions
Adverse reactions occurring in $\geq$ 3% of patients include dizziness, diarrhea, abdominal pain, dyspepsia, constipation, vomiting, fatigue, fever, pruritus.

The most frequent adverse events were headache and nausea.

VALACYCLOVIR HCl

Caplets: 500 mg, 1 g (*Rx*)	*Valtrex* (GlaxoSmithKline)

Indications
Herpes zoster: Treatment of herpes zoster (shingles) in immunocompetent adults.

Genital herpes: Treatment or suppression of genital herpes.

Administration and Dosage
Valacyclovir may be given without regard to meals.

Herpes zoster: The recommended dosage is 1 g 3 times daily for 7 days. Initiate therapy at the earliest sign or symptom of herpes zoster; it is most effective when started within 48 hours of the onset of zoster rash. No data are available on efficacy of treatment started > 72 hours after rash onset.

Genital herpes:
    Initial episodes – The recommended dosage is 1 g twice daily for 10 days. There are no data on the effectiveness of treatment when initiated > 72 hours after the onset of signs and symptoms. Therapy was most effective when administered within 48 hours of the onset of signs and symptoms.

    Recurrent episodes – The recommended dosage is 500 mg twice daily for 3 days. Advise patients to initiate therapy at the first sign or symptom of an episode. There are no data on the efficacy of treatment started > 24 hours after the onset of signs or symptoms.

    Suppressive therapy – The recommended dosage for chronic suppressive therapy of recurrent genital herpes is 1 g once daily. In patients with a history of $\leq$ 9 recurrences per year, an alternative dose is 500 mg once daily. The safety and efficacy of therapy with valacyclovir beyond 1 year have not been established.

Acute or chronic renal impairment:

Valacyclovir Dosage Adjustments for Renal Impairment				
	Normal dosage (Ccr ≥ 50)	Ccr (mL/min)		
Indication		30 to 49	10 to 29	< 10
Herpes zoster	1 g q 8 hr	1 g q 12 hr	1 g q 24 hr	500 mg q 24 hr
Genital herpes				
Initial treatment	1 g q 12 hr	No reduction	1 g q 24 hr	500 mg q 24 hr
Recurrent episodes	500 mg q 12 hr	No reduction	500 mg q 24 hr	500 mg q 24 hr
Suppressive therapy	1 g q 24 hr	No reduction	500 mg q 24 hr	500 mg q 24 hr
Suppressive therapy (≤ 9 recurrences/yr)	500 mg q 24 hr	No reduction	500 mg q 48 hr	500 mg q 48 hr

Hemodialysis: Following valacyclovir administration to volunteers with end-stage renal disease, the average acyclovir half-life is ≈ 14 hours. During hemodialysis, the half-life of acyclovir after administration of valacyclovir is ≈ 4 hours. About 33% of acyclovir in the body is removed by dialysis during a 4-hour hemodialysis session. Patients requiring hemodialysis should receive the recommended dose of valacyclovir after hemodialysis.

Peritoneal dialysis: Supplemental doses of valacyclovir should not be required following chronic ambulatory peritoneal dialysis (CAPD) or continuous arteriovenous hemofiltration/hemodialysis (CAVHD).

Actions

Pharmacology: Valacyclovir is the hydrochloride salt of L-valyl ester of the antiviral drug acyclovir. Valacyclovir is rapidly converted to acyclovir, which has in vitro and in vivo inhibitory activity against herpes simplex virus types I (HSV-1) and II (HSV-2), and varicella-zoster virus (VZV). In cell culture, acyclovir has the highest antiviral activity against HSV-1, followed by (in decreasing order of potency) HSV-2 and VZV.

In vitro, acyclovir triphosphate stops replication of herpes viral DNA in 3 ways: 1) Competitive inhibition of viral DNA polymerase; 2) incorporation and termination of the growing viral DNA chain; and 3) inactivation of the viral DNA polymerase.

Pharmacokinetics:

Absorption/Distribution – Valacyclovir is rapidly absorbed and is rapidly and nearly completely converted to acyclovir and L-valine by first-pass metabolism. The absolute bioavailability of acyclovir after administration of valacyclovir is 54.5%.

Metabolism – Neither valacyclovir nor acyclovir metabolism is metabolized by cytochrome P450 enzymes.

Excretion – Acyclovir accounted for 88.6% excreted in the urine. Renal clearance of acyclovir following the administration of a single 1 g valacyclovir dose to 12 healthy volunteers was ≈ 255 mL/min, which represents 41.9% of total acyclovir apparent plasma clearance.

The plasma elimination half-life of acyclovir typically averaged 2.5 to 3.3 hours in volunteers with normal renal function.

Contraindications

Hypersensitivity or intolerance to valacyclovir, acyclovir, or any component of the formulation.

Warnings

Thrombotic thrombocytopenic purpura/hemolytic uremic syndrome (TTP/HUS): TTP/HUS, in some cases resulting in death, has been reported in patients with advanced HIV disease and in bone marrow and renal transplant recipients. Valacyclovir is not indicated for the treatment of immunocompromised patients. TTP/HUS has not been seen in immunocompetent patients receiving valacyclovir in clinical trials.

Renal function impairment: Exercise caution when giving valacyclovir to patients with renal impairment or those receiving potentially nephrotoxic agents as this may increase the risk of renal dysfunction or the risk of reversible CNS symptoms such as those that occur infrequently in patients treated with IV acyclovir.

Hepatic function impairment: Administration of valacyclovir to patients with moderate (biopsy-proven cirrhosis) or severe (with and without ascites and biopsy-proven cirrhosis) liver disease indicated that the rate but not the extent of conversion of valacyclovir to acyclovir was reduced, and the acyclovir half-life was not affected. Dosage modification is not recommended for patients with cirrhosis.

Elderly: Dosage reduction may be required in geriatric patients, depending on the underlying renal status of the patient.

Pregnancy: Category B.

Lactation: Consider temporary discontinuation of nursing, as the safety of valacyclovir has not been established in infants.

Children: Safety and efficacy have not been established.

Drug Interactions
Drugs that may affect valacyclovir include cimetidine/probenecid.

Adverse Reactions
Adverse reactions occurring in ≥ 3% of patients include nausea, headache, vomiting, dizziness, abdominal pain, depression, AST abnormalities, dysmenorrhea, and arthralgia.

AMANTADINE HCl

Tablets: 100 mg (*Rx*)	*Symmetrel* (Endo)
Capsules: 100 mg (*Rx*)	Various
Syrup: 50 mg/5 mL (*Rx*)	Various, *Symmetrel* (Endo)

Indications
Influenza A viral infection: Amantadine is indicated for the prophylaxis and treatment of signs and symptoms of infection caused by various strains of influenza A virus.

   Prophylaxis – Chemoprophylaxis against influenza A virus infection when early vaccination is not feasible or when the vaccine is contraindicated or not available. Following vaccination during an influenza A outbreak, consider amantadine prophylaxis for the 2- to 4-week time period required to develop an antibody response.

   Treatment – Treatment of uncomplicated respiratory tract illness caused by influenza A virus, especially when administered early in the course of illness.

Prophylaxis recommendations:
1.) High-risk patients vaccinated after influenza outbreak has begun: Consider prophylaxis until immunity from the influenza vaccine has developed (up to 2 weeks).
2.) Caretakers of those at high risk: Consider prophylaxis for unvaccinated caretakers of high-risk patients during peak influenza activity.
3.) Patients with immune deficiency: Consider prophylaxis for high-risk patients who are expected to have inadequate antibody response to influenza vaccine (eg, HIV).
4.) Other: Consider prophylaxis in high-risk patients who should not be vaccinated. Prophylaxis also may be offered to those patients who desire to avoid influenza illness.

Parkinsonism and drug-induced extrapyramidal reactions: See amantadine in the Antiparkinson Agents section.

Administration and Dosage
Influenza A virus illness:
   Prophylaxis – Start in anticipation of contact or as soon as possible after exposure. Use daily for ≥ 10 days following a known exposure. The infectious period extends

from shortly before onset of symptoms to up to 1 week after. Because amantadine does not appear to suppress antibody response, it can be used in conjunction with inactivated influenza A virus vaccine until protective antibody responses develop; administer for 2 to 4 weeks after vaccine has been given. When the vaccine is unavailable or contraindicated, give amantadine for the duration of known influenza A in the community because of repeated and unknown exposure.

Symptomatic management – Start as soon as possible after onset of symptoms and continue for 24 to 48 hours after symptoms disappear.

Dosage:

| Amantadine Dosage by Patient Age and Renal Function ||
Renal function	Dosage
No recognized renal disease	
1 to 9 yrs[1]	4.4 to 8.8 mg/kg/day given once daily or divided twice daily, not to exceed 150 mg/day
9 to 12 yrs	100 mg twice daily
13 to 64 yrs	200 mg once daily or divided twice daily
≥ 65 yrs	100 mg once daily
Renal function impairment – Ccr (mL/min/1.73 m²)	
30 to 50	200 mg 1st day; 100 mg daily thereafter
15 to 29	200 mg 1st day; then 100 mg on alternate days
< 15	200 mg every 7 days
Hemodialysis patients	200 mg every 7 days

[1] Use in children < 1 year of age has not been evaluated adequately.

Dosage adjustments: For adults < 65 years of age, if CNS effects develop in a once-daily dosage, a split dosage schedule may reduce such complaints.

Special risk patients: Dose may need reduction in patients with CHF, peripheral edema, orthostatic hypotension, or impaired renal function.

Actions

Pharmacology: Inhibits the replication of influenza A virus isolates from each of the subtypes. Amantadine's antiviral activity is not completely understood. Its mode of action appears to be the prevention of the release of infectious viral nucleic acid into the host cell. Amantadine does not appear to interfere with the immunogenicity of inactivated influenza A virus vaccine.

Amantadine is 70% to 90% effective in preventing illnesses caused by type A influenza viruses.

Pharmacokinetics:

Absorption/Distribution – After administration of a single dose of 100 mg, maximum blood levels are reached in ≈ 4 hours, based on the mean time of the peak urinary excretion rate; the peak excretion rate is ≈ 5 mg/hr; the mean half-life of the excretion rate is ≈ 15 hours.

Clearance of amantadine is significantly reduced in adults with renal insufficiency. Elimination half-life increases 2- to 3-fold when Ccr < 40 mL/min/1.73 m² and averages 8 days in patients on chronic maintenance hemodialysis.

Metabolism/Excretion – Amantadine is readily absorbed, is not metabolized, and is excreted in the urine. The renal clearance of amantadine is reduced and plasma levels are increased in otherwise healthy elderly patients ≥ 65 years of age. The drug plasma levels in elderly patients receiving 100 mg daily have been reported to approximate those determined in younger adults taking 200 mg daily.

Contraindications

Hypersensitivity to amantadine.

Warnings

Deaths: Deaths have been reported from overdose with amantadine (see Overdosage).

Suicide attempts: Suicide attempts, some of which have been fatal, have been reported in patients treated with amantadine, many of whom received short courses for influenza treatment or prophylaxis. Suicide attempts and suicidal ideation have been reported in patients with and without prior history of psychiatric illness. Amantadine can exacerbate mental problems in patients with a history of psychiatric disorders or substance abuse. Patients who attempt suicide may exhibit abnormal mental states, which include disorientation, confusion, depression, personality changes, agitation, aggressive behavior, hallucinations, paranoia, other psychotic reactions, and somnolence or insomnia. Because of the possibility of serious adverse effects, observe caution when prescribing amantadine to patients being treated with drugs having CNS effects, or for whom the potential risks outweigh the benefit of treatment.

Seizures and other CNS effects: Closely observe patients with a history of seizures for increased seizure activity. Caution patients who note CNS effects or blurring of vision against driving or working in situations where alertness and adequate motor coordination are important.

CHF or peripheral edema: Closely follow patients with a history of CHF or peripheral edema as there are patients who developed CHF while receiving amantadine.

Glaucoma: Because amantadine has anticholinergic effects and may cause mydriasis, do not give to patients with untreated angle closure glaucoma.

Other: Exercise care when administering to patients with a history of recurrent eczematoid rash, or to patients with psychosis or severe psychoneurosis not controlled by chemotherapeutic agents.

Renal function impairment: Reduce the dose in renal impairment.

Elderly: Reduce dose in individuals ≥ 65 years of age.

Pregnancy: Category C.

Lactation: Amantadine is excreted in breast milk. Use is not recommended in nursing mothers.

Children: Safety and efficacy for use in neonates and infants < 1 year of age have not been established.

Precautions

Abrupt withdrawal: Do not discontinue amantadine abruptly in patients with Parkinson's disease. A few patients have experienced a parkinsonian crisis (a sudden marked clinical deterioration) when this medication was suddenly stopped. Abrupt discontinuation also may precipitate delirium, agitation, delusions, hallucinations, paranoid reaction, stupor, anxiety, depression, and slurred speech.

Neuroleptic malignant syndrome (NMS): Sporadic cases of possible NMS have been reported in association with dose reduction or withdrawal of amantadine therapy. Observe patients carefully when the dosage of amantadine is reduced abruptly or discontinued, especially if the patient is receiving neuroleptics.

Drug Interactions

Drugs that may affect amantadine include anticholinergic drugs, triamterene and thiazide diuretics, quinidine, quinine, and trimethoprim/sulfamethoxazole.

Drugs that may be affected by amantadine include CNS stimulants.

Adverse Reactions

Adverse reactions occurring in ≥ 3% of patients include nausea; dizziness; lightheadedness; insomnia; depression; anxiety; irritability; hallucinations; confusion; anorexia; dry mouth; constipation; ataxia; livedo reticularis; peripheral edema; orthostatic hypotension; headache.

RIBAVIRIN

Capsules: 200 mg (Rx)
Lyophilized powder for aerosol reconstitution: 6 g ribavirin/100 mL vial. Contains 20 mg/mL when reconstituted with 300 mL sterile water (Rx)

Rebetol (Schering)
Virazole (ICN)

Warning:

Capsules: Ribavirin monotherapy is not effective for the treatment of chronic hepatitis C virus infection and should not be used alone for this indication.

The primary toxicity of ribavirin is hemolytic anemia. The anemia associated with ribavirin therapy may result in worsening of cardiac disease that has led to fatal and nonfatal MIs. Do not treat patients with a history of significant or unstable cardiac disease with ribavirin.

Significant teratogenic or embryocidal effects have been demonstrated in all animal species exposed to ribavirin. In addition, ribavirin has a multiple-dose half-life of 12 days, and it may persist in nonplasma compartments for as long as 6 months. Therefore, ribavirin therapy is contraindicated in women who are pregnant and in the male partners of women who are pregnant. Extreme care must be taken to avoid pregnancy during therapy and for 6 months after completion of treatment in both female patients and in female partners of male patients who are taking ribavirin. At least 2 reliable forms of effective contraception must be utilized during treatment and during the 6-month posttreatment follow-up period.

Aerosol: In patients requiring mechanical ventilator assistance, pay strict attention to procedures that minimize the accumulation of drug precipitate that can result in mechanical ventilator dysfunction and associated increased pulmonary pressures.

Sudden deterioration of respiratory function has been associated with initiation of aerosolized ribavirin use in infants. Carefully monitor respiratory function during treatment. If initiation of aerosolized ribavirin treatment appears to produce sudden deterioration of respiratory function, stop treatment and reinstitute only with extreme caution, continuous monitoring, and consideration of concomitant administration of bronchodilators (see Warnings).

Ribavirin aerosol is not indicated for use in adults. Physicians and patients should be aware that ribavirin has been shown to produce testicular lesions in rodents and to be teratogenic in all animal species in which adequate studies have been conducted.

Indications

Capsules:

Chronic hepatitis C – Only in combination with *Intron A* (interferon alfa-2b, recombinant) injection for the treatment of chronic hepatitis C in patients with compensated liver disease previously untreated with alpha interferon or who have relapsed following alpha interferon therapy.

Aerosol:

Severe lower respiratory tract infections – Treatment of hospitalized infants and young children with severe lower respiratory tract infections caused by respiratory syncytial virus (RSV).

Administration and Dosage

Capsules: The recommended dose of ribavirin capsules depends on the patient's body weight.

Recommended Dosing	
Body weight	Ribavirin capsules
≤ 75 kg	2 × 200 mg capsules AM, 3 × 200 mg capsules PM daily PO
> 75 kg	3 × 200 mg capsules AM, 3 × 200 mg capsules PM daily PO

Ribavirin may be administered without regard to food but should be administered in a consistent manner with respect to food intake.

Treatment duration – The recommended duration of treatment for patients previously untreated with interferon is 24 to 48 weeks. Individualize the duration of treatment depending on baseline disease characteristics, response to therapy, and tolerability of the regimen. Assess virologic response after 24 weeks of treatment. Consider treatment discontinuation in any patient who has not achieved an HCV-RNA below the limit of detection by 24 weeks. There are no safety and efficacy data on treatment for > 48 weeks in the previously untreated patient population.

In patients who relapse following interferon therapy, the recommended duration of treatment is 24 weeks. There are no safety and efficacy data on treatment for > 24 weeks in the relapse patient population.

Dose modifications – In clinical trials, ≈ 26% of patients required modification of their dose of ribavirin capsules, *Intron A* injection, or both agents. If severe adverse reactions or laboratory abnormalities develop during combination therapy, modify or discontinue the dose, if appropriate, until the adverse reactions abate. If intolerance persists after dose adjustment, discontinue combination therapy.

A permanent dose reduction is required for patients with a history of stable cardiovascular disease if the hemoglobin decreases by ≥ 2 g/dL during any 4-week period. In addition, discontinue combination therapy in cardiac history patients if the hemoglobin remains < 12 g/dL after 4 weeks on a reduced dose.

It is recommended that a patient whose hemoglobin level falls below 10 g/dL have his/her ribavirin dose reduced to 600 mg daily (1 × 200 mg capsule AM, 2 × 200 mg capsules PM). Permanently discontinue ribavirin therapy in patients whose hemoglobin level falls below 8.5 g/dL.

Guidelines for Dose Modifications and Discontinuation for Anemia Based on Hemoglobin Levels		
	Dose reduction ribavirin capsules 600 mg daily	Permanent discontinuation of ribavirin treatment
No cardiac history	< 10 g/dL	< 8.5 g/dL
Cardiac history patients	≥ 2 g/dL decrease during any 4-wk period during treatment	< 12 g/dL after 4 wks of dose reduction

Special populations: Do not use ribavirin in patients with Ccr < 50 mL/min. Administer ribavirin with caution to patients with pre-existing cardiac disease. Assess patients before commencement of therapy and appropriately monitor them during therapy. Stop therapy if there is any deterioration of cardiovascular status.

Aerosol: For aerosol administration only. Ribavirin aerosol is not to be administered with any other aerosol-generating device or together with other aerosolized medications.

The recommended treatment regimen is 20 mg/mL as the starting solution in the drug reservoir of the Small Particle Aerosol Generator (SPAG-2) unit. Treatment is carried out for 12 to 18 hours/day for 3 to 7 days.

Mechanically ventilated infants – The recommended dose and administration schedule for infants who require mechanical ventilation is the same as for those who do not. Either a pressure or volume cycle ventilator may be used in conjunction with the

SPAG-2. In either case, suction endotracheal tubes every 1 to 2 hours and monitor pulmonary pressures frequently (every 2 to 4 hours). For both pressure and volume ventilators, heated wire connective tubing and bacteria filters in series in the expiratory limb of the system (which must be changed frequently, eg, every 4 hours) must be used to minimize the risk of ribavirin precipitation in the system and the subsequent risk of ventilator dysfunction. Use water column pressure release valves in the ventilator circuit for pressure-cycled ventilators. They also may be used with volume-cycled ventilators.

Nonmechanically ventilated infants – The aerosol is delivered to an infant oxygen hood from the SPAG-2 aerosol generator. Administration by face mask or oxygen tent may be necessary if a hood cannot be used. However, the volume and condensation area are larger in a tent, and this may alter the drug's delivery dynamics.

Reconstitution – Reconstitute drug with a minimum of 75 mL of Sterile Water for Injection or Inhalation in the original 100 mL vial. Shake well. Transfer to the clean, sterilized 500 mL wide-mouth Erlenmeyer flask (SPAG-2 Reservoir) and further dilute to a final volume of 300 mL with Sterile Water for Injection or Inhalation. The final concentration should be 20 mg/mL.

Important: This water should not have any antimicrobial agent or other substance added. Discard solutions placed in the SPAG-2 unit at least every 24 hours and when the liquid level is low before adding newly reconstituted solution. Using the recommended drug concentration of 20 mg/mL ribavirin as the starting solution in the SPAG-2 unit's drug reservoir, the average aerosol concentration for a 12-hour period is 190 mcg/L of air.

Actions

Pharmacology:

Antiviral effects – Ribavirin has antiviral inhibitory activity in vitro against RSV, influenza virus, and herpes simplex virus. The mechanism of action is unknown.

Immunologic effects – Neutralizing antibody responses to RSV were decreased in ribavirin-treated infants compared with placebo-treated infants; clinical significance of this observation is unknown.

Pharmacokinetics:

Absorption –

Capsules: Ribavirin was rapidly and extensively absorbed following oral administration. However, because of first-pass metabolism, the absolute bioavailability averaged 64%.

Aerosol: Ribavirin administered by aerosol is absorbed systemically. The plasma half-life was 9.5 hours.

Distribution –

Capsules: Following oral dosing with 600 mg twice daily, steady-state was reached by ≈ 4 weeks.

Aerosol: Bioavailability of the aerosol is unknown and may depend on mode of delivery. After aerosol use, peak plasma concentrations are less than the concentration that reduced RSV plaque formation in tissue culture by 85% to 98%. Respiratory tract secretions are likely to contain ribavirin in concentrations many times higher than those required to reduce plaque formation. However, RSV is an intracellular virus and serum concentrations may better reflect intracellular concentrations in the respiratory tract than respiratory secretion concentrations.

Accumulation of drug or metabolites in red blood cells occurs, with plateauing in red cells in ≈ 4 days. Accumulation gradually declines with an apparent half-life of 40 days.

Metabolism –

Capsules: Ribavirin is metabolized by a reversible phosphorylation pathway and a degradative pathway involving deribosylation and amide hydrolysis.

Excretion –

Capsules: Ribavirin and its metabolites are excreted renally. After oral administration of 600 mg ribavirin, ≈ 61% and 12% was eliminated in the urine and feces. Upon discontinuaton of dosing, the mean half-life was 298 hours.

Contraindications

Capsules: May cause birth defects or death of the exposed fetus. Ribavirin capsules are contraindicated in women who are pregnant or in men whose female partners are pregnant (see Warnings), and in patients with a history of hypersensitivity to ribavirin or any component of the capsule.

Patients with autoimmune hepatitis must not be treated with combination *Rebetol/Intron A* therapy because using these medicines can make the hepatitis worse.

Aerosol: Hypersensitivity to the drug or its components; pregnancy or the potential for pregnancy during exposure to the drug (see Warnings).

Warnings

Capsules:

Monotherapy – Ribavirin monotherapy is not effective for the treatment of chronic hepatitis C virus infection. Therefore, ribavirin capsules must not be used alone. The safety and efficacy of ribavirin capsules have only been established when used together with *Intron A* (interferon alfa-2b, recombinant) as *Rebetron* combination therapy.

Adverse events – There are significant adverse events caused by *Rebetol/Intron A*, including severe depression and suicidal ideation, hemolytic anemia, suppression of bone marrow function, pulmonary dysfunction, pancreatitis, and diabetes. Review the *Rebetron* combination therapy package insert in its entirety prior to initiation of combination treatment for additional safety information.

Hemoglobinopathies – Do not treat patients with hemoglobinopathies (eg, thalassemia major, sickle-cell anemia) with ribavirin.

Pancreatitis – Suspend ribavirin therapy in patients with signs and symptoms of pancreatitis and discontinue in patients with confirmed pancreatitis.

Renal function impairment – The multiple-dose pharmacokinetics of ribavirin cannot be accurately predicted in patients with renal dysfunction. Ribavirin is not effectively removed by hemodialysis. Do not treat patients with Ccr < 50 mL/min with ribavirin.

Hepatic function impairment – The mean C_{max} values increased with severity of hepatic dysfunction and was 2-fold greater in subjects with severe hepatic dysfunction when compared with control subjects.

Aerosol:

Underlying conditions – The presence of underlying conditions such as prematurity, immunosuppression, or cardiopulmonary disease may increase the severity of the infection and its risk to the patient.

Assisted ventilation – Some subjects requiring assisted ventilation have experienced serious difficulties because of inadequate ventilation and gas exchange. Drug precipitation within the ventilatory apparatus, including the endotracheal tube, has resulted in increased positive and expiratory pressure and increased positive inspiratory pressure. Accumulation of fluid in tubing ("rain out") also has been noted.

Respiratory function – Carefully monitor respiratory function during treatment. If ribavirin aerosol treatment produces sudden deterioration of respiratory function, stop treatment and reinstitute only with extreme caution, continuous monitoring, and consideration of concomitant administration of bronchodilators.

Deaths – Deaths during or shortly after treatment with aerosolized ribavirin have been reported in 20 cases.

Anemia: Although anemia has not been reported with aerosol use, it occurs frequently with oral and IV ribavirin.

Capsules – The primary toxicity of ribavirin is hemolytic anemia, which was observed in ≈ 10% of *Rebetol/Intron A*-treated patients in clinical trials. The anemia associated with ribavirin capsules occurs within 1 to 2 weeks of initiation of therapy. It is advised that hemoglobin or hematocrit be obtained pretreatment and at week 2 and 4 of therapy, or more frequently if clinically indicated. Then follow patients as clinically appropriate.

Mutagenesis:
    Capsules – Ribavirin demonstrated increased incidences of mutation and cell transformation in multiple genotoxicity assays.

Fertility impairment:
    Capsules – Use ribavirin with caution in fertile men. In studies in mice to evaluate the time course and reversibility of ribavirin-induced testicular degeneration at 0.1 to 0.8 × the maximum human 24-hour dose of ribavirin administered for 3 or 6 months, abnormalities in sperm occurred. Upon cessation of treatment, essentially total recovery from ribavirin-induced testicular toxicity was apparent within 1 or 2 spermatogenesis cycles.

Elderly:
    Capsules – In clinical trials, elderly subjects had a higher frequency of anemia (67%) than did younger patients (28%) (see Warnings).
    In general, cautiously administer ribavirin capsules to elderly patients, starting at the lower end of the dosing range, reflecting the greater frequency of decreased hepatic, renal, or cardiac function, and of concomitant disease or other drug therapy.
    Monitor renal function and make dosing adjustments accordingly. Do not use ribavirin in elderly patients with Ccr < 50 mL/min.

Pregnancy: Category X.

Lactation: Ribavirin is toxic to lactating animals and their offspring.
    It is not known whether ribavirin is excreted in human milk. Because of the potential for serious adverse reactions from the drug in nursing infants, a decision should be made whether to discontinue nursing or to delay or discontinue ribavirin.

Children:
    Capsules – Safety and effectiveness in pediatric patients have not been established.

Precautions

Monitoring:
    Capsules – The recommended monitoring for all patients treated with ribavirin prior to beginning treatment and then periodically thereafter:
- Standard hematologic tests: Including hemoglobin (pretreatment, week 2 and week 4 of therapy, and as clinically appropriate) (see Warnings), complete and differential white blood cell counts, and platelet count.
- Blood chemistries: Liver function tests and TSH.
- Pregnancy: Including monthly monitoring for women of childbearing potential.

    Aerosol – Monitor respiratory function and fluid status during treatment.

Health care personnel:
    Aerosol – Health care workers directly providing care to patients receiving aerosolized ribavirin should be aware that ribavirin is teratogenic in all animal species in which adequate studies have been conducted.
    Health care workers who are pregnant should consider avoiding direct care of patients receiving aerosolized ribavirin. If close patient contact cannot be avoided, take precautions to limit exposure.

Drug Interactions

Drugs that may interact with ribavirin capsules include antacids.

Adverse Reactions

Aerosol: Adverse reactions may include bacterial pneumonia; pneumothorax; apnea; ventilator dependence; cardiac arrest; hypotension; digitalis toxicity; rash; conjunctivitis; reticulocytosis; dyspnea; bigeminy; bradycardia; tachycardia; bronchospasm; pulmonary edema; hypoventilation; cyanosis; atelectasis; worsening of respiratory status.
    Healthcare workers: Headache (51%); conjunctivitis (32%); rhinitis, nausea, rash, dizziness, pharyngitis, lacrimation (10% to 20%).

Capsules: Adverse reactions occurring in ≥ 3% of patients include headache; dizziness; nausea; anorexia; dyspepsia; vomiting; myalgia; arthralgia; musculoskeletal pain; insomnia; irritability; depression; emotional lability; concentration impaired; nervousness; dyspnea; sinusitis; alopecia; rash; pruritus; injection site inflammation; injection site reaction; fatigue; rigors; fever; influenza-like symptoms; asthenia; chest pain; taste perversion.

RIMANTADINE HCl

Tablets: 100 mg *(Rx)*   *Flumadine* (Forest)
Syrup: 50 mg/5 mL *(Rx)*

Indications

Adults: Prophylaxis/treatment of illness caused by various strains of influenza A virus.

Children: Prophylaxis against influenza A virus.

Prophylaxis recommendations:
1.) High-risk patients vaccinated after influenza outbreak has begun: Consider prophylaxis until immunity from the influenza vaccine has developed (up to 2 weeks).
2.) Caretakers of those at high risk: Consider prophylaxis for unvaccinated caretakers of high-risk patients during peak influenza activity.
3.) Patients with immune deficiency: Consider prophylaxis for high-risk patients who are expected to have inadequate antibody response to influenza vaccine (eg, patients with HIV).
4.) Other: Consider prophylaxis in high-risk patients who should not be vaccinated. Prophylaxis also may be offered to those patients who desire to avoid influenza illness.

Administration and Dosage

Prophylaxis:

Adults – The recommended dose of rimantadine is 100 mg twice daily. In patients with severe hepatic dysfunction or renal failure (Ccr ≤ 10 mL/min) and in elderly nursing home patients, a dose reduction to 100 mg daily is recommended.

Children (< 10 years of age) – Administer once daily at a dose of 5 mg/kg, not exceeding 150 mg. For children ≥ 10 years of age, use the adult dose.

Treatment:

Adults – The recommended dose is 100 mg twice daily. In patients with severe hepatic dysfunction or renal failure (Ccr ≤ 10 mL/min) and in elderly nursing home patients, a dose reduction to 100 mg daily is recommended. Initiate therapy as soon as possible, preferably within 48 hours after onset of signs and symptoms of influenza A infection. Continue therapy for ≈ 7 days from the initial onset of symptoms.

Actions

Pharmacology: Rimantadine is a synthetic antiviral agent that appears to exert its inhibitory effect early in the viral replicative cycle, possibly inhibiting the uncoating of the virus.

Pharmacokinetics: The tablet and syrup formulations of rimantadine are equally absorbed after oral administration. The time to peak concentration was 6 hours in healthy adults. The single dose elimination half-life in this population was 25.4 hours. The single-dose elimination half-life in a group of healthy 71- to 79-year-old subjects was 32 hours.

In a group (n = 10) of children 4 to 8 years of age who were given a single dose (6.6 mg/kg) of syrup, plasma concentrations ranged from 446 to 988 ng/mL at 5 to 6 hours and from 170 to 424 ng/mL at 24 hours. In some children, the drug was detected in plasma 72 hours after the last dose. Following oral administration, rimantadine is extensively metabolized in the liver with < 25% of the dose excreted in the urine as unchanged drug. Three hydroxylated metabolites have been found in plasma. These metabolites, an additional conjugated metabolite and parent drug account for 74% of a single 200 mg dose excreted in urine over 72 hours.

Contraindications

Hypersensitivity to drugs of the adamantine class, including rimantadine and amantadine.

Warnings

Renal/Hepatic function impairment: The safety and pharmacokinetics of rimantadine in renal and hepatic insufficiency only have been evaluated after single dose administration. In a single dose study of patients with anuric renal failure, the apparent clearance was ≈ 40% lower and the elimination half-life was 1.6-fold greater than that in healthy controls. In a study of 14 people with chronic liver disease (mostly stabilized cirrhotics), no alterations in the pharmacokinetics were observed after a single dose of rimantadine. However, the apparent clearance of rimantadine following a single dose to 10 patients with severe liver dysfunction was 50% lower than that reported for healthy subjects. Because of the potential for accumulation of rimantadine and its metabolites in plasma, exercise caution when patients with renal or hepatic insufficiency are treated with rimantadine.

Pregnancy: Category C.

Lactation: Rimantadine should not be administered to nursing mothers because of the adverse affects noted in offspring of rats treated with rimantadine during the nursing period.

Children: In children, rimantadine is recommended for the prophylaxis of influenza A. Safety and efficacy of rimantadine in the treatment of symptomatic influenza infection in children have not been established. Prophylaxis studies with rimantadine have not been performed in children < 1 year of age.

Precautions

Seizures: An increased incidence of seizures has been reported in patients with a history of epilepsy who received the related drug amantadine. In clinical trials, the occurrence of seizure-like activity was observed in a small number of patients with a history of seizures who were not receiving anticonvulsant medication while taking rimantadine. If seizures develop, discontinue the drug.

Resistance: Consider transmission of rimantadine-resistant virus when treating patients whose contacts are at high risk for influenza A illness. Influenza A virus strains resistant to rimantadine can emerge during treatment and may be transmissible and cause typical influenza illness. Of patients with initially sensitive virus upon treatment with rimantadine, 10% to 30% shed rimantadine-resistant virus. Clinical response, although slower in those patients, was not significantly different from those who did not shed resistant virus.

Drug Interactions

Drugs that may affect rimantadine include acetaminophen, aspirin, and cimetidine.

Adverse Reactions

Adverse reactions occurring in ≥ 3% of patients included insomnia.

Geriatric subjects who received 200 or 400 mg of rimantadine daily experienced considerably more CNS and GI adverse events than comparable geriatric subjects receiving placebo. CNS events, including dizziness, headache, anxiety, asthenia, and fatigue occurred up to 2 times more often with rimantadine than with placebo. GI symptoms, particularly nausea, vomiting, and abdominal pain occurred at least twice as frequently with rimantadine than with receiving placebo. The GI symptoms appeared to be dose-related.

ZANAMIVIR

Blisters of powder for inhalation: 5 mg (*Rx*) *Relenza* (GlaxoSmithKline)

Indications

Influenza treatment: Treatment of uncomplicated acute illness caused by influenza A and B virus in adults and children ≥ 7 years of age who have been symptomatic for ≤ 2 days.

Administration and Dosage

Zanamivir is for administration to the respiratory tract by oral inhalation only, using the *Diskhaler* device provided. Instruct patients in the use of the delivery system. Include a demonstration whenever possible. If zanamivir is prescribed for children, it should be used only under adult supervision and instruction, and the supervising adult should first be instructed by a health care professional.

The recommended dose of zanamivir for the treatment of influenza in patients ≥ 7 years of age is 2 inhalations (one 5 mg blister per inhalation for a total dose of 10 mg) twice daily (≈ 12 hours apart) for 5 days. Two doses should be taken on the first day of treatment whenever possible, provided there is ≥ 2 hours between doses. On subsequent days, doses should be ≈ 12 hours apart (eg, morning and evening) at approximately the same time each day. There are no data on the effectiveness of treatment with zanamivir when initiated > 2 days after the onset of signs or symptoms. Safety and efficacy of repeated treatment courses have not been studied.

Patients scheduled to use an inhaled bronchodilator at the same time as zanamivir should use their bronchodilator before taking zanamivir.

Actions

Pharmacology: The proposed mechanism of action of zanamivir is via inhibition of influenza virus neuraminidase with the possibility of alteration of virus particle aggregation and release.

    Drug resistance – Influenza viruses with reduced susceptibility to zanamivir have been recovered in vitro by passage of the virus in the presence of increasing concentrations of the drug. Genetic analysis of these viruses showed that the reduced susceptibility in vitro to zanamivir is associated with mutations that result in amino acid changes in the viral neuraminidase or viral hemagglutinin or both.

Pharmacokinetics:

    Absorption – Approximately 4% to 17% of the inhaled dose is systemically absorbed. Peak serum concentrations ranged from 17 to 142 ng/mL within 1 to 2 hours after a 10 mg dose.

    Distribution – Zanamivir has limited plasma protein binding (< 10%).

    Metabolism – Zanamivir is renally excreted as unchanged drug. No metabolites have been detected.

    Excretion – The serum half-life of zanamivir following oral inhalation ranges from 2.5 to 5.1 hours. It is excreted unchanged in the urine with excretion of a single dose completed within 24 hours. Total clearance ranges from 2.5 to 10.9 L/hr. Unabsorbed drug is excreted in the feces.

Contraindications

Hypersensitivity to any component of the formulation.

Warnings

Elderly: No overall differences in safety or efficacy were observed between these subjects and younger patients, but greater sensitivity of some older individuals cannot be ruled out.

Pregnancy: Category C.

    There are no adequate and well-controlled studies in pregnant women. Use during pregnancy only if the potential benefit justifies the potential risk to the fetus.

Lactation: It is not known whether zanamivir is excreted in human breast milk. Exercise caution when zanamivir is administered to a nursing mother.

Children: Safety and efficacy of zanamivir have not been established in pediatric patients < 7 years of age.

Precautions

Allergic reactions: Allergic-like reactions, including oropharyngeal edema and serious skin rashes, have been reported in postmarketing experience with zanamivir. Stop zanamivir and institute appropriate treatment if an allergic reaction occurs or is suspected.

Bacterial infections: Serious bacterial infections may begin with influenza-like symptoms or may coexist with or occur as complications during the course of influenza. Zanamivir has not been shown to prevent such complications.

Other illness: There is no evidence for efficacy of zanamivir in any illness caused by agents other than influenza virus A and B.

Underlying respiratory disease: Safety and efficacy have not been demonstrated in patients with underlying chronic pulmonary disease. Instruct patients with underlying respiratory disease to have a fast-acting inhaled bronchodilator available when treated with zanamivir.

Prevention of influenza: Safety and efficacy of zanamivir have not been established for prophylactic use to prevent influenza. Use of zanamivir should not affect the evaluation of individuals for annual influenza vaccination in accordance with guidelines of the Centers for Disease Control and Prevention Advisory Committee on Immunization Practices.

High-risk patients: Safety and efficacy have not been demonstrated in patients with high-risk underlying medical conditions. No information is available regarding treatment of influenza in patients with any medical condition sufficiently severe or unstable to be considered at imminent risk of requiring inpatient management.

Drug Interactions

Zanamivir is not a substrate nor does it affect cytochrome P450 (CYP) isoenzymes (CYP1A1/2, 2A6, 2C9, 2C18, 2D6, 2E1, and 3A4) in human liver microsomes.

Adverse Reactions

Adverse reactions occurring in ≥ 3% of patients include diarrhea, nausea, nasal signs and symptoms, sinusitis, and ear, nose, and throat infections.

Lab test abnormalities: Elevations of liver enzymes and CPK, lymphopenia, and neutropenia. These were reported in similar proportions of zanamivir and lactose-vehicle placebo recipients with acute influenza-like illness.

OSELTAMIVIR PHOSPHATE

Capsules: 75 mg (75 mg free base equivalent of the phosphate salt) (*Rx*)   *Tamiflu* (Roche)

Powder for oral suspension: 12 mg/mL after reconstitution (*Rx*)   *Tamiflu* (Roche)

Indications

Influenza infection:

   Treatment – Treatment of uncomplicated acute illness caused by influenza infection in patients > 1 year of age who have been symptomatic for ≤ 2 days.

   Prophylaxis – For prophylaxis of influenza in adults and adolescents ≥ 13 years of age.

   Oseltamivir is not a substitute for early vaccination on an annual basis as recommended by the CDC Immunization Practices Advisory Committee.

Administration and Dosage

Standard dosage:

   Treatment of influenza –

   Adults and adolescents ≥ 13 years of age: The recommended oral dose of oseltamivir is 75 mg twice daily for 5 days. Begin treatment within 2 days of onset of symptoms of influenza. Oseltamivir may be taken without regard to food (see Pharmacokinetics). However, when taken with food, tolerability may be enhanced.

Children: The recommended oral dose of oseltamivir oral suspension for children ≥ 1 year of age or adults who cannot swallow a capsule is:

Oseltamivir Oral Suspension Dosing			
Body weight (kg)	Body weight (lbs)	Recommended dose for 5 days	Volume
≤ 15	≤ 33	30 mg twice daily	2.5 mL (½ tsp)
> 15 to 23	> 33 to 51	45 mg twice daily	3.8 mL (¾ tsp)
> 23 to 40	> 51 to 88	60 mg twice daily	5 mL (1 tsp)
> 40	> 88	75 mg twice daily	6.2 mL (1¼ tsp)

An oral dosing dispenser with 30, 45, and 60 mg graduations is provided with the oral suspension; the 75 mg dose can be measured using a combination of 30 and 45 mg. It is recommended that patients use this dispenser.

Influenza prophylaxis – The recommended oral dose of oseltamivir for influenza prophylaxis in adults and adolescents ≥ 13 years of age following close contact with an infected individual is 75 mg once daily for ≥ 7 days. Therapy should begin within 2 days of exposure. The recommended dose for prophylaxis during a community outbreak of influenza is 75 mg once daily. Safety and efficacy have been demonstrated for ≤ 6 weeks. The duration of protection lasts for as long as dosing is continued.

Renal function impairment: For plasma concentrations of oseltamivir carboxylate predicted to occur following various dosing schedules in patients with renal impairment, see Pharmacokinetics.

Influenza treatment – Dose adjustment is recommended for patients with Ccr between 10 and 30 mL/min receiving oseltamivir for treatment of influenza. In these patients, it is recommended that the dose be reduced to 75 mg oseltamivir once daily for 5 days.

Influenza prophylaxis – For prophylaxis of influenza, dose adjustment is recommended for patients with Ccr between 10 and 30 mL/min receiving oseltamivir. In these patients, it is recommended that the dose be reduced to 75 mg every other day.

Children: The safety and efficacy of oseltamivir for prophylaxis in children < 13 years of age have not been established. The safety and efficacy of oseltamivir for treatment in children < 1 year of age have not been established.

Elderly: No dose adjustment is required for geriatric patients.

Actions

Pharmacology: Oseltamivir is an ethyl ester prodrug requiring ester hydrolysis for conversion to the active form, oseltamivir carboxylate. The proposed mechanism of action of oseltamivir is via inhibition of influenza virus neuraminidase with the possibility of alteration of virus particle aggregation and release.

Drug resistance – In clinical studies of naturally acquired infection with influenza virus, 1.3% of posttreatment isolates in adults and adolescents, and 8.6% in children from 1 to 12 years of age showed emergence of influenza variants with decreased neuraminidase susceptibility to oseltamivir carboxylate.

The contribution of resistance because of alterations in the viral hemagglutinin has not been fully evaluated.

Pharmacokinetics:

Absorption – Oseltamivir phosphate is readily absorbed from the GI tract after oral administration.

The mean C_{max} of oseltamivir and oseltamivir carboxylate were 65.2 ng/mL and 348 ng/mL, respectively, after multiple doses of 75 mg twice daily. The mean $AUC_{(0\ to\ 12\ hr)}$ for oseltamivir was 112 ng•hr/mL and 2719 ng•hr/mL for oseltamivir carboxylate.

Coadministration with food has no significant effect on the peak plasma concentration and the area under the plasma concentration time curve of oseltamivir carboxylate.

Distribution – The binding of oseltamivir carboxylate to human plasma protein is low (3%). The binding of oseltamivir to human plasma protein is 42%, which is insufficient to cause significant displacement-based drug interactions.

Metabolism – Oseltamivir is extensively converted to oseltamivir carboxylate by esterases located predominantly in the liver. Neither oseltamivir nor oseltamivir carboxylate is a substrate for, or inhibitor of, cytochrome P450 isoforms.

Excretion – Absorbed oseltamivir is primarily (> 90%) eliminated by conversion to oseltamivir carboxylate. Plasma concentrations of oseltamivir declined with a half-life of 1 to 3 hours in most subjects after oral administration. Oseltamivir carboxylate is not further metabolized and is eliminated in the urine. Plasma concentrations of oseltamivir carboxylate declined with a half-life of 6 to 10 hours in most subjects. Oseltamivir carboxylate is eliminated entirely (> 99%) by renal excretion. Renal clearance (18.8 L/hr) exceeds glomerular filtration rate (7.5 L/hr) indicating that tubular secretion occurs, in addition to glomerular filtration. Less than 20% of an oral dose is eliminated in feces.

Contraindications
Hypersensitivity to any of the components of the product.

Warnings
Elderly: There was a reduction in the median time to improvement in the subjects receiving oseltamavir similar to that seen in younger adults. No overall difference in safety was observed between these subjects and younger adults.

Pregnancy: Category C.

Lactation: It is not known whether oseltamivir or oseltamivir carboxylate is excreted in human breast milk. Therefore, use oseltamivir only if the potential benefit for the lactating mother justifies the potential risk to the breast-fed infant.

Children: The safety and efficacy in children < 1 year of age have not been established.

Precautions
Other illnesses: There is no evidence for efficacy of oseltamivir in any illness caused by agents other than influenza viruses Types A and B.

Start of treatment: Efficacy of oseltamivir in patients who begin treatment after 40 hours of symptoms has not been established.

Underlying disease: Efficacy of oseltamivir in subjects with chronic cardiac disease or respiratory disease has not been established.

Prevention of influenza: Use of oseltamivir should not affect the evaluation of individuals for annual influenza vaccination in accordance with guidelines of the Center for Disease Controls and Prevention Advisory Committee on Immunization Practices. Efficacy of oseltamivir has not been established for prophylactic use to prevent influenza.

Repeated courses: Safety and efficacy of repeated treatment courses have not been established.

Drug Interactions
Clinically important drug interactions involving competition for renal tubular secretion are unlikely because of the known safety margin for most of these drugs, the elimination characteristics of oseltamivir carboxylate (glomerular filtration and anionic tubular secretion), and the excretion capacity of these pathways.

Adverse Reactions
Adverse reactions occurring in ≥ 3% of patients include nausea, vomiting, headache, abdominal pain, cough, fatigue, and diarrhea.

SAQUINAVIR MESYLATE

Capsules: 200 mg (as mesylate) (*Rx*)
Capsules, soft gelatin: 200 mg (*Rx*)

Invirase (Roche)
Fortovase (Roche)

> **Warning:**
> Saquinivir mesylate capsules (*Invirase*) and saquinavir soft gelatin capsules (*Fortovase*) are not bioequivalent and cannot be used interchangeably. When using saquinavir as part of an antiviral regimen, *Fortovase* is the recommended fomulation. In rare circumstances, *Invirase* may be considered if it is to be combined with antiretrovirals that significantly inhibit saquinavir's metabolism.

Indications
HIV infection: In combination with nucleoside analogs for the treatment of advanced HIV infection in selected patients.

Administration and Dosage
Saquinavir soft gelatin capsules (*Fortovase*) and saquinavir mesylate capsules (*Invirase*) are not bioequivalent and cannot be used interchangeably.

Invirase: Three 200 mg capsules 3 times daily taken within 2 hours after a full meal in combination with a nucleoside analog.

Use saquinavir mesylate only in combination with an active antiretroviral nucleoside analog regimen. Base concomitant therapy on a patient's prior drug exposure.

Fortovase: Six 200 mg capsules 3 times daily taken with a meal or up to 2 hours after a meal. When used in combination with nucleoside analogs, do not reduce the dosage of saquinavir, as this will lead to greater than dose-proportional decreases in saquinavir plasma levels.

Dose adjustment for combination therapy with saquinavir: For toxicities that may be associated with saquinavir, interrupt the drug. Saquinavir at doses < 600 mg 3 times daily are not recommended because lower doses have not shown antiviral activity. For recipients of combination therapy with saquinavir and nucleoside analogs, dose adjustment of the nucleoside analog should be based on the known toxicity profile of the individual drug.

Actions
Pharmacology: Saquinavir is an inhibitor of HIV protease which cleaves viral polyprotein precursors to generate functional proteins in HIV-infected cells. The cleavage of viral polyprotein precursors is essential for maturation of infectious virus. Saquinavir is a synthetic peptide-like substrate analog that inhibits the activity of HIV protease and prevents the cleavage of viral polyproteins.

Pharmacokinetics:
Absorption/Distribution – Saquinavir exhibits a low absolute bioavailability of 4% following a single dose of *Invirase* after a high-fat breakfast (48 g protein, 60 g carbohydrate, 57 g fat, 1006 kcal). This is considered to be the result of incomplete absorption and extensive first-pass metabolism. However, the relative bioavailability is ≈ 331% when saquinavir is administered as *Fortovase* compared with *Invirase*.

In HIV-infected patients, multiple dosing yields steady-state AUC values ≈ 2.5 times higher than a single *Invirase* dose and 80% higher than a single *Fortovase* dose. AUCs and peak levels in these patients are about twice those observed in healthy volunteers. Greater than dose-proportional increases in plasma levels occur following single and multiple doses when saquinavir is administered as *Fortovase*.

The mean steady-state Vd following 12 mg IV is 700 L, suggesting saquinavir partitions into tissues. Saquinavir is ≈ 98% bound to plasma proteins over a concentration range of 15 to 700 ng/mL. CSF levels are negligible.

Metabolism/Excretion – In vitro, the metabolism of saquinavir is cytochrome P450 mediated with specific isoenzyme, CYP3A4, responsible for > 90% of the hepatic metabolism. In vitro, saquinavir is rapidly metabolized to a range of mono- and di-hydroxylated inactive compounds; 88% and 1% of the oral dose was recovered in feces and urine, respectively, within 48 hours of dosing; 81% and 3% of an IV dose was recovered in feces and urine, respectively, within 48 hours of dosing. In mass balance studies, 13% of circulating radioactivity in plasma was attributed to unchanged drug after oral administration and the remainder attributed to saquinavir metabolites. Following IV administration, 66% of circulating radioactivity was attributed to unchanged drug and the remainder attributed to saquinavir metabolites, suggesting that saquinavir undergoes extensive first-pass metabolism.

Systemic clearance of saquinavir was rapid, 1.14 L/hr/kg after IV doses of 6, 36, and 72 mg. The mean residence time of saquinavir was 7 hours.

Contraindications

Clinically significant hypersensitivity to saquinavir or any components in the capsules; coadministration with terfenadine, cisapride, astemizole, triazolam, midazolam, or ergot derivatives.

Warnings

Diabetes mellitus, new onset: Exacerbation of pre-existing diabetes mellitus and hyperglycemia have been reported in HIV-infected patients receiving protease inhibitors.

Hepatic function impairment: Exercise caution when administering saquinavir to patients with hepatic insufficiency. Exacerbation of chronic liver dysfunction, including portal hypertension, in patients with underlying hepatitis B or C, cirrhosis or other underlying liver abnormalities have been reported.

Elderly: In general, take caution when dosing *Fortovase* in elderly patients because of the greater frequency of decreased hepatic, renal, or cardiac function, and of concomitant disease or other drug therapy.

Pregnancy: Category B.

Lactation: It is not known whether saquinavir is excreted in breast milk. Because of the potential for serious adverse reactions in nursing infants from saquinavir, decide whether to discontinue nursing or discontinue the drug, taking into account the importance of saquinavir to the mother.

The Centers for Disease Control and Prevention advises HIV-infected women not to breastfeed to avoid postnatal transmission of HIV to a child who may not be infected.

Children: Safety and efficacy in HIV-infected children or adolescents < 16 years of age have not been established.

Precautions

Monitoring: Perform clinical chemistry tests prior to initiating saquinavir therapy and at appropriate intervals thereafter. Periodically monitor triglyceride levels during therapy.

General: Saquinavir soft gelatin capsules (*Fortovase*) and saquinavir mesylate capsules (*Invirase*) are not bioequivalent and cannot be used interchangeably. Only *Fortovase* should be used for the initiation of saquinavir therapy (see Administration and Dosage) because *Fortovase* capsules provide greater bioavailability and efficacy than *Invirase*. For patients taking *Invirase* capsules with a viral load below the limit of quantification, a switch to *Fortovase* is recommended to maintain a virologic response. For patients taking *Invirase* capsules who have not had an adequate response or are failing therapy, if saquinavir resistance is clinically suspected, then do not use *Fortovase*. If resistance to saquinavir is not clinically suspected, consider a switch to *Fortovase*.

Hemophilia: There have been reports of spontaneous bleeding in patients with hemophilia A and B treated with protease inhibitors. In some patients, additional Factor VIII was required.

Fat redistribution: Redistribution/Accumulation of body fat, including central obesity, dorsocervical fat enlargement (buffalo hump), peripheral wasting, breast enlargement, and "cushingoid appearance" have been observed in patients receiving protease inhibitors.

Use with HMG-CoA reductase inhibitors: Concomitant use of saquinavir with lovastatin or simvastatin is not recommended. Exercise caution if HIV protease inhibitors, including saquinavir, are used concurrently with other HMG-CoA reductase inhibitors that are also metabolized by the CYP3A4 pathway (eg, atorvastatin, cerivastatin).

Toxicity: If a serious or severe toxicity occurs during treatment with saquinavir, interrupt therapy until the etiology of the event is identified or the toxicity resolves. At the time, resumption of treatment with full-dose saquinavir may be considered.

Photosensitization: Photosensitization (photoallergy or phototoxicity) may occur.

Drug Interactions

Drugs that may interact with saquinavir include ketoconazole, delavirdine, nevirapine, ritonavir, clarithromycin, indinavir, nelfinavir, and rifamycins.

Other drugs that induce CYP3A4 (eg, phenobarbital, phenytoin, dexamethasone, carbamazepine) may reduce saquinavir plasma concentrations.

Saquinavir may affect clarithromycin, nelfinavir, and sildenafil.

Competition for CYP3A by saquinavir could result in inhibition of the metabolism of astemizole, cisapride, ergot derivatives, midazolam, and triazolam and create the potential for serious or life-threatening reactions such as cardiac arrhythmias or prolonged sedation.

Drug/Food interactions: The mean 24-hour AUC after a single 600 mg oral dose in healthy volunteers was increased from 24 (under fasting conditions) to 161 ng•hr/mL when saquinavir was given following a high-fat breakfast. Saquinavir 24-hour AUC and C_{max} following the administration of a higher calorie meal (943 kcal, 54 g fat) were on average 2 times higher than after a lower calorie, lower fat meal. The effect of food persists for up to 2 hours.

Adverse Reactions

Adverse reactions occurring in ≥ 3% of patients include diarrhea, abdominal discomfort; nausea; buccal mucosa ulceration; paresthesia; peripheral neuropathy; asthenia; rash; headache; fatigue; pain; taste alteration; insomnia; dyspepsia; flatulence; vomiting; constipation; lab test abnormalities of creatine phosphokinase, glucose (low), AST, ALT, and neutrophils (low).

RITONAVIR

Capsules: 100 mg (*Rx*)	*Norvir* (Abbott)
Oral solution: 80 mg/mL (*Rx*)	

> **Warning:**
> Coadministration of ritonavir with certain nonsedating antihistamines, sedative hypnotics, or antiarrhythmics may result in potentially serious or life-threatening adverse events because of possible effects of ritonavir on the hepatic metabolism of certain drugs.

Indications

HIV infection: Combination with nucleoside analogs or as monotherapy for the treatment of HIV infection when therapy is warranted.

Administration and Dosage

The recommended dosage is 600 mg twice daily. If possible, take with food. Some patients experience nausea upon initiation of 600 mg twice daily dosing; dose escalation may provide some relief: 300 mg twice daily for 1 day, 400 mg twice daily for 2 days, 500 mg twice daily for 1 day and then 600 mg twice daily thereafter. In addition, patients initiating combination regimens with ritonavir and nucleosides may improve GI tolerance by initiating ritonavir alone and subsequently adding nucleosides before completing 2 weeks of ritonavir monotherapy.

Actions

Pharmacology: Ritonavir is an inhibitor of HIV protease with activity against HIV. Ritonavir is a petidomimetic inhibitor of the HIV-1 and HIV-2 proteases. Inhibition of HIV protease renders the enzyme incapable of processing the *gag-pol* polyprotein precursor which leads to production of noninfectious immature HIV particles. Cross-resistance between ritonavir and reverse transcriptase inhibitors is unlikely because of the different enzyme targets involved.

Pharmacokinetics: After a 600 mg dose of oral solution, peak concentrations of ritonavir were achieved ≈ 2 and 4 hours after dosing under fasting and nonfasting conditions, respectively. When the oral solution was given under nonfasting conditions, peak ritonavir concentrations decreased 23% and the extent of absorption decreased 7% relative to fasting conditions. Dilution of the oral solution, within 1 hour of administration, with 240 mL of chocolate milk, *Advera* or *Ensure* did not significantly affect the extent and rate of ritonavir absorption. After a single 600 mg dose under nonfasting conditions, in 2 separate studies, the capsule and oral solution formulations yielded mean areas under the plasma concentration-time curve (AUCs) of 129.5 and 129 mcg•hr/mL, respectively. Relative to fasting conditions, the extent of absorption of ritonavir from the capsule formulation was 15% higher when administered with a meal.

Nearly all of the plasma radioactivity after a single oral 600 mg dose of ^{14}C-ritonavir oral solution was attributed to unchanged ritonavir. Five ritonavir metabolites have been identified in urine and feces. The isopropylthiazole oxidation metabolite (M-2) is the major metabolite and has antiviral activity similar to that of the parent drug; however, the concentrations of this metabolite in plasma are low. Studies utilizing human liver microsomes demonstrate that cytochrome P450 3A (CYP3A) is a major isoform involved in ritonavir metabolism, although CYP2D6 also contributes to the formation of M-2.

Ritonavir Pharmacokinetic Characteristics			
Parameter	Values (mean)	Parameter	Values (mean)
C_{max} SS[1]	11.2 mcg/mL	CL/F[2]	4.6 L/h
C_{trough} SS[1]	3.7 mcg/mL	CL_R	< 0.1 L/h
V_β/F[2]	0.41 L/kg	RBC/Plasma ratio	0.14
CL/F[2]	8.8 L/h	Percent bound[3]	98% to 99%

[1] SS = Steady state; ritonavir doses of 600 mg q 12 h.
[2] Single ritonavir 600 mg dose.
[3] Primarily bound to human serum albumin and alpha-1 acid glycoprotein over the ritonavir concentration range of 0.01 to 30 μg/mL.

Contraindications

Hypersensitivity to the drug or any of its ingredients.

Ritonavir is expected to produce large increases in the plasma concentrations of amiodarone, astemizole, bepridil, bupropion, cisapride, clozapine, encainide, flecainide, meperidine, piroxicam, propafenone, propoxyphene, quinidine, rifabutin, and terfenadine. These agents have recognized risks of arrhythmias, hematologic abnormalities, seizures, or other potentially serious adverse effects. Do not administer these drugs concomitantly with ritonavir.

Coadministration is likely to produce large increases in the following highly metabolized sedatives and hypnotics: Alprazolam, clorazepate, diazepam, estazolam, flurazepam, midazolam, triazolam, and zolpidem. Because of the potential for extreme sedation and respiratory depression from these agents, do not administer with ritonavir.

Warnings

Hepatic function impairment: Ritonavir is principally metabolized by the liver. Exercise caution when administering this drug to patients with impaired hepatic function.

Pregnancy: Category B.

Lactation: It is not known whether this drug is excreted in breast milk. The CDC advises HIV-infected women not to breastfeed to avoid postnatal transmission of HIV to a child who may not be infected.

Children: Safety and efficacy in children < 12 years of age have not been established.

Precautions

Lab test abnormalities: Ritonavir has been associated with alterations in triglycerides, AST, ALT, GGT, CPK, and uric acid. Perform appropriate laboratory testing prior to initiating ritonavir therapy and at periodic intervals or if any clinical signs and symptoms occur during therapy.

Percentage of Patients with Marked Chemistry and Hematology Laboratory Value Abnormalities with Ritonavir Therapy						
		Naive patients			Advanced patients	
Variable	Limit	Ritonavir + AZT	Ritonavir	AZT	Ritonavir	Placebo
Chemistry values	high					
Uric acid	(> 12 mg/dL)	-	-	-	3.6	0.2
AST	(> 180 IU/L)	2.9	6.5	1.7	3.8	4.3
ALT	(> 215 IU/L)	3.9	3.6	2.6	6.1	2.6
GGT	(> 300 IU/L)	2	2.8	0.9	14.7	6.7
Triglycerides	(> 1500 mg/dL)	1	2.8	-	10.1	0.2
Triglycerides fasting	(> 1500 mg/dL)	2.1	1.4	-	7.9	0.4
CPK	(> 1000 IU/L)	7	7.5	7.1	8.6	4.5
Hematology values	low					
Hematocrit	(< 30%)	2	-	-	11.7	16
RBC	(< 3 x 10^{12}/L)	1	-	1.7	14.9	19.7
WBC	(< 2.5 x 10^9/L)	-	-	3.5	25.1	51.4
Neutrophils	(≤ 0.5 x 10^9/L)	-	-	-	4	6.9

- Indicates no events reported.

Drug Interactions

Drugs that may affect ritonavir include clarithromycin, didanosine, fluconazole, fluoxetine, and rifampin.

Drugs that may be affected by ritonavir include clarithromycin, didanosine, desipramine, disulfiram, metronidazole, ethinyl estradiol, narcotic analgesics, rifabutin, saquinavir, sulfamethoxazole, theophylline, trimethoprim, and zidovudine.

Agents Whose AUCs May be Increased by Ritonavir		
Alpha blockers	Antimalarials	Erythromycin
Antiarrhythmatics	Antineoplastics	Immunosuppressants
Antidepressants	Beta blockers	Methylphenidiate
Antiemetics	Calcium blockers	Pentoxifylline
Antifungals	Cimetidine	Phenothiazines
Antihyperlipidemics	Corticosteroids	Warfarin

Agents Whose AUCs May be Decreased by Ritonavir	
Atovaquone	Diphenoxylate
Clofibrate	Metoclopramide
Daunorubicin	Sedatives/Hypnotics

Drug/Food interactions: When the oral solution was given under nonfasting conditions, peak ritonavir concentrations decreased 23% and extent of absorption decreased 7% relative to fasting conditions. Extent of absorption of ritonavir from the capsule was 15% higher when given with a meal relative to fasting conditions. If possible, take ritonavir with meals.

Adverse Reactions

The most frequent clinical adverse events, other than asthenia, among patients receiving ritonavir were GI and neurological disturbances including nausea, diarrhea, vomiting, anorexia, abdominal pain, taste perversion, and circumoral and peripheral paresthesias.

INDINAVIR SULFATE

Capsules: 200 and 400 mg *(Rx)*   *Crixivan* (Merck)

Warning:
Indinavir is indicated for the treatment of HIV infection in adults when antiretroviral therapy is warranted. This indication is based on analyses of surrogate endpoints in studies of up to 24 weeks in duration. At present, there are no results from controlled clinical trials evaluating the effect of therapy with indinavir on clinical progression of HIV infection, such as survival or the incidence of opportunistic infections.

Indications

HIV infection: Treatment of HIV infection in adults when antiretroviral therapy is warranted.

Administration and Dosage

The recommended dosage is 800 mg (two 400 mg capsules) orally every 8 hours. The dosage is the same whether indinavir is used alone or in combination with other antiretroviral agents. The antiretroviral activity of indinavir may be increased when used in combination with approved reverse transcriptase inhibitors.

Administer at intervals of 8 hours. For optimal absorption, administer without food but with water 1 hour before or 2 hours after a meal or administer with other liquids such as skim milk, juice, coffee, or tea, or with a light meal (eg, dry toast with jelly, juice, and coffee with skim milk and sugar; or corn flakes, skim milk, and sugar).

If indinavir and didanosine are administered concomitantly, they should be administered at least 1 hour apart on an empty stomach.

In addition to adequate hydration, medical management in patients who experience nephrolithiasis may include temporary interruption of therapy (eg, 1 to 3 days) during the acute episode of nephrolithiasis or therapy discontinuation.

Cirrhosis: Reduce the dosage of indinavir to 600 mg every 8 hours in patients with mild to moderate hepatic insufficiency caused by cirrhosis.

Actions

Pharmacology: Indinavir is an inhibitor of the HIV protease. HIV protease is an enzyme required for the proteolytic cleavage of the viral polyprotein precursors into the individual functional proteins found in infectious HIV. Indinavir binds to the protease active site and inhibits the activity of the enzyme. This inhibition prevents cleavage of the viral polyproteins resulting in the formation of immature noninfectious viral particles. The relationship between in vitro susceptibility of HIV to indinavir and inhibition of HIV replication in humans has not been established.

Drug resistance – Isolates of HIV with reduced susceptibility to the drug have been recovered from some patients treated with indinavir.

Cross-resistance between indinavir and HIV reverse transcriptase inhibitors is unlikely because the enzyme targets involved are different. Cross-resistance was noted between indinavir and the protease inhibitor ritonavir. Varying degrees of cross-resistance have been observed between indinavir and other HIV-protease inhibitors.

Pharmacokinetics:

Absorption – Indinavir was rapidly absorbed in the fasted state with a time to peak plasma concentration (T_{max}) of 0.8 hours. A greater than dose-proportional increase in indinavir plasma concentrations was observed over the 200 to 1000 mg dose range. At a dosing regimen of 800 mg every 8 hours, steady-state AUC was 30,691 nM•hour, C_{max} was 12,617 nM, and plasma concentration 8 hours post-dose (trough) was 251 nM.

Distribution – Indinavir was ≈ 60% bound to human plasma proteins over a concentration range of 81 to 16,300 nM.

Metabolism – Following a 400 mg dose of ^{14}C-indinavir, 83% and 19% of the total radioactivity was recovered in feces and urine, respectively; radioactivity caused by parent drug in feces and urine was 19.1% and 9.4%, respectively. Seven metabolites have been identified, 1 glucuronide conjugate and 6 oxidative metabolites. In vitro studies indicate that cytochrome P450 3A4 (CYP3A4) is the major enzyme responsible for formation of the oxidative metabolites.

Excretion – Indinavir is excreted (< 20%) unchanged in the urine. Mean urinary excretion of unchanged drug was 10.4% and 12% following a single 700 and 1000 mg dose, respectively. Indinavir was rapidly eliminated with a half-life of 1.8 hours. Significant accumulation was not observed after multiple dosing at 800 mg every 8 hours.

Contraindications

Hypersensitivity to any component of the product.

Warnings

Concomitant agents: Do not administer indinavir concurrently with terfenadine, astemizole, cisapride, triazolam, and midazolam because competition for CYP3A4 by indinavir could result in inhibition of the metabolism of these drugs and create the potential for serious or life-threatening events.

Renal function impairment: Nephrolithiasis, including flank pain with or without hematuria (including microscopic hematuria), has been reported in ≈ 4% of patients. In general, these events were not associated with renal dysfunction and resolved with hydration and temporary interruption of therapy (eg, 1 to 3 days). Following the acute episode, 9.2% of patients discontinued therapy.

To ensure adequate hydration, it is recommended that the patient drink at least 1.5 liters (≈ 48 ounces) of liquids during the course of 24 hours.

Hepatic function impairment: Patients with mild to moderate hepatic insufficiency and clinical evidence of cirrhosis had evidence of decreased metabolism of indinavir resulting in ≈ 60% higher mean AUC following a single 400 mg dose. The half-life increased to 2.8 hours.

Pregnancy: Category C.

Lactation: Although it is not known whether indinavir is excreted in breast milk, there exists the potential for adverse effects from indinavir in nursing infants. Instruct mothers to discontinue nursing if they are receiving indinavir. This is consistent with the recommendation by the CDC that HIV-infected mothers not breast-feed their infants to avoid risking postnatal transmission of HIV.

Children: Safety and efficacy have not been established.

Precautions

Hyperbilirubinemia: Asymptomatic hyperbilirubinemia (total bilirubin ≥ 2.5 mg/dL), reported predominantly as elevated indirect bilirubin, has occurred in ≈ 10% of patients. In < 1%, this was associated with elevations in ALT or AST.

Drug Interactions

Drugs that may affect indinavir include clarithromycin, didanosine, fluconazole, ketoconazole, quinidine, rifampin, rifabutin, and zidovudine.

Drugs that may be affected by indinavir include astemizole, cisapride, midazolam, terfenadine, triazolam, clarithromycin, isoniazid, lamivudine, oral contraceptives, rifabutin, stavudine, TMP-SMZ, and zidovudine.

Drug/Food interactions: Administration of indinavir with a meal high in calories, fat, and protein (784 kcal, 48.6 g fat, 31.3 g protein) resulted in a 77% reduction in AUC and an 84% reduction in C_{max}. Administration with lighter meals resulted in little or no change in AUC, C_{max}, or trough concentration. A single 400 mg dose of indinavir with 8 oz of grapefruit juice resulted in a decrease in indinavir AUC (26%).

Adverse Reactions

Adverse reactions occurring in ≥ 3% of patients include abdominal pain; asthenia/fatigue; nausea; diarrhea; vomiting; headache; insomnia.

Indinavir vs Zidovudine: Selected Lab Test Abnormalities (%)			
Lab test abnormalities	Indinavir (n = 196)	Indinavir + zidovudine (n = 196)	Zidovudine (n = 195)
Hematology			
Decreased hemoglobin < 8 g/dL	0.5	1.1	0.5
Decreased platelet count < 50 THS/mm³	0.5	0.5	0
Decreased neutrophil < 0.75 THS/mm³	1.1	1.6	3.8
Blood chemistry			
Increased ALT > 500% ULN[1]	3.1	3.2	2.1
Increased AST > 500% ULN	2.1	2.1	1.1
Total serum bilirubin > 2.5 mg/dL	7.8	7.4	0.5
Increased serum amylase > 200% ULN	1	2.1	0.5

[1] Upper limit of the normal range.

NELFINAVIR MESYLATE

Tablets: 250 mg (*Rx*)
Powder: 50 mg/g (*Rx*)

Viracept (Agouron)

Warning:
Nelfinavir is indicated for the treatment of human immunodeficiency virus (HIV) infection when antiretroviral therapy is warranted. At present, there are no results from controlled trials evaluating the effect of therapy with nelfinavir on clinical progression of HIV infection, such as survival or the incidence of opportunistic infections.

Indications

HIV: For the treatment of HIV infection when antiretroviral therapy is warranted.

Administration and Dosage

Take with a meal or light snack.

Adults: The recommended dose is 750 mg (three 250 mg tablets) 3 times daily in combination with nucleoside analogs (antiretroviral activity is enhanced).

Pediatric patients (2 to 13 years of age): 20 to 30 mg/kg/dose 3 times/day.

Pediatric Dose of Nelfinavir (administered 3 times/day)				
Body weight		Number of level 1 g scoops	Number of level teaspoons	Number of tablets
kg	lbs			
7 to < 8.5	15.5 to < 18.5	4	1	
8.5 to < 10.5	18.5 to < 23	5	1¼	
10.5 to < 12	23 to < 26.5	6	1½	
12 to < 14	26.5 to < 31	7	1¾	
14 to < 16	31 to < 35	8	2	

Pediatric Dose of Nelfinavir (administered 3 times/day)				
Body weight		Number of level 1 g scoops	Number of level teaspoons	Number of tablets
kg	lbs			
16 to < 18	35 to < 39.5	9	2¼	-
18 to < 23	39.5 to < 50.5	10	2½	2
≥ 23	≥ 50.5	15	3¾	3

Oral powder – The oral powder may be mixed with a small amount of water, milk, formula, soy formula, soy milk, or dietary supplement; once mixed, the entire contents must be consumed in order to obtain the full dose. Acidic food or juice (eg, orange juice, apple juice, or apple sauce) are not recommended because of bitter taste. Do not reconstitute with water in its original container. Once mixed, store the oral powder for ≤ 6 hours.

Actions

Pharmacology: Nelfinavir is an inhibitor of the HIV-1 protease. Inhibition of the viral protease prevents cleavage of the gagpol polyprotein resulting in the production of immature, noninfectious virus.

Pharmacokinetics:

Absorption – After single and multiple oral doses of 500 to 750 mg with food, peak nelfinavir plasma concentrations were typically achieved in 2 to 4 hours. After multiple dosing with 750 mg 3 times daily for 28 days (steady-state), peak plasma concentrations averaged 3 to 4 mcg/mL and plasma concentrations prior to the morning dose were 1 to 3 mcg/mL.

Distribution – The apparent volume of distribution following oral administration of nelfinavir was 2 to 7 L/kg. Nelfinavir in serum is extensively protein-bound (> 98%).

Metabolism – Unchanged nelfinavir comprised 82% to 86% of the total plasma. In vitro multiple cytochrome P450 isoforms including CYP3A are responsible for metabolism of nelfinavir. One major and several minor oxidative metabolites were found in plasma. The major oxidative metabolite has in vitro antiviral activity comparable with the parent drug.

Excretion – The terminal half-life in plasma was typically 3.5 to 5 hours. The majority (87%) of an oral 750 mg dose was recovered in the feces, which consisted of numerous oxidative metabolites (78%) and unchanged nelfinavir (22%). Only 1% to 2% of the dose was recovered in the urine, of which unchanged nelfinavir was the major component.

Contraindications

Hypersensitivity to any components of the product; concurrent administration with astemizole, cisapride, rifampin, triazolam, or midazolam.

Warnings

Hepatic function impairment: Exercise caution when administering this drug to patients with hepatic impairment.

Pregnancy: Category B.

Lactation: The US Public Health Service Centers for Disease Control and Prevention advises HIV-infected women not to breastfeed to avoid postnatal transmission of HIV to a child who may not yet be infected. It is not known whether nelfinavir is excreted in breast milk.

Children: A similar adverse event profile was seen during the pediatric clinical trial as in adult patients. The evaluation of the antiviral activity of nelfinavir in pediatric patients is ongoing.

The safety, efficacy, and pharmacokinetics of nelfinavir have not been evaluated in pediatric patients < 2 years of age.

Precautions

Resistance/Cross-resistance: It is unknown what effect nelfinavir therapy will have on the activity of subsequently administered protease inhibitors.

Drug Interactions

Drugs that may affect nelfinavir include anticonvulsants, indinavir, ketoconazole, rifabutin, rifampin, ritonavir, and saquinavir.

Drugs that may be affected by nelfinavir include indinavir, rifabutin, saquinavir, nonsedating antihistamines, didanosine, oral contraceptives, zidovudine, and lamivudine.

Drug/Food interactions: Maximum plasma concentrations and AUC were 2- to 3-fold higher under fed conditions compared with fasting.

Adverse Reactions

Adverse effects occurring in ≥ 3% of patients include diarrhea, nausea, flatulence, and hematologic abnormalities.

AMPRENAVIR

Capsules: 50 and 150 mg (*Rx*)
Oral solution: 15 mg/mL (*Rx*)

Agenerase (GlaxoSmithKline)

> **Warning:**
> Amprenavir in combination with other antiretroviral agents is indicated for the treatment of human immunodeficiency virus type 1 (HIV-1) infection. This indication is based on analyses of plasma HIV RNA levels and CD4 cell counts in controlled studies of ≤ 24 weeks in duration. At present, there are no results from controlled trials evaluating long-term suppression of HIV RNA or disease progression with amprenavir.

Indications

HIV infection: In combination with other antiretroviral agents for the treatment of HIV-1 infection. This indication is based on analyses of plasma HIV RNA levels and CD4 cell counts in controlled studies of ≤ 24 weeks in duration. At present, there are no results from controlled trials evaluating long-term suppression of HIV RNA or disease progression with amprenavir.

Administration and Dosage

Amprenavir may be taken with or without food; however, a high-fat meal decreases the absorption of amprenavir and should be avoided. Advise adult and pediatric patients not to take supplemental vitamin E since the vitamin E content of amprenavir capsules and oral solution exceeds the Reference Daily Intake (adults, 30 IU; pediatrics, ≈ 10 IU).

Amprenavir capsules and oral solution are not interchangeable on a mg per mg basis.

Adults: The recommended oral dose of amprenavir capsules for adults is 1200 mg (eight 150 mg capsules) twice daily in combination with other antiretroviral agents.

Pediatric patients:

> *Capsules* – For adolescents (13 to 16 years of age), the recommended dose is 1200 mg (eight 150 mg capsules) twice daily in combination with other antiretroviral agents. For patients between 4 and 12 years of age or for patients 13 to 16 years of age with weight of < 50 kg, the recommended dose is 20 mg/kg twice daily or 15 mg/kg 3 times daily (to a maximum daily dose of 2400 mg) in combination with other antiretroviral agents.

> *Oral solution* – The recommended dose for patients between 4 and 12 years of age or for patients 13 to 16 years of age with weight < 50 kg is 22.5 mg/kg (1.5 mL/kg) twice daily or 17 mg/kg (1.1 mL/kg) 3 times daily (to a maximum daily dose of 2800 mg) in combination with other antiretroviral agents.

Hepatic function impairment: Use with caution in patients with moderate or severe hepatic impairment. Patients with Child-Pugh scores ranging from 5 to 8 should receive a reduced dose of amprenavir capsules of 450 mg twice daily, and patients with a

Child-Pugh score ranging from 9 to 12 should receive a reduced dose of amprenavir capsules of 300 mg twice daily.

Actions

Pharmacology: Amprenavir is an inhibitor of human immunodeficiency virus (HIV)-1 protease. Amprenavir binds to the active site of HIV-1 protease and thereby prevents the processing of viral gag and gag-pol polyprotein precursors, resulting in the formation of immature noninfectious viral particles.

Pharmacokinetics:

Absorption – Amprenavir was rapidly absorbed after oral administration in HIV-1 infected patients with a time to peak concentration (t_{max}) typically between 1 and 2 hours after a single oral dose.

Amprenavir oral solution was 14% less bioavailable compared to the capsules.

Distribution – The apparent volume of distribution is $\approx$ 430 L in healthy adult subjects. In vitro binding is $\approx$ 90% to plasma proteins.

Metabolism – Amprenavir is metabolized in the liver by the cytochrome CYP3A4 enzyme system.

Excretion – Excretion of unchanged amprenavir in urine and feces is minimal. The plasma elimination half-life of amprenavir ranged from 7.1 to 10.6 hours.

Contraindications

Concurrent use with astemizole, bepridil, cisapride, dihydroergotamine, ergotamine, midazolam, and triazolam. Although these drugs have not been specifically studied, coadministration may result in competitive inhibition of metabolism of these products and may cause serious or life-threatening adverse events.

Hypersensitivity to any of the components of this product.

Warnings

Drug interactions: See also Contraindications and Drug Interactions.

Serious or life-threatening drug interactions could occur between amprenavir and amiodarone, lidocaine (systemic), tricyclic antidepressants, and quinidine. Concentration monitoring of these agents is recommended if these agents are used concomitantly with amprenavir.

Do not use rifampin in combination with amprenavir because it reduces plasma concentrations and AUC of amprenavir by $\approx$ 90%.

Use particular caution when prescribing sildenafil in patients receiving amprenavir. Coadministration of amprenavir with sildenafil is expected to substantially increase sildenafil concentrations and may result in an increase in sildenafil-associated adverse events, including hypotension, visual changes, and priapism.

Skin reactions: Severe and life-threatening skin reactions, including Stevens-Johnson syndrome, have occurred in patients treated with amprenavir (see Adverse Reactions).

Anemia: Acute hemolytic anemia has occurred in a patient treated with amprenavir.

Diabetes mellitus/hyperglycemia: New-onset diabetes mellitus, exacerbation of pre-existing diabetes mellitus, and hyperglycemia have been reported during postmarketing surveillance in HIV-infected patients receiving protease inhibitor therapy.

Hepatic function impairment: Amprenavir is principally metabolized by the liver; exercise caution when administering this drug to patients with hepatic impairment.

Elderly: In general, dose selection for an elderly patient should be cautious, reflecting the greater frequency of decreased hepatic, renal, or cardiac function and of concomitant disease or other drug therapy.

Pregnancy: Category C.

Antiretroviral pregnancy registry – To monitor maternal-fetal outcomes of pregnant women exposed to amprenavir, an Antiretroviral Pregnancy Registry has been established. Physicians are encouraged to register patients by calling (800) 258-4263.

Lactation: The Centers for Disease Control and Prevention recommend that HIV-infected mothers not breastfeed their infants to avoid risking postnatal transmission of HIV. Because of both the potential for HIV transmission and any possible adverse effects of amprenavir, instruct mothers not to breastfeed if they are receiving amprenavir.

Children: One hundred eighteen patients 4 to 17 years of age have received amprenavir as single or multiple doses in studies. An adverse event profile similar to that seen in adults was seen in pediatric patients. The safety, efficacy, and pharmacokinetics of amprenavir have not been evaluated in pediatric patients < 4 years of age.

Precautions

Doseform interchangeability: Amprenavir capsules and oral solution are not interchangeable on a mg per mg basis.

Sulfonamide cross-sensitivity: Amprenavir is a sulfonamide. The potential for cross-sensitivity between drugs in the sulfonamide class and amprenavir is unknown. Treat patients with a known sulfonamide allergy with caution.

Vitamin E: Formulations of amprenavir provide high daily doses of vitamin E.

Hemophilia: There have been reports of spontaneous bleeding in patients with hemophilia A and B treated with protease inhibitors.

Fat redistribution: Redistribution/accumulation of body fat including central obesity, dorsocervical fat enlargement (buffalo hump), peripheral wasting, breast enlargement, and "cushingoid appearance" have been observed in patients receiving protease inhibitors.

Resistance/Cross-resistance: Because the potential for HIV cross-resistance among protease inhibitors has not been fully explored, it is unknown what effect amprenavir therapy will have on the activity of subsequently administered protease inhibitors.

Drug Interactions

Amprenavir is metabolized by the cytochrome P450 enzyme system and inhibits CYP3A4. Use caution when coadministering medications that are substrates, inhibitors, or inducers of CYP3A4, or potentially toxic medications that are metabolized by CYP3A4.

Drugs that might affect amprenavir include abacavir, rifampin, antacids, anticonvulsants, azole antifungals, cimetidine, macrolides, nonnucleoside reverse transcriptase inhibitors, and other protease inhibitors.

Drugs that might be affected by amprenavir include anticonvulsants, azole antifungals, astemizole, antiarrhythmics, benzodiazepines, calcium channel blockers, cisapride, clozapine, oral contraceptives, dapsone, ergot alkaloids, HMG-CoA reductase inhibitors, sildenafil, tricyclic antidepressants, and warfarin.

Adverse Reactions

Adverse reactions occurring in ≥ 3% of patients include paresthesia, nausea, vomiting, diarrhea, depression, taste disorder, and rash.

LOPINAVIR/RITONAVIR

Capsules: 133.3 mg lopinavir/33.3 mg ritonavir (*Rx*)   *Kaletra* (Abbott)
Solution, oral: 80 mg lopinavir/20 mg ritonavir per mL (*Rx*)

Indications

HIV treatment: In combination with other antiretroviral agents for the treatment of HIV infection. This indication is based on analyses of plasma HIV RNA levels and CD4 cell counts in a controlled study of lopinavir/ritonavir combination of 24 weeks duration and in smaller uncontrolled dose-ranging studies of 72 weeks duration. At present, there are no results from controlled trials evaluating the effect on clinical progression of HIV.

Administration and Dosage

Adults: The recommended dosage is 400/100 mg of lopinavir/ritonavir (3 capsules or 5 mL) twice daily taken with food.

Concomitant therapy with efavirenz or nevirapine – A dose increase to 533/133 mg lopinavir/ritonavir (4 capsules or 6.5 mL) twice daily taken with food should be considered when used in combination with efavirenz or nevirapine in treatment-experienced patients where reduced susceptibility to lopinavir is clinically suspected (by treatment history or laboratory evidence).

Children (6 months to 12 years of age):

Lopinavir/Ritonavir Pediatric Dosage without Efavirenz or Nevirapine		
Weight (kg)[1]	Dose (mg/kg)[2]	Volume of oral solution BID (80 mg lopinavir/20 mg ritonavir per mL)
7 to < 15	12 mg/kg BID	
7 to 10		1.25 mL
> 10 to < 15		1.75 mL
15 to 40	10 mg/kg BID	
15 to 20		2.25 mL
> 20 to 25		2.5 mL
> 25 to 30		3 mL
> 30 to 40		3.5 mL
> 40	Adult dose	5 mL (or 3 capsules)

[1] Note: Use adult dosage recommendation for children > 12 years of age.
[2] Dosing based on the lopinavir component of lopinavir/ritonavir solution (80 mg/20 mg per mL).

Concomitant therapy with efavirenz or nevirapine –

Lopinavir/Ritonavir Pediatric Dosing with Efavirenz or Nevirapine		
Weight (kg)[1]	Dose (mg/kg)[2]	Volume of oral solution BID (80 mg lopinavir/20 mg ritonavir per mL)
7 to < 15	13 mg/kg BID	
7 to 10		1.5 mL
> 10 to < 15		2 mL
15 to 50	11 mg/kg BID	
15 to 20		2.5 mL
> 20 to 25		3.25 mL
> 25 to 30		4 mL
> 30 to 40		4.5 mL
> 40 to 50		5 mL
> 50	Adult dose	6.5 mL (or 4 capsules)

[1] Note: Use adult dosage recommendation for children > 12 years of age.
[2] Dosing based on the lopinavir component of lopinavir/ritonavir solution (80 mg/20 mg per mL).

Actions

Pharmacology: Lopinavir, an HIV protease inhibitor, prevents cleavage of the Gag-Pol polyprotein, resulting in the production of immature, noninfectious viral particles. As coformulated in the lopinavir/ritonavir combination, ritonavir inhibits the CYP3A-mediated metabolism of lopinavir, providing increased lopinavir plasma levels.

Pharmacokinetics:

Absorption – Administration of a single 400/100 mg dose of lopinavir/ritonavir with a moderate fat meal was associated with a mean increase of 48% and 23% in lopinavir AUC and C_{max}, respectively, relative to fasting. To enhance bioavailability and minimize pharmacokinetic variability, take lopinavir/ritonavir with food.

Distribution – At steady state, lopinavir is ≈ 98% to 99% bound to plasma proteins. Lopinavir binds to alpha-1-acid glycoprotein (AAG) and albumin, but has a higher affinity for AAG.

Metabolism – In vitro experiments with human hepatic microsomes indicate that lopinavir primarily undergoes oxidative metabolism. Lopinavir is extensively metabolized by the hepatic cytochrome P450 system, almost exclusively by the CYP3A isozyme. Ritonavir is a potent CYP3A inhibitor that inhibits the metabolism of lopinavir, and therefore increases plasma levels of lopinavir.

Excretion – After multiple dosing, < 3% of the lopinavir dose is excreted unchanged in the urine. The half-life of lopinavir over a 12-hour dosing interval averaged 5 to 6 hours, and the apparent oral clearance (CL/F) of lopinavir is 6 to 7 L/hr.

Contraindications

Hypersensitivity to any of its ingredients, including ritonavir.

Coadministration of lopinavir/ritonavir is contraindicated with drugs that are highly dependent on CYP3A or CYP2D6 for clearance and for which elevated plasma concentrations are associated with serious or life-threatening events. These drugs include the following: Flecainide, propafenone, dihydroergotamine, ergonovine, ergotamine, methylergonovine, pimozide, midazolam, triazolam.

Warnings

Hepatic function impairment: Lopinavir/ritonavir is principally metabolized by the liver; therefore, exercise caution when administering this drug to patients with hepatic impairment, because lopinavir concentrations may be increased.

Elderly: Exercise appropriate caution in the administration and monitoring of lopinavir/ritonavir in elderly patients, reflecting the greater frequency of decreased hepatic, renal, or cardiac function, and of concomitant disease or other drug therapy.

Pregnancy: Category C. To monitor maternal-fetal outcomes of pregnant women exposed to lopinavir/ritonavir, an antiretroviral pregnancy registry has been established. Physicians are encouraged to register patients by calling (800) 258-4263.

Lactation: The Centers for Disease Control and Prevention recommend that HIV-infected mothers not breastfeed their infants to avoid risking postnatal transmission of HIV.

Children: The safety and pharmacokinetic profiles of lopinavir/ritonavir in children < 6 months of age have not been established. In HIV-infected patients 6 months to 12 years of age, the adverse event profile seen during a clinical trial was similar to that for adult patients. The evaluation of the antiviral activity of lopinavir/ritonavir in pediatric patients in clinical trials is ongoing.

Precautions

Pancreatitis: Pancreatitis has been observed in patients receiving lopinavir/ritonavir therapy, including those who developed marked triglyceride elevations. Fatalities have been observed. Although a causal relationship to lopinavir/ritonavir has not been established, marked triglyceride elevations is a risk factor for development of pancreatitis.

Evaluate patients who exhibit signs or symptoms of pancreatitis and suspend lopinavir/ritonavir or other antiretroviral therapy as clinically appropriate.

Diabetes mellitus/hyperglycemia: New onset diabetes mellitus, exacerbation of pre-existing diabetes mellitus, and hyperglycemia have been reported during postmarketing surveillance in HIV-infected patients receiving protease inhibitor therapy. Some patients required either initiation or dose adjustments of insulin or oral hypoglycemic agent for treatment of these events.

Hemophilia: There have been reports of increased bleeding, including spontaneous skin hematomas and hemarthrosis, in patients with hemophilia types A and B treated with protease inhibitors.

Fat redistribution: Redistribution/accumulation of body fat including central obesity, dorsocervical fat enlargement (buffalo hump), peripheral wasting, breast enlargement, and "cushingoid appearance" have been observed in patients receiving antiretroviral therapy.

Lipid elevations: Treatment with lopinavir/ritonavir has resulted in large increases in the concentration of total cholesterol and triglycerides. Perform triglyceride and cholesterol testing prior to initiating therapy and at periodic intervals during therapy. Manage lipid disorders as clinically appropriate.

Drug Interactions

CYP 450: Lopinavir/ritonavir is metabolized by CYP3A. Drugs that induce CYP3A activity would be expected to increase the clearance of lopinavir, resulting in lowered plasma concentrations of lopinavir. Although not noted with concurrent ketoconazole, co-administration of lopinavir/ritonavir and other drugs that inhibit CYP3A may increase lopinavir plasma concentrations.

Drugs that might decrease plasma concentrations of lopinavir/ritonavir include rifampin, phenobarbital, carbamazepine, St. John's wort, efavirenz, nevirapine, and corticosteroids.

Drugs that might be affected by lopinavir/ritonavir include ergot derivatives, oral contraceptives, antiarrhythmics, HMG-CoA reductase inhibitors, and HIV protease inhibitors.

Drug/Food interactions:

Didanosine – It is recommended that didanosine be administered on an empty stomach; therefore, give didanosine 1 hour before or 2 hours after lopinavir/ritonavir (give with food).

Adverse Reactions

Adverse reactions occurring in ≥ 3% of patients include the following: Abdominal pain, nausea, diarrhea, and asthenia. Lab abnormalities include the following: Elevations of AST, ALT, GGT, total cholesterol, triglycerides, and amylase.

Children – Lab abnormalities occurring in ≥ 3% of patients include the following: Total bilirubin, AST, ALT, amylase, sodium, and platelet count.

TENOFOVIR DISOPROXIL FUMARATE (PMPA)

Tablets: 300 mg (equivalent to 245 mg tenofovir disoproxil)   *Viread* (Gilead Sciences)
(Rx)

> **Warning:**
> Lactic acidosis and severe hepatomegaly with steatosis, including fatal cases, have been reported with the use of nucleoside analogs alone or in combination with other antiretrovirals. A majority of these cases have been in women. Obesity and prolonged nucleoside exposure may be risk factors. Exercise particular caution when administering nucleoside analogs to any patient with known risk factors for liver disease. Cases also have been reported in patients with no known risk factors. Suspend treatment with tenofovir in any patient who develops clinical or laboratory findings suggestive of lactic acidosis or pronounced hepatotoxicity, which may include hepatomegaly and steatosis even in the absence of marked transaminase elevations.

Indications

HIV infection: In combination with other antiretroviral agents for the treatment of HIV-1 infection. This indication is based on studies conducted in treatment-experienced adults with evidence of HIV-1 viral replication despite ongoing antiretroviral therapy. Studies in antiretroviral naïve patients are ongoing. Consider the use of tenofovir for treating adult patients with HIV strains that are expected to be susceptible to tenofovir as assessed by laboratory testing or treatment history.

Administration and Dosage

The recommended dose is 300 mg once daily taken orally with a meal.

When administered with didanosine, give tenofovir 2 hours before or 1 hour after didanosine administration.

Actions

Pharmacology: Tenofovir disoproxil, an acyclic nucleoside phosphonate diester analog of adenosine monophosphate, inhibits the activity of HIV reverse transcriptase by competing with the natural substrate deoxyadenosine 5'-triphosphate and, after incorporation into DNA, by DNA chain termination.

Pharmacokinetics:

Absorption – The oral bioavailability of tenofovir in fasted patients is ≈ 25%. Maximum serum concentrations (C_{max}) are achieved in ≈ 1 hour. C_{max} and AUC values are ≈ 296 ng/mL and ≈ 2287 ng•hr/mL, respectively.

Administration of tenofovir disoproxil following a high-fat meal increases the oral biovavailability with an increase in tenofovir $AUC_{0-\infty}$ of ≈ 40% and an increase in C_{max} of ≈ 14%. Take tenofovir with a meal to enhance its bioavailability.

Distribution – In vitro binding of tenofovir to human plasma or serum proteins is < 0.7 and 7.2%, respectively. The volume of distribution at steady state is ≈ 1.3 L/kg.

Metabolism/Excretion – In vitro studies indicate that neither tenofovir disoproxil nor tenofovir are substrates of CYP450 enzymes. Tenofovir is eliminated by a combination of glomerular filtration and active tubular secretion. There may be competition for elimination with other compounds that are also renally eliminated.

Special populations –

Renal function impairment: Because tenofovir is primarily renally eliminated, tenofovir pharmacokinetics are likely to be affected by renal impairment.

Warnings

Lactic acidosis/severe hepatomegaly with steatosis: Lactic acidosis and severe hepatomegaly with steatosis, including fatal cases, have been reported with the use of nucleoside analogs alone or in combination with other antiretrovirals. A majority of these cases have been in women. Obesity and prolonged nucleoside exposure may be risk factors. Exercise particular caution when administering nucleoside analogs to any patient with known risk factors for liver disease. Cases also have been reported in patients with no known risk factors. Suspend treatment with tenofovir in any patient who develops clinical or laboratory findings suggestive of lactic acidosis or pronounced hepatotoxicity, which may include hepatomegaly and steatosis even in the absence of marked transaminase elevations (see Warning Box).

Renal function impairment: Do not administer tenofovir to patients with renal insufficiency (Ccr < 60 mL/min) until data become available describing the disposition of tenofovir in these patients.

Hepatic function impairment: The pharmacokinetics of tenofovir have not been studied in patients with hepatic impairment. Tenofovir pharmacokinetics may be altered in patients with hepatic insufficiency.

Mutagenesis: Tenofovir was mutagenic in the in vitro mouse lymphoma assay and negative in an in vitro bacterial mutagenicity test (Ames test).

Fertility impairment: In female rats, there was an alteration of the estrous cycle.

Elderly: In general, dose selection for the elderly patient should be cautious, keeping in mind the greater frequency of decreased hepatic, renal, or cardiac function, and of concomitant disease or other drug therapy.

Pregnancy: Category B.

Antiretroviral Pregnancy Registry – To monitor fetal outcomes of pregnant women exposed to tenofovir, an Antiretroviral Pregnancy Registry has been established. Health care providers are encouraged to register patients by calling (800) 258-4263.

Lactation: The Centers for Disease Control and Prevention recommend that HIV-infected mothers not breastfeed their infants to avoid risking postnatal transmission of HIV.

Precautions

Monitoring:

Bone toxicity – It is not known if long-term administration of tenofovir (> 1 year) will cause bone abnormalities. Therefore, if bone abnormalities are suspected, obtain appropriate consultation.

Renal toxicity – Long-term renal effects are unknown. Consider monitoring for changes in serum creatinine and serum phosphorus in patients at risk or with a history of renal dysfunction.

Fat redistribution: Redistribution and accumulation of body fat have been observed in patients receiving antiretroviral therapy.

Drug Interactions

Drugs that may interact with tenofovir include didanosine and drugs eliminated by the kidneys (eg, cidofovir, acyclovir, valacyclovir, ganciclovir, valganciclovir).

Adverse Reactions

Adverse reactions occurring in ≥ 3% of patients include the following: Nausea, diarrhea, asthenia, headache, vomiting, flatulence, abdominal pain, anorexia, creatine kinase > 782 U/L, triglycerides > 750 mg/dL, serum amylase > 175 U/L, AST, urine glucose 3+ or 4+.

DIDANOSINE (ddI; dideoxyinosine)

Tablets, buffered, chewable/dispersible: 25, 50, 100, 150, and 200 mg (*Rx*)	*Videx* (Bristol-Myers Squibb)
Capsules, delayed release (with enteric-coated beadlets): 125, 200, 250, and 400 mg (*Rx*)	*Videx EC* (Bristol-Myers Squibb)
Powder for oral solution, buffered: 100, 167, and 250 mg (*Rx*)	*Videx* (Bristol-Myers Squibb)
Powder for oral solution, pediatric: 2 and 4 g (*Rx*)	*Videx* (Bristol-Myers Squibb)

Warning:
  Fatal and nonfatal pancreatitis has occurred during therapy with didanosine alone or in combination regimens in treatment-naive and treatment-experienced patients, regardless of degree of immunosuppression. Suspend didanosine in patients with suspected pancreatitis, and discontinue therapy in patients with confirmed pancreatitis (see Warnings).

  Lactic acidosis and severe hepatomegaly with steatosis, including fatal cases, have been reported with the use of nucleoside analogs alone or in combination, including didanosine and other antiretrovirals. Fatal lactic acidosis has been reported in pregnant women who received the combination of didanosine and stavudine with other antiretroviral agents. The combination of didanosine and stavudine should be used with caution during pregnancy and is recommended only if the potential benefit clearly outweighs the potential risk (see Warnings).

Indications

Didanosine (Videx): In combination with other antiretroviral agents for treatment of HIV-1 infection.

Didanosine EC (Videx EC): In combination with other antiretroviral agents for treatment of HIV-1 infection in adults whose management requires once-daily administration of didanosine or an alternative didanosine formulation. There are limited data to date to support the long-term durability of response with a once-daily regimen of didanosine.

Administration and Dosage

Dosage:
  Didanosine (Videx) – Administer all didanosine formulations on an empty stomach, at least 30 minutes before or 2 hours after eating. For either a once-daily or twice-daily regimen, patients must take at least 2 of the appropriate strength tablets at each dose to provide adequate buffering and prevent gastric acid degradation of didanosine. Because of the need for adequate buffering, use the 200 mg strength buffered tablet only as a component of the once-daily regimen. To reduce the risk of GI side effects, patients should take no more than 4 tablets at each dose.

Adults:

Didanosine (Videx) – The preferred dosing frequency of didanosine buffered is twice daily because there is more evidence to support the effectiveness of this dosing regimen. Once-daily dosing should be considered only for adult patients whose management requires once-daily dosing of didanosine.

Didanosine EC (Videx EC) – Didanosine EC should be administered on an empty stomach and should be swallowed intact.

Adult Didanosine Dosing			
Patient weight (kg)	Tablets[1]	Buffered powder[2]	Enteric-coated capsules
≥ 60	400 mg qd or 200 mg bid	250 mg bid	400 mg qd
< 60	250 mg qd or 125 mg bid	167 mg bid	250 mg qd

[1] Use the 200 mg strength tablet only as a component of the once-daily regimen.
[2] Not suitable for once-daily dosing except for patients with renal impairment.

Children:

Didanosine (Videx) – The recommended dose of didanosine in pediatric patients is 120 mg/m^2 twice daily. There are no data on once-daily dosing of didanosine in pediatric patients.

Didanosine EC (Videx EC) – Didanosine EC has not been studied in pediatric patients. Please consult the complete prescribing information for didanosine buffered formulation and pediatric powder for oral solution for dosage and administration of didanosine to pediatric patients.

Dose adjustment: If clinical and laboratory signs suggest pancreatitis, promptly suspend dose and carefully evaluate the possibility of pancreatitis. Discontinue in patients with confirmed pancreatitis.

Based on data with buffered didanosine formulations, patients with symptoms of peripheral neuropathy may tolerate a reduced dose after resolution of these symptoms following drug discontinuation. If neuropathy recurs after resumption of didanosine, consider permanent discontinuation.

Renal function impairment – In adult patients with impaired renal function, adjust the dose of didanosine to compensate for the slower rate of elimination.

Recommended Dose (mg) of Didanosine by Body Weight in Renal Function Impairment						
	≥ 60 kg			< 60 kg		
Ccr (mL/min)	Tablet (mg)[1]	Buffered powder (mg)[2]	Enteric-coated capsules	Tablet (mg)[1]	Buffered powder (mg)[2]	Enteric-coated capsules
≥ 60	400 qd or 200 bid	250 bid	400 mg qd	250 qd or 125 bid	167 bid	250 mg qd
30 to 59	200 qd or 100 bid	100 bid	200 mg qd	150 qd or 75 bid	100 bid	125 mg qd
10 to 29	150 qd	167 qd	125 mg qd	100 qd	100 qd	125 mg qd
< 10	100 qd	100 qd	125 mg qd	75 qd	100 qd	—[3]

[1] Didanosine chewable/dispersible buffered tablets. Two didanosine tablets must be taken with each dose; different strengths of tablets may be combined to yield the recommended dose.
[2] Didanosine buffered powder for oral solution.
[3] Didanosine EC capsules are not suitable for patients < 60 kg with Ccr < 10 mL/min. An alternate didanosine formulation should be used.

Didanosine (Videx): Urinary excretion is also a major route of didanosine elimination in pediatric patients; therefore, the clearance of didanosine may be altered in children with renal impairment. Although there are insufficient data to recommend a specific dose adjustment in this patient population, consider a reduction in the dose or an increase in the interval between doses.

Patients requiring continuous ambulatory peritoneal dialysis (CAPD) or hemodialysis –

Didanosine (Videx): It is recommended that ¼ of the total daily dose of didanosine be administered once daily. For patients with Ccr < 10 mL/min, it is not necessary to administer a supplemental dose of didanosine following hemodialysis.

Didanosine EC (Videx EC): For patients ≥ 60 kg, administer 125 mg once daily. Didanosine EC is not suitable for use in patients < 60 kg with Ccr < 10 mL/min. It is not necessary to administer a supplemental dose of didanosine EC following hemodialysis.

Method of preparation:
  Adults –
    Chewable/Dispersible buffered tablets: To provide adequate buffering, thoroughly chew at least 2 of the appropriate strength tablets, but no more than 4 tablets, or disperse in ≥ 1 ounce of water prior to consumption. To disperse tablets, add 2 tablets to ≥ 1 ounce of water. Stir until a uniform dispersion forms, and drink entire dispersion immediately. If additional flavoring is desired, the dispersion may be diluted with 1 ounce of clear apple juice. Stir the further diluted dispersion just prior to consumption. The dispersion with clear apple juice is stable at room temperature for up to 1 hour.
    Buffered powder for oral solution:
1.) Open packet carefully and pour contents into ≈ 4 ounces of water. Do not mix with fruit juice or other acid-containing liquid.
2.) Stir until the powder completely dissolves (≈ 2 to 3 minutes).
3.) Drink the entire solution immediately.
  Children –
    Chewable/Dispersible buffered tablets: Chew tablets or manually crush or disperse 1 or 2 tablets in water prior to consumption, as described for adults.
    Pediatric powder for oral solution: Prior to dispensing, the pharmacist must constitute dry powder with Purified Water, USP, to an initial concentration of 20 mg/mL and immediately mix the resulting solution with antacid to a final concentration of 10 mg/mL as follows:
      20 mg/mL initial solution – Reconstitute the product to 20 mg/mL by adding 100 or 200 mL Purified Water, USP, to the 2 or 4 g of powder, respectively, in the product bottle. Prepare final admixture as described below.
      10 mg/mL final admixture –
1.) Immediately mix 1 part of the 20 mg/mL initial solution with 1 part of either *Mylanta Double Strength Liquid, Extra Strength Maalox Plus Suspension,* or *Maalox TC Suspension* for a final dispensing concentration of 10 mg/mL. For patient home use, dispense the admixture in flint-glass or plastic bottles with child-resistant closures. This admixture is stable for 30 days under refrigeration at 2° to 8°C (36° to 46°F).
2.) Instruct the patient or caregiver to shake the admixture thoroughly prior to use and to store the tightly closed container in the refrigerator at 2° to 8°C (36° to 46°F) up to 30 days.

Actions
Pharmacology: Didanosine is a synthetic purine nucleoside analog of deoxyadenosine, in which the 3'-hydroxyl group is replaced by hydrogen. Intracellularly, it is converted by cellular enzymes to the active metabolite, dideoxyadenosine 5'-triphosphate. It inhibits the activity of HIV-1 reverse transcriptase by competing with the natural substrate, deoxyadenosine 5'-triphosphate, and by incorporating in viral DNA causing termination of viral DNA chain elongation.

Pharmacokinetics:
  Effect of food on oral absorption – Didanosine C_{max} and AUC were decreased by ≈ 55% when didanosine tablets were administered up to 2 hours after a meal. Administration of didanosine tablets up to 30 minutes before a meal did not result in any significant changes in bioavailability.
    Enteric-coated capsules: In the presence of food, C_{max} and AUC for didanosine capsules were reduced by ≈ 46% and 19%, respectively, compared with the fasting state. Take didanosine capsules on an empty stomach.

Pharmacokinetic Parameters of Didanosine in Adult and Pediatric Patients		
Parameter	Adult patients[1]	Pediatric patients
Oral bioavailability	$\approx$ 42%	$\approx$ 25%
Apparent volume of distribution[2]	$\approx$ 1.08 L/kg	$\approx$ 28 L/m^2
CSF[3]-plasma ratio[4]	$\approx$ 21%	46% (range, 12% to 85%)
Systemic clearance[2]	$\approx$ 13 mL/min/kg	$\approx$ 516 mL/min/m^2
Renal clearance[5]	$\approx$ 5.5 mL/min/kg	$\approx$ 240 mL/min/m^2
Elimination half-life[5]	$\approx$ 1.5 hr	$\approx$ 0.8 hr
Urine recovery of didanosine[5]	$\approx$ 18%	$\approx$ 18%

[1] Administered as buffered formulation.
[2] Following IV administration.
[3] CSF = cerebrospinal fluid.
[4] Following IV administration in adults and IV or oral administration in pediatric patients.
[5] Following oral administration.

Children – The pharmacokinetics of didanosine administered as *Videx EC* has not been studied in pediatric patients.

Comparison of didanosine formulations – In didanosine EC (*Videx EC*), the active ingredient, didanosine, is protected against degradation by stomach acid by the use of an enteric coating on the beadlets in the capsule. The enteric coating dissolves when the beadlets empty into the small intestine, the site of drug absorption. With buffered formulations of didanosine, administration with antacid provides protection from degradation by stomach acid.

Contraindications
Hypersensitivity to any of the components of the formulations.

Warnings
Pancreatitis: Fatal and nonfatal pancreatitis has occurred during didanosine therapy used alone or in combination regimens in treatment-naive and treatment-experienced patients regardless of degree of immunosuppression (see Warning Box).

Lactic acidosis/Severe hepatomegaly with steatosis: Lactic acidosis and severe hepatomegaly with steatosis, including fatal cases, have been reported with the use of nucleoside analogs alone or in combination, including didanosine and other antiretrovirals. A majority of these cases have been in women. Obesity and prolonged nucleoside exposure may be risk factors (see Warning Box).

Retinal changes and optic neuritis: Retinal changes and optic neuritis have been reported in adult and pediatric patients. Consider periodic retinal examinations for patients receiving didanosine.

Peripheral neuropathy: Peripheral neuropathy, manifested by numbness, tingling, or pain in the hands or feet, has been reported in patients receiving didanosine therapy.

Myopathy: Human myopathy has been associated with administration of other nucleoside analogs.

Renal function impairment: Patients with renal impairment (serum creatinine > 1.5 mg/dL or Ccr < 60 mL/min) may be at greater risk of toxicity from didanosine because of decreased drug clearance; consider a dose reduction. The magnesium hydroxide content of each buffered tablet (8.6 mEq) may present an excessive magnesium load to patients with significant renal impairment, particularly after prolonged dosing.

Hepatic function impairment: It is unknown if hepatic impairment significantly affects didanosine pharmacokinetics. Therefore, monitor these patients closely for evidence of didanosine toxicity.

Elderly: In an expanded access program using a buffered formulation of didanosine for the treatment of advanced HIV infection, patients $\geq$ 65 years of age had a higher frequency of pancreatitis (10%) than younger patients (5%).

Pregnancy: Category B.

To monitor maternal-fetal outcomes of pregnant women exposed to didanosine and other antiretroviral agents, an Antiretroviral Pregnancy Registry has been established. Physicians are encouraged to register patients by calling (800) 258-4263.

Lactation: It is not known whether didanosine is excreted in breast milk. Because of the potential for serious adverse reactions from didanosine in nursing infants, instruct mothers to discontinue nursing when taking didanosine; this is consistent with the CDC's recommendation that HIV-infected mothers not breastfeed their infants to avoid risking postnatal transmission of HIV infection.

Children: Safety and efficacy of didanosine EC have not been established in pediatric patients (see Administration and Dosage).

Precautions

Frequency of dosing: The preferred dosing frequency of didanosine is twice daily because there is more evidence to support the effectiveness of this dosing frequency. Once daily dosing should be considered only for adult patients whose management requires once daily dosing of didanosine.

Phenylketonuria: Didanosine chewable/dispersible buffered tablets contain the following quantities of phenylalanine: 73 mg phenylalanine per 2-tablet dose (36.5 mg phenylalanine per tablet).

Sodium-restricted diets: Each buffered tablet contains 264.5 mg sodium. Each single-dose packet of buffered powder for oral solution contains 1380 mg sodium.

Hyperuricemia: Didanosine has been associated with asymptomatic hyperuricemia; consider suspending treatment if clinical measures aimed at reducing uric acid levels fail.

Drug Interactions

Drugs that may affect didanosine include allopurinol, methadone, and ganciclovir.

Drugs that may be affected by didanosine include ganciclovir, antacids, antifungal agents, antiretroviral drugs, fluoroquinolones, and stavudine.

Coadministration of didanosine buffered tablets, buffered powder for oral solution, and pediatric powder for oral solution with drugs that are known to cause peripheral neuropathy or pancreatitis or patients who have a history of neuropathy or neurotoxic drug therapy may have increased risk of toxicities. Closely observe patients who receive these drugs or have a history of neuropathy or neurotoxic drug therapy.

Drug/Food interactions: Ingestion of didanosine with food reduces the absorption of didanosine by as much as 50%. Therefore, administer on an empty stomach, ≥ 30 minutes before or 2 hours after eating.

Adverse Reactions

A serious toxicity of didanosine is pancreatitis, which may be fatal (see Warnings). Other important toxicities include lactic acidosis/severe hepatomegaly with steatosis; retinal changes and optic neuritis; and peripheral neuropathy (see Warnings and Precautions).

When didanosine is used in combination with other agents with similar toxicities, the incidence of these toxicities may be higher than when didanosine is used alone. Thus, patients treated with didanosine in combination with stavudine, with or without hydroxyurea, may be at increased risk for pancreatitis and liver function abnormalities (see Warnings). Patients treated with didanosine in combination with stavudine may also be at increased risk for peripheral neuropathy (see Precautions).

Adverse reactions occurring in ≥ 3% of patients include diarrhea, neuropathy (all grades), rash/pruritus, abdominal pain, headache, pain, nausea/vomiting, pancreatitis, and laboratory abnormalities including amylase, ALT, AST, and uric acid.

LAMIVUDINE (3TC)

Tablets: 100 mg (*Rx*)	*Epivir-HBV* (GlaxoSmithKline)
Tablets: 150 mg (*Rx*)	*Epivir* (GlaxoSmithKline)
Oral solution: 5 mg/mL (*Rx*)	*Epivir-HBV* (GlaxoSmithKline)
Oral solution: 10 mg/mL (*Rx*)	*Epivir* (GlaxoSmithKline)

> **Warning:**
>
> Lactic acidosis and severe hepatomegaly with steatosis, including fatal cases, have been reported with the use of antiretroviral nucleoside analogs alone or in combination, including lamivudine and other antiretroviral agents (see Warnings).
>
> Offer human immunodeficiency virus (HIV) counseling and testing to patients before beginning *Epivir-HBV* and periodically during treatment because *Epivir-HBV* tablets and oral solution contain a lower dose of the same active ingredient (lamivudine) as the *Epivir* tablets and oral solution used to treat HIV infection. If treatment with *Epivir-HBV* is prescribed for chronic hepatitis B for a patient with unrecognized or untreated HIV infection, rapid emergence of HIV resistance is likely because of subtherapeutic dose and inappropriate monotherapy.
>
> *Epivir* tablets and oral solution (used to treat HIV infection) contain a higher dose of the active ingredient (lamivudine) than *Epivir-HBV* tablets and oral solution (used to treat chronic hepatitis B). Patients with HIV infection should receive only dosing forms appropriate for the treatment of HIV (see Warnings and Precautions).

Indications

HIV infection (Epivir): Lamivudine in combination with other antiretroviral agents is indicated for the treatment of HIV infection.

Chronic hepatitis B (Epivir-HBV): Treatment of chronic hepatitis B associated with evidence of hepatitis B viral replication and active liver inflammation.

Administration and Dosage

HIV infection:

Adults – 150 mg twice daily in combination with other antiretroviral agents. Lamivudine may be administered with or without food.

Children (3 months to ≤ 16 years of age) – 4 mg/kg twice daily (up to a maximum of 150 mg twice a day) administered with other antiretroviral agents.

Renal function impairment – Adjust lamivudine dose in accordance with renal function. Insufficient data are available to recommend a dosage of lamivudine in dialysis.

Adjustment of Lamivudine Dosage in HIV-Infected Adult and Adolescent Patients with Renal Function Impairment	
Ccr (mL/min)	Recommended lamivudine dosage
≥ 50	150 mg twice daily
30 to 49	150 mg once daily
15 to 29	150 mg first dose, then 100 mg once daily
5 to 14	150 mg first dose, then 50 mg once daily
< 5	50 mg first dose, then 25 mg once daily

Chronic hepatitis B: 100 mg once daily in adults. Safety and efficacy of treatment > 1 year have not been established, and the optimum duration of treatment is not known.

Children (2 to 17 years of age) – 3 mg/kg once daily up to a maximum daily dose of 100 mg. Safety and effectiveness of treatment beyond 1 year have not been established, and the optimum duration of treatment is not known.

HIV co-infection – The formulation and dosage of lamivudine in *Epivir-HBV* are not appropriate for patients dually infected with HBV and HIV. If lamivudine is administered to such patients, use the higher dosage indicated for HIV therapy as part of an appropriate combination regimen.

Renal function impairment – Adjust the dose of lamivudine in accordance with renal function. No additional dosing of lamivudine is required after routine (4-hour) hemodialysis. Insufficient data are available to recommend a dosage of lamivudine in patients undergoing peritoneal dialysis.

Adjustment of Lamivudine Dosage in Chronic Hepatitis B Adult Patients with Renal Function Impairment	
Ccr (mL/min)	Recommended lamivudine dosage
≥ 50	100 mg once daily
30 to 49	100 mg first dose, then 50 mg once daily
15 to 29	100 mg first dose, then 25 mg once daily
5 to 14	35 mg first dose, then 15 mg once daily
< 5	35 mg first dose, then 10 mg once daily

Actions
Pharmacology: Lamivudine is a synthetic nucleoside analog with activity against HIV and hepatitis B virus (HBV). Lamivudine is phosphorylated intracellularly to lamivudine 5'-triphosphate (L-TP). Incorporation of the monophosphate form into viral DNA by HBV polymerase results in DNA chain termination. L-TP also inhibits the RNA- and DNA-dependent DNA polymerase activities of HIV-1 reverse transcriptase.

Pharmacokinetics:

Absorption/Distribution – Lamivudine is rapidly absorbed after oral administration in HIV- and HBV-infected patients and phosphorylated to its active form, L-TP. Absolute bioavailability as demonstrated in HIV-infected patients is 86% for the tablet and 87% for the oral solution. Although the solution demonstrates a slightly higher C_{max} than the tablet, no significant difference exists in AUC; therefore, the solution and tablet may be used interchangeably.

The apparent volume of distribution (V_d) is 1.3 L/kg suggesting distribution into extravascular spaces. C_{max} reported in HBV-infected patients was 0.5 to 2 hours. Binding of lamivudine to plasma proteins is < 36% and independent of dose.

Metabolism/Excretion – Metabolism is a minor route of elimination; the only known metabolite is the trans-sulfoxide metabolite. The mean elimination half-life of lamivudine ranges from 5 to 7 hours. In HIV-infected patients, renal clearance is 280.4 mL/min, representing 71% of total clearance; total clearance is 398.5 mL/min. The majority of the dose is eliminated in the urine as unchanged drug, with ≈ 5% excreted as the metabolite within 12 hours of dose administration.

Special populations:

Children – In HIV-infected pediatric patients ≈ 4 months to 16 years of age and chronic hepatitis B pediatric patients 2 to 12 years of age, lamivudine was rapidly absorbed with a T_{max} of 0.5 to 1 hour and an absolute bioavailability of 66%. After 8 mg/kg/day, C_{max} was 1.1 mcg/mL and half-life was 2 hours (vs 3.7 hours in adults). Weight-corrected oral clearances were higher, resulting in lower AUCs compared with adults. Total exposure to lamivudine, as reflected by mean AUC values, was comparable between pediatric patients receiving 8 mg/kg/day and adults receiving 4 mg/kg/day. Age-stratified oral clearance was highest at 2 years of age and declined from 2 to 12 years of age, where values were then similar to those seen in adults. In 8 patients, CSF lamivudine concentrations (0.04 to 0.3 mcg/mL) ranged from 5.6% to 30.9% of the concentration in a simultaneous serum sample.

Contraindications
Hypersensitivity to any of the components of the products.

Warnings
Lactic acidosis/severe hepatomegaly with steatosis: Lactic acidosis and severe hepatomegaly with steatosis, including fatal cases, have occurred with the use of antiretroviral nucleoside analogs alone or in combination, including lamivudine and other antiretrovirals. A majority of these cases have been in women. Obesity and prolonged nucleoside exposure may be risk factors. Most of these reports have described

patients receiving nucleoside analogs for treatment of HIV infection, but there have been reports of lactic acidosis in patients receiving lamivudine for hepatitis B. Exercise caution when administering lamivudine to any patient, particularly to those with known risk factors for liver disease. Suspend treatment with lamivudine in any patient who develops clinical or laboratory findings suggestive of lactic acidosis or pronounced hepatotoxicity (which may include hepatomegaly and steatosis even in the absence of marked transaminase elevations).

HIV-HBV co-infection: Epivir-HBV tablets and oral solution contain a lower dose of the same active ingredient (lamivudine) as *Epivir* tablets and oral solution (and lamivudine/zidovudine tablets) used to treat HIV infection. The formulation and dosage of lamivudine in *Epivir-HBV* are not appropriate for patients infected with both HBV and HIV. If a decision is made to administer lamivudine to patients dually infected with HIV and HBV, *Epivir* tablets or oral solution or *Combivir* (lamivudine/zidovudine) tablets should be used as a part of an appropriate combination regimen and prescribing information should be consulted. *Combivir* (a fixed-dose combination tablet of lamivudine and zidovudine) should not be administered concomitantly with either *Epivir, Epivir-HBV,* or *Retrovir* (zidovudine).

Posttreatment exacerbations of hepatitis: Clinical and laboratory evidence of exacerbations of hepatitis have occurred after discontinuation of lamivudine (these have been primarily detected by serum ALT elevations in addition to the re-emergence of HBV DNA commonly observed after stopping treatment). Although most events appear to have been self-limited, fatalities have been reported in some cases. Similar events have been reported from postmarketing experience after changes from lamivudine-containing HIV treatment regimens to non-lamivudine-containing regimens in patients infected with both HIV and HBV. The causal relationship to discontinuation of lamivudine treatment is unknown. Closely monitor patients with clinical and laboratory follow-up for at least several months after stopping treatment. There is insufficient evidence to determine whether reinitiation of therapy alters the course of posttreatment exacerbations of hepatitis.

Elderly: Because elderly patients are more likely to have decreased renal function, take care in dose selection and monitor renal function.

Pregnancy: Category C.

Lamivudine has not affected the transmission of HBV from mother to infant; immunize infants appropriately to prevent neonatal acquisition of HBV.

Antiretroviral pregnancy registry – To monitor maternal-fetal outcomes of women exposed to lamivudine, an Antiretroviral Pregnancy Registry has been established. Physicians are encouraged to register patients by calling (800) 258-4263.

Lactation: Instruct mothers to discontinue nursing if they are receiving lamivudine, which is consistent with the CDC recommendation that HIV-infected mothers not breastfeed their infants to avoid risking postnatal transmission of HIV infection.

Children:

Hepatitis B – Safety and efficacy of lamivudine for treatment of chronic hepatitis B in children have been studied in pediatric patients from 2 to 17 years of age in a controlled clinical trial. Safety and efficacy in pediatric patients < 2 years of age have not been established.

HIV infection – The safety and effectiveness of lamivudine in combination with other antiretroviral agents have been established in pediatric patients ≥ 3 months of age.

Total exposure to lamivudine, as reflected by mean AUC values, was comparable between pediatric patients receiving an 8 mg/kg/day dose and adults receiving a 4 mg/kg/day dose.

Pancreatitis – Pancreatitis, which has been fatal in some cases, has been observed in antiretroviral nucleoside-experienced pediatric patients receiving lamivudine alone or in combination with other antiretroviral agents. Stop lamivudine treatment immediately if clinical signs, symptoms, or lab abnormalities suggestive of pancreatitis occur (see Adverse Reactions).

Precautions

Monitoring:

Epivir-HBV – Monitor patients regularly during treatment. The safety and efficacy of treatment with *Epivir-HBV* > 1 year have not been established. During treatment, combinations of events such as return of persistently elevated ALT, increasing levels of HBV DNA over time after an initial decline below assay limit, progression of clinical signs or symptoms of hepatic disease, and worsening of hepatic necroinflammatory findings may be considered as potentially reflecting loss of therapeutic response. Consider such observations when determining the advisability of continuing therapy.

Emergence of resistance-associated HBV mutations: Progression of hepatitis B, including death, has been reported in some patients with YMDD-mutant HBV, including patients from the liver transplant setting and from other clinical trials. The long-term clinical significance of YMDD-mutant HBV is not known. Increased clinical and laboratory monitoring may aid in treatment decisions if emergence of viral mutants is suspected.

Special risk: Safety and efficacy of *Epivir-HBV* have not been established in patients with decompensated liver disease or organ transplants; pediatric patients < 2 years of age (use appropriate infant immunizations to prevent HBV); patients dually infected with HBV and HCV, hepatitis delta, or HIV; or other populations not included in the principal Phase III controlled studies.

Drug Interactions

Drugs that may interact with lamivudine include zidovudine, zalcitabine, and trimethoprim/sulfamethoxazole.

Adverse Reactions

HIV – Adverse reactions occurring in ≥ 5% of patients include neuropathy, insomnia, dizziness, depression, nausea, diarrhea, vomiting, anorexia, abdominal pain/cramps, dyspepsia, myalgia, arthralgia, nasal symptoms, cough, headache, malaise, fatigue, fever, chills, and rash. Lab abnormalitites may include neutropenia, thrombocytopenia, anemia, and elevations in amylase, AST, ALT, and bilirubin.

Chronic hepatitis B – Adverse reactions occurring in ≥ 3% of patients include the following: Abdominal discomfort/pain; nausea/vomiting; diarrhea; myalgia; arthralgia; ear, nose, and throat infections; sore throat; malaise/fatigue; headache; fever or chills; rash. Lab abnormalitites may include platelets and elevations in ALT, serum lipase, and CPK.

Children – Adverse reactions in children are similar to adults and include pancreatitis, hepatomegaly, splenomegaly, stomatitis, and ear pain/swelling.

Pancreatitis, which has been fatal in some cases, has been observed in antiretroviral nucleoside-experienced pediatric patients receiving lamivudine alone or in combination with other antiretroviral agents. In 1 study, 14% of patients developed pancreatitis while receiving monotherapy with lamivudine. Three of these patients died of complications of pancreatitis. In a second study, 18% of patients developed pancreatitis.

Paresthesias and peripheral neuropathies were reported in < 1% to 15%.

In a 1-month pharmacokinetic study in children (2 to 12 years of age) and adolescents (13 to 17 years of age) with chronic hepatitis B receiving *Epivir-HBV*, the most commonly observed adverse events were malaise, fatigue, cough, fever, diarrhea, headache, and viral respiratory tract infections.

STAVUDINE (d4T)

Capsules: 15, 20, 30, and 40 mg (*Rx*)
Powder for oral solution: 1 mg/mL (*Rx*)

Zerit (Bristol-Myers Squibb)

Warning:

Lactic acidosis and severe hepatomegaly with steatosis, including fatal cases, have been reported with the use of nucleoside analogs alone or in combination, including stavudine and other antiretrovirals (see Warnings). Fatal lactic acidosis has been reported in pregnant women who received the combination of stavudine and didanosine with other antiretroviral agents. Use the combination of stavudine and didanosine with caution during pregnancy and is recommended only if the potential benefit clearly outweighs the potential risk (see Warnings).

Fatal and nonfatal pancreatitis have occurred during therapy when stavudine was part of a combination regimen that included didanosine, with or without hydroxyurea, in both treatment-naive and treatment-experienced patients, regardless of degree of immunosuppression (see Warnings).

Indications

HIV infection: For the treament of HIV-1 infection in combination with other antiretroviral agents.

Administration and Dosage

Adults: The interval between oral doses should be 12 hours. C_{max} was decreased by ≈ 45% when stavudine was administered with food; however, the systemic availability (AUC) was unchanged. Thus, stavudine may be taken without regard to meals. The recommended starting dose based on body weight is as follows:

Patients ≥ 60 kg – 40 mg every 12 hours.
Patients < 60 kg – 30 mg every 12 hours.

Children: The recommended dose for pediatric patients weighing < 30 kg is 1 mg/kg/dose, given every 12 hours. Pediatric patients weighing ≥ 30 kg should receive the recommended adult dosage.

Dosage adjustment: Monitor patients for the development of peripheral neuropathy which is usually characterized by numbness, tingling, or pain in the feet or hands. These symptoms may be difficult to detect in young children. If these symptoms develop, interrupt stavudine therapy. Symptoms may resolve if therapy is withdrawn promptly. In some cases, symptoms may worsen temporarily following discontinuation of therapy. If symptoms resolve completely, resumption of treatment may be considered at 50% the recommended dose using the following dosage schedule:

Patients ≥ 60 kg – 20 mg twice daily.
Patients < 60 kg – 15 mg twice daily.

If neuropathy recurs after resumption of stavudine, consider permanent discontinuation.

Manage clinically significant elevations of hepatic transaminases in the same way.

Renal function impairment – Stavudine may be administered to adult patients with impaired renal function. The following schedule is recommended:

Stavudine Dosage in Renal Function Impairment		
	Recommended stavudine dose by patient weight	
Ccr (mL/min)	≥ 60 kg	< 60 kg
26 to 50	20 mg every 12 hours	15 mg every 12 hours
10 to 25	20 mg every 24 hours	15 mg every 24 hours

Because urinary excretion is a major route of elimination of stavudine in pediatric patients, the clearance may be altered in children with renal impairment. Although there are insufficient data to recommend a specific dose adjustment in this patient population, consider a reduction in the dose or an increase in the interval between doses.

Hemodialysis patients – The recommended dose is 20 mg every 24 hours (≥ 60 kg) or 15 mg every 24 hours (< 60 kg) administered after the completion of hemodialysis and at the same time of day on nondialysis days.

Preparation of stavudine oral solution: Prior to dispensing, reconstitute the dry powder with purified water to a concentration of 1 mg/mL of solution as follows:

1.) Add 202 mL of purified water to the container.
2.) Shake container vigorously until the powder dissolves completely. Constitution in this way produces 200 mL (deliverable volume) of 1 mg/mL stavudine solution. The solution may appear slightly hazy.
3.) Dispense solution in original container with measuring cup provided. Instruct patient to shake the container vigorously prior to measuring each dose and to store the tightly-closed container in a refrigerator, 36° to 46°F (2° to 8°C). Discard any unused portion after 30 days.

Actions

Pharmacology: Stavudine is a synthetic thymidine nucleoside analog active against the human immunodeficiency virus (HIV). It inhibits the replication of HIV in human cells in vitro. Stavudine is phosphorylated by cellular kinases to stavudine triphosphate, which exerts antiviral activity and inhibits HIV replication by 2 known mechanisms:

1.) It inhibits HIV reverse transcriptase by competing with the natural substrate deoxythymidine triphosphate; and
2.) it inhibits viral DNA synthesis by causing DNA chain termination because stavudine lacks the 3'-hydroxyl group necessary for DNA elongation. Stavudine triphosphate also inhibits cellular DNA polymerase beta and gamma, and markedly reduces mitochondrial DNA synthesis.

Pharmacokinetics:

Absorption – Following oral administration, stavudine is rapidly absorbed, with peak plasma concentrations occurring within 1 hour after dosing. The systemic exposure to stavudine is the same following administration as capsules or solution.

Distribution – Binding to serum proteins was negligible over the concentration range of 0.01 to 11.4 mcg/mL. Stavudine distributes equally between red blood cells and plasma.

Excretion – Renal elimination accounted for ≈ 40% of the overall clearance regardless of the route of administration; there is active tubular secretion in addition to glomerular filtration.

Pharmacokinetic Parameters of Stavudine in Adult and Pediatric HIV-infected Patients		
Parameter	Adult patients	Pediatric patients
Oral bioavailability (F)	≈ 86.4%	≈ 76.9%
Volume of distribution[1] (VD)	≈ 58 L	≈ 18.5 L/m^2
Apparant oral volume of distribution[2] (VD/F)	≈ 66 L	not determined
Ratio of CSF:plama concentrations (as %)[3]	not determined	≈ 59%
Total body clearance[1] (CL)	≈ 8.3 mL/min/kg	≈ 247 mL/min/m^2
Apparent oral clearance[2] (CL/F)	≈ 8 mL/min/kg	≈ 333 mL/min/m^2
Elimination half-life (T½), IV dose[1]	≈ 1.15 hr	≈ 1.11 hr
Elimination half-life (T½), oral dose[2]	≈ 1.44 hr	≈ 0.96 hr
Urinary recovery of stavudine (% of dose)	≈ 39%	≈ 34%

[1] Following 1 hour IV infusion.
[2] Following single oral dose.
[3] Following multiple oral doses.

Contraindications

Hypersensitivity to stavudine or to any components of the formulation.

Warnings

Lactic acidosis/severe hepatomegaly with steatosis: Lactic acidosis and severe hepatomegaly with steatosis, including fatal cases, have been reported with the use of nucleoside analogs alone or in combination, including stavudine and other antiretrovirals. A majority of these cases have been in women. Obesity and prolonged nucleoside exposure may be risk factors. Fatal lactic acidosis has been reported in pregnant women who received the combination of stavudine and didanosine with other antiretroviral agents. The combination of stavudine and didanosine should be used with caution during pregnancy and is recommended only if the potential benefit clearly outweighs the potential risk. In addition, deaths attributed to hepatotoxicity have occurred in patients receiving the combination of stavudine, didanosine, and hydroxyurea. Exercise caution when administering stavudine to any patient with known risk factors for liver disease; however, cases also have been reported in patients with no known risk factors. Suspend treatment with stavudine in any patient who develops clinical or laboratory findings suggestive of lactic acidosis or pronounced hepatotoxicity (which may include hepatomegaly and steatosis even in the absence of marked transaminase elevations). An increased risk of hepatotoxicity, which may be fatal, may occur in patients treated with stavudine in combination with didanosine and hydroxyurea compared to when stavudine is used alone. Closely monitor patients treated with this combination for signs of liver toxicity.

Peripheral neuropathy: Stavudine therapy has been associated with peripheral neuropathy, which can be severe and is dose-related. Monitor patients for development of neuropathy, usually characterized by numbness, tingling, or pain in feet or hands. Stavudine-related peripheral neuropathy may resolve if therapy is withdrawn promptly. Symptoms may worsen temporarily following therapy discontinuation. If symptoms resolve completely, resumption of treatment may be considered at 50% of the dose (see Administration and Dosage). Patients with advanced HIV disease, a history of peripheral neuropathy, or concurrent neurotoxic drug therapy, including didanosine, are at increased risk for developing neuropathy. If stavudine must be given in this clinical setting, careful monitoring is essential. If neuropathy recurs after resumption of stavudine, consider permanent discontinuation.

Pancreatitis: Fatal and nonfatal pancreatitis have occurred during therapy when stavudine was part of a combination regimen that included didanosine, with or without hydroxyurea, in treatment-naive and treatment-experienced patients, regardless of degree of immunosuppression. The combination of stavudine and didanosine (with or without hydroxyurea) and any other agents that are toxic to the pancreas should be suspended in patients with suspected pancreatitis. Reinstitution of stavudine after a confirmed diagnosis of pancreatitis should be undertaken with particular caution and close patient monitoring. The new regimen should not contain either didanosine or hydroxyurea.

Elderly: Clinical studies of stavudine did not include sufficient numbers of patients ≥ 65 years of age to determine whether they respond differently than younger patients.

Closely monitor elderly patients for signs and symptoms of peripheral neuropathy.

Because elderly patients are more likely to have decreased renal function, it may be useful to monitor renal function.

Pregnancy: Category C.

To monitor maternal-fetal outcomes of pregnant women exposed to stavudine and other antiretroviral agents, an Antiretroviral Pregnancy Registry has been established. Physicians are encouraged to register patients by calling (800) 258-4263.

Fatal lactic acidosis has been reported in pregnant women who received the combination of stavudine and didanosine with other antiretroviral agents (see Warning Box).

Lactation: It is not known whether stavudine is excreted in human breast milk. Because of the potential for adverse reactions in nursing infants, instruct mothers to discontinue nursing if they are receiving stavudine. To avoid risking postnatal transmission of HIV infection, instruct HIV-infected mothers not to breastfeed their infants; this is consistent with the CDC's recommendation.

Children: Use of stavudine in pediatric patients is supported by evidence from adequate and well-controlled studies of stavudine in adults with additional pharmacokinetic and safety data in pediatric patients.

Drug Interactions

Zidovudine: Zidovudine may competitively inhibit the intracellular phosphorylation of stavudine. Therefore, use of zidovudine in combination with stavudine is not recommended.

Methadone: Coadministration produced a 25% decrease in AUC and a 44% decrease in peak drug concentration for stavudine. This may be secondary to decreased GI motility associated with methadone, resulting in decreased rate of absorption of stavudine.

Adverse Reactions

When stavudine is used in combination with other agents with similar toxicities, the incidence of adverse events may be higher than when stavudine is used alone. Pancreatitis, peripheral neuropathy, and liver function abnormalities occur more frequently in patients treated with the combination of stavudine and didanosine, with or without hydroxyurea. Fatal pancreatitis and hepatotoxicity may occur more frequently in patients treated with stavudine in combination with didanosine and hydroxyurea (see Warnings).

Adverse reactions occurring in ≥ 3% of patients include headache, diarrhea, neuropathy, rash, nausea, and vomiting. Lab abnormalities include elevations in bilirubin, AST, ALT, GGT, lipase, and amylase.

ZALCITABINE (Dideoxycytidine; ddC)

Tablets: 0.375 and 0.75 mg (*Rx*)   *Hivid* (Roche)

Warning:
The use of zalcitabine has been associated with significant clinical adverse reactions, some of which are potentially fatal. Zalcitabine can cause severe peripheral neuropathy; therefore, use with extreme caution in patients with pre-existing neuropathy. Zalcitabine may also rarely cause pancreatitis, and patients who develop any symptoms suggestive of pancreatitis while using zalcitabine should have therapy suspended immediately until this diagnosis is excluded.

Lactic acidosis and severe hepatomegaly with steatosis, including fatal cases, have been reported with the use of antiretroviral nucleoside analogs alone or in combination, including zalcitabine. In addition, rare cases of hepatic failure and death, considered possibly related to underlying hepatitis B and zalcitabine have been reported (see Warnings).

Indications

Combination therapy with antiretrovirals: For the treatment of human immunodeficiency virus (HIV) infection.

Administration and Dosage

Combination therapy with antiretrovirals: The recommended regimen is one 0.75 mg tablet of zalcitabine orally every 8 hours (2.25 mg zalcitabine total daily dose) in combination with other antiretroviral agents.

Renal function impairment: Dosage reduction is recommended: Ccr 10 to 40 mL/min, 0.75 mg every 12 hours; Ccr < 10 mL/min, 0.75 mg every 24 hours.

Dose adjustment:

Combination therapy – For toxicities likely to be associated with zalcitabine (eg, peripheral neuropathy, severe oral ulcers, pancreatitis, elevated liver function tests, especially in patients with chronic hepatitis B; see Warnings and Precautions), interrupt or reduce dose. For severe toxicities or those persisting after dose reduction, interrupt zalcitabine therapy. For recipients of combination therapy with zalcitabine and other antiretrovirals, base dose adjustments or interruption for either drug on the known toxicity profile of the individual drugs.

Peripheral neuropathy – Patients developing moderate discomfort with signs or symptoms of peripheral neuropathy should stop zalcitabine. Zalcitabine-associated peripheral neuropathy may continue to worsen despite interruption of therapy. Reintroduce the drug at 50% dose (0.375 mg every 8 hours) only if all findings related to peripheral neuropathy have improved to mild symptoms. Permanently discontinue the drug when patients experience severe discomfort related to peripheral neuropathy or moderate discomfort progresses. If other moderate to severe clinical adverse reactions or lab abnormalities (eg, increased liver function tests) occur, interrupt zalcitabine (or both zalcitabine and the other potential causative agent(s) in combination therapy) until the adverse reaction abates. Carefully reintroduce zalcitabine or the other agent at lower doses if appropriate. If adverse reactions recur, discontinue therapy. The minimum effective dose of zalcitabine in combination with zidovudine for the treatment of adults with advanced HIV infection has not been established.

Hematologic toxicities – Significant toxicities, such as anemia (hemoglobin < 7.5 g/dL or reduction of > 25% of baseline) or granulocytopenia (granulocyte count of < 750/mm^3 or reduction of > 50% from baseline), may require a treatment interruption of zalcitabine and zidovudine until evidence of marrow recovery is observed (see Warnings). For less severe anemia or granulocytopenia, a reduction in the daily dose of zidovudine in those patients receiving combination therapy may be adequate. In patients who develop significant anemia, dose modification does not necessarily eliminate the need for transfusion. If marrow recovery occurs following dose modification, gradual increases in dose may be appropriate, depending on hematologic indices and patient intolerance.

Actions

Pharmacology: Zalcitabine, active against HIV, is a synthetic pyrimidine nucleoside analog of the naturally occurring nucleoside deoxycytidine in which the 3′-hydroxyl group is replaced by hydrogen. Within cells, zalcitabine is converted to the active metabolite, dideoxycytidine 5′-triphosphate (ddCTP), by cellular enzymes. ddCTP inhibits the activity of the HIV-reverse transcriptase both by competing for utilization of the natural substrate, deoxycytidine 5′-triphosphate (dCTP), and by its incorporation into viral DNA.

Pharmacokinetics:

Adults –

Absorption/Distribution: Following oral administration to HIV-infected patients, the mean absolute bioavailability of zalcitabine was > 80%. The absorption rate of a 1.5 mg oral dose was reduced when administered with food. This resulted in a 39% decrease in mean maximum plasma concentrations (C_{max}) from 25.2 to 15.5 ng/mL, and a 2-fold increase in time to achieve C_{max} from a mean of 0.8 hours under fasting conditions to 1.6 hours when the drug was given with food. The extent of absorption was decreased by 14% (from 72 to 62 ng•hr/mL).

The steady-state volume of distribution following IV administration of a 1.5 mg dose averaged 0.534 L/kg. Cerebrospinal fluid obtained from 9 patients at 2 to 3.5 hours following 0.06 or 0.09 mg/kg IV infusion showed measurable concentrations of zalcitabine. The CSF:plasma concentration ratio ranged from 9% to 37% (mean, 20%), demonstrating drug penetration through the blood-brain barrier.

Metabolism/Excretion: Zalcitabine is phosphorylated intracellularly to zalcitabine triphosphate, the active substrate for HIV-reverse transcriptase. Concentrations of zalcitabine triphosphate are too low for quantitation. Metabolism has not been fully evaluated. Zalcitabine does not appear to undergo a significant degree of metabolism by the liver. Renal excretion appears to be the primary route of elimination, and accounted for ≈ 70% of an orally administered dose within 24 hours after dosing. The mean elimination half-life is 2 hours. Total body clearance following an IV dose averages 285 mL/min. Less than 10% of a dose appears in the feces.

Children – Limited pharmacokinetic data have been reported for 5 HIV-positive children using doses of 0.03 and 0.04 mg/kg administered orally every 6 hours. The mean bioavailability of zalcitabine in this study was 54% and mean apparent systemic clearance was 150 mL/min/m².

Contraindications

Hypersensitivity to zalcitabine or any components of the product.

Warnings

Significant clinical adverse reactions, some of which are potentially fatal, have been reported with zalcitabine. Patients with decreased CD₄ cell counts appear to have an increased incidence of adverse events.

Peripheral neuropathy: The major clinical toxicity is peripheral neuropathy (22% to 35%) of subjects.

In some patients, symptoms of neuropathy may initially progress despite discontinuation of zalcitabine. With prompt discontinuation, the neuropathy is usually slowly reversible.

Use with extreme caution in patients with pre-existing peripheral neuropathy. Avoid zalcitabine in individuals with moderate or severe peripheral neuropathy, as evidenced by symptoms accompanied by objective findings.

Zalcitabine should be used with caution in the following patients with a risk of developing peripheral neuropathy: Patients with low CD4 cell counts (CD4 < 50 cells/mm³), diabetes, weight loss, or patients receiving zalcitabine concomitantly with drugs that have the potential to cause peripheral neuropathy. Careful monitoring is strongly recommended for these individuals.

Stop zalcitabine promptly if signs or symptoms of peripheral neuropathy occurs, such as when moderate discomfort from numbness, tingling, burning, or pain of the extremities progresses, or any related symptoms occur that are accompanied by an objective finding (see Administration and Dosage).

Pancreatitis: Pancreatitis, fatal in some cases, has been observed with zalcitabine administration. Pancreatitis is an uncommon complication of zalcitabine therapy, occurring in up to 1.1% of patients.

Lactic acidosis/severe hepatomegaly with steatosis/hepatic toxicity: Lactic acidosis and severe hepatomegaly with steatosis, including fatal cases, have been reported with the use of nucleoside analogs alone or in combination, including zalcitabine and other antiretrovirals. A majority of these cases have been in women. Obesity and prolonged nucleoside exposure may be risk factors. Exercise particular caution when administering zalcitabine to any patient with known risk factors for liver disease; however, cases also have been reported in patients with no known risk factors. Suspend treatment with zalcitabine in any patient who develops clinical or laboratory findings suggestive of lactic acidosis or pronounced hepatotoxicity (which may include hepatomegaly and steatosis even in the absence of marked transaminase elevations).

Suspend treatment with zalcitabine in any patient who develops clinical or laboratory findings suggestive of pronounced hepatotoxicity. In clinical trials, drug interruption was recommended if liver function tests exceeded 5 times the upper limit of normal.

Hematologic toxicities: In patients with poor bone marrow reserve, particularly those patients with advanced symptomatic HIV disease, frequent monitoring of hematologic indices is recommended to detect serious anemia or granulocytopenia. In patients who experience hematologic toxicity, reduction in hemoglobin may occur as early as 2 to 4 weeks after initiation of therapy and granulocytopenia usually occurs after 6 to 8 weeks of therapy.

Oral ulcers: Severe oral ulcers occurred in ≈ 3% of patients in 2 trials. Less severe oral ulcerations occurred at higher frequencies in other clinical trials.

Esophageal ulcers: Infrequent cases of esophageal ulcers have been attributed to zalcitabine therapy. Consider interruption of therapy in patients who develop esophageal ulcers that do not respond to specific treatment for opportunistic pathogens in order to assess a possible relationship to zalcitabine.

Cardiomyopathy/CHF: Cardiomyopathy and CHF have occurred with the use of nucleoside antiretroviral agents in AIDS patients; infrequent cases have occurred in patients receiving zalcitabine. Approach treatment with caution in patients with baseline cardiomyopathy or history of CHF.

Anaphylactoid reaction: There has been 1 report of an anaphylactoid reaction occurring in a patient receiving zalcitabine and zidovudine. In addition, there have been several reports of urticaria without other signs of anaphylaxis.

Carcinogenesis: No increase in tumor incidence was observed in rats or male mice treated with zalcitabine.

Mutagenesis: Human peripheral blood lymphocytes were exposed to zalcitabine, and at ≥ 1.5 mcg/mL, dose-related increases in chromosomal aberrations were seen. Oral doses of zalcitabine at 2500 and 4500 mg/kg were clastogenic in the mouse micronucleus assay.

Elderly: Clinical studies of zalcitabine did not include sufficient numbers of subjects ≥ 65 years of age to determine whether they respond differently than younger subjects. In general, dose selection for an elderly patient should be cautious, reflecting the greater frequency of decreased hepatic, renal, or cardiac function, and of concomitant disease or other drug therapy.

Pregnancy: Category C.

Lactation: It is not known whether zalcitabine is excreted in breast milk. Decide whether to discontinue nursing or the drug, taking into account the importance of the drug to the mother. In the US, it currently is recommended that HIV-infected women do not breastfeed infants regardless of the use of antiretroviral agents.

Children: Safety and efficacy of zalcitabine in combination with zidovudine or as monotherapy in HIV-infected children < 13 years of age have not been established.

Precautions

Monitoring: Perform periodic complete blood counts and clinical chemistry tests. Monitor serum amylase levels in those individuals who have a history of elevated amylase, pancreatitis, ethanol abuse, who are on parenteral nutrition, or who are otherwise at high risk of pancreatitis.

Drug Interactions

Drugs that may interact with zalcitabine include antacids, chloramphenicol, cisplatin, dapsone, didanosine, disulfiram, ethionamide, glutethimide, gold, hydralazine, iodoquinol, isoniazid, metronidazole, nitrofurantoin, phenytoin, ribavirin, vincristine, cimetidine, metoclopramide, amphotericin, aminoglycosides, foscarnet, antiretroviral nucleoside analogs, pentamidine, and probenecid.

Drug/Food interactions: The absorption rate of a 1.5 mg dose is reduced when administered with food resulting in a 39% decrease in mean C_{max} and a 2-fold increase in time to achieve C_{max}. The extent of absorption is decreased by 14%.

Adverse Reactions

Adverse reactions occurring in ≥ 3% of patients include malaise/fatigue; abdominal pain; oral lesions/stomatitis; vomiting/nausea; peripheral neuropathy; elevated amylase; rash/pruritus/urticaria; diarrhea; oral ulcers; dysphagia; hypoglycemia; hyponatremia; bilirubin increased; loss of appetite; abnormal weight loss; abnormal hepatic function; hyperglycemia; myalgia; headache; nasal discharge; cough; pruritic disorder; fever; thrombocytopenia; neutropenia; leukopenia; eosinophilia; anemia.

ZIDOVUDINE (Azidothymidine; AZT; Compound S)

Capsules: 100 mg (*Rx*)
Syrup: 50 mg/5 mL (*Rx*)
Injection: 10 mg/mL (*Rx*)

Retrovir (GlaxoSmithKline)

Warning:
Zidovudine may be associated with hematologic toxicity including granulocytopenia and severe anemia particularly in patients with advanced human immunodeficiency (HIV) disease. Prolonged use of zidovudine has been associated with symptomatic myopathy similar to that produced by HIV.

Rare occurrences of lactic acidosis in the absence of hypoxemia, and severe hepatomegaly with steatosis have occurred with antiretroviral nucleoside analogs, including zidovudine and zalcitabine, and are potentially fatal.

Indications
Oral:
   Monotherapy –
     Adults: Initial treatment of HIV-infected adults with CD4 cell count ≤ 500/mm³. Monotherapy with zidovudine was found to be clinically superior to didanosine or zalcitabine monotherapy for the initial management of HIV-infected patients who have not received previous antiretroviral treatment. However, for some patients with advanced disease on prolonged zidovudine therapy, modifying the antiviral regimen may be more effective in delaying disease progression than remaining on zidovudine monotherapy.

     Children: For HIV-infected children > 3 months of age who have HIV-related symptoms or who are asymptomatic with abnormal laboratory values indicating significant HIV-related immunosuppression.

     Maternal-Fetal HIV transmission: Prevention of maternal-fetal HIV transmission as part of a regimen that includes oral zidovudine beginning between 14 and 34 weeks of gestation, IV zidovudine during labor, and zidovudine syrup to the newborn after birth. However, transmission to infants may still occur in some cases despite the use of this regimen.

     Combination therapy with zalcitabine – Treatment of selected patients with advanced HIV disease (CD4 cell count ≤ 300 cells/mm³). In patients without prior exposure to zidovudine, this indication is based on greater increases in CD4 cell counts that were maintained longer for patients treated with combination therapy vs monotherapy with zidovudine.

  IV: For the management of certain adult patients with symptomatic HIV infection (AIDS and advanced ARC) who have a history of cytologically confirmed *Pneumocystis carinii* pneumonia (PCP) or an absolute CD4 lymphocyte count of < 200/mm³ in the peripheral blood before therapy is begun.

Administration and Dosage
Oral:
   Monotherapy –
     Adults:
     Symptomatic HIV infection (including AIDS) – 100 mg (one 100 mg capsule or 2 teaspoonfuls [10 mL] syrup) every 4 hours (600 mg daily dose). The effectiveness of this dose compared with higher dosing regimens in improving neurologic dysfunction associated with HIV disease is unknown. A small study found a greater effect of higher doses on improvement of neurological symptoms in patients with pre-existing neurological disease.

     Asymptomatic HIV infection – 100 mg every 4 hours while awake (500 mg/day).

    Children (3 months to 12 years of age): The recommended starting dose is 180 mg/m² every 6 hours (720 mg/m²/day), not to exceed 200 mg every 6 hours.

Maternal-Fetal HIV transmission:

Maternal dosing (> 14 weeks of pregnancy) – 100 mg orally 5 times/day until the start of labor. During labor and delivery, administer IV zidovudine at 2 mg/kg over 1 hour followed by a continuous IV infusion of 1 mg/kg/hr until clamping of the umbilical cord.

Infant dosing – 2 mg/kg orally every 6 hours starting within 12 hours after birth and continuing through 6 weeks of age. Infants unable to receive oral dosing may be given zidovudine IV at 1.5 mg/kg, infused over 30 minutes, every 6 hours.

Combination therapy with zalcitabine – Zidovudine 200 mg orally with zalcitabine 0.75 mg every 8 hours.

Monitor – Monitor hematologic indices every 2 weeks to detect serious anemia or granulocytopenia. In patients with hematologic toxicity, reduction in hemoglobin may occur as early as 2 to 4 weeks, and granulocytopenia usually occurs after 6 to 8 weeks. Hematologic toxicities appear to be related to pretreatment bone marrow reserve and to dose and duration of therapy.

Dose adjustment – Significant anemia (hemoglobin of < 7.5 g/dL or reduction of > 25% of baseline) or significant granulocytopenia (granulocyte count of < 750/mm^3 or reduction of > 50% from baseline) may require a dose interruption until evidence of marrow recovery is observed. For less severe anemia or granulocytopenia, dose reduction may be adequate. In patients who develop significant anemia, dose modification does not necessarily eliminate the need for transfusion. If marrow recovery occurs following dose modification, gradual increases in dose may be appropriate depending on hematologic indices and patient tolerance.

Renal function impairment: In end-stage renal disease patients maintained on hemodialysis or peritoneal dialysis, recommended dosing is 100 mg every 6 to 8 hours.

IV: 1 to 2 mg/kg infused over 1 hour at a constant rate; administer every 4 hours around the clock (6 times daily). Avoid rapid infusion or bolus injection. Do not give IM. Patients should receive the IV infusion only until oral therapy can be administered. The IV dosing regimen equivalent to the oral administration of 100 mg every 4 hours is ≈ 1 mg/kg IV every 4 hours.

Actions

Pharmacology: Zidovudine is a thymidine analog and an inhibitor of the in vitro replication of some retroviruses, including HIV. Cellular thymidine kinase converts zidovudine into zidovudine monophosphate and finally to the triphosphate derivative by other cellular enzymes. Zidovudine triphosphate interferes with the HIV viral RNA-dependent DNA polymerase (reverse transcriptase) and inhibits viral replication. It also inhibits cellular α-DNA polymerase, but at concentrations 100-fold higher than those required to inhibit reverse transcriptase. In vitro, zidovudine triphosphate is incorporated into growing chains of DNA by viral reverse transcriptase, and the DNA chain is terminated.

Pharmacokinetics:

Absorption/Distribution – Overall, the pharmacokinetics in pediatric patients> 3 months of age are similar to that in adults. Zidovudine is rapidly absorbed from the GI tract with peak serum concentrations occurring within 0.5 to 1.5 hours. As a result of first-pass metabolism, the average oral capsule bioavailability is 65% (range, 52% to 75%). The rate of absorption of the syrup is greater than that of the capsules. Dose-dependent kinetics were observed over the range of 2 mg/kg every 8 hours to 10 mg/kg every 4 hours. Zidovudine plasma protein binding is 34% to 38%. Mean steady-state predose and 1.5 hours postdose concentrations were 0.16 mcg/mL (range, 0 to 0.84 mcg/mL) and 0.62 mcg/mL (range, 0.05 to 1.46 mcg/mL), respectively, following chronic oral use of 250 mg every 4 hours (n = 21; 3 to 5.4 mg/kg).

Metabolism/Excretion – Zidovudine is rapidly metabolized in the liver to an inactive metabolite which has an apparent elimination half-life of 1 hour (range, 0.61 to 1.73). The mean zidovudine half-life was ≈ 1 hour (range, 0.78 to 1.93). Urinary recovery of zidovudine and its metabolite was 14% and 74% of an oral dose, respectively, and the total urinary recovery averaged 90% (range, 63% to 95%).

Following IV dosing (1 to 5 mg/kg) total body clearance averaged 1900 mL/min/70 kg and the apparent volume of distribution was 1.6 L/kg. Renal clearance is ≈ 400 mL/min/70 kg, indicating glomerular filtration and active tubular secretion by the kidneys. The zidovudine CSF/plasma concentration ratios measured at 2 to 4 hours following IV dosing of 2.5 and 5 mg/kg were 0.2 and 0.64, respectively.

Contraindications
Life-threatening allergic reactions to any of the components of the product.

Warnings
Hematologic effects: Use with extreme caution in patients who have bone marrow compromise evidenced by granulocyte count < 1000/mm^3 or hemoglobin < 9.5 g/dL. Anemia and granulocytopenia are the most significant adverse events observed. Reversible pancytopenia has been reported.

Myopathy: Myopathy and myositis with pathological changes, similar to that produced by HIV disease, have been associated with prolonged use of zidovudine.

Lactic acidosis/severe hepatomegaly with steatosis: Rare occurrences of lactic acidosis in the absence of hypoxemia, and severe hepatomegaly with steatosis have been reported with the use of antiretroviral nucleoside analogs, including zidovudine and zalcitabine, and are potentially fatal.

Combination therapy: No benefit from combination therapy with zalcitabine has been observed in a study of patients with extensive prior exposure to zidovudine (median, 18 months) and CD4 cell counts < 150 cells/mm^3; combination therapy is therefore not recommended for these patients.

Hypersensitivity reactions: Sensitization reactions, including anaphylaxis in 1 patient, have occurred with zidovudine therapy. Patients experiencing a rash should undergo medical evaluation.

Renal/Hepatic function impairment: Zidovudine is eliminated from the body primarily by renal excretion following metabolism in the liver (glucuronidation). In patients with severely impaired renal function, dosage reduction is recommended. Although very little data are available, patients with severely impaired hepatic function may be at greater risk of toxicity.

Carcinogenesis: In cultured human lymphocytes, zidovudine caused dose-related structural chromosomal abnormalities at concentrations ≥ 3 mcg/mL.

Pregnancy: Category C.

Lactation: It is not known whether zidovudine is excreted in breast milk or whether zidovudine reduces the potential for transmission of HIV in breast milk. The US Public Health Centers for Disease Control and Prevention advises HIV-infected women not to breastfeed to avoid postnatal transmission of HIV to a child who may not yet be infected.

Children: A positive test for HIV-antibody in children < 15 months of age may represent passively acquired maternal antibodies, rather than an active antibody response to infection in the infant. Thus, the presence of HIV-antibody in a child < 15 months of age must be interpreted with caution, especially in the asymptomatic infant. Pursue confirmatory tests such as serum P_{24} antigen or viral culture in such children.

Drug Interactions
Drugs that may affect zidovudine include acetaminophen, bone marrow, suppressive/cytotoxic agents (eg, adriamycin, dapsone), fluconazole, ganciclovir, interferon alfa, interferon beta-1b, nucleoside analogs, probenecid, rifamycins, trimethoprim, and phenytoin.

Drugs that may be affected by zidovudine include acyclovir and phenytoin.

Drug/Food interactions: Administration of capsules with food decreased peak plasma concentrations by > 50%; however, bioavailability as determined by AUC may not be affected.

Adverse Reactions

The most frequent adverse events and abnormal laboratory values reported in the placebo controlled clinical trial of oral zidovudine were granulocytopenia and anemia. Several serious adverse reactions have been reported in clinical practice. Myopathy and myositis with pathological changes, similar to these produced by HIV disease, have been associated with prolonged use. Reports of hepatomegaly with steatosis, hepatitis, pancreatitis, lactic acidosis, sensitization reactions (including anaphylaxis in 1 patient), hyperbilirubinemia, vasculitis, and seizures have been rare. A single case of macular edema has been reported.

Adverse reactions occurring in ≥ 3% of patients include asthenia; diaphoresis; fever; headache; malaise; dizziness; insomnia; paresthesia; somnolence; anorexia; diarrhea; dyspepsia; GI pain; nausea; vomiting; dyspnea; myalgia; rash; taste perversion.

ABACAVIR SULFATE

Tablets: 300 mg (Rx)
Oral solution: 20 mg/mL (Rx)

Ziagen (GlaxoSmithKline)

> **Warning:**
> Fatal hypersensitivity reactions have been associated with abacavir sulfate therapy. Discontinue abacavir in patients developing signs or symptoms of hypersensitivity (eg, fever, rash, fatigue; GI symptoms such as nausea, vomiting, diarrhea, abdominal pain; respiratory symptoms such as pharyngitis, dyspnea, cough) as soon as a hypersensitivity reaction is suspected. To avoid a delay in diagnosis and minimize the risk of a life-threatening hypersensitivity reaction, permanently discontinue abacavir therapy if hypersensitivity cannot be ruled out, even when other diagnoses are possible (eg, acute onset respiratory diseases, gastroenteritis, reactions to other medications). Do not restart abacavir following a hypersensitivity reaction because more severe symptoms will recur within hours and may include life-threatening hypotension and death. Severe or fatal hypersensitivity reactions can occur within hours after reintroduction of abacavir in patients who have no identified history or unrecognized symptoms of hypersensitivity to abacavir therapy (see Warnings).
>
> Lactic acidosis and severe hepatomegaly with steatosis, including fatal cases, have been reported with the use of nucleoside analogs alone or in combination, including abacavir and other antiretrovirals (see Warnings).
>
> Abacavir in combination with other antiretroviral agents is indicated for the treatment of HIV-1 infection. This indication is based on analyses of surrogate markers in controlled studies of ≤ 24 weeks in duration. At present, there are no results from controlled trials evaluating long-term suppression of HIV RNA or disease progression with abacavir.

Indications

HIV infection: In combination with other antiretroviral agents for the treatment of HIV-1 infection.

Administration and Dosage

Dispense Medication Guide and Warning Card that provide information about recognition of hypersensitivity reactions with each new prescription and refill.

Always use abacavir in combination with other antiretroviral agents. Do not add abacavir as a single agent when antiretroviral regimens are changed because of loss of virologic response.

Abacavir may be taken with or without food.

Adults: The recommended dose is 300 mg twice daily in combination with other antiretroviral agents.

Adolescents and children (3 months to ≤ 16 years of age): 8 mg/kg twice daily (up to a maximum of 300 mg twice daily) in combination with other antiretroviral agents.

Actions

Pharmacology: Abacavir is a synthetic carbocyclic synthetic nucleoside analog with inhibitory activity against HIV. Intracellularly, abacavir is converted by cellular enzymes to the active metabolite carbovir triphosphate. Carbovir triphosphate is an analog of deoxyguanosine-5'-triphosphate (dGTP). Carbovir triphosphate inhibits the activity of HIV-1 reverse transcriptase both by competing with the natural substrate dGTP and by its incorporation into viral DNA. Abacavir has synergistic activity in combination with amprenavir, nevirapine, and zidovudine, and additive activity in combination with didanosine, lamivudine, stavudine, and zalcitabine in vitro.

Cross-resistance – In vitro, recombinant laboratory strains of HIV-1 (HXB2) containing multiple reverse transcriptase mutations conferring abacavir resistance exhibited cross-resistance to lamivudine, didanosine, and zalcitabine.

Cross-resistance between abacavir and HIV protease inhibitors is unlikely because of the different enzyme targets involved. Cross-resistance between abacavir and nonnucleoside reverse transcriptase inhibitors is unlikely because of different binding sites on reverse transcriptase.

Pharmacokinetics:

Absorption – Abacavir was rapidly and extensively absorbed after oral administration with bioavailability at 83%. Systemic exposure to abacavir was comparable after administration of oral solution and tablets. Therefore, these products may be used interchangeably.

Distribution – The apparent volume of distribution after IV administration of abacavir was 0.86 ± 0.15 L/kg, suggesting that abacavir distributes into extravascular space. Binding to human plasma proteins is ≈ 50% and was independent of concentration.

Metabolism – In single-dose studies, the observed elimination half-life was 1.54 ± 0.63 hr. Abacavir is not significantly metabolized by cytochrome P450 enzymes.

Excretion – Of the 99% of the total abacavir dose recovered, 1.2% was excreted in the urine as abacavir. Fecal elimination accounted for 16% of the dose.

Contraindications

Hypersensitivity to any of the components of the product (see Warnings and Warning Box).

Warnings

Lactic acidosis/severe hepatomegaly with steatosis: Lactic acidosis and severe hepatomegaly with steatosis, including fatal cases, have been reported with the use of nucleoside analogs alone or in combination, including abacavir and other antiretrovirals. A majority of these cases have been in women. Obesity and prolonged nucleoside exposure may be risk factors. Suspend treatment with abacavir in any patient who develops clinical or laboratory findings suggestive of lactic acidosis or pronounced hepatotoxicity (which may include hepatomegaly and steatosis even in the absence of marked transaminase elevations).

Hypersensitivity reactions: Fatal hypersensitivity reactions have been associated with abacavir therapy. Discontinue abacavir in patients developing signs or symptoms of hypersensitivity as soon as a hypersensitivity reaction is first suspected; seek medical attention immediately. Do not restart abacavir following a hypersensitivity reaction because more severe symptoms will recur within hours and may include life-threatening hypotension and death.

In ongoing clinical studies, ≈ 5% of adult and pediatric patients receiving abacavir developed a hypersensitivity reaction. This reaction is characterized by the appearance of symptoms indicating multi-organ/body system involvement. Symptoms usually appear within the first 6 weeks of treatment, although these reactions may occur at any time during therapy. Frequently observed signs and symptoms include fever, rash, fatigue, and GI symptoms such as nausea, vomiting, diarrhea, or abdominal pain. Other signs and symptoms include malaise, lethargy, myalgia, arthralgia, edema, myolysis, pharyngitis, cough, dyspnea, headache, and paresthesia. Some patients who experienced a hypersensitivity reaction were initially thought to have acute onset or worsening respiratory disease. Physical findings include lymphadenopathy, mucous membrane lesions (conjunctivitis and mouth ulcerations), and rash. The rash usually appears maculopapular or urticarial but may be variable in appearance. Hypersensitivity reactions have occurred without rash. Laboratory abnormalities include elevated liver function tests, increased creatine phosphokinase or creatinine, and lymphopenia. Anaphylaxis, liver failure, renal failure, hypotension, and death have occurred in association with hypersensitivity reactions. Symptoms worsen with continued therapy but often resolve upon discontinuation of therapy.

Risk factors that may predict the occurrence or severity of hypersensitivity to abacavir have not been identified.

Abacavir hypersensitivity reaction registry – To facilitate reporting of hypersensitivity reactions and collection of information on each case, an Abacavir Hypersensitivity Registry has been established. Physicians should register patients by calling (800) 270-0425.

Mutagenesis: Abacavir induced chromosomal aberrations in the presence and absence of metabolic activation in an in vitro cytogenetic study in human lymphocytes.

Pregnancy: Category C.

Antiretroviral pregnancy registry – To monitor maternal-fetal outcomes of pregnant women exposed to abacavir, an Antiretroviral Pregnancy Registry has been established. Physicians are encouraged to register patients by calling (800) 258-4263.

Lactation: The Centers for Disease Control and Prevention recommend that HIV-infected mothers not breastfeed their infants to avoid risking postnatal transmission of HIV infection.

Because of the potential for HIV transmission and any possible adverse effects of abacavir, instruct mothers not to breastfeed if they are receiving abacavir.

Children: Use of abacavir in pediatric patients 3 months to 13 years of age is safe and effective and is supported by pharmacokinetic studies and evidence from adequate and well-controlled studies of abacavir in adults and pediatric patients.

Precautions

Cross-resistance: In clinical trials, patients with prolonged prior nucleoside reverse transcriptase inhibitor (NRTI) exposure or who had HIV-1 isolates that contained multiple mutations conferring resistance to NRTIs, had limited response to abacavir. Consider the potential for cross-resistance between abacavir and other NRTIs when choosing new therapeutic regimens in therapy-experienced patients.

Drug Interactions

Ethanol: It decreases the elimination of abacavir causing an increase in overall exposure.

Adverse Reactions

Adults: Adverse effects occurring in ≥ 5% of adults include the following: Nausea; nausea and vomiting; diarrhea; loss of appetite/anorexia; insomnia and other sleep disorders.

Children: Adverse effects occurring in ≥ 5% of children include the following: Nausea and vomiting; fever; headache; diarrhea; rash; loss of appetite/anorexia.

Hypersensitivity: Fatal hypersensitivity reactions have been associated with abacavir therapy (see Warnings and Warning Box).

Lab test abnormalities: Mild elevations of blood glucose were more frequent in subjects receiving abacavir. In 1 study, triglyceride elevations (all grades) were more common in the abacavir patients (25%) than placebo (11%).

Miscellaneous: Other adverse events observed in the expanded access program were pancreatitis and increased GGT.

LAMIVUDINE/ZIDOVUDINE (3TC/ZDV, 3TC/AZT)

Tablets: 150 mg lamivudine/300 mg zidovudine (*Rx*)   *Combivir* (GlaxoSmithKline)

Consult the complete prescribing information for each agent, lamivudine and zidovudine, prior to administration of lamivudine/zidovudine combination tablets.

> **Warning:**
> Zidovudine may result in hematologic toxicity (eg, neutropenia, severe anemia) especially in patients with advanced human immunodeficiency virus (HIV). Prolonged use has been associated with symptomatic myopathy (see zidovudine Warnings section).
>
> Lactic acidosis and severe hepatomegaly with steatosis, including fatal cases, have been reported with use of nucleoside analogs alone or in combination.

Indications
HIV infection: In combination with other antiretrovirals for the treatment of HIV infection.

Administration and Dosage
Adults and children > 12 years of age : One lamivudine/zidovudine combination tablet (150 mg/300 mg) orally twice daily.

Actions
Pharmacology: Lamivudine/zidovudine combination tablets contain 2 synthetic nucleoside analog reverse transcriptase inhibitors with activity against human immunodeficiency virus (HIV). Lamivudine in combination with zidovudine has exhibited synergistic antiretroviral activity. Refer to lamivudine and zidovudine individual monographs.

Pharmacokinetics: One combination lamivudine/zidovudine (150 mg/300 mg) tablet is bioequivalent to a 150 mg lamivudine tablet plus a 300 mg zidovudine tablet.

Contraindications
Hypersensitivity to any of the components of this product.

Because this product is a fixed-dose combination doseform, avoid use in patients requiring dosage reduction.

Warnings
Fixed-dose combination: Lamivudine/zidovudine tablets are a fixed-dose combination doseform that does not allow for dose reduction. Avoid use in patients requiring lamivudine or zidovudine dosage reduction including children < 12 years of age, renally impaired patients with Ccr ≤ 50 mL/min, patients with low body weight (< 50 kg or 110 lbs), or those experiencing dose-limiting adverse effects.

Hematologic: Use lamivudine/zidovudine with caution in patients who have bone marrow compromise evidenced by granulocyte count < 1000 cells/mm^3 or hemoglobin < 9.5 g/dL.

Lactic acidosis/severe hepatomegaly with steatosis: Lactic acidosis and severe hepatomegaly with steatosis, including fatal cases, have been reported with the use of nucleoside analogs alone or in combination, including lamivudine, zidovudine, and other antiretrovirals. Suspend treatment with lamivudine/zidovudine in any patient who develops clinical or laboratory findings suggestive of lactic acidosis or pronounced hepatotoxicity (which may include hepatomegaly and steatosis even in the absence of marked transaminase elevations).

Precautions
Monitoring: Blood counts are recommended frequently for patients with advanced HIV disease and periodically for patients with asymptomatic or early HIV disease.

ABACAVIR SULFATE/LAMIVUDINE/ZIDOVUDINE

Tablets: 300 mg abacavir sulfate/150 mg lamivudine/300 mg zidovudine (*Rx*)   *Trizivir* (GlaxoSmithKline)

Warning:

This product contains 3 nucleoside analogs (abacavir sulfate, lamivudine, and zidovudine) and is intended only for patients whose regimen would otherwise include these 3 components.

Abacavir sulfate has been associated with fatal hypersensitivity reactions (see Warnings). Patients developing signs or symptoms of hypersensitivity (eg, fever; skin rash; fatigue; GI symptoms such as nausea, vomiting, diarrhea, or abdominal pain; respiratory symptoms such as pharyngitis, dyspnea, or cough) should discontinue abacavir/lamivudine/zidovudine as soon as a hypersensitivity reaction is suspected. To avoid a delay in diagnosis and minimize the risk of a life-threatening hypersensitivity reaction, permanently discontinue abacavir/lamivudine/zidovudine if hypersensitivity cannot be ruled out, even when other diagnoses are possible (eg, acute onset respiratory diseases, gastroenteritis, or reactions to other medications).

Abacavir should not be restarted following a hypersensitivity reaction to abacavir because more severe symptoms will recur within hours and may include life-threatening hypotension and death.

Severe or fatal hypersensitivity reactions can occur within hours after reintroduction of abacavir in patients who have no identified history or unrecognized symptoms of hypersensitivity to abacavir therapy (see Warnings and Adverse Reactions).

Zidovudine has been associated with hematologic toxicity including neutropenia and severe anemia, particularly in patients with advanced HIV disease (see Warnings). Prolonged use of zidovudine has been associated with symptomatic myopathy.

Lactic acidosis and severe hepatomegaly with steatosis, including fatal cases, have been reported with the use of nucleoside analogs alone or in combination, including abacavir, lamivudine, zidovudine, and other antiretrovirals (see Warnings).

Abacavir/lamivudine/zidovudine alone or in combination with other antiretroviral agents is indicated for the treatment of HIV-1 infection. The indication is based on analyses of surrogate markers in controlled studies with abacavir of up to 24 weeks in duration. At present, there are no results from controlled trials evaluating long-term suppression of HIV RNA or disease progression with abacavir.

There are limited data on the use of this triple-combination regimen in patients with higher viral load levels (> 100,000 copies/mL) at baseline.

Indications

HIV infection: For use alone or in combination with other antiretroviral agents for the treatment of HIV-1 infection.

Administration and Dosage

Dispense a Medication Guide and Warning Card that provide information about recognition of hypersensitivity reactions with each new prescription or refill. To facilitate reporting hypersensitivity reactions and collection of information on each case, an Abacavir Hypersensitivity Registry has been established. Physicians should register patients by calling 1-800-270-0425.

Adults and adolescents (≥ 40 kg): 1 tablet twice daily. Not recommended in adults or adolescents who weigh < 40 kg because it is a fixed-dose tablet.

Dose adjustment: Because it is a fixed-dose tablet, do not prescribe for patients requiring dosage adjustments such as those with Ccr ≤ 50 mL/min or those experiencing dose-limiting adverse events.

Actions

Pharmacology: The combination tablets contain the following 3 synthetic nucleoside analogs: Abacavir sulfate, lamivudine, and zidovudine. Abacavir is a carbocyclic synthetic nucleoside analog. Lamivudine and zidovudine are synthetic nucleoside analogs.

Cross-resistance – Cross-resistance among certain reverse transcriptase inhibitors has been recognized, including abacavir, lamivudine, and zidovudine.

Pharmacokinetics:

Metabolism – In humans, abacavir, lamivudine, and zidovudine are not significantly metabolized by cytochrome P450 enzymes.

Abacavir – Following oral administration, abacavir is rapidly absorbed and extensively distributed. Binding of abacavir to human plasma proteins is $\approx$ 50%. Total blood and plasma drug-related radioactivity concentrations are identical, demonstrating that abacavir readily distributes into erythrocytes. The primary routes of elimination of abacavir are metabolism by alcohol dehydrogenase to form the 5'-carboxylic acid and glucuronyl transferase to form the 5'-glucuronide.

Lamivudine – Following oral administration, lamivudine is rapidly absorbed and extensively distributed. Binding to plasma protein is low. Approximately 70% of an IV dose of lamivudine is recovered as unchanged drug in the urine. Metabolism of lamivudine is a minor route of elimination. In humans, the only known metabolite is the trans-sulfoxide metabolite ($\approx$ 5% of an oral dose after 12 hours).

Zidovudine – Following oral administration, zidovudine is rapidly absorbed and extensively distributed. Binding to plasma protein is low. Zidovudine is eliminated primarily by hepatic metabolism.

The pharmacokinetic properties of abacavir, lamivudine, and zidovudine in fasting patients are summarized below.

Pharmacokinetic Parameters[1] for Abacavir, Lamivudine, and Zidovudine in Adults						
Parameter	Abacavir		Lamivudine		Zidovudine	
Oral bioavailability (%)	86 ± 25	n = 6	86 ± 16	n = 12	64 ± 10	n = 5
Apparent volume of distribution (L/kg)	0.86 ± 0.15	n = 6	1.3 ± 0.4	n = 20	1.6 ± 0.6	n = 8
Systemic clearance (L/hr/kg)	0.80 ± 0.24	n = 6	0.33 ± 0.06	n = 20	1.6 ± 0.6	n = 6
Renal clearance (L/hr/kg)	0.007 ± 0.008	n = 6	0.22 ± 0.06	n = 20	0.34 ± 0.05	n = 9
Elimination half-life (hr)[2]	1.45 ± 0.32	n = 20	5 to 7		0.5 to 3	

[1] Data presented as mean ± standard deviation except where noted.
[2] Approximate range.

Contraindications

Abacavir sulfate has been associated with fatal hypersensitivity reactions. Abacavir should not be restarted following a hypersensitivity reaction to abacavir (see Warnings and Adverse Reactions).

Abacavir/lamivudine/zidovudine tablets are contraindicated in patients with previously demonstrated hypersensitivity to any of the components of the product (see Warnings).

Warnings

Lactic acidosis/severe hepatomegaly with steatosis: Lactic acidosis and severe hepatomegaly with steatosis, including fatal cases, have been reported with the use of nucleoside analogs alone or in combination, including abacavir, lamivudine, zidovudine, and other antiretrovirals. A majority of these cases have been in women. Obesity and prolonged nucleoside exposure may be risk factors. Exercise particular caution when administering abacavir/lamivudine/zidovudine to any patient with known risk factors for liver disease; however, cases have also been reported in patients with no known risk factors. Suspend treatment in any patient who develops clinical or laboratory findings suggestive of lactic acidosis or pronounced hepatotoxicity (which may include heptomegaly and steatosis even in the absence of marked transaminase elevations).

Hematologic effects: Because the combination contains zidovudine, use with caution in patients who have bone marrow compromise evidenced by granulocyte count < 1000 cells/mm^3 or hemoglobin < 9.5 g/dL.

Myopathy: Myopathy and myositis, with pathological changes similar to that produced by HIV disease, have been associated with prolonged use of zidovudine, and therefore may occur with therapy with abacavir/lamivudine/zidovudine.

Hypersensitivity reactions: Abacavir sulfate has been associated with fatal hypersensitivity reactions. Patients developing signs or symptoms of hypersensitivity (eg, fever; skin rash; fatigue; GI symptoms such as nausea, vomiting, diarrhea, or abdominal pain; and respiratory symptoms such as pharyngitis, dyspnea, or cough) should discontinue abacavir/lamivudine/zidovudine combination tablets as soon as a hypersensitivity reaction is first suspected, and should seek medical evaluation immediately. To avoid a delay in diagnosis and minimize the risk of a life-threatening hypersensitivity reaction, permanently discontinue the combination tablets if hypersensitivity cannot be ruled out, even when other diagnoses are possible (eg, acute onset respiratory diseases, gastroenteritis, or reactions to other medications). Abacavir should not be restarted following a hypersensitivity reaction because more severe symptoms will recur within hours and may include life-threatening hypotension and death.

Renal function impairment: Since the dosage of individual components cannot be altered, do not administer to patients with Ccr ≤ 50 mL/min.

Pregnancy: Category C.

Lactation: The Centers for Disease Control and Prevention recommend that HIV-infected mothers not breastfeed their infants to avoid risking postnatal transmission of HIV infection.

Zidovudine is excreted in breast milk; abacavir is secreted into the milk of lactating rats; there are no data on lamivudine.

Children: Abacavir/lamivudine/zidovudine combination tablets are not intended for use in pediatric patients. Do not administer to adolescents who weigh < 40 kg because it is a fixed-dose tablet that cannot be adjusted for this patient population.

Precautions

Cross-resistance:

Abacavir – The potential for cross-resistance between abacavir and other nucleoside reverse transcriptase inhibitors (NRTIs) should be considered when choosing new therapeutic regimens in therapy-experienced patients.

HIV-HBV co-infection:

Lamivudine – Some patients with HIV infection who have chronic liver disease due to hepatitis B virus infection experienced clinical or laboratory evidence of recurrent hepatitis upon discontinuation of lamivudine. Consequences may be more severe in patients with decompensated liver disease.

Drug Interactions

Ethanol may interact with abacavir. Trimethoprim/sulfamethoxazole may interact with lamivudine. Drugs that may affect zidovudine include the following: Acetaminophen, atovaquone, bone marrow suppressive/cytotoxic agents, clarithromycin, fluconazole, ganciclovir, interferon alfa, interferon beta-1b, lamivudine, methadone, nucleoside analogs, zidovudine, phenytoin, probenecid, rifamycins, trimethoprim, and valproic acid. Acyclovir may be affected by zidovudine.

Adverse Reactions

Adverse Reactions Associated with Individual Agents and Combination Therapy (%)[1]				
Adverse reaction	Abacavir	Zidovudine	Lamivudine[2]/ Zidovudine	Abacavir/ Lamivudine/ Zidovudine
CNS				
Headache	✓[3]	27	35	✓[3]
Paresthesias	✓[3]	-	-	✓[3]
Neuropathy	-	10	12	-
Insomnia and other sleep disorders	-	7	11	7
Dizziness	-	4	10	-
Depressive disorders	-	4	9	-
GI				
Nausea	✓[3]	29	33	47
Nausea and vomiting	✓[3]	12	13	16
Diarrhea	✓[3]	22	18	12
Loss of appetite/anorexia	-	7	10	11
Abdominal pain	✓[3]	11	9	✓[3]
Mouth ulcerations	✓[3]	-	-	✓[3]
Abdominal cramps	-	3	6	-
Dyspepsia	-	5	5	-
Hematologic/Lymphatic				
Lymphadenopathy	✓[3]	-	-	✓[3]
Neutropenia	-	5.4	7.2	-
Anemia (Hb < 8 g/dL)	-	1.8	2.9	-
Thrombocytopenia	-	1.3	0.4	-
Lymphopenia	✓[3]	-	-	✓[3]
Lab test abnormalities				
Liver function tests, increased	✓[3]	-	-	✓[3]
ALT (> 5 × ULN[4])	✓[3]	3.6	3.7	✓[3]
AST (> 5 × ULN[4])	✓[3]	1.8	1.7	✓[3]
CPK, increased	✓[3]	-	-	✓[3]
Creatinine, increased	✓[3]	-	-	✓[3]
Bilirubin (> 2.5 × ULN[4])	-	0.4	0.8	-
Amylase (> 2 × ULN[4])	-	1.5	4.2	-
Glucose	✓	-	-	-
Triglyceride	25	-	-	-
Musculoskeletal				
Myalgia	✓[3]	6	8	✓[3]
Myolysis	✓[3]	-	-	✓[3]
Arthralgia	✓[3]	5	5	✓[3]
Musculoskeletal pain	-	10	12	-
Respiratory				
Pharyngitis	✓[3]	-	-	✓[3]
Cough	✓[3]	13	18	✓[3]
Dyspnea	✓[3]	-	-	✓[3]
Nasal signs and symptoms	-	11	20	-
Miscellaneous				
Fever	✓[3]	-	-	✓[3]
Fever or chills	-	12	10	-
Fatigue	✓[3]	-	-	✓[3]
Malaise	✓[3]	-	-	✓[3]
Malaise and fatigue	-	23	27	-
Lethargy	✓[3]	-	-	✓[3]
Edema	✓[3]	-	-	✓[3]

Adverse Reactions Associated with Individual Agents and Combination Therapy (%)[1]				
Adverse reaction	Abacavir	Zidovudine	Lamivudine[2]/ Zidovudine	Abacavir/ Lamivudine/ Zidovudine
Renal failure	✓[3]	-	-	✓[3]
Liver failure	✓[3]	-	-	✓[3]
Hypotension	✓[3]	-	-	✓[3]
Conjunctivitis	✓[3]	-	-	✓[3]
Skin rash	✓[3]	6	9	✓[3]
Anaphylaxis	✓[3]	-	-	✓[3]
Death	✓[3]	-	-	✓[3]

[1] Data are pooled from separate studies and are not necessarily comparable; different dosing and combinations affect reporting.
[2] Reports of adverse reactions to lamivudine alone are not available; lamivudine is indicated only for the treatment of HIV when given in combination therapy.
[3] Symptom is associated with hypersensitivity reaction to abacavir; incidence not reported.
[4] ULN = Upper limit of normal.

Hypersensitivity: This product contains abacavir sulfate, which has been associated with fatal hypersensitivity reactions (see Warnings and Warning Box).

In clinical studies, ≈ 5% of adult and pediatric patients receiving abacavir developed a hypersensitivity reaction. This reaction is characterized by the appearance of symptoms indicating multi-organ/body system involvement. Symptoms usually appear within the first 6 weeks of treatment with abacavir, although these reactions may occur at any time during therapy. Some patients who experienced a hypersensitivity reaction were initially thought to have acute onset or worsening respiratory disease.

NEVIRAPINE

Tablets: 200 mg (*Rx*)
Oral suspension: 50 mg/5 mL (as nevirapine hemihydrate) (*Rx*)

Viramune (Roxane)

Warning:
The duration of benefit from antiretroviral therapy may be limited. Consider alteration of antiretroviral therapies if disease progression occurs while patients are receiving nevirapine.

Resistant HIV virus emerges rapidly and uniformly when nevirapine is administered as monotherapy. Therefore, always administer nevirapine in combination with ≥ 1 additional antiretroviral agent.

Nevirapine has been associated with severe rash (Stevens-Johnson syndrome, toxic epidermal necrolysis), which in some cases, has been life-threatening. When severe rash occurs, discontinue nevirapine.

Severe and life-threatening hepatotoxicity, including fatal hepatic necrosis, has occurred in patients treated with nevirapine (see Warnings).

Indications
HIV-1 infection: In combination with nucleoside analogs for the treatment of HIV-1 infected adults and pediatric patients ≥ 2 months of age who have experienced clinical and immunologic deterioration.

Administration and Dosage
Adults:

Initial therapy – 200 mg tablet daily for 14 days. May administer with or without food.

Maintenance – 200 mg tablet twice daily in combination with nucleoside analog antiretroviral agents. For concomitantly administered nucleoside therapy, the manufacturer's recommended dosage and monitoring should be followed.

Pediatric:
2 *months to 8 years of age* – 4 mg/kg once daily for 14 days followed by 7 mg/kg twice daily.

≥ 8 *years of age* – 4 mg/kg once daily for 14 days followed by 4 mg/kg twice daily. The total daily dose should not exceed 400 mg for any patient.

Suspension – Shake nevirapine suspension gently prior to administration. It is important to administer the entire measured dose of suspension by using an oral dosing syringe or dosing cup. If a dosing cup is used, thoroughly rinse with water and administer the rinse to the patient.

Missed doses: Patients who interrupt nevirapine dosing for > 7 days should restart the recommended dosing, using one 200 mg tablet daily (4 mg/kg/day in pediatric patients) for the first 14 days (lead-in), followed by one 200 mg tablet twice daily (4 or 7 mg/kg twice daily, according to age, for pediatric patients).

Actions
Pharmacology: Nevirapine is a nonnucleoside reverse transcriptase inhibitor (NNRTI) with activity against human immunodeficiency virus type 1 (HIV-1).

Nevirapine binds directly to reverse transcriptase (RT) and blocks the RNA-dependent and DNA-dependent DNA polymerase activities by causing a disruption of the enzyme's catalytic site. The activity of nevirapine does not compete with template or nucleoside triphosphates. HIV-2 RT and eukaryotic DNA polymerases are not inhibited by nevirapine.

Pharmacokinetics:
Absorption – Nevirapine is readily absorbed (> 90%) after oral administration. Peak plasma nevirapine concentrations of 2 mcg/mL (7.5 µM) were attained within 4 hours following a single 200 mg dose. Following multiple doses, nevirapine peak concentrations appear to increase linearly in the dose range of 200 to 400 mg/day. Steady-state trough nevirapine concentrations of 4.5 mcg/mL were attained at 400 mg/day. Nevirapine tablets and suspension have been shown to be comparably bioavailable and interchangeable at doses ≤ 200 mg.

Distribution – Nevirapine is highly lipophilic and is essentially nonionized at physiologic pH. Following IV administration to healthy adults, the volume of distribution of nevirapine was 1.21 L/kg, suggesting that nevirapine is widely distributed in humans.

Metabolism/Excretion – Nevirapine is extensively biotransformed via cytochrome P450 (oxidative) metabolism to several hydroxylated metabolites.

Nevirapine has been shown to be an inducer of hepatic cytochrome P450 metabolic enzymes. The pharmacokinetics of autoinduction are characterized by an ≈ 1.5- to 2-fold increase in the apparent oral clearance of nevirapine as treatment continues from a single dose to 2 to 4 weeks of dosing with 200 to 400 mg/day. Auto-induction also results in a corresponding decrease in the terminal phase half-life of nevirapine in plasma from ≈ 45 hours (single dose) to ≈ 25 to 30 hours following multiple dosing with 200 to 400 mg/day.

Contraindications
Hypersensitivity to any of the components contained in the product.

Warnings
Skin reactions: Severe and life-threatening skin reactions have occurred in patients treated with nevirapine including Stevens-Johnson syndrome (SJS) and toxic epidermal necrolysis. Discontinue nevirapine in patients developing a severe rash accompanied by constitutional symptoms such as fever, blistering, oral lesions, conjunctivitis, swelling muscle or joint aches, or general malaise. The majority of rashes associated with nevirapine occur within the first 6 weeks of initiation of therapy. Instruct patients not to increase the 200 mg/day (4 mg/kg/day in pediatric patients) dosage if any rash occurs during the 2-week lead-in dosing period until the rash resolves.

Rashes are usually mild to moderate, maculopapular, erythematous cutaneous eruptions with or without pruritus, located on the trunk, face, and extremities.

Renal/Hepatic function impairment: Use with caution in these patient populations.

Hepatotoxicity – Abnormal liver function tests have been reported with nevirapine, some in the first few weeks of therapy, including cases of fatal fulminant hepatitis. Interrupt administration in patients experiencing moderate or severe liver function test abnormalities until liver function tests return to baseline values. Discontinue treatment permanently if liver function abnormalities recur on readministration.

Pregnancy: Category C.

Lactation: Nevirapine readily crosses the placenta and is found in breast milk. Instruct patients receiving nevirapine to discontinue nursing, consistent with the recommendation by the US Public Health Service Centers for Disease Control and Prevention that HIV-infected mothers not breastfeed their infants to avoid risking postnatal transmission of HIV.

Children: Nevirapine apparent clearance adjusted for body weight was at least 2-fold greater in children < 8 years of age compared with adults.

Precautions

Monitoring: Perform clinical chemistry tests, which include liver function tests, prior to initiating nevirapine therapy and at appropriate intervals during therapy.

Drug Interactions

Drugs that may affect nevirapine include rifampin and rifabutin.

Nevirapine may affect protease inhibitors, ketoconazole, and oral contraceptives.

Adverse Reactions

The most frequent adverse events related to nevirapine therapy are rash, fever, nausea, headache, and abnormal liver function tests.

Lab test abnormalities: Decreased H_2, platelets, and neutrophils. Increase ALT, AST, GGT, and total bilirubin.

Pediatric patients – The most frequently reported adverse events related to nevirapine in pediatric patients were similar to those observed in adults, with the exception of granulocytopenia which was more commonly observed in children. The safety profile of nevirapine in neonates has not been established.

DELAVIRDINE MESYLATE

Tablets: 100 and 200 mg (*Rx*)   *Rescriptor* (Agouron)

> **Warning:**
> Delavirdine tablets are indicated for the treatment of HIV-1 infection in combination with appropriate antiretroviral agents when therapy is warranted. This indication is based on surrogate marker changes in clinical studies. Clinical benefit was not demonstrated for delavirdine based on survival or incidence of AIDS-defining clinical events in a completed trial comparing delavirdine plus didanosine with didanosine monotherapy.
>
> Resistant virus emerges rapidly when delavirdine is administered as monotherapy. Therefore, always administer delavirdine in combination with appropriate antiretroviral therapy.

Indications

Human immunodeficiency virus-1 (HIV-1): For the treatment of HIV-1 infection in combination with appropriate antiretroviral agents when therapy is warranted.

Administration and Dosage

The recommended dosage for delavirdine is 400 mg (four 100 mg or two 200 mg tablets) 3 times daily. Use delavirdine in combination with appropriate other antiretroviral therapy. Consult the complete prescribing information for other antiretroviral agents for information on dosage and administration.

The 100 mg delavirdine tablets may be dispersed in water prior to consumption. To prepare a dispersion, add four 100 mg tablets to ≥ 3 ounces of water, allow to stand for a few minutes, and then stir until a uniform dispersion occurs. Consume the dispersion promptly. Rinse the glass and swallow the rinse to ensure the entire dose is consumed. Take the 200 mg tablets intact because they are not readily dispersed in water.

Administer delavirdine with or without food. Patients with achlorhydria should take delavirdine with an acidic beverage (eg, orange or cranberry juice). However, the effect of an acidic beverage on the absorption of delavirdine in patients with achlorhydria has not been investigated.

Actions

Pharmacology: Delavirdine is a nonnucleoside reverse transcriptase inhibitor (NNRTI) of HIV-1. Delavirdine binds directly to reverse transcriptase (RT) and blocks RNA-dependent and DNA-dependent DNA polymerase activities.

Cross-resistance – Rapid emergence of HIV strains that are cross-resistant to certain NNRTIs has been observed in vitro. Delavirdine may confer cross-resistance to other non-nucleoside reverse transcriptase inhibitors when used alone or in combination. The potential for cross-resistance between delavirdine and protease inhibitors and between NNRTIs and nucleoside analog RT inhibitors is low.

Pharmacokinetics:

Absorption – Delavirdine is rapidly absorbed following oral administration with peak plasma concentrations occurring at ≈ 1 hour. The single-dose bioavailability of delavirdine tablets was increased by ≈ 20% when a slurry of drug was prepared by allowing the tablets to disintegrate in water before administration.

Distribution – Delavirdine is extensively bound (≈ 98%) to plasma proteins, primarily albumin. CSF concentrations of delavirdine averaged 0.4% of the corresponding plasma delavirdine concentrations.

Metabolism/Excretion – Delavirdine is extensively converted to several inactive metabolites. Delavirdine is primarily metabolized by cytochrome P450 3A (CYP3A), but in vitro data suggest that delavirdine may also be metabolized by CYP2D6. The apparent plasma half-life of delavirdine increases with dose; mean half-life following 400 mg 3 times daily is 5.8 hours (range, 2 to 11 hours).

Delavirdine reduces CYP3A activitiy and inhibits its own metabolism. In vitro studies have also shown that delavirdine reduces CYP2C9 and CYP2C19 activity. Inhibition of CYP3A by delavirdine is reversible within 1 week after discontinuation of the drug.

Gender – Following administration of delavirdine (400 mg every 8 hours), median delavirdine AUC was 31% higher in female patients than in male patients.

Contraindications

Hypersensitivity to any of the components of the formulation.

Warnings

Cytochrome P450 inhibition: Coadministration of delavirdine tablets with certain nonsedating antihistamines, sedative hypnotics, antiarrhythmics, calcium channel blockers, ergot alkaloid preparations, amphetamines, and cisapride may result in potentially serious or life-threatening adverse events caused by possible effects of delavirdine on the hepatic metabolism of certain drugs metabolized by CYP3A and CYP2C9.

Hepatic function impairment: Delavirdine is metabolized primarily by the liver. Therefore, exercise caution when administering to patients with impaired hepatic function.

Pregnancy: Category C.

Lactation: The US Public Health Services Centers for Disease Control and Prevention advises HIV-infected women not to breastfeed to avoid postnatal transmission of HIV to a child who may not yet be infected.

Children: Safety and efficacy of delavirdine in combination with other antiretroviral agents has not been established in HIV-1-infected individuals < 16 years of age.

Precautions

Monitor: Monitor hepatocellular enzymes (ALT/AST) frequently if delavirdine is prescribed with saquinavir.

Resistance/Cross-resistance: NNRTIs, when used alone or in combination, may confer cross-resistance to other NNRTIs.

Skin rash: Skin rash attributable to delavirdine has occurred in 18% of patients in combination regimens in clinical trials who received delavirdine 400 mg 3 times daily.

Drug Interactions

Drugs that may affect delavirdine include the following: Anticonvulsants, antacids, clarithromycin, didanosine, fluoxetine, histamine H_2 antagonists, ketoconazole, rifabutin, rifampin, and saquinavir.

Drugs that may be affected by delavirdine include the following: Clarithromycin, indinavir, amprenavir, benzodiazepines, cisapride, dihydropyridine calcium channel blockers, ergot derivatives, quinidine, sildenafil, warfarin, saquinavir, and didanosine.

Adverse Reactions

Adverse reactions occurring in ≥ 3% of patients include the following: Headache; fatigue; nausea; diarrhea; increased ALT and AST; rash; maculopapular rash; neutropenia; increased amylase; pruritus.

EFAVIRENZ

Capsules: 50, 100, and 200 mg (*Rx*) *Sustiva* (DuPont)

Indications

Human immunodeficiency virus (HIV) infection: In combination with other antiretroviral agents for the treatment of HIV-1 infection.

Administration and Dosage

Adults: The recommended dosage is 600 mg once daily in combination with a protease inhibitor or nucleoside analog reverse transcriptase inhibitors (NRTIs). It may be taken with or without food; however, a high-fat meal may increase the absorption of efavirenz and should be avoided.

In order to improve the tolerability of nervous system side effects, bedtime dosing is recommended during the first 2 to 4 weeks of therapy and in patients who continue to experience these symptoms.

Concomitant antiretroviral therapy: Efavirenz must be given in combination with other antiretroviral medications.

Children: The following table describes the recommended dose for pediatric patients ≥ 3 years of age and weighing between 10 and 40 kg (22 and 88 lbs). The recommended dosage for pediatric patients weighing > 40 kg (88 lbs) is 600 mg once daily.

Pediatric Dose of Efavirenz to be Administered Once Daily		
Body weight		Efavirenz dose (mg)
kg	lbs	
10 to < 15	22 to < 33	200
15 to < 20	33 to < 44	250
20 to < 25	44 to < 55	300
25 to < 32.5	55 to < 71.5	350
32.5 to < 40	71.5 to < 88	400
≥ 40	≥ 88	600

Actions

Pharmacology: Efavirenz is a nonnucleoside reverse transcriptase inhibitor (NNRTI) of HIV-1. Its activity is mediated predominantly by noncompetitive inhibition of HIV-1 reverse transcriptase (RT). It does not inhibit HIV-2 RT and human cellular DNA polymerases alpha, beta, gamma, and delta.

Pharmacokinetics:

Absorption – Time-to-peak plasma concentrations were ≈ 3 to 5 hours and steady-state plasma concentrations were reached in 6 to 10 days.

Distribution – Efavirenz is highly protein-bound (≈ 99.5% to 99.75%), predominantly to albumin. In HIV-1-infected patients (n = 9) who received efavirenz 200 to 600 mg once daily for ≥ 1 month, CSF concentrations ranged from 0.26% to 1.19% (mean 0.69%) of the corresponding plasma concentration.

Metabolism – Efavirenz is principally metabolized by the cytochrome P450 system to hydroxylated metabolites with subsequent glucuronidation of these hydroxylated metabolites. These metabolites are essentially inactive against HIV-1.

Efavirenz induces P450 enzymes, resulting in the induction of its own metabolism.

Excretion – Efavirenz has a terminal half-life of 52 to 76 hours after single doses and 40 to 55 hours after multiple doses. Approximately 14% to 34% of a radiolabeled dose was recovered in the urine and 16% to 61% was recovered in the feces. Nearly all of the urinary excretion of the radiolabeled drug was in the form of metabolites. Efavirenz accounted for the majority of the total radioactivity measured in feces.

Contraindications

Do not administer concurrently with cisapride, midazolam, triazolam, or ergot derivatives. Competition for CYP3A4 by efavirenz could result in inhibition of metabolism of these drugs and create the potential for serious or life-threatening adverse events (eg, cardiac arrhythmias, prolonged sedation, respiratory depression; see Drug Interactions).

Clinically significant hypersensitivity to any components of the product.

Warnings

Monotherapy: Resistant virus emerges rapidly when NNRTIs are administered as monotherapy. Always initiate therapy in combination with ≥ 1 other new antiretroviral agent to which the patient has not been previously exposed.

Psychiatric symptoms: Serious psychiatric adverse experiences have been reported in patients treated with efavirenz. Patients with a prior history of psychiatric disorders appear to be at greater risk for serious psychiatric adverse experiences.

CNS symptoms: Patients should be informed that common symptoms were likely to improve with continued therapy and were not predictive of subsequent onset of the less frequent psychiatric symptoms. Dosing at bedtime improves the tolerability of these nervous system symptoms and is recommended during the first weeks of therapy and for patients who continue to experience these symptoms (see Adverse Reactions).

Alert patients to the potential for additive CNS effects when efavirenz is used concomitantly with alcohol or psychoactive drugs.

Pregnancy: Category C.

Antiretroviral Pregnancy Registry – To monitor fetal outcomes of pregnant women exposed to efavirenz, an Antiretroviral Pregnancy Registry has been established. Physicians are encouraged to register patients by calling (800) 258-4263.

Lactation: The Centers for Disease Control and Prevention recommend that HIV-infected mothers not breastfeed their infants to avoid risking postnatal transmission of HIV infection. Instruct mothers not to breastfeed during treatment.

Children: Efavirenz has not been studied in pediatric patients < 3 years of age or who weigh < 13 kg (29 lbs). The combination of efavirenz and nelfinavir caused the same type and frequency of adverse experiences as those of adult patients with the exception of a higher incidence of rash, which was reported in 40% of pediatric patients compared with 28% of adults. A higher frequency of Grade 3 or 4 rash was reported in 7% of pediatric patients, compared with 0.9% of adults.

Precautions

Skin rash: In controlled clinical trials, 27% of patients treated with 600 mg efavirenz experienced new onset skin rash compared with 17% of patients treated in control groups. The median time to onset of rash in adults was 11 days and the median duration, 14 days. Rash was reported in 40% of pediatric patients treated with efavirenz with the median time to onset of 8 days.

Hepatic enzymes: Monitor liver enzymes in patients with known or suspected history of hepatitis B or C infection and in patients treated with other medications associated with liver toxicity. In patients with persistent elevations of serum transaminases to > 5 times the upper limit of the normal range, the benefit of continued therapy needs to be weighed against the unknown risks of significant liver toxicity. Because of the extensive cytochrome P450-mediated metabolism of efavirenz and limited clinical experience in patients with hepatic impairment, exercise caution in administering efavirenz to these patients.

Cholesterol: Consider monitoring of cholesterol in patients treated with efavirenz.

Drug Interactions

P450 system: Efavirenz induces CYP3A4 in vitro. Other compounds that are substrates of CYP3A4 may have decreased plasma concentrations when coadministered with efavirenz. Drugs that induce CYP3A4 activity (eg, phenobarbital, rifampin, rifabutin) would be expected to increase the clearance of efavirenz, resulting in lowered plasma concentrations.

In vitro, efavirenz inhibits 2C9, 2C19, and 3A4 isozymes in the range of observed efavirenz plasma levels. Coadministration with drugs primarily metabolized by these isozymes may result in altered plasma concentrations of the coadministered drug. Therefore, appropriate dose adjustments may be necessary for these drugs.

Drugs that may affect efavirenz include rifampin, rifabutin, and ritonavir. Drugs that may be affected by efavirenz include ritonavir, amprenavir, benzodiazepines, clarithromycin, ethinyl estradiol, indinavir, nelfinavir, saquinavir, and warfarin.

Drug/Lab test interactions:

Cannabinoid test interaction – False-positive urine cannabinoid test results have been reported in uninfected volunteers who received efavirenz. False-positive test results have only been observed in assay tests used for screening, and have not been observed with tests used for confirmation of positive results. Efavirenz does not bind to cannabinoid receptors.

Drug/Food interactions: The relative bioavailability of a single 1200 mg dose in uninfected volunteers (n = 5) was increased 50% (range, 11% to 126%) following a high-fat meal.

Adverse Reactions

The most significant adverse events with efavirenz are nervous system symptoms and rash. Of patients receiving efavirenz, 52% reported CNS and psychiatric symptoms.

Adverse events occurring in ≥ 3% of patients include dizziness, fatigue, headache, concentration impaired, insomnia, abnormal dreams, somnolence, depression, anxiety, pruritus, nervousness, rash, nausea, vomiting, diarrhea, dyspepsia, abdominal pain.

Skin rash – Rashes are usually mild to moderate maculopapular skin eruptions that occur within the first 2 weeks of initiating therapy. Rash is more common in children and more often of higher grade (ie, more severe). In most patients, rash resolves with continuing therapy within 1 month. Efavirenz can be reinitiated in patients interrupting therapy because of rash. Use of appropriate antihistamines or corticosteroids is recommended when it is restarted. Discontinue in patients developing severe rash associated with blistering, desquamation, mucosal involvement, or fever.

Lab test abnormalities:

Hepatic enzymes – Patients treated with 600 mg of efavirenz had similar elevations in AST and ALT as patients in the control regimen.

Monitor liver function tests in patients with a history of hepatitis B or C.

Lipids – Increases in total cholesterol of 10% to 20% have been observed in some uninfected volunteers receiving efavirenz. Modest elevations of serum triglycerides and cholesterol have also been observed in nonfasting patients receiving efavirenz; however, the significance of these findings is unknown. The effect of efavirenz on total, LDL, and HDL cholesterol in patients receiving therapy has not been well characterized.

Serum amylase – Asymptomatic elevations in serum amylase greater than 1.5 times the upper limit of normal were seen in 10% of patients treated with efavirenz and in 6% of patients treated with control regimens. The clinical significance of asymptomatic increases in serum amylase is unknown.

TRIMETHOPRIM AND SULFAMETHOXAZOLE (Co-Trimoxazole; TMP-SMZ)

Tablets: 80 mg trimethoprim and 400 mg sulfamethoxazole (*Rx*)	Various, *Bactrim* (Roche), *Septra* (GlaxoSmithKline)
Tablets, double strength: 160 mg trimethoprim and 800 mg sulfamethoxazole (*Rx*)	Various, *Bactrim DS* (Roche), *Septra DS* (GlaxoSmithKline)
Oral suspension: 40 mg trimethoprim and 200 mg sulfamethoxazole/5 mL (*Rx*)	Various, *Bactrim Pediatric* (Roche), *Septra* (GlaxoSmithKline)
Injection: 80 mg trimethoprim and 400 mg sulfamethoxazol/5 mL (*Rx*)	Various, *Bactrim IV* (Roche), *Septra IV* (GlaxoSmithKline)

Indications

Oral and parenteral:

Urinary tract infections (UTIs) – Urinary tract infections (UTIs) caused by susceptible strains of *Escherichia coli*, *Klebsiella* and *Enterobacter* sp., *Morganella morganii*, *Proteus mirabilis*, and *Proteus vulgaris*.

Shigellosis – Shigellosis enteritis caused by susceptible strains of *Shigella flexneri* and *Shigella sonnei* in children and adults.

Pneumocystis carinii pneumonia (PCP) – Treatment in children and adults.

Oral:

Pneumocystis carinii pneumonia – Prophylaxis in individuals who are immunosuppressed and considered to be at increased risk.

Acute otitis media in children – Acute otitis media in children due to susceptible strains of *Haemophilus influenzae* or *Streptococcus pneumoniae*. There are limited data on the safety of repeated use in children < 2 years of age. Not indicated for prophylactic use or prolonged administration.

Acute exacerbations of chronic bronchitis in adults – Acute exacerbations of chronic bronchitis in adults caused by susceptible strains of *H. influenzae* and *S. pneumoniae*.

Travelers' diarrhea in adults – Travelers' diarrhea in adults caused by susceptible strains of enterotoxigenic *E. coli*.

Unlabeled uses: TMP 40 mg and SMZ 200 mg daily at bedtime, a minimum of 3 times weekly or postcoitally has been used to prevent recurrent UTIs in females.

Treatment of acute and chronic prostatitis – 160 mg TMP/800 mg SMZ twice daily has been used for chronic bacterial prostatitis for up to 12 weeks.

Administration and Dosage

Administration and Dosage of TMP-SMZ	
Organisms/Infections	Dosage
Urinary tract infections, shigellosis and acute otitis media:	
Adults:	160 mg TMP/800 mg SMZ every 12 hours for 10 to 14 days (5 days for shigellosis).
Children (≥ 2 months of age):	8 mg/kg TMP/40 mg/kg SMZ per day given in 2 divided doses every 12 hours for 10 days (5 days for shigellosis).

Guideline for proper dosage:		Dose every 12 hours:	
Weight (kg)	Teaspoonfuls		Tablets
10	1 (5 mL)		-
20	2 (10 mL)		1
30	3 (15 mL)		1½
40	4 (20 mL)		2 (or 1 double strength tablet)

Patients with impaired renal function Ccr (mL/min):	Recommended dosage regimen:
> 30	Usual regimen
15 to 30	½ usual regimen
< 15	Not recommended
IV: Adults and children > 2 months with normal renal function for severe UTIs and shigellosis.	8 to 10 mg/kg/day (based on TMP) in 2 to 4 divided doses every 6, 8 or 12 hours for up to 14 days for severe UTIs and 5 days for shigellosis.

Administration and Dosage of TMP-SMZ	
Organisms/Infections	Dosage
Travelers' diarrhea in adults:	160 mg TMP/800 mg SMZ every 12 hrs for 5 days.
Acute exacerbations of chronic bronchitis in adults:	160 mg TMP/800 mg SMZ every 12 hrs for 14 days.
Pneumocystis carinii pneumonia:	
Treatment:	15 to 20 mg/kg TMP/100 mg/kg SMZ per day in divided doses every 6 hours for 14 to 21 days.

Guideline for proper dosage in children — Dose every 6 hours:

Weight (kg)	Teaspoonfuls	Tablets
8	1 (5 mL)	-
16	2 (10 mL)	1
24	3 (15 mL)	1½
32	4 (20 mL)	2 (or 1 double strength tablet)

IV for adults and children > 2 months:	15 to 20 mg/kg/day (based on TMP) in 3 or 4 divided doses every 6 to 8 hours for up to 14 days.
Prophylaxis:	
Adults:	160 mg TMP/800 mg SMZ given orally every 24 hours.
Children:	150 mg/m^2 TMP/ 750 mg/m^2 SMZ per day given orally in equally divided doses twice a day, on 3 consecutive days per week. The total daily dose should not exceed 320 mg TMP/1600 mg SMZ.

Guideline for proper dosage in children — Dose every 12 hours:

Body surface area (m^2)	Teaspoonfuls	Tablets
0.26	½ (2.5 mL)	-
0.53	1 (5 mL)	½
1.06	2 (10 mL)	1

Parenteral:
   IV – Administer over 60 to 90 minutes. Avoid rapid infusion or bolus injection. Do not give IM.

Actions
   Pharmacology: SMZ inhibits bacterial synthesis of dihydrofolic acid by competing with para-aminobenzoic acid. TMP blocks the production of tetrahydrofolic acid by inhibiting the enzyme dihydrofolate reductase.

   Pharmacokinetics:
      Absorption/Distribution – TMP-SMZ is rapidly and completely absorbed following oral administration. Approximately 44% of TMP and 70% of SMZ are protein bound. Following oral administration, the half-lives of TMP (8 to 11 hours) and SMZ (10 to 12 hours) are similar. Following IV administration, the mean plasma half-life was 11.3 hours for TMP and 12.8 hours for SMZ.
      Metabolism/Excretion – TMP is metabolized to a small extent; SMZ undergoes bio-transformation to inactive compounds.
         Urine concentrations are considerably higher than serum concentrations.

Contraindications
   Hypersensitivity to TMP or SMZ; megaloblastic anemia caused by folate deficiency; pregnancy at term and lactation; infants < 2 months of age.

   The sulfonamides are chemically similar to some goitrogens, diuretics (acetazolamide and the thiazides) and oral hypoglycemic agents. Goiter production, diuresis, and hypoglycemia occur rarely in patients receiving sulfonamides. Cross-sensitivity may exist with these agents.

Warnings
   Streptococcal pharyngitis: Do not use to treat streptococcal pharyngitis.

Hematologic effects: Sulfonamide-associated deaths, although rare, have occurred from hypersensitivity of the respiratory tract, Stevens-Johnson syndrome, toxic epidermal necrolysis, fulminant hepatic necrosis, agranulocytosis, aplastic anemia, and other blood dyscrasias.

IV use at high doses or for extended periods of time may cause bone marrow depression manifested as thrombocytopenia, leukopenia, or megaloblastic anemia.

PCP in patients with Acquired Immunodeficiency Syndrome (AIDS): AIDS patients may not tolerate or respond to TMP-SMZ.

Renal/Hepatic function impairment: Use with caution. Maintain adequate fluid intake to prevent crystalluria and stone formation. Patients with severely impaired renal function exhibit an increase in the half-lives of both TMP and SMZ, requiring dosage regimen adjustment.

Elderly: There may be an increased risk of severe adverse reactions, particularly when complicating conditions exist.

Pregnancy: Category C.

Lactation: TMP-SMZ is not recommended in the nursing period because sulfonamides are excreted in breast milk and may cause kernicterus. Premature infants and infants with hyperbilirubinemia or G-6-PD deficiency are also at risk for adverse effects.

Children: Not recommended for infants < 2 months of age. See Indications.

Precautions

Extravascular infiltration: If local irritation and inflammation caused by extravascular infiltration of the infusion occurs, discontinue the infusion and restart at another site.

Benzyl alcohol: Benzyl alcohol, contained in some of these products as a preservative, has been associated with a fatal "gasping syndrome" in premature infants.

Special risk: Use with caution in patients with possible folate deficiency, severe allergy or bronchial asthma. In G-6-PD deficient individuals, hemolysis may occur; it is frequently dose-related.

Drug Interactions

Drugs that may be affected by TMP-SMZ include anticoagulants, cyclosporine, dapsone, diuretics, hydantoins, methotrexate, sulfonylureas, and zidovudine. Drugs that may affect TMP-SMZ include dapsone.

Adverse Reactions

Adverse reactions may include GI disturbances; allergic skin reactions; agranulocytosis; aplastic, hemolytic or megaloblastic anemia; thrombocytopenia; leukopenia; neutropenia; hypoprothrombinemia; eosinophilia; methemoglobinemia; hyperkalemia; hyponatremia; erythema multiforme; Stevens-Johnson syndrome; generalized skin eruptions; rash; toxic epidermal necrolysis; urticaria; pruritus; exfoliative dermatitis; anaphylactoid reactions; photosensitization; allergic myocarditis; angioedema; drug fever; chills; systemic lupus erythematosus; generalized allergic reactions; glossitis; anorexia; stomatitis; pancreatitis; elevation of serum transaminase and bilirubin; headache; mental depression; convulsions; ataxia; hallucinations; tinnitus; vertigo; insomnia; apathy; fatigue; weakness; nervousness; peripheral neuritis; renal failure; interstitial nephritis; BUN and serum creatinine elevation; toxic nephrosis with oliguria and anuria; crystalluria; arthralgia; myalgia.

ERYTHROMYCIN ETHYLSUCCINATE AND SULFISOXAZOLE

Granules for oral suspension: Erythromycin ethylsuccinate (equivalent to 200 mg erythromycin activity) and sulfisoxazole acetyl (equivalent to 600 mg sulfisoxazole)/5 mL when reconstituted (*Rx*)

Various, *Eryzole* (Alra), *Pediazole* (Ross)

Indications
Children: Acute otitis media caused by susceptible strains of *Haemophilus influenzae*.

Administration and Dosage
Do not administer to infants < 2 months of age; systemic sulfonamides are contraindicated in this age group.

Acute otitis media: 50 mg/kg/day erythromycin and 150 mg/kg/day (to a maximum of 6 g/day) sulfisoxazole. Give in equally divided doses 4 times daily for 10 days. Administer without regard to meals.

Erythromycin/Sulfisoxazole Dosage Based on Weight		
Weight		
kg	lb	Dose (every 6 hours)
< 8	< 18	Adjust dosage by body weight
8	18	2.5 mL
16	35	5 mL
24	53	7.5 mL
> 45	> 100	10 mL

PENTAMIDINE ISETHIONATE

Injection: 300 mg (*Rx*)
Powder for injection, lyophilized: 300 mg (*Rx*)
Aerosol: 300 mg (*Rx*)

Pentam 300 (Lyphomed), *Pentacarinat* (Armour)
Pentamidine Isethionate (Abbott)
NebuPent (Lyphomed)

Indications
Injection: Treatment of *Pneumocystis carinii* pneumonia (PCP).

Inhalation: Prevention of PCP in high-risk, HIV-infected patients defined by one or both of the following criteria: History of ≥ 1 episodes of PCP; a peripheral CD4+ (T4 helper/inducer) lymphocyte count ≤ 200 mm^3.

Administration and Dosage
Injection:
Adults and children – 4 mg/kg once a day for 14 days administered deep IM or IV only. The benefits and risks of therapy for > 14 days are not well defined. Dosage in renal failure should be patient-specific. If necessary, reduce dosage, use a longer infusion time or extend the dosing interval.

Preparation of solution:
IM – Dissolve the contents of 1 vial in 3 mL of Sterile Water for Injection.
IV – Dissolve the contents of 1 vial in 3 to 5 mL of Sterile Water for Injection or 5% Dextrose Injection. Further dilute the calculated dose in 50 to 250 mL of 5% Dextrose Injection.
Infuse the diluted IV solution over 60 minutes.

Aerosol:
Prevention of PCP – 300 mg once every 4 weeks administered via the *Respirgard II* nebulizer by Marquest.
Deliver the dose until the nebulizer chamber is empty (≈ 30 to 45 minutes). The flow rate should be 5 to 7 L/min from a 40 to 50 lbs/in^2 (PSI) air or oxygen source. Alternatively, a 40 to 50 PSI air compressor can be used with flow limited by setting the flowmeter at 5 to 7 L/min or by setting the pressure at 22 to 25 PSI. Do not use low pressure (< 20 PSI) compressors.
Reconstitution – The contents of 1 vial must be dissolved in 6 mL Sterile Water for Injection, USP. It is important to use *only* sterile water; saline solution will cause the drug to precipitate. Place the entire reconstituted contents of the vial into the

Respirgard II nebulizer reservoir for administration. Do not mix the pentamidine solution with any other drugs.

Actions

Pharmacology: Pentamidine isethionate, an aromatic diamidine antiprotozoal agent, has activity against *P. carinii*. In vitro studies indicate that the drug interferes with nuclear metabolism and inhibits the synthesis of DNA, RNA, phospholipids, and protein synthesis.

Pharmacokinetics:

Absorption/Distribution – Pentamidine is well absorbed after IM administration.

Metabolism/Excretion – Pentamidine may accumulate in renal failure.

Plasma concentrations after aerosol administration are substantially lower than those observed after a comparable IV dose. The extent of pentamidine accumulation and distribution following chronic inhalation therapy are not known.

Contraindications

Injection: Once the diagnosis of PCP has been established, there are no absolute contraindications to the use of pentamidine.

Inhalation: Patients with a history of an anaphylactic reaction to inhaled or parenteral pentamidine isethionate.

Warnings

Development of acute PCP: Development of acute PCP still exists in patients receiving pentamidine prophylaxis. The use of pentamidine may alter the clinical and radiographic features of PCP and could result in an atypical presentation, including but not limited to mild diseases or focal infection.

Prior to initiating pentamidine prophylaxis, evaluate symptomatic patients to exclude the presence of PCP. The recommended dose for the prevention of PCP is insufficient to treat acute PCP.

Fatalities: Fatalities caused by severe hypotension, hypoglycemia, and cardiac arrhythmias have been reported, both by the IM and IV routes. Severe hypotension may result after a single dose. Limit administration of the drug to patients in whom *P. carinii* has been demonstrated.

Pregnancy: Category C.

Lactation: It is not known whether pentamidine is excreted in breast milk. Because of the potential for serious adverse reactions in nursing infants, decide whether to discontinue nursing or to discontinue the drug, taking into account the importance of the drug to the mother.

Children: Safety and efficacy of inhalation solution have not been established.

Precautions

Use with caution: Use with caution in patients with hypertension, hypotension, hypoglycemia, hyperglycemia, hypocalcemia, leukopenia, thrombocytopenia, anemia, hepatic or renal dysfunction, ventricular tachycardia, pancreatitis, and Stevens-Johnson syndrome.

Hypotension: Patients may develop sudden, severe hypotension after a single dose, whether given IV or IM. Therefore, patients receiving the drug should be supine; monitor blood pressure closely during drug administration and several times thereafter until the blood pressure is stable. Have equipment for emergency resuscitation readily available. If pentamidine is administered IV, infuse over 60 minutes.

Hypoglycemia: Pentamidine-induced hypoglycemia has been associated with pancreatic islet cell necrosis and inappropriately high plasma insulin concentrations. Hyperglycemia and diabetes mellitus, with or without preceding hypoglycemia, also have occurred, sometimes several months after therapy. Therefore, monitor blood glucose levels daily during therapy and several times thereafter.

Pulmonary: Inhalation of pentamidine isethionate may induce bronchospasm or cough, particularly in patients who have a history of smoking or asthma. In patients who experience bronchospasm or cough, administration of an inhaled bronchodilator prior to giving each pentamidine dose may minimize recurrence of the symptoms.

Extrapulmonary infection with *P. carinii* has been reported infrequently with inhalation use.

Laboratory tests – Laboratory tests to perform before, during, and after therapy:

1.) Daily BUN, serum creatinine and blood glucose.
2.) Complete blood count and platelet counts.
3.) Liver function test, including bilirubin, alkaline phosphatase, AST, and ALT.
4.) Serum calcium.
5.) ECG at regular intervals.

Adverse Reactions

Injection – 244 of 424 (57.5%) patients treated with pentamidine injection developed some adverse reaction. Most of the patients had acquired immunodeficiency syndrome (AIDS). In the following, "severe" refers to life-threatening reactions or reactions that required immediate corrective measures and led to discontinuation of pentamidine.

Severe – Leukopenia (< 1000/mm^3) 2.8%; hypoglycemia (< 25 mg/dL) 2.4%; thrombocytopenia (< 20,000/mm^3) 1.7%; hypotension (< 60 mm Hg systolic) 0.9%; acute renal failure (serum creatinine > 6 mg/dL) 0.5%; hypocalcemia (0.2%); Stevens-Johnson syndrome and ventricular tachycardia (0.2%); fatalities caused by severe hypotension, hypoglycemia, and cardiac arrhythmias.

Adverse reactions occurring in ≥ 3 % of patients include elevated serum creatinine; sterile abscess, pain, or induration at the IM injection site; elevated liver function tests; leukopenia; nausea; anorexia; hypotension; fever; hypoglycemia; rash; bad taste in mouth; shortness of breath; dizziness; cough; pharyngitis; chest pain/congestion; night sweats; chills; vomiting; bronchospasm; pneumothorax; diarrhea; headache; anemia (generally associated with zidovudine use), myalgia; abdominal pain; edema.

Adverse reactions may also include tachycardia; hypertension; palpitations; syncope; cerebrovascular accident; vasodilation; vasculitis; gingivitis; dyspepsia; oral ulcer/abscess; gastritis; gastric ulcer; hypersalivation; dry mouth; splenomegaly; melena; hematochezia; esophagitis; colitis; pancreatitis; pancytopenia; neutropenia; eosinophilia; thrombocytopenia; hepatitis; hepatomegaly; hepatic dysfunction; renal failure; flank pain; nephritis; tremors; confusion; anxiety; memory loss; seizure; neuropathy; paresthesia; insomnia; hypesthesia; drowsiness; emotional lability; vertigo; paranoia; neuralgia; hallucination; depression; unsteady gait; rhinitis; laryngitis; pneumonitis; pleuritis; cyanosis; tachypnea; rales; pruritus; erythema; dry skin; desquamation; urticaria; eye discomfort; conjunctivitis; blurred vision; blepharitis; loss of taste and smell; incontinence; miscarriage; arthralgia; allergic reactions; extrapulmonary pneumocystosis.

ATOVAQUONE

Suspension: 750 mg/5 mL (*Rx*)   Mepron (GlaxoSmithKline)

Indications

Pneumocystitis carinii pneumonia (PCP): Prevention of PCP in patients who are intolerant to trimethoprim-sulfamethoxazole (TMP-SMZ).

Acute oral treatment of mild to moderate PCP in patients who are intolerant to TMP-SMZ.

Administration and Dosage

Prevention of PCP:

Adults and adolescents 13 to 16 years of age – 1500 mg once daily with a meal.

Treatment of mild to moderate PCP:

Adults and adolescents 13 to 16 years of age – 750 mg administered with food twice daily for 21 days (total daily dose 1500 mg).

Failure to administer with food may result in lower atovaquone plasma concentrations and may limit response to therapy.

Actions

Pharmacology: Atovaquone, an analog of ubiquinone, is an antiprotozoal with antipneumocystis activity.

Pharmacokinetics: Absorption is enhanced ≈ 2-fold when given with food. Atovaquone is extensively bound to plasma proteins (> 99.9%). CSF concentratons are < 1% of plasma concentrations. Half-life ranged from 67 to 77.6 hours following the suspension. The long half-life is caused by presumed enterohepatic cycling and eventual fecal elimination. There is indirect evidence that atovaquone may undergo limited metabolism; however, a specific metabolite has not been identified.

Contraindications

Development or history of potentially life-threatening allergic reactions to any of the components of the formulation.

Warnings

Severe PCP: Clinical experience has been limited to patients with mild to moderate PCP. Treatment of more severe episodes of PCP has not been systematically studied. Atovaquone efficacy in patients who are failing therapy with TMP-SMZ has not been systematically studied.

Hepatic function impairment: Use caution in patients with severe hepatic impairment, and closely monitor administration.

Elderly: Dose selection for an elderly patient should be cautious. Exercise caution when treating elderly patients reflecting the greater frequency of decreased hepatic, renal, and cardiac function.

Pregnancy: Category C.

Lactation: It is not known whether atovaquone is excreted into breast milk.

Children: Safety and efficacy have not been established. Preliminary analysis suggests that the pharmacokinetics are age-dependent.

Precautions

Absorption: Absorption of atovaquone is limited but can be significantly increased when the drug is taken with food. Plasma concentrations correlate with the likelihood of successful treatment and survival. GI disorders may limit absorption of orally administered drugs. Patients with these disorders also may not achieve plasma concentrations of atovaquone associated with response to therapy in controlled trials.

Concurrent pulmonary conditions: Atovaquone is not effective therapy for concurrent pulmonary conditions such as bacterial, viral, or fungal pneumonia or mycobacterial diseases. Clinical deterioration in patients may be due to infections with other pathogens, as well as progressive PCP.

Drug Interactions

Use caution when administering atovaquone concurrently with other highly plasma protein bound drugs with narrow therapeutic indices as competition for binding sites may occur.

Drugs that may interact include rifamycins, TMP-SMZ, and zidovudine.

Drug/Food interactions: Administering atovaquone with food enhances its absorption by ≈ 2-fold.

Adverse Reactions

Adverse reactions occurring in ≥ 3% of patients include rash (including maculopapular), nausea, diarrhea, headache, vomiting, fever, cough, insomnia, asthenia, pruritus, monilia (oral), abdominal pain, constipation, dizziness, anemia, neutropenia, elevated ALT and AST, elevated alkaline phosphatase, elevated amylase, hyponatremia, pain, sweating, anxiety, anorexia, sinusitis, dyspepsia, rhinitis, and taste perversion.

TRIMETREXATE GLUCURONATE

Powder for injection, lyophilized: 25 mg trimetrexate (*Rx*)   *Neutrexin* (US Bioscience)

Warning:
Trimetrexate must be used with concurrent leucovorin (leucovorin protection) to avoid potentially serious or life-threatening toxicities.

Indications
As an alternative therapy with concurrent leucovorin administration (leucovorin protection) for the treatment of moderate to severe *Pneumocystis carinii* pneumonia (PCP) in immunocompromised patients, including patients with acquired immunodeficiency syndrome (AIDS), who are intolerant of or refractory to TMP-SMZ therapy, or for whom TMP-SMZ is contraindicated.

Administration and Dosage
Trimetrexate must be given with concurrent leucovorin (leucovorin protection) to avoid potentially serious or life-threatening toxicities. Leucovorin must be given daily during trimetrexate treatment and for 72 hours past the last trimetrexate dose.

Trimetrexate is administered at a dose of 45 mg/m^2 once daily by IV infusion over 60 to 90 minutes. Leucovorin may be administered IV at a dose of 20 mg/m^2 over 5 to 10 minutes every 6 hours for a total daily dose of 80 mg/m^2, or orally as 4 doses of 20 mg/m^2 spaced equally throughout the day. Round up the oral dose to the next higher 25 mg increment. The recommended course of therapy is 21 days of trimetrexate and 24 days of leucovorin.

Dosage modifications:
  Hematologic toxicity – Modify trimetrexate and leucovorin doses based on the worst hematologic toxicity according to the following table. If leucovorin is given orally, round up doses to the next higher 25 mg increment.

Dose Modifications for Hematologic Toxicity				
Toxicity grade	Neutrophils/ mm^3	Platelets/ mm^3	Trimetrexate	Leucovorin
1	> 1000	> 75,000	45 mg/m^2 once daily	20 mg/m^2 every 6 hours
2	750 to 1000	50,000 to 75,000	45 mg/m^2 once daily	40 mg/m^2 every 6 hours
3	500 to 749	25,000 to 49,999	22 mg/m^2 once daily	40 mg/m^2 every 6 hours
4	< 500	< 25,000	Day 1 to 9 discontinue Day 10 to 21 interrupt up to 96 hours[1]	40 mg/m^2 every 6 hours

[1] If Grade 4 hematologic toxicity occurs prior to day 10, discontinue trimetrexate. Administer leucovorin (40 mg/m^2 every 6 hours) for an additional 72 hours. If Grade 4 hematologic toxicity occurs at day 10 or later, trimetrexate may be held up to 96 hours to allow counts to recover. If counts recover to Grade 3 within 96 hours, administer trimetrexate at a dose of 22 mg/m^2 and maintain leucovorin at 40 mg/m^2 every 6 hours. When counts recover to Grade 2 toxicity, trimetrexate dose may be increased to 45 mg/m^2, but the leucovorin dose should be maintained at 40 mg/m^2 for the duration of treatment. If counts do not improve to ≤ Grade 3 toxicity within 96 hours, discontinue trimetrexate. Administer leucovorin at a dose of 40 mg/m^2 every 6 hours for 72 hours following the last dose of trimetrexate.

Actions
Pharmacology: Trimetrexate, a 2.4-diaminoquinazoline, nonclassical folate antagonist, is a synthetic inhibitor of the enzyme dihydrofolate reductase. The end result is disruption of DNA, RNA, and protein synthesis, with consequent cell death.

Pharmacokinetics: Clearance was 38 ± 15 mL/min/m^2 and volume of distribution at steady state (Vd$_{ss}$) was 20 ± 8 L/m^2. The plasma concentration time profile declined in a biphasic manner over 24 hours with a terminal half-life of 11 ± 4 hours.

Renal clearance in cancer patients has varied from about 4 ± 2 to 10 ± 6 mL/min/m^2 and 10% and 30% is excreted unchanged in the urine. Considering the free fraction of trimetrexate, active tubular secretion may possibly contribute to the renal clearance.

Contraindications

Clinically significant sensitivity to trimetrexate, leucovorin, or methotrexate.

Warnings

Concurrent leucovorin: Trimetrexate must be used with concurrent leucovorin to avoid potentially serious or life-threatening complications, including bone marrow suppression, oral and GI mucosal ulceration, and renal and hepatic dysfunction. Leucovorin therapy must extend for 72 hours past the last dose of trimetrexate. Inform patients that failure to take the recommended dose and duration of leucovorin can lead to fatal toxicity. Closely monitor patients for the development of serious hematologic adverse reactions.

Pregnancy: Category D.

Lactation: It is not known if trimetrexate is excreted in breast milk.

Children: Safety and efficacy of trimetrexate for the treatment of histologically confirmed PCP has not been established for patients < 18 years of age.

Precautions

Monitoring: Perform blood tests at least twice a week during therapy to assess the following parameters: Hematology (absolute neutrophil counts [ANC], platelets); renal function (serum creatinine, BUN); hepatic function (AST, ALT, alkaline phosphatase).

Pulmonary conditions: Trimetrexate has not been evaluated clinically for the treatment of concurrent pulmonary conditions such as bacterial, viral, or fungal pneumonia or mycobacterial diseases.

Special risk: Patients receiving trimetrexate may experience hematologic, hepatic, renal, and GI toxicities. Use caution in treating patients with impaired hematologic, renal, or hepatic function.

Drug Interactions

Because trimetrexate is metabolized by a P450 enzyme system, drugs that induce or inhibit this drug metabolizing enzyme system may elicit important drug interactions that may alter trimetrexate plasma concentrations, which include erythromycin, rifampin, rifabutin, ketoconazole, fluconazole, cimetidine, nitrogen substituted imidazole drugs (eg, clotrimazole, ketoconazole, miconazole).

Adverse Reactions

Adverse reactions occurring in ≥ 3% of patients include fever, rash/pruritus, nausea/vomiting, neutropenia, thrombocytopenia, anemia, increased AST and ALT, increased alkaline phosphatase, hyponatremia.

ANTHELMINTICS

The following table lists the major parasitic infections, causative organisms, and drugs of choice for treatment.

Major Parasite Infections		
Infection (common name)	Organism	Drug(s) of Choice
Intestinal Nematodes		
Ascariasis[1] (Roundworm)	*Ascaris lumbricoides*	Mebendazole, Pyrantel pamoate, or Diethylcarbamazine
Uncinariasis (Hookworm)	*Ancylostoma duodenale Necator americanus*	Mebendazole or Pyrantel pamoate[2]
Strongyloidiasis (Threadworm)	*Strongyloides stercoralis*	Thiabendazole
Trichuriasis (Whipworm)	*Trichuris trichiura*	Mebendazole
Enterobiasis[3] (Pinworm)	*Enterobius vermicularis*	Mebendazole, Pyrantel pamoate, or Albendazole
Capillariasis	*Capillaria philippinensis*	Mebendazole or Thiabendazole
Tissue Nematodes		
Trichinosis	*Trichinella spiralis*	Steroids for severe symptoms plus Thiabendazole, Albendazole, Flubendazole[4], or Mebendazole[2]
Cutaneous larva migrans (creeping eruption)	*Ancylostoma braziliense* and others	Thiabendazole, Albendazole, or Ivermectin[5]
Onchocerciasis (River blindness)	*Onchocerca volvulus*	Suramin,[6] Diethylcarbamazine, or Ivermectin[5]
Dracontiasis (guinea worm)	*Dracunculus medinensis*	Thiabendazole or Mebendazole
Angiostrongyliasis (rat lungworm)	*Angiostrongylus cantonensis*	Thiabendazole or Mebendazole
Loiasis	*Loa loa*	Diethylcarbamazine
Cestodes		
Taeniasis (Beef tapeworm)	*Taenia saginata*	Praziquantel[2] or Niclosamide
(Pork tapeworm)	*Taenia solium*	Praziquantel,[2] Niclosamide, or Albendazole
Diphyllobothriasis (Fish tapeworm)	*Diphyllobothrium latum*	Praziquantel[2] or Niclosamide
Dog tapeworm	*Dipylidium caninum*	Praziquantel[2]
Hymenolepiasis (Dwarf tapeworm)	*Hymenolepis nana*	Praziquantel[2] or Niclosamide[4]
Hydatid cysts	*Echinococcus granulosus*	Albendazole or Praziquantel
Trematodes		
Schistosomiasis	*Schistosoma mansoni*	Praziquantel or Oxamniquine
	Schistosoma japonicum	Praziquantel
	Schistosoma haematobium	Praziquantel
	Schistosoma mekongi	Praziquantel
Hermaphroditic Flukes Fasciolopsiasis (Intestinal fluke)	*Fasciolopsis buski*	Praziquantel
	Heterophyes heterophyes Metagonimus yokogawai	Praziquantel
Clonorchiasis (Chinese liver fluke)	*Clonorchis sinensis*	Praziquantel
Fascioliasis (Sheep liver fluke)	*Fasciola hepatica*	Praziquantel or Bithionol[5]
Opisthorchiasis (Liver fluke)	*Opisthorchis viverrini*	Praziquantel
Paragonimiasis (Lung fluke)	*Paragonimus westermani*	Praziquantel or Bithionol[5] (alternate)

[1] The following drugs also are indicated in *Ascariasis*: Piperazine citrate (if intestinal or biliary obstruction); thiabendazole.
[2] Unlabeled use.
[3] The following drugs also are indicated in *Enterobiasis*: Piperazine and thiabendazole.
[4] Not available in the US.
[5] Available from the CDC.
[6] Available from the CDC, although generally not recommended.

Chapter 10

BIOLOGIC AND IMMUNOLOGIC AGENTS

Immune Serums, 983
  Immune Globulin IV, 983
  Immune Globulin IM, 985
  Hepatitis B Immune Globulin, 986
  Tetanus Immune Globulin, 987
  Cytomegalovirus Immune Globulin IV, Human, 988
  Varicella-Zoster Immune Globulin, 989
Agents for Active Immunization, 990
  Bacterial Vaccines, 993
    Haemophilus b Conjugate, 993
    Pneumococcal 7-Valent Conjugate, 996
  Viral Vaccines, 998
    Hepatitis B, 998
    Hepatitis A, 1002
    Varicella Virus, 1003
Interferon Gamma-1B, 1005
Interferon Beta, 1007
Etanercept, 1009
Immunosuppressive Drugs, 1012
  Azathioprine, 1012
  Tacrolimus, 1013
  Sirolimus, 1016
  Mycophenolate Mofetil, 1019
  Cyclosporine, 1024
  Muromonab-CD3, 1029
Immunomodulators, 1032
  Peginterferon Alfa-2B, 1032

IMMUNE SERUMS

Indications
To provide passive immunization to ≥ 1 infectious disease. Protection derived will be of rapid onset but short duration (1 to 3 months).

Actions
Pharmacology: Standard immune globulins contain ≈ 16.5% gamma globulin. Immune globulin IV contains 5% immune globulins. These products are obtained, purified, and standardized from human serum or plasma. They are obtained from pooled plasma of donors from the general population or of hyperimmunized donors (for immune globulins for specific diseases).

Contraindications
Allergic response to gamma globulin or anti-immunoglobulin A (IgA) antibodies; allergic response to thimerosal; people with isolated immunoglobulin A (IgA) deficiency.

Immune globulin, IM: Patients who have severe thrombocytopenia or any coagulation disorder that would contraindicate IM use.

Warnings
Route of administration: Do not give these products IV (except immune globulin IV). IV injections can cause a precipitous fall in blood pressure and a picture similar to anaphylaxis. Give IM.

Hypersensitivity reactions:
    Anaphylactic reactions – Anaphylactic reactions (rare) may occur following injection of human immune globulin preparations. Anaphylaxis is more likely if immune globulin is given IV.
    Give with caution to patients with prior systemic allergic reactions following use of human immunoglobulin preparations.

Pregnancy: Category C.

Lactation: It is not known whether immune globulin is excreted in breast milk.

Precautions
Skin testing: Do not perform skin testing because intradermal injection of concentrated gamma globulin causes a localized area of inflammation that can be misinterpreted as a positive allergic reaction.

Drug Interactions
Live virus vaccines may interact with immune globulins.

Adverse Reactions
Adverse reactions may include tenderness; pain; muscle stiffness at injection site; urticaria; angioedema.

IMMUNE GLOBULIN INTRAVENOUS (IGIV)

IGIV provides immediate antibody levels, whereas IM administration involves a 2- to 5-day delay before adequate serum levels are attained. Half-life is ≈ 3 weeks.

Injection: 5% and 10% (*Rx*)	*Gamimune N* (Bayer)
Powder for injection: 5% and 10% immune globulin IV (human) (*Rx*)	*Venoglobulin-S* (Alpha Therapeutic)
Powder for injection (freeze-dried, solvent/detergent treated): 50 mg/mL (*Rx*)	*Gammagard S/D* (Baxter)
Powder for injection (freeze-dried): 50 mg/mL; 90% gammaglobulin (*Rx*)	*Polygam S/D* (American Red Cross)
Powder for injection (lyophilized): 1, 3, 6, and 12 g immune globulin G (*Rx*)	*Sandoglobulin* (Novartis), *Panglobulin* (American Red Cross)
Powder for injection, lyophilized: 5% IgG, 3% human albumin (*Rx*)	*Gammar-P I.V.* (Aventis)
Powder for injection (freeze-dried): 50 mg/mL (*Rx*)	*Iveegam* (Immuno)

Warning:

Immune globulin IV (human) products have been associated with renal dysfunction, acute renal failure, osmotic nephrosis, and death. Patients predisposed to acute renal failure include patients with any degree of pre-existing renal insufficiency, diabetes mellitus, > 65 years of age, volume depletion, sepsis, paraproteinemia, or patients receiving known nephrotoxic drugs. Especially in such patients, administer IGIV products at the minimum concentration available and the minimum rate of infusion practicable. While these reports of renal dysfunction and acute renal failure have been associated with the use of many of the licensed IGIV products, those containing sucrose as a stabilizer accounted for a disproportionate share of the total number.

Administration and Dosage

Administer IV only.

Sandoglobulin:

Immunodeficiency syndrome – 100 to 400 mg/kg once a month by IV infusion. If clinical response or the IgG level achieved is insufficient (minimum serum level, 300 mg/dL), increase to 300 mg/kg or repeat the infusion more frequently.

Idiopathic thrombocytopenic purpura –

Induction: 400 mg/kg for 2 to 5 consecutive days.

Maintenance-chronic ITP: In adults and children, if after induction therapy the platelet count falls to < 30,000/mcL or the patient manifests clinically significant bleeding, 0.4 g/kg of body weight may be given as a single infusion. If an adequate response does not result, the dose can be increased to 0.8 to 1 g/kg of body weight given as a single infusion.

Gammagard S/D:

Immunodeficiency syndrome – 200 to 400 mg/kg. Monthly doses of at least 100 mg/kg are recommended.

B-cell chronic lymphocytic leukemia (CLL) – 400 mg/kg every 3 to 4 weeks.

Kawasaki disease – Either a single 1 g/kg dose or a dose of 400 mg/kg for 4 consecutive days beginning within 7 days of the onset of fever, administered concomitantly with appropriate aspirin therapy (80 to 100 mg/kg/day in 4 divided doses) is recommended.

Idiopathic thrombocytopenic purpura – 1000 mg/kg. Give up to 3 doses on alternate days if required.

Gammar-P.I.V.:

Immunodeficiency syndrome – Starting doses of 200 mg/kg body weight every 3 to 4 weeks are recommended in children and adolescents. Slightly higher doses of 200 to 400 mg/kg every 3 to 4 weeks are recommended in adults. Individualize treatment.

Gamimune N:

Immunodeficiency syndrome – 100 to 200 mg/kg administered once a month by IV infusion. If clinical response or the level of IgG achieved is insufficient, increase to 400 mg/kg or repeat the infusion more frequently than once a month.

Idiopathic thrombocytopenic purpura – 400 mg/kg for 5 consecutive days or 1000 mg/kg/day for 1 day or 2 consecutive days.

BMT – 500 mg/kg (10 mL/kg) beginning on days 7 and 2 pretransplant or at the time conditioning therapy for transplantation is begun, then weekly through the 90-day posttransplant period.

Pediatric HIV infection – 400 mg/kg (8 mL/kg) every 28 days.

Iveegam:

Immunodeficiency syndrome – 200 mg/kg/month. If desired clinical results are not obtained, the dosage may be increased up to 4-fold or intervals shortened. Doses up to 800 mg/kg/month have been tolerated.

Kawasaki disease – 400 mg/kg/day for 4 consecutive days or a single dose of 2000 mg/kg given over a 10-hour period. Initiate treatment within 10 days of onset of the disease. Treatment regimen should include aspirin (100 mg/kg each day through the 14th day of illness, then 3 to 5 mg/kg/day thereafter for 5 weeks).

Panglobulin:
> *Immunodeficiency syndrome –*
>> *Adult and child substitution therapy:* The usual dose of *Panglobulin* in immunodeficiency syndromes is 0.2 g/kg of body weight administered once a month IV. If the clinical response is inadequate, the dose may be increased to 0.3 g/kg or the infusion may be repeated more frequently than once a month.
>
>> *Idiopathic thrombocytopenic purpura –* Initiate 0.4 g/kg of body weight on 2 to 5 consecutive days.

Polygam S/D:
> *Immunodeficiency syndrome –* 100 mg/kg/month. An initial dose of 200 to 400 mg/kg may be administered.
>
>> *B-cell CLL –* 400 mg/kg every 3 to 4 weeks.
>
>> *Kawasaki disease –* For patients with Kawasaki disease, either a single 1 g/kg dose or a dose of 400 mg/kg for 4 consecutive days beginning within 7 days of the onset of fever, administered concomitantly with appropriate aspirin therapy (80 to 100 mg/kg/day in 4 divided doses is recommended).
>
>> *Idiopathic thrombocytopenic purpura –* 1 g/kg. Give up to 3 separate doses on alternate days as required.

Venoglobulin-S:
> *Immunodeficiency syndrome –* 200 mg/kg/month. If clinical response or the level of IgG achieved is insufficient, increase to 300 to 400 mg/kg or repeat the infusion more frequently than once a month.
>
>> *Idiopathic thrombocytopenic purpura –* 2000 mg/kg over a maximum of 5 days for induction therapy.
>
>> *Maintenance therapy –* 1000 mg/kg may be given as needed to maintain platelet counts of 30,000/mm^3 in children and 20,000/mm^3 in adults, or to prevent bleeding episodes in the interval between infusions.
>
>> *Kawasaki disease –* Initiate treatment within 10 days of the onset of symptoms. Give a single dose of 2 g/kg (40 mL/kg) over a 10- to 12-hour period. The treatment regimen should include the administration of aspirin (100 mg/kg/day) until the patient becomes afebrile or through the fourteenth day after the onset of symptoms. Administer 3 to 10 mg/kg/day of aspirin for the following 5 weeks. If symptoms persist or recur because of active Kawasaki disease, retreatment with the same dose level may be useful.

IMMUNE GLOBULIN IM (IG; Gamma Globulin; ISG)

Solution for injection (*Rx*)	BayGam (Bayer)

Administration and Dosage
For IM injection only.

Hepatitis A: A dose of 0.02 mL/kg (0.01 mL/lb) is recommended for household and institutional hepatitis A case contacts and for people who plan to travel for < 3 months in areas where hepatitis A is common; for prolonged travel (> 3 months), the dose is 0.06 mL/kg (repeat every 4 to 6 months).

Measles (Rubeola): To prevent or modify measles in a susceptible person exposed < 6 days previously, give 0.25 mL/kg (0.11 mL/lb). If a susceptible child who is also immunocompromised is exposed to measles, give 0.5 mL/kg (15 mL maximum) immediately.

Immunoglobulin deficiency: The usual dosage consists of an initial dose of 1.3 mL/kg followed in 3 or 4 weeks by 0.66 mL/kg (at least 100 mg/kg) to be given every 3 to 4 weeks. Some patients may require more frequent injections.

Varicella: Give 0.6 to 1.2 mL/kg promptly, if zoster immune globulin is unavailable.

Rubella: Some studies suggest that the use of IG in exposed susceptible women can lessen the likelihood of infection and fetal damage; therefore, a dose of 0.55 mL/kg within 72 hours of exposure has been recommended and may benefit those women who do not consider a therapeutic abortion.

HEPATITIS B IMMUNE GLOBULIN (HBIG)

Solution for injection *(Rx)*   *BayHep B* (Bayer), *Nabi-HB* (Nabi)

Administration and Dosage

Give injections IM. IM injections are preferably administered in the anterolateral aspects of the upper thigh and the deltoid muscle of the upper arm. The gluteal region should not be used routinely as an injection site because of the risk of injury to the sciatic nerve. An individual decision as to which muscle is injected must be made for each patient based on the volume of material to be administered. If the gluteal region is used when very large volumes are to be injected or multiple doses are necessary, the central region must be avoided; use only the upper, outer quadrant.

Postexposure prophylaxis: The recommended dose is 0.06 mL/kg; the usual adult dose is 3 to 5 mL. Administer the appropriate dose as soon after exposure as possible (preferably within 7 days) and repeat 28 to 30 days after exposure.

Recommendations for Hepatitis B Prophylaxis Following Percutaneous or Permucosal Exposure		
	Exposed person	
Source	Unvaccinated	Vaccinated
Hepatitis B surface antigen (HBsAg)-positive	1. HBIG × 1 immediately[1] 2. Initiate HB vaccine series[2]	1. Test exposed person for anti-HBs. 2. If inadequate antibody,[3] HBIG (× 1) immediately plus HB vaccine booster dose, or 2 doses of HBIG,[1] one as soon as possible after exposure and the second 1 month later.
Known source (high risk)	1. Initiate HV vaccine series 2. Test source for HBsAg. If positive, HBIG × 1	1. Test source for HBsAg only if exposed is vaccine nonresponder; if source is HBsAg-positive, give HBIG (× 1) immediately plus HB vaccine booster dose, or 2 doses of HBIG,[1] one as soon as possible after exposure and the second 1 month later.
Low risk HBsAg-positive	Initiate HB vaccine series.	Nothing required.
Unknown source	Initiate HB vaccine series within 7 days of exposure.	Nothing required.

[1] HBIG, dose 0.06 mL/kg IM.
[2] HB vaccine dose 20 mcg IM for adults; 10 mcg IM for infants or children < 10 years of age. First dose within 1 week; second and third doses, 1 and 6 months later.
[3] < 10 sample ratio units (SRU) by radioimmunoassay (RIA), negative by enzyme immunoassay (EIA).

Prophylaxis of infants born to HBsAG- and hepatitis B early antigen (HBeAg)-positive mothers: The recommended dose for at-risk newborns is 0.5 mL IM into the anterolateral thigh, as soon after birth as possible, preferably within 12 hours. Administer hepatitis B vaccine IM in 3 doses of 0.5 mL of vaccine (10 mcg) each. Give the first dose within 7 days of birth and give concurrently with HBIG but at a separate site. Give the second and third doses of vaccine 1 month and 6 months, respectively, after the first. If administration of the first dose of hepatitis B vaccine is delayed for as long as 3 months, then repeat a 0.5 mL dose of HBIG at 3 months. If hepatitis B vaccine is refused, repeat the 0.5 mL dose of HBIG at 3 and 6 months.

Recommended Schedule of Hepatitis B Immunoprophylaxis to Prevent Perinatal Transmission of Hepatitis B Virus Infection		
	Age of infant	
Administer	Infant born to mother known to be HBsAg positive	Infant born to mother not screened for HBsAg
First vaccination[1]	Birth (within 12 hours)	Birth (within 12 hours)
Hepatitis B Immune Globulin (human)[2]	Birth (within 12 hours)	If mother is found to be HBsAg positive, administer dose to infant as soon as possible, not later than 1 week after birth.
Second vaccination[1]	1 month	1 to 2 months
Third vaccination[1]	6 months[3]	6 months[3]

[1] See manufacturer's recommendations for appropriate dose.
[2] 0.5 mL administered IM at a site different from that used for the vaccine.
[3] See ACIP recommendations.

Sexual exposure to an HBsAg-positive person: All susceptible people whose sex partners have acute hepatitis B infection should receive a single dose of HBIG (0.06 mL/kg) and should begin the hepatitis B vaccine series if prophylaxis can be started within 14 days of the last sexual contact or if sexual contact with the infected person will continue (see table below). Administering the vaccine with HBIG may improve the efficacy of postexposure treatment. The vaccine has the added advantage of conferring long-lasting protection.

Recommendations for Postexposure Prophylaxis for Sexual Exposure to Hepatitis B			
HBIG		Vaccine	
Dose	Recommended timing	Dose	Recommended timing
0.06 mL/kg IM	Single dose within 14 days of last sexual contact.	1 mL IM	First dose at time of HBIG[1] treatment.

[1] The first dose can be administered the same time as the HBIG dose but at a different site; subsequent doses should be administered as recommended for specific vaccine.

Household exposure to people with acute HBV infection: Prophylactic treatment with a 0.5 mL dose of HBIG and hepatitis B vaccine is indicated for infants < 12 months of age who have been exposed to a primary care-giver who has acute hepatitis B. Prophylaxis for other household contacts of people with acute HBV infection is not indicated unless they have had identifiable blood exposure to the index patient (eg, sharing toothbrushes or razors). Such exposures should be treated like sexual exposures. If the index patient becomes an HBV carrier, all household contacts should receive hepatitis B vaccine.

HBIG may be administered at the same time (but at a different site), or ≤ 1 month preceding hepatitis B vaccination without impairing the active immune response from hepatitis B vaccination.

TETANUS IMMUNE GLOBULIN

Solution for injection: (Rx)   *BayTet* (Bayer)

Administration and Dosage
Administer IM. Do NOT inject IV.

Prophylaxis:
 Adults and children ≥ 7 years of age – 250 units.
  Children < 7 years of age – In small children, the dose may be calculated by the body weight (4 units/kg). However, it may be advisable to administer the entire contents

of the vial or syringe (250 units) regardless of the child's size, because theoretically the same amount of toxin will be produced in his body by the infecting tetanus organisms as in an adult.

Therapy: Several studies suggest the value of human tetanus antitoxin in the actual treatment of active tetanus using single doses of 3000 to 6000 units in combination with other accepted clinical procedures.

Guide to Tetanus Prophylaxis in Wound Management				
	Clean, minor wounds		All other wounds[1]	
History of tetanus immunization (doses)	Td[2]	TIG[3]	Td	TIG
Uncertain or < 3	Yes	No	Yes	Yes
≥ 3[4]	No[5]	No	No[6]	No

[1] Such as, but not limited to, wounds contaminated with dirt, feces, soil, and saliva; puncture wounds; avulsions; and wounds resulting from missiles, crushing, burns, and frostbite.
[2] Adult type tetanus and diphtheria toxoids. If the patient is < 7 years of age, DT or DTP is preferred to tetanus toxoid alone. For people ≥ 7 years of age, Td is preferred to tetanus toxoid alone.
[3] Tetanus immune globulin (human).
[4] If only 3 doses of fluid tetanus toxoid have been received, a fourth dose of toxoid, preferably an adsorbed toxoid, should be given.
[5] Yes, if > 10 years since the last dose.
[6] Yes, if > 5 years since the last dose. (More frequent boosters are not needed and can accentuate side effects.)

CYTOMEGALOVIRUS IMMUNE GLOBULIN IV, HUMAN (CMV-IGIV)

Solution for injection (*Rx*)   *CytoGam* (MedImmune)

Administration and Dosage

The maximum recommended total dosage per infusion is 150 mg/kg, administered according to the following schedule:

Dosage Schedule for CMV-IGIV in Transplantation		
	Dosage (mg/kg)	
Time of infusion	Kidney	Liver, pancreas, lung, heart
Within 72 hours of transplant	150	150
2 weeks posttransplant	100	150
4 weeks posttransplant	100	150
6 weeks posttransplant	100	150
8 weeks posttransplant	100	150
12 weeks posttransplant	50	100
16 weeks posttransplant	50	100

Initial dose: Administer IV at 15 mg Ig/kg/hr. If no untoward reactions occur after 30 minutes, the rate may be increased to 30 mg Ig/kg/hr; if no untoward reactions occur after a subsequent 30 minutes, the infusion may be increased to 60 mg Ig/kg/hr (volume not to exceed 75 mL/hour). Do not exceed this rate of administration. Monitor the patient closely during and after each rate change.

Subsequent doses: Administer at 15 mg Ig/kg/hr for 15 minutes. If no untoward reactions occur, increase to 30 mg Ig/kg/hr for 15 minutes and then increase to a maximum rate of 60 mg Ig/kg/hr (volume not to exceed 75 mL/hr). Do not exceed this rate of administration. Monitor the patient closely during each rate change.

Renal insufficiency – Use with caution in patients with pre-existing renal insufficiency and in patients judged to be at increased risk of developing renal insufficiency (including, but not limited to, those with diabetes mellitus, > 65 years of age, volume depletion, paraproteinemia, sepsis, and patients receiving known nephrotoxic drugs). In these cases especially, it is important to ensure that patients are not volume depleted prior to CMV-IGIV infusion. While most cases of renal insufficiency have occurred in patients receiving total doses of ≥ 400 mg Ig/kg, no pro-spective data are presently available to identify a maximum safe dose, concentration, or rate of infusion in patients determined to be at increased risk of acute renal fail-ure. In the absence of prospective data, do not exceed recommended doses and select the minimum practicable concentration and infusion rate. Infuse the prod-uct at a rate of ≤ 180 mg Ig/kg/hr.

Potential adverse reactions are flushing; chills; muscle cramps; back pain; fever; nausea; vomiting; wheezing; drop in blood pressure. Minor adverse reactions have been infusion-rate related. If the patient develops a minor side effect (eg, nau-sea, back pain, flushing), slow the rate or temporarily interrupt the infusion. If ana-phylaxis or drop in blood pressure occurs, discontinue infusion and use an antidote such as diphenhydramine and epinephrine. Refer to Management of Acute Hypersensitivity Reactions.

Infusion: Begin infusion within 6 hours of entering the vial and complete within 12 hours of entering the vial. Monitor vital signs pre-infusion, midway, and post-infusion, as well as before any rate increase. Administer through an IV line using an administration set that contains an in-line filter (pore size 15 micron) and a con-stant infusion pump (eg, IVAC pump or equivalent). A smaller in-line filter (0.2 micron) is also acceptable. Predilution of CMV-IGIV before infusion is not rec-ommended. Administer through a separate IV line. If this is not possible, it may be "piggybacked" into a preexisting line if that line contains either Sodium Chlor-ide Injection or one of the following dextrose solutions (with or without NaCl added): 2.5%, 5%, 10%, or 20% Dextrose in Water. If a pre-existing line must be used, do not dilute the CMV-IGIV more than 1:2 with any of the above solu-tions. Admixtures of CMV-IGIV with any other solutions have not been evalu-ated.

VARICELLA-ZOSTER IMMUNE GLOBULIN (HUMAN) (VZIG)

Injection (*Rx*)   *Varicella-Zoster Immune Globulin (Human)*
                                     (American Red Cross)[1]

[1] Within MA, VZIG is distributed by the MA Public Health Biologic Laboratories.

Administration and Dosage

Greatest efficacy of treatment is to be expected when begun within 96 hours after exposure. High-risk susceptible patients who are exposed after a prior dose of VZIG should receive another full dose.

Do not inject IV: Administer by deep IM injection in the gluteal muscle, or in another large muscle mass.

VZIG Dose Based on Weight			
Weight of patient			Dose
Kilograms	Pounds	Units	Number of Vials
0 to 10	0 to 22	125	1 @ 125 units
10.1 to 20	22.1 to 44	250	2 @ 125 units
20.1 to 30	44.1 to 66	375	3 @ 125 units
30.1 to 40	66.1 to 88	500	4 @ 125 units
> 40	> 88	625	1 @ 625 units or 5 @ 125 units

Administer entire contents of each vial. For patients ≤ 10 kg, administer 1.25 mL at a single site. For patients > 10 kg, give no more than 2.5 mL at a single site. Each vial of varicella-zoster virus antibody contains 125 units in a volume of ≈ 1.25 mL and each 625 unit vial contains 625 units of antibody in a volume of ≈ 6.25 mL.

The regimen effectively modifies severity of chickenpox and reduces frequency of death, pneumonia, and encephalitis to < 25% expected without treatment.

AGENTS FOR ACTIVE IMMUNIZATION

In contrast to the immune serums and antitoxins that contain exogenous antibodies to provide passive immunity, the Agents for Active Immunization include specific antigens that induce the endogenous production of antibodies. Agents that induce active immunity include vaccines and toxoids.

Vaccines contain whole (killed or attenuated live) or partial microorganisms capable of inducing antibody formation that are not pathogenic. Toxoids are detoxified byproducts derived from organisms that induce disease primarily through the elaboration of exotoxins. Although toxoids are not toxic, they are antigenic, and therefore, stimulate specific antibody production. Active immunization induced through administration of vaccines and toxoids provides prolonged immunity, whereas passive immunization with immune sera or antitoxins is of short duration.

Vaccination with any vaccine may not result in a protective antibody response in all individuals given the vaccine.

The table below indicates the recommended immunization schedule for infants and children. This schedule has been approved by the Advisory Committee on Immunization Practices (ACIP), The American Academy of Pediatrics (AAP), and the American Academy of Family Physicians (AAFP).

Recommended Childhood Immunization Schedule[1] - United States, 2000												
Vaccine	Birth	1 mo.	2 mos.	4 mos.	6 mos.	12 mos.	15 mos.	18 mos.	24 mos.	4-6 yrs.	11-12 yrs.	14-16 yrs.
Hepatitis B[2]	Hep B-1[3]											
		Hep B-2[3]			Hep B-3[3]						Hep B[4]	
Diphtheria, tetanus, and pertussis[5]			DTaP	DTaP	DTaP		DTaP[3]			DTaP	Td[3]	
Haemophilus influenzae type b[6]			Hib	Hib	Hib	Hib[3]						
Polio[7]			IPV	IPV		IPV[3,7]				IPV[7]		
Measles, mumps, rubella[8]						MMR[3]				MMR[8]	MMR[4]	
Varicella[9]						Var[3]					Var[4,9]	
Hepatitis A[10]										Hep A (in selected areas)[3,10]		

[1] This schedule indicates the recommended age for routine administration of currently licensed childhood vaccines as of November 1, 1999. Additional vaccines may be licensed and recommended during the year. Combination vaccines may be used whenever any components of the combination are indicated and its other components are not contraindicated. Give catch-up immunizations whenever feasible. Consult the manufacturers' package inserts for detailed recommendations.

[2] **Infants born to HBsAg-negative mothers** should receive the first dose of hepatitis B vaccine by 2 months of age. The second dose of hepatitis B (Hep B) vaccine should be given ≥ 1 month after the first dose. The third dose should be administered ≥ 4 months after the first dose and ≥ 2 months after the second dose but not before 6 months of age.

Infants born to HBsAg-positive mothers should receive hepatitis B vaccine and 0.5 mL hepatitis B immune globulin (HBIG) within 12 hours of birth at separate sites. The second dose is recommended at 1 month of age and the third dose at 6 months of age.

Infants born to mothers whose HBsAg status is unknown should receive hepatitis B vaccine within 12 hours of birth. Maternal blood should be drawn at the time of delivery to determine the mother's HBsAg status; if the HBsAg test is positive, the infant should receive HBIG as soon as possible (≤ 1 week of age).

All children and adolescents (≤ 18 years of age) who have not been immunized against hepatitis B may begin the series during any visit. Special efforts should be made to immunize children who were born in or whose parents were born in areas of the world with moderate or high endemicity of hepatitis B virus infection.

[3] Range of acceptable ages for vaccination.

[4] Vaccines to be assessed and administered if necessary.

[5] The fourth dose of DTaP may be administered as early as 12 months of age, provided 6 months have elapsed since the third dose and the child is unlikely to return at 15 to 18 months of age. Tetanus and diphtheria toxoids (Td) is recommended at 11 to 12 years of age if ≥ 5 years have elapsed since the last dose of DTP, DTaP, or diphtheria and tetanus toxoids (DT). Subsequent routine Td boosters are recommended every 10 years.

[6] Three *Haemophilus influenzae* type b (Hib) conjugate vaccines are licensed for infant use. If PRP-OMP (*Pedvax-HIB* or *ComVax*, Merck) is administered at 2 and 4 months of age, a dose at 6 months of age is not required. Because clinical studies in infants have demonstrated that using some combination products may induce a lower immune response to the Hib vaccine component, DTaP/Hib combination products should not be used for primary immunization in infants at 2, 4, or 6 months of age, unless FDA-approved for these ages.

[7] To eliminate the risk of vaccine-associated paralytic polio (VAPP), an all-IPV schedule now is recommended for routine childhood polio vaccination in the US. All children should receive 4 doses of IPV at 2, 4, and 6 to 18 months of age and 4 to 6 years of age. OPV (if available) may be used only for the following special circumstances: 1) Mass vaccination campaigns to control outbreaks of paralytic polio, 2) Unvaccinated children who will be traveling in < 4 weeks to areas where polio is endemic or epidemic, 3) Children of parents who do not accept the recommended number of vaccine injections. These children may receive OPV only for the third or fourth dose or both; in this situation, health care providers should administer OPV only after discussing the risks for VAPP with parents or caregivers. 4) During the transition to an all-IPV schedule, recommendations for the use of remaining OPV supplies in physicians' offices and clinics have been issued by the AAP (see *Pediatrics*, December 1999) and the AAFP.

[8] The second dose of measles-mumps-rubella vaccine is routinely recommended at 4 to 6 years of age but may be administered duing any visit provided ≥ 4 weeks have elapsed since receipt of the first dose and that both doses are administered at or after 12 months of age. Those who have not previously received the second dose should complete the schedule by 11 to 12 years of age.

[9] Varicella (Var) vaccine is recommended at any visit on or after the first birthday for susceptible children, ie, those who lack a reliable history of chickenpox (as judged by a health care provider) and who have not been immunized. Susceptible people ≥ 13 years of age should receive 2 doses given ≥ 4 weeks apart.

[10] Hepatitis A is included to indicate its recommended use in selected states of regions; consult the local public health authority. (Also see *MMWR*. 1999;48:1-37.)

Concomitant vaccination: Several routine pediatric vaccines may safely and effectively be administered simultaneously at separate injection sites. National authorities recommend simultaneous immunization at separate sites as indicated by age or health risk if return of a vaccine recipient for a subsequent visit is doubtful.

Immunization for other diseases: Immunization for other diseases is recommended for people with a risk of exposure. Specific immunization requirements and recommendations for international travel can be obtained from the CDC website (www.cdc.gov), including their online publication "Health Information for International Travel."

Hypersensitivity to vaccine components: Vaccine antigens produced in systems containing allergenic substances, (ie, embryonated chicken eggs) may cause hypersensitivity reactions including anaphylaxis. In contrast, influenza vaccine antigens (whole or split), although prepared in embryonated eggs, are highly purified and only rarely are associated with hypersensitivity reactions.

Live virus vaccines prepared by growing viruses in cell cultures essentially are devoid of allergenic substances.

Some vaccines contain preservatives (eg, thimerosal) or trace amounts of antibiotics (eg, neomycin) to which patients may be hypersensitive.

Before the injection of any biological, take all precautions known for prevention of allergic or other side effects, including a review of the patient's history regarding possible sensitivity, occurrence of any adverse event-related symptoms or signs to determine any contraindication to immunization, and a knowledge of the recent literature pertaining to the use of the biological concerned. Have epinephrine 1:1000 available for immediate use when this product is injected.

Altered immunocompetence: Microbial replication after administration of live, attenuated virus vaccines may be enhanced in people with immune deficiency diseases, and in those with suppressed capability for immune response (eg, leukemia, lymphoma, generalized malignancy or therapy with corticosteroids, alkylating agents, antimetabolites, or radiation). Do not give live, attenuated virus vaccines to such patients. Do not give live, attenuated virus vaccines to a member of a household in which there is a family history of congenital or hereditary immunodeficiency until the immune competence of the recipient is known.

HIV infection: Special immunization recommendations are appropriate for people infected with HIV.

Live bacterial or viral vaccines – People infected with HIV and those who have developed AIDS are theoretically at risk of disseminated infection following immunization with a live, albeit attenuated, bacterial or viral vaccine.

Inactivated vaccines or toxoids – In general, immunization with an inactivated vaccine or toxoid poses no additional risk to people infected with HIV and people who have developed AIDS. But these people may be less likely to develop an adequate immune response to vaccination and may remain susceptible to the disease at issue.

Immunization of HIV-infected people – No clinical data have substantiated the concern about antigenic stimulation causing deterioration of clinical status. CDC and WHO continue to recommend immunization of HIV-infected people when the benefits of immunization outweigh the risks of infection.

Summary Recommendations for Routine Immunization of HIV-infected People in the US		
Drug	Known asymptomatic	Symptomatic
DTP/Td	yes	yes
OPV	no	no
e-IPV[1]	yes	yes
MMR	yes	yes
Hib[2]	yes	yes[2]
Pneumococcal	yes	yes
Influenza	yes[3]	yes

[1] For adults ≥ 18 years of age, use only if indicated.
[2] Consider for HIV-infected adults also.
[3] Consider risk and benefit.

Severe febrile illnesses: Immunization of people with severe febrile illnesses generally should be deferred until they have recovered.

Vaccination during pregnancy: On the grounds of a theoretical risk to the developing fetus, live, attenuated virus vaccines generally are not given to pregnant women or to those likely to become pregnant within 3 months after receiving vaccine(s). With some of these vaccines, particularly rubella, measles, and mumps, pregnancy is a contraindication. When vaccine is to be given during pregnancy, waiting until the second or third trimester to minimize any concern over teratogenicity is a reasonable precaution.

Measles, mumps, rubella, or oral polio vaccines may be safely administered to children of pregnant women.

There is no convincing evidence of risk to the fetus from immunization of pregnant women using inactivated virus vaccines, bacterial vaccines, or toxoids. Give tetanus and diphtheria toxoid (Td) to inadequately immunized pregnant women because it affords protection against neonatal tetanus. Similarly, hepatitis B, influenza, and meningococcal vaccines may be indicated during pregnancy.

HAEMOPHILUS b CONJUGATE VACCINE

Injection: 10 mcg purified *Haemophilus* b saccharide capsular oligosaccharide, ≈ 25 mcg diphtheria CRM$_{197}$ protein/0.5 mL dose (*Rx*)

HibTITER (Wyeth-Lederle)

Powder for injection, lyophilized: 10 mcg purified capsular polysaccharide and 24 mcg tetanus toxoid/0.5 mL (*Rx*)

ActHIB (Aventis Pasteur)

Injection: 7.5 mcg *Haemophilus* B PRP, 125 mcg *Neisseria meningitidis* OMPC, and 225 mcg aluminum (as aluminum hydroxide)/0.5 mL (*Rx*)

Liquid PedvaxHIB (Merck)

Injection: 7.5 mcg *Haemophilus* b PRP purified capsular polysaccharide, 125 mcg *Neisseria meningitidis* OMPC and 5 mcg hepatitis B surface antigen, ≈ 225 mcg aluminum (as aluminum hydroxide), 35 mcg sodium borate (decahydrate)/0.5 mL (*Rx*)

Comvax (Merck)

Indications

For the routine immunization of children 2 to 71 months of age (*HibTITER*, *Pedvax-HIB*), 6 weeks to 15 months of age born of HBsAg negative mothers (*Comvax*), 2 through 18 months of age (*ActHIB* and *ActHIB* reconstituted with Aventis Pasteur DTP), and 15 to 18 months of age (*ActHIB* reconstituted with *Tripedia* [*Tri-HIBiT*]) against invasive diseases caused by *Haemophilus influenzae* type b.

The Advisory Committee on Immunization Practices (ACIP) recommends that all children receive one of the conjugate vaccines licensed for infant use beginning routinely at 2 months of age. The vaccine series may be initiated as early as 6 weeks of age.

Children < 24 months of age who have had invasive *H. influenzae* type b (Hib) disease should still receive the vaccine, since many children of that age fail to develop adequate immunity following natural disease. The vaccine can be initiated (or continued) at the time of hospital discharge.

Conjugate vaccines may be given simultaneously with diphtheria and tetanus toxoids and pertussis vaccine adsorbed (DTP); combined measles, mumps, and rubella vaccine (MMR); oral poliovirus vaccine (OPV); or inactivated poliovirus vaccine (IPV).

Haemophilus b conjugate vaccines will not protect children against *H. influenzae* other than type b or other microorganisms that cause meningitis or septic disease.

Administration and Dosage

Administer IM doses in the outer aspect area of the vastus lateralis (mid-thigh) or deltoid. Do not inject IV.

Data are incomplete regarding interchangeability of *Haemophilus* b conjugate vaccines with regard to safety, immunogenicity, or efficacy. Ideally, use the same conjugate vaccine throughout entire vaccination series. Situations will arise in which the vaccine provider does not know which vaccine was previously used. It is prudent for vaccine providers to ensure that, at a minimum, an infant 2 to 6 months of age receives a primary series of 3 doses of conjugate vaccine.

HibTITER:

2 to 6 months of age – Three separate IM injections of 0.5 mL given at ≈ 2 month intervals.

7 to 11 months of age – Previously unvaccinated – 2 separate IM injections of 0.5 mL given ≈ 2 months apart.

12 to 14 months of age – Previously unvaccinated – One IM injection.

All vaccinated children receive single booster dose at ≥ 15 months of age, not < 2 months after the previous dose. Previously unvaccinated children 15 to 71 months of age receive a single 0.5 mL IM injection in mid-thigh or deltoid muscle.

PedvaxHIB: Shake well before withdrawal and use.

2 to 14 months of age – Two separate IM injections of 0.5 mL given at 2 months of age and 2 months later (or as soon as possible thereafter). When the primary 2-dose regimen is completed before 12 months of age, a 0.5 mL booster dose is required at 12 months of age but not earlier than 2 months after the second dose.

≥ 15 months of age (previously unvaccinated) – Give a single 0.5 mL IM injection.

COMVAX: Shake well before withdrawal and use.

Infants born to HBsAg negative mothers – Three 0.5 mL doses administered IM ideally at 2, 4, and 12 to 15 months of age. If the recommended schedule cannot be followed exactly, the interval between the first 2 doses should be ≥ 2 months and the interval between the second and third doses should be as close as possible to 8 to 11 months.

Children previously vaccinated with ≥ 1 dose of either hepatitis B vaccine or Haemophilus b conjugate vaccine – Children who receive 1 dose of hepatitis B vaccine at or shortly after birth may receive COMVAX on the schedule of 2, 4, and 12 to 15 months of age. There are no data to support the use of a 3-dose series of COMVAX in infants who previously received > 1 dose of hepatitis B vaccine; however, COMVAX may be given to children otherwise scheduled to receive concurrent *Recombivax HB* and *PedvaxHIB*.

Children not vaccinated according to recommended schedule – Consider vaccination schedules on an individual basis. The number of doses of a PRP-OMPC-containing product (ie, COMVAX, *PedvaxHIB*) depends on the age that vaccination is begun. An infant 2 to 10 months of age should receive 3 doses of a product containing PRP-OMPC. An infant 11 to 14 months of age should receive 2 doses of a product containing PRP-OMPC. A child 15 to 71 months of age should receive one dose of a product containing PRP-OMPC. Infants and children, regardless of age, should receive 3 doses of an HBsAg-containing product.

ActHIB: Use only Aventis Pasteur whole-cell DTP, *Tripedia*, or 0.4% sodium chloride diluent for reconstitution of lyophilized *ActHIB*.

Reconstitution with DTP or Tripedia – Thoroughly agitate the DTP or *Tripedia* vials, withdraw a 0.6 mL dose and inject into the vial of *ActHIB*. After reconstitution and thorough agitation, the combined vaccines will appear whitish in color. Withdraw and administer a 0.5 mL dose IM.

ActHIB/DTP: Use reconstituted vaccine within 24 hours.

ActHIB/Tripedia (TriHIBiT): Use reconstituted vaccine immediately (within 30 minutes).

Reconstitution with 0.4% sodium chloride – Inject the entire volume of diluent in the vial or syringe into the vial of *ActHIB*. Thoroughly agitate to ensure complete reconstitution. Draw back the entire volume of reconstituted vaccine into the syringe before injecting 0.5 mL IM. Vaccine will appear clear and colorless. Use within 24 hours.

ActHIB reconstituted with saline, Tripedia, or DTP (previously unvaccinated) –

2 to 6 months of age: 3 separate 0.5 mL IM injections given at 2, 4, and 6 months of age, then at 15 to 18 months of age. A fifth immunization of DTP should be given at 4 to 6 years of age.

7 to 11 months of age: Two 0.5 mL IM doses of *Haemophilus* b conjugate vaccine at 8-week intervals and a booster dose at 15 to 18 months of age.

12 to 14 months of age: One 0.5 mL IM dose of *Haemophilus* b conjugate vaccine followed by a booster 2 months later.

15 to 18 months of age: One 0.5 mL dose injected IM. An immunization of *Tripedia* should be given at 4 to 6 years of age.

Vaccination Schedule for Haemophilus b Conjugate Vaccines					
	HibTITER		PedvaxHIB		ActHIB
Age at first dose (mos)	Primary series	Booster	Primary series	Booster	Primary series	Booster
2 to 6	3 doses, 2 mos. apart	15 mos.[1]	2 doses, 2 mos. apart	12 mos.[1]	3 doses, 2 mos. apart	12 to 18 mos[1]

Vaccination Schedule for Haemophilus b Conjugate Vaccines						
	HibTITER		PedvaxHIB		ActHIB	
Age at first dose (mos)	Primary series	Booster	Primary series	Booster	Primary series	Booster
7 to 11	2 doses, 2 mos. apart	15 mos.[1]	2 doses, 2 mos. apart	15 mos.[1]	2 doses, 2 mos. apart	12 to 15 mos.[1]
12 to 14	1 dose	15 mos.[1]	1 dose	15 mos.[1]	1 dose	15 mos.[1]
15 to 71	1 dose	-	1 dose	-	1 dose[2]	-

[1] At least 2 months after previous dose.
[2] One dose at 15 to 59 months.

Actions

Pharmacology: An antibody concentration of ≥ 0.15 mcg/mL is correlated with protection; in 3-week postvaccination serum, antibody levels ≥ 1 mcg/mL were correlated with long-term protection.

Contraindications

Hypersensitivity to diphtheria toxoid, the diluent, or any component of the vaccines to be administered, including thimerosal. Any contraindication for DTP or *Tripedia* is a contraindication for use of ActHIB reconstituted with those respective vaccines.

Warnings

Deficient antibodies: The expected immune response may not be attained in people deficient in producing antibody, whether caused by genetic defect or immunosuppressive therapy.

Illness or infection: Any febrile illness or active infection is reason for delaying vaccine.

Haemophilus b disease: Haemophilus b disease may occur in the week after vaccination, prior to the onset of the protective effects of the vaccine.

Although some immune response to the diphtheria toxoid component of the conjugate vaccine may occur, it does not substitute for routine diphtheria immunization.

Hypersensitivity reactions: Have epinephrine 1:1000 available for immediate use if an anaphylactoid reaction occurs. Refer to Management of Acute Hypersensitivity Reactions.

Pregnancy: Category C. These vaccines are not recommended for use in pregnant patients.

Children: PedvaxHIB and COMVAX are not recommended for use in infants < 6 weeks of age. Safety and efficacy not established for use in infants < 6 weeks of age (HibTITER, ActHIB reconstituted with AP DTP or 0.4% sodium chloride), < 2 months of age (*Pedvax HIB*), < 15 months of age (ActHIB reconstituted with *Tripedia*), > 15 months of age (COMVAX), or ≥ 6 years of age (*Pedvax HIB*).

Drug Interactions

Drug/Lab test interactions: Sensitive tests (eg, *Latex Agglutination Kits*) may detect PRP derived from the vaccine in urine of some vaccinees for up to 30 days following vaccination.

Adverse Reactions

Adverse reactions may include fever, erythema, and tenderness.

PNEUMOCOCCAL 7-VALENT CONJUGATE VACCINE (DIPHTHERIA CRM$_{197}$ PROTEIN)

Injection: 2 mcg each of 6 polysaccharide isolates; 4 mcg of   *Prevnar* (Wyeth Lederle)
1 polysaccharide isolate per 0.5 mL dose

Indications

Immunization against Streptococcus pneumoniae: Active immunization of infants and toddlers against invasive disease caused by *S. pneumoniae* because of the capsular serotypes included in the vaccine (4, 6B, 9V, 14, 18C, 19F, and 23F).

This vaccine is not intended to be used for treatment of active infection.

Administration and Dosage

Administer as one 0.5 mL IM injection. Do not inject IV.

Vaccination schedule: For infants, the immunization series of pneumococcal 7-valent conjugate vaccine consists of 3 doses of 0.5 mL each, at ≈ 2-month intervals, followed by a fourth dose of 0.5 mL at 12 to 15 months of age. The customary age for the first dose is 2 months of age, but it can be given as young as 6 weeks of age. The recommended dosing interval is 4 to 8 weeks. Administer the fourth dose ≥ 2 months after the third dose.

Previously unvaccinated older infants and children: For previously unvaccinated older infants and children who are beyond the age of the routine infant schedule, the following schedule applies:

Pneumococcal Vaccine Dosage in Previously Unvaccinated Older Infants and Children	
Age at first dose	Total number of 0.5 mL doses
7 to 11 months of age	3[1]
12 to 23 months of age	2[2]
≥ 24 months through 9 years of age	1

[1] Two doses ≥ 4 weeks apart; third dose after the 1-year birthday, separated from the second dose by ≥ 2 months.
[2] Two doses ≥ 2 months apart.

Safety and immunogenicity data are either limited or not available for children in specific high-risk groups for invasive pneumococcal disease (eg, individuals with sickle cell disease, asplenia, HIV infection).

Actions

Pharmacology: Pneumococcal 7-valent conjugate vaccine is a sterile solution of saccharides of the capsular antigens of *S. pneumoniae* serotypes 4, 6B, 9V, 14, 18C, 19F, and 23F individually conjugated to diphtheria CRM$_{197}$ protein.

Contraindications

Hypersensitivity to any component of the vaccine, including diphtheria toxoid.

Infections: Severe or even a moderate febrile illness is sufficient reason to postpone vaccinations. Minor illnesses, such as a mild upper respiratory tract infection, with or without low-grade fever, are not generally contraindications.

Warnings

Efficacy: This vaccine will not protect against *S. pneumoniae* disease other than that caused by the 7 serotypes included in the vaccine, nor will it protect against other microorganisms that cause invasive infection such as bacteremia and meningitis.

Immunization with pneumococcal 7-valent conjugate vaccine does not substitute for routine diphtheria immunization.

Hematologic disorders: Do not give to infants or children with thrombocytopenia or any coagulation disorder that would contraindicate IM injection unless the potential benefit clearly outweighs the risk of administration. Use caution if administering this vaccine to children with coagulation disorders (see Drug Interactions).

Immunosuppressed patients: Children with impaired immune responsiveness, whether caused by the use of immunosuppressive therapy (including irradiation, corticosteroids, antimetabolites, alkylating agents, and cytotoxic agents), a genetic defect, HIV infection, or other causes, may have reduced antibody response to active immunization (see Drug Interactions).

Immunocompromised patients: The use of pneumococcal conjugate vaccine does not replace the use of 23-valent pneumococcal polysaccharide vaccination in children ≥ 24 months of age with sickle cell disease, asplenia, HIV infection, chronic illness, or those who are immunocompromised.

Latex sensitivity: Use caution in patients with a possible history of latex sensitivity; the packaging contains dry natural rubber.

Hypersensitivity reactions: Epinephrine 1:1000 must be available to control immediate allergic reaction. Refer to Management of Acute Hypersensitivity Reactions.

Elderly: This vaccine is not recommended for use in adult populations.

Pregnancy: Category C.

Lactation: This vaccine is not recommended for use in nursing mothers.

Children: Pneumococcal 7-valent conjugate vaccine has been shown to be usually well-tolerated and immunogenic in infants. The safety and efficacy of pneumococcal 7-valent conjugate vaccine in children < 6 weeks of age have not been established. Immune responses elicited by pneumococcal 7-valent conjugate vaccine among infants born prematurely have not been studied. See Administration and Dosage for the recommended pediatric dosage.

Precautions
Route of administration: Pneumococcal 7-valent conjugate vaccine is for IM use only. Do not administer IV under any circumstances. The safety and immunogenicity for other routes of administration (eg, SC) have not been evaluated. Take special care to prevent injection into or near a blood vessel or nerve.

Drug Interactions
Immunosuppressive agents may interfere with vaccine. The vaccine should be used cautiously in children receiving anticoagulants.

Adverse Reactions
Adverse reactions occurring in ≥ 3% of patients include the following: Decreased appetite; vomiting; diarrhea; fever; drowsiness; irritability; restless sleep.

With vaccines in general, including pneumococcal 7-valent conjugate vaccine, it is not uncommon for patients to note within 48 to 72 hours at or around the injection site the following minor reactions: Edema; pain or tenderness; redness, inflammation, or skin discoloration; mass; or local hypersensitivity reaction. Such local reactions are usually self-limited and require no therapy.

As with other aluminum-containing vaccines, a nodule may occasionally be palpable at the injection site for several weeks.

HEPATITIS B VACCINE

Injection (adult formulation): 10 mcg/mL (*Rx*) **Injection (pediatric/adolescent formulation):** 5 mcg/0.5 mL (*Rx*)	*Recombivax HB* (Merck)
Injection (dialysis formulation): 40 mcg/mL (*Rx*) **Injection (adult formulation):** 20 mcg/mL (*Rx*) **Injection (pediatric formulation):** 10 mcg/0.5 mL (*Rx*)	*Engerix-B* (GlaxoSmithKline)

Indications

For immunization against infection caused by all known subtypes of hepatitis B virus. Because hepatitis D virus (caused by the delta virus) can only infect and cause illness in people infected with hepatitis B, immunity to hepatitis B also protects against hepatitis D.

Vaccination: Vaccination is recommended in people of all ages, especially in those at increased risk of infection with hepatitis B virus.

Healthcare personnel – Dentists; oral surgeons; physicians; surgeons; podiatrists; nurses; paramedical personnel and custodial staff who may be exposed via blood or patient specimens; dental hygienists and nurses; blood bank and plasma fractionation workers; laboratory personnel handling blood, blood products, and patient specimens; dental, medical, and nursing students; hospital cleaning staff who handle potentially infectious waste.

Selected patients and patient contacts – Patients and staff in hemodialysis units and hematology/oncology units; patients requiring frequent or large volume blood transfusions or clotting factor concentrates; residents and staff of institutions for the mentally challenged; classroom contacts of deinstitutionalized mentally challenged people who have persistent hepatitis B antigenemia and who show aggressive behavior; household and other intimate contacts of people with persistent hepatitis B antigenemia.

Adolescents – Because a vaccination strategy limited to high-risk individuals has failed to substantially lower the overall incidence of hepatitis B infection, the Immunization Practices Advisory Committee (ACIP) and the Committee on Infectious Diseases of the American Academy of Pediatrics (AAP) have endorsed universal infant immunization as part of a comprehensive strategy for the control of hepatitis B infection. These advisory groups further recommend broad-based vaccination of adolescents. All individuals not receiving the hepatitis B vaccine are recommended to be vaccinated at 11 to 12 years of age. In addition, vaccination is recommended in older unvaccinated adolescents at high-risk.

Infants, including those born to hepatitis B surface antigen (HBsAg)-positive mothers whether hepatitis B early antigen (HBeAg)-positive or -negative – CDC, ACIP, and AAP recommend routine vaccination of all infants against hepatitis B.

Populations with high incidence of the disease – Alaskan Eskimos; Pacific islanders; Indochinese immigrants; Haitian immigrants; immigrants from other HBV-endemic areas; all infants of women born in areas where the infection is highly endemic.

Individuals with chronic hepatitis C – Risk factors for hepatitis C are similar to those for hepatitis B. Consequently, immunization with hepatitis B vaccine is recommended for individuals with chronic hepatitis C.

Persons at increased risk because of their sexual practices – People who have heterosexual activity with multiple partners (eg, > 1 partner in a 6-month period), people who repeatedly contract sexually transmitted diseases, homosexually active males, and prostitutes.

Others at increased risk – Certain military personnel; morticians and embalmers; prisoners; users of illicit injectable drugs; police and fire department personnel who render first aid or medical assistance; blood bank and plasma-fractionation workers; adoptees from countries of high HBV endemicity; and any others who through their work or personal lifestyle may be exposed to the hepatitis B virus.

Unlabeled uses: Hepatitis B vaccination is appropriate for people expected to receive human alpha-1 proteinase inhibitor that is produced from heat-treated, pooled human plasma that may contain the causative agents of hepatitis and other viral diseases.

Administration and Dosage

Route and site: For IM use. Never inject IV or intradermally. The deltoid muscle is the preferred site in adults. Injections given in the buttocks frequently are given into fatty tissue instead of into muscle and have resulted in a lower seroconversion rate than expected. The anterolateral thigh is the recommended site in infants and young children. May be given SC to people at risk of hemorrhage following IM injection (eg, hemophiliacs). However, the SC route may produce a less than optimal response, and an increased incidence of local reactions, including SC nodules, may occur.

Immunization Regimen of Hepatitis B Vaccine Doses				
	Engerix-B		Recombivax HB	
Age group	Dose	Schedule[1]	Dose[2]	Schedule[1]
Infants[3] born of HBsAg-negative mothers HBsAg-positive mothers	10 mcg/0.5 mL 10 mcg/0.5 mL	Usual Either	5 mcg/0.5 mL[4] 5 mcg/0.5 mL[4]	Usual Usual
Children 0 to 10 years of age	10 mcg/0.5 mL	Either	5 mcg/0.5 mL[4]	Usual
Adolescents 11 to 19 years of age	10 mcg/0.5 mL	Usual	5 mcg/0.5 mL	Usual
Adults ≥ 20 years of age	20 mcg/1 mL	Either	10 mcg/1 mL	Usual
Adult predialysis, dialysis patients	40 mcg/2 mL[5]	0, 1, 2, 6 months	40 mcg/1 mL	Usual

[1] Usual dosing schedule is 0, 1, 6 months; alternate dosing schedule is 0, 1, 2, 12 months.
[2] If the suggested formulation is not available, the appropriate dosage can be achieved from another formulation provided that the total volume of vaccine administered does not exceed 1 mL. However, the dialysis formulation may only be used in adult dialysis patients.
[3] If the mother is determined to be HBsAg-positive within 7 days of delivery, immediately administer HBIG (0.5 mL) in the opposite antilateral thigh of the infant. The vaccine and HBIG can be administered at the same time as long as they are injected at different sites. If the 4-dose schedule for *Engerix-B* is used, give the third dose at 2 months of age and the fourth dose at 12 to 18 months of age.
[4] Infants and children who initiated their vaccination series with the 2.5 mcg dose may complete the 3-dose regimen with either the 2.5 mcg or 5 mcg dose. Begin all new vaccine regimens with the 5 mcg dose for infants and children.
[5] Two × 20 mcg in 1 or 2 injections.

Alternate schedule:
  Engerix-B – Designed for certain populations (eg, neonates born of hepatitis B infected mothers, others who have or might have been recently exposed to the virus, certain travelers to high-risk areas). On this alternate schedule, an additional dose at 12 months is recommended for infants born of infected mothers and for others for whom prolonged maintenance of protective titers is desired.
  Recombivax HB – An alternate schedule has been recommended. Give doses at 0, 1, and 2 months to provide rapid induction of immunity. On this alternate schedule, give an additional dose 12 months after the first dose if prolonged protection is needed.

Postexposure prophylaxis: In response to known or presumed exposure to hepatitis B surface antigen, give previously unvaccinated people postexposure prophylaxis. This consists of 0.06 mL/kg hepatitis B immune globulin (HBIG) as soon as possible or within 24 hours after exposure, if possible (within 14 days in the case of sexual contact). Give the appropriate volume of either hepatitis B vaccine based on age within 7 days of exposure, with additional vaccine doses either 1 and 6 months after the first dose or 1, 2, and 12 months later.

Revaccination (booster doses):
  Adults and children with normal immune status – The antibody response to properly administered vaccine is excellent, and protection lasts for ≥ 10 years. Booster doses

are not routinely recommended, nor is routine serologic testing to assess antibody levels in vaccine recipients necessary during this period.

Hemodialysis patients – The vaccine-induced protection is less complete and may persist only as long as antibody levels remain > 10 mIU/mL. Assess the need for booster doses by annual antibody testing; give booster doses when antibody levels are < 10 mIU/mL.

Vaccinated people who experience percutaneous or needle exposure to HBsAg-positive blood – Serologic testing to assess immune status is recommended unless tests have previously indicated adequate antibody levels. If inadequate levels exist, treat with HBIG or a booster dose of vaccine.

Nonresponders – Most people who do not initially respond to the primary series may develop adequate antibody concentrations after revaccination with a fourth or fifth dose or a new complete vaccine series. Give additional doses of vaccine to people who do not develop protective levels of anti-HBs antibodies after an initial 3-dose series.

Routine infant immunization:

Recombivax HB – From birth through 10 years of age, each dose consists of 5 mcg/ 0.5 mL.

Engerix-B – From birth through 10 years of age, each dose consists of 10 mcg/ 0.5 mL.

Revaccination (booster): See Pharmacology.

Hemodialysis patients (Engerix-B) – Assess need by annual antibody testing. Give 40 mcg (two 20 mcg doses) when antibody levels decline below 10 mIU/mL.

Recombivax HB dialysis formulation: Recombivax HB dialysis formulation is only for adult predialysis/dialysis patients.

Dosage – Recommended vaccination schedule is as follows: 40 mcg/mL initially, then 40 mcg/mL at 1 and 6 months.

Revaccination – A booster dose may be considered if the anti-HBs level is < 10 mIU/ mL 1 to 2 months after the third dose.

Preparation: Shake well before use to maintain suspension of the vaccine. After thorough agitation, the vaccine is a slightly opaque, white suspension. Use as supplied; no dilution or reconstitution is necessary.

Actions

Pharmacology: The recombinant hepatitis B vaccine is derived from HBsAg produced in yeast cells.

Antibody titers ≥ 10 mIU/mL against HBsAg are recognized as conferring protection against hepatitis B. Seroconversion is defined as antibody titers ≥ 1 mIU/mL. Duration of protective effect is unknown.

The vaccine induces protective anti-HBs antibody levels in 95% to 99% of healthy infants, children, and young adults who received the recommended regimen; lack of responsiveness to the vaccine can be attributed to genetic predisposition (eg, recessive trait associated with the major histocompatibility complex, male gender, obesity, smoking, gluteal vaccination, SC injection, freezing of vaccine, accelerated schedule, age > 40 years, immunocompromised and immunosuppressed individuals).

Interchangeability with hepatitis B vaccines – It is possible to interchange the use of vaccines for completion of a series or for booster doses because studies indicate the antibody produced in response to each type of vaccine is comparable. However, the quantity of antigen or the dosage volume will vary.

Contraindications

Hypersensitivity to yeast or any component of the vaccines.

Warnings

Hypersensitivity: Refer to Management of Acute Hypersensitivity Reactions.

Immunosuppressed patients: Immunosuppressed patients may require larger vaccine doses and may not respond as well as healthy individuals.

Unrecognized hepatitis B infection: Unrecognized hepatitis B infection may be present at the time the vaccine is given, and the vaccine may not prevent hepatitis B in such patients because of the long incubation period.

Limitations: No hepatitis B vaccine will protect against hepatitis A, C, and E viruses or other viruses known to infect the liver.

Elderly: Immunogenicity of hepatitis B vaccine is somewhat reduced in people > 40 years of age.

Pregnancy: Category C.

Lactation: Safety for use in the nursing mother has not been established. Empirical evidence suggests no harm.

Children: Hepatitis B vaccine is well-tolerated and highly immunogenic in infants and children of all ages. Newborns also respond well; maternally transferred antibodies do not interfere with the active immune response to the vaccine.

Precautions

Infection: Serious active infection is reason to delay use of hepatitis B vaccine, except when withholding the vaccine entails a greater risk.

Multiple sclerosis: Although no causal relationship has been established, rare instances of multiple sclerosis (MS) exacerbation have been reported following administration of hepatitis B vaccines and other vaccines. In people with MS, the benefit of immunization for prevention of hepatitis B infection and sequelae must be weighed against the risk of disease exacerbation.

Special risk: Give cautiously in severely compromised cardiopulmonary status or when a febrile or systemic reaction could be a significant risk.

Drug Interactions

Other vaccines: ACIP states that, in general, simultaneous administration of certain live and inactivated pediatric vaccines has not resulted in impaired antibody responses or increased rates of adverse reactions. Use separate sites and syringes for simultaneous administration of injectable vaccines.

HBIG, administered with hepatitis B vaccine at separate sites, does not interfere with induction of protective antibodies against hepatitis B virus.

Drugs that may interact with hepatitis B vaccine include immunosuppressants, yellow fever vaccine, anticoagulants, and interleukin-2.

Adverse Reactions

Adverse reactions may include the following: Erythema; swelling; warmth; induration; pain; tenderness; pruritus; rash; urticaria; petechiae; eczema; purpura; herpes zoster; alopecia; flushing; angioedema; nausea; vomiting; abdominal pain/cramps; dyspepsia; diminished appetite; anorexia; diarrhea; abnormal liver function tests; headache; lightheadedness; vertigo; dizziness; insomnia; disturbed sleep; somnolence; irritability; agitation; migraine; syncope; paresis; neuropathy including hypoesthesia, seizures, Guillain-Barré syndrome, Bell's palsy; transverse myelitis; arthralgia; myalgia; back/neck/arm/shoulder pain; neck stiffness; upper respiratory tract infection; influenza-like symptoms; bronchospasm; pharyngitis; fatigue/weakness; lymphadenopathy; tinnitus; earache; dysuria; hypertension; thrombocytopenia; conjunctivitis; keratitis; fever; malaise; hypotension; tachycardia/palpitations; visual disturbances; optic neuritis; multiple sclerosis; asthma-like symptoms; serum-sickness-like reactions of delayed onset days to weeks after vaccination.

HEPATITIS A VACCINE, INACTIVATED

Injection (pediatric formulation): 360 ELU/0.5 mL or 25 U/0.5 mL of viral antigen (*Rx*)	*Havrix* (GlaxoSmithKline), *Vaqta* (Merck)
Injection (adult formulation): 1440 ELU/1 mL or 50 U/1 mL of viral antigen (*Rx*)	

Indications

Hepatitis A virus (HAV): For active immunization of people ≥ 2 years of age against disease caused by HAV.

Primary immunization: Primary immunization should be completed at least 2 weeks prior to expected exposure to HAV. Immunization with hepatitis A vaccine is indicated for those people desiring protection against hepatitis A who are, or will be, at increased risk of infection by HAV:

Travelers – People traveling to areas of higher endemicity for hepatitis A.

Populations with high incidence of the disease – Native people of Alaska and the Americas.

People at increased risk because of their employment – Certain institutional workers (eg, caretakers for the developmentally challenged); employees of child day care centers; laboratory workers who handle live hepatitis A virus; handlers of primate animals that may be harboring HAV.

Others – People engaging in high-risk sexual activity (such as homosexually active males); users of illicit injectable drugs; residents of a community experiencing an outbreak of hepatitis A; military personnel; people living in or relocating to areas of high endemicity.

Administration and Dosage

Route and site: For IM use. Do not inject IV, ID, or SC. In adults, give the injection in the deltoid region. It should not be administered in the gluteal region; such injections may result in suboptimal response.

Primary immunization regimen:

Adults – A single dose of 1440 EL.U.

Children (2 to 18 years of age) – 2 doses, each containing 360 EL.U. given 1 month apart.

Booster dose – A booster dose is recommended anytime between 6 and 12 months after the initiation of the primary course in order to ensure the highest antibody titers.

In those with an impaired immune system, adequate anti-HAV response may not be obtained after the primary immunization course. Such patients may therefore require administration of additional doses of vaccine.

Contraindications

Hypersensitivity to any component of the vaccine.

Warnings

Hepatitis: Hepatitis A vaccine will not prevent hepatitis caused by other agents such as hepatitis B, C, or E virus or other pathogens known to infect the liver.

Hypersensitivity reactions: Epinephrine should be available for use in case of anaphylaxis or anaphylactoid reaction.

Pregnancy: Category C.

Lactation: It is not known whether the vaccine is excreted in breast milk.

Children: Hepatitis A vaccine is well tolerated and highly immunogenic and effective in children ≥ 2 years of age.

Precautions

Febrile illness: Febrile illness is reason to delay use of hepatitis A vaccine, except when withholding the vaccine entails a greater risk.

Bleeding disorders: Administer cautiously to people with thrombocytopenia or a bleeding disorder as bleeding may occur following IM use.

Immunosuppressed people: Immunosuppressed people or people receiving immunosuppressive therapy may not obtain the expected immune response.

Injection site: Do not inject into a blood vessel.

Drug Interactions

When concomitant administration of other vaccines or immune globulin is required, they should be given with different syringes and at different injection sites.

Adverse Reactions

Adverse reactions occurring in ≥ 3% of patients include injection site soreness/pain, tenderness, induration, redness, swelling, fatigue, fever, malaise, anorexia, nausea, and headache.

VARICELLA VIRUS VACCINE

Powder for injection: 1350 PFU of Oka/Merck varicella virus (live) (*Rx*)   *Varivax* (Merck)

Indications

Varicella: Vaccination against varicella in individuals ≥ 12 months of age.

Administration and Dosage

For SC administration; the outer aspect of the upper arm (deltoid) is the preferred site of injection. Do not inject IV. During clinical trials, some children received varicella vaccine IM resulting in seroconversion rates similar to those in children who received the vaccine by the SC route.

Children (1 to 12 years of age): A single 0.5 mL dose administered SC.

Adults and adolescents (≥ 13 years of age): A 0.5 mL dose administered SC at elected date and a second 0.5 mL dose 4 to 8 weeks later.

Actions

Pharmacology: Varicella virus vaccine is a preparation of the Oka/Merck strain of live, attenuated varicella virus.

Contraindications

Hypersensitivity to any component of the vaccine, including gelatin; history of anaphylactoid reaction to neomycin; individuals with blood dyscrasia, leukemia, lymphomas of any type, or other malignant neoplasms affecting the bone marrow or lymphatic systems; concomitant immunosuppressive therapy; individuals with primary and acquired immunodeficiency states, including those who are immunosuppressed in association with AIDS or other clinical manifestations of infection with HIV, cellular immune deficiencies, and hypogammaglobulinemic and dysgammaglobulinemic states; family history of congenital or hereditary immunodeficiency, unless the immune competence of the potential vaccine recipient is demonstrated; active untreated tuberculosis; any febrile respiratory illness or other active febrile infection; pregnancy.

Warnings

Booster doses: The duration of protection of varicella vaccine is unknown at present and the need for booster doses is not defined. Postmarketing surveillance studies are ongoing to evaluate the need and timing for booster vaccination.

Protection/Prevention: Vaccination with varicella vaccine may not result in protection of all healthy, susceptible children, adolescents, and adults. It is not known whether varicella vaccine given immediately after exposure to natural varicella virus will prevent illness.

Acute lymphoblastic leukemia (ALL): Children and adolescents with ALL in remission can receive the vaccine under an investigational protocol.

Hypersensitivity reactions: Have adequate treatment provisions, including epinephrine injection (1:1000), available for immediate use should an anaphylactoid reaction occur.

Pregnancy: Category C.

Lactation: It is not known whether varicella vaccine virus is excreted in breast milk.

Children: Administration to infants < 1 year of age is not recommended.

Precautions

Reye's syndrome: Vaccine recipients should avoid use of salicylates for 6 weeks after vaccination with varicella vaccine as Reye's syndrome has been reported following the use of salicylates during natural varicella infections.

Transmission: Individuals vaccinated with varicella vaccine potentially may be capable of transmitting the vaccine virus to close contacts. Therefore, vaccine recipients should avoid close association with susceptible high-risk individuals.

Immunodeficiency: The safety and efficacy of varicella vaccine have not been established in children and young adults who are known to be infected with HIV with and without evidence of immunosuppression. Vaccination should be deferred in patients with a family history of congenital or hereditary immunodeficiency until the patient's own immune system has been evaluated.

Drug Interactions

Drugs that may interact with varicella vaccine include immune globulins, immunosuppressants, and salicylates.

Concomitant vaccines: Results from clinical studies indicate that varicella vaccine can be administered concomitantly with MMR II.

Limited data from an experimental product containing varicella vaccine suggest that varicella vaccine can be administered concomitantly with DTaP and *Pedvax-HIB* (Haemophilus b conjugate vaccine) using separate sites and syringes.

Adverse Reactions

Adverse reactions occurring in ≥ 3% of patients include fever, injection site complaints, and varicella-like rash.

INTERFERON GAMMA-1B

Injection: 100 mcg (2 million IU/0.5 mL) (*Rx*)   *Actimmune* (InterMune Pharm.)

Indications
Chronic granulomatous disease (GCD): For reducing the frequency and severity of serious infections associated with chronic granulomatous disease.

Osteopetrosis: For delaying time to disease progression in patients with severe, malignant osteopetrosis.

Administration and Dosage
Chronic granulomatous disease: 50 mcg/m² (1 million IU/m²) for patients whose body surface area is > 0.5 m² and 1.5 mcg/kg/dose for patients whose body surface area is ≤ 0.5 m². Administer SC 3 times/week (eg, Monday, Wednesday, Friday). The optimum sites of injection are the right and left deltoid and anterior thigh.

Higher doses are not recommended. Safety and efficacy have not been established for interferon gamma given in doses greater or less than the recommended dose of 50 mcg/m². The minimum effective dose has not been established.

If severe reactions occur, modify the dosage (50% reduction) or discontinue therapy until the adverse reaction abates.

The formulation does not contain a preservative. Discard the unused portion of any vial.

Actions
Pharmacology: Interferon gamma-1b, a biologic response modifier, is a single-chain polypeptide containing 140 amino acids. Interferon gamma has potent phagocyte-activating effects not seen with other interferon preparations, including generation of toxic oxygen metabolites within phagocytes, which are capable of mediating the killing of microorganisms such as *Staphylococcus aureus*, *Toxoplasma gondii*, *Leishmania donovani*, *Listeria monocytogenes*, and *Mycobacterium avium intracellulare*. Interferon gamma-1b was found to enhance osteoclast function in vitro.

Pharmacokinetics: After IM or SC injection, the apparent fraction of dose absorbed was > 89%. The mean elimination half-life after IV administration was 38 minutes. The mean elimination half-lives for IM and SC dosing were 2.9 and 5.9 hours, respectively. Peak plasma concentrations occurred ≈ 4 hours after IM dosing and 7 hours after SC dosing.

Contraindications
Hypersensitivity to interferon gamma, *Escherichia coli* derived products, or any component of the product.

Warnings
CNS disorders: CNS adverse reactions including decreased mental status, gait disturbance, and dizziness have been observed, particularly in patients receiving doses > 250 mcg/m²/day. Most of these abnormalities were mild and reversible within a few days upon dose reduction or discontinuation of therapy. Exercise caution in patients with seizure disorders and compromised CNS function.

Cardiac disease: Use with caution in patients with pre-existing cardiac disease, including symptoms of ischemia, CHF, or arrhythmia.

Myelosuppression: Exercise caution in patients with myelosuppression. Reversible neutropenia and elevation of hepatic enzymes can be dose-limiting at doses > 250 mcg/m²/day.

Hypersensitivity reactions: Acute serious hypersensitivity reactions have not been observed in patients receiving interferon gamma; however, if such an acute reaction develops, discontinue the drug immediately and institute appropriate medical therapy. Refer to Management of Acute Hypersensitivity Reactions.

Pregnancy: Category C.

Lactation: It is not known whether interferon gamma is excreted in breast milk.

Children: Safety and efficacy in children < 1 year of age has not been established.

Precautions

Monitoring: In addition to tests normally required for monitoring patients with chronic granulomatous disease, the following laboratory tests are recommended for all patients prior to beginning therapy and at 3-month intervals during treatment: Hematologic tests including complete blood counts, differential and platelet counts; blood chemistries including renal and liver function tests; urinalysis.

Drug Interactions

Exercise caution when administering interferon gamma in combination with other potentially myelosuppressive agents. Possible depression of CYP450 hepatic metabolism of drugs.

Adverse Reactions

Adverse reactions may include fever, headache, rash, chills, injection site erythema or tenderness, fatigue, diarrhea, vomiting, nausea, abdominal pain, myalgia, and depression.

INTERFERON BETA

INTERFERON BETA-1a
Powder for injection, lyophilized: 33 mcg (6.6 mIU) (*Rx*)   *Avonex* (Biogen)
INTERFERON BETA-1b
Powder for injection, lyophilized: 0.3 mg (9.6 mIU) (*Rx*)   *Betaseron* (Berlex)

Indications
Interferon beta-1a:
> *Multiple sclerosis (MS)* – For the treatment of relapsing forms of MS to slow the accumulation of physical disability and decrease the frequency of clinical exacerbations.

Interferon beta-1b:
> *Multiple sclerosis (MS)* – For use in ambulatory patients with relapsing-remitting MS to reduce the frequency of clinical exacerbations. Relapsing-remitting MS is characterized by recurrent attacks of neurologic dysfunction followed by complete or incomplete recovery.

Administration and Dosage
Interferon beta-1a:
> *Relapsing/Remitting MS* – 30 mcg IM once/week.

Interferon beta-1b:
> *Relapsing/Remitting MS* – 0.25 mg SC every other day. Evidence of efficacy > 2 years is not known.

Administration: Withdraw 1 mL of reconstituted solution from the vial into a sterile syringe fitted with a 27-gauge needle and inject the solution SC. Sites for self-injection include arms, abdomen, hips, and thighs.

Actions
Pharmacology: Interferon beta-1a and beta-1b have antiviral and immunoregulatory activities. The mechanisms by which they exert their actions in MS are not clearly understood.

Pharmacokinetics:
> *Interferon beta-1a* – Biological response marker levels increase within 12 hours of dosing and remain elevated for ≥ 4 days. Peak biological response marker levels typically are observed 48 hours after dosing.

Pharmacokinetic Parameters Following 60 mcg Administration of Interferon Beta-1a				
Route	AUC (IU-hr/mL)	C_{max} (IU/mL)	T_{max} (range [hr])	Elimination half-life (hr)
IM	1352	45	9.8 (3 to 15)	10
SC	478	30	7.8 (3 to 18)	8.6

> *Interferon beta-1b* – Peak serum concentrations occurred between 1 and 8 hours. Bioavailability, based on a total dose of 0.5 mg given as 2 SC injections at different sites, was ≈ 50%.
> Mean serum clearance values ranged from 9.4 to 28.9 mL/min/kg and were independent of dose. Mean terminal elimination half-life values ranged from 8 minutes to 4.3 hours and mean steady-state volume of distribution values ranged from 0.25 to 2.88 L/kg. IV dosing 3 times/week for 2 weeks resulted in no accumulation of interferon beta-1a or beta-1b in the serum of patients.

Contraindications
Hypersensitivity to natural or recombinant interferon beta, albumin human, or any other component of the formulation.

Warnings
Chronic progressive MS: The safety and efficacy of interferon beta in chronic progressive MS have not been evaluated.

Suicide/Mental disorders: Inform patients to be treated with interferon beta that depression and suicidal ideation can be a side effect of the treatment and that they should report these symptoms immediately. Other mental disorders have been observed and can include anxiety, emotional lability, depersonalization, and confusion.

Seizures: Exercise caution when administering interferon beta to patients with pre-exisiting seizure disorder. It is not known whether these events were related to the effects of MS alone, to interferon beta or to a combination of both.

Cardiac disease: Closely monitor patients with cardiac disease, such as angina, CHF, or arrhythmia, for worsening of their clinical condition during initiation. Interferon beta does not have any known direct-acting cardiac toxicity; however, symptoms of flu syndrome seen with interferon beta therapy may prove stressful to patients with severe cardiac conditions.

Pregnancy: Category C.

Lactation: It is not known whether interferon beta is excreted in breast milk.

Children: Safety and efficacy in children < 18 years of age have not been established.

Precautions

Monitoring: The following laboratory tests are recommended prior to initiating therapy and at periodic intervals thereafter: Hemoglobin; complete and differential white blood cell counts; platelet counts; and blood chemistries including liver function tests.

Self-administration: Instruct patients in injection techniques to ensure the safe self-administration of interferon beta.

Flu-like symptoms complex: Flu-like symptoms complex was reported in 61% to 76% of the patients treated with interferon beta. A patient was defined as having a flu-like symptom complex if ≥ 2 of the following symptoms were concurrently reported: Fever, chills, myalgia, malaise, sweating, or flu-like syndrome. Only myalgia, fever, and chills were reported as severe in > 5% of the patients.

Photosensitivity: Photosensitization (photoallergy or phototoxicity) may occur.

Adverse Reactions

Adverse reactions occurring in ≥ 3% of patients may include injection site reaction, headache, fever, flu-like symptoms, pain, asthenia, chills, infection, abdominal pain, chest pain, malaise, generalized edema, pelvic pain, injection site necrosis/inflammation, cyst/ovarian cyst, suicide attempt, hypersensitivity reaction, migraine, palpitation, hypertension, tachycardia, peripheral vascular disorder, hemorrhage, syncope, vasodilation, lymphocytes < 1500/mm^3, ANC < 3000/mm^3, lymphadenopathy, anemia, eosinophils ≥ 10%, HCT (%) ≤ 37, sinusitis, upper respiratory tract infection, dyspnea, laryngitis, myalgia, myasthenia, arthralgia, nausea, diarrhea, constipation, vomiting, dyspepsia, anorexia, GI disorder, ALT > 5 × baseline, glucose < 55 mg/dL, total bilirubin > 2.5 × baseline, urine protein > 1 +, AST > 5 × baseline, weight gain/loss, AST ≥ 3 × ULN, mental symptoms, hypertonia, sleep difficulty, dizziness, muscle spasm, somnolence, speech disorder, convulsion, sweating, urticaria, alopecia, nevus, herpes zoster, conjunctivitis, abnormal vision, otitis media, hearing decreased, dysmenorrhea, menstrual disorder, metrorrhagia, cystitis, breast pain, menorrhagia, urinary urgency, vaginitis, fibrocystic breast.

ETANERCEPT

Powder for Injection, lyophilized: 25 mg (*Rx*)	*Enbrel*[1] (Immunex)

[1] Because of a probable temporary limited supply of etanercept, beginning January 1, 2001, patients must register for an *Enbrel Enrollment Card*. The enrollment cards will be needed by the pharmacy to order etanercept to fill prescriptions. Without prior enrollment, patients will be unable to receive the drug beginning January 1, 2001. To register, patients need to call 1-888-4ENBREL (1-888-436-2735) 24 hours/day, 7 days/week.

Indications

Rheumatoid arthritis (RA): For reduction in signs and symptoms and inhibiting the progression of structural damage in moderately to severely active RA. It can be used in combination with methotrexate (MTX) in patients who do not respond adequately to MTX alone.

Polyarticular-course juvenile rheumatoid arthritis (JRA): For reducing signs and symptoms of moderately to severely active polyarticular-course JRA in patients who have had an inadequate response to ≥ 1 disease-modifying antirheumatic drug (DMARD).

Administration and Dosage

Adults: 25 mg given twice weekly as an SC injection 72 to 96 hours apart. MTX, glucocorticoids, salicylates, nonsteroidal anti-inflammatory drugs (NSAIDs), or analgesics may be continued during treatment. Higher doses have not been studied.

Children (4 to 17 years of age): The recommended dose of etanercept for children 4 to 17 years of age with active polyarticular-course JRA is 0.4 mg/kg (up to a maximum of 25 mg/dose) given SC twice weekly 72 to 96 hours apart. Glucocorticoids, NSAIDs, or analgesics may be continued during treatment with etanercept. Concurrent use with MTX and higher doses of etanercept have not been studied in pediatric patients.

Admixture incompatibilities: Do not add other medications to solutions containing etanercept, and do not reconstitute with other diluents. Do not filter reconstituted solution during preparation or administration.

Self-administration: Etanercept is intended for use under the guidance and supervision of a physician. Patients may self-inject only if the physician determines that it is appropriate and medical follow-up is provided, as necessary, after proper training in injection technique and how to measure the correct dose.

Rotate injection sites (thigh, abdomen, or upper arm). Give new injections ≥ 1 inch from an old site and never into areas where the skin is tender, bruised, red, or hard.

Actions

Pharmacology: Etanercept, used for RA, is a dimeric fusion protein consisting of the extracellular ligand-binding portion of the human 75 kd (p75) tumor necrosis factor receptor (TNFR) linked to the Fc portion of human IgG1. Etanercept binds specifically to tumor necrosis factor (TNF) and blocks its interaction with cell surface TNFRs. TNF is a naturally occurring cytokine that is involved in normal inflammatory and immune responses. It plays an important role in the inflammatory processes of RA, polyarticular-course JRA, and the resulting joint pathology.

Pharmacokinetics:

Absorption/Distribution – After administration of 25 mg of etanercept by a single SC injection to 25 patients with RA, a mean half-life of ≈ 102 hours was observed with a clearance of ≈ 160 mL/hr. A maximum serum concentration (C_{max}) of ≈ 1.1 mcg/mL and time to C_{max} of ≈ 69 hours was observed in these patients. Patients exhibited a 2- to 7-fold increase in peak serum concentrations and an ≈ 4-fold increase in $AUC_{0-72\ hr}$ (range, 1- to 17-fold) with repeated dosing.

Pediatric patients 4 to 17 years of age with JRA were administered 0.4 mg/kg of etanercept twice weekly for ≤ 18 weeks. The mean serum concentration after repeated SC dosing was 2.1 mcg/mL (range, 0.7 to 4.3 mcg/mL).

Contraindications

Sepsis; hypersensitivity to etanercept or any of its components.

Warnings

Infections: In postmarketing reports, serious infections and sepsis, including fatalities, have been reported with the use of etanercept. Many of these serious infections have occurred in patients on concomitant immunosuppressive therapy that, in addition to their underlying disease, could predispose them to infections. Rare cases of tuberculosis (TB) have been observed in patients treated with TNF antagonists, including etanercept.

Neurologic events: Treatment with etanercept and other agents that inhibit TNF have been associated with rare cases of new onset or exacerbation of CNS demyelinating disorders, some presenting with mental status changes and some associated with permanent disability. Rare cases of transverse myelitis, optic neuritis, and new onset or exacerbation of seizure disorders have been observed in association with etanercept therapy. Other TNF antagonists administered to patients with MS have been associated with increases in disease activity. Exercise caution in considering the use of etanercept in patients with pre-existing or recent-onset CNS demyelinating disorders.

Hematologic events: Rare reports of pancytopenia including aplastic anemia, some fatal, have been reported in patients with RA treated with etanercept. Advise all patients to seek immediate medical attention if they develop signs and symptoms suggestive of blood dyscrasias or infection (eg, persistent fever, bruising, bleeding, pallor) while on etanercept.

Hypersensitivity reactions: Allergic reactions associated with etanercept during clinical trials have been reported in < 2% of patients.

Elderly: No overall differences in safety or effectiveness were observed in clinical trials between elderly and younger patients. However, because there is a higher incidence of infections in the elderly population in general, use caution in treating the elderly.

Pregnancy: Category B.

Lactation: It is not known whether etanercept is excreted in breast milk or absorbed systemically after ingestion. Because many drugs and immunoglobulins are excreted in breast milk and because of the potential for serious adverse reactions in nursing infants from etanercept, decide whether to discontinue nursing or to discontinue the drug.

Children: Etanercept has not been studied in children < 4 years of age. Preliminary data suggest the clearance of etanercept is reduced slightly in children 4 to 8 years of age.

Precautions

Immunogenicity: Antibodies, all nonneutralizing, were detected at least once in sera of 5% of adult RA patients. No apparent correlation of antibody development to clinical response or adverse events was observed.

Injection site reactions: In controlled trials, 37% of patients developed injection site reactions. Reactions were mild to moderate (erythema or itching, pain, or swelling) and generally did not necessitate drug discontinuation.

Malignancies/Infections: The possibility exists for anti-TNF therapies, including etanercept, to affect host defenses against infections and malignancies because TNF mediates inflammation and modulates cellular immune responses.

Vaccinations: Do not give live vaccines concurrently with etanercept.

It is recommended that JRA patients, if possible, be brought up to date with all immunizations in agreement with current immunization guidelines prior to initiating therapy.

Autoantibodies: Treatment with etanercept may result in the formation of autoimmune antibodies.

Latex allergies: The needle cover of the diluent syringe contains dry natural rubber (latex), which should not be handled by people sensitive to this substance.

Benzyl alcohol: Benzyl alcohol, a preservative contained in the diluent supplied, has been associated with a fatal "gasping syndrome" in premature infants.

Adverse Reactions

The following adverse events were reported in ≥ 3% of all patients: Infection; headache; rhinitis; nausea; dizziness; pharyngitis; cough; asthenia; abdominal pain; rash; respiratory disorder; dyspepsia; sinusitis; vomiting; peripheral edema; mouth ulcer; alopecia; injection site reaction.

Children:

Miscellaneous – Adverse events in children were similar in frequency and type as those in adults. Differences from adults and other special considerations are discussed below.

Severe adverse reactions reported in 69 JRA patients from 4 to 17 years of age included varicella, gastroenteritis, depression/personality disorder, cutaneous ulcer, esophagitis/gastritis, group A streptococcal septic shock, type I diabetes mellitus, and soft tissue and postoperative wound infection.

The following adverse reactions were reported more commonly in 69 JRA patients receiving 3 months of etanercept compared with the 349 adult RA patients in placebo-controlled trials. These included headache (19%; 1.7 events per patient year), nausea (9%; 1 event per patient year), abdominal pain (19%; 0.74 events per patient year), and vomiting (13%; 0.74 events per patient year).

AZATHIOPRINE

Tablets: 50 mg (*Rx*)
Injection: 100 mg (as sodium)/vial (*Rx*)

Imuran (GlaxoSmithKline)
Various, *Imuran* (GlaxoSmithKline)

Warning:
> Chronic immunosuppression with azathioprine increases the risk of neoplasia. Physicians using this drug should be familiar with this risk as well as with the mutagenic potential to men and women and with possible hematologic toxicities.

Indications
Renal homotransplantation: As an adjunct for the prevention of rejection in renal homotransplantation.

Rheumatoid arthritis: Indicated only in adult patients meeting criteria for classic or definite rheumatoid arthritis as specified by the American Rheumatism Association. Restrict use to patients with severe, active, and erosive disease not responsive to conventional management.

Administration and Dosage
Renal homotransplantation: Initial dose is usually 3 to 5 mg/kg/day, given as a single daily dose on the day of transplantation, and in a minority of cases, 1 to 3 days before transplantation. It is often initiated IV, with subsequent use of tablets (at the same dose level) after the postoperative period. Reserve IV administration for patients unable to tolerate oral medications. Maintenance levels are 1 to 3 mg/kg/day.

  Children – An initial dose of 3 to 5 mg/kg/day IV or orally followed by a maintenance dose of 1 to 3 mg/kg/day has been recommended.

Rheumatoid arthritis: Initial dose is ≈ 1 mg/kg (50 to 100 mg) given as a single dose or twice daily. The dose may be increased, beginning at 6 to 8 weeks and thereafter by steps at 4-week intervals, if there are no serious toxicities and if initial response is unsatisfactory. Use dose increments of 0.5 mg/kg/day, up to a maximum dose of 2.5 mg/kg/day.

  Use the lowest effective dose for maintenance therapy; lower decrementally with changes of 0.5 mg/kg or ≈ 25 mg/day every 4 weeks while other therapy is kept constant.

Renal function impairment: Relatively oliguric patients, especially those with tubular necrosis in the immediate postcadaveric transplant period, may have delayed clearance of azathioprine or its metabolites.

Use with allopurinol: Reduce dose of azathioprine to ≈ 25% to 33% of the usual dose.

Actions
Pharmacology: Azathioprine, an imidazoyl derivative of 6-mercaptopurine (6-MP), has many biological effects similar to those of the parent compound.

  Homograft survival – Although the use of azathioprine for inhibition of renal homograft rejection is well established, the mechanism(s) for this action are obscure.

  Immuno-inflammatory response – The severity of adjuvant arthritis is reduced by azathioprine. The mechanisms whereby it affects autoimmune diseases are not known.

Pharmacokinetics: Azathioprine is well absorbed following oral administration. Blood levels are of little value for therapy because the magnitude and duration of clinical effects correlate with thiopurine nucleotide levels in tissues rather than with plasma drug levels.

Contraindications
Hypersensitivity to azathioprine; pregnancy in rheumatoid arthritis patients.

Warnings
Hematologic effects: Severe leukopenia or thrombocytopenia, macrocytic anemia, severe bone marrow depression, and selective erythrocyte aplasia may occur in patients on azathioprine. Hematologic toxicities are dose-related, may occur late in the course of therapy, and may be more severe in renal transplant patients whose homo-

graft is undergoing rejection. Perform complete blood counts, including platelet counts, weekly during the first month, twice monthly for the second and third months of treatment, then monthly or more frequently if dosage alterations or other therapy changes are necessary.

Infections: Serious infections are a constant hazard for patients on chronic immunosuppression, especially for homograft recipients. The incidence of infection in renal homotransplantation is 30 to 60 times that in rheumatoid arthritis. Fungal, viral, bacterial, and protozoal infections may be fatal and should be treated vigorously.

GI toxicity: A GI hypersensitivity reaction characterized by severe nausea and vomiting has been reported. These symptoms also may be accompanied by diarrhea, rash, fever, malaise, myalgias, elevations in liver enzymes, and, occasionally, hypotension.

Hepatotoxicity: Hepatotoxicity with elevated serum alkaline phosphatase and bilirubin may occur primarily in allograft recipients. Periodically measure serum transaminases, alkaline phosphatase and bilirubin for early detection of hepatotoxicity.

Carcinogenesis: Azathioprine is carcinogenic in animals and may increase the patient's risk of neoplasia.

Mutagenesis: Azathioprine is mutagenic in animals and humans.

Pregnancy: Category D.

Lactation: Use of azathioprine in nursing mothers is not recommended.

Children: Safety and efficacy in children have not been established. However, azathioprine has been used in children.

Drug Interactions
Drugs that may affect azathioprine include ACE inhibitors, allopurinol, and methotrexate.

Drugs that may be affected by azathioprine include anticoagulants, cyclosporine, and nondepolarizing neuromuscular blockers.

Adverse Reactions
The principal and potentially serious toxic effects are hematologic and GI. Adverse reactions may include leukopenia, infections, and neoplasia.

TACROLIMUS (FK506)

Capsules: 0.5, 1, and 5 mg *(Rx)*   *Prograf* (Fujisawa)
Injection: 5 mg/mL *(Rx)*

Tacrolimus also is available as a cream for moderate to severe atopic dermatitis; refer to Dermatologics chapter.

> **Warning:**
> Increased susceptibility to infection and the possible development of lymphoma may result from immunosuppression. Manage patients receiving the drug in facilities equipped and staffed with adequate laboratory and supportive medical resources.

Indications
Organ (liver) rejection prophylaxis: Prophylaxis of organ rejection in patients receiving allogeneic liver transplants. It is recommended that tacrolimus be used concomitantly with adrenal corticosteroids.

Administration and Dosage
Injection: For IV infusion only.

In patients unable to take the capsules, therapy may be initiated with the injection. Administer the initial dose no sooner than 6 hours after transplantation. The recommended starting dose is 0.05 to 0.1 mg/kg/day as a continuous IV infusion.

Give adult patients doses at the lower end of the dosing range. Concomitant adrenal corticosteroid therapy is recommended early posttransplantation. Proceed with continuous IV infusion only until the patient can tolerate oral administration.

Oral: It is recommended that patients be converted from IV to oral therapy as soon as oral therapy can be tolerated. This usually occurs within 2 to 3 days. Give the first dose of oral therapy 8 to 12 hours after discontinuing the IV infusion. The recommended starting oral dose is 0.15 to 0.3 mg/kg/day administered in 2 divided daily doses every 12 hours. Administer the initial dose no sooner than 6 hours after transplantation. Give adult patients doses at the lower end of the dosing range.

Children (< 12 years of age): It is recommended that therapy be initiated in pediatric patients at the high end of the recommended adult IV and oral dosing ranges (0.1 mg/kg/day IV and 0.3 mg/kg/day oral).

Hepatic/Renal function impairment: Because of the potential for nephrotoxicity, give patients with renal or hepatic impairment doses at the lowest value of the recommended IV and oral dosing ranges.

Conversion from one immunosuppressive regimen to another: Do not use tacrolimus simultaneously with cyclosporine. Discontinue either agent ≥ 24 hours before initiating the other.

Actions

Pharmacology: Tacrolimus is a macrolide immunosuppressant that prolongs the survival of the host and transplanted graft and inhibits T-lymphocyte activation, although the exact mechanism of action is not known.

Pharmacokinetics:

Pharmacokinetic Parameters of Tacrolimus in Whole Blood After Oral Administration					
Population	Dose (mg/kg/12 h)	C_{max} (ng/mL)	T_{max} (hr)	AUC (ng/mL•hr)	Absolute bioavailability
Liver transplant patients (n = 17)	0.15	68.5	2.3	519	21.8
Food	0.15	27.1	3.2	223	-
Fasting	0.15	52.4	1.5	290	-

The disposition of tacrolimus from whole blood was biphasic with a terminal elimination half-life of 11.7 hours in liver transplant patients.

Contraindications

Hypersensitivity to tacrolimus; hypersensitivity to HCO-60 polyoxyl 60 hydrogenated castor oil (used in vehicle for injection).

Warnings

Nephrotoxicity: Tacrolimus can cause nephrotoxicity, particularly when used in high doses. Nephrotoxicity has been noted in 33% to 40% of liver transplantation patients receiving the drug.

Hyperkalemia: Mild to severe hyperkalemia has been noted in liver transplant recipients treated with tacrolimus and may require treatment.

Neurotoxicity: Neurotoxicity, including tremor, headache, and other changes in motor function, mental status, and sensory function occurred in ≈ 55% of liver transplant recipients. Tremor and headache have been associated with high whole-blood concentrations of tacrolimus and may respond to dosage adjustment. Seizures have occurred in adult and pediatric patients. Coma and delirium also have been associated with high plasma concentrations of tacrolimus.

Lymphomas: As with other immunosuppressants, patients receiving tacrolimus are at increased risk of developing lymphomas and other malignancies, particularly of the skin.

Hypersensitivity reactions: A few patients receiving the injection have experienced anaphylactic reactions. Although the exact cause of these reactions is not known, other drugs with castor oil derivatives in the formulation have been associated with anaphylaxis in a small percentage of patients.

Continuously observe patients receiving the injection for at least the first 30 minutes following the start of the infusion and at frequent intervals thereafter.

Renal/Hepatic function impairment: The use of tacrolimus in liver transplant recipients experiencing posttransplant hepatic impairment may be associated with increased risk of developing renal insufficiency related to high whole-blood levels of tacrolimus.

Carcinogenesis: An increased incidence of malignancy is a recognized complication of immunosuppression in recipients of organ transplants.

Pregnancy: Category C. The use of tacrolimus during pregnancy has been associated with neonatal hyperkalemia and renal dysfunction.

Lactation: Tacrolimus is excreted in breast milk; avoid nursing.

Precautions

Monitoring: Regularly assess serum creatinine and potassium. Perform routine monitoring of metabolic and hematologic systems as clinically warranted.

Hypertension: Hypertension is a common adverse effect of tacrolimus therapy. Mild or moderate hypertension is more frequently reported than severe hypertension.

Hyperglycemia: Hyperglycemia was associated with the use of tacrolimus in 29% to 47% of liver transplant recipients and may require treatment.

Drug Interactions

Drugs that may affect tacrolimus include nephrotoxic agents (aminoglycosides, amphotericin B, cisplatin, cyclosporine), antifungals, bromocriptine, calcium channel blockers, cimetidine, clarithromycin, danazol, diltiazem, erythromycin, methylprednisolone, metoclopramide, carbamazepine, phenobarbital, phenytoin, and rifamycins.

Drugs that may be affected by tacrolimus include vaccines.

Because tacrolimus is metabolized mainly by the cytochrome P450 IIIA enzyme systems, substances known to inhibit or induce these enzymes may affect the metabolism of tacrolimus with resultant increases or decreases in whole blood or plasma levels.

Drug/Food interactions: The presence of food reduced the absorption of tacrolimus (decrease in AUC and C_{max} and increase in T_{max}). The relative oral bioavailability (whole blood) was reduced by 27% compared with the fasting state.

Adverse Reactions

The principal adverse reactions of tacrolimus are tremor, headache, diarrhea, hypertension, nausea, and renal dysfunction. Other reactions may include insomnia, paresthesia, constipation, anorexia, vomiting, anemia, leukocytosis, thrombocytopenia, hyperglycemia, dyspnea, prutitus, rash, abdominal pain, fever, asthenia, back pain, ascites and peripheral edema, abnormal dreams, agitation, anxiety, confusion, convulsion, depression, dizziness, hallucinations, incoordination, nervousness, somnolence, abnormal thinking, abnormal vision, tinnitus, dyspepsia, flatulence, GI hemorrhage, GI perforation, hepatitis, increased appetite, jaundice, liver damage, oral moniliasis, chest pain, hypotension, tachycardia, hematuria, hyperlipemia, hyperphosphatemia, hyperuricemia, hypocalcemia, hypophosphatemia, hyponatremia, diabetes mellitus, coagulation disorder, ecchymosis, leukopenia, prothrombin decreased, abdomen enlarged, chills, peritonitis, photosensitivity reaction, arthralgia, generalized spasm, leg cramps, myalgia, asthma, bronchitis, cough increased, pulmonary edema, pharyngitis, rhinitis, sinusitis, voice alteration, alopecia, hirsutism, sweating.

SIROLIMUS

Tablets: 1 mg (*Rx*)   *Rapamune* (Wyeth Labs.)
Solution, oral: 1 mg/mL (*Rx*)   *Rapamune* (Wyeth Labs.)

Warning:

Increased susceptibility to infection and the possible development of lymphoma may result from immunosuppression. Only physicians experienced in immunosuppressive therapy and management of renal transplant patients should use sirolimus. Manage patients receiving the drug in facilities equipped and staffed with adequate laboratory and supportive medical resources. The physician responsible for maintenance therapy should have complete information needed for the follow-up of the patient.

Indications

Organ rejection: Prophylaxis of organ rejection in patients receiving renal transplants. It is recommended that sirolimus be used in a regimen with cyclosporine and corticosteroids.

Administration and Dosage

It is recommended that sirolimus be used in a regimen with cyclosporine and corticosteroids. Coadministration of sirolimus and cyclosporine A reduces rejection episode frequency, permits reductions in cyclosporine dosage, and facilitates corticosteroid withdrawal. Sirolimus is to be administered orally once daily. Administer the initial dose of sirolimus as soon as possible after transplantation. For de novo transplant recipients, give a loading dose of sirolimus 3 times the maintenance dose. A daily maintenance dose of 2 mg with a 6 mg loading dose is recommended for use in renal transplant patients. A 5 mg daily maintenance dose with a 15 mg loading dose was shown to be safe and effective. No efficacy advantage over the 2 mg dose could be established for renal transplant patients. Patients receiving 2 mg/day demonstrated an overall better safety profile than did patients receiving 5 mg/day. It is recommended that sirolimus be taken 4 hours after cyclosporine.

To minimize the variability of exposure to sirolimus, this drug should be taken consistently with or without food. Grapefruit juice reduces CYP3A4-mediated metabolism of sirolimus and must not be administered with sirolimus or used for dilution.

Oral solution: 2 mg of oral solution has been demonstrated to be clinically equivalent to 2 mg oral tablets, making them interchangeable on a milligram-to-milligram basis. However, it is not known if higher doses of oral solution are clinically equivalent to higher doses of tablets on a milligram-to-milligram basis. Patients receiving 2 mg/day oral solution demonstrated an overall better safety profile than did patients receiving 5 mg/day oral solution.

Patients ≥ 13 years of age weighing < 40 kg (88 lb): Adjust the initial dosage based on body surface area to 1 mg/m^2/day. The loading dose should be 3 mg/m^2 in this population.

Hepatic function impairment: Reduce the maintenance dose of sirolimus by ≈ 33% in patients with hepatic function impairment. It is not necessary to modify the sirolimus loading dose.

Renal function impairment: Dosage need not be adjusted.

Blood concentration monitoring: Routine therapeutic drug level monitoring is not required in most patients. Monitor blood sirolimus levels in pediatric patients; in patients with hepatic function impairment, during concurrent administration of strong CYP3A4 inducers and inhibitors; and if cyclosporine dosing is markedly reduced or discontinued. In controlled clinical trials with concomitant cyclosporine, mean sirolimus whole blood trough levels, as measured by immunoassay, were 9 ng/mL for the 2 mg/day treatment group, and 17 ng/mL for the 5 mg/day dose. Results from other assays may differ from those with an immunoassay.

Instructions for dilution and administration:

Bottles – Use the amber oral dose syringe to withdraw the prescribed amount of sirolimus oral solution from the bottle. Empty the correct amount of sirolimus from the syringe into a glass or plastic container holding ≥ 2 ounces (¼ cup, 60 mL) of water or orange juice. No other liquids, including grapefruit juice, should be used for dilution. Stir vigorously and drink at once. Refill the container with an additional volume (minimum of 4 ounces [½ cup, 120 mL]) of water or orange juice, stir vigorously, and drink at once.

Pouches – When using the pouch, squeeze the entire contents of the pouch into a glass or plastic container holding ≥ 2 ounces (¼ cup, 60 mL) of water or orange juice. No other liquids, including grapefruit juice, should be used for dilution. Stir vigorously and drink at once. Refill the container with an additional volume (minimum of 4 ounces [½ cup, 120 mL]) of water or orange juice, stir vigorously, and drink at once.

Actions

Pharmacology: Sirolimus, a macrolide immunosuppressive agent, inhibits both T-lymphocyte activation and proliferation that occurs in response to antigenic and cytokine (interleukin-2, -4, and -15) stimulation and also inhibits antibody production. In cells, sirolimus binds to the immunophilin, FK binding protein-12 (FKBP-12), to generate an immunosuppressive complex.

Pharmacokinetics:

Absorption – Sirolimus is rapidly absorbed following oral administration, with a mean time-to-peak concentration of ≈ 1 hour after a single dose in healthy subjects and ≈ 2 hours after multiple oral doses in renal transplant recipients. The systemic bioavailability of sirolimus was estimated to be ≈ 14%.

Distribution – The mean volume of distribution is 12 L/kg. Sirolimus is extensively bound (≈ 92%) to human plasma proteins. The binding of sirolimus was shown mainly to be associated with serum albumin (97%), α_1-acid glycoprotein, and lipoproteins. The majority of sirolimus is sequestered in erythrocytes, resulting in considerably higher whole blood concentrations vs plasma concentrations. Sirolimus also is distributed in high concentrations to the heart, intestines, kidneys, liver, lungs, muscle, spleen, and testes.

Metabolism – Sirolimus is a substrate for both cytochrome P450 IIIA4 (CYP3A4) and P-glycoprotein. Sirolimus is extensively metabolized by O-demethylation and hydroxylation. Seven major metabolites, including hydroxy, demethyl, and hydroxydemethyl, are identifiable in whole blood. Some of these metabolites are also detectable in plasma, fecal, and urine samples. Glucuronide and sulfate conjugates are not present in any of the biologic matrices. Sirolimus is the major component in human whole blood and contributes to > 90% of the immunosuppressive activity.

Excretion – After a single dose of sirolimus in healthy volunteers, 91% was recovered from the feces and 2.2% was excreted in urine.

Contraindications

Hypersensitivity to sirolimus, its derivatives, or any component of the drug product.

Warnings

Infection/Lymphoma: Increased susceptibility to infection and the possible development of lymphoma may result from immunosuppression.

Lipids: Increased serum cholesterol and triglycerides that may require treatment occurred more frequently in patients treated with sirolimus compared to azathioprine or placebo controls.

Renal transplant patients have a higher prevalence of clinically significant hyperlipidemia. Accordingly, carefully consider the risk/benefit in patients with established hyperlipidemia before initiating an immunosuppressive regimen including sirolimus.

Monitor patients who are administered sirolimus for hyperlipidemia using laboratory tests. If hyperlipidemia is detected, initiate subsequent interventions such as diet, exercise, and lipid-lowering agents, as outlined by the National Cholesterol Education Program guidelines.

Concurrent immunosuppressants: Sirolimus has been administered concurrently with cyclosporine and corticosteroids. The efficacy and safety of the use of sirolimus in combination with other immunosuppressive agents have not been determined.

Renal function impairment: In phase III studies, mean serum creatinine was increased and mean glomerular filtration rate was decreased in patients treated with sirolimus and cyclosporine compared with those treated with cyclosporine and placebo or azathioprine controls. Monitor renal function during the administration of maintenance immunosuppression regimens including sirolimus in combination with cyclosporine, and consider appropriate adjustment of the immunosuppression regimen in patients with elevated serum creatinine levels. Exercise caution when using agents that are known to impair renal function (eg, aminoglycosides, amphotericin B).

Carcinogenesis: Animal studies have shown that sirolimus caused an increase in malignant lymphoma and testicular adenoma.

Fertility impairment: Animal studies have shown that sirolimus caused a reduction of testicular weight and histological lesions and reduced sperm counts.

Pregnancy: Category C.

Lactation: It is not known whether sirolimus is excreted in human breast milk. The pharmacokinetic and safety profiles of sirolimus in infants are not known. Because of the potential for adverse reactions in nursing infants from sirolimus, decide whether to discontinue nursing or to discontinue the drug, taking into account the importance of the drug to the mother.

Children: The safety and efficacy of sirolimus in pediatric patients < 3 years of age have not been established.

Precautions

Monitoring: It is prudent to monitor blood sirolimus levels in patients likely to have altered drug metabolism, patients ≥ 13 years of age who weigh < 40 kg, hepatically impaired patients, and during concurrent administration of potent CYP3A4 inducers and inhibitors. Trough concentrations ≥ 15 ng/mL are associated with an increased frequency of adverse effects.

Lymphocele: Lymphocele, a known surgical complication of renal transplantation, occurred significantly more often in a dose-related fashion in sirolimus-treated patients. Consider appropriate postoperative measures to minimize this complication.

Antimicrobial prophylaxis: Cases of *Pneumocystis carinii* pneumonia (PCP) have been reported in patients not receiving antimicrobial prophylaxis. Therefore, administer antimicrobial prophylaxis for PCP for 1 year following transplantation. Cytomegalovirus (CMV) prophylaxis is recommended for 3 months after transplantation, particularly for patients at increased risk for CMV disease.

Drug Interactions

P450 system: Sirolimus is extensively metabolized by the CYP3A4 isoenzyme in the gut wall and liver. Therefore, absorption and the subsequent elimination of systemically absorbed sirolimus may be influenced by drugs that affect this isoenzyme. Inhibitors of CYP3A4 may decrease the metabolism of sirolimus and increase sirolimus levels, while inducers of CYP3A4 may increase the metabolism of sirolimus and decrease sirolimus levels. Exercise care when concomitantly administering drugs metabolized by CYP3A4 with sirolimus.

Drugs that may increase sirolimus blood concentrations include the following: Nicardipine, verapamil, clotrimazole, fluconazole, itraconazole, clarithromycin, erythromycin, troleandomycin, cisapride, metoclopramide, bromocriptine, cimetidine, danazol, HIV-protease inhibitors, cyclosporine, diltiazem, ketoconazole.

Drugs that may decrease sirolimus levels include the following: Carbamazepine, phenobarbital, phenytoin, rifabutin, rifapentine, rifampin.

Drugs that may be affected by sirolimus include vaccines.

Drug/Food interactions: To minimize variability, sirolimus should be taken consistently with or without food (see Administration and Dosage).

Grapefruit juice reduced CYP3A4-mediated metabolism of sirolimus and must not be used for dilution.

Adverse Reactions

Adverse reactions occurring in ≥ 3% of patients include tremor, acne, constipation, diarrhea, nausea, increased serum creatinine, edema, hypercholesterolemia, hyperkalemia, hyperlipemia, hyperphosphatemia, peripheral edema, weight gain, rash, dyspepsia, vomiting, anemia, thrombocytopenia, leukopenia, dyspnea, pharyngitis, upper respiratory tract infection, abdominal pain, asthenia, back/chest pain, fever, headache, pain, arthralgia, urinary tract infection, hypertension.

Among the adverse events that were reported at a rate of ≥ 3% and < 20%, the following were more prominent in patients maintained on sirolimus 5 mg/day vs 2 mg/day: Epistaxis, lymphocele, insomnia, thrombotic thrombocytopenic purpura (hemolytic-uremic syndrome), skin ulcer, increased LDH, hypotension, facial edema.

MYCOPHENOLATE MOFETIL

Tablets: 500 mg (*Rx*)	*CellCept* (Roche)
Capsules: 250 mg (*Rx*)	*CellCept* (Roche)
Powder for Oral Suspension: 200 mg/mL (constituted) (*Rx*)	*CellCept* (Roche)
Powder for Injection, lyophilized: 500 mg (as HCl)	*CellCept* (Roche)

> **Warning:**
> Increased susceptibility to infection and the possible development of lymphoma may result from immunosuppression. Only physicians experienced in immunosuppressive therapy and management of renal, hepatic, or cardiac transplant patients should use mycophenolate. Manage patients receiving the drug in facilities equipped and staffed with adequate laboratory and supportive medical resources. The physician responsible for maintenance therapy should have complete information requisite for the follow-up of the patient.

Indications

Allogeneic transplants: For the prophylaxis of organ rejection in patients receiving allogeneic renal, hepatic, or cardiac transplants. Use mycophenolate concomitantly with cyclosporine and corticosteroids.

Unlabeled uses: Refractory uveitis (2 g/day alone or in combination with previous corticosteroid, cyclosporine, or tacrolimus therapy).

Administration and Dosage

Renal transplantation: 1 g administered orally or IV (over ≥ 2 hours) twice a day (daily dose of 2 g). Although a dose of 1.5 g twice daily (daily dose of 3 g) was used in clinical trials and was shown to be safe and effective, no efficacy advantage could be established for renal transplant patients. Patients receiving 2 g/day demonstrate an overall better safety profile than patients receiving 3 g/day.

Cardiac transplantation: 1.5 g administered orally or IV (over ≥ 2 hours) twice daily (daily dose of 3 g) is recommended.

Hepatic transplantation: 1 g twice daily administered IV (over ≥ 2 hours) or 1.5 g twice daily orally (daily dose of 3 g) is recommended.

Capsules, oral suspension, and tablets: Give the initial oral dose as soon as possible following transplantation. It is recommended that mycophenolate be administered on an empty stomach. However, in stable renal transplant patients, it may be administered with food if necessary.

If required, the oral suspension can be administered via a nasogastric tube with a minimum size of 8 French (minimum 1.7 mm interior diameter).

IV administration: Do not administer IV solution by rapid or bolus IV injection. Mycophenolate IV is recommended for patients unable to take capsules or tablets. Administer ≤ 24 hours following transplantation and for ≤ 14 days; switch patients to oral mychophenolate as soon as they can tolerate oral medication. Following reconstitution, administer by slow IV infusion over a period of ≥ 2 hours by peripheral or central vein.

Preparation of oral suspension: Tap the closed bottle several times to loosen the powder. Measure 94 mL of water in a graduated cylinder. Add ≈ ½ the total amount of water for constitution to the bottle and shake the closed bottle well for ≈ 1 minute. Add the remainder of water and shake the closed bottle well for ≈ 1 minute. Remove the child-resistant cap and push bottle adapter into neck of bottle. Close bottle with child-resistant cap tightly. This will assure the proper seating of the bottle adapter in the bottle and child-resistant status of the cap.

Preparation of infusion solution (6 mg/mL): Mycophenolate IV must be reconstituted and diluted to a concentration of 6 mg/mL using 5% Dextrose Injection. Mycophenolate IV is incompatible with other IV infusion solutions.

Mycophenolate IV does not contain an antibacterial preservative; use within 4 hours of reconstitution and dilution.

Reconstitute the contents of each vial with 14 mL of 5% Dextrose Injection. Gently shake the vial to dissolve the drug. The resulting solution is slightly yellow. Discard the vial if particulate matter or discoloration is observed.

Further dilute the contents of 2 reconstituted vials (for a 1 g dose) into 140 mL of 5% Dextrose Injection or 3 reconstituted vials (for a 1.5 g dose) into 210 mL of 5% Dextrose Injection. The final concentration of both solutions is 6 mg/mL. Discard the infusion solution if particulate matter or discoloration is observed.

Dosage adjustments: In patients with severe chronic renal impairment (GFR < 25 mL/min/1.73 m^2) outside of the immediate post-transplant period, avoid doses > 1 g administered twice a day; carefully observe these patients. No dose adjustments are needed in patients experiencing delayed graft function postoperatively. If neutropenia develops (ANC < 1.3 x 10^3/mcL), interrupt dosing or reduce the dose, perform appropriate diagnostic tests, and appropriately manage the patient.

Handling/Disposal: Because mycophenolate has demonstrated teratogenic effects in rats and rabbits, do not crush tablets, and do not open or crush the capsules. Avoid inhalation or direct contact with skin or mucous membranes of the powder contained in mycophenolate capsules, oral suspension, and injection (before or after constitution). If such contact occurs, wash thoroughly with soap and water; rinse eyes with plain water. Should a spill occur, wipe up using paper towels wetted with water to remove spilled powder or suspension.

Admixture incompatibility: Do not mix or administer mycophenolate IV concurrently via the same infusion catheter with other IV drugs or infusion admixtures.

Actions

Pharmacology: Mycophenolate is rapidly absorbed following oral administration and hydrolyzed to form MPA, which is the active metabolite. MPA is a potent, selective, uncompetitive and reversible inhibitor of inosine monophosphate dehydrogenase (IMPDH), and therefore inhibits the de novo pathway of guanosine nucleotide synthesis without incorporation into DNA.

Pharmacokinetics:

Absorption/Distribution – Following oral and IV administration, mycophenolate undergoes rapid and extensive absorption and complete presystemic metabolism to MPA, the active metabolite.

In 12 healthy volunteers, the mean absolute bioavailability of oral mycophenolate relative to IV mycophenolate (based on MPA AUC) was 94%. The AUC for MPA appears to increase in a dose-proportional fashion in renal trasplant patients receiving multiple doses of mycophenolate up to a daily dose of 3 g.

Immediately post-transplant (< 40 days), mean AUC and C_{max} are $\approx$ 45% to 50% and 20% to 30% lower, respectively, as compared with healthy volunteers or with stable renal and cardiac transplant patients.

Metabolism – In addition to MPA, other metabolites of the 2-hydroxyethyl-morpholino moiety are also recovered in the urine.

Excretion – Negligible amount of drug is excreted as MPA (< 1% of dose) in the urine. Oral administration resulted in complete recovery of the administered dose; 93% was recovered in the urine and 6% recovered in feces. Most (about 87%) of the administered dose is excreted in the urine as MPAG (phenolic glucuronide of MPA).

Mean Pharmacokinetic Parameters for MPA Following Mycophenolate Administration				
Parameter	Dose/ Route	T_{max} (hr)	C_{max} (mcg/mL)	AUC (mcg•hr/mL)
Healthy volunteers (n = 129) (single dose)	1 g/oral	$\approx$ 0.8	$\approx$ 24.5	$\approx$ 63.9 (n = 117)
Renal transplant patients				
Time after renal transplantation				
5 days (n = 31)	1 g bid/IV	$\approx$ 1.58	$\approx$ 12	$\approx$ 40.8[1]
6 days (n = 31)	1 g bid/oral	$\approx$ 1.33	$\approx$ 10.7	$\approx$ 32.9[1]
Early (< 40 days; n = 25)	1 g bid/oral	$\approx$ 1.31	$\approx$ 8.16	$\approx$ 27.3[1]
Early (< 40 days; n = 27)	1.5 g bid/oral	$\approx$ 1.21	$\approx$ 13.5	$\approx$ 38.4[1]
Late (> 3 months; n = 23)	1.5 g bid/oral	$\approx$ 0.9	$\approx$ 24.1	$\approx$ 65.3[1]
Cardiac transplant patients				
Time after cardiac transplantation				
Early (day before discharge)	1.5 g bid/oral	$\approx$ 1.8 (n = 11)	$\approx$ 11.5 (n = 11)	$\approx$ 43.3 (n = 9)[1]
Late (> 6 months)	1.5 g bid/oral	$\approx$ 1.1 (n = 52)	$\approx$ 20 (n = 52)	$\approx$ 54.1 (n = 49)[2]
Hepatic transplant patients				
Time after hepatic transplantation				
4 to 9 days (n = 22)	1 g bid/IV	$\approx$ 1.5	$\approx$ 17	$\approx$ 34[1]
Early (5 to 8 days) (n = 20)	1.5 g bid/oral	$\approx$ 1.15	$\approx$ 13.1	$\approx$ 29.2[1]
Late (> 6 months) (n = 6)	1.5 g bid/oral	$\approx$ 1.54	$\approx$ 19.3	$\approx$ 49.3[1]
Renal impairment (single dose) ($GFR, mL/min/1.73 m^2$)				
Healthy volunteers (GFR > 80; n = 6)	1 g/oral	$\approx$ 0.75	$\approx$ 25.3	$\approx$ 45[3]
Mild renal impairment (GFR 50 to 80; n = 6)	1 g/oral	$\approx$ 0.75	$\approx$ 26	$\approx$ 59.9[3]
Moderate renal impairment (GFR 25 to 49; n = 6)	1 g/oral	$\approx$ 0.75	$\approx$ 19	$\approx$ 52.9[3]
Severe renal impairment (GFR < 25; n = 7)	1 g/oral	$\approx$ 1	$\approx$ 16.3	$\approx$ 78.6[3]
Hepatic impairment (single dose)				
Healthy volunteers (n = 6)	1 g/oral	$\approx$ 0.63	$\approx$ 24.3	$\approx$ 29[4]
Alcoholic cirrhosis (n = 18)	1 g/oral	$\approx$ 0.85	$\approx$ 22.4	$\approx$ 29.8[4]

[1] Interdosing interval AUC_{0-12}.
[2] AUC_{0-12} values quoted are extrapolated from data from samples collected over 4 hours.
[3] Interdosing interval AUC_{0-96}.
[4] Interdosing interval AUC_{0-48}.

Contraindications

Hypersensitivity to the drug, mycophenolic acid, or any component of the drug product; people with a sensitivity to polysorbate 80 (*Tween*) (IV only).

Warnings

Lymphomas/Malignancies: Patients receiving immunosuppressive regimens involving combinations of drugs, including mycophenolate, as part of an immunosuppressive regimen are at increased risk of developing lymphomas and other malignancies, particularly of the skin. Lymphoproliferative disease or lymphoma developed in 0.4% to 1% of patients in the controlled studies of prevention of rejection.

Instruct patients to limit exposure to sunlight and UV light by wearing protective clothing and using a strong sunscreen.

Neutropenia: Up to 2% of renal transplant patients, up to 3.6% of hepatic transplant patients, and up to 2.8% of cardiac transplant patients receiving mycophenolate developed severe neutropenia. Neutropenia has been observed most frequently in the period from 31 to 180 days posttransplant in patients treated for prevention of rejection.

Renal function impairment: Avoid mycophenolate doses > 1 g administered twice a day and carefully observe patients.

No data are available for cardiac or hepatic transplant patients with severe chronic renal impairment. Mycophenolate may be used for cardiac or hepatic transplant patients with severe chronic renal impairment if the potential benefits outweigh the potential risks.

Elderly: Elderly patients, particularly those who are receiving mycophenolate as part of a combination immunosuppressive regimen, may be at increased risk of certain infections (including CMV tissue invasive disease) and possibly GI hemorrhage and pulmonary edema, compared with younger individuals.

Pregnancy: Category C.

Lactation: It is not known whether this drug is excreted in human milk. Because of the potential for serious adverse reactions in nursing infants from mycophenolate, decide whether to discontinue nursing or discontinue the drug, taking into account the importance of the drug to the mother.

Children: Safety and efficacy have not been established.

Precautions

Monitoring: Perform CBCs weekly during the first month of treatment, twice monthly for the second and third months, then monthly through the first year.

GI hemorrhage: GI tract hemorrhage has been observed in ≈ 3% of renal transplants, 5.4% of hepatic transplants, and 1.7% of cardiac transplants treated with mycophenolate 3 g/day. GI tract perforations rarely have been observed.

Delayed graft function: In patients with delayed graft function posttransplant, mean MPA AUC was comparable, but MPAG AUC was 2- to 3-fold higher, compared to that seen in posttransplant patients without delayed graft function. No dose adjustment is recommended for these patients; however, they should be carefully observed.

Rare hereditary deficiency: On theoretical grounds, because mycophenolate is an inosine monophosphate dehydrogenase (IMPDH) inhibitor, avoid in patients with rare hereditary deficiency of hypoxanthine-guanine phosphoribosyl-transferase (HGPRT), such as Lesch-Nyhan and Kelley-Seegmiller syndromes.

Phenylketonuria: Mycophenolate oral suspension contains aspartame, a source of phenylalanine (0.56 mg phenylalanine/mL suspension). Therefore, take care if the oral suspension is administered to patients with phenylketonuria.

Drug Interactions

Drugs that alter the GI flora: Drugs that alter the GI flora may interact with mycophenolate by disrupting enterohepatic recirculation. Interference of MPAG hydrolysis may lead to less MPA available for absorption.

Drugs that may be affected by mycophenolate include acyclovir, ganciclovir, live attenuated vaccines, oral contraceptives, phenytoin, and theophylline.

Drugs that may affect mycophenolate include acyclovir, antacids, azathioprine, cholestyramine, ganciclovir, iron, probenecid, and salicylates.

Drug/Food interactions: Food (27 g fat, 650 calories) had no effect on the extent of absorption (MPA AUC) of mycophenolate when administered at doses of 1.5 g twice daily to renal transplant patients. However, MPA C_{max} was decreased by 40% in the presence of food.

Adverse Reactions

The principal adverse reactions associated with mycophenolate include diarrhea, leukopenia, sepsis, and vomiting, and there is evidence of a higher frequency of certain types of infections.

Adverse reactions occurring in ≥ 10% of patients include pain; abdominal pain; fever; headache; infection; pain; accidental injury; chills; ascites; hernia; amblyopia; peritonitis; sepsis; asthenia; chest pain; back pain; hypertension; hypotension; cardiovascular disorder; tachycardia; arrhythmia; bradycardia; pericardial effusion; heart failure; anemia; leukopenia; ecchymosis; thrombocytopenia; hypochromic anemia; leukocytosis; urinary tract infection; oliguria; kidney tubular necrosis; hematuria; kidney tubular necrosis; peripheral edema; hypercholesterolemia; hypophosphatemia; edema; hyperglycemia; liver function tests, abnormal; creatinine increased; BUN increased; LDH increased; bilirubinemia; hypervolemia; hyperuricemia; AST increased; hypomagnesemia; acidosis; weight gain; ALT increased; hyponatremia; hyperlipemia; hypocalcemia; hypoproteinemia; hypoglycemia; healing abnormal; hypokalemia; hyperkalemia; diarrhea; constipation; nausea; dyspepsia; vomiting; flatulence; abdomen enlarged; anorexia; cholangitis; hepatitis; cholestatic jaundice; oral moniliasis; dyspnea; cough increased; lung disorder; sinusitis; rhinitis; pleural effusion; asthma; atelectasis; pharyngitis; pneumonia; acne; rash; skin disorder; pruritus; sweating; tremor; insomnia; anxiety; paresthesia; hypertonia; depression; agitation; somnolence; confusion; nervousness; dizziness; leg cramps; myasthenia; myalgia.

Patients receiving mycophenolate 2 g/day had an overall better safety profile than did patients receiving 3 g/day. Sepsis, which was generally CMV viremia, was slightly more common in renal transplant patients treated with mycophenolate, compared with patients receiving azathioprine. The incidence of sepsis was comparable to mycophenolate and in azathioprine-treated patients in cardiac and hepatic studies. In the digestive system, diarrhea was increased in renal and cardiac transplant patients receiving mycophenolate compared with patients receiving azathioprine, but was comparable in hepatic transplant patients treated with mycophenolate or azathioprine. Severe neutropenia developed in ≤ 2% of renal transplant patients, ≤ 2.8% of cardiac transplant patients, and ≤ 3.6% of hepatic transplant patients receiving mycophenolate 3 g daily (see Warnings).

Viral and Fungal Infections in Prevention of Renal, Cardiac, or Hepatic Transplant Rejection with Mycophenolate (%)[1]							
	Renal studies			Cardiac study		Hepatic study	
Infection	Mycophenolate 2 g/day (n = 336)	Mycophenolate 3 g/day (n = 330)	Azathioprine 1 to 2 mg/ kg/day or 100 to 150 mg/day (n = 326)	Mycophenolate 3 g/day (n = 289)	Azathioprine 1.5 to 3 mg/ kg/day (n = 289)	Mycophenolate 3 g/day (n = 277)	Azathioprine 1 to 2 mg/ kg/day (n = 287)
Herpes simplex	16.7	20	19	20.8	14.5	10.1	5.9
CMV							
Viremia/ Syndrome	13.4	12.4	13.8	12.1	10	14.1	12.2
Tissue invasive disease	8.3	11.5	6.1	11.4	8.7	5.8	8
Herpes zoster	6	7.6	5.8	10.7	5.9	4.3	4.9
Cutaneous disease	6	7.3	5.5	10	5.5	4.3	4.9
Candida	17	17.3	18.1	18.7	17.6	22.4	24.4
Mucocutaneous	15.5	16.4	15.3	18	17.3	18.4	17.4

[1] Data pooled from 3 separate studies and are not necessarily comparable.

CYCLOSPORINE (Cyclosporin A)

Capsules, soft gelatin: 25 and 50 mg (Rx)	*Sandimmune* (Sandoz)
Capsules, soft gelatin for microemulsion: 25 and 100 mg (Rx)	*Neoral* (Sandoz)
Oral solution: 100 mg/mL (Rx)	*Sandimmune* (Sandoz)
Oral solution for microemulsion: 100 mg/mL (Rx)	*Neoral* (Sandoz)
IV solution: 50 mg/mL (Rx)	*Sandimmune* (Sandoz)

Warning:

Administer *Sandimmune* with adrenal corticosteroids but not with other immuno-suppressants. Increased susceptibility to infection and the possible development of lymphoma may result from immunosuppression. Cyclosporine for micro-emulsion (*Neoral*) may be given with other immunosuppressants.

Sandimmune capsules and oral solution have decreased bioavailability compared with *Neoral*. *Sandimmune* and *Neoral* are not bioequivalent and cannot be used inter-changeably without physician supervision.

Absorption during chronic *Sandimmune* use is erratic. Monitor blood levels at repeated intervals and make dose adjustments to avoid toxicity (high levels) or possible organ rejection (low absorption). This is of special importance in liver transplants. For a given trough concentration, cyclosporine exposure will be greater with *Neoral* than with *Sandimmune*. If a patient who is receiving exceptionally high doses of *Sandimmune* is converted to *Neoral*, use particular caution.

Psoriasis patients: Psoriasis patients previously treated with PUVA and, to a lesser extent, methotrexate or other immunosuppressive agents, UVB, coal tar, or radiation therapy, are at an increased risk of developing skin malignancies when taking *Neoral*.

Cyclosporine in recommended dosages can cause systemic hypertension and nephrotoxicity. The risk increases with increasing dose and duration of cyclosporine therapy. Renal dysfunction, including structural kidney damage, is a potential consequence of therapy; therefore, monitor renal function during therapy. Susceptibility to infection and the development of neoplasia also is increased.

Indications

Allogeneic transplants: Prophylaxis of organ rejection in kidney, liver, and heart alloge-neic transplants. *Sandimmune* is always to be taken in conjunction with adrenal corticosteroids; *Neoral* has been used in combination with azathioprine and cortico-steroids. *Sandimmune* also may be used to treat chronic rejection in patients pre-viously treated with other immunosuppressants. Because of the risk of anaphylaxis, reserve the injection for patients unable to take the capsule or oral solution.

Rheumatoid arthritis (Neoral only): Alone or in combination with methotrexate for the treatment of patients with severe, active rheumatoid arthritis when the disease has not adequately responded to methotrexate.

Psoriasis (Neoral only): Treatment of adult, nonimmunocompromised patients with severe (eg, extensive or disabling), recalcitrant plaque psoriasis who failed to respond to ≥ 1 systemic therapy (eg, PUVA, retinoids, methotrexate) or patients for whom other systemic therapies are contraindicated or cannot be tolerated.

Unlabeled uses: The following conditions have been treated with cyclosporine (oral dos-ages have ranged from 1 to 10 mg/kg/day): Alopecia areata; aplastic anemia; atopic dermatitis; Behcet's disease; biliary cirrhosis; corneal transplantation or other eye diseases which have an autoimmune component (compounded into ophthalmic drops; cyclosporine has orphan drug status for ophthalmic use); Crohn's disease; ulcerative colitis; dermatomyositis; Graves' ophthalmopathy; type 1 diabetes melli-tus (see Glucose metabolism in Warnings); lichen planus (topical preparation);

lupus nephritis; multiple sclerosis; myasthenia gravis; nephrotic syndrome; pemphigus and pemphigoid; polymyositis; psoriatic arthritis; pulmonary sarcoidosis; pyoderma gangrenosum; uveitis.

Administration and Dosage

Bioequivalency: Sandimmune capsules and oral solution have decreased bioavailability compared with Neoral. Sandimmune and Neoral are not bioequivalent and cannot be used interchangeably without physician supervision. Neoral capsules and oral solution are bioequivalent. Sandimmune capsules and oral solution are bioequivalent.

Adjunct therapy: Adjunct therapy with adrenal corticosteroids is recommended.

Sandimmune:

Initial – 15 mg/kg/day 4 to 12 hours prior to transplantation. There is a trend toward use of even lower initial doses for renal transplantation in the ranges of 10 to 14 mg/kg/day. Continue dose postoperatively for 1 to 2 weeks, then taper by 5% per week to a maintenance level of 5 to 10 mg/kg/day. Some centers successfully tapered the dose to as low as 3 mg/kg/day in selected renal transplant patients without an apparent rise in rejection rate.

Parenteral – For infusion only. Patients unable to take the oral solution or capsules preoperatively or postoperatively may be given the IV concentrate. Use the IV form at ⅓ the oral dose.

Initial dose: 5 to 6 mg/kg/day given 4 to 12 hours prior to transplantation as a single IV dose. Continue this daily single dose postoperatively until the patient can tolerate the oral doseforms. Switch patients to oral therapy as soon as possible.

Children – May use same dose and dosing regimen, but higher doses may be required.

Neoral:

Initial dose – The initial dose of Neoral can be given 4 to 12 hours prior to transplantation or postoperatively. In newly transplanted patients, the initial dose of Neoral is the same as the initial oral dose of Sandimmune. The mean doses were 9 mg/kg/day for heart transplant patients, 8 mg/kg/day for liver transplant patients and 7 mg/kg/day for heart transplant patients. Divide total daily dose into 2 equal daily doses. The Neoral dose is subsequently adjusted to achieve a predefined cyclosporine blood concentration. If cyclosporine trough blood concentrations are used, the target range is the same for Neoral as for Sandimmune. Using the same trough concentration target range as for Sandimmune results in greater cyclosporine exposure when Neoral is administered. Titrate dosing based on clinical assessments of rejection and tolerability. Lower Neoral doses may be sufficient as maintenance therapy.

Conversion from Sandimmune to Neoral – In transplanted patients who are considered for conversion to Neoral from Sandimmune, start Neoral with the same daily dose as was previously used with Sandimmune (1:1 dose conversion). Subsequently adjust Neoral to attain the preconversion cyclosporine blood trough concentration. Using the same trough concentration target range for Neoral as for Sandimmune results in greater cyclosporine exposure when Neoral is administered. Monitor blood trough concentration every 4 to 7 days until preconversion value is obtained.

Poor Sandimmune absorption – Patients with lower than expected cyclosporine blood trough concentrations in relation to the oral dose of Sandimmune may have poor or inconsistent absorption. After conversion to Neoral, patients tend to have higher cyclosporine concentrations. Because of the increase in bioavailability following conversion to Neoral, the cyclosporine blood trough concentration may exceed the target range. Exercise particular caution when converting patients to Neoral at doses > 10 mg/kg/day. Individually titrate Neoral dose based on cyclosporine trough concentrations, tolerability, and clinical response. Measure cyclosporine blood trough concentration more frequently, at least twice a week (daily, if initial dose exceeds 10 mg/kg/day) until concentration stabilizes within desired range.

Rheumatoid arthritis (Neoral only) – Initial dose of *Neoral* is 2.5 mg/kg/day, taken twice daily as a divided oral dose. Salicylates, NSAIDs and oral corticosteroids may be continued. Onset of action generally occurs between 4 and 8 weeks. If insufficient benefit is seen and tolerability is good (including serum creatinine < 30% above baseline), the dose may be increased by 0.5 to 0.75 mg/kg/day after 8 weeks and again after 12 weeks to a maximum of 4 mg/kg/day. If no benefit is seen by 16 weeks of therapy, discontinue. There is limited long-term treatment data. Recurrence of disease activity is generally apparent within 4 weeks after stopping cyclosporine.

With methotrexate: The same initial dose and dosage range should be used if *Neoral* is combined with the recommended dose of methotrexate. Most patients can be treated with *Neoral* doses of ≤ 3 mg/kg/day when combined with methotrexate doses of ≤ 15 mg/week.

Psoriasis (Neoral only) – The initial dose of *Neoral* is 2.5 mg/kg/day. Take *Neoral* twice daily, as a 1.25 mg/kg oral dose. Keep patients at that dose for ≥ 4 weeks, barring adverse events. If significant clinical improvement has not occurred in patients by that time, increase the patient's dosage at 2-week intervals. Based on patient response, make dose increases of ≈ 0.5 mg/kg/day to a maximum of 4 mg/kg/day.

Patients generally show some improvement in the clinical manifestations of psoriasis in 2 weeks. Satisfactory control and stabilization of the disease may take 12 to 16 weeks to achieve. Discontinue treatment if satisfactory response cannot be achieved after 6 weeks at 4 mg/kg/day or the patient's maximum tolerated dose. Once a patient is adequately controlled and appears stable the dose should be lowered.

Upon stopping treatment with cyclosporine, relapse will occur in ≈ 6 weeks (50% of patients) to 16 weeks (75% of patients). In the majority of patients, rebound does not occur after cessation of treatment with cyclosporine. Continuous treatment for extended periods > 1 year is not recommended. Consider alternation with other forms of treatment in the long-term management of patients with this disease.

Admixture compatibility/incompatibility:

Magnesium sulfate – Magnesium sulfate and cyclosporine in 5% Dextrose stored in glass bottles at room temperature is stable for 6 hours.

Actions

Pharmacology: Cyclosporine is a cyclic polypeptide immunosuppressant consisting of 11 amino acids. The exact mechanism of action is unknown.

Pharmacokinetics:

Absorption –

Select Pharmacokinetic Parameters of Cyclosporine Formulations				
	Absolute bioavailability (%)	T_{max} (hours)	C_{max} (ng/mL/mg of dose)	t½ (hours)
Conventional: *Sandimmune*	30[1]	3.5	≈ 1 (2.7 to 1.4)[2]	19 (10 to 27)
Lipid microemulsion: *Neoral*	60	1.5 to 2	↑ (40% to 106%)[3]	8.4 (5 to 18)

[1] < 10% in liver transplant and ≈ 89% in renal transplant patients.

[2] Blood levels for low to high doses, respectively.

[3] In renal transplant patients treated with *Neoral*, peak levels were 40% to 106% greater than those following *Sandimmune* administration.

Absorption from the GI tract is incomplete and variable. Peak blood and plasma concentrations are achieved at ≈ 3.5 hours. *Neoral* has increased bioavailability compared with *Sandimmune*. Factors that may affect bioavailability include: 1) Food that may delay and impair absorption; 2) enterohepatic recirculation; 3) radioimmunoassay (RIA) vs high pressure liquid chromatography (HPLC) assay (RIA cross-reacts w/metabolites); and 4) whole blood vs plasma specimen.

Ingestion of conventional cyclosporine with food may increase its bioavailability, although the effect only appears to be significant when the meal is high in fat.

However, the administration of food with *Neoral* (a lipid microemulsion) decreases the AUC and C_{max} (see Drug Interactions).

Distribution – Largely outside the blood volume; $\approx$ 33% to 47% is in plasma, 4% to 9% in lymphocytes, 5% to 12% in granulocytes and 41% to 58% in erythrocytes. In plasma, $\approx$ 90% is bound to proteins, primarily lipoproteins. Blood level monitoring is useful in patient management.

Metabolism – Cyclosporine is metabolized by the cytochrome P450 hepatic enzyme system. The disposition from blood is biphasic with a terminal half-life of $\approx$ 19 hours (*Sandimmune*) or 8.4 hours (*Neoral*).

Excretion – Primarily biliary. Only 6% of the dose is excreted in urine.

Contraindications

Hypersensitivity to cyclosporine, polyoxyethylated castor oil, or any component of the products; *Neoral* in psoriasis or rheumatoid arthritis patients with abnormal renal function, uncontrolled hypertension, or malignancies; *Neoral* concomitantly with PUVA or UVB in psoriasis patients.

Warnings

Nephrotoxicity: Based on *Sandimmune* oral solution experience, nephrotoxicity has been noted in 25%, 38%, and 37% of renal, cardiac, and liver transplantation cases, respectively. Mild nephrotoxicity was generally noted 2 to 3 months after transplant and consisted of an arrest in the fall of preoperative elevations of BUN and creatinine. These elevations were often responsive to dosage reduction. More overt nephrotoxicity was seen early after transplantation and was characterized by a rapidly rising BUN and creatinine. This form of nephrotoxicity is usually responsive to *Sandimmune* dosage reduction.

Hepatotoxicity: Hepatotoxicity has been noted in 4%, 7%, and 4% of renal, cardiac, and liver transplantation cases, respectively. This usually occurred during the first month of therapy when high doses were used, and consisted of elevated hepatic enzymes and bilirubin.

Glomerular capillary thrombosis: Glomerular capillary thrombosis, which may result in graft failure, occasionally develops.

Convulsions: Convulsions have occurred in adult and pediatric patients receiving cyclosporine, particularly in combination with high-dose methylprednisolone.

Bioequivalency: Sandimmune is not bioequivalent to *Neoral.*

CNS toxicity: CNS toxicity may include headache; flushing; confusion; seizures; ataxia; hallucinations; mania; depression; encephalopathy; sleep problems; blurred vision.

Glucose metabolism: There are conflicting reports of the drug's effects on glucose metabolism.

Malignancies: Warn patients to protect themselves appropriately when in the sun and to avoid excessive sun exposure while taking *Neoral.*

Hypersensitivity reactions: Anaphylactic reactions are rare ($\approx$ 1 in 1000) in patients on cyclosporine injection. Continuously observe patients on IV cyclosporine for at least the first 30 minutes after start of infusion and frequently thereafter. If anaphylaxis occurs, stop infusion.

Renal function impairment: Requires close monitoring and possibly frequent dosage adjustment. In patients with persistent high elevations of BUN and creatinine who are unresponsive to dosage adjustments, consider switching to other immunosuppressive therapy.

Carcinogenesis: The risk of malignancies in cyclosporine recipients is higher than in the healthy population but similar to that in patients receiving other immunosuppressive therapies.

With cyclosporine, some patients have developed a lymphoproliferative disorder, which regresses when the drug is discontinued. Patients receiving cyclosporine are at increased risk for development of lymphomas and other malignancies, particularly those of the skin. The increased risk appears related to the intensity and duration of immunosuppression rather than to the use of specific agents. Because of the danger of oversuppression of the immune system, which can also increase susceptibility to infection, do not give *Sandimmune* with other immunosuppressive agents except adrenal corticosteroids. Because of the danger of oversuppression of the immune system resulting in increased risk of infection or malignancy caused by *Neoral*, use a treatment regimen containing multiple immunosuppressants with caution.

Pregnancy: Category C.

Lactation: Avoid nursing; cyclosporine is excreted in breast milk.

Children: Patients as young as 6 months of age have received *Sandimmune* with no unusual adverse effects. Transplant recipients as young as 1 year of age have received *Neoral* with no unusual adverse effects. The safety and efficacy of *Neoral* treatment in children < 18 years of age with juvenile rheumatoid arthritis or psoriasis have not been established.

Precautions

Monitoring:

Blood levels – Blood level monitoring of cyclosporine is a useful and essential component in patient management. While no fixed relationships have yet been established, blood concentration monitoring may assist in the clinical evaluation of rejection and toxicity, dose adjustments, and the assessment of compliance.

Of major importance to blood level analysis are the type of assay used, the transplanted organ, and the other immunosuppressant agents being administered.

While several assays and assay matrices are available, there is a consensus that parent-compound-specific assays correlate best with clinical events. Of these, HPLC is the standard reference, but the monoclonal antibody RIAs and the monoclonal antibody FPIA offer sensitivity, reproducibility, and convenience.

Repeatedly assess renal and liver functions by measurement of BUN, serum creatinine, serum bilirubin, and liver enzymes.

Malabsorption: Patients with malabsorption may have difficulty achieving therapeutic levels with oral *Sandimmune* use.

Hypertension: Hypertension is a fairly common side effect. Mild or moderate hypertension, which may occur in ≈ 50% of patients following renal transplantation and in most cardiac transplant patients, is more frequently encountered than severe hypertension and the incidence decreases over time. Control of blood pressure can be accomplished with any of the common antihypertensive agents. Because cyclosporine may cause hyperkalemia, do not use potassium-sparing diuretics. While calcium antagonists can be effective agents in treating cyclosporine-associated hypertension, use care because interference with cyclosporine metabolism may require a dosage adjustment.

Drug Interactions

P450 system: Monitoring of circulating cyclosporine levels and appropriate dosage adjustment are essential when drugs that affect hepatic microsomal enzymes, particularly the cytochrome P450 III-A enzymes, are used concomitantly (eg, HIV protease inhibitors, anticonvulsants, azole antifungals).

Nephrotoxic drugs: Use with caution in patients receiving cyclosporine. The following drugs may potentiate renal dysfunction: Antibiotics: Gentamicin, tobramycin, vancomycin, TMP-SMZ; Antineoplastics: Melphalan; Antifungals: Amphotericin B, ketoconazole; Anti-inflammatory drugs: Diclofenac, naproxen, sulindac; GI agents: Cimetidine, ranitidine; Immunosuppressives: Tacrolimus.

Drugs that may affect cyclosporine include amiodarone, androgens (eg, danazol, methyltestosterone), anticonvulsants (eg, carbamazepine, phenobarbital, phenytoin), azole antifungals (eg, fluconazole, ketoconazole), calcium channel blockers, colchicine, oral contraceptives, corticosteroids, foscarnet, imipenem-cilastatin, macrolide antibiotics, metoclopramide, probucol, rifamycins (rifampin, rifabutin), sulfamethoxazole/trimethoprim, and terbinafine.

Drugs that may be affected by cyclosporine include digoxin, etoposide, and lovastatin.

Drug/Food interactions: Administration of food with *Neoral* decreases the AUC and C_{max} of cyclosporine. A high-fat meal consumed within 30 minutes of *Neoral* administration decreased the AUC by 13% and C_{max} by 33%. The effects of a low-fat meal were similar. In addition, do not take cyclosporine simultaneously with grapefruit juice unless specifically instructed to do so; trough cyclosporine concentrations may be increased.

Adverse Reactions
Adverse reactions may include renal dysfunction; tremor; infectious complications; hirsutism; hypertension; gum hyperplasia; cramps; acne; convulsions; paresthesia.

MUROMONAB-CD3

Injection: 5 mg/5 mL (*Rx*)   *Orthoclone OKT3 (Ortho Biotech)*

Warning:
Anaphylactic or anaphylactoid reactions may occur following administration of any dose or course of muromonab-CD3. Serious and occasionally life-threatening systemic, cardiovascular, and CNS reactions have been reported. These have included the following: Pulmonary edema, especially in patients with volume overload; shock; cardiovascular collapse; cardiac or respiratory arrest; seizures; coma.

Indications
Renal allograft rejection: Treatment of acute allograft rejection in renal transplant patients.

Cardiac/Hepatic allograft rejection: Treatment of steroid-resistant acute allograft rejection in cardiac and hepatic transplant patients.

Administration and Dosage
Muromonab-CD3 is for IV use only.

Administer as an IV bolus in < 1 minute. Do not give by IV infusion or in conjunction with other drug solutions.

Renal allograft rejection, acute: 5 mg/day for 10 to 14 days. Begin treatment once acute renal rejection is diagnosed.

Cardiac/hepatic allograft rejection, steroid resistant: 5 mg/day for 10 to 14 days. Begin treatment when it is determined that a rejection has not been reversed by an adequate course of corticosteroid therapy.

Actions
Pharmacology: Muromonab-CD3 is a murine monoclonal antibody to the T3 (CD3) antigen of human T cells which functions as an immunosuppressant. The antibody is a biochemically purified IgG_{2a} immunoglobulin. It reverses graft rejection, probably by blocking the T-cell function, which plays a major role in acute renal rejection.

Pharmacokinetics: Serum levels are measured with an enzyme-linked immunosorbent assay (ELISA). During treatment with 5 mg/day for 14 days, mean serum trough levels rose over the first 3 days and then averaged 0.9 mcg/mL on days 3 to 14. Circulating serum levels > 0.8 mcg/mL block the function of cytotoxic T cells in vitro and in vivo.

Contraindications
Hypersensitivity to this or any product of murine origin; anti–mouse antibody titers ≥ 1:1000; patients in fluid overload or uncompensated heart failure, as evidenced by chest x-ray or > 3% weight gain within the week prior to treatment; history of seizures or predisposition to seizures; pregnancy; breastfeeding.

Warnings

Cytokine release syndrome (CRS): Temporally associated with the administration of the first few doses of muromonab-CD3 (particularly, the first 2 to 3 doses), most patients have developed CRS that has been attributed to the release of cytokines by activated lymphocytes or monocytes. This clinical syndrome has ranged from a more frequently reported mild, self-limited, "flu-like" illness to a less frequently reported severe, life-threatening shock-like reaction, which may include serious cardiovascular and CNS manifestations. The syndrome typically begins ≈ 30 to 60 minutes after administration of a dose (but may occur later) and may persist for several hours. The frequency and severity of this symptom complex usually are greatest with the first dose.

Pulmonary edema – Severe pulmonary edema has occurred in patients who appeared to be euvolemic. The pathogenesis of pulmonary edema may involve some or all of the following: Volume overload; increased pulmonary vascular permeability; reduced left ventricular compliance/contractility.

Serum creatinine – During the first 1 to 3 days of therapy, some patients have experienced an acute and transient decline in the glomerular filtration rate (GFR) and diminished urine output with a resulting increase in the level of serum creatinine.

Patients at risk – Patients at risk for more serious complications of the CRS may include those with the following conditions: Unstable angina; recent MI or symptomatic ischemic heart disease; heart failure of any etiology; pulmonary edema of any etiology; any form of chronic obstructive pulmonary disease; intravascular volume overload or depletion of any etiology (eg, excessive dialysis, recent intensive diuresis, blood loss); cerebrovascular disease; patients with advanced symptomatic vascular disease or neuropathy; history of seizures; septic shock.

Fluid status – Prior to administration, assess the patient's volume (fluid) status carefully. It is imperative, especially prior to the first few doses, that there be no clinical evidence of volume overload or uncompensated heart failure, including a clear chest X-ray and weight restriction of ≤ 3% above the patient's minimum weight during the week prior to injection.

Prevention/Minimization – Manifestations of the CRS may be prevented or minimized by pretreatment with 8 mg/kg methylprednisolone, given 1 to 4 hours prior to administration of the first dose of muromonab-CD3 and by closely following recommendations for dosage and treatment duration.

Neuropsychiatric events: Seizures, encephalopathy, cerebral edema, aseptic meningitis, and headaches have occurred during therapy with muromonab-CD3, even following the first dose, resulting in part from T-cell activation and subsequent systemic release of cytokines.

Aseptic meningitis syndrome – The incidence of this syndrome was 6%. Fever, headache, meningismus, and photophobia were the most commonly reported symptoms; a combination of these 4 symptoms occurred in 5% of patients.

Headache – Headache is frequently seen after any of the first few doses and may occur in any of the aforementioned neurologic syndromes or by itself.

Patients who may be at greater risk for CNS adverse experiences – Patients who may be at greater risk for CNS adverse experiences include the following: Known or suspected CNS disorders; cerebrovascular disease (small or large vessel); conditions having associated neurologic problems; underlying vascular diseases; concomitant medication that may, by itself, affect the CNS.

Infections: Muromonab-CD3 is usually added to immunosuppressive therapeutic regimens, thereby augmenting the degree of immunosuppression. This increase in the total burden of immunosuppression may alter the spectrum of infections observed and increase the risk, the severity and the potential gravity (morbidity) of infectious complications.

Neoplasia: As a result of depressed cell-mediated immunity, organ transplant patients have an increased risk of developing malignancies.

Hypersensitivity reactions: Serious and occasionally fatal, immediate (usually within 10 minutes) hypersensitivity reactions have occurred. Manifestations of anaphylaxis may appear similar to manifestations of the CRS.

Pregnancy: Category C.

Lactation: It is not known whether muromonab-CD3 is excreted in breast milk.

Children: Safety and efficacy in children have not been established. Muromonab-CD3 has been used in infants/children, beginning with a dose of ≤ 5 mg.

Precautions

Monitoring: Monitor the following tests prior to and during therapy:

- *Renal:* BUN, serum creatinine, etc.;
- *Hepatic:* Transaminases, alkaline phosphatase, bilirubin;
- *Hematopoietic:* WBCs and differential, platelet count, etc.;
- *Chest X-ray:* within 24 hours before initiating treatment, which should be free of any evidence of heart failure or fluid overload.

Monitor one of the following immunologic tests during therapy:

- Plasma levels determined by an ELISA; (target levels should be ≥ 800 ng/mL); or
- Quantitative T lymphocyte surface phenotyping (CD3, CD4, CD8); target CD3 positive T cells < 25 cells/mm^3.

Testing for human-mouse antibody titers is strongly recommended; a titer ≥ 1:1000 is a contraindication for use.

Intravascular thrombosis: As with other immunosuppressive therapies, arterial or venous thromboses of allografts and other vascular beds have been reported.

Drug Interactions

Drugs that may affect muromonab include other immunosuppressants (eg, azathioprine, corticosteroids, cyclosporine) and indomethacin.

Adverse Reactions

Adverse reactions associated with CRS may include high (often spiking, up to 107°F) fever, chills/rigors, abdominal pain, malaise, muscle/joint aches and pains, dyspnea, shortness of breath, tachypnea, respiratory arrest/failure/distress, cardiovascular collapse, cardiac arrest, angina/MI, nausea, vomiting, chest pain/tightness, hemodynamic instability, heart failure, pulmonary edema, adult respiratory distress syndrome, hypoxemia, apnea, arrhythmias, diarrhea, tremor, bronchospasm/wheezing, headache, tachycardia, rigor, and hypertension.

Other adverse events may include pancytopenia, aplastic anemia, neutropenia, leukopenia, thrombocytopenia, lymphopenia, leukocytosis, lymphademopathy, coagulation disturbances, hypotension/shock, heart failure, angina/MI, tachycardia, bradycardia, tachypnea/hyperventilation, abnormal chest sounds, pneumonia/pneumonitis, rash, urticaria, pruritus, erythema, flushing, diaphoresis, diarrhea, bowel infarction, arthralgia, arthritis, blindness, blurred vision, diplopia, hearing loss, otitis media, tinnitus, vertigo, photophobia, conjunctivitis, nasal/ear stuffiness, and anuria/oliguria.

PEGINTERFERON ALFA-2B

Powder for injection, lyophilized: 100, 160, 240, and 300 mcg/mL (*Rx*)   *PEG-Intron* (Schering)

> **Warning:**
>   Alpha interferons, including peginterferon alfa-2b, cause or aggravate fatal or life-threatening neuropsychiatric, autoimmune, ischemic, and infectious disorders. Closely monitor patients with periodic clinical and laboratory evaluations. Withdraw from therapy patients with persistently severe or worsening signs or symptoms of these conditions. In many but not all cases, these disorders resolve after stopping peginterferon alfa-2b therapy.

Indications

Chronic hepatitis C: As monotherapy for the treatment of chronic hepatitis C in patients not previously treated with interferon alpha who have compensated liver disease and are ≥ 18 years of age. The safety and effectiveness of peginterferon alfa-2b in combination with ribavirin for the treatment of chronic hepatitis C have not been established.

Unlabeled uses: Renal carcinoma.

Administration and Dosage

Patients should self-inject only if the physician determines that it is appropriate and patients agree to medical follow-up as necessary and receive training in proper injection technique.

Peginterferon alfa-2b is administered SC once weekly for 1 year. Administer the dose on the same day of each week. Base initial dosing on weight, as described in the following table.

Recommended Dosing of Peginterferon Alfa-2b			
Vial strength[1] to use (mcg/mL)	Weight (kg)	Amount of peginterferon alfa-2b to administer (mcg)	Volume of peginterferon alfa-2b to administer (mL)
100	37 to 45	40	0.4
	46 to 56	50	0.5
160	57 to 72	64	0.4
	73 to 88	80	0.5
240	89 to 106	96	0.4
	107 to 136	120	0.5
300	137 to 160	150	0.5

[1] When reconstituted as directed.

Assess serum hepatitis C virus (HCV) RNA levels after 24 weeks of treatment. Consider discontinuation of treatment in any patient who has not achieved an HCV RNA below the limit of detection of the assay after 24 weeks of therapy with peginterferon alfa-2b.

There are no safety and efficacy data for treatment ≥ 48 weeks or for retreatment of patients who relapse following peginterferon alfa-2b therapy.

Dose reduction: If a serious adverse reaction develops during the course of treatment discontinue or modify the dosage of peginterferon alfa-2b to 50% of the starting dosage until the adverse reaction abates or decreases in severity. If persistent or recurrent intolerance develops despite adequate dosage adjustment, discontinue treatment with peginterferon alfa-2b. For dose modification in the event of neutropenia and thrombocytopenia, refer to the following table.

Guidelines for Dose Modifications of Peginterferon Alfa-2b for Neutropenia and Thrombocytopenia		
	Dose reduction	Permanent discontinuation
Neutrophil count	< 0.75 × 10⁹/L	< 0.50 × 10⁹/L
Platelet count	< 80 × 10⁹/L	< 50 × 10⁹/L

Actions

Pharmacology: The biological activity of peginterferon alfa-2b is derived from its interferon alfa-2b moiety. Interferons exert their cellular activities by binding to specific membrane receptors on the cell surface and initiate a complex sequence of intracellular events.

Pharmacokinetics:

   Absorption/Distribution – Maximal serum concentrations (C_{max}) occur between 15 and 44 hours postdose and are sustained for ≤ 48 to 72 hours.

   Metabolism/Excretion – The mean peginterferon alfa-2b elimination half-life is ≈ 40 hours (range, 22 to 60 hours) in patients with HCV infection. The apparent clearance of peginterferon alfa-2b is estimated to be ≈ 22 mL/hr•kg. Renal elimination accounts for 30% of the clearance.

   Pegylation of interferon alfa-2b produces a product (peginterferon alfa-2b) whose clearance is lower than that of nonpegylated interferon alfa-2b. When compared to interferon alfa-2b, peginterferon alfa-2b (1 mcg/kg) has an ≈ 7-fold lower mean apparent clearance and a 5-fold greater mean half life permitting a reduced dosing frequency.

Contraindications

Hypersensitivity to peginterferon alfa-2b or any component of the product; autoimmune hepatitis; decompensated liver disease.

Warnings

Hypersensitivity reactions: Serious, acute hypersensitivity reactions (eg, urticaria, angioedema, bronchoconstriction, anaphylaxis) have been rarely observed during alpha interferon therapy.

Renal function impairment: Closely monitor patients with impairment of renal function for signs and symptoms of interferon toxicity and adjust doses of peginterferon alfa-2b accordingly. Use peginterferon alfa-2b with caution in patients with Ccr < 50 mL/min.

Elderly: Treatment with alpha interferons, including peginterferon alfa-2b, is associated with CNS, cardiac, and systemic (flu-like) adverse effects. Because these adverse reactions may be more severe in the elderly, exercise caution in the use of interferon alfa-2b in this population.

Pregnancy: Category C. Peginterferon alfa-2b should be assumed to have abortifacient potential. Use during pregnancy only if the potential benefit justifies the potential risk to the fetus. Therefore, peginterferon alfa-2b is recommended for use in fertile women only when they are using effective contraception during the treatment period.

Lactation: It is not known whether the components of interferon alfa-2b are excreted in human milk.

Children: Safety and efficacy in pediatric patients < 18 years of age have not been established.

Precautions

Neuropsychiatric events: Life-threatening or fatal neuropsychiatric events, including suicide, suicidal and homicidal ideation, depression, relapse of drug addiction/overdose, and aggressive behavior have occurred in patients with and without a previous psychiatric disorder during peginterferon alfa-2b treatment and follow-up. Psychoses and hallucinations have been observed in patients treated with alpha interferons.

Bone marrow toxicity: Peginterferon alfa-2b suppresses bone marrow function, sometimes resulting in severe cytopenias. Discontinue peginterferon alfa-2b in patients who develop severe decreases in neutrophil or platelet counts. Very rarely, alpha interferons may be associated with aplastic anemia.

Colitis: Fatal and nonfatal ulcerative and hemorrhagic colitis have been observed within 12 weeks of the start of alpha-interferon treatment. Abdominal pain, bloody diarrhea, and fever are the typical manifestations. Immediately discontinue peginterferon alfa-2b in patients who develop these symptoms and signs. The colitis usually resolves within 1 to 3 weeks of discontinuation of alpha interferons.

Pancreatitis: Fatal and nonfatal pancreatitis have been observed in patients treated with alpha interferon. Suspend peginterferon alfa-2b therapy in patients with signs and symptoms suggestive of pancreatitis and discontinue in patients diagnosed with pancreatitis.

Pulmonary disorders: Dyspnea, pulmonary infiltrates, pneumonitis, and pneumonia, some resulting in patient deaths, have been associated with peginterferon alfa-2b or alpha-interferon therapy. Closely monitor patients with pulmonary infiltrates or pulmonary function impairment.

Immunogenicity: One percent of patients receiving peginterferon alfa-2b developed low-titer (≤ 64) neutralizing antibodies to interferon alfa-2b. The clinical and pathological significance of the appearance of serum neutralizing antibodies is unknown.

Special risk:

Endocrine disorders – Peginterferon alfa-2b causes or aggravates hypothyroidism and hyperthyroidism. Hyperglycemia has been observed in patients treated with interferon alfa-2b. Diabetes mellitus has been observed in patients treated with alpha interferons.

Cardiovascular events – Cardiovascular events, including hypotension, arrhythmia, tachycardia, cardiomyopathy, and MI, have been observed in patients treated with peginterferon alfa-2b.

Autoimmune disorders – Development or exacerbation of autoimmune disorders (eg, thyroiditis, thrombocytopenia, rheumatoid arthritis, interstitial nephritis, systemic lupus erythematosus, psoriasis) have been observed in patients receiving peginterferon alfa-2b.

Ophthalmologic disorders – Retinal hemorrhages, cotton wool spots, and retinal artery or vein obstruction have been observed after treatment with peginterferon alfa-2b or alpha interferons.

Lab test abnormalities: Peginterferon alfa-2b may cause severe decreases in neutrophil and platelet counts and abnormality of TSH. In 10% of patients treated with peginterferon alfa-2b, ALT levels rose 2- to 5-fold above baseline. The elevations were transient and were not associated with deterioration of other liver functions.

Patients on peginterferon alfa-2b therapy should have hematology and blood chemistry testing before the start of treatment and then periodically thereafter.

Drug Interactions
It is not known if peginterferon alfa-2b therapy causes clinically significant drug interactions with drugs metabolized by the liver in patients with hepatitis C.

Adverse Reactions
Adverse reactions occurring in ≥ 3% of patients include the following: Headache; depression; anxiety/emotional lability/irritability; insomnia; dizziness; alopecia; pruritus; dry skin; sweating increased; rash; flushing; nausea; anorexia; diarrhea; abdominal pain; vomiting; dyspepsia; thrombocytopenia; neutropenia; pharyngitis; sinusitis; coughing; musculoskeletal pain; fatigue; injection site inflammation/reaction; influenza-like symptoms; rigors; fever; weight decrease; viral infection; right upper quadrant pain; malaise; hepatomegaly; hypertonia; hypothyroidism.

Chapter 11

DERMATOLOGICAL AGENTS

Acne Products, 1037
   Isotretinoin, 1037
Corticosteroids, Topical, 1044
Miscellaneous Topical Drugs, 1049
   Tretinoin, 1049
   Capsaicin, 1051
   Penciclovir, 1052
Immunomodulators, Topical, 1053
   Imiquimod, 1053
   Tacrolimus, 1054

ISOTRETINOIN (13-cis-Retinoic Acid)

Capsules: 10, 20, and 40 mg (Rx)	*Accutane* (Roche)

Warning:
Isotretinoin must not be used by females who are pregnant. Although not every fetus exposed to isotretinoin has resulted in a deformed child, there is an extremely high risk that a deformed infant can result if pregnancy occurs while taking isotretinoin in any amount even for short periods of time. Potentially any fetus exposed during pregnancy can be affected. Presently, there are no accurate means of determining, after isotretinoin exposure, which fetus has been affected and which has not.

Major human fetal abnormalities related to isotretinoin administration in females have been documented. There is an increased risk of spontaneous abortion. In addition, premature births have been reported.

Documented external abnormalities include the following: Skull abnormality; ear abnormalities (including anotia, micropinna, small or absent external auditory canals); eye abnormalities (including microphthalmia), facial dysmorphia; cleft palate. Documented internal abnormalities include the following: CNS abnormalities (including cerebral abnormalities, cerebellar malformation, hydrocephalus, microcephaly, cranial nerve deficit); cardiovascular abnormalities; thymus gland abnormality; parathyroid hormone deficiency. In some cases death has occurred with certain previously noted abnormalities.

Cases of IQ scores < 85 with or without obvious CNS abnormalities also have been reported.

Isotretinoin is contraindicated in females of childbearing potential unless the patient meets all of the following conditions:
- Must not be pregnant or breastfeeding,
- Must be capable of complying with mandatory contraceptive measures required for isotretinoin therapy and understand behaviors associated with an increased risk of pregnancy, and
- Must be reliable in understanding and carrying out instructions.

Accutane must be prescribed under the System to Manage Accutane-Related Teratogenicity (SMART). The prescriber must obtain a supply of yellow self-adhesive *Accutane* qualification stickers. To obtain these stickers: 1) Read the booklet entitled *SMART Guide to Best Practices*; 2) sign and return the completed SMART letter of understanding containing the prescriber checklist; and 3) use the yellow self-adhesive *Accutane* qualification sticker. *Accutane* should not be prescribed or dispensed to any patient (male or female) without a yellow self-adhesive *Accutane* qualification sticker.

Warning: (cont.)

Female patients: For female patients, the yellow self-adhesive *Accutane* qualification sticker signifies that she understands the following:

- Must have had 2 negative urine or serum pregnancy tests with a sensitivity of ≥ 25 mIU/mL before receiving the initial isotretinoin prescription. The first test (a screening test) is obtained by the prescriber when the decision is made to pursue qualification of the patient for isotretinoin. The second pregnancy test (a confirmation test) should be done during the first 5 days of the menstrual period immediately preceding the beginning of isotretinoin therapy. For patients with amenorrhea, the second test should be done at least 11 days after the last act of unprotected sexual intercourse (without using 2 effective forms of contraception). Each month of therapy, the patient must have a negative result from a urine or serum pregnancy test. A pregnancy test must be repeated every month prior to the female patient receiving each prescription. The manufacturer will make available urine pregnancy test kits for female isotretinoin patients for the initial, second, and monthly testing during therapy.

- Must have selected and has committed to using 2 forms of effective contraception simultaneously, ≥ 1 of which must be a primary form, unless absolute abstinence is the chosen method, or the patient has undergone a hysterectomy. Patients must use 2 forms of effective contraception for ≥ 1 month prior to initiation of isotretinoin therapy, during isotretinoin therapy, and for 1 month after discontinuing isotretinoin therapy. Counseling about contraception and behaviors associated with an increased risk of pregnancy must be repeated on a monthly basis.

Effective forms of contraception include both primary and secondary forms of contraception. Primary forms of contraception include the following: Tubal ligation, partner's vasectomy, intrauterine devices, birth control pills, and injectable/implantable/insertable hormonal birth control products. Secondary forms of contraception include diaphragms, latex condoms, and cervical caps; each must be used with a spermicide.

Any birth control method can fail. Therefore, it is critically important that women of childbearing potential use 2 effective forms of contraception simultaneously. A drug interaction that decreases effectiveness of hormonal contraceptives has not been entirely ruled out for isotretinoin. Although hormonal contraceptives are highly effective, there have been reports of pregnancy from women who have used oral contraceptives, as well as injectable/implantable contraceptive products. These reports occurred while these patients were taking isotretinoin. These reports are more frequent for women who use only a single method of contraception. Patients must receive written warnings about the rates of possible contraception failure (included in patient education kits).

Prescribers are advised to consult the package insert of any medication administered concomitantly with hormonal contraceptives, because some medications may decrease the effectiveness of these birth control products. Patients should be prospectively cautioned not to self-medicate with the herbal supplement St. John's wort because a possible interaction has been suggested with hormonal contraceptives based on reports of breakthrough bleeding on oral contraceptives shortly after starting St. John's wort. Pregnancies have been reported by users of combined hormonal contraceptives who also used some form of St. John's wort.

- Must have signed a patient information/consent form that contains warnings about the risk of potential birth defects if the fetus is exposed to isotretinoin.

Warning: (cont.)
- Must have been informed of the purpose and importance of participating in the *Accutane* survey and has been given the opportunity to enroll.

The yellow self-adhesive *Accutane* qualification sticker documents that the female patient is qualified and includes the date of qualification, patient gender, cut-off date for filling the prescription, and up to a 30-day supply limit with no refills.

Male patients: These yellow self-adhesive *Accutane* qualification stickers also should be used for male patients: Check off the male gender box without checking the qualification statement.

If a pregnancy does occur during treatment with isotretinoin, the prescriber and patient should discuss the desirability of continuing the pregnancy. Prescribers are strongly encouraged to report all cases of pregnancy to Roche at 1-800-526-6367 where a Roche pregnancy prevention program specialist will be available to discuss Roche pregnancy information, or prescribers may contact the FDA MedWatch program at 1-800-FDA-1088.

Isotretinoin should be prescribed only by those who have demonstrated special competence in the diagnosis and treatment of severe recalcitrant nodular acne, are experienced in the use of systemic retinoids, have read the *SMART Guide to Best Practices*, signed and returned the completed SMART letter of understanding, and obtained self-adhesive *Accutane* qualification stickers. Do not prescribe or dispense *Accutane* without a yellow self-adhesive *Accutane* qualification sticker.

Information for pharmacists: Isotretinoin must only be dispensed as follows:
- In no more than 1-month supply.
- Only on presentation of an *Accutane* prescription with a yellow self-adhesive *Accutane* qualification sticker.
- Prescription written within the previous 7 days.
- Refills require a new prescription with a yellow self-adhesive *Accutane* qualification sticker.
- No telephone or computerized prescriptions are permitted.

An *Accutane* medication guide must be given to the patient each time isotretinoin is dispensed, as required by law. This guide is an important part of the risk management program for the patient.

Indications
Severe recalcitrant nodular acne: Nodules are inflammatory lesions with a diameter of ≥ 5 mm. The nodules may become suppurative or hemorrhagic. "Severe," by definition, means "many" as opposed to "few or several" nodules.

Adverse effects are significant; reserve treatment for patients unresponsive to conventional therapy, including systemic antibiotics. In addition, for female patients of childbearing potential, isotretinoin is indicated only for those who are not pregnant (see Contraindications, Warnings). A single course of therapy for 15 to 20 weeks has resulted in complete, prolonged remission in many patients. If a second course is needed, do not initiate therapy until ≥ 8 weeks after completion of the first course. Patients may continue to improve while not receiving the drug. The optimal interval before retreatment has not been defined for patients who have not completed skeletal growth.

Administration and Dosage
Individualize dosage. Adjust the dose according to side effects and disease response. Administer with food.

Recommended course of therapy: Initial dose is 0.5 to 1 mg/kg/day (range, 0.5 to 2 mg/kg/day) divided into 2 doses, for 15 to 20 weeks. Patients whose disease is very severe or is primarily manifest on the body may require up to the maximum recommended dose, 2 mg/kg/day. If the total nodule count decreases by > 70% prior to this time, the drug may be discontinued. After ≥ 2 months off therapy, and if warranted by persistent or recurring severe nodular acne, a second course of therapy may be initiated.

In studies comparing 0.1, 0.5, and 1 mg/kg/day, all doses provided initial clearing of disease, but there was a greater need for retreatment with the lower doses.

Actions

Pharmacology: Isotretinoin is a retinoid which, when administered in pharmacologic dosages of 0.5 to 2 mg/kg/day, inhibits sebaceous gland function and keratinization. The exact mechanism of action of isotretinoin is unknown.

Clinical improvement in nodular acne occurs in association with a reduction in sebum secretion. The decrease in sebum secretion is temporary and is related to the dose and duration of treatment with isotretinoin, and reflects a reduction in sebaceous gland size and an inhibition of sebaceous gland differentiation.

Pharmacokinetics:

Absorption/Distribution – Oral bioavailability from oil-filled capsules is ≈ 23% to 25%. Food and milk increase GI absorption of isotretinoin. The drug is 99.9% bound to plasma albumin. Maximum concentrations of 4-oxo-isotretinoin, the major metabolite, were 87 to 399 ng/mL, and were reached in 6 to 20 hours.

Metabolism/Excretion – The major metabolite in blood, 4-oxo-isotretinoin, generally exceeds the concentration of isotretinoin after 6 hours. Terminal elimination half-life of isotretinoin is 10 to 20 hours. Elimination half-life of 4-oxo-isotretinoin ranges from 17 to 50 hours (average, 25 hours).

Relatively equal amounts of radioactivity were recovered in the urine and feces with 65% to 83% of the dose recovered.

Contraindications

Pregnancy; hypersensitivity to this medication or any of its components; hypersensitivity to parabens (used as preservatives in the formulation).

Warnings

Psychiatric disorders: Isotretinoin may cause depression, psychosis, and rarely, suicidal ideation, suicide attempts, and suicide.

Pseudotumor cerebri (benign intracranial hypertension): Isotretinoin use has been associated with a number of cases of pseudotumor cerebri, some of which involved concomitant use of tetracycline. Therefore, avoid concomitant treatment with tetracyclines. Early signs and symptoms include papilledema, headache, nausea, vomiting, and visual disturbances. Screen patients with these symptoms for papilledema; if present, discontinue drug immediately and consult a neurologist. Minocycline and tetracycline have been associated with pseudotumor cerebri or papilledema in isotretinoin patients.

Pancreatitis: Acute pancreatitis has been reported in patients with elevated or normal serum triglyceride levels.

Visual impairment: Carefully monitor visual problems.

Inflammatory bowel disease: Inflammatory bowel disease (including regional ileitis) has been temporally associated with isotretinoin in patients with no history of intestinal disorders. In some instances, symptoms have been reported to persist after isotretinoin therapy has been stopped. Discontinue treatment immediately if abdominal pain, rectal bleeding, or severe diarrhea occurs.

Hypertriglyceridemia: Hypertriglyceridemia in excess of 800 mg/dL occurred in ≈ 25% of patients; 15% develop a decrease in high density lipoproteins (HDL) and ≈ 7% show an increase in cholesterol. Obtain baseline values, then perform tests weekly or biweekly until lipid response is established (usually 4 weeks).

These effects are reversible generally within 8 weeks after cessation of therapy. Patients with increased tendency to develop hypertriglyceridemia include those with diabetes mellitus, obesity, increased alcohol intake, lipid metabolism disorder, and a familial history.

Reduction of weight, dietary fat, alcohol intake, and dose may reverse serum triglycerides, allowing patients to continue therapy.

Musculoskeletal symptoms: Musculoskeletal symptoms (including arthralgia) develop in ≈ 16% of patients. In general, these are mild to moderate and occasionally require discontinuation. They generally clear rapidly after discontinuing isotretinoin, and rarely persist.

Hepatotoxicity: Mild to moderate elevations of liver enzymes have been seen in ≈ 15% of patients, some of which normalized with dosage reduction or continued administration of the drug.

Hearing impairment: Impaired hearing has been reported in patients taking isotretinoin; in some cases, the hearing impairment has been reported to persist after therapy has been discontinued.

Hormonal contraceptives: Microdosed progesterone preparations (minipills) may be an inadequate method of contraception during isotretinoin therapy.

Hypersensitivity reactions: Anaphylactic reactions and other allergic reactions have been reported. Cutaneous allergic reactions and serious cases of allergic vasculitis, often with purpura (bruises and red patches), of the extremities and extracutaneous involvement (including renal) have been reported.

Pregnancy: Category X.

Lactation: It is not known whether this drug is excreted in breast milk. Because of the potential for adverse effects, do not give to a nursing mother.

Children: Safety and efficacy have not been established.

Precautions
Monitoring:
    Pregnancy test – Female patients of childbearing potential must have negative results from 2 urine or serum pregnancy tests with a sensitivity of ≥ 50 mIU/mL before a prescription is given.

    Lipids – Obtain pretreatment and follow-up blood lipids under fasting conditions.

    Liver function tests – Perform pretreatment and follow-up liver function tests at weekly or biweekly intervals until the response to isotretinoin has been established.

Monitoring:
    Pregnancy test – Female patients of childbearing potential must have negative results from 2 urine or serum pregnancy tests with a sensitivity of ≥ 25 mIU/mL before receiving the initial isotretinoin prescription. The first test is obtained by the prescriber when the decision is made to pursue qualification of the patient for isotretinoin (a screening test). The second pregnancy test (a confirmation test) should be done during the first 5 days of the menstrual period immediately preceding the beginning of isotretinoin therapy. For patients with amenorrhea, the second test should be done at least 11 days after the last act of unprotected sexual intercourse (without using 2 effective forms of contraception).

    Each month of therapy, the patient must have a negative result from a urine or serum pregnancy test. Repeat the pregnancy test each month prior to the female patient receiving each prescription.

    Lipids – Obtain pretreatment and follow-up blood lipids under fasting conditions. After consumption of alcohol, ≥ 36 hours should elapse before these determinations are made. It is recommended that these tests be performed at weekly or biweekly intervals until the lipid response to isotretinoin is established. The incidence of hypertriglyceridemia is 1 patient in 4 on isotretinoin therapy.

    Liver function tests – Because elevations of liver enzymes have been observed during clinical trials, and hepatitis has been reported, perform pretreatment and follow-up liver function tests at weekly or biweekly intervals until the response to isotretinoin has been established.

Exacerbation of acne: Exacerbation of acne (transient) has occurred, generally during initial therapy period.

Contact lens: Contact lens tolerance may decrease.

Diabetes: Certain patients have experienced problems in the control of their blood sugar.

Blood donation: Because of isotretinoin's teratogenic potential, patients receiving the drug should not donate blood for transfusion during treatment and for 1 month after discontinuing therapy.

Neutropenia/Agranulocytosis: Neutropenia and rare cases of agranulocytosis have been reported.

Photosensitivity: Photosensitization (photoallergy or phototoxicity) may occur; caution patients to take protective measures (ie, sunscreens, protective clothing) against exposure to ultraviolet light or sunlight until tolerance is determined.

Drug Interactions

Drugs that may interact with isotretinoin include vitamin A, tetracycline, and minocycline.

Drug/Food interactions: When taken with food or milk, the absorption of isotretinoin is increased.

Adverse Reactions

Most adverse reactions are reversible upon discontinuation; however, some have persisted after cessation of therapy. Many are similar to those described in patients taking high doses of vitamin A.

Cardiovascular: Palpitation; tachycardia; vascular thrombotic disease; stroke.

CNS: Fatigue; headache; pseudotumor cerebri, including headache, visual disturbances, and papilledema; dizziness; drowsiness; insomnia; lethargy; malaise; nervousness; paresthesias; seizures; stroke; syncope; weakness; suicidal ideation; suicide attempts; suicide; psychosis; emotional instability. Depression has occurred and has subsided with discontinuation of therapy and recurred upon reinstitution.

Dermatologic: Cheilitis, usually dose-related; dry skin; pruritus; skin fragility; drying of mucous membranes; rash (including erythema, seborrhea, and eczema); thinning of hair that rarely has persisted; peeling of palms and soles; skin infections; photosensitivity; erythema nodosum, paronychia, hypo- or hyperpigmentation; urticaria; hirsutism; nail dystrophy; pyogenic granuloma; bruising; acne fulminans; sweating.

GI: Dry mouth; nausea, vomiting; nonspecific GI symptoms; inflammatory bowel disease (see Warnings); weight loss; bleeding and inflammation of the gums; hepatitis; pancreatitis; colitis; ileitis.

GU: White cells in urine; proteinuria, microscopic or gross hematuria; nonspecific urogenital findings; abnormal menses; glomerulonephritis.

Hematologic: Thrombocytopenia; neutropenia; agranulocytosis (rare).

Hypersensitivity: Allergic reactions; systemic hypersensitivity.

Musculoskeletal: Mild to moderate musculoskeletal symptoms that occasionally require drug discontinuation and rarely persist after discontinuation (16%); skeletal hyperostosis (see Warnings); calcification of tendons and ligaments; premature epiphyseal closure; arthritis; tendonitis; other bone abnormalities.

Ophthalmic: Conjunctivitis; optic neuritis, photophobia, eyelid inflammation; corneal opacities (see Warnings); cataracts; visual disturbances; color vision disorder; keratitis. Dry eyes and decreased night vision have occurred and, in rare instances, have persisted.

Respiratory: Bronchospasms, with or without a history of asthma; respiratory infections; voice alterations.

Miscellaneous: Epistaxis; dry nose; transient chest pain (rarely persists after discontinuation); vasculitis (including Wegener's granulomatosis); flushing; anemia; lymphadenopathy; disseminated herpes simplex; edema; tinnitus; hearing impairment.

Lab test abnormalities: Elevated sedimentation rate; decreased red blood cell parameters and white blood cell counts, including severe neutropenia and rare reports of agranulocytosis; elevated platelet counts; increased alkaline phosphatase, AST, ALT,

GGTP, and LDH; increased fasting blood sugar; hyperuricemia; thrombocytopenia; elevated CPK levels in patients who undergo vigorous physical activity.

Patient Information

Patient information leaflet available with product.

Prior to use, have patients complete a consent form included with package insert.

Report depression, visual disturbances, abdominal pain, rectal bleeding, severe diarrhea, difficulty in controlling blood sugar, and decreased tolerance to contact lens wear to physician immediately.

Do not donate blood for transfusion during therapy or for 1 month after stopping therapy because the blood might be given to a pregnant woman whose fetus must not be exposed to isotretinoin.

Do not share isotretinoin with anyone else because of the risk of birth defects and other serious adverse events.

CORTICOSTEROIDS, TOPICAL

ACLOMETASONE DIPROPIONATE
Ointment: 0.05% (*Rx*) *Aclovate* (GlaxoSmithKline)
Cream: 0.05% (*Rx*)

AMCINONIDE
Ointment: 0.01% (*Rx*) *Cyclocort* (Fujisawa)
Cream: 0.1% (*Rx*)
Lotion: 0.1% (*Rx*)

AUGMENTED BETAMETHASONE DIPROPIONATE
Ointment: 0.05% (*Rx*) *Diprolene* (Schering)
Cream: 0.05% (*Rx*) *Diprolene AF* (Schering)
Lotion: 0.05% (*Rx*) *Diprolene* (Schering)
Gel: 0.05% (*Rx*) *Diprolene* (Schering)

BETAMETHASONE BENZOATE
Cream: 0.025% (*Rx*) *Uticort* (Parke-Davis)
Lotion: 0.025% (*Rx*)
Gel: 0.025% (*Rx*)

BETAMETHASONE DIPROPIONATE
Ointment: 0.05% (*Rx*) Various, *Diprosone* (Schering), *Maxivate* (West-
Cream: 0.05% (*Rx*) wood-Squibb)
Lotion: 0.05% (*Rx*)
Aerosol: 0.1% (*Rx*)

BETAMETHASONE VALERATE
Ointment: 0.1% (*Rx*) Various, *Betatrex* (Savage), *Valisone* (Schering)
Cream: 0.01%, 0.05%, 0.1% (*Rx*) Various, *Valisone* (Schering)
Lotion: 0.1% (*Rx*) Various, *Valisone* (Schering), *Betatrex* (Savage)
Powder for compounding (*Rx*) *Betamethasone Valerate* (Paddock)

CLOBETASOL PROPIONATE
Ointment: 0.05% (*Rx*) Various, *Temovate* (GlaxoSmithKline)
Cream: 0.05% (*Rx*)
Scalp application: 0.05% (*Rx*) *Temovate* (GlaxoSmithKline)
Gel: 0.05% (*Rx*)

CLOCORTOLONE PIVALATE
Cream: 0.1% (*Rx*) *Cloderm* (Hermal)

DESONIDE
Ointment: 0.05% (*Rx*) Various, *DesOwen* (Owen/Galderma), *Tridesilon*
(Miles Inc)
Cream: 0.05% and 0.25% (*Rx*) *DesOwen* (Owen/Galderma), *Tridesilon* (Miles
Inc)
Lotion: 0.05% (*Rx*) *DesOwen* (Owen/Galderma)

DESOXIMETASONE
Ointment: 0.25% (*Rx*) *Topicort* (Aventis)
Cream: 0.05% and 0.25% (*Rx*) Various, *Topicort* (Aventis)
Gel: 0.05% (*Rx*) *Topicort* (Aventis)

DEXAMETHASONE SODIUM PHOSPHATE
Aerosol: 0.01% and 0.04% (*Rx*) *Aeroseb-Dex* (Herbert)

DIFLORASONE DIACETATE
Ointment: 0.05% (*Rx*) *Florone* (Dermik), *Maxiflor* (Herbert), *Psorcon*
Cream: 0.05% (*Rx*) (Dermik)

FLUOCINOLONE ACETONIDE
Ointment: 0.025% (*Rx*) Various, *Flurosyn* (Rugby), *Synalar* (Syntex)
Cream: 0.01%, 0.025%, 0.2% (*Rx*)
Solution: 0.01% (*Rx*) Various, *Synalar* (Syntex)
Shampoo: 0.01% (*Rx*) *FS Shampoo* (Hill)
Oil: 0.01% (*Rx*) *Derma-Smoothe/FS* (Hill)

FLUOCINONIDE
Cream: 0.05% (*Rx*) — Various, *Fluonex* (ICN), *Lidex* (Syntex)
Ointment: 0.05% (*Rx*) — Various, *Lidex* (Syntex)
Solution: 0.05% (*Rx*)
Gel: 0.05% (*Rx*)

FLURANDRENOLIDE
Ointment: 0.025% and 0.05% (*Rx*) — *Cordran* (Oclassen)
Cream: 0.025% and 0.05% (*Rx*) — *Cordran SP* (Oclassen)
Lotion: 0.05% (*Rx*) — Various, *Cordran* (Oclassen)
Tape: 4 mcg/cm² (*Rx*) — *Cordran* (Oclassen)

FLUTICASONE PROPIONATE
Cream: 0.05% (*Rx*) — *Cutivate* (GlaxoSmithKline)
Ointment: 0.005% (*Rx*)

HALCINONIDE
Ointment: 0.1% (*Rx*) — *Halog* (Princeton)
Cream: 0.025% and 0.1% (*Rx*) — *Halog* (Princeton), *Halog-E* (Princeton)
Solution: 0.1% (*Rx*) — *Halog* (Princeton)

HALOBETASOL PROPIONATE
Ointment: 0.05% (*Rx*) — *Ultravate* (Westwood-Squibb)
Cream: 0.05% (*Rx*)

HYDROCORTISONE
Ointment: 0.5%, 1%, 2.5% (*Rx and otc*) — Various, *Cortizone•5* (Thompson), *Cortizone•10* (Thompson), *Hytone* (Dermik)
Cream: 0.5%, 1%, 2.5% (*Rx and otc*) — Various, *Dermolate* (Schering-Plough), *Dermacort* (Solvay), *Procort* (Roberts)
Lotion: 0.25%, 0.5%, 1%, 2%, 2.5% (*Rx*) — Various, *Cetacort* (Owen/Galderma), *Ala-Scalp* (Del-Ray)
Liquid: 1% (*otc*) — *Scalpicin* (Combe), *T/Scalp* (Neutrogena)
Gel: 0.5% and 1% (*otc*) — *Extra Strength CortaGel* (Norstar)
Solution: 1% (*Rx*) — *Penecort* (Herbert), *Texacort* (GenDerm)
Aerosol/Pump spray: 0.5% (*Rx and otc*) — *Aeroseb-HC* (Herbert), *Cortaid* (Pharmacia)
Pump spray: 1% (*otc*) — *Maximum Strength Cortaid* (Pharmacia)
Stick, roll-on: 1% (*otc*) — *Maximum Strength Cortaid Faststick* (Pharmacia)

HYDROCORTISONE ACETATE
Ointment: 0.5% and 1% (*otc*) — *Lanacort-5* (Combe), *Maximum Strength Lanacort 10* (Combe), *Anusol HC-1* (Parke-Davis)
Cream: 0.5% and 1% (*Rx*) — *Cortaid with Aloe* (Pharmacia), *U-Cort* (Thames)

HYDROCORTISONE BUTEPRATE
Cream: 1% (*Rx*) — *Pandel* (Savage)

HYDROCORTISONE BUTYRATE
Solution: (*Rx*) — *Locoid* (Ferndale)

HYDROCORTISONE VALERATE
Ointment: 0.2% (*Rx*) — *Westcort* (Westwood-Squibb)
Cream: 0.2% (*Rx*)

MOMETASONE FUROATE
Ointment: 0.1% (*Rx*) — *Elocon* (Schering)
Cream: 0.1% (*Rx*)
Lotion: 0.1% (*Rx*)

PREDNICARBATE
Cream: 0.1% (*Rx*) — *Dermatop* (Aventis)

TRIAMCINOLONE ACETONIDE
Ointment: 0.025%, 0.1%, 0.5% (*Rx*) — Various, *Kenalog* (Westwood-Squibb), *Aristocort* (Fujisawa)
Cream: 0.025%, 0.1%, 0.5% (*Rx*)
Lotion: 0.025% and 0.1% (*Rx*) — Various, *Kenalog* (Westwood-Squibb)
Aerosol: (2 sec. spray) (*Rx*) — *Kenalog* (Westwood-Squibb)

Indications
Pruritus:
    Relief of inflammatory and pruritic manifestations of corticosteroid-responsive dermatoses – Contact dermatitis, atopic dermatitis, nummular eczema, stasis eczema, asteatotic

eczema, lichen planus, lichen simplex chronicus, insect and arthropod bite reactions, first- and second-degree localized burns, and sunburns.

Alternative/Adjunctive treatment: Psoriasis, seborrheic dermatitis, severe diaper rash, dishidrosis, nodular prurigo, chronic discoid lupus erythematosus, alopecia areata, lymphocytic infiltration of the skin, mycosis fungoides, and familial benign pemphigus of Hailey-Hailey.

Possibly effective: Possibly effective in the following conditions: Bullous pemphigoid, cutaneous mastocytosis, lichen sclerosus et atrophicus, and vitiligo.

Nonprescription hydrocortisone preparations: Temporary relief of itching associated with minor skin irritations, inflammation, and rashes caused by eczema, insect bites, poison ivy, poison oak, poison sumac, soaps, detergents, cosmetics, jewelry, seborrheic dermatitis, psoriasis, and external genital and anal itching.

Administration and Dosage
Usual dose: Apply sparingly to affected areas 1 to 4 times daily.

Actions
Pharmacology: The primary therapeutic effects of the topical corticosteroids are caused by their anti-inflammatory activity, which is nonspecific (eg, they act against most causes of inflammation including mechanical, chemical, microbiological, and immunological).

Pharmacokinetics: The amount of corticosteroid absorbed from the skin depends on the intrinsic properties of the drug itself, the vehicle used, the duration of exposure, and the surface area and condition of the skin to which it is applied.

    Vehicles – Ointments are more occlusive and are preferred for dry scaly lesions. Use creams on oozing lesions or in intertriginous areas where the occlusive effects of ointments may cause maceration and folliculitis.

    Relative potency – The relative potency of a product depends on several factors including the characteristics and concentration of the drug and the vehicle used.

Relative Potency of Selected Topical Corticosteroid Products		
Drug	Dosage Form	Strength
I. Very high potency		
Augmented betamethasone dipropionate	Ointment	0.05%
Clobetasol propionate	Cream, Ointment	0.05%
Diflorasone diacetate	Ointment	0.05%
Halobetasol propionate	Cream, Ointment	0.05%
II. High potency		
Amcinonide	Cream, Lotion, Ointment	0.1%
Augmented betamethasone dipropionate	Cream	0.05%
Betamethasone dipropionate	Cream, Ointment	0.05%
Betamethasone valerate	Ointment	0.1%
Desoximetasone	Cream, Ointment	0.25%
	Gel	0.05%
Diflorasone diacetate	Cream, Ointment (emollient base)	0.05%
Fluocinolone acetonide	Cream	0.2%
Fluocinonide	Cream, Ointment, Gel	0.05%
Halcinonide	Cream, Ointment	0.1%
Triamcinolone acetonide	Cream, Ointment	0.5%
III. Medium potency		
Betamethasone benzoate	Cream, Gel, Lotion	0.025%
Betamethasone dipropionate	Lotion	0.05%
Betamethasone valerate	Cream	0.1%
Clocortolone pivalate	Cream	0.1%
Desoximetasone	Cream	0.05%
Fluocinolone acetonide	Cream, Ointment	0.025%
Flurandrenolide	Cream, Ointment	0.025%
	Cream, Ointment, Lotion	0.05%
	Tape	4 mcg/cm^2

Relative Potency of Selected Topical Corticosteroid Products		
Drug	Dosage Form	Strength
III. Fluticasone propionate	Cream	0.05%
	Ointment	0.005%
Hydrocortisone butyrate	Ointment, Solution	0.1%
Hydrocortisone valerate	Cream, Ointment	0.2%
Mometasone furoate	Cream, Ointment, Lotion	0.1%
Triamcinolone acetonide	Cream, Ointment, Lotion	0.025%
	Cream, Ointment, Lotion	0.1%
IV. *Low potency*		
Aclometasone dipropionate	Cream, Ointment	0.05%
Desonide	Cream	0.05%
Dexamethasone	Aerosol	0.01%
	Aerosol	0.04%
Dexamethasone sodium phosphate	Cream	0.1%
Fluocinolone acetonide	Cream, Solution	0.01%
Hydrocortisone	Lotion	0.25%
	Cream, Ointment, Lotion, Aerosol	0.5%
	Cream, Ointment, Lotion, Solution	1%
	Cream, Ointment, Lotion	2.5%
Hydrocortisone acetate	Cream, Ointment	0.5%
	Cream, Ointment	1%

Contraindications

Hypersensitivity to any component; monotherapy in primary bacterial infections such as impetigo, paryonchia, erysipelas, cellulitis, angular cheilitis, erythrasma (clobetasol), treatment of rosacea, perioral dermatitis, or acne; use on the face, groin, or axilla (very high or high potency agents); ophthalmic use.

Warnings

Pregnancy: Category C.

Lactation: It is not known whether topical corticosteroids could result in sufficient systemic absorption to produce detectable quantities in breast milk.

Children: Children may be more susceptible to topical corticosteroid-induced hypothalamic-pituitary-adrenal (HPA) axis suppression and Cushing's syndrome than adults because of a larger skin surface area to body weight ratio.

Precautions

Systemic effects: Systemic absorption of topical corticosteroids has produced reversible HPA axis suppression, Cushing's syndrome, hyperglycemia, and glycosuria.

As a general rule, little effect on the HPA axis will occur with a potent topical corticosteroid in amounts of < 50 g weekly for an adult and 15 g weekly for a small child, without occlusion. To cover the adult body 1 time requires 12 to 26 g.

Local irritation: If local irritation develops, discontinue use and institute appropriate therapy.

Psoriasis: Do not use topical corticosteroids as sole therapy in widespread plaque psoriasis.

Atrophic changes: Skin atrophy is common and may be clinically significant in 3 to 4 weeks with potent preparations. Certain areas of the body, such as the face, groin, and axillae, are more prone to atrophic changes than other areas of the body following treatment with corticosteroids.

Infections: Treating skin infections with topical corticosteroids can extensively worsen the infection.

Occlusive therapy: Occlusive dressings such as a plastic wrap increase skin penetration by 10-fold. Discontinue the use of occlusive dressings if infection develops and institute appropriate antimicrobial therapy.

Do not use occlusive dressings in augmented betamethasone dipropionate, betamethasone dipropionate, clobetasol, halobetasol propionate, and mometasone treatment regimens.

Adverse Reactions

Adverse reactions may include burning; itching; irritation; erythema; dryness; folliculitis; hypertrichosis; pruritus; acneiform eruptions; hypopigmentation; perioral dermatitis; allergic contact dermatitis; numbness of fingers; stinging and cracking/tightening of skin; maceration of the skin; secondary infection; skin atrophy; striae; miliaria; telangiectasia. These may occur more frequently with occlusive dressings.

TRETINOIN (trans-Retinoic Acid; Vitamin A Acid)

Cream: 0.02%, 0.05% (*Rx*)	Renova (Ortho Dermatological)
Cream: 0.025%, 0.05%, 0.1% (*Rx*)	Retin-A (Ortho)
Gel: 0.025%, 0.1% (*Rx*)	Retin-A (Ortho)
Liquid: 0.05% (*Rx*)	Retin-A (Ortho)

Indications

Retin-A:

   Acne – Topical treatment of acne vulgaris.

Renova:

   Dermatologic conditions –

      0.02% cream: Adjunctive agent for use in the mitigation (palliation) of the fine wrinkles in patients who do not achieve such palliation using comprehensive skin care and sun avoidance programs alone.

      0.05% cream: Adjunctive agent for use in the mitigation (palliation) of the fine wrinkles, mottled hyperpigmentation, and tactile roughness of facial skin in patients who do not achieve such palliation using comprehensive skin care and sun avoidance programs alone.

Administration and Dosage

Retin-A: Apply once a day, before bedtime. Cover the entire affected area lightly. Thoroughly wash hands immediately after applying tretinoin.

   Liquid – Apply with fingertip, gauze pad, or cotton swab. Do not oversaturate gauze or cotton to the extent that liquid will run into unaffected areas.

   Gel – Excessive application results in "pilling" of the gel, which minimizes the likelihood of overapplication by the patient.

      Closely monitor alterations of vehicle, drug concentration, or dose frequency. During the early weeks of therapy, an apparent exacerbation of inflammatory lesions may occur because of the action of the medication on deep, previously undetected lesions; this is not a reason to discontinue therapy.

      Therapeutic results should be seen after 2 to 3 weeks, but may not be optimal until after 6 weeks. Once lesions have responded satisfactorily, maintain therapy with less frequent applications or other dosage forms.

      Patients may use cosmetics but should thoroughly cleanse area to be treated before applying medication.

Renova: Apply tretinoin to the face once a day at bedtime, using only enough to cover the entire affected area lightly. Gently wash face with a mild soap, pat the skin dry, and wait 20 to 30 minutes before applying. Apply a pea-sized amount of cream to cover the entire face. Take caution to avoid contact with eyes, ears, nostrils, and mouth.

   For best results, do not apply another skin care product or cosmetic for ≥ 1 hour after applying tretinoin.

   Do not wash face for ≥ 1 hour after applying tretinoin.

   Application of tretinoin may cause a transitory feeling of warmth or slight stinging.

   Mitigation (palliation) of fine facial wrinkling, mottled hyperpigmentation, and tactile roughness may occur gradually over the course of therapy. Up to 6 months of therapy may be required before the effects are seen. Most of the improvement noted with tretinoin is seen during the first 24 weeks of therapy. Thereafter, therapy primarily maintains the improvement noticed during the first 24 weeks.

Actions

Pharmacology: Although the exact mode of action of tretinoin is unknown, current evidence suggests that topical tretinoin decreases cohesiveness of follicular epithelial cells with decreased microcomedone formation. Additionally, tretinoin stimulates mitotic activity and increases turnover of follicular epithelial cells, causing extrusion of the comedones.

   Retinoids are believed to exert an effect on the growth and differentiation of various epithelial cells.

Pharmacokinetics: The transdermal absorption of tretinoin from various topical formulations ranged from 1% to 31% of applied dose, depending on whether it was applied to healthy skin or dermatatic skin.

Contraindications

Hypersensitivity to any component of the product.

Warnings

For external use only: Keep tretinoin away from the eyes, mouth, angles of the nose, and mucous membranes.

Irritation: Tretinoin may induce severe local erythema, pruritus, burning, stinging, and peeling at the application site. Tretinoin may cause severe irritation to eczematous skin; use with caution in patients with this condition.

Mitigating effects: Tretinoin has shown no mitigating effects on significant signs of chronic sun exposure. Tretinoin does not eliminate wrinkles, repair sun damaged skin, reverse photoaging, or restore a more youthful or younger dermal histologic pattern.

Tretinoin 0.02% cream has shown no mitigating effects on tactile roughness or mottled hyperpigmentation.

Long-term use: There is evidence of atypical changes in melanocytes and keratinocytes and of increased dermal elastosis in some patients treated for > 48 weeks.

Photosensitivity: Because of heightened burning susceptibility, avoid or minimize exposure to sunlight (including sunlamps) during use of tretinoin. Warn patients to use sunscreens (minimum SPF of 15) and protective clothing when using tretinoin. Advise patients with sunburn not to use tretinoin until fully recovered. Patients who may have considerable sun exposure because of their occupations and those with inherent sensitivity to sunlight should exercise particular caution when using tretinoin.

Eczematous skin: Tretinoin has been reported to cause severe irritation on eczematous skin; use with utmost caution.

Pregnancy: Category C.

Lactation: It is not known whether this drug is excreted in breast milk.

Children: Safety and efficacy in patients < 18 years of age have not been established.

Precautions

Excessive application: Redness, peeling, or discomfort may occur if medication is applied excessively, and results will not be improved.

Photosensitivity: Minimize exposure to sunlight and sunlamps and advise patients with sunburn not to use tretinoin until fully recovered. Patients who undergo considerable sun exposure because of occupation and those with inherent sun sensitivity should exercise particular caution. Use sunscreen products and protective clothing over treated areas. Other weather extremes, such as wind and cold, also may be irritating.

Drug Interactions

Drugs that may interact with tretinoin include sulfur, resorcinol, benzoyl peroxide, and salicylic acid.

Topical preparations: Use caution with concomitant topical medications, medicated or abrasive soaps, shampoos, cleansers, cosmetics with a strong drying effect, products with high concentrations of alcohol, astringents, spices or lime, permanent wave solutions, electrolysis, hair depilatories or waxes, and products that may irritate the skin in patients being treated with tretinoin because they may increase irritation.

Photosensitizers: Do not use tretinoin if the patient is also taking drugs known to be photosensitizers (eg, thiazides, tetracyclines, fluoroquinolones, phenothiazines, sulfonamides) because of the possibility of augmented phototoxicity.

Adverse Reactions
Adverse reactions may include excessively red, edematous, blistered, or crusted skin; hyperpigmentation, hypopigmentation; peeling; dry skin; burning; stinging; erythema; pruritus.

CAPSAICIN

Cream: 0.025% and 0.075% in an emollient base (*otc*)	*Zostrix* (GenDerm), *Zostrix-HP* (GenDerm)
Cream: 0.025% (*otc*)	*Capzasin•P* (Thompson Medical)
Gel: 0.025% (*otc*)	*R-Gel* (Healthline Labs)
Lotion: 0.025% and 0.075% (*otc*)	*Capsin* (Fleming)
Roll-on: 0.075% (*otc*)	*No pain-HP* (Young Again Products)

Indications
Temporary relief of pain from rheumatoid arthritis, osteoarthritis, and relief of neuralgias such as the pain following shingles (herpes zoster) or painful diabetic neuropathy.

Administration and Dosage
Adults and children ≥ 2 years of age: Apply to affected area not more than 3 or 4 times daily. May cause transient burning on application. This is observed more frequently when application schedules of < 3 or 4 times daily are used. If applied with the fingers, wash hands immediately after application.

Actions
Pharmacology: Capsaicin is a natural chemical derived from plants. Although the precise mechanism of action is not fully understood, evidence suggests that the drug renders skin and joints insensitive to pain by depleting and preventing reaccumulation of substance P in peripheral sensory neurons.

Warnings
For external use only: Avoid contact with eyes or broken or irritated skin. Use care when handling contact lenses following application of capsaicin.

Bandage use: Do not bandage tightly.

Worsened condition: If condition worsens or if symptoms persist 14 to 28 days, discontinue use and consult physician.

Adverse Reactions
Adverse reactions include burning; stinging; erythema; cough; respiratory irritation.

PENCICLOVIR

Cream: 10 mg/kg (*Rx*) *Denavir* (GlaxoSmithKline)

Indications

Herpes labialis: For the treatment of recurrent herpes labialis (cold sores) in adults.

Administration and Dosage

Apply penciclovir every 2 hours while awake for 4 days. Start treatment as early as possible (eg, during the prodrome or when lesions appear).

Actions

Pharmacology: Penciclovir is an antiviral agent active against herpes viruses. It has in vitro inhibitory activity against herpes simplex virus types 1 (HSV-1) and 2 (HSV-2).

Pharmacokinetics: Measurable penciclovir concentrations were not detected in plasma or urine of healthy male volunteers following single or repeat application of the 1% cream at a dose of 180 mg penciclovir daily ($\approx$ 67 times the estimated usual clinical dose).

Contraindications

Hypersensitivity to the product or any of its components.

Warnings

Pregnancy: Category B.

Lactation: There is no information on whether penciclovir is excreted in breast milk after topical administration.

Children: Safety and efficacy in pediatric patients have not been established.

Precautions

Mucous membranes: Use penciclovir on herpes labialis on the lips and face only. Application to human mucous membranes is not recommended. Avoid application in or near the eyes because it may cause irritation.

Immunocompromised patients: Penciclovir's effect in immunocompromised patients has not been established.

Adverse Reactions

Adverse reactions occurring in $\geq$ 3% of patients include headache.

IMIQUIMOD

Cream: 5% (Rx)	Aldara (3M Pharm)

Indications

Genital and perianal warts: Treatment of external genital and perianal warts/condyloma acuminata in adults.

Unlabeled uses: May be effective for the treatment of basal cell carcinoma.

Administration and Dosage

Apply imiquimod 3 times per week, prior to normal sleeping hours, and leave on the skin for 6 to 10 hours. Following the treatment period, remove cream by washing the treated area with mild soap and water. Examples of 3 times per week application schedules are Monday/Wednesday/Friday or Tuesday/Thursday/Saturday. Continue imiquimod treatment until there is total clearance of the genital/perianal warts or for ≤ 16 weeks. A rest period of several days may be taken if required by the patient's discomfort or severity of the local skin reaction. Treatment may resume once the reaction subsides.

Nonocclusive dressings such as cotton gauze or cotton underwear may be used in the management of skin reactions. Hand-washing before and after cream application is recommended. Imiquimod is packaged in single-use packets that contain sufficient cream to cover a wart area of up to 20 cm²; avoid use of excessive amounts of cream. Instruct patients to apply imiquimod to external, genital, or perianal warts. Apply a thin layer to the wart area and rub in until the cream is no longer visible. Do not occlude the application site.

Actions

Pharmacology: Imiquimod is an immune response modifier. The mechanism of action of imiquimod in treating genital/perianal warts is unknown. Imiquimod has no direct antiviral activity in cell culture.

Pharmacokinetics: Less than 0.9% of the dose was excreted in the urine and feces following topical application.

Contraindications

None known.

Warnings

Other conditions: Imiquimod has not been evaluated for the treatment of urethral, intravaginal, cervical, rectal, or intra-anal human papilloma viral disease and is not recommended for these conditions.

Pregnancy: Category B.

Lactation: It is not known whether imiquimod is excreted in breast milk.

Children: Safety and efficacy in patients < 18 years of age have not been established.

Precautions

Skin reactions: The most frequently reported adverse reactions were local skin and application site reactions. These reactions were usually mild to moderate in intensity. These reactions were more frequent and more intense with daily application than with 3 times/week application.

Local skin reactions such as erythema, erosion, excoriation/flaking, and edema are common. Should severe local skin reaction occur, remove the cream by washing the treatment area with mild soap and water. Treatment with imiquimod cream can be resumed after the skin reaction has subsided. There is no clinical experience with imiquimod cream therapy immediately following the treatment of genital/perianal warts with other cutaneously applied drugs; therefore, imiquimod cream administration is not recommended until genital/perianal tissue is healed from any previous drug or surgical treatment. Imiquimod has the potential to exacerbate inflammatory conditions of the skin.

Adverse Reactions

The adverse reactions with an incidence of ≥ 3% include erythema, erosion, excoriation, flaking, edema, induration, ulceration, scabbing, vesicles, itching, burning, local pain, soreness, fungal infection, headache, and influenza-like symptoms.

TACROLIMUS

Ointment: 0.03%, 0.1% (*Rx*)   *Protopic* (Fujisawa)

Tacrolimus also is available as a capsule for organ rejection prophylaxis. Refer to the Biological and Immunologic Agents chapter.

Indications

Moderate to severe atopic dermatitis: Tacrolimus ointment, both 0.03% and 0.1% for adults, and only 0.03% for children 2 to 15 years of age, is indicated for short-term and intermittent long-term therapy in the treatment of patients with moderate to severe atopic dermatitis.

Administration and Dosage

Adults:

0.03% and 0.1% – Apply a thin layer to the affected skin areas twice daily and rub in gently and completely. Continue treatment for 1 week after clearing of signs and symptoms of atopic dermatitis.

Children:

0.03% – Apply a thin layer to the affected skin areas twice daily and rub in gently and completely. Continue treatment for 1 week after clearing of signs and symptoms of atopic dermatitis.

The safety of tacrolimus ointment under occlusion, which may promote systemic exposure, has not been evaluated. Do not use tacrolimus ointment with occlusive dressings.

Actions

Pharmacology: Tacrolimus is a macrolide immunosuppressant produced by *Streptomyces tsukubaensis*. The mechanism of action of tacrolimus in atopic dermatitis is not known. It has been demonstrated that tacrolimus inhibits T-lymphocyte activation by first binding to an intracellular protein, FKBP-12.

Pharmacokinetics:

Absorption/Distribution – In atopic dermatitis patients, tacrolimus is absorbed after topical application of 0.1% tacrolimus ointment.

There was no evidence based on blood concentrations that tacrolimus accumulates systemically upon intermittent topical application for periods of up to 1 year. The absolute bioavailability of topical tacrolimus is unknown.

Contraindications

A history of hypersensitivity to tacrolimus or any other component of the preparation.

Warnings

Pregnancy: Category C.

Lactation: Tacrolimus is excreted in human milk. A decision should be made whether to discontinue nursing or to discontinue the drug, taking into account the importance of the drug to the mother.

Children: Tacrolimus 0.03% ointment may be used in children ≥ 2 years of age.

Precautions

Infected atopic dermatitis: Before commencing treatment with tacrolimus ointment, clear clinical infections at treatment sites.

Viral infection: Treatment with tacrolimus ointment may be associated with an increased risk of varicella zoster virus infection (chicken pox or shingles), herpes simplex virus infection, or eczema herpeticum.

Lymphadenopathy: Patients who receive tacrolimus ointment and who develop lymphadenopathy should have the etiology of their lymphadenopathy investigated. In the absence of a clear etiology for the lymphadenopathy, or in the presence of acute infectious mononucleosis, consider discontinuation of tacrolimus ointment. Monitor patients who develop lymphadenopathy to ensure that the lymphadenopathy resolves.

Phototoxicity: It is prudent for patients to minimize or avoid natural or artificial sunlight exposure.

Other skin disorders: The use of tacrolimus ointment in patients with Netherton's syndrome is not recommended because of the potential for increased systemic absorption of tacrolimus. The safety of tacrolimus ointment has not been established in patients with generalized erythroderma.

Drug Interactions
Coadminister known CYP3A4 inhibitors (eg, erythromycin, itraconazole, ketoconazole, fluconazole, calcium channel blockers, cimetidine) with caution in patients with widespread or erythrodermic disease.

Adverse Reactions
Adverse events that occurred in ≥ 3% of patients include the following: Skin burning, pruritus, skin erythema, skin infection, herpes simplex, pustular rash, folliculitis, urticaria, maculopapular rash, rash, fungal dermatitis, acne, sunburn, skin disorder, vesiculobullous rash, skin tingling, dry skin, benign skin neoplasm, contact dermatitis, eczema, exfoliative dermatitis, diarrhea, vomiting, abdominal pain, gastroenteritis, nausea, cough increased, asthma, pharyngitis, rhinitis, sinusitis, bronchitis, flu-like symptoms, allergic reaction, headache, fever, infection, accidental injury, otitis media, lack of drug effect, alcohol intolerance, conjunctivitis, pain, lymphadenopathy, face edema, hyperesthesia, back pain, peripheral edema, varicella zoster/herpes zoster, asthenia, insomnia, dysmenorrhea, periodontal abscess, myalgia, cyst.

Chapter 12

OPHTHALMIC AND OTIC AGENTS

Topical Ophthalmics, 1059
Agents for Glaucoma, 1061
    Brimonidine Tartrate, 1062
    Epinephrine, 1063
    Dipivefrin HCl, 1064
    Apraclonidine HCl, 1065
    Beta-Adrenergic Blocking Agents, 1066
    Miotics, Direct-Acting, 1068
    Miotics, Cholinesterase Inhibitors, 1070
    Carbonic Anhydrase Inhibitors, 1072
    Prostaglandin Agonists, 1074
Ophthalmics, 1076
    Corticosteroids, 1076
    Lodoxamide Tromethamine, 1079
    Levocabastine HCl, 1079
    Antibiotics, 1080
    Natamycin, 1082
Antiviral Agents, 1084
    Vidarabine, 1084
    Trifluridine, 1085

TOPICAL OPHTHALMICS

General considerations in topical ophthalmic drug therapy: Proper administration is essential to optimal therapeutic response. In many instances, health professionals may be too casual when instructing patients on proper use of ophthalmics. The administration technique used often determines drug safety and efficacy.

- The normal eye retains ≈ 10 mcL of fluid (adjusted for blinking). The average dropper delivers 25 to 50 mcL/drop. The value of > 1 drop is questionable.
- Minimize systemic absorption of ophthalmic drops by compressing lacrimal sac for 3 to 5 minutes after instillation. This retards passage of drops via nasolacrimal duct into areas of potential absorption such as nasal and pharyngeal mucosa.
- Because of rapid lacrimal drainage and limited eye capacity, if multiple drop therapy is indicated, the best interval between drops is 5 minutes. This ensures the first drop is not flushed away by the second or the second is not diluted by the first.
- Topical anesthesia will increase the bioavailability of ophthalmic agents by decreasing the blink reflex and the production and turnover of tears.
- Factors that may increase absorption from ophthalmic dosage forms include lax eyelids of some patients, usually the elderly, which creates a greater reservoir for retention of drops, and hyperemic or diseased eyes.
- Eyecup use is discouraged because of the risk of contamination and spreading disease.
- Ophthalmic suspensions mix with tears less rapidly and remain in the cul-de-sac longer than solutions.
- Ophthalmic ointments maintain contact between the drug and ocular tissues by slowing the clearance rate to as little as 0.5%/min. Ophthalmic ointments provide maximum contact between drug and external ocular tissues.
- Ophthalmic ointments may impede delivery of other ophthalmic drugs to the affected side by serving as a barrier to contact.
- Ointments may blur vision during waking hours. Use with caution in conditions where visual clarity is critical (eg, operating motor equipment, reading).
- Monitor expiration dates closely. Do not use outdated medication.
- Solutions and ointments are frequently misused. Do not assume that patients know how to maximize safe and effective use of these agents. Combine appropriate patient education and counseling with prescribing and dispensing of ophthalmics.

Topical application is the most common route of administration for ophthalmic drugs. Advantages include convenience, simplicity, noninvasive nature, and the ability of the patient to self-administer. Because of blood and aqueous losses of drug, topical medications typically do not penetrate in useful concentrations to posterior ocular structures and therefore are of no therapeutic benefit for diseases of the retina, optic nerve, and other posterior segment structures.

Medications:

Solutions and suspensions – Most topical ocular preparations are commercially available as solutions or suspensions that are applied directly to the eye from the bottle, which serves as the eye dropper. Avoid touching the dropper tip to the eye because this can lead to contamination of the medication and also may cause ocular injury. Resuspend suspensions (notably, many ocular steroids) by shaking to provide an accurate dosage of drug.

Recommended procedures for administration of solutions or suspensions –

- Wash hands thoroughly before administration.
- Tilt head backward or lie down and gaze upward.
- Gently grasp lower eyelid below eyelashes and pull the eyelid away from the eye to form a pouch.

- Place dropper directly over eye. Avoid contact of the dropper with the eye, finger or any surface.
- Look upward just before applying a drop.
- After instilling the drop, look downward for several seconds.
- Release the lid slowly.
- With eyes closed, apply gentle pressure with fingers to the inside corner of eye for 3 to 5 minutes. This retards drainage of solution from intended solution.
- Do not rub the eye. Minimize blinking.
- Do not rinse the dropper.
- Do not use eye drops that have changed color.
- If > 1 type of ophthalmic drop is used, wait ≥ 5 minutes before administering the second agent.
- When the instillation of eye drops is difficult (eg, pediatric patients, adults with particularly strong blink reflex), the close-eye method may be used. This involves lying down, placing the prescribed number of drops on the eyelid in the inner corner of the eye, then opening eye so that drops will fall into the eye by gravity.

Ointments – The primary purpose for an ophthalmic ointment vehicle is to prolong drug contact time with the external ocular surface. This is particularly useful for treating children, who may "cry out" topically applied solutions, and for medicating ocular injuries, such as corneal abrasions, when the eye is to be patched. Administer solutions before ointments. Ointments preclude entry of subsequent drops.

Recommended procedures for administration of ointments –
- Wash hands thoroughly before administration.
- Holding the ointment tube in the hand for a few minutes will warm the ointment and facilitate flow.
- When opening the ointment tube for the first time, squeeze out and discard the first 0.25 inch of ointment as it may be too dry.
- Tilt head backward or lie down and gaze upward.
- Gently pull down the lower lid to form a pouch.
- Place 0.25 to 0.5 inch of ointment with a sweeping motion inside the lower lid by squeezing the tube gently.
- Close the eye for 1 to 2 minutes and roll the eyeball in all directions.
- Temporary blurring of vision may occur. Avoid activities requiring visual acuity until blurring clears.
- Remove excessive ointment around the eye or ointment tube tip with a tissue.
- If using > 1 kind of ointment, wait about 10 minutes before applying the second drug.

AGENTS FOR GLAUCOMA

Glaucoma is a condition of the eye in which an elevation of the intraocular pressure (IOP) leads to progressive cupping and atrophy of the optic nerve head, deterioration of the visual fields, and, ultimately, to blindness. Primary open-angle glaucoma is the most common type of glaucoma. Angle-closure glaucoma and congenital glaucoma are treated primarily by surgical methods, although short-term drug therapy is used to decrease IOP prior to surgery.

Drugs used in the therapy of primary open-angle glaucoma include a variety of agents with different mechanisms of action. The therapeutic goal in treating glaucoma is reducing the elevated IOP, a major risk factor in the pathogenesis of glaucomatous visual field loss. The higher the level of IOP, the greater the likelihood of glaucomatous visual field loss and optic nerve damage. Reduction of IOP may be accomplished by: 1) Decreasing the rate of production of aqueous humor or 2) increasing the rate of outflow (drainage) of aqueous humor from the anterior chamber of the eye.

The 5 groups of agents used in therapy of primary open-angle glaucoma are listed in the table, which summarizes their mechanism of decreasing IOP, effects on pupil size and ciliary muscle and duration of action.

Agents for Glaucoma						
Drug	Strength	Duration (hrs)	Decrease aqueous production	Increase aqueous outflow	Effect on pupil	Effect on ciliary muscle
Sympathomimetics						
Apraclonidine[1]	0.5 to 1%	7 to 12	+++	NR	NR	NR
Brimonidine	0.2%	12	++	++	NR	NR
Dipivefrin	0.1%	12	+	++	mydriasis	NR
Epinephrine	0.1% to 2%	12 to 24	+	++	mydriasis	NR
Beta blockers						
Betaxolol	0.25% to 0.5%	12	+++	NR	NR	NR
Carteolol	1%	12	+++	nd	NR	NR
Levobunolol	0.25% to 0.5%	12 to 24	+++	NR	NR	NR
Metipranolol	0.3%	12 to 24	+++	+	NR	NR
Timolol	0.25% to 0.5%	12 to 24	+++	+	NR	NR
Miotics, direct-acting						
Acetylcholine[2]	1%	10 to 20 min	NR	+++	miosis	accommodation
Carbachol[2]	0.75% to 3%	6 to 8	NR	+++	miosis	accommodation
Pilocarpine[3]	0.25% to 10%	4 to 8	NR	+++	miosis	accommodation
Miotics, cholinesterase inhibitors						
Demecarium	0.125% to 0.25%	days/wks	NR	+++	miosis	accommodation
Echothiophate	0.03% to 0.25%	days/wks	NR	+++	miosis	accommodation
Physostigmine	0.25% to 0.5%	12 to 36	NR	+++	miosis	accommodation
Carbonic anhydrase inhibitors[3]						
Acetazolamide	125 to 500 mg	8 to 12	+++	NR	NR	NR
Dichlorphenamide	50 mg	6 to 12	+++	NR	NR	NR
Dorzolamide	2%	≈ 8	+++	NR	NR	NR
Methazolamide	25 to 50 mg	10 to 18	+++	NR	NR	NR
Prostaglandin analog						
Latanoprost	0.0005%	24	NR	+++	NR	NR

+++ = significant activity   ++ = moderate activity   + = some activity   NR = no activity reported

nd = No data available

[1] 1% used only to decrease IOP in surgery.

[2] Intraocular administration only for miosis during surgery; carbachol also available as a topical agent.

[3] Also available as a gel and an insert; the duration of these doseforms is longer (18 to 24 hours and 1 week, respectively) than the solution.

[4] Systemic agents; for detailed information, see group monograph in Cardiovascular section.

[5] Topical ophthalmic agent.

Prostaglandin analogs: Prostaglandin analogs increase uveoscleral outflow through a new mechanism of action; selective prostanoid receptor agonism. Latanoprost, currently the only agent available in this class, can be used concurrently with other topical ophthalmic drug products to reduce IOP.

BRIMONIDINE TARTRATE

Solution: 0.2% (*Rx*)   *Alphagan* (Allergan)

Indications

Intraocular pressure (IOP): Lowering IOP in patients with open-angle glaucoma or ocular hypertension.

Administration and Dosage

The recommended dose is 1 drop of brimonidine tartrate in the affected eye(s) 3 times daily, ≈ 8 hours apart.

Actions

Pharmacology: Brimonidine tartrate is an alpha-2 adrenergic receptor agonist. It has a peak ocular hypotensive effect occurring at 2 hours postdose. Brimonidine has a dual mechanism of action by reducing aqueous humor production and increasing uveoscleral outflow.

Pharmacokinetics: After ocular administration of a 0.2% solution, plasma concentrations peaked within 1 to 4 hours and declined with a systemic half-life of ≈ 3 hours.

It is metabolized primarily by the liver. Urinary excretion is the major route of elimination of the drug and its metabolites. Approximately 87% of an orally administered radioactive dose was eliminated within 120 hours, with 74% found in the urine.

Contraindications

Hypersensitivity to brimonidine tartrate or any component of this medication; patients receiving monoamine oxidase (MAO) inhibitor therapy.

Warnings

Soft contact lenses: The preservative in brimonidine tartrate, benzalkonium chloride, may be absorbed by soft contact lenses. Instruct patients wearing soft contact lenses to wait at least 15 minutes after instilling brimonidine tartrate to insert soft contact lenses.

Renal/Hepatic function impairment: Use caution when treating patients with hepatic or renal impairment.

Pregnancy: Category B.

Lactation: It is not known whether brimonidine tartrate is excreted in breast milk.

Children: Safety and efficacy in pediatric patients have not been established.

Precautions

Cardiovascular disease: Exercise caution in treating patients with severe cardiovascular disease.

Caution: Use with caution in patients with depression, cerebral or coronary insufficiency, Raynaud's phenomenon, orthostatic hypotension, or thromboangiitis obliterans.

Loss of effect: Loss of effect in some patients may occur. The IOP-lowering efficacy observed with brimonidine tartrate during the first month of therapy may not always reflect the long-term level of IOP reduction. Therefore, routinely monitor IOP.

Drug Interactions

Drugs that may be affected by brimonidine tartrate include CNS depressants, beta-blockers, antihypertensives, and cardiac glycosides.

Drugs that may affect brimonidine tartrate include tricyclic antidepressants.

Adverse Reactions

Adverse events occurring in ≈ 10% to 30% of patients in descending order include oral dryness, ocular hyperemia, burning and stinging, headache, blurring, foreign body sensation, fatigue/drowsiness, conjunctival follicles, ocular allergic reactions, and ocular pruritus.

Adverse events occurring in ≈ 3% to 9% in descending order include corneal staining/erosion, photophobia, eyelid erythema, ocular ache/pain, ocular dryness, tearing, upper respiratory symptoms, eyelid edema, conjunctival edema, dizziness, blepharitis, ocular irritation, GI symptoms, asthenia, conjunctival blanching, abnormal vision, and muscular pain.

EPINEPHRINE

EPINEPHRINE (as HCl)	
Solution: 0.1%, 1%, and 2% (*Rx*)	*Epinephrine HCl* (Novartis Ophthalmic), *Glaucon* (Alcon)
Solution: 0.5%, 1%, and 2% (as base) (*Rx*)	*Epifrin* (Allergan)
EPINEPHRINE (as Borate)	
Solution: 0.5%, 1%, and 2% (*Rx*)	*Epinal* (Alcon)

Indications

Glaucoma: Management of open-angle (chronic simple) glaucoma; may be used in combination with miotics, beta blockers, hyperosmotic agents, or carbonic anhydrase inhibitors.

Administration and Dosage

Instill 1 drop into affected eye(s) once or twice daily. Determine frequency of instillation by tonometry.

More frequent instillation than 1 drop twice daily does not usually elicit any further improvement in therapeutic response.

When used in conjunction with miotics, instill the miotic first.

Actions

Pharmacology: Epinephrine, a direct-acting sympathomimetic agent, acts on α and β receptors. Topical application, therefore, causes conjunctival decongestion (vasoconstriction), transient mydriasis (pupillary dilation), and reduction in intraocular pressure (IOP). It is believed IOP reduction primarily is caused by reduced aqueous production and increased aqueous outflow. The duration of decrease in IOP is 12 to 24 hours.

Contraindications

Hypersensitivity to epinephrine or any component of the formulation; narrow- or shallow-angle (angle Y closure) glaucoma; aphakia; patients with a narrow angle but no glaucoma; if the nature of the glaucoma is not clearly established. Do not use while wearing soft contact lenses; discoloration of lenses may occur.

Warnings

For ophthalmic use only: Not for injection or intraocular use.

Gonioscopy: Because pupil dilation may precipitate an acute attack of narrow-angle glaucoma, evaluate anterior chamber angle by gonioscopy prior to beginning therapy.

Anesthesia: Discontinue use prior to general anesthesia with anesthetics that sensitize the myocardium to sympathomimetics (eg, cyclopropane, halothane).

Aphakic patients: Maculopathy with associated decrease in visual acuity may occur in the aphakic eye; if this occurs, promptly discontinue use.

Elderly: Use with caution.

Pregnancy: Category C.

Lactation: It is not known whether this drug is excreted in breast milk.

Children: Safety and efficacy for use in children have not been established.

Precautions

Instillation discomfort: Epinephrine is relatively uncomfortable upon instillation. Discomfort lessens as concentration of epinephrine decreases.

Special risk: Use with caution in the presence or history of the following: Hypertension; diabetes; hyperthyroidism; heart disease; cerebral arteriosclerosis; bronchial asthma.

Hazardous tasks: Epinephrine may cause temporarily blurred or unstable vision after instillation; observe caution while driving, operating machinery, or performing other tasks requiring physical dexterity.

Drug Interactions

Consider interactions that occur with systemic use of epinephrine, including beta blockers and chymotrypsin.

Adverse Reactions

Adverse reactions may include transient stinging and burning; eye pain/ache; browache; headache; allergic lid reaction; conjunctival hyperemia; conjunctival or corneal pigmentation; ocular irritation (hypersensitivity); localized adrenochrome deposits in conjunctiva and cornea (prolonged use); reversible cystoid macular edema (may result from use in aphakic patients); palpitations; tachycardia; extrasystoles; cardiac arrhythmia; hypertension; faintness.

DIPIVEFRIN HCl (Dipivalyl epinephrine)

Solution: 0.1% (*Rx*)   Various, *Propine* (Allergan), *AKPro* (Akorn)

Indications

Glaucoma: Initial therapy or as an adjunct with other antiglaucoma agents for the control of intraocular pressure (IOP) in chronic open-angle glaucoma.

Administration and Dosage

Initial glaucoma therapy: Instill 1 drop into the eye(s) every 12 hours.

Actions

Pharmacology: Dipivefrin is a prodrug of epinephrine. Dipivefrin, converted to epinephrine in the eye by enzymatic hydrolysis, appears to act by decreasing aqueous production and enhancing outflow facility. It has the same therapeutic effects as epinephrine with fewer local and systemic side effects.

Pharmacokinetics: The onset of action with 1 drop occurs $\approx$ 30 minutes after treatment, with maximum effect seen at $\approx$ 1 hour.

Contraindications

Hypersensitivity to dipivefrin or any formulation component; narrow-angle glaucoma.

Warnings

Pregnancy: Category B.

Lactation: It is not known whether this drug is excreted in breast milk.

Children: Safety and efficacy for use in children have not been established.

Precautions

Aphakic patients: Macular edema occurs in up to 30% of aphakic patients treated with epinephrine. Discontinuation generally results in reversal of the maculopathy.

Adverse Reactions

Adverse reactions may include tachycardia; arrhythmias; hypertension; burning and stinging; conjunctival injection.

APRACLONIDINE HYDROCHLORIDE

Solution: 0.5% and 0.01% *(Rx)*   *Iopidine* (Alcon)

Indications
1%: To control or prevent postsurgical elevations in IOP that occur in patients after argon laser trabeculoplasty or iridotomy.

0.5%: Short-term adjunctive therapy in patients on maximally tolerated medical therapy who require additional IOP reduction.

Administration and Dosage
0.5%: Instill 1 to 2 drops in the affected eye(s) 3 times daily. Because apraclonidine 0.5% will be used with other ocular glaucoma therapies, use an approximate 5-minute interval between instillation of each medication to prevent washout of the previous dose. Not for injection into the eye.

1%: Instill 1 drop in scheduled operative eye 1 hour before initiating anterior segment laser surgery. Instill second drop into same eye immediately upon completion of surgery.

Actions
Pharmacology: Apraclonidine HCl is a relatively selective α-adrenergic agonist. When instilled into the eyes, apraclonidine reduces intraocular pressure (IOP) and has minimal effect on cardiovascular parameters.

Pharmacokinetics: Topical use of apraclonidine 0.5% leads to systemic absorption. The onset of action is usually within 1 hour and the maximum IOP reduction occurs 3 to 5 hours after application of a single dose.

Contraindications
Hypersensitivity to any component of this medication or to clonidine; concurrent monamine oxidase inhibitor therapy.

Warnings
Concomitant therapy: The addition of 0.5% apraclonidine to patients already using 2 aqueous suppressing drugs (eg, beta blocker plus carbonic anhydrase inhibitor) as part of their maximally tolerated medical therapy may not provide additional benefit.

Tachyphylaxis: The IOP-lowering efficacy of 0.5% apraclonidine diminishes over time in some patients. The benefit for most patients is < 1 month.

Hypersensitivity reactions: Apraclonidine can lead to an allergic-like reaction characterized wholly or in part by the symptoms of hyperemia, pruritus, discomfort, tearing, foreign body sensation, and edema of the lids and conjunctiva. If ocular allergic-like symptoms occur, discontinue therapy.

Renal/Hepatic function impairment: Although the topical use of apraclonidine has not been studied in renal failure patients, structurally related clonidine undergoes a significant increase in half-life in patients with severe renal impairment. Close monitoring of cardiovascular parameters in patients with impaired renal function is advised if they are candidates for topical apraclonidine therapy. Close monitoring of cardiovascular parameters in patients with impaired liver function is also advised as the systemic dosage form of clonidine is partly metabolized in the liver.

Pregnancy: Category C.

Lactation: Consider discontinuing nursing for the day on which apraclonidine is used.

Children: Safety and efficacy for use in children have not been established.

Precautions
Monitoring: Glaucoma patients on maximally tolerated medical therapy who are treated with 0.5% apraclonidine to delay surgery should have their visual fields monitored periodically. Discontinue treatment if IOP rises significantly.

IOP reduction: Because apraclonidine is a potent depressor of IOP, closely monitor patients who develop exaggerated reductions in IOP.

Cardiovascular disease: Acute administration of 2 drops of apraclonidine has had minimal effect on heart rate or blood pressure; however, observe caution in treating patients with severe cardiovascular disease, including hypertension.

Use 0.5% apraclonidine with caution in patients with coronary insufficiency, recent MI, cerebrovascular disease, chronic renal failure, Raynaud's disease, or thromboangiitis obliterans.

Depression: Use caution and monitor depressed patients because apraclonidine has been infrequently associated with depression.

Drug Interactions

Drugs that may interact include cardiovascular agents and MAOIs.

Adverse Reactions

Adverse reactions from 1% solution may include upper lid elevation; conjunctival blanching; mydriasis; burning; discomfort; foreign body sensation; dryness; itching; hypotony; blurred or dimmed vision; allergic response; conjunctival microhemorrhage; dry mouth; bradycardia; vasovagal attack; palpitations; orthostatic episode; headache; taste abnormalities; nasal burning or head-cold sensation; shortness of breath.

Adverse reactions from 0.5% solution may include hyperemia; pruritus; discomfort; tearing; taste perversion; use can lead to an allergic-type reaction.

BETA-ADRENERGIC BLOCKING AGENTS

BETAXOLOL HCl	
Solution: 5.6 mg (equiv. to 5 mg base) per mL (0.5%) (*Rx*)	Various, *Betoptic* (Alcon)
Suspension: 2.8 mg (equiv. to 2.5 mg base) per mL (0.25%) (*Rx*)	*Betoptic S* (Alcon)
CARTEOLOL HCl	
Solution: 1% (*Rx*)	Various, *Ocupress* (Otsuka America)
LEVOBETAXOLOL HCl	
Suspension: 0.5% as base (5.6 mg/mL) (*Rx*)	*Betaxon* (Alcon)
LEVOBUNOLOL HCl	
Solution: 0.25% and 0.5% (*Rx*)	Various, *AKBeta* (Akorn), *Betagan Liquifilm* (Allergan)
METIPRANOLOL HCl	
Solution: 0.3% (*Rx*)	*OptiPranolol* (Bausch & Lomb)
TIMOLOL MALEATE	
Solution: 0.25% and 0.5% (*Rx*)	Various, *Timoptic* (Merck)
Gel: 0.25% and 0.5% (*Rx*)	Various, *Timoptic-XE* (Merck)

Indications

Glaucoma: Lowering intraocular pressure (IOP) in patients with chronic open-angle glaucoma and intraocular hypertension.

Administration and Dosage

BETAXOLOL HCl: Instill 1 to 2 drops twice daily.

CARTEOLOL HCl: One drop in the affected eye(s) twice daily.

LEVOBETAXOLOL HCl: Instill 1 drop in the affected eye(s) twice daily. In some patients, the IOP-lowering responses may require a few weeks to stabilize.

LEVOBUNOLOL HCl:

0.5% – 1 to 2 drops in the affected eye(s) once daily.

0.25% – 1 to 2 drops in the affected eye(s) twice daily.

In patients with more severe or uncontrolled glaucoma, the 0.5% solution can be administered twice daily.

METIPRANOLOL HCl: One drop in the affected eye(s) twice a day. If the patient's IOP is not at a satisfactory level on this regimen, more frequent administration or a larger dose is not known to be of benefit.

TIMOLOL MALEATE:
  Solution –
     Initial therapy: 1 drop of 0.25% or 0.5% twice daily. If clinical response is not adequate, change the dosage to 1 drop of 0.5% solution twice a day. If the IOP is maintained at satisfactory levels, change the dosage to 1 drop once a day.
     Gel – Administer other ophthalmics at least 10 minutes before the gel. Dose is 1 drop (0.25% or 0.5%) once daily. Dosages > 1 drop of 0.5% have not been studied. Consider concomitant therapy if IOP is not at a satisfactory level.

Actions

Pharmacology: The exact mechanism of ocular antihypertensive action is not established, but it appears to be a reduction of aqueous production. However, some studies show a slight increase in outflow facility with **timolol** and **metipranolol**.

Pharmacokinetics:

Pharmacokinetics of Ophthalmic β-Adrenergic Blocking Agents				
Drug	β-receptor selectivity	Onset (min)	Maximum effect (hr)	Duration (hr)
Carteolol	β_1 and β_2	nd[1]	2	12
Betaxolol	β_1	≤ 30	2	12
Levobunolol	β_1 and β_2	< 60	2 to 6	≤ 24
Metipranolol	β_1 and β_2	≤ 30	≈ 2	24
Timolol	β_1 and β_2	≤ 30	1 to 2	≤ 24
Levobetaxolol	β_1	≤ 30	2	≈ 12

[1] nd = No data

Contraindications

Bronchial asthma, a history of bronchial asthma, or severe chronic obstructive pulmonary disease; sinus bradycardia; second- and third-degree AV block; overt cardiac failure; cardiogenic shock; hypersensitivity to any component of the products.

Warnings

Systemic absorption: These agents may be absorbed systemically. The same adverse reactions found with systemic β-blockers may occur with topical use.

Cardiovascular: These agents can decrease resting and maximal exercise heart rate, even in healthy subjects.

Cardiac failure: Sympathetic stimulation may be essential for circulation support in diminished myocardial contractility; its inhibition by β-receptor blockade may precipitate more severe failure.

Bronchospasm: Nonallergic bronchospasm patients or patients with a history of chronic bronchitis, emphysema, etc., should receive β-blockers with caution; they may block bronchodilation produced by catecholamine stimulation of β_2-receptors.

Diabetes mellitus: Administer with caution to patients subject to spontaneous hypoglycemia or to diabetic patients (especially labile diabetics). Beta-blocking agents may mask signs and symptoms of acute hypoglycemia.

Thyroid: Beta-adrenergic blocking agents may mask clinical signs of hyperthyroidism (eg, tachycardia).

Cerebrovascular insufficiency: Because of potential effects of β-blockers on blood pressure and pulse, use with caution in patients with cerebrovascular insufficiency.

Pregnancy: Category C.

Lactation: It is not known whether these agents are excreted in human breast milk.

Children: Safety and efficacy for use in children have not been established.

Precautions

Angle-closure glaucoma: The immediate objective is to reopen the angle, requiring constriction of the pupil with a miotic. These agents have little or no effect on the pupil.

Muscle weakness: Beta-blockade may potentiate muscle weakness consistent with certain myasthenic symptoms (eg, diplopia, ptosis, generalized weakness).

Long-term therapy: In long-term studies (2 and 3 years), no significant differences in mean IOP were observed after initial stabilization.

Drug Interactions

Ophthalmic beta blockers may affect oral beta blockers, catecholamine-depleting drugs, calcium antagonists, digitalis, and phenothiazines.

Drugs that may affect ophthalmic beta blockers include catecholamine-depleting drugs, digitalis, and quinidine.

Other drugs that may interact with systemic β-adrenergic blocking agents also may interact with ophthalmic agents.

Adverse Reactions

Adverse reactions may include headache; depression; arrhythmia; syncope; heart block; cerebral vascular accident; cerebral ischemia; CHF; palpitation; nausea; hypersensitivity, including localized and generalized rash; bronchospasm; respiratory failure; eratitis; bleparoptosis; visual disturbances including refractive changes; diplopia; ptosis.

Systemic β-adrenergic blocker-associated reactions – Consider potential effects with ophthalmic use. The following adverse reactions have occurred with each individual agent:

Carteolol –

Ophthalmic: Transient irritation, burning, tearing, conjunctival hyperemia, edema ($\approx$ 25%).

Betaxolol –

Ophthalmic: Brief discomfort (> 25%); occasional tearing (5%).

Metipranolol –

Ophthalmic: Transient local discomfort; conjunctivitis; eyelid dermatitis; blepharitis; blurred vision; tearing; browache; abnormal vision; photophobia; edema; uveitis.

Levobetaxolol –

Ophthalmic: Transient ocular discomfort upon installation (11%).

Levobunolol –

Ophthalmic: Transient burning/stinging ($\leq$ 33%); blepharoconjunctivitis ($\leq$ 5%).

Timolol –

Ophthalmic: Ocular irritation including conjunctivitis; blepharitis; keratitis; blepharoptosis; decreased corneal sensitivity; visual disturbaces including refractive changes; diplopia; ptosis.

MIOTICS, DIRECT-ACTING

ACETYLCHOLINE CHLORIDE, INTRAOCULAR	
Solution: 1:100 acetylcholine chloride when reconstituted (*Rx*)	*Miochol-E* (Novartis Ophthalmic)
CARBACHOL, INTRAOCULAR	
Solution: 0.01% (*Rx*)	*Miostat* (Alcon), *Carbastat* (Novartis Ophthalmic)
CARBACHOL, TOPICAL	
Solution: 0.75%, 1.5%, 2.25%, and 3% (*Rx*)	*Isopto Carbachol* (Alcon), *Carboptic* (Optopics)
PILOCARPINE HCl	
Solution: 0.25%, 0.5%, 1%, 2%, 3%, 4%, 5%, 6%, 8%, and 10% (*Rx*)	Various, *Pilocar* (Novartis Ophthalmic), *Isopto Carpine* (Alcon)
Gel: 4% (*Rx*)	*Pilopine HS* (Alcon)
PILOCARPINE NITRATE	
Solution: 1%, 2%, and 4% (*Rx*)	*Pilagan* (Allergan)
PILOCARPINE OCULAR THERAPEUTIC SYSTEM	
Ocular Therapeutic System: Releases 20 or 40 mcg pilocarpine/hour for 1 week (*Rx*)	*Ocusert Pilo-20, Ocusert Pilo-40* (Alza)

Indications

Carbachol, topical; pilocarpine:
   Glaucoma – To decrease elevated intraocular pressure (IOP) in glaucoma.

Acetylcholine; carbachol, intraocular:
   Miosis – To induce miosis during surgery.

Administration and Dosage

ACETYLCHOLINE CHLORIDE, INTRAOCULAR:
   Solution – 0.5 to 2 mL produces satisfactory miosis. Solution need not be flushed from the chamber after miosis occurs.

CARBACHOL, INTRAOCULAR: Gently instill no more than 0.5 mL into the anterior chamber before or after securing sutures. Miosis is usually maximal 2 to 5 minutes after application.

CARBACHOL, TOPICAL: Instill 2 drops into eye(s) up to 3 times daily.

PILOCARPINE:
   Solution –
      Initial: 1 or 2 drops 3 to 4 times daily. Individuals with heavily pigmented irides may require higher strengths.
      Gel – Apply a 0.5 inch ribbon in the lower conjunctival sac of affected eye(s) once daily at bedtime.

PILOCARPINE NITRATE:
   Glaucoma – 1 to 2 drops 2 to 4 times daily.
   Emergency miosis – 1 to 2 drops of higher concentrations.
   Reversal of mydriasis – Dosage and strength required are dependent on the cycloplegic used.

PILOCARPINE OCULAR THERAPEUTIC SYSTEM:
   Initiation of therapy – It has been estimated that 20 mcg Ocusert is roughly equal to 0.5% or 1% drops and 40 mcg is roughly equal to 2% or 3% drops. Therapy may be started with the 20 mcg system, regardless of the strength of pilocarpine solution the patient previously required. Because of the patient's age, family history, and disease status or progression, however, therapy may be started with the 40 mcg system.
      If pressure is satisfactorily reduced with the 30 mcg system, the patient should continue its use, replacing each unit every 7 days. If IOP reduction greater than that achieved by 20 mcg is needed, transfer the patient to the 40 mcg system.

Actions

Pharmacology: Direct-acting miotics are parasympathomimetic (cholinergic) drugs which duplicate the muscarinic effects of **acetylcholine**. When applied topically, these drugs produce pupillary constriction, stimulate ciliary muscles, and increase aqueous humor outflow facility. With the increase in outflow facility, there is a decrease in IOP. Topical ophthalmic instillation of acetylcholine causes no discernible response, as cholinesterase destroys the molecule more rapidly than it can penetrate the cornea; therefore, acetylcholine only is used intraocularly.

Pharmacokinetics:

Miosis Induction of Direct-Acting Miotics			
Miotic	Onset	Peak	Duration
Acetylcholine, intraocular	seconds	—	10 min
Carbachol			
Intraocular	seconds	2 to 5 min	1 to 2 days
Topical	10 to 20 min	—	4 to 8 hours
Pilocarpine, topical	10 to 30 min	—	4 to 8 hours

Contraindications

Hypersensitivity to any component of the formulation; where constriction is undesirable (eg, acute iritis, acute or anterior uveitis, some forms of secondary glaucoma, pupillary block glaucoma, acute inflammatory disease of the anterior chamber).

Warnings

Corneal abrasion: Use carbachol with caution in the presence of corneal abrasion to avoid excessive penetration.

Pregnancy: Category C (carbachol, pilocarpine).

Lactation: It is not known whether these drugs are excreted in breast milk.

Children: Safety and efficacy for use in children have not been established.

Precautions

Systemic reactions: Caution is advised in patients with acute cardiac failure, bronchial asthma, peptic ulcer, hyperthyroidism, GI spasm, urinary tract obstruction, Parkinson's disease, recent MI, hypertension, or hypotension.

Retinal detachment: Retinal detachment has been caused by miotics in susceptible individuals, in individuals with pre-existing retinal disease, or in those who are predisposed to retinal tears.

Miosis: Miosis usually causes difficulty in dark adaptation. Advise patients to use caution while night driving or performing hazardous tasks in poor light.

Angle-closure: Although withdrawal of the peripheral iris from the anterior chamber angle by miosis may reduce the tendency for narrow-angle closure, miotics occasionally can precipitate angle closure by increasing resistance to aqueous flow from posterior to anterior chamber.

Pilocarpine ocular therapeutic system (Ocusert): Carefully consider and evaluate patients with acute infectious conjunctivitis or keratitis prior to use.

Adverse Reactions

Acetylcholine:
> *Ophthalmic* – Corneal edema; corneal clouding; corneal decompensation.
> *Systemic* – Bradycardia; hypotension; flushing; breathing difficulties; sweating.

Carbachol:
> *Ophthalmic* – Transient stinging and burning; corneal clouding; persistent bullous keratopathy; retinal detachment; transient ciliary and conjunctival injection; ciliary spasm with resultant temporary decrease of visual acuity.
> *Systemic* – Headache; salivation; GI cramps; vomiting; diarrhea; asthma; syncope; cardiac arrhythmia; flushing; sweating; epigastric distress; tightness in bladder; hypotension; frequent urge to urinate.

Pilocarpine:
> *Ophthalmic* – Transient stinging and burning; tearing; ciliary spasm; conjunctival vascular congestion; temporal, peri-, or supra-orbital headache; superficial keratitis-induced myopia; blurred vision; poor dark adaptation; reduced visual acuity in poor illumination in older individuals and in individuals with lens opacity.

MIOTICS, CHOLINESTERASE INHIBITORS

DEMECARIUM BROMIDE
Solution: 0.125% and 0.25% (*Rx*) — Humorsol (Merck)

ECHOTHIOPHATE IODIDE
Powder for Reconstitution: 1.5 mg to make 0.03%, 3 mg to make 0.06%, 6.25 mg to make 0.125%, 12.5 mg to make 0.25% (*Rx*) — Phospholine Iodide (Wyeth-Ayerst)

PHYSOSTIGMINE (Eserine)
Ointment: 0.25% (as sulfate) (*Rx*) — Eserine Sulfate (Novartis Ophthalmic)

Indications

Glaucoma: Therapy of open-angle glaucoma.

Administration and Dosage

PHYSOSTIGMINE (ESERINE):
> *Ointment* – Apply small quantity to lower fornix, up to 3 times daily.

DEMECARIUM BROMIDE:

   Glaucoma –

      Initial: Place 1 or 2 drops into eye(s).

      Usual dose: 1 or 2 drops twice a week to 1 or 2 drops twice a day. The 0.125% strength used twice daily usually results in smooth control of the physiologic diurnal variation in intraocular pressure (IOP).

   Strabismus –

      Diagnosis: Instill 1 drop daily for 2 weeks, then 1 drop every 2 days for 2 to 3 weeks. If the eyes become straighter, an accommodative factor is demonstrated.

      Therapy: In esotropia uncomplicated by amblyopia or anisometropia, instill not more than 1 drop at a time in both eyes every day for 2 to 3 weeks; too severe a degree of miosis may interfere with vision. Then reduce dosage to 1 drop every other day for 3 to 4 weeks and reevaluate the patient's status. Continue with a dosage of 1 drop every 2 days 1 drop twice a week. If improvement continues, reduce to 1 drop once a week and eventually to trial without medication.

ECHOTHIOPHATE IODIDE:

   Glaucoma – Two doses per day are preferred to maintain as smooth a diurnal tension curve as possible, although 1 dose/day or every other day has been used with satisfactory results. Instill the daily dose or 1 of the 2 daily doses just before bedtime to avoid inconvenience due to miosis.

      Early chronic simple glaucoma: Instill a 0.03% solution just before retiring and in the morning in cases not controlled with pilocarpine.

      Advanced chronic simple glaucoma and glaucoma secondary to cataract surgery: Instill 0.03% solution twice daily, as above.

   Accommodative esotropia –

      Diagnosis: Instill 1 drop of 0.125% solution once a day into both eyes at bedtime for 2 or 3 weeks. If the esotropia is accommodative, a favorable response may begin within a few hours.

      Treatment: After initial period of treatent for diagnostic purposes, reduce schedule to 0.125% every other day or 0.06% every day. The 0.03% strength has proven effective in some cases. The maximum recommended dose is 0.125% once a day, although more intensive therapy has been used for short periods.

Actions

Pharmacology: Topical application to the eye produces intense miosis and muscle contraction. IOP is reduced by a decreased resistance to aqueous outflow.

Cholinesterase-Inhibiting Miotics					
	Miosis		IOP reduction		
Miotics	Onset (minutes)	Duration	Onset (hours)	Peak (hours)	Duration
Reversible					
Physostigmine	20 to 30	12 to 36 hrs	—	2 to 6	12 to 36 hrs
Demecarium	15 to 60	3 to 10 days	—	24	7 to 28 days
Irreversible					
Echothiophate	10 to 30	1 to 4 weeks	4 to 8	24	7 to 28 days

Contraindications

Hypersensitivity to cholinesterase inhibitors or any component of the formulation; active uveal inflammation or any inflammatory disease of the iris or ciliary body; glaucoma associated with iridocyclitis.

Demecarium: Pregnancy.

Echothiophate: Most cases of angle-closure glaucoma (because of the possibility of increasing angle-block).

Warnings

Myasthenia gravis: Because of possible additive adverse effects, administer **demecarium** and **echothiophate** only with extreme caution to patients with myasthenia gravis who are receiving systemic anticholinesterase therapy.

Surgery: In patients receiving cholinesterase inhibitors, administer succinylcholine with extreme caution before and during general anesthesia. Use prior to ophthalmic surgery only as a considered risk because of the possible occurrence of hyphema.

Pregnancy: Category X (demecarium).

Category C (physostigmine, echothiophate).

Lactation: It is not known whether these drugs are excreted in breast milk.

Children: The occurrence of iris cysts is more frequent in children. Exercise extreme caution in children receiving **demecarium** and isoflurophate who may require general anesthesia. Safety and efficacy for use of **physostigmine** have not been established.

Precautions

Concomitant therapy: Cholinesterase inhibitors may be used in combination with adrenergic agents, β-blockers, carbonic anhydrase inhibitors, or hyperosmotic agents.

Narrow-angle glaucoma: Use with caution in patients with chronic angle-closure (narrow-angle) glaucoma or in patients with narrow angles, because of the possibility of producing pupillary block and increasing angle blockage. Temporarily discontinue if cardiac irregularities occur.

Ophthalmic ointments: Ophthalmic ointments may retard corneal healing.

Miosis: Miosis usually causes difficulty in dark adaptation. Use caution while driving at night or performing hazardous tasks in poor light.

Gonioscopy: Use only when shorter-acting miotics have proven inadequate. Gonioscopy is recommended prior to use of medication.

Concomitant ocular conditions: When an intraocular inflammatory process is present, breakdown of the blood-aqueous barrier from anticholinesterase therapy requires abstention from, or cautious use of, these drugs. Use with great caution where there is a history of quiescent uveitis.

Systemic effects: Repeated administration may cause depression of the concentration of cholinesterase in the serum and erythrocytes, with resultant systemic effects.

Iris cysts: Iris cysts may form, enlarge, and obscure vision (more frequent in children).

Special risk: Use caution in patients with marked vagotonia, bronchial asthma, spastic GI disturbances, peptic ulcer, pronounced bradycardia/hypotension, recent MI, epilepsy, parkinsonism, and other disorders that may respond adversely to vagotonic effects.

Drug Interactions

Drugs that may interact with cholinesterase inhibitors include carbamate/organophosphate insecticides and pesticides, succinylcholine, and systemic anticholinesterases.

Adverse Reactions

Ophthalmic: Iris cysts; burning; lacrimation; lid muscle twitching; conjunctival and ciliary redness; browache; headache; activation of latent iritis or uveitis; induced myopia with visual blurring.

Systemic: Nausea; vomiting; abdominal cramps; diarrhea; urinary incontinence; fainting; sweating; salivation; difficulty in breathing; cardiac irregularities.

CARBONIC ANHYDRASE INHIBITORS

DORZOLAMIDE	
Solution: 2% (*Rx*)	*Trusopt* (Merck)
BRINZOLAMIDE	
Suspension: 1% (*Rx*)	*Azopt* (Alcon)

Indications

Elevated intraocular pressure (IOP): Treatment of elevated IOP in patients with ocular hypertension or open-angle glaucoma.

Administration and Dosage

Dosage: One drop in the affected eye(s) 3 times daily.

Concomitant therapy: If more than one ophthalmic drug is being used, administer the drugs at least 10 minutes apart.

Actions

Pharmacology: **Dorzolamide** and **brinzolamide** are carbonic anhydrase inhibitors formulated for topical ophthalmic use.

Pharmacokinetics: When topically applied, **dorzolamide** and **brinzolamide** reach the systemic circulation and accumulate in RBCs during chronic dosing. Extensive distribution into RBCs yields a long half-life, ≈ 3.5 to 4 months. The drugs primarily are excreted unchanged in the urine and the metabolite also is excreted in urine.

Contraindications

Hypersensitivity to any component of this product.

Warnings

Systemic effects: These agents are sulfonamides and, although administered topically, are absorbed systemically. Therefore, the same types of adverse reactions attributable to sulfonamides may occur with topical administration of **dorzolamide** and **brinzolamide**.

Renal function impairment: These agents have not been studied in patients with severe renal impairment (Ccr < 30 mL/min). However, because the drugs and their metabolites are excreted predominantly by the kidney, these agents are not recommended in such patients.

Elderly: No overall differences in efficacy or safety were observed between these patients and younger patients.

Pregnancy: Category C.

Lactation: It is not known whether these drugs are excreted in breast milk.

Children: Safety and efficacy in children have not been established.

Precautions

Corneal endothelium effects: The effect of continued administration of **dorzolamide** and **brinzolamide** on the corneal endothelium has not been fully evaluated.

Acute angle-closure glaucoma: The management of patients with acute angle-closure glaucoma requires therapeutic interventions in addition to ocular hypotensive agents. These agents have not been studied in patients with acute angle-closure glaucoma.

Ocular effects: Local ocular adverse effects, primarily conjunctivitis and lid reactions, were reported with chronic administration.

Concomitant oral carbonic anhydrase inhibitors: There is a potential for an additive effect of the known systemic effects of carbonic anhydrase (CA) inhibition in patients receiving an oral and ophthalmic CA inhibitor. The concomitant administration of ocular and oral CA inhibitors is not recommended.

Contact lenses: The preservative in these products, benzalkonium chloride, may be absorbed by soft contact lenses. Do not administer these agents while wearing soft contact lenses; reinsert lenses ≥ 15 minutes after drug administration.

Drug Interactions

Although acid-base and electrolyte disturbances were not reported in the clinical trials, these disturbances have been reported with oral CA inhibitors and have, in some instances, resulted in drug interactions (eg, toxicity associated with high-dose salicylate therapy).

Adverse Reactions

Adverse reactions occurring in ≥ 3% of patients include ocular burning, stinging, or discomfort immediately following administration; bitter taste following administration; superficial punctate keratitis; signs and symptoms of ocular allergic reaction; blurred vision; tearing; dryness; photophobia; blepharitis; dermatitis, foreign body sensation, hyperemia, ocular discharge/keratitis/pain/pruritus; rhinitis.

PROSTAGLANDIN AGONISTS

BIMATOPROST
Solution: 0.03% (*Rx*)   *Lumigan* (Allergan)
LATANOPROST
Solution: 0.005% (50 mcg/mL) (*Rx*)   *Xalatan* (Pharmacia)
TRAVOPROST
Solution: 0.004% (*Rx*)   *Travatan* (Alcon)
UNOPROSTONE ISOPROPYL
Solution: 0.15% (*Rx*)   *Rescula* (Novartis Ophthalmics)

Indications
Elevated intraocular pressure (IOP): For reduction of elevated IOP in patients with open-angle glaucoma and ocular hypertension who are intolerant of other IOP-lowering medications or insufficiently responsive to another IOP-lowering medication.

Administration and Dosage
BIMATOPROST, LATANOPROST, TRAVOPROST: The recommended dosage is 1 drop in the affected eye(s) once daily in the evening. Do not exceed once-daily dosage because it has been shown that more frequent administration may decrease the IOP-lowering effect. Reduction of IOP starts ≈ 2 to 4 hours after administration and the maximum effect is reached after 8 to 12 hours.

UNOPROSTONE: The recommended dosage is 1 drop in the affected eye(s) twice daily.

Bimatoprost, latanoprost, travoprost, or **unoprostone** may be used concomitantly with other topical ophthalmic drug products to lower IOP. If > 1 topical ophthalmic drug is being used, administer the drugs ≥ 5 minutes apart.

Actions
Pharmacology: Prostaglandin agonists lower IOP by increasing outflow of aqueous humor, although the exact mechanism is unknown at this time.

Contraindications
Hypersensitivity to any component of these products, including benzalkonium chloride. **Travoprost** may interfere with the maintenance of pregnancy and should not be used by women during pregnancy or by women attempting to become pregnant.

Warnings
Eye pigment changes: Prostaglandin agonists may gradually change eye color, increasing the amount of brown pigment in the iris by increasing the number of melanosomas (pigment granules) in melanocytes.

Pregnancy: Category C. Because prostaglandins are biologically active and may be absorbed through the skin, women who are pregnant or attempting to become pregnant should exercise appropriate precautions to avoid direct exposure to the contents of the bottle.

Lactation: It is not known whether these drugs or their metabolites are excreted in breast milk.

Children: Safety and efficacy in children have not been established.

Precautions
Bacterial keratitis: There have been reports of bacterial keratitis associated with the use of multiple-dose containers of topical ophthalmic products. These containers had been inadvertently contaminated by patients who, in most cases, had a concurrent corneal disease or a disruption of the ocular epithelial surface.

Contact lenses: Do not administer prostaglandin agonists while wearing contact lenses.

Macular edema: Macular edema, including cystoid edema, has been reported during treatment with prostaglandin agonists. These reports mainly have occurred in aphakic patients, pseudoaphakic patients with torn posterior lens capsule, or patients with known risk factors for macular edema.

Cornea: **Latanoprost** is hydrolyzed in the cornea. The effect of continued administration of latanoprost on the corneal endothelium has not been fully evaluated.

Active intraocular inflammation: Use **bimatoprost** or **unoprostone** with caution in patients with active intraocular inflammation (eg, uveitis).

Drug Interactions
In vitro studies have shown that precipitation occurs when eye drops containing thimerosal are mixed with **latanoprost**. If such drugs are used, administer with an interval of ≥ 5 minutes between applications.

Adverse Reactions
Prostaglandin agonists:
> *Systemic* – The most common systemic adverse events seen with prostaglandin agonists were upper respiratory tract infection/cold/flu (4% to 10%).

Bimatoprost:
> *Ophthalmic* – Bimatoprost-associated ocular adverse events that occurred in 3% to 10% of patients, in descending order of incidence, included the following: Ocular dryness, visual disturbances, ocular burning, foreign body sensation, eye pain, pigmentation of the periocular skin, blepharitis, cataract, superficial punctate keratitis, eyelid erythema, ocular irritation, eyelash darkening.

Latanoprost:
> *Ophthalmic* – Latanoprost-associated ocular adverse events reported at an incidence of 5% to 15% included the following: Blurred vision, burning and stinging, conjunctival hyperemia, foreign body sensation, itching, increased pigmentation of the iris, punctate epithelial keratopathy.

Travoprost:
> *Ophthalmic* – Travoprost-associated ocular adverse events reported at an incidence of 5% to 15% included the following: Decreased visual acuity, eye discomfort, foreign body sensation, pain, pruritus.

Unoprostone:
> *Ophthalmic* – Unoprostone-associated ocular adverse events occurring in 10% to 25% of patients included the following: Burning/stinging, burning/stinging upon drug instillation, dry eyes, itching, increased number of eyelashes. Other ocular adverse events occurring at 5% to 10% of patients were abnormal vision, eyelid disorder, foreign body sensation, and lacrimation disorder.

CORTICOSTEROIDS

FLUOROMETHOLONE

Suspension: 0.1% and 0.25% (*Rx*)	Various, *Fluor-Op* (Novartis Ophthalmic), *FML* (Allergan), *FML Forte* (Allergan)
Suspension: 0.1% fluorometholone acetate (*Rx*)	*Flarex* (Alcon)
Ointment: 0.1% (*Rx*)	*FML S.O.P.* (Allergan)

MEDRYSONE

Suspension: 1% (*Rx*)	*HMS* (Allergan)

PREDNISOLONE

Suspension: 0.12%, 0.125%, 1% prednisolone acetate (*Rx*)	*Econopred* (Alcon), *Econopred Plus* (Alcon), *Pred Mild* (Allergan), *Pred Forte* (Allergan), *Prednisolone Acetate Ophthalmic* (Falcon)
Solution: 0.125% and 1% prednisolone sodium phosphate (*Rx*)	Various, *AK-Pred* (Akorn), *Inflamase Mild* (Novartis Ophthalmic), *Inflamase Forte* (Novartis Ophthalmic)

DEXAMETHASONE

Solution: 0.1% dexamethasone phosphate (*Rx*)	Various, *AK-Dex* (Akorn), *Decadron Phosphate* (Merck)
Suspension: 0.1% (*Rx*)	*Maxidex* (Alcon)
Ointment: 0.05% dexamethasone phosphate (*Rx*)	Various, *Decadron Phosphate* (Merck)

RIMEXOLONE

Suspension: 1% (*Rx*)	*Vexol* (Alcon)

LOTEPREDNOL ETABONATE

Suspension: 0.5% (*Rx*)	*Lotemax* (Bausch & Lomb)
Suspension: 0.2% (*Rx*)	*Alrex* (Bausch & Lomb)

Indications

Inflammatory conditions: Treatment of steroid-responsive inflammatory conditions of the palpebral and bulbar conjunctiva, lid, sclera, cornea, and anterior segment of the globe, such as: Allergic conjunctivitis; acne rosacea; superficial punctate keratitis; herpes zoster keratitis; iritis; cyclitis; and selected infective conjunctivitis (when the inherent hazard of steroid use is accepted to obtain an advisable diminution in edema and inflammation [prednisolone]); vernal conjunctivitis; episcleritis; epinephrine sensitivity; and anterior uveitis.

Mild to moderate – For the treatment of mild to moderate noninfectious allergic and inflammatory disorders of the lid, conjunctiva, cornea, and sclera (including chemical and thermal burns) (**prednisolone**).

Moderate to severe – Use higher strengths for moderate to severe inflammations. In difficult cases of anterior segment eye disease, systemic therapy may be required. When deeper ocular structures are involved, use systemic therapy (**prednisolone**).

Ocular surgery – For treatment of postoperative inflammation following ocular surgery.

Corneal injury: For corneal injury from chemical, radiation, or thermal burns, or from penetration of foreign bodies.

Administration and Dosage

Treatment duration varies with type of lesion and may extend from a few days to several weeks, depending on therapeutic response. If signs and symptoms fail to improve after 2 days, re-evaluate the patient. Relapse may occur if therapy is reduced too rapidly; taper over several days. Relapses, more common in chronic active lesions than in self-limited conditions, usually respond to retreatment.

FLUOROMETHALONE: Consult a physician if there is no improvement after 2 days. Do not discontinue therapy prematurely. In chronic conditions, withdraw treatment by gradually decreasing the frequency of applications.

Suspension – Shake well before using. Instill 1 to 2 drops into the conjunctival sac(s) 2 to 4 times daily. During the initial 24 to 48 hours, the dosage may be increased to 2 drops every 2 hours.

Ointment – Apply a small amount (≈ ½ inch ribbon) of ointment to the conjunctival sac 1 to 3 times daily. During the first 24 to 48 hours, the dosing frequency may be increased to one application every 4 hours.

MEDRYSONE: Shake well before using. Instill 1 drop into the conjunctival sac up to every 4 hours.

PREDNISOLONE:

Solutions – Depending on the severity of inflammation, instill 1 or 2 drops of solution into the conjunctival sac up to every hour during the day and every 2 hours during the night as necessary as initial therapy.

When a favorable response is observed, reduce dosage to 1 drop every 4 hours. Further reduction in dosage to 1 drop 3 to 4 times daily may suffice to control symptoms.

Suspensions – Shake well before using. Instill 1 to 2 drops into the conjunctival sac 2 to 4 times daily. During the initial 24 to 48 hours, the dosing frequency may be increased if necessary.

In cases of bacterial infections, concomitant use of anti-infective agents is mandatory.

If signs and symptoms do not improve after 2 days, re-evaluate the patient.

Dosing may be reduced, but advise patients not to discontinue therapy prematurely. In chronic conditions, withdraw treatment by gradually decreasing the frequency of applications.

DEXAMETHASONE:

Solutions – Instill 1 to 2 drops into the conjunctival sac every hour during the day and every 2 hours during the night as initial therapy. When a favorable response is observed, reduce dosage to 1 drop every 4 hours. Further reduction in dosage to 1 drop 3 or 4 times daily may suffice to control symptoms.

Suspension – Shake well before using. Instill 1 or 2 drops in the conjunctival sac(s). In severe disease, drops may be used hourly, being tapered to discontinuation as inflammation subsides. In mild disease, drops may be used ≤ 4 to 6 times daily.

Ointment – Apply a thin coating of ointment 3 to 4 times a day. When a favorable response is observed, reduce the number of daily applications to twice daily and later to once daily as a maintenance dose if this is sufficient to control symptoms.

The ointment is particularly convenient when an eye pad is used. It also may be the preparation of choice for patients in whom therapeutic benefit depends on prolonged contact of the active ingredients with ocular tissues.

RIMEXOLONE: Shake well before using.

Postoperative inflammation – Apply 1 to 2 drops into the conjunctival sac of the affected eye(s) 4 times daily begining 24 hours after surgery and continuing throughout the first 2 weeks of the postoperative period.

Anterior uveitis – Apply 1 to 2 drops into the conjunctival sac of the affected eye every hour during waking hours for the first week, 1 drop every 2 hours during waking hours of the second week, and then taper until uveitis is resolved.

LOTEPREDNOL ETABONATE: Shake well before using.

0.2% suspension – Instill 1 drop into the affected eye(s) 4 times daily.

0.5% suspension –

Steroid responsive disease: Apply 1 to 2 drops into the conjunctival sac of the affected eye(s) 4 times daily. During the initial treatment within the first week, the dosing may be increased up to 1 drop every hour. Advise patients not to discontinue therapy prematurely. If signs and symptoms fail to improve after 2 days, re-evaluate the patient.

Postoperative inflammation: Apply 1 to 2 drops into the conjunctival sac of the operated eye(s) 4 times daily beginning 24 hours after surgery and continuing throughout the first 2 weeks of the postoperative period.

Actions

Pharmacology: Topical corticosteroids exert an anti-inflammatory action. Steroids inhibit inflammatory response to inciting agents of mechanical, chemical, or immunological nature.

Contraindications

Acute epithelial herpes simplex keratitis (dendritic keratitis); fungal diseases of ocular structures; vaccinia, varicella and most other viral diseases of the cornea and conjunctiva; ocular tuberculosis; hypersensitivity; after uncomplicated removal of a superficial corneal foreign body; mycobacterial eye infection; acute, purulent, untreated eye infections that may be masked or enhanced by the presence of steroids.

Medrysone: Medrysone is not for use in iritis and uveitis; its efficacy has not been demonstrated.

Warnings

Moderate to severe inflammation: Use higher strengths for moderate to severe inflammations. In difficult cases of anterior segment eye disease, systemic therapy may be required. When deeper ocular structures are involved, use systemic therapy.

Ocular damage: Prolonged use may result in glaucoma, elevated IOP, optic nerve damage, defects in visual acuity and fields of vision, posterior subcapsular cataract formation or secondary ocular infections from pathogens liberated from ocular tissues.

Cataract surgery: The use of steroids after cataract surgery may delay healing and increase the incidence of bleb formation.

Mustard gas keratitis or Sjogren's keratoconjunctivitis: Topical steroids are not effective.

Infections: Prolonged use may result in secondary ocular infections caused by suppression of host response. Acute, purulent, untreated eye infections may be masked or activity enhanced by steroids. Fungal infections of the cornea have been reported with long-term local steroid applications.

Pregnancy: Category C.

Lactation: It is not known whether topical steroids are excreted in breast milk.

Children: Safety and efficacy have not been established in children.

Precautions

Bacterial keratitis: Bacterial keratitis associated with the use of multiple-dose containers of topical ophthalmic products has been reported. Serious damage to the eye and subsequent loss of vision may result from using contaminated preparations.

Benzalkonium chloride: Benzalkonium chloride is a preservative used in some of these products that may be absorbed by soft contact lenses. Patients wearing soft contact lenses should wait ≥ 15 minutes after instilling products containing this preservative before inserting their lenses.

Adverse Reactions

Glaucoma (elevated IOP) with optic nerve damage, loss of visual acuity and field defects; posterior subcapsular cataract formation; delayed wound healing; secondary ocular infection from pathogens, including herpes simplex and fungi liberated from ocular tissues; acute uveitis; perforation of globe where there is corneal or scleral thinning; exacerbation of viral, bacterial, and fungal corneal infections; transient stinging or burning; chemosis; dry eyes; epiphora; photophobia; keratitis; conjunctivitis; corneal ulcers; mydriasis; ptosis; blurred vision, discharge, discomfort, ocular pain, foreign body sensation, hyperemia, pruritus (**rimexolone**).

Systemic: Systemic side effects may occur with extensive use.

LODOXAMIDE TROMETHAMINE

Solution: 0.1% (*Rx*)   *Alomide* (Alcon)

Indications
Treatment of the ocular disorders referred to by the terms vernal keratoconjunctivitis, vernal conjunctivitis, and vernal keratitis.

Administration and Dosage
Adults and children > 2 years of age: 1 to 2 drops in each affected eye 4 times daily for up to 3 months.

Actions
Pharmacology: Lodoxamide is a mast cell stabilizer that inhibits the in vivo Type I immediate hypersensitivity reaction. Although lodoxamide's precise mechanism of action is unknown, the drug may prevent calcium influx into mast cells upon antigen stimulation.

Pharmacokinetics: The disposition of lodoxamide was studied in 6 healthy adult volunteers receiving a 3 mg oral dose. Urinary excretion was the major route of elimination. The elimination half-life was 8.5 hours in urine. In a study in 12 healthy adult volunteers, topical administration of 1 drop in each eye 4 times/day for 10 days did not result in any measurable lodoxamide plasma levels at a detection limit of 2.5 ng/mL.

Contraindications
Hypersensitivity to any component of this product.

Warnings
For ophthalmic use only. Not for injection.

Contact lenses: As with all ophthalmic preparations containing benzalkonium chloride, instruct patients not to wear soft contact lenses during treatment with lodoxamide.

Pregnancy: Category B.

Lactation: It is not known whether lodoxamide is excreted in breast milk.

Children: Safety and efficacy in children < 2 years of age have not been established.

Precautions
Burning/Stinging: Patients may experience a transient burning or stinging upon instillation of lodoxamide. Should these symptoms persist, advise patients to contact their physicians.

Adverse Reactions
Adverse reactions occurring in ≥ 3% of patients include transient burning, stinging or discomfort upon instillation; ocular itching/pruritus; blurred vision; dry eye; tearing/discharge; hyperemia; crystalline deposits; and foreign body sensation.

LEVOCABASTINE HCl

Ophthalmic suspension: 0.05% (*Rx*)   *Livostin* (Iolab)

Indications
Allergic conjunctivitis: For the temporary relief of the signs and symptoms of seasonal allergic conjunctivitis.

Administration and Dosage
Shake well before using.

The usual dose is 1 drop instilled in affected eyes 4 times daily. Treatment may be continued for up to 2 weeks.

Actions
Pharmacology: Levocabastine is a potent, selective histamine H_1-receptor antagonist for topical ophthalmic use. Antigen challenge studies performed 2 and 4 hours after initial drug instillation indicated activity was maintained for at least 2 hours.

Pharmacokinetics: After instillation in the eye, levocabastine is systemically absorbed. However, the amount of systemically absorbed levocabastine after therapeutic ocular doses is low.

Contraindications

Hypersensitivity to any components of the product; while soft contact lenses are being worn.

Warnings

For ophthalmic use only: Not for injection.

Pregnancy: Category C.

Lactation: Levocabastine is excreted in breast milk.

Children: Safety and efficacy in children < 12 years of age have not been established.

Adverse Reactions

Adverse reactions occurring in ≥ 3% of patients include mild, transient stinging and burning; headache; visual disturbances; dry mouth; fatigue; pharyngitis; eye pain/dryness; somnolence; red eyes; lacrimation/discharge; cough; nausea; rash/erythema; eyelid edema; dyspnea.

ANTIBIOTICS

CHLORAMPHENICOL	
Ointment: 10 mg/g (*Rx*)	Various, *Chloroptic S.O.P.* (Allergan)
Solution: 5 mg/mL (*Rx*)	Various, *Chloroptic* (Allergan), *AK-Chlor* (Akorn)
ERYTHROMYCIN	
Ointment: 5 mg/g (*Rx*)	Various, *Ilotycin* (Dista)
GENTAMICIN SULFATE	
Ointment: 3 mg/g (*Rx*)	Various, *Garamycin* (Schering), *Genoptic S.O.P.* (Allergan)
Solution: 3 mg/mL (*Rx*)	Various, *Garamycin* (Schering), *Genoptic* (Allergan)
TOBRAMYCIN	
Ointment: 3 mg/g (*Rx*)	Various, *Tobrex* (Alcon)
Solution: 0.3% (*Rx*)	Various, *AKTob* (Akorn), *Tobrex* (Alcon)
POLYMYXIN B SULFATE	
Powder for solution: 500,000 units (*Rx*)	*Polymyxin B Sulfate Sterile* (Roerig)
BACITRACIN	
Ointment: 500 units/g (*Rx*)	Various, *AK-Tracin* (Akorn)
CIPROFLOXACIN	
Solution: 3.5 mg/mL (equivalent to 3 mg base) (*Rx*)	*Ciloxan* (Alcon)
NORFLOXACIN	
Solution: 3 mg/mL (*Rx*)	*Chibroxin* (Merck)
OFLOXACIN	
Solution: 3 mg/mL (*Rx*)	*Ocuflox* (Allergan)
LEVOFLOXACIN	
Solution: 5 mg/mL (*Rx*)	*Quixin* (Santen)

Indications

Infections: Treatment of superficial ocular infections involving the conjunctiva or cornea (eg, conjunctivitis, keratitis, keratoconjunctivitis, corneal ulcers, blepharitis, blepharoconjunctivitis, acute meibomianitis, dacryocystitis) caused by strains of microorganisms susceptible to antibiotics.

Tetracycline and erythromycin: Tetracycline and erythromycin also are indicated for the prophylaxis of ophthalmia neonatorum caused by *Neisseria gonorrhoeae* or *Chlamydia trachomatis*.

Chloramphenicol: Use chloramphenicol only in those serious infections for which less potentially dangerous drugs are ineffective or contraindicated (see Warnings).

Topical Ophthalmic Antibiotic Preparations

Organism/Infection	Bacitracin	Gramicidin	Polymyxin B	Erythromycin	Chloramphenicol	Trimethoprim	Norfloxacin	Ciprofloxacin	Levofloxacin	Ofloxacin	Neomycin	Gentamicin	Tobramycin	Tetracycline	Chlortetracycline	Oxytetracycline	Sodium sulfacetamide	Sulfisoxazole
Gram-Positive																		
Staphylococcus sp.	✓	✓					✓	✓	✓	✓		✓	✓	✓				
S. aureus	✓	✓		✓	✓	✓	✓	✓	✓	✓	✓	✓	✓	✓	✓		✓	
Streptococcus sp.	✓	✓			✓			✓	✓	✓			✓	✓			✓	
S. pneumoniae	✓	✓		✓	✓	✓	✓	✓	✓	✓		✓[1]	✓	✓				
α-hemolytic streptococci (viridans group)				✓						✓								
β-hemolytic streptococci	✓											✓[1]	✓					
S. pyogenes	✓			✓		✓		✓		✓		✓			✓			
Corynebacterium sp.	✓	✓		✓							✓	✓	✓					
Gram-Negative																		
Escherichia coli			✓		✓	✓	✓	✓			✓	✓	✓	✓	✓	✓	✓	✓
Haemophilus aegyptius					✓	✓	✓					✓	✓				✓	✓
H. ducreyi					✓			✓				✓	✓		✓	✓		
H. influenzae			✓	✓	✓	✓	✓	✓	✓	✓	✓	✓	✓		✓	✓		
Klebsiella sp.					✓			✓	✓			✓	✓			✓		
K. pneumoniae			✓			✓	✓	✓	✓			✓	✓		✓			
Neisseria sp.	✓				✓			✓			✓	✓	✓	✓				
N. gonorrhoeae	✓		✓[2]				✓	✓		✓		✓		✓[2]	✓		✓	
Proteus sp.						✓	✓	✓			✓	✓	✓	✓				
Acinetobacter calcoaceticus							✓	✓		✓		✓	✓					
A. lwoffi									✓									
Enterobacter aerogenes			✓				✓	✓			✓	✓	✓			✓		
Enterobacter sp.					✓		✓	✓		✓	✓	✓	✓					
Serratia marcescens							✓	✓	✓	✓		✓	✓					
Moraxella sp.					✓					✓		✓	✓					
Chlamydia trachomatis				✓[2]				✓		✓					✓[3]	✓[3]	✓[4]	✓
Pasteurella tularensis															✓	✓		
Pseudomonas aeruginosa			✓		✓			✓	✓		✓	✓[1]	✓					
Bartonella bacilliformis																✓		
Bacteroides sp.					✓									✓	✓	✓		
Vibrio sp.					✓		✓	✓				✓	✓			✓		
Yersinia pestis															✓	✓		

[1] Increasing resistance has been seen.
[2] For prophylaxis.
[3] In conjunction with oral therapy
[4] Adjunct in systemic sulfonamide therapy.

Administration and Dosage

Administration and dosage varies for the individual products. Refer to individual manufacturer inserts.

Contraindications

Hypersensitivity to any component of these products; epithelial herpes simplex keratitis (dendritic keratitis); vaccinia; varicella; mycobacterial infections of the eye; fungal diseases of the ocular structure; use of steroid combinations after uncomplicated removal of a corneal foreign body.

Warnings

Sensitization: Sensitization from the topical use of an antibiotic may contraindicate the drug's later systemic use in serious infections.

Cross-sensitivity: Allergic cross-reactions may occur that could prevent future use of any or all of these antibiotics – Kanamycin, neomycin, paromomycin, streptomycin, and possibly, gentamicin.

> *Chloramphenicol* – Hematopoietic toxicity has occurred occasionally with the systemic use of chloramphenicol and rarely with topical administration.

Pregnancy: Category B (tobramycin); Category C (gentamicin, ciprofloxacin, norfloxacin, ofloxacin).

Lactation: It is not known whether **ciprofloxacin**, **norfloxacin**, or **ofloxacin** appears in breast milk following ophthalmic use. Exercise caution when administering ciprofloxacin to a nursing mother.

Children: **Tobramycin** is safe and effective in children. Safety and efficacy of **ciprofloxacin** in children < 12 years of age and **norfloxacin** and **ofloxacin** in infants < 1 year of age have not been established.

Precautions

Superinfection: Do not use topical antibiotics in deep-seated ocular infections or in those that are likely to become systemic.

> *Systemic antibiotics* – In all except very superficial infections, supplement the topical use of antibiotics with appropriate systemic medication.

> *Crystalline precipitate* – A white crystalline precipitate located in the superficial portion of the corneal defect was observed in ≈ 17% of patients on **ciprofloxacin**.

Adverse Reactions

Sensitivity reactions such as transient irritation, burning, stinging, itching, inflammation, angioneurotic edema, urticaria, and vesicular and maculopapular dermatitis have occurred in some patients.

Chloramphenicol: Hematological events (including aplastic anemia) have been reported.

Ciprofloxacin: White crystalline precipitates; lid margin crusting; crystals/scales; foreign body sensation; itching; conjunctival hyperemia; bad taste in mouth; corneal staining; keratopathy/keratitis; allergic reactions; lid edema; tearing; photophobia; corneal infiltrates; nausea; decreased vision.

Norfloxacin: Conjunctival hyperemia; chemosis; photophobia; bitter taste in mouth.

NATAMYCIN

Suspension: 5% (Rx)	Natacyn (Alcon)

Indications

Fungal infections: Fungal blepharitis, conjunctivitis, and keratitis caused by susceptible organisms. Natamycin is the initial drug of choice in Fusarium solani keratitis.

Administration and Dosage

Fungal keratitis: Instill 1 drop into the conjunctival sac at 1 or 2 hour intervals. The frequency of application can usually be reduced to 1 drop 6 to 8 times daily after the first 3 to 4 days. Generally, continue therapy for 14 to 21 days, or until there is resolution of active fungal keratitis. In many cases, it may help to reduce the dosage gradually at 4 to 7 day intervals to ensure that the organism has been eliminated.

Fungal blepharitis and conjunctivitis: 4 to 6 daily applications may be sufficient.

Actions

Pharmacology: Natamycin, a tetraene polyene antibiotic, is derived from *Streptomyces natalensis*.

It possesses in vitro activity against a variety of yeast and filamentous fungi, including *Candida, Aspergillus, Cephalosporium, Fusarium,* and *Penicillium*. The mechanism of action appears to be through binding of the molecule to the fungal cell membrane. The polyenesterol complex alters membrane permeability, depleting essential cellular constituents. Although activity against fungi is dose-related, natamycin is predominantly fungicidal.

Pharmacokinetics: Topical administration appears to produce effective concentrations within the corneal stroma, but not in intraocular fluid. Absorption from the GI tract is very poor. Systemic absorption should not occur after topical administration.

Contraindications
Hypersensitivity to any component of the formulation.

Warnings
Pregnancy: Safety for use during pregnancy has not been established.

Precautions
For topical use only: Not for injection.

Fungal endophthalmitis: The effectiveness of topical natamycin as a single agent in fungal endophthalmitis has not been established.

Resistance: Failure of keratitis to improve following 7 to 10 days of administration suggests that the infection may be caused by a microorganism not susceptible to natamycin. Base continuation of therapy on clinical reevaluation and additional laboratory studies.

Toxicity: Adherence of the suspension to areas of epithelial ulceration or retention in the fornices occurs regularly. Should suspicion of drug toxicity occur, discontinue the drug.

Diagnosis/Monitoring: Determine initial and sustained therapy of fungal keratitis by the clinical diagnosis (laboratory diagnosis by smear and culture of corneal scrapings) and by response to the drug. Whenever possible, determine the in vitro activity of natamycin against the responsible fungus. Monitor tolerance to natamycin at least twice weekly.

Adverse Reactions
One case of conjunctival chemosis and hyperemia, thought to be allergic in nature, was reported.

INTRODUCTION

The topical ophthalmic antiviral preparations appear to interfere with viral reproduction by altering DNA synthesis. Idoxuridine, vidarabine, and trifluridine are effective treatment for herpes simplex infections of the conjunctiva and cornea. Ganciclovir is indicated for use in immunocompromised patients with cytomegalovirus (CMV) retinitis and for prevention of CMV retinitis in transplant patients. Foscarnet is indicated for use only in AIDS patients with CMV retinitis.

Monographs for idoxuridine, vidarabine, and trifluridine follow this introduction. Prescribing information for foscarnet and ganciclovir appear in the Antivirals section of the Anti-Infectives chapter.

Viral infection, especially epidemic keratoconjunctivitis (EKC), more often is associated with a follicular conjunctivitis, a serous conjunctival discharge, and preuricular lymphadenopathy. The exceptionally contagious organism causing EKC is not susceptible to antiviral therapy at this time.

VIDARABINE (Adenine Arabinoside; Ara-A)

Ophthalmic ointment: 3% vidarabine monohydrate (equivalent to 2.8% vidarabine) (*Rx*)	*Vira-A* (Parke-Davis)

Indications

Acute keratoconjunctivitis and recurrent epithelial keratitis: Acute keratoconjunctivitis and recurrent epithelial keratitis caused by herpes simplex virus types 1 and 2.

Superficial keratitis: Superficial keratitis caused by herpes simplex virus that has not responded to topical idoxuridine, or when toxic or hypersensitivity reactions to idoxuridine have occurred.

Administration and Dosage

Administer ≈ 0.5 inch of ointment into the lower conjunctival sac(s) 5 times daily at 3-hour intervals.

If there are no signs of improvement after 7 days, or if complete re-epithelialization has not occurred in 21 days, consider other forms of therapy. Some severe cases may require longer treatment.

After re-epithelialization has occurred, treat for an additional 7 days at a reduced dosage to prevent recurrence.

Concomitant therapy: Topical antibiotics or topical steroids have been administered concurrently with vidarabine without an increase in adverse reactions, although their advantages and disadvantages must be considered.

Actions

Pharmacology: The antiviral mechanism of action has not been established. Vidarabine appears to interfere with the early steps of viral DNA synthesis. It is rapidly deaminated to arabinosylhypoxanthine (Ara-Hx), the principal metabolite. Ara-Hx also possesses in vitro antiviral activity less than vidarabine's.

Pharmacokinetics:

Absorption – Systemic absorption is not expected to occur following ocular administration and swallowing lacrimal secretions.

Distribution – Because of its low solubility, trace amounts of both vidarabine and Ara-Hx can be detected in the aqueous humor only if there is an epithelial defect in the cornea. If the cornea is normal, only trace amounts of Ara-Hx can be recovered from the aqueous humor.

Contraindications

Hypersensitivity to vidarabine; sterile trophic ulcers.

Warnings

Efficacy in other conditions: Vidarabine is not effective against RNA virus; adenoviral ocular infections; bacterial, fungal, or chlamydial infections of the cornea; or trophic ulcers. Effectiveness against stromal keratitis and uveitis caused by herpes simplex virus has not been established.

Corticosteroids: Corticosteroids alone are normally contraindicated in herpes simplex virus eye infections. If vidarabine is coadministered with topical corticosteroid therapy, consider corticosteroid-induced ocular side effects such as glaucoma or cataract formation and progression of bacterial or viral infection.

Visual haze: Temporary visual haze may be produced with vidarabine.

Pregnancy: Category C.

Lactation: It is not known whether vidarabine is excreted in breast milk.

Precautions
Viral resistance: Viral resistance to vidarabine has not been observed, although this possibility exists.

Adverse Reactions
Adverse reactions may include the following: Lacrimation; foreign body sensation; conjunctival infection; burning; irritation; superficial punctate keratitis; pain; photophobia; punctal occlusion; sensitivity; uveitis; stromal edema; secondary glaucoma; trophic defects; corneal vascularization; hyphema.

TRIFLURIDINE (Trifluorothymidine)

Ophthalmic solution: 1% (*Rx*)	*Viroptic* (Burroughs Wellcome)

Indications
Primary keratoconjunctivitis and recurrent epithelial keratitis caused by herpes simplex virus types 1 and 2.

Epithelial keratitis that has not responded clinically to topical idoxuridine, or when ocular toxicity or hypersensitivity to idoxuridine has occurred. In a smaller number of patients resistant to topical vidarabine, trifluridine was also effective.

Administration and Dosage
Instill 1 drop onto the cornea of the affected eye(s) every 2 hours while awake for a maximum daily dosage of 9 drops until the corneal ulcer has completely re-epithelialized. Following re-epithelialization, treat for an additional 7 days with 1 drop every 4 hours while awake for a minimum daily dosage of 5 drops.

If there are no signs of improvement after 7 days, or if complete re-epithelialization has not occurred after 14 days, consider other forms of therapy. Avoid continuous administration for periods exceeding 21 days because of potential ocular toxicity.

Actions
Pharmacology: A fluorinated pyrimidine nucleoside with in vitro and in vivo activity against herpes simplex virus types 1 and 2, and vaccinia virus. Some strains of adenovirus are also inhibited in vitro. Its antiviral mechanism of action is not completely known.

Pharmacokinetics:
  Absorption – Intraocular penetration occurs after topical instillation. Decreased corneal integrity or stromal or uveal inflammation may enhance the penetration into the aqueous humor. Systemic absorption following therapeutic dosing appears negligible.

Contraindications
Hypersensitivity reactions or chemical intolerance to trifluridine.

Warnings
Efficacy in other conditions: The clinical efficacy in the treatment of stromal keratitis and uveitis caused by herpes simplex or ophthalmic infections caused by vaccinia virus and adenovirus, or in the prophylaxis of herpes simplex virus keratoconjunctivi-

tis and epithelial keratitis has not been established by well-controlled clinical trials. Not effective against bacterial, fungal, or chlamydial infections of the cornea or trophic lesions.

Dosage/Frequency: Do not exceed the recommended dosage or frequency of administration.

Pregnancy: Safety for use during pregnancy has not been established.

Lactation: Safety and efficacy have not been established.

Precautions

Viral resistance: Viral resistance, although documented in vitro, has not been reported following multiple exposure to trifluridine; this possibility may exist.

Adverse Reactions

Adverse reactions may include mild, transient burning or stinging upon instillation; palpebral edema; superficial punctate keratopathy; epithelial keratopathy; hypersensitivity reaction; stromal edema; irritation; keratitis sicca; hyperemia and increased intraocular pressure.

Chapter 13
ANTINEOPLASTIC AGENTS

Antineoplastics Introduction, 1089
Hormones, 1093
    Tamoxifen, 1093
Miscellaneous Antineoplastics, 1095
    Interferon Alfa-2a, 1095
    Interferon Alfa-2b, 1098
    Interferon Alfa-2b, Recombinant and Ribavirin Combination, 1102

ANTINEOPLASTICS INTRODUCTION

The chemotherapeutic agents include a wide range of compounds that work by various mechanisms. Although development has been directed toward agents capable of selective actions on neoplastic tissues, those presently available manifest significant toxicity on normal tissues as a major complication of therapy. Thoroughly consider the risks vs benefits of therapy when using these agents.

Because of the complexities and dangers in cancer chemotherapy, use should be restricted to, or under the direct supervision of, physicians experienced in its use. In addition to drug therapy, surgical excision and radiation therapy also are employed when appropriate.

Handling of cytotoxic agents: Most antineoplastics are toxic compounds known to be carcinogenic, mutagenic, or teratogenic. Direct contact may cause irritation of the skin, eyes, and mucous membranes. Safe and aseptic handling of parenteral chemotherapeutic drugs by medical personnel involved in preparation and administration of these agents is mandatory. Potential risks from repeated contact with parenteral antineoplastics can be controlled by a combination of specific containment equipment and proper work techniques. The NIH Division of Safety brochure outlines recommendations for safe handling of these agents.

Mechanisms of action: The mechanism of action by which these agents suppress proliferation of neoplasms is not fully understood. Generally, they affect ≥ 1 stages of cell growth or replication. Those more active at one specific phase of cellular growth are referred to as *cell cycle specific* agents; those that are active on both proliferating and resting cells are *cell cycle nonspecific* agents. The selectivity of cytotoxic agents inversely follows cell cycle specificity. Rapidly dividing normal tissues including bone marrow, blood components, hair follicles, and mucous membranes of the GI tract also may experience major adverse effects.

Alkylating agents: Alkylating agents form highly reactive carbonium ions that react with essential cellular components, thereby altering normal biological function. Alkylating agents replace hydrogen atoms with an alkyl radical causing cross-linking and abnormal base pairing in deoxyribonucleic acid (DNA) molecules. They also react with sulfhydryl, phosphate, and amine groups, resulting in multiple lesions in dividing and nondividing cells. The resultant defective DNA molecules are unable to carry out normal cellular reproductive functions. Examples of alkylating agents include the following:

>   busulfan
>   carboplatin
>   carmustine
>   chlorambucil
>   cisplatin
>   cyclophosphamide
>   dacarbazine
>   estramustine
>   ifosfamide
>   lomustine
>   mechlorethamine
>   melphalan
>   pipobroman
>   streptozocin
>   thiotepa
>   uracil mustard

Antimetabolites: Antimetabolites include a diverse group of compounds that interfere with various metabolic processes, thereby disrupting normal cellular functions. These agents may act by the following 2 general mechanisms: By incorporating the drug, rather than a normal cellular constituent, into an essential chemical compound; or by inhibiting a key enzyme from functioning normally. Their primary benefit is the ability to disrupt nucleic acid synthesis. These agents work only on dividing cells during the S phase of nucleic acid synthesis and are most effective on rapidly proliferating neoplasms. Examples of antimetabolites include the following:

> cytarabine
> floxuridine
> 5-fluorouracil
> fludarabine
> gemcitabine
> hydroxyurea
> mercaptopurine
> methotrexate
> thioguanine

Hormones: Hormones have been used to treat several types of neoplasms. Hormonal therapy interferes at the cellular membrane level with growth stimulatory receptor proteins. The mechanism of action, however, is still unclear. Adrenocortical steroids are used primarily for their suppressant effect on lymphocytes in leukemias and lymphomas and as a component in many combination regimens. The counterbalancing effect of androgens, estrogens, and progestins has been used to advantage in the therapy of malignancies of tissues dependent upon these sex-related hormones (eg, tumors of the breast, endometrium, prostate). These agents have the advantage of greater specificity for tissues responsive to their effects, thus inhibiting proliferation without a direct cytotoxic action.

Examples of hormone agents include the following:

> aminoglutethimide
> anastrozole
> bicalutamide
> diethylstilbestrol
> estramustine
> flutamide
> goserelin
> leuprolide
> medroxyprogesterone
> megestrol
> mitotane
> polyestradiol
> tamoxifen
> testolactone

Antibiotic: Antibiotic-type agents, unlike their anti-infective relatives, are capable of disrupting cellular functions of host (mammalian) tissues. Their primary mechanisms of action are to inhibit DNA-dependent RNA synthesis and to delay or inhibit mitosis. The antibiotics are cell cycle nonspecific. Examples of antineoplastic antibiotics include the following:

> bleomycin
> dactinomycin
> daunorubicin
> doxorubicin
> idarubicin
> mitomycin
> mitoxantrone
> pentostatin
> plicamycin.

Mitotic inhibitors: Mitotic inhibitor mechanisms are not fully understood. Podophyllotoxin derivatives inhibit DNA synthesis at specific phases of the cell cycle. Vinca alkaloids bind to tubulin, the subunits of the microtubules that form the mitotic spindle. This complex inhibits microtubule assembly, causing metaphase arrest. In contrast, paclitaxel enhances the polymerization of tubulin and induces the production of stable, nonfunctional microtubules, thus inhibiting cell replication. Podophyllotoxin derivatives include etoposide and teniposide. Vinca alkaloids include vinblastine, vincristine, and vinorelbine. A new class of agents called taxanes includes paclitaxel and docetaxel.

Radiopharmaceuticals: Radiopharmaceuticals exert direct toxic effects on exposed tissue via radiation emission. Primary activity is against metastatic disease. Examples include strontium-89, sodium iodide I 131, and chromic phosphate P 32.

Biological response modifiers: Biological response modifiers have complex antineoplastic, antiviral, and immunomodulating activities. It is believed that the antitumor activity of interferons is a result of a direct antiproliferative action against tumor cells and modulation of the host immune response. Examples of biological agents include the following:

        aldesleukin (human interleukin-2)
        interferon alfa-2a (recombinant DNA)
        interferon alfa-2b (recombinant DNA)
        interferon alfa-n3 (human leukocyte)
        interferon gamma-1B (recombinant DNA)

Miscellaneous: Metabolism of altretamine is required for cytotoxicity, although the mechanisms are not clear. Asparaginase is an enzyme that inhibits protein synthesis of malignant cells by inhibiting asparagine, which is required for protein synthesis. Intravesical BCG is a suspension of *Mycobacterium bovis* that promotes a local inflammatory reaction in the urinary bladder and reduces cancerous lesions. Cladribine inhibits DNA synthesis and repair through a complex mechanism. Levamisole is an immunomodulator with complex effects. Procarbazine produces toxic metabolites, which induce chromosomal breakage. Tretinoin is a retinoid related to retinol (vitamin A), which induces cytodifferentiation. Porfimer is a photosensitivity agent. Topotecan and irinotecan are topoisomerase I inhibitors.

Extravasation: This occurs when IV fluid and medication leak into interstitial tissue. Damage resulting from extravasation of certain antineoplastic agents can range from painful erythematous swelling to full-thickness injury with deep necrotic lesions requiring surgical debridement and skin grafting.

    Prevention of extravasation injury – This is based on careful, accurate IV drug administration. Avoid areas of previous irradiation and extremities with poor venous circulation for IV cannula placement. Dilute drugs properly and give at an appropriate rate.

    Treatment – Treatment of extravasation includes immediate discontinuation of infusion and appropriate antidote administration. Goals of treatment are palliation and prevention of severe tissue damage. For further information regarding the instillation of a specific antidote, refer to individual product monographs. Consider surgical evaluation if an open wound occurs. Some practitioners recommend leaving the IV cannula in place to aspirate some of the chemotherapeutic agent and administering an antidote to the injured site. Others recommend immediate removal of the cannula and administration of the antidote by intradermal or SC injections. Immediate removal of the cannula followed by application of ice also has been recommended for all agents except etoposide, vinblastine, and vincristine (warm compresses are recommended for these agents). Apply the ice for 15 to 20 minutes every 4 to 6 hours for the first 72 hours. Elevate the affected area.

    Hydrocortisone sodium succinate or dexamethasone sodium phosphate have been used on the extravasated site for their anti-inflammatory activity. However, these agents, as well as other drugs (sodium bicarbonate, DMSO), are unproven for antidote use. Specific antidotes that are recommended include sodium thiosulfate for mechlorethamine and hyaluronidase for vincristine and vinblastine.

    Drugs associated with severe local necrosis (vesicants) include the following –

        dacarbazine
        dactinomycin
        daunorubicin
        doxorubicin
        epirubicin
        idarubicin
        mechlorethamine
        mitomycin

streptozocin
vinblastine
vincristine
vinorelbine

Nausea and vomiting: These may be the most prominent adverse reactions of cancer chemotherapy from the patient's perspective. In clinical trials, 17% to 98% of patients reported emesis. At least 30% of patients experience acute emesis despite anti-emetic therapy. Uncontrolled emesis may cause serious complications, including dehydration, malnutrition, metabolic disorders, esophageal injury, and aspiration. In addition, the patient's quality of life may be reduced significantly. Prevention and management of nausea and vomiting is an important aspect of cancer treatment.

Antineoplastics can be categorized according to their emetogenic potential based on the frequency of emesis. Level 1 is the least emetogenic, while Level 5 is the most emetogenic. Combining antineoplastic agents may increase the overall risk for emesis. For example, a combination of drugs with the risks factors of 2 + 2 + 2 may give a combined emetogenic risk of Level 3 (or 2 + 2 + 3 = 4 and 3 + 3 + 3 = 5).

Emetogenic Potential of Antineoplastics		
Level	Frequency of emesis	Chemotherapeutic agent
1	< 10%	Bleomycin Busulfan (oral, < 4 mg/kg/day) Chlorambucil (oral) Cladribine Doxorubicin, liposomal Estramustine Floxuridine Fludarabine Hydroxyurea	Inteferon alfa Melphalan (oral) Mercaptopurine Methotrexate $\leq$ 50 mg/m^2 Pentostatin Thioguanine (oral) Tretinoin Vinblastine Vincristine Vinorelbine
2	10% to 30%	Asparaginase Cytarabine (< 1000 mg/m^2) Daunorubicin, liposomal Docetaxel Doxorubicin HCl (< 20 mg/m^2) Etoposide Fluorouracil (< 1000 mg/m^2) Denileukin diftitox	Gemcitabine Methotrexate (50 to 250 mg/m^2) Mitomycin Paclitaxel Pegaspargase Teniposide Thiotepa Topotecan
3	30% to 60%	Aldesleukin Altretamine (oral) Capecitabine (oral) Cyclophosphamide ($\leq$ 750 mg/m^2) Cyclophosphamide (oral) Dactinomycin ($\leq$ 1.5 mg/m^2) Daunorubicin ($\leq$ 50 mg/m^2)	Doxorubicin HCl (20 to 60 mg/m^2) Epirubicin Idarubicin Ifosfamide ($\leq$ 1500 mg/m^2) Methotrexate (250 to 1000 mg/m^2) Mitoxantrone (< 15 mg/m^2) Temozolomide
4	60% to 90%	Carboplatin Carmustine ($\leq$ 250 mg/m^2) Cisplatin (< 50 mg/m^2) Cyclophosphamide (750 to 1500 mg/m^2) Cytarabine ($\geq$ 1000 mg/m^2) Dactinomycin (> 1.5 mg/m^2) Daunorubicin (> 50 mg/m^2)	Doxorubicin HCl (> 60 mg/m^2) Irinotecan Lomustine ($\leq$ 60 mg/m^2) Melphalan (IV) Methotrexate ($\geq$ 1000 mg/m^2) Mitoxantrone ($\geq$ 15 mg/m^2) Procarbazine
5	> 90%	Carmustine (> 250 mg/m^2) Cisplatin ($\geq$ 50 mg/m^2) Cyclophosphamide (> 1500 mg/m^2) Dacarbazine	Ifosfamide (> 1500 mg/m^2) Lomustine (> 60 mg/m^2) Mechlorethamine Streptozocin

The incidence of emesis with these and other agents varies greatly among individuals. Dose, schedule, concomitant therapy, other medical complications, and psychologic parameters may affect the incidence as well.

Prevention and treatment – Prevention and treatment of nausea and vomiting should include measures such as dietary adjustment, restriction of activity, and positive support. However, if pharmacologic management is necessary, several agents or groups of agents may prove useful. Some drugs that have been used with varying degrees of success, either alone or in combination, include 5-HT$_3$ receptor antagonists (such as ondansetron, dolasetron, and granisetron), phenothiazines, butyrophenones, cannabinoids, corticosteroids, antihistamines, benzodiazepines, metoclopramide, and scopolamine.

TAMOXIFEN CITRATE

Tablets: 10 and 20 mg (*Rx*)　　　　　Various, *Nolvadex* (AstraZeneca)

Indications

Breast cancer:

　　Adjuvant therapy – For treatment of axillary node-negative breast cancer in women following total mastectomy or segmental mastectomy, axillary dissection, and breast irradiation.

　　For treatment of node-positive breast cancer in postmenopausal women following total mastectomy or segmental mastectomy, axillary dissection, and breast irradiation.

　　Advanced disease therapy – Effective in the treatment of metastatic breast cancer in women and men. In premenopausal women with metastatic breast cancer, tamoxifen is an alternative to oophorectomy or ovarian irradiation. Estrogen receptor positive tumors are most likely to benefit.

Reduction in breast cancer incidence in high-risk women: To reduce the incidence of breast cancer in women at high risk for breast cancer. "High risk" is defined as women ≥ 35 years of age with a 5-year predicted risk of breast cancer ≥ 1.67% as calculated by the Gail model. (Refer to the Package Insert for examples of risk factor combinations.)

Ductal carcinoma in situ (DCIS): In women with DCIS, following breast surgery and radiation, tamoxifen is indicated to reduce the risk of invasive breast cancer.

Unlabeled uses: Tamoxifen has been used in the treatment of mastalgia (10 mg/day for 4 months).

Administration and Dosage

Breast cancer patients: 20 to 40 mg daily. Give doses > 20 mg/day in divided doses (morning and evening).

　　Some studies have used dosages of 10 mg 2 or 3 times/day for 2 years, and 10 mg twice daily for 5 years. The reduction in recurrence and mortality was greater in those studies that used the drug for ≈ 5 years than in those that used it for a shorter period. There was no indication that doses > 20 mg/day were more effective. Current data from clinical trials support 5 years of adjuvant tamoxifen therapy for patients with breast cancer.

Reduction in breast cancer incidence in high-risk women: 20 mg daily for 5 years. There are no data to support the use of tamoxifen other than for 5 years.

　　For sexually active women of childbearing potential, initiate tamoxifen therapy during menstruation. In women with menstrual irregularity, a negative B-HCG immediately prior to the initiation of therapy is sufficient.

DCIS: 20 mg daily for 5 years.

Actions

Pharmacology: Tamoxifen is a nonsteroidal agent with potent antiestrogenic properties.

Pharmacokinetics: Tamoxifen is extensively metabolized after oral administration. Approximately 65% of an administered dose was excreted from the body over a period of 2 weeks with fecal excretion as the primary route of elimination.

　　After initiation of therapy, steady-state concentrations for tamoxifen are achieved in ≈ 4 weeks and steady-state concentrations for N-desmethyl tamoxifen are achieved in ≈ 8 weeks, suggesting a half-life of ≈14 days for this metabolite.

Contraindications

Hypersensitivity to the drug; women who require concomitant coumarin-type anticoagulant therapy; women with a history of deep vein thrombosis or pulmonary embolus (reduction in breast cancer incidence and DCIS indications).

Warnings

Thromboembolic effects: Consider the risks and benefits of tamoxifen carefully in women with a history of thromboembolic events. Among women receiving tamoxifen, the events appeared between 2 and 60 months from the start of treatment.

Visual disturbances: Visual disturbances, including corneal changes, cataracts, the need for cataract surgery, decrement in color vision perception, retinal vein thrombosis, and retinopathy have occurred with tamoxifen use.

Disease of bone: Increased bone pain, tumor pain, and local disease flare sometimes are associated with a good tumor response shortly after starting tamoxifen, and generally subside rapidly. Lesion size may increase suddenly in soft tissue disease, sometimes with new lesions, or with erythema in or around the lesion.

Hypercalcemia: Hypercalcemia has occurred in some breast cancer patients with bone metastases within a few weeks of starting therapy with tamoxifen.

Hepatic effects: Tamoxifen has been associated with changes in liver enzyme levels and, on rare occasions, fatty liver, cholestasis, hepatitis, and hepatic necrosis.

Pregnancy: Category D.

Lactation: It is not known whether this drug is excreted in breast milk.

Children: Safety and efficacy in pediatric patients have not been established.

Precautions

Monitoring: Perform periodic complete blood counts, including platelet counts, and liver function tests. Perform a breast examination, a mammogram, and a gynecologic examination prior to the initiation of therapy. Repeat these studies at regular intervals while on therapy.

Leukopenia/Thrombocytopenia: Use cautiously in patients with existing leukopenia or thrombocytopenia.

Hyperlipidemias: Hyperlipidemias have occurred infrequently.

Drug Interactions

Drugs that may interact with tamoxifen include bromocriptine, anticoagulants, and cytotoxic agents.

Drug/Lab test interactions: T_4 elevations occurred in a few postmenopausal patients but were not accompanied by clinical hyperthyroidism. Variations in the karyopyknotic index on vaginal smears and various degrees of estrogen effect on Pap smears have been infrequently seen in postmenopausal patients.

Adverse Reactions

Adverse reactions occuring in ≥ 3% of patients after 5-year therapy include the following: Hot flashes, fluid retention, vaginal discharge, nausea, irregular menses, weight loss, skin changes, increased AST.

Adverse reactions occurring in ≥ 3% of patients taking tamoxifen vs ovarian ablation include the following: Flushing, amenorrhea, altered menses, oligomenorrhea, bone pain, menstrual disorder, nausea, coughing, edema, fatigue, musculoskeletal pain, pain, ovarian cyst(s).

INTERFERON ALFA-2a (rIFN-A; IFLrA)

Injection Solution: 3 million IU/mL, 6 million IU/mL, 9 million IU/0.9 mL, 36 million IU/mL *(Rx)*   *Roferon*-A (Roche)

Powder for Injection: 6 million IU/mL when reconstituted *(Rx)*

Indications

Hairy-cell leukemia: In select patients ≥ 18 years of age.

AIDS-related Kaposi's sarcoma: In select patients ≥ 18 years of age.

Chronic myelogenous leukemia (CML): In chronic phase, Philadelphia chromosome (Ph) positive CML patients who are minimally pretreated (within 1 year of diagnosis).

Administration and Dosage

Give SC or IM. SC administration is suggested for, but not limited to, patients who are thrombocytopenic (platelet count < 50,000/mm^3) or who are at risk for bleeding.

Hairy-cell leukemia:
 Induction dose – 3 million IU daily for 16 to 24 weeks, SC or IM.

 Maintenance dose – 3 million IU 3 times/week. Dosage reduction by one-half or withholding of individual doses may be needed when severe adverse reactions occur. The use of doses higher than 3 million IU is not recommended.

 Treat patients for ≈ 6 months before determining whether to continue therapy. Patients with hairy-cell leukemia have been treated for up to 20 consecutive months. The optimal duration of treatment for this disease has not been determined.

AIDS-related Kaposi's sarcoma:
 Induction dose – 36 million IU daily for 10 to 12 weeks, administered IM or SC.

 Maintenance dose – 36 million IU 3 times/week. Dose reductions by one-half or withholding of individual doses may be required when severe adverse reactions occur. An escalating schedule of 3, 9, and 18 million IU daily for 3 days followed by 36 million IU daily for the remainder of the 10- to 12-week induction period also has produced equivalent therapeutic benefit with some amelioration of the acute toxicity in some patients.

 When disease stabilization or a response to treatment occurs, treatment should continue until there is no further evidence of tumor or until discontinuation is required because of a severe opportunistic infection or adverse effects. The optimal duration of treatment for this disease has not been determined.

 If severe reactions occur, modify dosage (50% reduction) or temporarily discontinue therapy until the adverse reactions abate. The need for dosage reduction should take into account effects of prior x-ray therapy or chemotherapy that may have compromised bone marrow reserve. Minimum effective doses have not been established.

CML:
 Chronic phase Ph-positive CML – Prior to initiation of therapy, make a diagnosis of Ph-positive CML in chronic phase by the appropriate peripheral blood, bone marrow and other diagnostic testing. Regularly monitor hematologic parameters (eg, monthly). Because significant cytogenic changes are not readily apparent until after hematologic response has occurred, and usually not until several months of therapy have elapsed, cytogenic monitoring may be performed at less frequent intervals. Achievement of complete cytogenic response has been observed up to 2 years following the start of interferon alfa-2a treatment.

 Induction dose – 9 million units daily administered SC or IM. Based on clinical experience, short-term tolerance may be improved by gradually increasing the dose of interferon alfa-2a over the first week of administration from 3 million IU daily for 3 days to 6 million IU daily for 3 days to the target dose of 9 million IU daily for the duration of the treatment period.

 Maintenance – Optimal dose and duration of therapy have not been determined.

Even though the median time to achieve the complete hematologic response was 5 months in clinical studies, hematologic responses have been observed up to 18 months after starting treatment. Continue therapy until disease progression. If severe side effects occur, a treatment interruption or reduction in either the dose or the frequency of injections may be necessary to achieve the individual maximally tolerated dose.

Children – Limited data are available on the use of interferon alfa-2a in children with CML. In one report of 15 children with Ph-positive, adult-type CML, doses between 2.5 and 5 million IU/m²/day given IM were tolerated. In another study, severe adverse effects including death were noted in children with previously untreated, Ph-negative juvenile CML who received interferon doses of 30 million IU/m²/day.

Actions

Pharmacology: Interferon alfa-2a is a sterile protein product manufactured by recombinant DNA technology that employs a genetically engineered *Escherichia coli* bacterium. The mechanism by which interferons exert antitumor activity is not clearly understood. However, direct antiproliferative action against tumor cells and modulation of the host immune response may play important roles.

Pharmacokinetics:

Absorption/Distribution – In healthy people, interferon alfa-2a exhibited an elimination half-life of 3.7 to 8.5 hours (mean, 5.1 hours), volume of distribution at steady state of 0.223 to 0.748 L/kg (mean, 0.4 L/kg), and a total body clearance of 2.14 to 3.62 mL/min/kg (mean, 2.79 mL/min/kg) after a 36 million IU (2.2 x 10⁸ pg) IV infusion. After IM and SC administrations of 36 million IU, peak serum concentrations ranged from 1500 to 2580 pg/mL (mean, 2020 pg/mL) at a mean time to peak of 3.8 hours and from 1250 to 2320 pg/mL (mean, 1730 pg/mL) at a mean time to peak of 7.3 hours, respectively. Multiple IM doses resulted in accumulation of 2 to 4 times the single dose serum concentrations. The apparent fraction of the dose absorbed after IM injection was greater than 80%.

Metabolism/Excretion – Alfa interferons are filtered through the glomeruli and undergo rapid proteolytic degradation during tubular reabsorption, rendering a negligible reappearance of intact alpha interferon in the systemic circulation, suggesting near complete reabsorption of interferon alfa-2a catabolites. Liver metabolism and subsequent biliary excretion are minor pathways of elimination.

Contraindications

Hypersensitivity to alpha interferon or any component of the product.

Warnings

GI hemorrhage: Infrequently, severe or fatal GI hemorrhage has been reported in association with alfa interferon therapy.

Laboratory tests: Prior to initiation of therapy, perform tests to quantitate peripheral blood hemoglobin, platelets, granulocytes, and hairy cells and bone marrow hairy cells. Monitor periodically (eg, monthly) during treatment to determine response to treatment. If a patient does not respond within 6 months, discontinue treatment. If a response occurs, continue treatment until no further improvement is observed and these laboratory parameters have been stable for ≈ 3 months. It is not known whether continued treatment after that time is beneficial.

Exercise caution in the following: In patients with severe renal or hepatic disease, seizure disorders, or compromised CNS function or myelosuppression.

Administer with caution to patients with cardiac disease or with any history of cardiac illness. Acute, self-limited toxicities (eg, fever, chills) frequently associated with interferon alfa administration may exacerbate preexisting cardiac conditions.

Exercise caution when administering to patients with myelosuppression.

CNS reactions: CNS reactions have occurred in a number of patients and included decreased mental status, exaggerated CNS function, and dizziness. Careful periodic neuropsychiatric monitoring of all patients is recommended.

Leukopenia and elevation of hepatic enzymes: Leukopenia and elevation of hepatic enzymes occurred frequently but were rarely dose-limiting. Thrombocytopenia occurred less frequently. Proteinuria and increased cells in urinary sediment also were seen infrequently.

Neutralizing antibodies: Neutralizing antibodies were detected in ≈ 27% of all patients (3.4% for patients with hairy cell leukemia). No clinical sequelae have been documented.

Anemia: In CML patients, a severe or life-threatening anemia was seen in 15% of patients. A severe life-threatening leukopenia and thrombocytopenia were seen in ≤ 27%. Changes usually were reversible when therapy was discontinued.

Renal/Hepatic function impairment: Transient increases in liver transaminases or alkaline phosphatase of any intensity were seen in up to 50% of patients during treatment with interferon alfa-2a. Only 5% of patients had a severe or life-threatening increase in AST.

Dose-limiting hepatic or renal toxicities are unusual.

Pregnancy: Category C.

Lactation: It is not known whether this drug is excreted in breast milk. Because of the potential for serious adverse reactions in nursing infants, decide whether to discontinue nursing or to discontinue the drug, taking into account the importance of the drug to the mother.

Children: Safety and efficacy in children < 18 years of age have not been established.

Precautions
Monitoring: Prior to initiation of therapy, perform tests to quantitate peripheral blood hemoglobin, platelets, granulocytes, hairy cells, and bone marrow hairy cells. Monitor periodically (eg, monthly) during treatment to determine response to treatment. If a patient does not respond within 6 months, discontinue treatment. If a response occurs, continue treatment until no further improvement is observed and these laboratory parameters have been stable for ≈ 3 months. It is not known whether continued treatment after that time is beneficial.

Because responses of hairy-cell leukemia generally are not observed for 1 to 3 months after initiation of treatment, very careful monitoring for severe depression of blood cell counts is warranted during the initial phase of treatment.

Patients who have preexisting cardiac abnormalities or who are in advanced stages of cancer should have ECGs taken prior to and during the course of treatment.

Drug Interactions
Drugs that may be affected by interferon alfa-2a include aminophylline; theophylline; neurotoxic, hematotoxic, or cardiotoxic drugs; interleukin-2; and CNS drugs.

Adverse Reactions
Most adverse reactions are reversible if detected early. If severe reactions occur, reduce dosage or discontinue the drug; take appropriate corrective measures according to physician's clinical judgment. Reinstitute therapy with caution; consider further need for the drug, and be alert to possible recurrence of toxicity.

Adverse reactions occurring in ≥ 3% of patients include fever; fatigue; myalgias; headache; chills; arthralgia; coughing; dyspnea; hypotension; edema; chest pain; anorexia; nausea; diarrhea; emesis; abdominal pain; dizziness; decreased mental status; depression; confusion; diaphoresis; paresthesias; numbness; lethargy; visual or sleep disturbances; partial alopecia; rash; dryness or inflammation of the oropharynx; dry skin or pruritus; weight loss; change in taste; reactivation of herpes labialis; transient impotence; night sweats; rhinorrhea; lab test abnormalities including leukopenia; neutropenia; thrombocytopenia; decreased hemoglobin; abnormal AST-alkaline phosphatase, LDH, and BUN; hypocalcemia; elevated fasting serum glucose and elevated serum phosphorus and serum uric acid neutralizing antibodies.

INTERFERON ALFA-2b (IFN-alpha 2; rIFN-α2; α-2-interferon)

Powder for injection, lyophilized: 3, 5, 10, 18, 25, and 50 million IU/vial *(Rx)*　　*Intron A (Schering)*

Solution for injection: 3, 5, 10, 18, and 25 million IU/vial *(Rx)*　　*Intron A (Schering)*

Indications

Hairy-cell leukemia: In select patients, previously splenectomized and nonsplenectomized.

Malignant melanoma: Adjuvant to surgical treatment in patients with malignant melanoma who are free of disease but at high risk for systemic recurrence within 56 days of surgery.

Condylomata acuminata: Intralesional treatment of genital or venereal warts in select patients who do not respond to other treatment modalities or whose lesions are more readily treatable by interferon alfa-2b.

AIDS-related Kaposi's sarcoma: In select patients.

Chronic hepatitis C: In patients with compensated liver disease and a history of blood or blood product exposure or are HCV antibody positive.

Chronic hepatitis B: In patients with compensated liver disease and HBV replication. Patients must be serum HBsAg-positive for ≥ 6 months and have HBV replication (serum HBeAg-positive) with elevated serum ALT.

Administration and Dosage

Patients should be well hydrated, especially during the initial stages of treatment.

Hairy-cell leukemia: 2 million IU/m², IM or SC 3 times/week.

　　Maintain this dosage regimen unless the disease progresses rapidly or severe intolerance occurs.

　　The patient may self-administer at bedtime.

Malignant melanoma: 20 million IU/m² IV on 5 consecutive days/week for 4 weeks. Maintenance dosage is 10 million IU/m² SC 3 times/week for 48 weeks.

　　Perform regular laboratory testing to monitor abnormalities for the purpose of dose modification. If adverse reactions develop during interferon alfa-2b treatment, particularly if granulocytes decrease to < 500/mm³ or ALT/AST rises to > 5 × upper limit of normal (ULN), temporarily discontinue treatment until adverse reactions abate.

　　Restart interferon alfa-2b at 50% of the previous dose. If intolerance persists or if granulocytes decrease to < 250/mm³ or ALT/AST rises to > 10 × ULN, discontinue interferon alfa-2b therapy.

　　Maintain therapy for 1 year unless there is a progression of disease.

Condylomata acuminata: 1 million IU/lesion 3 times/week for 3 weeks intralesionally. Use only 10 million IU vial because dilution of other strengths required for intralesional use results in a hypertonic solution. Do not reconstitute 10 million IU vial with > 1 mL diluent. Use tuberculin or similar syringe and 25- to 30-gauge needle. Do not go beneath lesion too deeply or inject too superficially. As many as 5 lesions can be treated at one time.

　　Maximum response usually occurs 4 to 8 weeks after therapy initiation. If results are not satisfactory after 12 to 16 weeks, a second course may be instituted.

　　Drug delivery – Direct the needle at the center of the base of the wart and at an angle almost parallel to the plane of the skin. This will deliver the interferon to the dermal core of the lesion, infiltrating the lesion and causing a small wheal.

AIDS-related Kaposi's sarcoma: 30 million IU/m² 3 times/week administered SC or IM. Use only 50 million IU vial. Maintain the selected dosage regimen unless the disease progresses rapidly or severe intolerance occurs. When patients initiate therapy at 30 million IU/m² 3 times/week, the average dose tolerated at the end of 12 weeks therapy is 110 million IU/week and 75 million IU/week at the end of 24 weeks therapy.

Chronic hepatitis non-A, non-B/C (NANB/C): 3 million IU 3 times/week SC or IM. Normalization of ALT levels may occur in some patients as early as 2 weeks after treatment initiation; however, current experience suggests completing a 6-month course of therapy in responding patients. Patients who relapse may be retreated with the same dosage regimen to which they had previously responded.

Chronic hepatitis B: 30 to 35 million IU/week SC or IM, either as 5 million IU/day or 10 million IU 3 times/week for 16 weeks.

Decreased granulocyte or platelet counts – Use the following guidelines:

Interferon Alfa-2b Dose with Decreased Granulocyte or Platelet Counts		
Granulocyte count	Platelet count	Interferon alfa-2b dose
< 750/mm³	< 50,000/mm³	Reduce by 50%
< 500/mm³	< 30,000/mm³	Interrupt

When platelet or granulocyte counts return to normal or baseline values, reinstitute therapy at up to 100% of initial dose.

Actions

Pharmacology: Interferon alfa is a protein produced by recombinant DNA techniques. Interferons exert their cellular activities by binding to specific membrane receptors on the cell surface. Once bound to the cell membrane, interferon initiates a complex sequence of intracellular events that includes the induction of certain enzymes. This process, at least in part, may be responsible for the various cellular responses to interferon, including inhibition of virus replication in virus-infected cells, suppression of cell proliferation, and such immunomodulating activities as enhancement of the phagocytic activity of macrophages and augmentation of the specific cytotoxicity of lymphocytes for target cells.

Pharmacokinetics: Mean serum concentrations following IM and SC injections were comparable. Elimination half-lives were ≈ 2 to 3 hours. Serum concentrations were below the detection limit by 16 hours after the injections.

After IV use, serum concentrations peaked by the end of infusion, then declined at a slightly more rapid rate than after IM or SC administration, becoming undetectable 4 hours after infusion. Elimination half-life was ≈ 2 hours.

Interferon could not be detected in urine; the kidney may be the main site of interferon catabolism.

Contraindications

Hypersensitivity to interferon alfa-2b or any components of the product.

Warnings

Hairy-cell leukemia:

Monitoring – Before initiating therapy, perform tests to quantitate peripheral blood hemoglobin, platelets, granulocytes, and hairy cells, and bone marrow hairy cells. Monitor periodically to determine response.

IM use – Do not give IM to patients with platelet counts < 50,000/mm³. Instead, give SC.

Cardiovascular – Use therapy cautiously in patients with a history of cardiovascular disease. Cardiovascular adverse experiences, which include hypotension, arrhythmia, or tachycardia of ≥ 150 beats/min and, rarely, cardiomyopathy and MI, have been observed. Hypotension may occur during administration, or ≤ 2 days post-therapy, and may require supportive therapy, including fluid replacement to maintain intravascular volume.

CNS effects – CNS effects (eg, depression, confusion, other alterations of mental status) were seen in ≈ 2% of hairy-cell leukemia patients. Overall incidence in a larger patient population with other malignancies treated with higher doses was 10%.

Condylomata acuminata:

    Do not use – Do not use 3, 5, 18, 25, or 50 million IU vials of powder for injection or the 3 or 18 million IU multidose vials intralesionally to treat condylomata acuminata; concentrations are inappropriate.

AIDS-related Kaposi's sarcoma: Use only the 50 million IU vial size. Do not use in patients with rapidly progressive visceral disease. There may be synergistic adverse effects between interferon alfa-2b and zidovudine. Patients have had a higher incidence of neutropenia than that expected with zidovudine alone. Careful monitoring of the WBC count is indicated.

Thyroid abnormalities: Patients may develop thyroid abnormalities during interferon therapy. Discontinuation of therapy has not always reversed thyroid dysfunction.

Chronic hepatitis – NANB/C:

    Monitoring – Before treatment, establish and consider the following criteria: Bilirubin ≤ 2 mg/dL; albumin stable and within normal limits; prothrombin time (PT) < 3 seconds prolonged; WBC ≥ 3000/mm^3; platelets > 70,000/mm^3; serum creatinine normal or near normal. Evaluate CBC and platelet counts; repeat at weeks 1 and 2 after therapy initiation, monthly thereafter. Evaluate ALT levels after 2, 16, and 24 weeks.

    Pre-existing psychiatric condition/history of severe psychiatric disorder – Do not treat; discontinue therapy in any patient developing severe depression.

    Pre-existing thyroid abnormalities – Do not treat patients whose thyroid function cannot be maintained in the normal range by medication.

Chronic hepatitis B:

    Monitoring – Before treatment, establish and consider the following criteria: Bilirubin normal; albumin stable and within normal limits; PT < 3 seconds prolonged; WBC ≥ 4000/mm^3; platelets ≥ 100,000/mm^3. Evaluate CBC and platelet counts, then repeat at weeks 1, 2, 4, 8, 12, and 16. Evaluate liver function tests, including serum ALT, albumin and bilirubin at treatment weeks 1, 2, 4, 8, 12, and 16. Evaluate HBeAg, HBsAg, and ALT at the end of therapy and 3 and 6 months posttherapy.

    ALT increase – A transient increase in ALT ≥ 2 times baseline (flare) can occur, generally 8 to 12 weeks after therapy initiation, and is more frequent in responders. Continue therapy unless signs and symptoms of hepatic failure occur.

Chronic hepatitis C and B: Do not treat patients with decompensated liver disease, autoimmune hepatitis; history of autoimmune disease, or immunosuppressed transplant recipients. In these patients, worsening liver disease, including jaundice, hepatic encephalopathy, hepatic failure, and death have occurred following therapy.

Adverse experiences: Moderate to severe adverse experiences may require modification of the patient's dosage regimen, or, in some cases, termination of therapy.

Fever/"Flu-like" symptoms: Because of fever and other "flu-like" symptoms associated with this drug, use cautiously in debilitating medical conditions, such as those with a history of cardiovascular disease, pulmonary disease, or diabetes mellitus prone to ketoacidosis. Observe caution in coagulation disorders or severe myelosuppression.

Rare adverse events: Pulmonary infiltrates, pneumonitis, and pneumonia, including fatality, have been observed rarely. Take chest X-rays of any patient developing fever, cough, dyspnea, or other respiratory symptoms.

Other rare adverse events: Retinal hemorrhages, cotton wool spots, and retinal artery or vein obstruction have been observed rarely.

Hepatotoxicity: Hepatotoxicity, including fatality, has been observed.

Autoimmune disease: Rare cases of autoimmune diseases including thrombocytopenia, vasculitis, Raynaud's phenomenon, rheumatoid arthritis, lupus erythematosus, and rhabdomyolysis have been observed.

Hyperglycemia: Diabetes mellitus and hyperglycemia have been observed rarely in patients treated with interferon alpha-2b. Symptomatic patients should have their blood glucose measured and followed up accordingly. Patients with diabetes mellitus may require adjustment of their antidiabetic regimen.

Hypersensitivity reactions: Hypersensitivity reactions (eg, urticaria, angioedema, bronchoconstriction, anaphylaxis) have been observed in treated patients.

Hepatic function impairment: Do not treat patients with decompensated liver disease, autoimmune hepatitis, history of autoimmune disease, or immunocompromised transplant recipients. In these patients, worsening liver disease, including jaundice, hepatic encephalopathy, hepatic failure, and death have occurred following therapy.

Discontinue therapy for any patient developing signs and symptoms of liver failure.

Fertility impairment: Interferon may impair fertility.

Pregnancy: Category C.

Lactation: It is not known if this drug is excreted in breast milk.

Children: Safety and efficacy in children < 18 years of age have not been established.

Precautions

Monitoring: Prior to beginning treatment and periodically thereafter perform the following: Standard hematologic tests with complete blood counts and differential, platelet counts, blood chemistries, electrolytes, and liver function tests. Patients with pre-existing cardiac abnormalities or those in advanced stages of cancer should have ECGs taken before and during treatment. Refer also to the monitoring sections under Warnings for each indication.

Baseline chest X-rays are suggested; repeat if clinically indicated.

For malignant melanoma patients, monitor differential, WBC count, and liver function tests weekly during the induction phase of therapy and monthly during the maintenance phase of therapy.

Photosensitivity: Photosensitivity may occur.

Drug Interactions

Drugs that may be affected by inteferon alfa-2b include aminophylline and zidovudine.

Adverse Reactions

The most frequently reported reactions are "flu-like" symptoms, particularly fever, headache, chills, myalgia, and fatigue. Other adverse reactions include the following: Dizziness; paresthesia; depression; anxiety; confusion; hypoesthesia; amnesia; impaired concentration; nervousness; irritability; somnolence; decreased libido; nausea; diarrhea; vomiting; anorexia; dyspnea; constipation; loose stools; abdominal pain; pharyngitis; nasal congestion; dyspnea; coughing; sinusitis; dry mouth/thirst; arthralgia; asthenia; rigors; back pain; muscle pain/weakness; rash; pruritus; dry skin; dermatitis; alopecia; moniliasis; edema/facial edema; chest pain; increased sweating; malaise; taste alteration; insomnia; weight loss; herpes simplex; gingivitis; "flu-like" symptoms; back pain; thinning hair; lab test abnormalities including hemoglobin, WBC count, platelet count, serum creatinine, alkaline phosphatase, AST, ALT, and granulocyte count.

INTERFERON ALFA-2b, RECOMBINANT AND RIBAVIRIN COMBINATION

Injection/Capsules: 3 million IU interferon alfa-2b, recombinant/0.5 mL and 200 mg ribavirin (*Rx*)   *Rebetron* (Schering)

Injection/Capsules: 3 million IU interferon alfa-2b, recombinant/0.2 mL and 200 mg ribavirin (*Rx*)   *Rebetron* (Schering)

Warning:

Combination ribavirin/interferon alfa-2b therapy is contraindicated in women who are pregnant. Women of childbearing potential and men must use effective contraception during treatment and during the 6-month posttreatment follow-up period. Significant teratogenic or embryocidal potential has been demonstrated for ribavirin in all animal species studied.

Indications

Hepatitis C: Treatment of chronic hepatitis C in patients with compensated liver disease who have relapsed following alpha interferon therapy.

Ribavirin monotherapy is not effective for the treatment of chronic hepatitis C and should not be used for this indication.

Administration and Dosage

Administer interferon alfa-2b SC and ribavirin orally without regard to food. Hydrate patients well, especially during initial treatment stages.

The recommended ribavirin dose depends on the patient's body weight. Administer doses of ribavirin and interferon alfa-2b according to the following table for 6 months (24 weeks). The safety and efficacy of the combination therapy has not been established for > 6 months of treatment.

Recommended Interferon Alfa-2b/Ribavirin Combination Dosing		
Body weight	Ribavirin	Interferon alfa-2b injection
≤ 75 kg	400 mg am	3 million IU 3 times weekly SC
	600 mg pm	
> 75 kg	600 mg am	
	600 mg pm	

Dose modifications: It is recommended that patients who experience moderate depression (persistent low mood, loss of interest, poor self image, or hopelessness) have their interferon alfa-2b dose temporarily reduced or be considered for medical therapy. Discontinue treatment in patients experiencing severe depression or suicidal ideation/attempt from combination therapy and follow closely with appropriate medical management.

Interferon Alfa-2b/Ribavirin Combination Dose Modification Guidelines		
Parameter	Dose reduction[1] Ribavirin - 600 mg daily Interferon alfa-2b - 1.5 million IU TIW	Permanent discontinuation of combination treatment
Hemoglobin	< 10 g/dL (reduce ribavirin) *Cardiac history patients only:* ≥ 2 g/dL decrease during any 4-week period during treatment (reduce ribavirin/interferon alfa-2b)	< 8.5 g/dL *Cardiac history patients only:* < 12 g/dL after 4 weeks of dose reduction
White blood count	< 1.5 × 10⁹/L (reduce interferon alfa-2b)	< 1 × 10⁹/L
Neutrophil count	< 0.75 × 10⁹/L (reduce interferon alfa-2b)	< 0.5 × 10⁹/L
Platelet count	< 50 × 10⁹/L (reduce interferon alfa-2b)	< 25 × 10⁹/L

[1] Medication to have a dose reduction is shown in parentheses.

Administration of interferon alfa-2b injection: At the discretion of the physician, the patient may self-administer interferon alfa-2b.

Withdraw the appropriate dose from the vial or set on the multidose pen and inject SC. After administration, follow the procedure for proper disposal of syringes and needles.

Administration of Interferon Alfa-2b Injection		
Vial/Pen label strength	Fill volume	Concentration
3 million IU vial	0.5 mL	3 million IU/0.5 mL
18 million IU multidose vial[1]	3.8 mL	3 million IU/0.5 mL
18 million IU multidose pen[2]	1.5 mL	3 million IU/0.2 mL

[1] This is a multidose vial that contains 22.8 million IU of interferon alfa-2b/3.8 mL in order to provide the delivery of six 0.5 mL doses, each containing 3 million IU of interferon alfa-2b (for a label strength of 18 million IU).

[2] This is a multidose pen that contains a 22.5 million IU of interferon alfa-2b/1.5 mL in order to provide the delivery of six 0.2 mL doses, each containing 3 million IU of interferon alfa-2b (for a label strength of 18 million IU).

Precautions

Monitoring: The following laboratory tests are recommended for all patients on combination therapy, prior to beginning treatment and then periodically thereafter: Standard hematologic tests including hemoglobin (pretreatment, week 2 and week 4 of therapy, and as clinically appropriate), complete and differential white blood cell counts, and platelet count; liver function tests and TSH; pregnancy including monthly monitoring for women of childbearing potential.

Cardiac disease: Administer therapy with caution to patients with pre-existing cardiac disease. Assess patients before commencement of therapy and appropriately monitor them during therapy. If there is any deterioration of cardiovascular status, stop therapy.

Renal function impairment: Administer with caution in patients with Ccr < 50 mL/min.

APPENDIX

FDA Pregnancy Categories, 1107
Controlled Substances, 1108
Management of Acute Hypersensitivity Reactions, 1109
Calculations, 1111
Normal Laboratory Values, 1112
General Management of Acute Overdosage, 1118

FDA PREGNANCY CATEGORIES

The rational use of any medication requires a risk versus benefit assessment. Among the myriad of risk factors that complicate this assessment, pregnancy is one of the most perplexing.

The FDA has established five categories to indicate the potential of a systemically absorbed drug for causing birth defects. The key differentiation among the categories rests upon the degree (reliability) of documentation and the risk versus benefit ratio. Pregnancy *Category* X is particularly notable in that if any data exists that may implicate a drug as a teratogen and the risk versus benefit ratio does not support use of the drug, the drug is contraindicated during pregnancy. These categories are summarized below:

FDA Pregnancy Categories	
Pregnancy Category	Definition
A	Controlled studies show no risk. Adequate, well-controlled studies in pregnant women have failed to demonstrate risk to the fetus.
B	No evidence of risk in humans. Either animal findings show risk, but human findings do not; or if no adequate human studies have been done, animal findings are negative.
C	Risk cannot be ruled out. Human studies are lacking, and animal studies are either positive for fetal risk or lacking. However, potential benefits may justify the potential risks.
D	Positive evidence of risk. Investigational or post-marketing data show risk to the fetus. Nevertheless, potential benefits may outweigh the potential risks. If needed in a life-threatening situation or a serious disease, the drug may be acceptable if safer drugs cannot be used or are ineffective.
X	Contraindicated in pregnancy. Studies in animals or human, or investigational or post-marketing reports have shown fetal risk which clearly outweighs any possible benefit to the patient.

Regardless of the designated Pregnancy Category or presumed safety, no drug should be administered during pregnancy unless it is clearly needed and potential benefits outweigh potential hazards to the fetus.

CONTROLLED SUBSTANCES

The Controlled Substances Act of 1970 regulates the manufacturing, distribution and dispensing of drugs that have abuse potential. The Drug Enforcement Administration (DEA) within the US Department of Justice is the chief federal agency responsible for enforcing the act.

DEA Schedules: Drugs under jurisdiction of the Controlled Substances Act are divided into five schedules based on their potential for abuse and physical and psychological dependence. All controlled substances listed in *Drug Facts and Comparisons*® are identified by schedule as follows:

Schedule I *(c-i)* – High abuse potential and no accepted medical use (eg, heroin, marijuana, LSD).

Schedule II *(c-ii)* – High abuse potential with severe dependence liability (eg, narcotics, amphetamines, dronabinol, some barbiturates).

Schedule III *(c-iii)* – Less abuse potential than schedule II drugs and moderate dependence liability (eg, nonbarbiturate sedatives, nonamphetamine stimulants, limited amounts of certain narcotics).

Schedule IV *(c-iv)* – Less abuse potential than schedule III drugs and limited dependence liability (eg, some sedatives, antianxiety agents, nonnarcotic analgesics).

Schedule V *(c-v)* – Limited abuse potential. Primarily small amounts of narcotics (codeine) used as antitussives or antidiarrheals. Under federal law, limited quantities of certain *c-v* drugs may be purchased without a prescription directly from a pharmacist if allowed under state statutes. The purchaser must be at least 18 years of age and must furnish suitable identification. All such transactions must be recorded by the dispensing pharmacist.

Registration: Prescribing physicians and dispensing pharmacies must be registered with the DEA, PO Box 28083, Central Station, Washington, DC 20005.

Inventory: Separate records must be kept of purchases and dispensing of controlled substances. An inventory of controlled substances must be made every 2 years.

Prescriptions: Prescriptions for controlled substances must be written in ink and include the following: Date; name and address of the patient; name, address, and DEA number of the physician. Oral prescriptions must be promptly committed to writing. Controlled substance prescriptions may not be dispensed or refilled more than 6 months after the date issued or be refilled more than 5 times. A written prescription signed by the physician is required for schedule II drugs. In case of emergency, oral prescriptions for schedule II substances may be filled; however, the physician must provide a signed prescription within 72 hours. Schedule II prescriptions cannot be refilled. A triplicate order form is necessary for the transfer of controlled substances in schedule II. Forms are available for the individual prescriber at no charge from the DEA.

State Laws: In many cases, state laws are more restrictive than federal laws and therefore impose additional requirements (eg, triplicate prescription forms).

MANAGEMENT OF ACUTE HYPERSENSITIVITY REACTIONS

Type I hypersensitivity reactions (immediate hypersensitivity or anaphylaxis) are immunologic responses to a foreign antigen to which a patient has been previously sensitized. Anaphylactoid reactions are not immunoogically mediated; however, symptoms and treatment are similar.

Signs and Symptoms

Acute hypersensitivity reactions typically begin within 1 to 30 minutes of exposure to the offending antigen. Tingling sensations and a generalized flush may proceed to a fullness in the throat, chest tightness, or a "feeling of impending doom." Generalized urticaria and sweating are common. *Severe* reactions include life-threatening involvement of the airway and cardiovascular system.

Treatment

Appropriate and immediate treatment is imperative. The following general measures are commonly employed:

Epinephrine: 1:1000, 0.2 to 0.5 mg (0.2 to 0.5 mL) SC is the primary treatment. In children, administer 0.01 mg/kg or 0.1 mg. Doses may be repeated every 5 to 15 minutes if needed. A succession of small doses is more effective and less dangerous than a single large dose. Additionally, 0.1 mg may be introduced into an injection site where the offending drug was administered. If appropriate, the use of a tourniquet above the site of injection of the causative agent may slow its absorption and distribution. However, remove or loosen the tourniquet every 10 to 15 minutes to maintain circulation.

Epinephrine IV (generally indicated in the presence of hypotension) is often recommended in a 1:10,000 dilution, 0.3 to 0.5 mg over 5 minutes; repeat every 15 minutes, if necessary. In children, inject 0.1 to 0.2 mg or 0.01 mg/kg/dose over 5 minutes; repeat every 30 minutes.

A conservative IV epinephrine protocol includes 0.1 mg of a 1:100,000 dilution (0.1 mg of a 1:1000 dilution mixed in 10 mL normal saline) given over 5 to 10 minutes. If an IV infusion is necessary, administer at a rate of 1 to 4 mcg/min. In children, infuse 0.1 to 1.5 (maximum) mcg/kg/min.

Dilute epinephrine 1:10,000 may be administered through an endotracheal tube, if no other parenteral access is available, directly into the bronchial tree. It is rapidly absorbed there from the capillary bed of the lung.

Airway: Ensure a patent airway via endotracheal intubation or cricothyrotomy (ie, inferior laryngotomy, used prior to tracheotomy) and administer oxygen. Severe respiratory difficulty may respond to IV aminophylline or to other bronchodilators.

Hypotension: The patient should be recumbent with feet elevated. Depending upon the severity, consider the following measures:
- Establish a patent IV catheter in a suitable vein.
- Administer IV fluids (eg, Normal Saline, Lactated Ringer's).
- Administer plasma expanders.

◆ Administer cardioactive agents (see group and individual monographs). Commonly recommended agents include dopamine, dobutamine, norepinephrine, and phenylephrine.

Adjunctive therapy: Adjunctive therapy does not alter acute reactions, but may modify an ongoing or slow-onset process and shorten the course of the reaction.

◆ *Antihistamines:* Diphenhydramine – 50 to 100 mg IM or IV, continued orally at 5 mg/kg/day or 50 mg every 6 hours for 1 to 2 days. For children, give 5 mg/kg/day, maximum 300 mg/day.

   Chlorpheniramine – (adults, 10 to 20 mg; children, 5 to 10 mg) IM or slowly IV.

   Hydroxyzine – 10 to 25 mg orally or 25 to 50 mg IM 3 to 4 times daily.

◆ *Corticosteroids,* eg, hydrocortisone IV 100 to 1000 mg or equivalent, followed by 7 mg/kg/day IV or oral for 1 to 2 days. The role of corticosteroids is controversial.

◆ H_2 *antagonists:* Cimetidine – Children, 25 to 30 mg/kg/day IV in 6 divided doses; *adults,* 300 mg every 6 hours.

   Ranitidine – 50 mg IV over 3 to 5 minutes. May be of value in addition to H_1 antihistamines, although this opinion is not universally shared.

CALCULATIONS

To calculate *milliequivalent weight*: $mEq = \dfrac{\text{gram molecular weight/valence}}{1000}$

$mEq = \dfrac{mg}{eq\ wt}$ equivalent weight or eq wt $= \dfrac{\text{gram molecular weight}}{\text{valence}}$

Commonly used mEq weights			
Chloride	35.5 mg = 1 mEq	Magnesium	12 mg = 1 mEq
Sodium	23 mg = 1 mEq	Potassium	39 mg = 1 mEq
Calcium	20 mg = 1 mEq		

To convert *temperature* °C ↔ °F: $\dfrac{°C}{°F-32} = \dfrac{5}{9}$ or $°C = \dfrac{5}{9}\ (°F - 32)$

$$°F = 32 + \dfrac{9}{5}\ °C$$

To calculate *creatinine clearance* (Ccr) *from serum creatinine*:

Male: $Ccr = \dfrac{\text{weight (kg)} \times (140 - \text{age})}{72 \times \text{serum creatinine (mg/dL)}}$ Female: Ccr = 0.85 × calculation for males

To calculate *ideal body weight* (kg):

Male = 50 kg + 2.3 kg (each inch > 5 ft)   Female = 45.5 kg + 2.3 kg (each inch > 5 ft)

To calculate *body surface area* (BSA) *in adults and children*:

1) *Dubois method*:

SA (cm^2) = wt $(kg)^{0.425}$ × ht $(cm)^{0.725}$ × 71.84

SA (m^2) = K × $\sqrt[3]{wt^2}$ (kg) (common K value 0.1 for toddlers, 0.103 for neonates)

2) *Simplified method*:

$$BSA\ (m^2) = \sqrt{\dfrac{\text{ht (cm)} \times \text{wt (kg)}}{3600}}$$

To approximate *surface area* (m^2) *of children from weight* (kg):

Weight range (kg)	≈ Surface area (m^2)
1 to 5	(0.05 x kg) + 0.05
6 to 10	(0.04 x kg) + 0.10
11 to 20	(0.03 x kg) + 0.20
21 to 40	(0.02 x kg) + 0.40

Suggested Weights for Adults	
Height*	Weight in pounds†
4'10"	91-119
4'11"	94-124
5'0"	97-128
5'1"	101-132
5'2"	104-137
5'3"	107-141
5'4"	111-146
5'5"	114-150
5'6"	118-155
5'7"	121-160
5'8"	125-164
5'9"	129-169
5'10"	132-174
5'11"	136-179
6'0"	140-184
6'1"	144-189
6'2"	148-195
6'3"	152-200
6'4"	156-205
6'5"	160-211
6'6"	164-216

* Without shoes.   † Without clothes.

The higher weights in the ranges generally apply to people with more muscle and bone. Source: Nutrition and Your Health: Dietary Guidelines for Americans, 4th ed, 1995. US Department of Agriculture, US Department of Health and Human Services. At press time, these new guidelines had not been officially released. It is possible some changes to this chart will occur.

NORMAL LABORATORY VALUES

In the following tables, normal reference values for commonly requested laboratory tests are listed in traditional units and in SI units. The tables are a guideline only. Values are method dependent and "normal values" may vary between laboratories.

Blood, Plasma, or Serum		
	Reference Value	
Determination	Conventional Units	SI Units
Ammonia (NH_3) – diffusion	20-120 mcg/dL	12-70 mcmol/L
Ammonia Nitrogen	15–45 µg/dL	11–32 µmol/L
Amylase	35-118 IU/L	0.58-1.97 mckat/L
Anion Gap ($Na^+ - [Cl^- + HCO_3^-]$) (P)	7–16 mEq/L	7–16 mmol/L
Antinuclear antibodies	negative at 1:10 dilution of serum	negative at 1:10 dilution of serum
Antithrombin III (AT III)	80-120 U/dL	800-1200 U/L
Bicarbonate: Arterial	21–28 mEq/L	21–28 mmol/L
Venous	22–29 mEq/L	22–29 mmol/L
Bilirubin: Conjugated (direct)	≤ 0.2 mg/dL	≤ 4 mcmol/L
Total	0.1-1 mg/dL	2-18 mcmol/L
Calcitonin	< 100 pg/mL	< 100 ng/L
Calcium: Total	8.6-10.3 mg/dL	2.2-2.74 mmol/L
Ionized	4.4-5.1 mg/dL	1-1.3 mmol/L
Carbon dioxide content (plasma)	21-32 mmol/L	21-32 mmol/L
Carcinoembryonic antigen	< 3 ng/mL	< 3 mcg/L
Chloride	95-110 mEq/L	95-110 mmol/L
Coagulation screen:		
Bleeding time	3-9.5 min	180-570 sec
Prothrombin time	10-13 sec	10-13 sec
Partial thromboplastin time (activated)	22-37 sec	22-37 sec
Protein C	0.7-1.4 µ/mL	700-1400 U/mL
Protein S	0.7-1.4 µ/mL	700-1400 U/mL
Copper, total	70-160 mcg/dL	11-25 mcmol/L
Corticotropin (ACTH adrenocorticotropic hormone) – 0800 hr	< 60 pg/mL	< 13.2 pmol/L
Cortisol: 0800 hr	5-30 mcg/dL	138-810 nmol/L
1800 hr	2-15 mcg/dL	50-410 nmol/L
2000 hr	≤ 50% of 0800 hr	≤ 50% of 0800 hr
Creatine kinase: Female	20-170 IU/L	0.33-2.83 mckat/L
Male	30-220 IU/L	0.5-3.67 mckat/L
Creatine kinase isoenzymes, MB fraction	0-12 IU/L	0-0.2 mckat/L
Creatinine	0.5-1.7 mg/dL	44-150 mcmol/L
Fibrinogen (coagulation factor I)	150-360 mg/dL	1.5-3.6 g/L
Follicle-stimulating hormone (FSH):		
Female	2-13 mIU/mL	2-13 IU/L
Midcycle	5-22 mIU/mL	5-22 IU/L
Male	1-8 mIU/mL	1-8 IU/L
Glucose, fasting	65-115 mg/dL	3.6-6.3 mmol/L

Glucose Tolerance Test (Oral)	mg/dL		mmol/L	
	Normal	Diabetic	Normal	Diabetic
Fasting	70-105	> 140	3.9-5.8	> 7.8
60 min	120-170	≥ 200	6.7-9.4	≥11.1
90 min	100-140	≥ 200	5.6-7.8	≥ 11.1
120 min	70-120	≥ 140	3.9-6.7	≥ 7.8

(γ) - Glutamyltransferase (GGT): Male	9-50 units/L	9-50 units/L
Female	8-40 units/L	8-40 units/L
Haptoglobin	44-303 mg/dL	0.44-3.03 g/L

Blood, Plasma, or Serum		
	Reference Value	
Determination	Conventional Units	SI Units
Hematologic tests:		
Fibrinogen	200-400 mg/dL	2-4 g/L
Hematocrit (Hct), female	36%-44.6%	0.36-0.446 fraction of 1
male	40.7%-50.3%	0.4-0.503 fraction of 1
Hemoglobin A_{1C}	5.3%-7.5% of total Hgb	0.053-0.075
Hemoglobin (Hb), female	12.1-15.3 g/dL	121-153 g/L
male	13.8-17.5 g/dL	138-175 g/L
Leukocyte count (WBC)	3800-9800/mcL	$3.8-9.8 \times 10^9$/L
Erythrocyte count (RBC), female	$3.5-5 \times 10^6$/mcL	$3.5-5 \times 10^{12}$/L
male	$4.3-5.9 \times 10^6$/mcL	$4.3-5.9 \times 10^{12}$/L
Mean corpuscular volume (MCV)	80-97.6 mcm^3	80-97.6 fl
Mean corpuscular hemoglobin (MCH)	27-33 pg/cell	1.66-2.09 fmol/cell
Mean corpuscular hemoglobin concentrate (MCHC)	33-36 g/dL	20.3-22 mmol/L
Erythrocyte sedimentation rate (sedrate, ESR)	≤ 30 mm/hr	≤ 30 mm/hr
Erythrocyte enzymes: Glucose-6-phosphate dehydroge nase (G-6-PD)	250-5000 units/10^6 cells	250-5000 mcunits/cell
Ferritin	10-383 ng/mL	23-862 pmol/L
Folic acid: normal	> 3.1-12.4 ng/mL	7-28.1 nmol/L
Platelet count	$150-450 \times 10^3$/mcL	$150-450 \times 10^9$/L
Reticulocytes	0.5%-1.5% of erythrocytes	0.005-0.015
Vitamin B_{12}	223-1132 pg/mL	165-835 pmol/L
Iron: Female	30-160 mcg/dL	5.4-31.3 mcmol/L
Male	45-160 mcg/dL	8.1-31.3 mcmol/L
Iron binding capacity	220-420 mcg/dL	39.4-75.2 mcmol/L
Isocitrate Dehydrogenase	1.2-7 units/L	1.2-7 units/L
Isoenzymes		
Fraction 1	14%-26% of total	0.14-0.26 fraction of total
Fraction 2	29%-39% of total	0.29-0.39 fraction of total
Fraction 3	20%-26% of total	0.20-0.26 fraction of total
Fraction 4	8%-16% of total	0.08-0.16 fraction of total
Fraction 5	6%-16% of total	0.06-0.16 fraction of total
Lactate dehydrogenase	100-250 IU/L	1.67-4.17 mckat/L
Lactic acid (lactate)	6-19 mg/dL	0.7-2.1 mmol/L
Lead	≤ 50 mcg/dL	≤ 2.41 mcmol/L
Lipase	10-150 units/L	10-150 units/L
Lipids:		
Total Cholesterol		
Desirable	< 200 mg/dL	< 5.2 mmol/L
Borderline-high	200-239 mg/dL	< 5.2-6.2 mmol/L
High	> 239 mg/dL	> 6.2 mmol/L
LDL		
Desirable	< 130 mg/dL	< 3.36 mmol/L
Borderline-high	130-159 mg/dL	3.36-4.11 mmol/L
High	> 159 mg/dL	> 4.11 mmol/L

Blood, Plasma, or Serum		
Determination	Reference Value	
	Conventional Units	SI Units
HDL (low)	< 35 mg/dL	< 0.91 mmol/L
Triglycerides		
Desirable	< 200 mg/dL	< 2.26 mmol/L
Borderline-high	200-400 mg/dL	2.26-4.52 mmol/L
High	400-1000 mg/dL	4.52-11.3 mmol/L
Very high	> 1000 mg/dL	> 11.3 mmol/L
Magnesium	1.3-2.2 mEq/L	0.65-1.1 mmol/L
Osmolality	280-300 mOsm/kg	280-300 mmol/kg
Oxygen saturation (arterial)	94%-100%	0.94-1 fraction of 1
PCO_2, arterial	35-45 mm Hg	4.7-6 kPa
pH, arterial	7.35-7.45	7.35-7.45
PO_2, arterial: Breathing room air[1]	80-105 mm Hg	10.6-14 kPa
On 100% O_2	> 500 mm Hg	
Phosphatase (acid), total at 37°C	0.13-0.63 IU/L	2.2-10.5 IU/L or 2.2-10.5 mckat/L
Phosphatase alkaline[2]	20-130 IU/L	20-130 IU/L or 0.33-2.17 mckat/L
Phosphorus, inorganic,[3] (phosphate)	2.5-5 mg/dL	0.8-1.6 mmol/L
Potassium	3.5-5 mEq/L	3.5-5 mmol/L
Progesterone		
Female	0.1-1.5 ng/mL	0.32-4.8 nmol/L
Follicular phase	0.1-1.5 ng/mL	0.32-4.8 nmol/L
Luteal phase	2.5-28 ng/mL	8-89 nmol/L
Male	< 0.5 ng/mL	< 1.6 nmol/L
Prolactin	1.4-24.2 ng/mL	1.4-24.2 mcg/L
Prostate specific antigen	0-4 ng/mL	0-4 ng/mL
Protein: Total	6-8 g/dL	60-80 g/L
Albumin	3.6-5 g/dL	36-50 g/L
Globulin	2.3-3.5 g/dL	23-35 g/L
Rheumatoid factor	< 60 IU/mL	< 60 kIU/L
Sodium	135-147 mEq/L	135-147 mmol/L
Testosterone: Female	6-86 ng/dL	0.21-3 nmol/L
Male	270-1070 ng/dL	9.3-37 nmol/L
Thyroid Hormone Function Tests:		
Thyroid-stimulating hormone (TSH)	0.35-6.2 mcU/mL	0.35-6.2 mU/L
Thyroxine-binding globulin capacity	10-26 mcg/dL	100-260 mcg/L
Total triiodothyronine (T_3)	75-220 ng/dL	1.2-3.4 nmol/L
Total thyroxine by RIA (T_4)	4-11 mcg/dL	51-142 nmol/L
T_3 resin uptake	25%-38%	0.25-0.38 fraction of 1
Transaminase, AST (aspartate aminotransferase, SGOT)	11-47 IU/L	0.18-0.78 mckat/L
Transaminase, ALT (alanine aminotransferase, SGPT)	7-53 IU/L	0.12-0.88 mckat/L
Transferrin	220-400 mg/dL	2.20-4.00 g/L
Urea nitrogen (BUN)	8-25 mg/dL	2.9-8.9 mmol/L
Uric acid	3-8 mg/dL	179-476 mcmol/L
Vitamin A (retinol)	15-60 mcg/dL	0.52-2.09 mcmol/L
Zinc	50-150 mcg/dL	7.7-23 mcmol/L

[1] Age dependent   [2] Infants and adolescents up to 104 U/L   [3] Infants in the first year up to 6 mg/dL

Urine		
	Reference Value	
Determination	Conventional Units	SI Units
Calcium[1]	50-250 mcg/day	1.25-6.25 mmol/day
Catecholamines: Epinephrine	< 20 mcg/day	< 109 nmol/day
Norepinephrine	< 100 mcg/day	< 590 nmol/day
Catecholamines, 24-hr	< 110 µg	< 650 nmol
Copper[1]	15-60 mcg/day	0.24-0.95 mcmol/day
Creatinine: Child	8-22 mg/kg	71-195 µmol/kg
Adolescent	8-30 mg/kg	71-265 µmol/kg
Female	0.6-1.5 g/day	5.3-13.3 mmol/day
Male	0.8-1.8 g/day	7.1-15.9 mmol/day
pH	4.5-8	4.5-8
Phosphate[1]	0.9-1.3 g/day	29-42 mmol/day
Potassium[1]	25-100 mEq/day	25-100 mmol/day
Protein		
Total	1-14 mg/dL	10-140 mg/L
At rest	50-80 mg/day	50-80 mg/day
Protein, quantitative	< 150 mg/day	< 0.15 g/day
Sodium[1]	100-250 mEq/day	100-250 mmol/day
Specific Gravity, random	1.002-1.030	1.002-1.030
Uric Acid, 24-hr	250-750 mg	1.48-4.43 mmol

[1] Diet dependent

Drug Levels†			
		Reference Value	
Drug Determination		Conventional Units	SI Units
Aminoglycosides	Amikacin		
	(trough)	1-8 mcg/mL	1.7-13.7 mcmol/L
	(peak)	20-30 mcg/mL	34-51 mcmol/L
	Gentamicin		
	(trough)	0.5-2 mcg/mL	1-4.2 mcmol/L
	(peak)	6-10 mcg/mL	12.5-20.9 mcmol/L
	Kanamycin		
	(trough)	5-10 mcg/mL	nd
	(peak)	20-25 mcg/mL	nd
	Netilmicin		
	(trough)	0.5-2 mcg/mL	nd
	(peak)	6-10 mcg/mL	nd
	Streptomycin		
	(trough)	< 5 mcg/mL	nd
	(peak)	5-20 mcg/mL	nd
	Tobramycin		
	(trough)	0.5-2 mcg/mL	1.1-4.3 mcmol/L
	(peak)	5-20 mcg/mL	12.8-21.8 mcmol/L

Drug Levels†		
Drug Determination	Reference Value	
	Conventional Units	SI Units
Antiarrhythmics Amiodarone	0.5-2.5 mcg/mL	1.5-4 mcmol/L
Bretylium	0.5-1.5 mcg/mL	nd
Digitoxin	9-25 mcg/L	11.8-32.8 nmol/L
Digoxin	0.8-2 ng/mL	0.9-2.5 nmol/L
Disopyramide	2-8 mcg/mL	6-18 mcmol/L
Flecainide	0.2-1 mcg/mL	nd
Lidocaine	1.5-6 mcg/mL	4.5-21.5 mcmol/L
Mexiletine	0.5-2 mcg/mL	nd
Procainamide	4-8 mcg/mL	17-34 mcmol/mL
Propranolol	50-200 ng/mL	190-770 nmol/L
Quinidine	2-6 mcg/mL	4.6-9.2 mcmol/L
Tocainide	4-10 mcg/mL	nd
Verapamil	0.08-0.3 mcg/mL	nd
Anticonvulsants Carbamazepine	4-12 mcg/mL	17-51 mcmol/L
Phenobarbital	10-40 mcg/mL	43-172 mcmol/L
Phenytoin	10-20 mcg/mL	40-80 mcmol/L
Primidone	4-12 mcg/mL	18-55 mcmol/L
Valproic acid	40-100 mcg/mL	280-700 mcmol/L
Antidepressants Amitriptyline	110-250 ng/mL[3]	500-900 nmol/L
Amoxapine	200-500 ng/mL	nd
Bupropion	25-100 ng/mL	nd
Clomipramine	80-100 ng/mL	nd
Desipramine	115-300 ng/mL	nd
Doxepin	110-250 ng/mL[3]	nd
Imipramine	225-350 ng/mL[3]	nd
Maprotiline	200-300 ng/mL	nd
Nortriptyline	50-150 ng/mL	nd
Protriptyline	70-250 ng/mL	nd
Trazodone	800-1600 ng/mL	nd
Antipsychotics Chlorpromazine	50-300 ng/mL	150-950 nmol/L
Fluphenazine	0.13-2.8 ng/mL	nd
Haloperidol	5-20 ng/mL	nd
Perphenazine	0.8-1.2 ng/mL	nd
Thiothixene	2-57 ng/mL	nd
Miscellaneous Amantadine	300 ng/mL	nd
Amrinone	3.7 mcg/mL	nd
Chloramphenicol	10-20 mcg/mL	31-62 mcmol/L
Cyclosporine[1]	250-800 ng/mL (whole blood, RIA)	nd
	50-300 ng/mL (plasma, RIA)	nd
Ethanol[2]	0 mg/dL	0 mmol/L
Hydralazine	100 ng/mL	nd
Lithium	0.6-1.2 mEq/L	0.6-1.2 mmol/L
Salicylate	100-300 mg/L	724-2172 mcmol/L
Sulfonamide	5-15 mg/dL	nd
Terbutaline	0.5-4.1 ng/mL	nd
Theophylline	10-20 mcg/mL	55-110 mcmol/L
Vancomycin		
(trough)	5-15 ng/mL	nd
(peak)	20-40 mcg/mL	nd

† The values given are generally accepted as desirable for treatment without toxicity for most patients. However, exceptions are not uncommon.

[1] 24 hour trough values   [2] Toxic: 50-100 mg/dL (10.9-21.7 mmol/L)   [3] Parent drug plus N-desmethyl metabolite

nd – No data available

Classification of Blood Pressure*			
	Reference Value		
Category	Systolic (mm Hg)		Diastolic (mm Hg)
Optimal†	< 120	and	< 80
Normal	< 130	and	< 85
High-normal	130-139	or	85-89
Hypertension‡			
Stage 1	140-159	or	90-99
Stage 2	160-179	or	100-109
Stage 3	≥ 180	or	≥ 110

Adopted from the Sixth Report of the Joint National Committee on Prevention, Detection, Evaluation, and Treatment of High Blood Pressure, National Institutes of Health

* For adults age 18 and older who are not taking antihypertensive drugs and not acutely ill. When systolic and diastolic blood pressures fall into different categories, the higher category should be selected to classify the individual's blood pressure status. In addition to classifying stages of hypertension on the basis of average blood pressure levels, clinicians should specify presence or absence of target organ disease and additional risk factors.

† Optimal blood pressure with respect to cardiovascular risk is below 120/88 mm Hg. However, unusually low readings should be evaluated for clinical significance.

‡ Based on the average of two or more readings taken at each of two or more visits after an initial screening.

GENERAL MANAGEMENT OF ACUTE OVERDOSAGE

Rapid intervention is essential to minimize morbidity and mortality in an acute toxic ingestion. Institute measures to prevent absorption and hasten elimination as soon as possible; however, symptomatic and supportive care takes precedence over other therapy. It is assumed that basic life support measures, (eg, cardiopulmonary resuscitation [CPR]) have been instituted. Specific antidotes are discussed in the overdosage section of individual or group monographs. The discussion below outlines procedures used in the management of acute overdosage of orally ingested systemic drugs.

Advanced Life Support Measures

Adequate Airway: Adequate airway must be established and maintained, generally via oropharyngeal or endotracheal airways, cricothyrotomy, or tracheostomy.

Ventilation: Ventilation may then be performed via mouth-to-mouth insufflation, hand-operated bag (ambu bag) or by mechanical ventilator.

Circulation: Circulation must be maintained.
- *Hypotension:* If hypotension/hypoperfusion occurs, place the patient in shock position (head lowered, feet elevated); specific therapy may include:
    Establish IV access and initiate IV fluids (eg, 0.9% or 0.45% Saline, Lactated Ringer's, Dextrose). A maintenance flow rate is generally 100 to 200 mL/hour; individualize as necessary.
    Plasma, plasma protein fractions, whole blood or plasma expanders may be required.
    Severe hypotension may require judicious use of cardiovascular active agents. The most commonly recommended agents are dopamine, dobutamine and norepinephrine.
- *Arrhythmia* treatment is dictated by the offending drug.
- *Hypertension,* sometimes severe, may occur. (See Nitroprusside and Diazoxide, Parenteral in the Agents for Hypertensive Emergencies section.)

Seizures: Simple isolated seizures may require only observation and supportive care. Repetitive seizures or status epilepticus require therapy. Give IV diazepam or lorazepam followed by fosphenytoin and/or phenobarbital. Pancuronium may also be considered.

Reduction of Absorption

Gastric emptying is generally recommended as soon as possible; however, this is generally not very effective unless employed within the first 1 to 2 hours after ingestion. Syrup of ipecac and gastric lavage are the two most commonly employed methods for gastric emptying.
- *Syrup of ipecac* is the method of choice outside the hospital. Do not induce vomiting if the medication is caustic or a petroleum or if the patient is in a coma or having seizures. Syrup of ipecac takes 20 to 30 minutes to work. Consider gastric lavage if response is needed immediately.
    6 months to 1 year – 10 mL
    1 year to 12 years – 15 mL
    > 12 years – 30 mL

May be followed by a glass of water. A second dose may be given if results do not occur within 20 to 30 minutes.

♦ *Gastric lavage* is indicated in the comatose patient or for those in whom syrup of ipecac fails to produce emesis. Gastric lavage is immediate and does not have a delay reaction, and is preferred over forced emesis. Airway protection via endotracheal intubation is appropriate for the patient without a gag reflex or comatose patients. Position the patient on left side, face down and use a large bore tube. Instill warm water or saline 300 to 360 mL for adults. Avoid water for infants and children; use warm saline or 5% to 6% polyethylene glycol solution. Give until lavage solution becomes clear. Add charcoal before removing the tube.

Adsorption: Adsorption, using activated charcoal alone or after completion of emesis or lavage, is indicated for virtually all significant toxic ingestions. It adsorbs a wide variety of toxins and there are no contraindications. However, it adsorbs many orally administered antidotes as well, so space dosage properly. Give an adult 50 to 100 g of activated charcoal mixed in 240 mL of water; the pediatric dose is 1 g/kg, or 25 to 50 g in 120 mL of water.

Cathartics: Cathartics increase the elimination of charcoal-poison complex. Generally using a saline or osmotic cathartic (eg, magnesium sulfate or citrate or sorbitol) with 3 mL/kg of a 35% to 75% solution of sorbitol has the most rapid effect.

Whole bowel irrigation (WBI): Whole bowel irrigation utilizes rapid administration of large volumes of lavage solutions, such as PEG. The dose is 4 to 6 L over 1 to 2 hours for adults and 0.5 L/hr for children. It may be most useful to remove iron tablets, sustained-release capsules or cocaine-containing condoms or balloons.

Elimination of Absorbed Drug

Interruption of enterohepatic circulation: Interruption of enterohepatic circulation by "gastric dialysis" uses scheduled doses of activated charcoal for 1 to 2 days. Gastric dialysis not only interrupts the enterohepatic cycle of some drugs, but also creates an osmotic gradient, drawing drug from the plasma back into the gastrointestinal lumen where it is bound by the charcoal and excreted in the feces.

Diuresis: Diuresis may be effective as identified in the individual drug monographs.

♦ *Forced diuresis* is occasionally useful. It may cause volume overload or electrolyte disturbances. Forced diuresis is useful for phenobarbital, bromides, lithium, salicylate, or amphetamines overdoses. Do not use for tricyclic antidepressants, sedative-hypnotics, or highly protein-bound medications. The most common agents employed are furosemide and osmotic diuretics with mannitol.

♦ *Alkaline diuresis* promotes elimination of weak acids (eg, barbiturates, salicylates) and is accomplished by the administration of IV sodium bicarbonate.

♦ *Acid diuresis* may be indicated in overdoses with weak bases (eg, amphetamines, fenfluramine, quinine), but use with caution in patients with renal or liver disease. It is usually accomplished with oral or IV ascorbic acid or ammonium chloride.

Dialysis: Dialysis is indicated in a minority of severe overdose cases. Drug factors that alter dialysis effectiveness include volume of distribution, drug compartmentalization, protein binding and lipid/water solubility.

♦ *Hemodialysis* may be used after an overdose and when the patient is having complications (eg, severe metabolic acidosis, electrolyte imbalances, renal failure).

♦ *Peritoneal dialysis* is even less effective than hemodialysis.

♦ *Charcoal hemoperfusion* is useful when a drug can be adsorbed by charcoal (eg, theophylline, barbiturates).

Poison Control Center:

Consultation with a regional poison control center is highly recommended.

INDEX

1/2 Halfprin, 455
3TC, 940
3TC/AZT, 957
3TC/ZDV, 957
4-Way Fast Acting Original, 387
4-Way Long Lasting Nasal, 386
8-hour Bayer Timed-Release Caplets, 455

A

A-Hydrocort, 132
A-Methapred, 132
A-Spas S/L, 669
Abacavir Sulfate, 954
Abacavir Sulfate/ Lamivudine/Zidovudine, 958
Abelcet, 848
Acarbose, 147
Accolate, 408
AccuNeb, 353
Accupril, 290
Accurbron, 365
Accutane, 1037
ACE Inhibitors, 289
Acebutolol HCl, 255
Aceon, 290
Acephen, 453
Acetaminophen, 453
Acetaminophen, Buffered, 453
Acetaminophen Uniserts, 453
Acetate and Betamethasone, 132
Acetazolamide, 347
Acetohexamide, 156
N-acetyl-p-aminophenol, 453
Acetylcholine Chloride, Intraocular, 1068
Acetylcysteine, Antidotes, 185
Respiratory Inhalants, 378
N-acetylcysteine, 378
Acetylsalicyclic Acid, 455
Achromycin V, 804
Aciphex, 682

Aclometasone Dipropionate, 1044
Aclovate, 1044
Acne Products, 1037
Acova, 82
ActHIB, 993
Actimmune, 1005
Actiq, 423
Activated Charcoal, 186
Activella, 99
Actonel, 179
Actos, 167
Acycloguanosine, 898
Acyclovir, 898
Adalat, 241
Adalat CC, 241
Adderall, 417
Adenine Arabinoside, 1084
Adenocard, 239
Adenosine, 239
Adipex-P, 420
Adlone, 132
Adprin-B, 455
Adprin-B, Extra Strength, 455
Adrenal Cortical Steroids, 132
Adrenalin Chloride, 386
Adrenalin Chloride Solution, 353
Advair Diskus, 412
Advil, 463
Advil, Children's, 463
Advil, Junior Strength, 463
Advil Liqui-Gels, 463
AeroBid, 371
AeroBid-M, 371
Aerolate, 365
Aeroseb-Dex, 1044
Aeroseb-HC, 1045
Afrin, 386
Afrin Children's Nose Drops, 386
Afrin Sinus, 386
Agenerase, 928
Agents for Active Immunization, 990
Agents for Glaucoma, 1061
Agents for Gout, 478
Agents for Impotence, 317
Agents for Migraine, 485
Aggrenox, 54
Agoral, 693

Airet, 353
AK-Chlor, 1080
AK-Dex, 1076
AK-Pred, 1076
AK-Tracin, 1080
AKBeta, 1066
Akineton, 642
AKPro, 1064
AKTob, 1080
Ala-Scalp, 1045
Alatrofloxacin Mesylate, 781
Albuterol, 353
Albuterol and Ipratropium, 381
Alconefrin, 386
Alconefrin 12, 386
Alconefrin 25, 386
Aldactone, 343
Aldara, 1053
Aldomet, 278
Alendronate, 179
Alesse, 106
Aleve, 463
Alfenta, 423
Alfentanil HCl, 423
Alka-Mints, 665
Alka-Seltzer Extra Strength with Aspirin, 455
Alka-Seltzer with Aspirin, 455
Alkets Antacid, Extra Strength, 665
Allegra, 394
Aller-Chlor, 394
Allerest 12 Hour Nasal, 386
Allergy, 394
AllerMax Allergy & Cough Formula, 394
AllerMax Caplets, 394
Allermed, 386
Allopurinol, 480
Almora, 13
Almotriptan Malate, 485
Alomide, 1079
Alora, 91
Alosetron, 503
Alpha-1-Adrenergic Blockers, 283
Alpha/Beta-Adrenergic Blocking Agents, 269
Alphagan, 1062
Alprazolam, 509

Alprostadil, 317
Alrex, 1076
Altace, 290
AlternaGEL, 665
Alu-Cap, 665
Alu-Tab, 665
Aluminum Carbonate Gel, Basic, 665
Aluminum Hydroxide Gel, 665
Alupent, 353
Alurate, 592
Amantadine HCl,
    Antiparkinson Agents, 649
    Antiviral Agents, 905
Amaryl, 156
Ambien, 585
AmBisome, 848
Amcinonide, 1044
Amen, 102
Amerge, 485
Amigesic, 455
Amikacin Sulfate, 832
Amikin, 832
Amiloride HCl, 342
Aminoglycosides,
    Oral, 840
    Parenteral, 832
Aminophylline, 364
Aminosalicylate Sodium, 878
5-aminosalicylic acid, 706
Amiodarone HCl, 233
Amitone, 665
Amitriptyline, 519
Amlodipine, 241
Amobarbital Sodium, 592
Amoxapine, 519
Amoxicillin, 719
Amoxicillin and Potassium Clavulanate, 719
Amoxil, 719
Amoxil Pediatric Drops, 719
Amphetamine Sulfate, 417
Amphetamines,
    CNS Agents, 417
    Miscellaneous Psychotherapeutics, 583
    Mixtures, 417
Amphocin, 848
Amphojel, 665
Amphotec, 848
Amphotericin B, 848
Ampicillin, 719
Ampicillin Sodium and Sulbactam Sodium, 719
Ampicillin Sodium, Parenteral, 719

Amprenavir, 928
Amyl Nitrite,
    Antianginal Agents, 205
    Antidotes, 185
Amyl Nitrite Vaporole, 205
Amytal Sodium, 592
Anacin, Aspirin Free Maximum Strength, 453
Anafranil, 519
Anaprox, 463
Ancef, 740
Androderm, 122
AndroGel 1%, 122
Androgen Hormone Inhibitor, 128
Androgens, 122
Android, 122
Anergan 50, 395
Angiomax, 84
Angiotensin II Receptor Antagonists, 298
Angiotensin-Converting Enzyme Inhibitors, 289
Anisindione, 73
Anisotropine Methylbromide, 669
Anorexiants, 420
Ansaid, 463
Antabuse, 655
Antacids, 665
Anthelmintics, 979
Anti-infectives,
    Miscellaneous, 970
    Systemic, 717
    Topical, 1052
Antialcoholic Agents, 655
Antianginal Agents, 205
Antianxiety Agents, 508
Antiarrhythmic Agents, 209
Antibiotics, Ophthalmic, 1080
Anticholinergics,
    Antiparkinson Disease Agents, 642
    Gastrointestinal, 669
    Renal/Genitourinary, 325
Anticholinesterases, Antidotes, 185
Anticoagulants, 61
Anticonvulsants, 597
Antidepressants, 518
Antidiabetic Agents, 141
Antidiabetic Combination Products, 171
Antidiarrheals, 701
Antidotes, 185
Antiemetic/Antivertigo Agents, 494

Antifungal Agents, 845
Antihist-1, 394
Antihistamines, 394
Antihyperlipidemic Agents, 302
Antihypertensives, 274
Antilirium, 185
Antineoplastics, 1087
Antiparkinson Disease Agents, 642
Antiplatelet Agents, 53
Antipsychotic Agents, 548
Antiretroviral Agents, 919
Antispasmodics, 669
Antithyroid Agents, 177
Antituberculosis Drugs, 867
Antitussives,
    Narcotic, 403
    Nonnarcotic, 405
Antivert, 498
Antivertigo/Antiemetic Agents, 494
Antiviral Agents,
    Anti-infectives, 888
    Topicals, 1084
Antizol, 185
Anusol HC-1, 1045
Anzemet, 503
APAP, 453
Apomorphine, 186
Apraclonidine HCl, 1065
Apresoline, 285
Apri, 106
Aprobarbital, 592
AquaMEPHYTON, 42
Aquaphyllin, 365
Aquatensen, 330
Ara-A, 1084
Aranesp, 49
Aredia, 179
Argatroban, 82
Aricept, 582
Aristocort,
    Systemic, 133
    Topical, 1045
Aristocort Forte, 133
Aristocort Intralesional, 133
Aristospan Intra-articular, 133
Aristospan Intralesional, 133
Armour Thyroid, 172
Aromatic Cascara Fluid Extract, 692
Artane, 642
Artane Sequels, 642
Arthritis Pain Formula, 455
Arthropan, 455
Arthrotec, 461

5-ASA, 706
ASA, 455
Asacol, 706
Ascorbic Acid, 7
Ascorbicap, 7
Ascriptin Extra Strength, 455
Ascriptin, Regular Strength, 455
Asendin, 519
Asmalix, 365
Aspergum, 455
Aspirin, 455
Aspirin and Dipyridamole, 54
Aspirin, Buffered, 455
Aspirin Free Anacin Maximum Strength, 453
Asprimox, 455
Asprimox Extra Protection for Arthritis Pain, 455
Astelin, 394
Astramorph PF, 423
Atacand, 298
Atarax,
   Antianxiety Agents, 515
   Antihistamines, 395
Atarax 100, 395
Atenolol, 255
Ativan, 509
Atorvastatin Calcium, 306
Atovaquone, 975
Atropine, Antidotes, 185
Atropine Sulfate,
   Anticholinergic/
      Antispasmodic, 669
   with Difenoxin, 701
   with Diphenoxylate, 702
Atrovent, 380
Augmented Betamethasone Dipropionate, 1044
Augmentin, 719
Avandia, 167
Avapro, 298
Avelox, 781
Aventyl HCl, 519
Aventyl HCl Pulvules, 519
Aviane, 106
Avonex, 1007
Axert, 485
Axid AR, 674
Axid Pulvules, 674
Aygestin, 102
Azactam, 775
Azatadine Maleate, 394
Azathioprine, 1012
Azelastine HCl, 394
Azidothymidine, 951
Azithromycin, 811

Azmacort, 371
Azopt, 1072
AZT, 951
Aztreonam, 775
Azulfidine,
   Antirheumatic Agents, 477
   GI, 710
Azulfidine EN-tabs,
   Antirheumatic Agents, 477
   GI, 710

B

B_{12}, 39
Bacampicillin HCl, 719
Bacitracin, 1080
Backache Maximum Strength Relief, 455
Baclofen, 637
Bacterial Vaccines, 993
Bactocill, 719
Bactrim, 970
Bactrim DS, 970
Bactrim IV, 970
Bactrim Pediatric, 970
BAL in Oil, 185
Balsalazide Disodium, 709
Banophen, 394
Banophen Caplets, 394
Banthine, 669
Basaljel, 665
Bayer Aspirin Tablets and Caplets, Genuine, 455
Bayer Aspirin Tablets and Caplets, Maximum, 455
Bayer Buffered Aspirin, 455
Bayer Children's Aspirin, 455
Bayer Enteric 500 Aspirin, Extra Strength, 455
Bayer Enteric Coated Caplets, Regular Strength, 455
Bayer Low Adult Strength, 455
Bayer Plus Caplets, Extra Strength, 455
Bayer Select Maximum Strength Backache, 455
Bayer Timed-Release Caplets, 8-hour, 455
BayGam, 985
BayHep B, 986
BayTet, 987
Beclomethasone, 371
Beclomethasone Dipropionate, 390
Beconase, 390
Beconase AQ, 390

Beepen-VK, 720
Bell/ans, 665
Belladonna, 669
Bellafoline, 669
Benadryl, 394
Benadryl Allergy, 394
Benadryl Allergy Kapseals, 394
Benadryl Allergy Ultratabs, 394
Benadryl Dye-Free Allergy, 394
Benadryl Dye-Free Allergy Liqui-Gels, 394
Benazepril HCl, 289
Bendroflumethiazide, 330
Benemid, 478
Bentyl, 669
Benylin Adult, 405
Benylin DM, 405
Benylin Pediatric, 405
Benzedrex, 386
Benzisoxazole Derivatives, 565
Benzocaine and Dextro-methorphan HBr, 407
Benzodiazepines,
   Antianxiety Agents, 509
   Sedatives and Hypnot-ics, 589
Benzonatate, 406
Benzphetamine HCl, 420
Benzthiazide, 330
Benztropine Mesylate, 642
Bepridil HCl, 241
Beta-adrenergic Blocking Agents,
   Ophthalmic, 1066
   Systemic, 255
Betagan Liquifilm, 1066
Betamethasone, 132
Betamethasone Benzoate, 1044
Betamethasone Dipropionate, 1044
Betamethasone Sodium Phosphate, 132
Betamethasone Sodium Phosphate and Ace-tate, 132
Betamethasone Valerate, 1044
Betapace, 255
Betapace AF, 255
Betaseron, 1007
Betatrex, 1044

Betaxolol HCl,
  Ophthalmic, 1066
  Systemic, 255
Betaxon, 1066
Betoptic, 1066
Betoptic S, 1066
Bextra, 464
Biaxin, 811
Biaxin XL, 811
Bicillin C-R, 720
Bicillin C-R 900/300, 720
Bicillin L-A, 720
Bile Acid Sequestrants, 304
Bimatoprost, 1074
Bio-Tab, 804
Biocef, 741
Biologic and Immunologic
  Agents, 981
Biperiden, 642
Biphasic Oral Contraceptives,
  106
Bisac-Evac, 692
Bisacodyl, 692
Bisacodyl Uniserts, 692
Bismuth Subsalicylate, 705
Bisoprolol Fumarate, 255
Bisphosphonates, 179
Bitolterol, 353
Bivalirudin, 84
Black-Draught, 693
Blocadren, 255
Bonine, 498
Bontril PDM, 420
Bontril Slow-Release, 420
Bowel Evacuants,
  Miscellaneous, 693
Brethine, 353
Bretylium Tosylate, 231
Bretylol, 231
Brevibloc, 255
Brevicon, 106
Brimonidine Tartrate, 1062
Brinzolamide, 1072
Bromo Seltzer, 453
Bromocriptine Mesylate,
  650
Bronchodilators, 353
Bronkodyl, 365
BSS, 705
Bucladin-S Softabs, 499
Buclizine HCl, 499
Budesonide,
  Corticosteroids, 371
  Glucocorticoids, 132
  Intranasal Steroids, 390
Bufferin, 455
Buffex, 455

Bulk Forming Fiber
  Laxative, 692
Bulk-Producing Laxatives,
  Miscellaneous, 693
Bumetanide, 336
Bumex, 336
Buprenex, 449
Buprenorphine HCl, 449
Bupropion HCl,
  Antidepressants, 529
  Smoking Deterrents, 660
BuSpar, 514
Buspirone HCl, 514
Butabarbital Sodium, 592
Butisol Sodium, 592

C

Cal Carb-HD, 9
Cal-Guard Softgels, 9
Cal-Plus, 9
Calan, 241
Calan SR, 241
Calci-Chew, 9
Calci-Mix, 9
Calcium, 9
Calcium Acetate, 9
Calcium Ascorbate, 7
Calcium Carbonate,
  Antacids, 665
  Minerals/Electrolytes, 9
Calcium Channel Blocking
  Agents, 241
Calcium Chloride, 9
Calcium Citrate, 9
Calcium Disodium
  Versenate, 185
Calcium Glubionate, 9
Calcium Gluceptate, 9
Calcium Gluconate, 9
Calcium Lactate, 9
Calcium Salt Combinations,
  9
Calculations, 1111
Calm-X, 500
Calphosan, 9
Calphron, 9
Caltrate 600, 9
Caltrate, Jr., 9
Cama Arthritis Pain
  Reliever, 455
Candesartan Cilexetil, 298
Cantil, 669
Capastat Sulfate, 884
Capoten, 289
Capreomycin, 884
Capsaicin, 1051
Capsin, 1051

Captopril, 289
Capzasin•P, 1051
Carafate, 668
Carbachol, Intraocular, 1068
Carbachol, Topical, 1068
Carbamazepine, 621
Carbapenem, 766
Carbastat, 1068
Carbatrol, 621
Carbenicillin Indanyl
  Sodium, 719
Carbidopa and Levodopa,
  645
Carbonic Anhydrase
  Inhibitors,
  Diuretics, 347
  Ophthalmic, 1072
Carbonyl Iron, 27
Carboptic, 1068
Cardene, 241
Cardene I.V., 241
Cardene SR, 241
Cardiac Glycosides, 197
Cardioquin, 212
Cardiovascular Agents, 195
Cardizem, 241
Cardizem CD, 241
Cardizem SR, 241
Cardura, 283
Caroid, 692
Carteolol HCl,
  Ophthalmic, 1066
  Systemic, 255
Cartrol, 255
Carvedilol, 271
Cascara Aromatic, 692
Cascara Sagrada, 692
Castor Oil, 692
Cataflam, 463
Catapres, 280
Catapres-TTS-1, 280
Catapres-TTS-2, 280
Catapres-TTS-3, 280
Cathartics, Antidotes, 186
Caverject, 317
Ceclor, 740
Ceclor CD, 740
Ceclor Pulvules, 740
Cecon, 7
Cedax, 741
Cefaclor, 740
Cefadroxil, 740
Cefadyl, 741
Cefamandole Nafate, 740
Cefazolin Sodium, 740
Cefdinir, 740
Cefditoren Pivoxil, 740
Cefepime HCl, 740

Cefixime, 740
Cefizox, 741
Cefmetazole Sodium, 740
Cefobid, 740
Cefonicid Sodium, 740
Cefoperazone Sodium, 740
Cefotan, 740
Cefotaxime Sodium, 740
Cefotetan Disodium, 740
Cefoxitin Sodium, 740
Cefpodoxime Proxetil, 740
Cefprozil, 740
Ceftazidime, 740
Ceftibuten, 741
Ceftin, 741
Ceftizoxime Sodium, 741
Ceftriaxone Sodium, 741
Cefuroxime, 741
Cefzil, 740
Celebrex, 463
Celecoxib, 463
Celestone, 132
Celestone Phosphate, 132
Celestone Soluspan, 132
Celexa, 537
CellCept, 1019
Cena-K, 15, 16
Cenafed, 386
Cenafed Syrup, 386
Cenestin, 91
Cenolate, 7
Central Analgesics, 451
Central Nervous System
    Agents, 415
Centrax, 509
Ceo-Two, 692
Cephalexin, 741
Cephalexin HCl
    Monohydrate, 741
Cephalosporins and Related
    Antibiotics, 740
Cephapirin Sodium, 741
Cephradine, 741
Cephulac, 692
Ceptaz, 740
Cerebyx, 598
Cetacort, 1045
Cetirizine HCl, 394
Ce-Vi-Sol, 7
Cevi-Bid, 7
Cevi-Fer, 27
Charcoal, Activated, 186
Chelated Magnesium, 13
Chemet, 185
Cheracol Nasal, 386
Chibroxin, 1080
Children's Advil, 463
Children's Dramamine, 500

Children's Hold, 405
Children's Motrin, 463
Children's Nostril, 386
Children's Sudafed, 386
Chlo-Amine, 394
Chlor-Trimeton Allergy 4
    Hour, 394
Chlor-Trimeton Allergy 8
    Hour, 394
Chlor-Trimeton Allergy 12
    Hour, 394
Chloramphenicol,
    Ophthalmic, 1080
    Systemic, 778
Chlordiazepoxide, 509
Chloromycetin Kapseals, 778
Chloromycetin Sodium
    Succinate, 778
Chloroptic, 1080
Chloroptic S.O.P., 1080
Chlorothiazide, 330
Chlorphed-LA, 386
Chlorpheniramine Maleate,
    394
Chlorpromazine, 494
Chlorpromazine HCl,
    Antiemetics, 494
    Antipsychotics, 553
Chlorpropamide, 156
Chlorthalidone, 330
Cholac, 692
Choledyl, 364
Choledyl SA, 364
Cholestyramine, 304
Choline Magnesium
    Trisalicylate, 455
Choline Salicylate, 455
Cholinesterase Inhibitors,
    1070
Chooz, 665
Chronulac, 692
Ciloxan, 1080
Cimetidine, 674
Cimetidine Oral Solution,
    674
Cipro, 781
Cipro IV, 781
Ciprofloxacin,
    Fluoroquinolones, 781
    Ophthalmics, 1080
Citalopram HBr, 537
Citra pH, 665
Citracal, 9
Citracal Liquitab, 9
Citrovorum Factor, 36
Citrucel, 693
Citrucel Sugar Free, 693
Claforan, 740

Clarinex, 394
Clarithromycin, 811
Claritin, 395
Claritin Reditabs, 395
Clavulanate Potassium and
    Ticarcillin, 720
Clemastine Fumarate, 394
Cleocin, 828
Cleocin Pediatric, 828
Cleocin Phosphate, 828
Clidinium Bromide, 669
Climara, 91
Clindamycin, 828
Clinoril, 464
Clobetasol Propionate, 1044
Clocortolone Pivalate, 1044
Cloderm, 1044
Clomipramine HCl, 519
Clonazepam, 605
Clonidine HCl, 280
Clopidogrel, 59
Clopra, 494
Clorazepate Dipotassium,
    Antianxiety Agents, 509
    Anticonvulsants, 605
Cloxacillin Sodium, 719
Cloxapen, 719
Clozapine, 562
Clozaril, 562
CMV-IGIV, 988
CNS Drugs, 415
Co-trimoxazole, 970
CO_2 Releasing Suppositories,
    692
Codeine,
    Analgesics, 423
    Antitussives, 403
Cogentin, 642
Cognex, 576
Colace, 692
Colazal, 709
Colchicine, 483
Colesevelam, 304
Colestid, 304
Colestipol HCl, 304
CoLyte, 699
CombiPatch, 99
Combivent, 381
Combivir, 957
Compazine,
    Antiemetics, 494
    Antipsychotics, 553
Compazine Spansules, 494
Compound S, 951
Comtan, 646
Comvax, 993
Concentrated Milk of
    Magnesia-Cascara, 693

Concerta, 571
Conjugated Estrogens,
  Oral, 91
  Parenteral, 91
  Synthetic, 91
Constilac, 692
Constulose, 692
Contraceptive Products, 106
Controlled Substances, 1108
Cordarone, 233
Cordran, 1045
Cordran SP, 1045
Coreg, 271
Corgard, 255
Correctol, 692
CortaGel, Extra Strength,
  1045
Cortaid, 1045
Cortaid, Maximum
  Strength, 1045
Cortaid with Aloe, 1045
Cortaid Faststick, Maximum
  Strength, 1045
Cortef, 132
Corticosteroids,
  Ophthalmic, 1076
  Respiratory Inhalants, 371
  Topical, 1044
Cortisol, 132
Cortisone, 132
Cortisone Acetate, 132
Cortizone•5, 1045
Cortizone•10, 1045
Cortone Acetate, 132
Cough-X, 407
Coumadin, 73
Coumarin Derivatives, 73
Covera-HS, 241
Cozaar, 298
Creo-Terpin, 405
Crinone, 102
Crixivan, 924
Cromolyn Sodium, 382
Crysti 1000, 39
Cuprimine, 322
Curretab, 102
Cutivate, 1045
Cyanide Antidote Kit, 185
Cyanocobalamin, 39
Cyanoject, 39
Cyclizine, 498
Cyclobenzaprine HCl, 635
Cyclocort, 1044
Cycloserine, 880
Cyclosporin A, 1024
Cyclosporine, 1024
Cycrin, 102
Cylert, 574

Cyproheptadine HCl, 394
Cystospaz, 669
Cystospaz-M, 669
CytoGam, 988
Cytomegalovirus Immune
  Globulin IV, Human,
  988
Cytomel, 172
Cytotec, 680
Cytovene, 891

D

d4T, 944
Dalalone, 132
Dalalone D.P., 132
Dalalone L.A., 132
Dalmane, 589
Dalteparin Sodium, 63
Danazol, 130
Danocrine, 130
Dantrium, 639
Dantrium Intravenous, 639
Dantrolene Sodium, 639
Dapa Extra Strength, 453
Daranide, 347
Darbepoetin Alfa, 49
Daricon, 669
Darvon-N, 424
Darvon Pulvules, 424
Daypro, 464
DC Softgels, 692
ddC, 947
ddI, 935
Decadron, 132
Decadron-LA, 132
Decadron Phosphate,
  Injection, 132
  Ophthalmic, 1076
Declomycin, 804
Deferoxamine Mesylate, 185
Delatestryl, 122
Delavirdine Mesylate, 964
Delestrogen, 91
Delsym, 405
Delta-Cortef, 132
Deltasone, 133
Demadex, 336
Demecarium Bromide, 1070
Demeclocycline HCl, 804
Demerol, 423
Demulen, 106
Denavir, 1052
Depacon, 615
Depakene, 615
Depakote, 615
Depakote ER, 615
Depen, 322

depGynogen, 91
depMedalone, 132
Depo-Estradiol Cypionate, 91
Depo-Medrol, 132
Depo-Provera, 120
Depo-Testosterone, 122
DepoGen, 91
L-Deprenyl, 650
Derma-Smoothe/FS, 1044
Dermacort, 1045
Dermatological Agents, 1035
Dermatop, 1045
Dermolate, 1045
Desferal Mesylate, 185
Desipramine HCl, 519
Desloratadine, 394
Desogen, 106
Desonide, 1044
DesOwen, 1044
Desoximetasone, 1044
Desoxyephedrine HCl, 417
Desoxyn, 417
Desoxyn Gradumet, 417
Desyrel, 528
Desyrel Dividose, 528
Detrol, 327
Detrol LA, 327
Dexamethasone,
  Ophthalmic, 1076
  Systemic, 132
Dexamethasone Acetate, 132
Dexamethasone Sodium
  Phosphate,
  Systemic, 132
  Topical, 1044
Dexchlorpheniramine, 394
Dexedrine, 417
Dexedrine Spansules, 417
DexFerrum, 30
Dexmethylphenidate HCl,
  569
Dexone, 132
Dextroamphetamine
  Sulfate, 417
Dextromethorphan HBr, 405
  with Benzocaine, 407
Dextrose and Theophylline,
  365
D.H.E. 45, 491
DHPG, 891
DiaBeta, 156
Diabinese, 156
Dialume, 665
Diamox, 347
Diamox Sequels, 347
Diastat, 606

Diazepam,
  Antianxiety Agents, 509
  Anticonvulsants, 606
  Skeletal Muscle Relaxants, 636
Diazepam Intensol,
  Antianxiety Agents, 509
  Anticonvulsants, 606
  Skeletal Muscle Relaxants, 636
Dibenzapine Derivatives, 562
Dicarbosil, 665
Dichlorphenamide, 347
Diclofenac, 463
Diclofenac Sodium and Misoprostol, 461
Dicloxacillin Sodium, 719
Dicumarol, 73
Dicyclomine HCl, 669
Didanosine, 935
Dideoxycytidine, 947
Dideoxyinosine, 935
Didrex, 420
Didronel, 179
Didronel IV, 179
Diethylpropion HCl, 420
Difenoxin HCl with Atropine Sulfate, 701
Diflorasone Diacetate, 1044
Diflucan, 854
Diflunisal, 459
Digibind, 185
Digitek, 197
Digoxin, 197
Digoxin Immune Fab, 185
Dihydroergotamine, 491
Dihydroergotoxine, 583
Dihydrogenated Ergot Alkaloids, 583
Dilacor XR, 241
Dilantin, 598
Dilantin-30, 598
Dilantin-125, 598
Dilantin Infatab, 598
Dilantin Kapseals, 598
Dilantin with Phenobarbital Kapseals, 598
Dilatrate-SR, 205
Dilaudid, 423
Dilaudid-HP, 423
Dilor, 364
Diltiazem HCl, 241
Dimenhydrinate, 500
Dimercaprol, 185
Dimetabs, 500
Dinate, 500
Diocto, 692

Diocto C, 693
Dioctyl Calcium Sulfosuccinate, 692
Dioctyl Sodium Sulfosuccinate, 692
Diovan, 298
Dipentum, 708
Diphen AF, 394
Diphen Cough, 394
Diphenhist, 394
Diphenhist Captabs, 394
Diphenhydramine, 499
Diphenhydramine HCl,
  Antihistamines, 394
  Antitussives, 406
Diphenoxylate HCl with Atropine Sulfate, 702
Diphenylan Sodium, 598
Diphtheria CRM_{197} Protein, 996
Dipivalyl Epinephrine, 1064
Dipivefrin HCl, 1064
Diprolene, 1044
Diprolene AF, 1044
Diprosone, 1044
Dipyridamole, 53
Dipyridamole and Aspirin, 54
Direct-Acting Miotics, 1068
Dirithromycin, 811
Disalcid, 455
Disodium Cromoglycate, 382
Disopyramide, 219
Disulfiram, 655
Ditropan, 325
Ditropan XL, 325
Diucardin, 330
Diurese, 330
Diuretics,
  Antidotes, 186
  Loop, 336
  Potassium-sparing, 341
  Thiazide, 330
Diurigen, 330
Diuril, 330
Dizac,
  Antianxiety Agents, 509
  Skeletal Muscle Relaxants, 636
Dizac Emulsified, 606
Doan's, Extra Strength, 455
Doan's, Original, 455
Docu, 692
Docusate Calcium, 692
Docusate Sodium, 692
DOK-Plus, 693
Dolanex, 453
Dolasetron, 503

Dolobid, 459
Dolophine HCl, 423
Donepezil HCl, 582
Donnamar, 669
Dopamine Receptor Agonists, Non-ergot, 652
Doral, 589
Dorcol Children's Decongestant, 386
Doryx, 804
Dorzolamide, 1072
D.O.S., 692
Doxazosin Mesylate, 283
Doxepin HCl,
  Antianxiety Agents, 517
  Antidepressants, 519
Doxidan Capsules, 693
Doxycycline, 804
Dramamine, 500
Dramamine II, 498
Dramamine, Children's, 500
Dristan 12 Hr Nasal, 386
Dristan Nasal, 387
Drixoral Cough Liquid Caps, 405
Drixoral Non-Drowsy Formula, 386
Dronabinol, 502
DSS, 692
D-S-S, 692
DSS 100 Plus, 693
Dulcolax, 692
Dull-C, 7
Duphalac, 692
Duragesic-25, 423
Duragesic-50, 423
Duragesic-75, 423
Duragesic-100, 423
Duramist Plus, 386
Duramorph, 423
Duration, 386
Duricef, 740
Dycill, 719
Dymelor, 156
Dymenate, 500
Dynabac, 811
Dynacin, 804
DynaCirc, 241
Dynapen, 719
Dyphylline, 364
Dyrenium, 345

E

E-Base, 811
E-Mycin, 811
Easprin, 455
EC-Naprosyn, 463
Echothiophate Iodide, 1070

Econopred, 1076
Econopred Plus, 1076
Ecotrin Maximum Strength Tablets and Caplets, 455
Ecotrin Tablets and Caplets, 455
ED-SPAZ, 669
Edecrin, 336
Edecrin Sodium, 336
Edetate Calcium Disodium, 185
Edetate Disodium, 185
Edex, 317
Edrophonium Cl, 185
E.E.S. 200, 811
E.E.S. 400, 811
E.E.S. Granules, 811
Efavirenz, 966
Effer-K, 15
Effexor, 532
Effexor XR, 532
Efidac/24, 386
Elavil, 519
Eldepryl, 650
Electrolytes, Oral, 9
Elixomin, 365
Elixophyllin, 365
Elocon, 1045
Eltroxin, 172
Emergency Contraceptives, 106
Emetics, Antidotes, 186
Empirin, 455
Emulsoil, 692
Enalapril, 289
Enbrel, 1009
Endocodone, 424
Endocrine and Metabolic Agents, 89
Enduron, 330
Enemas, 693
Engerix-B, 998
Enoxacin, 781
Enoxaparin Sodium, 63
Entacapone, 646
Entocort EC, 132
Enulose, 692
Ephedrine Sulfate,
  Bronchodilators, 353
  Decongestants, 386
Epifrin, 1063
Epinal, 1063
Epinephrine,
  Bronchodilators, 353
  Decongestants, 386
  Glaucoma, Agents for, 1063
Epinephrine HCl, 1063

Epitol, 621
Epivir, 940
Epivir-HBV, 940
EPO, 45
Epoetin Alfa, 45
Epogen, 45
Eprosartan Mesylate, 298
Epsom Salt, 693
Equalactin, 692
Equanil, 508
Ergoloid Mesylates, 583
Ergomar, 491
Ergotamine Derivatives, 491
Ergotamine Tartrate, 491
Ertapenem, 772
Ery-Tab, 811
Eryc, 811
EryPed, 811
EryPed 200, 811
EryPed 400, 811
EryPed Drops, 811
Erythrocin, 811
Erythrocin Stearate, 811
Erythromycin,
  Ophthalmic, 1080
  Systemic, 811
Erythromycin Estolate, 811
Erythromycin Ethylsuccinate,
  Anti-infectives, 811
  with Sulfisoxazole, 973
Erythromycin Filmtabs, 811
Erythromycin Gluceptate, 811
Erythromycin Lactobionate, 811
Erythromycin Stearate, 811
Erythropoietin, 45
Eryzole, 973
Esclim, 91
Eserine Sulfate, 1070
Esidrix, 330
Eskalith, 566
Eskalith CR, 566
Esmolol HCl, 255
Esomeprazole, 682
Estazolam, 589
Esterified Estrogens, 91
Estinyl, 91
Estra-L 40, 91
Estrace,
  Systemic, 91
  Vaginal, 98
Estraderm, 91
Estradiol Cypionate in Oil, 91
Estradiol Hemihydrate, 91
Estradiol, Oral, 91

Estradiol Transdermal System, 91
Estradiol Valerate in Oil, 91
Estratab, 91
Estring, 98
Estrogen Receptor Modulator, Selective, 100
Estrogens,
  Combined with Progestins, 99
  Systemic, 91
  Vaginal, 98
Estrone Aqueous, 91
Estropipate, 91
Estrostep 21, 106
Estrostep Fe, 106
Etanercept, 1009
Ethacrynic Acid, 336
Ethambutol HCl, 875
Ethinyl Estradiol, 91
Ethionamide, 879
Ethopropazine HCl, 642
Ethotoin, 598
Etidronate Disodium, 179
Etodolac, 463
Evac-Q-Kwik, 693
Evista, 100
ex•lax, 693
ex•lax Chocolated, 693
ex•lax Maximum Relief, 693
ex-lax Stool Softener, 692
Exelon, 578
Exna, 330
Extra Strength Adprin-B, 455
Extra Strength Alkets Antacid, 665
Extra Strength Bayer Enteric 500 Aspirin, 455
Extra Strength Bayer Plus Caplets, 455
Extra Strength CortaGel, 1045
Extra Strength Doan's, 455
Extra Strength Tums E-X, 665
Ezide, 330

F

Famciclovir, 901
Famotidine, 674
Famvir, 901
FDA Pregnancy Categories, 1107
Fe⁵⁰, 27
Feen-a-Mint, 692
Feldene, 464
Felodipine, 241

Femhrt, 99
Femiron, 27
FemPatch, 91
Fenofibrate, 312
Fenoprofen Calcium, 463
Fentanyl, 423
Fentanyl Oralet, 423
Fentanyl Transdermal
    System, 423
Fentanyl Transmucosal
    System, 423
Feosol, 27
Feostat, 27
Fer-gen-sol, 27
Fer-In-Sol, 27
Fer-Iron, 27
Feratab, 27
Fergon, 27
Fero-Grad-500, 27
Ferrex 150, 27
Ferro-Sequels, 27
Ferrous Fumarate, 27
Ferrous Gluconate, 27
Ferrous Sulfate, 27
Ferrous Sulfate Exsiccated, 27
Feverall Sprinkle Caps, 453
Fexofenadine HCl, 394
Fiber-Lax, 692
Fiberall Orange Flavor, 693
Fiberall Tropical Fruit
    Flavor, 693
FiberCon, 692
FiberNorm, 692
Finasteride, 128
FK506, 1013
Flagyl, 842
Flagyl 375, 842
Flagyl I.V., 842
Flagyl I.V. RTU, 842
Flarex, 1076
Flavoxate, 325
Flecainide Acetate, 228
Fleet, 693
Fleet Babylax, 692
Fleet Bisacodyl, 693
Fleet Laxative, 692
Fleet Mineral Oil, 693
Fleet Phospho-Soda, 693
Fleet Prep Kit 1, 693
Fleet Prep Kit 2, 693
Fleet Prep Kit 3, 693
Fletcher's Castoria, 693
Flexeril, 635
Flomax, 283
Flonase, 390
Florone, 1044
Flovent, 371
Flovent Rotadisk, 371

Floxin, 781
Fluconazole, 854
Flumadine, 913
Flumazenil, 192
Flunisolide,
    Intranasal Steroids, 390
    Respiratory Inhalants, 371
Fluocinolone Acetonide,
    1044
Fluocinonide, 1045
Fluonex, 1045
Fluor-Op, 1076
Fluorometholone, 1076
Fluoroquinolones, 781
Fluoxetine HCl, 537
Fluoxymesterone, 122
Fluphenazine, 553
Flurandrenolide, 1045
Flurazepam HCl, 589
Flurbiprofen, 463
Flurosyn, 1044
Fluticasone,
    Corticosteroids, 371
    Intranasal Steroids, 390
Fluticasone Propionate, 1045
Fluticasone Propionate/
    Salmeterol, 412
Fluvastatin, 306
Fluvoxamine Maleate, 537
FML, 1076
FML Forte, 1076
FML S.O.P., 1076
Focalin, 569
Folacin, 35
Folate, 35
Folic Acid, 35
Folic Acid Derivatives, 35
Folinic acid, 36
Folvite, 35
Fomepizole, 185
Foradil Aerolizer, 353
Formoterol Fumarate, 353
Fortaz, 740
Fortovase, 919
Fosamax, 179
Foscarnet Sodium, 888
Foscavir, 888
Fosinopril Sodium, 289
Fosphenytoin Sodium, 598
Fragmin, 63
Frova, 485
Frovatriptan Succinate, 485
FS Shampoo, 1044
Fulvicin P/G, 853
Fulvicin U/F, 853
Fungizone Intravenous, 848
Furosemide, 336

G

Gabapentin, 624
Gabitril Filmtabs, 625
Galantamine HBr, 580
Gamimune N, 983
Gamma Globulin, 985
Gammagard S/D, 983
Gammar-P I.V., 983
Ganciclovir, 891
Gantanol, 864
Gantrisin, 864
Garamycin,
    Injection, 832
    Topical, 1080
Gastrocrom, 382
Gastrointestinal Agents, 663
Gastrointestinal
    Anticholinergics/
    Antispasmodics, 669
Gastrointestinal Stimulants,
    688
Gastrosed, 669
Gatifloxacin, 781
Gemcor, 310
Gemfibrozil, 310
Gen-K, 16
Genahist, 394
Genasoft, 692
Genasoft Plus Softgels, 693
General Management of
    Acute Overdosage, 1118
Genfiber, 693
Genfiber, Orange Flavor, 693
Genitourinary Agents, 315
Genoptic, 1080
Genoptic S.O.P., 1080
Genpril, 463
Genprin, 455
Gentamicin, 832
Gentamicin Sulfate, 1080
Genuine Bayer Aspirin
    Tablets and Caplets, 455
Geocillin, 719
Geodon, 565
Gerimal, 583
GI Stimulants, 688
Glaucoma, Agents for, 1061
Glaucon, 1063
GlaucTabs, 347
Glimepiride, 156
Glipizide, 156
Glucagon, 185
Glucocorticoids, 132
Glucophage, 163
Glucophage XR, 163
Glucotrol, 156
Glucotrol XL, 156

Glucovance, 171
Glyburide, 156
Glyburide/Metformin HCl, 171
Glycerin, 692
Glycopyrrolate, 669
Glynase PresTab, 156
Glyset, 141
GoLYTELY, 699
Gout, Agents for, 478
Granisetron, 503
Grifulvin V, 853
Grisactin 250, 853
Grisactin 500, 853
Grisactin Ultra, 853
Griseofulvin, 853
Griseofulvin Microsize, 853
Griseofulvin Ultramicro-size, 853
Gris-PEG, 853
Gynogen L.A. 20, 91

H

Habitrol, 657
Haemophilus b Conjugate Vaccine, 993
Halcinonide, 1045
Halcion, 589
Haldol, 559
Haldol Decanoate 50, 559
Haldol Decanoate 100, 559
Haley's M-O, 693
Halobetasol Propionate, 1045
Halofed, 386
Halog, 1045
Halog-E, 1045
Haloperidol, 559
Halotestin, 122
Haltran, 463
Havrix, 1002
HBIG, 986
Helicobacter Pylori Agents, 713
Hemaspan, 27
Hematological Agents, 25
Hemocyte, 27
Hep-Lock, 69
Heparin, 69
Heparin Sodium, 69
Heparin Sodium and 0.09% Sodium Chloride, 69
Heparin Sodium and 0.45% Sodium Chloride, 69
Heparin Sodium and Sodium Chloride, 69
Heparin Sodium Lock Flush, 69

Hepatitis A Vaccine, Inactivated, 1002
Hepatitis B Immune Globulin, 986
Hepatitis B Vaccine, 998
Hexadrol, 132
Hexadrol Phosphate, 132
HibTITER, 993
Histamine H_2 Antagonist Combinations, 674
Histamine H_2 Antagonists, 674
Hivid, 947
HMG-CoA Reductase Inhibitors, 306
HMS, 1076
Hold, Children's, 405
Hold DM, 405
Hormones,
  Antineoplastics, 1093
  Thyroid, 172
5-HT$_3$ Receptor Antagonists, 503
Humalog, 149
Humalog Mix 50/50, 149
Humalog Mix 75/25, 149
Human Insulin Lispro with Protamine, 149
Humatin, 840
Humorsol, 1070
Humulin 50/50, 148
Humulin 70/30, 148
Humulin L, 149
Humulin N, 148
Humulin R, 148
Humulin U Ultralente, 149
Hydantoins, 598
Hydeltra-T.B.A., 132
Hydeltrasol, 132
Hydergine, 583
Hydergine LC, 583
Hydralazine HCl, 285
Hydrate, 500
Hydro-Crysti-12, 39
Hydro-Par, 330
Hydrochlorothiazide, 330
Hydrocil Instant, 693
Hydrocortisone,
  Systemic, 132
  Topicals, 1045
Hydrocortisone Acetate,
  Systemic, 132
  Topicals, 1045
Hydrocortisone Buteprate, 1045
Hydrocortisone Butyrate, 1045

Hydrocortisone Cypionate, 132
Hydrocortisone Sodium Phosphate, 132
Hydrocortisone Sodium Succinate, 132
Hydrocortisone Valerate, 1045
Hydrocortone, 132
Hydrocortone Acetate, 132
Hydrocortone Phosphate, 132
HydroDIURIL, 330
Hydroflumethiazide, 330
Hydromorphone HCl, 423
Hydromox, 330
Hydroxocobalamin,
  Antidotes, 185
  Vitamins, 39
Hydroxyprogesterone in Oil, 102
Hydroxyzine,
  Antianxiety Agents, 515
  Antihistamines, 395
Hygroton, 330
Hylutin, 102
Hyoscine HBr, 669
Hyoscyamine Sulfate, 669
L-Hyoscyamine Sulfate, 669
Hypersensitivity Reactions, Management of Acute, 1109
Hypnotics/Sedatives, Barbiturates, 592
Hypnotics/Sedatives, Nonbarbiturates, 585
Hyprogest 250, 102
Hyrexin-50, 394
Hytinic, 27
Hytone, 1045
Hytrin, 283
Hyzine-50, 515

I

Ibuprofen, 463
Icar, 27
IFLrA, 1095
IFN-alpha 2, 1098
IG, 985
IGIV, 983
Iletin II Regular, 148
Iletin II U-500, Regular (Concentrated), 155
Ilosone, 811
Ilosone Pulvules, 811
Ilotycin, 1080
Ilotycin Gluceptate, 811

Imdur, 205
Imipenem-Cilastatin, 768
Imipramine HCl, 519
Imipramine Pamoate, 519
Imiquimod, 1053
Imitrex, 485
Immune Globulin
    Intramuscular, 985
Immune Globulin
    Intravenous, 983
Immune Serums, 983
Immunization, Agents for,
    990
Immunologic and Biologic
    Agents, 981
Immunomodulators,
    Injection, 1032
    Topical, 1053
Immunosuppressive Drugs,
    1012
Imodium, 703
Imodium A-D, 703
Imodium A-D Caplets, 703
Impotence, Agents for,
    317
Imuran, 1012
Indandione Derivatives, 73
Indapamide, 330
Inderal, 255
Inderal LA, 255
Indinavir Sulfate, 924
Indocin, 463
Indocin SR, 463
Indomethacin, 463
Infants' Motrin, 463
InFeD, 30
Inflamase Forte, 1076
Inflamase Mild, 1076
Infumorph 200, 423
INH, 869
Innohep, 63
Insulin, 148
Insulin Analog Injection,
    149
Insulin Combined with
    Protamine and Zinc,
    148
Insulin Glargine, 149
Insulin Injection, 148
Insulin Injection
    Concentrated, 155
Insulin Lispro (Human)
    with Protamine, 149
Insulin Zinc Suspension,
    149
Insulin Zinc Suspension,
    Extended, 149
Intal, 382

α-2-Interferon, 1098
Interferon alfa-2a, 1095
Interferon alfa-2b, 1098
Interferon alfa-2b,
    Recombinant and
    Ribavirin Combination,
    1102
Interferon beta, 1007
Interferon beta-1a, 1007
Interferon beta-1b, 1007
Interferon gamma-1B, 1005
Intranasal Steroids, 390
Intron A, 1098
Invanz, 772
Invirase, 919
Ionamin, 420
Iopidine, 1065
Iosopan, 665
Ipecac, Syrup of, 186
Ipratropium Bromide, 380
Ipratropium Bromide and
    Albuterol Sulfate, 381
Irbesartan, 298
Ircon, 27
Iron-Containing Products,
    Oral, 27
Iron-Containing Products,
    Parenteral, 30
Iron Dextran, 30
Iron Sucrose, 33
Iron with Vitamin C, 27
Irospan, 27
ISG, 985
ISMO, 205
Isocarboxazid, 545
Isocom, 493
Isoetharine HCl, 353
Isometheptene
    Mucate/Dichloral-
    Phenazone/Acetam-
    inophen, 493
Isoniazid, 869
Isonicotinic Acid Hydrazide,
    869
Isopap, 493
Isophane Insulin Suspension,
    148
Isophane Insulin
    Suspension and Insulin
    Injection, 148
Isoproterenol, 353
Isoptin, 241
Isoptin SR, 241
Isopto Carbachol, 1068
Isopto Carpine, 1068
Isordil, 205
Isordil Tembids, 205
Isordil Titradose, 205

Isosorbide Dinitrate (Oral),
    205
Isosorbide Dinitrate
    (Sublingual and
    Chewable), 205
Isosorbide Mononitrate
    (Oral), 205
Isotretinoin, 1037
Isradipine, 241
Isuprel, 353
Itraconazole, 857
Iveegam, 983

J

Jenest-28, 106
Junior Strength Advil, 463
Junior Strength Motrin, 463
Junior Strength Panadol,
    453

K

K + Care, 16
K + Care ET, 15
K-Dur 10, 15
K-Dur 20, 15
K-G Elixir, 16
K-Lease, 15
K-Lor, 16
K•Lyte, 15
K•Lyte/Cl, 15, 16
K•Lyte/Cl 50, 15
K•Lyte DS, 15
K-Norm, 15
K-Tab, 15
K_1, 42
Kadian, 423
Kaletra, 930
Kanamycin Sulfate,
    Injection, 832
    Oral, 840
Kantrex,
    Injection, 832
    Oral, 840
Kaochlor 10%, 15
Kaochlor S-F, 15
Kaon, 16
Kaon-Cl, 15
Kaon Cl-10, 15
Kaon-Cl 20%, 16
Kaopectate II Caplets, 703
Kay Ciel, 15, 16
Keflex, 741
Keftab, 741
Kefurox, 741
Kefzol, 740
Kemadrin, 642
Kenalog, 1045

Kenalog-10, 133
Kenalog-40, 133
Keppra, 611
Kerlone, 255
Kestrone 5, 91
Ketoconazole, 846
Ketoprofen, 463
Ketorolac Tromethamine, 463
Key-Pred 25, 132
Key-Pred 50, 132
Klonopin, 605
Klor-Con, 16
Klor-Con 8, 15
Klor-Con 10, 15
Klor-Con/EF, 15
Klorvess, 15
Klorvess Effervescent Granules, 16
Klotrix, 15
Kolyum, 16
Konakion, 42
Kondremul Plain, 692
Konsyl, 693
Konsyl-D, 693
Konsyl Easy Mix Formula, 693
Konsyl Fiber, 692
Konsyl-Orange, 693
Kytril, 503

L

LA-12, 39
Labetalol HCl, 269
Laboratory Values, Normal, 1112
Lactulose, 692
Lamictal, 607
Lamictal Chewable Dispersible Tablets, 607
Lamisil, 862
Lamivudine, 940
Lamivudine/Zidovudine, 957
Lamotrigine, 607
Lanacort-5, 1045
Lanacort 10, Maximum Strength, 1045
Lanophyllin, 365
Lanoxicaps, 197
Lanoxin, 197
Lansoprazole, 682
Lantus, 149
Lasix, 336
Latanoprost, 1074
Laxative Combinations, 693
Laxatives, 692
Lente, 149

Lente Iletin II, 149
Lepirudin, 78
Lescol, 306
Lescol XL, 306
Leucovorin Calcium, Antidotes, 185
Folic Acid Derivative, 36
Leukotriene Receptor Inhibitors, 408
Levalbuterol HCl, 353
Levaquin, 781
Levatol, 255
Levbid, 669
Levetiracetam, 611
Levlen, 106
Levlite, 106
Levo-Dromoran, 423
Levo-T, 172
Levobetaxolol HCl, 1066
Levobunolol HCl, 1066
Levocabastine HCl, 1079
Levodopa and Carbidopa, 645
Levofloxacin,
Fluoroquinolones, 781
Ophthalmic, 1080
Levomethadyl Acetate HCl, 423
Levonorgestrel Implant Contraceptive System, 117
Levonorgestrel Implants, 117
Levora, 106
Levorotatory Alkaloids of Belladonna, 669
Levorphanol Tartrate, 423
Levothroid, 172
Levothyroxine Sodium, 172
Levoxine, 172
Levoxyl, 172
Levsin, 669
Levsin Drops, 669
Levsin/SL, 669
Levsinex Timecaps, 669
Libritabs, 509
Librium, 509
Lidex, 1045
Lidocaine HCl, 222
LidoPen Auto-Injector, 222
Lincocin, 828
Lincomycin, 828
Lincorex, 828
Lincosamides, 828
Linezolid, 825
Lioresal, 637
Liothyronine Sodium, 172
Liotrix, 172

Lipase Inhibitors, 686
Lipitor, 306
Liquaemin Sodium, 69
Liquaemin Sodium Preservative Free, 69
Liqui-Doss, 693
Liquid PedvaxHIB, 993
Liquid Pred, 133
Liquiprin Infants' Drops, 453
Lisinopril, 289
Lithane, 566
Lithium, 566
Lithium Carbonate, 566
Lithobid, 566
Lithonate, 566
Lithotabs, 566
Livostin, 1079
Lo/Ovral, 106
LoCHOLEST, 304
LoCHOLEST Light, 304
Locoid, 1045
Lodine, 463
Lodine XL, 463
Lodoxamide Tromethamine, 1079
Loestrin, 106
Logen, 702
Lomefloxacin HCl, 781
Lomotil, 702
Loniten, 287
Lonox, 702
Loop Diuretics, 336
Loperamide HCl, 703
Lopid, 310
Lopinavir/Ritonavir, 930
Lopressor, 255
Lorabid, 741
Loracarbef, 741
Loratadine, 395
Lorazepam, 509
Lorazepam Intensol, 509
Losartan Potassium, 298
Lotemax, 1076
Lotensin, 289
Loteprednol Etabonate, 1076
Lotronex, 503
Lovastatin, 306
Lovenox, 63
Low Molecular Weight Heparins, 63
Low-Ogestrel, 106
Loxapine, 562
Loxitane, 562
Loxitane C, 562
Loxitane IM, 562
Lozol, 330
Lufyllin, 364
Lumigan, 1074

Luminal Sodium, 592
Luvox, 537

M

M-oxy, 424
Maalox Antacid Caplets, 665
Maalox Anti-Diarrheal Caplets, 703
Macrolides, 811
Mag-200, 13
Mag-Ox 400,
  Antacids, 665
  Minerals and Electrolytes, 13
Mag-Tab SR, 13
Magaldrate, 665
Magan, 455
Magnaprin, 455
Magnesia, 665
Magnesium, 13
Magnesium Citrate Solution, 693
Magnesium Hydroxide, 665
Magnesium Oxide, 665
Magnesium Salicylate, 455
Magnesium Sulfate, 630
Magonate, 13
Magtrate, 13
Mallamint, 665
Maltsupex, 693, 694
Management of Acute Hypersensitivity Reactions, 1109
Management of Acute Overdosage, General, 1118
Mandol, 740
MAOIs, see Monoamine Oxidase Inhibitors
Maox 420, 665
Maprotiline, 525
Marcillin, 719
Marezine, 498
Marinol, 502
Marplan, 545
Marthritic, 455
Mavik, 290
Maxair Autohaler, 353
Maxair Inhaler, 353
Maxalt, 485
Maxalt-MLT, 485
Maxaquin, 781
Maxidex, 1076
Maxiflor, 1044
Maximum Bayer Aspirin Tablets and Caplets, 455
Maximum Relief ex•lax, 693

Maximum Strength Cortaid, 1045
Maximum Strength Cortaid Faststick, 1045
Maximum Strength Lanacort 10, 1045
Maximum Strength Midol, 463
Maxipime, 740
Maxivate, 1044
Maxolon,
  Antiemetic/Antivertigo Agents, 494
  GI Stimulants, 688
Mebaral, 592
Meclizine, 498
Meclofenamate Sodium, 463
Medrol, 132
Medroxyprogesterone, 102
Medroxyprogesterone Acetate, 120
Medroxyprogesterone Contraceptive Injection, 120
Medrysone, 1076
Mefenamic Acid, 463
Mefoxin, 740
Megace, 102
Megestrol Acetate, 102
Melfiat-105 Unicelles, 420
Mellaril, 553
Mellaril-S, 553
Meloxicam, 463
Menadol, 463
Menest, 91
Meni-D, 498
Mepenzolate Bromide, 669
Meperidine HCl, 423
Mephenytoin, 598
Mephobarbital, 592
Mephyton, 42
Meprobamate, 508
Mepron, 975
Meridia, 420
Meropenem, 766
Merrem IV, 766
Mesalamine, 706
Mesantoin, 598
Mesoridazine, 553
Mestinon, 185
Metabolic Agents, 89
Metadate CD, 571
Metadate ER, 571
Metahydrin, 330
Metamucil, 693
Metamucil Orange Flavor, 693
Metamucil Sugar Free, 693

Metaproterenol, 353
Metformin HCl, 163
Metformin HCl/Glyburide, 171
Methadone HCl, 423
Methadone HCl Diskets, 423
Methadone HCl Intensol, 423
Methadose, 423
Methamphetamine HCl, 417
Methantheline Bromide, 669
Methazolamide, 347
Methimazole, 177
Methitest, 122
Methscopolamine Bromide, 669
Methyclothiazide, 330
Methyldopa, 278
Methyldopate HCl, 278
Methylene Blue, 185
Methylin, 571
Methylin ER, 571
Methylphenidate HCl, 571
Methylphytyl Naphthoquinone, 42
Methylprednisolone, 132
Methylprednisolone Acetate, 132
Methylprednisolone Sodium Succinate, 132
Methyltestosterone, 122
Methysergide Maleate, 490
Meticorten, 133
Metipranolol HCl, 1066
Metoclopramide,
  Antiemetic/Antivertigo Agents, 494
  GI Stimulants, 688
Metoclopramide Intensol,
  Antiemetic/Antivertigo Agents, 494
  GI Stimulants, 688
Metolazone, 330
Metoprolol, 255
Metronidazole, 842
Mevacor, 306
Mezlin, 719
Mezlocillin Sodium, 719
Mibefradil, 241
Micardis, 298
Miconazole, 845
Micro-K 10 Extencaps, 15
Micro-K Extencaps, 15
Micro-K LS, 16
Microgestin Fe, 106
Micronase, 156
microNefrin, 353

Micronor, 106
Midamor, 342
Midchlor, 493
Midol, Maximum Strength, 463
Midrin, 493
Miglitol, 141
Migraine, Agents for, 485
Migraine Combinations, 493
Migratine, 493
Milk of Magnesia, 693
Milk of Magnesia, Concentrated, 693
Miltown, 508
Mineral Oil, 692
Minerals, Oral, 9
Minipress, 283
Minocin, 804
Minocin IV, 804
Minocycline, 804
Minoxidil, 287
Miochol-E, 1068
Miostat, 1068
Miotics,
  Cholinesterase Inhibitors, 1070
  Direct-Acting, 1068
Miradon, 73
MiraLax, 700
Mirapex, 652
Mircette, 106
Mirtazapine, 525
Misoprostol, 680
Misoprostol and Diclofenac Sodium, 461
Mitrolan, 692
Moban, 561
Mobic, 463
Mobidin, 455
Modane, 692
Modane Bulk, 693
Modane Soft, 692
Modicon, 106
Modified Iron Products, 27
Moexipril HCl, 290
Molindone HCl, 561
Mometasone Furoate,
  Corticosteroids, 1045
  Intranasal Steroids, 390
Monistat i.v., 845
Monoamine Oxidase Inhibitors, 545
Monobactams, 775
Monocid, 740
Monodox, 804
Monoket, 205

Monophasic Oral Contraceptives, 106
Monopril, 289
Montelukast Sodium, 410
Morphine Sulfate, 423
Motofen, 701
Motrin, 463
Motrin, Children's, 463
Motrin IB, 463
Motrin, Junior Strength, 463
Mouth/Throat Products, 715
Moxifloxacin, 781
MS Contin, 423
MSIR, 423
Mucomyst,
  Antidotes, 185
  Respiratory Inhalants, 378
Mucosil-10, 378
Mucosol, 185
Muromonab-CD3, 1029
Muse, 317
Myambutol, 875
Myci-Spray, 387
Mycifradin, 840
Mycobutin, 873
Mycophenolate Mofetil, 1019
Mycostatin, 845
Mykrox, 330
Mylanta, 665
Mysoline, 613

N

Na Nitrite, 185
Na Thiosulfate, 185
Nabi-HB, 986
Nabumetone, 463
Nadolol, 255
Nafcillin Sodium, 719
Nalbuphine HCl, 447
Nalfon Pulvules, 463
Nallpen, 719
Nalmefene HCl, 186
Naloxone HCl, 189
Naltrexone HCl, 190
Naphazoline, 386
Naprelan, 464
Naprosyn, 463, 464
Naproxen, 463, 464
Naqua, 330
Naratriptan, 485
Narcan, 189
Narcotic Agonist Analgesics, 423

Narcotic Agonist-Antagonist Analgesics, 445
Narcotic Antagonists, Antidotes, 185
Narcotic Antitussives, 403
Nardil, 545
Nasacort, 390
Nasacort AQ, 390
Nasal Decongestant Combinations, 387
Nasal Decongestant Inhalers, 386
Nasal Decongestants, 386
Nasalcrom, 382
Nasalide, 390
Nasarel, 390
Natacyn, 1082
Natamycin, 1082
Nateglinide, 145
Natural Fiber Laxative, 693
Nature's Remedy, 693
Nature's Remedy Tablets, 693
Naturetin, 330
Navane, 554
Naxonex, 390
Nebcin, 832
Nebcin Pediatric, 832
NebuPent, 973
Necon, 106
Necon 10/11, 106
Nedocromil Sodium, 384
Nefazodone HCl, 535
Nelfinavir Mesylate, 926
Nembutal Sodium, 592
Neo-Calglucon, 9
Neo-Fradin, 840
Neo-Synephrine, 386
Neo-Tabs, 840
Neoloid, 692
Neomycin Sulfate, 840
Neopap, 453
Neoral, 1024
Neostigmine, 185
Nephro-Fer, 27
Nephron, 353
Neptazane, 347
Netilmicin Sulfate, 832
Netromycin, 832
Neurontin, 624
Neut, 22
Neutrexin, 977
Nevirapine, 962
Nexium, 682
Nicardipine HCl, 241
N'ice Vitamin C Drops, 7
Nicoderm CQ, 657
Nicorette, 657

Nicotine, 657
Nicotine Inhalation System, 657
Nicotine Nasal Spray, 657
Nicotine Polacrilex, 657
Nicotine Transdermal, 657
Nicotrol, 657
Nicotrol Inhaler, 657
Nicotrol NS, 657
Nifedipine, 241
Niferex, 27
Niferex-150, 27
Nighttime Sleep Aid, 394
Nimodipine, 241
Nimotop, 241
Nisoldipine, 241
Nitrates, 205
Nitro-Dur, 205
Nitro-Time, 205
Nitrogard, 205
Nitroglycerin (IV), 205
Nitroglycerin (Sublingual), 205
Nitroglycerin (Sustained Release), 205
Nitroglycerin (Topical), 205
Nitroglycerin Transdermal Systems, 205
Nitroglycerin (Translingual), 205
Nitroglycerin (Transmucosal), 205
Nitroglyn, 205
Nitrol, 205
Nitrolingual, 205
Nitrong, 205
NitroQuick, 205
Nitrostat, 205
Nizatidine, 674
Nizoral, 846
No-Hist, 386
No Pain-HP, 1051
Nolahist, 395
Nolvadex, 1093
Non-Habit Forming Stool Softener, 692
Nonnarcotic Analgesic Combinations, 461
Nonnarcotic Antitussives, 405
Nonsteroidal Anti-inflammatory Agents, 463
Nor-QD, 106
Nordette, 106

Norelgestromin/Ethinyl Estradiol Transdermal System, 106
Norethindrone Acetate, 102
Norfloxacin,
   Ophthalmic, 1080
   Systemic, 781
Norinyl, 106
Normal Laboratory Values, 1112
Normodyne, 269
Norpace, 219
Norpace CR, 219
Norplant System, 117
Norpramin, 519
Norrel, 106
Nortriptyline HCl, 519
Norvasc, 241
Norvir, 921
Norwich Extra-Strength, 455
Norzine, 494
Nostril, 386
Nostril, Children's, 386
Nostrilla, 386
Novafed, 386
Novolin 70/30, 148
Novolin 70/30 PenFill, 148
Novolin 70/30 Prefilled, 148
Novolin L, 149
Novolin N, 148
Novolin N PenFill, 148
Novolin N Prefilled, 148
Novolin R, 148
Novolin R PenFill, 148
Novolin R Prefilled, 148
Novolog, 149
NPH Iletin II, 148
NPH Insulin, 148
NSAIDs, see Nonsteroidal Anti-inflammatory Agents
NTZ Long Acting Nasal, 386
Nu-Iron, 27
Nu-Iron 150, 27
Nubain, 447
NuLytely, 699
Numorphan, 424
Nuprin, 463
Nutrients and Nutritional Agents, 1
Nutritional therapy, 20
Nydrazid, 869
Nystatin, oral, 845

Octamide, 494
Octamide PFS,
   Antiemetic/Antivertigo Agents, 494
   GI Stimulants, 688
Ocuflox, 1080
Ocupress, 1066
Ocusert Pilo-20, 1068
Ocusert Pilo-40, 1068
Ofloxacin,
   Fluoroquinolones, 781
   Ophthalmic, 1080
Ogen,
   Systemic, 91
   Vaginal, 98
Ogestrel, 106
Olanzapine, 562
Olsalazine Sodium, 708
Omeprazole, 682
Omnicef, 740
Omnipen, 719
Omnipen-N, 719
Ondansetron, 503
One A Day Extras Vitamin C, 7
Ophthalmic/Otic Agents, 1057
Ophthalmics, Topical, 1059
Opium, 424
Opium Tincture, Deodorized, 424
Optimine, 394
OptiPranolol, 1066
Oral Contraceptives, 106
Oramorph SR, 423
Orap, 559
Oraphen-PD, 453
Orasone, 133
Oretic, 330
Original Doan's, 455
Orinase, 156
ORLAAM, 423
Orlistat, 686
Ormazine, 494
Ortho-Cept, 106
Ortho-Cyclen, 106
Ortho Dienestrol, 98
Ortho-Est, 91
Ortho Evra, 106
Ortho-Novum, 106
Ortho-Novum 10/11, 106
Ortho-Novum 777, 106
Ortho-Prefest, 99
Ortho Tri-Cyclen, 106
Orthoclone OKT3, 1029
Orudis, 463
Orudis KT, 463
Oruvail, 463

O

OCL, 699

Os-Cal 500, 9
Oseltamivir Phosphate, 916
Osmotic Diuretics, 186
Otic Agents, 1057
Otrivin, 386
Otrivin Pediatric Nasal
    Drops, 386
Ovcon, 106
Overdosage, General
    Management of
    Acute, 1118
Ovral, 106
Ovrette, 106
Oxacillin Sodium, 719
Oxacillin Sodium,
    Parenteral, 719
Oxalodinones, 825
Oxaprozin, 464
Oxazepam, 509
Oxcarbazepine, 631
Oxtriphylline, 364
Oxybutynin Chloride, 325
Oxycodone HCl, 424
OxyContin, 424
Oxydose, 424
OxyFAST, 424
OxyIR, 424
Oxymetazoline, 386
Oxymorphone HCl, 424
Oxyphencyclimine HCl, 669
Oxytetracycline, 804
Oyster Shell Calcium-500, 9

P

Pacerone, 233
Pamelor, 519
Pamidronate Disodium, 179
Pamine, 669
Panadol, Junior Strength,
    453
Pandel, 1045
Panglobulin, 983
Pantoprazole, 682
Para-aminosalicylate Sodium,
    878
Paregoric, 424
Parkinson's Disease Agents,
    642
Parlodel, 650
Parlodel SnapTabs, 650
Parnate, 545
Paromomycin Sulfate, 840
Paroxetine HCl, 537
Parsidol, 642
Paser, 878
Pathilon, 669
Pathocil, 719

Paxil, 537
PBZ, 395
PBZ-SR, 395
PCE Dispertab, 811
PediaCare Fever, 463
PediaCare Infants'
    Decongestant, 386
Pediapred, 132
Pediatric Advil Drops, 463
Pediatric Triban, 501
Pediazole, 973
PEG, 700
PEG-ES, 699
PEG-Intron, 1032
Peganone, 598
Peginterferon alfa-2B, 1032
PemADD, 574
PemADD CT, 574
Pemoline, 574
Pen•Vee K, 720
Penbutolol Sulfate, 255
Penciclovir, 1052
Penecort, 1045
Penetrex, 781
Penicillamine, 322
Penicillin G (Aqueous),
    720
Penicillin G Benzathine,
    Intramuscular, 720
Penicillin G Benzathine
    and Procaine
    Combined,
    Intramuscular, 720
Penicillin G Potassium, 720
Penicillin G Procaine,
    Intramuscular, 720
Penicillin G Sodium, 720
Penicillin V, 720
Penicillins, 719
Pentacarinat, 973
Pentam 300, 973
Pentamidine Isethionate, 973
Pentasa, 706
Pentazocine, 445
Pentazocine Combinations,
    447
Pentobarbital Sodium, 592
Pepcid, 674
Pepcid AC, 674
Pepcid AC Acid Controller,
    674
Pepcid Complete, 674
Pepcid RPD, 674
Pepto-Bismol, 705
Pepto Diarrhea Control, 703
Percolone, 424
Perdiem Overnight Relief,
    693

Pergolide Mesylate, 651
Peri-Colace, 693
Peri-Dos Softgels, 693
Periactin, 394
Perindopril Erbumine, 290
Peritoneal Dialysis
    Solutions, 186
Permapen, 720
Permax, 651
Permitil, 553
Perphenazine,
    Antiemetic/Antivertigo
    Agents, 494
    Antipsychotics, 553
Persantine, 53
Pertussin CS, 405
Pertussin ES, 405
Pfizerpen, 720
PGE₁, 317
Phendimetrazine Tartrate,
    420
Phenelzine, 545
Phenergan, 395
Phenergan Fortis, 395
Phenergan Plain, 395
Phenindamine Tartrate, 395
Phenobarbital, 592
Phenothiazine Derivatives,
    553
Phenoxymethyl Penicillin,
    720
Phentermine HCl, 420
Phenylbutylpiperadine
    Derivatives, 559
Phenylephrine, 386
Phenytoin, Oral, 598
Phenytoin Sodium,
    Extended, 598
Phenytoin Sodium, Oral,
    Prompt, 598
Phenytoin Sodium,
    Parenteral, 598
Phenytoin Sodium with
    Phenobarbital, 598
Phillips' Chewable, 665
Phillips' Liqui-Gels, 692
Phillips' Milk of Magnesia,
    Antacids, 665
    Laxatives, 693
Phillips' Milk of Magnesia,
    Concentrated,
    Antacids, 665
    Laxatives, 693
PhosLo, 9
Pholine Iodide, 1070
Phosphonoformic Acid, 888
Phyllocontin, 364
Phylloquinone, 42

Physostigmine, 1070
Physostigmine Salicylate, 185
Phytonadione, 42
Pilagan, 1068
Pilocar, 1068
Pilocarpine HCl,
   Mouth/Throat
      Preparations, 715
   Ophthalmic, 1068
Pilocarpine Nitrate, 1068
Pilocarpine Ocular
   Therapeutic System,
   1068
Pilopine HS, 1068
Pimozide, 559
Pindolol, 255
Pioglitazone HCl, 167
Piperacillin Sodium, 720
Piperacillin Sodium and
   Tazobactam Sodium, 720
Pipracil, 720
Pirbuterol, 353
Piroxicam, 464
Plan B, 106
Plavix, 59
Plendil, 241
PMPA, 933
Pneumococcal 7-Valent
   Conjugate Vaccine, 996
Polaramine, 394
Polaramine Repetabs, 394
Polycarbophil, 692
Polyethylene
   Glycol-Electrolyte
      Solution, 699
Polyethylene Glycol
   Solution, 700
Polygam S/D, 983
Polymyxin B Sulfate, 1080
Polymyxin B Sulfate Ster-
   ile, 1080
Polysaccharide-Iron
   Complex, 27
Polythiazide, 330
Ponstel, 463
Posicor, 241
Posture, 9
Potassium Acetate, 16
Potassium Chloride
   Concentrate, 16
Potassium Clavulanate and
   Amoxicillin, 719
Potassium Replacement
   Products, 15
Potassium-Sparing Diuretics,
   341
Pralidoxime Cl, 185

Pramipexole, 652
Prandin, 142
Pravachol, 306
Pravastatin Sodium, 306
Prazepam, 509
Prazosin, 283
Precose, 147
Pred Forte, 1076
Pred Mild, 1076
Prednicarbate, 1045
Prednisolone,
   Ophthalmic, 1076
   Systemic, 132
Prednisolone Acetate,
   Ophthalmic, 1076
   Systemic, 132
Prednisolone Sodium
   Phosphate, 132
Prednisolone Tebutate, 132
Prednisone, 133
Pregnancy Categories,
   FDA, 1107
Prelone, 132
Prelu-2, 420
Premarin,
   Systemic, 91
   Vaginal, 98
Premarin Intravenous, 91
Premphase, 99
Prempro, 99
Pretz-D, 386
Prevacid, 682
Prevalite, 304
Preven, 106
Prevnar, 996
Priftin, 886
Prilosec, 682
Primatene Mist, 353
Primaxin I.M., 768
Primaxin I.V., 768
Primidone, 613
Principen, 719
Prinivil, 289
Privine, 386
Pro-Banthine, 669
Pro-Fast HS, 420
Pro-Fast SA, 420
Pro-Fast SR, 420
Probalan, 478
Probenecid, 478
Procainamide, 215
Procaine, Combined with
   Penicillin, 720
Procan SR, 215
Procardia, 241
Procardia XL, 241

Prochlorperazine,
   Antiemetic/Antivertigo
      Agents, 494
   Antipsychotic Agents, 553
Procort, 1045
Procrit, 45
Procyclidine, 642
Progesterone Gel, 102
Progesterone in Oil, 102
Progesterone Powder, 102
Progestin-only Products
   (Contraceptive
      Products), 106
Progestins, 102
Progestins and Estrogens,
   Combined, 99
Prograf, 1013
Prolixin, 553
Prolixin Decanoate, 553
Promazine HCl, 553
Promethazine HCl, 395
Pronestyl, 215
Pronestyl-SR, 215
Propafenone HCl, 226
Propantheline Bromide, 669
Propecia, 128
Propine, 1064
Propoxyphene HCl, 424
Propoxyphene Napsylate, 424
Propranolol, 255
Propranolol Intensol, 255
Propylthiouracil, 177
Proscar, 128
ProSom, 589
Prostaglandin Agonists, 1074
Prostaglandin E_1, 317
Prostaglandins, 680
Prostigmin, 185
Protamine Sulfate, 185
Proton Pump Inhibitors, 682
Protonix, 682
Protonix I.V., 682
Protopam, 185
Protopic, 1054
Protriptyline HCl, 519
Proventil, 353
Proventil Repetabs, 353
Provera, 102
Prozac, 537
Prozac Weekly, 537
Pseudoephedrine HCl, 386
Pseudoephedrine Sulfate,
   386
Psorcon, 1044
Psychotherapeutic Agents,
   Miscellaneous, 569
Psyllium, 693
Pteroylglutamic Acid, 35

Pulmicort Respules, 371
Pulmicort Turbuhaler, 371
Purge, 692
Pyrazinamide, 876
Pyridostigmine Br, 185

Q

Quarzan, 669
Quazepam, 589
Questran, 304
Questran Light, 304
Quetiapine Fumarate, 562
Quibron-T Dividose, 365
Quibron-T/SR, 365
Quiess, 515
Quinaglute Dura-Tabs, 212
Quinapril HCl, 290
Quinethazone, 330
Quinidex Extentabs, 212
Quinidine, 212
Quinidine Gluconate, 212
Quinidine
    Polygalacturonate, 212
Quinidine Sulfate, 212
Quinora, 212
Quixin, 1080
QVAR, 371

R

R-Gel, 1051
Rabeprazole, 682
Racemic Amphetamine
    Sulfate, 417
Raloxifene, 100
Ramipril, 290
Ranitidine, 674
Rapamune, 1016
Rebetol, 908
Rebetron, 1102
Reclomide, 494
Recombinant Human
    Erythropoietin, 45
Recombivax HB, 998
Recommended Dietary
    Allowances of Vitamins
    and Minerals, 3
Refludan, 78
Reglan,
    Antiemetic/Antivertigo
    Agents, 494
    GI Stimulants, 688
Regonol, 185
Regular (Concentrated)
    Iletin II U-500, 155
Regular Strength Ascriptin,
    455

Regular Strength Bayer
    Enteric Coated Caplets,
    455
Regulax SS, 692
Reguloid, 693
Reguloid, Orange, 693
Reguloid, Sugar Free
    Orange, 693
Relafen, 463
Relenza, 915
Reliable Gentle Laxative, 692
Remeron, 525
Remeron SolTab, 525
Remifentanil HCl, 424
Reminyl, 580
Renal and Genitourinary
    Agents, 315
Renese, 330
Renova, 1049
Repaglinide, 142
Requip, 652
Rescriptor, 964
Rescula, 1074
Respbid, 365
Respiratory Agents, 351
Respiratory Inhalant
    Combinations, 412
Respiratory Inhalant
    Products, 371
Restoril, 589
Retin-A, 1049
13-cis-Retinoic Acid, 1037
Retrovir, 951
Revex, 186
ReVia, 190
Rexolate, 455
Rhinall, 386
Rhinocort, 390
Rhinocort Aqua, 390
Ribavirin, 908
Ridenol, 453
Rifabutin, 873
Rifadin, 871
Rifampin, 871
Rifapentine, 886
rIFN-A, 1095
rIFN-α2, 1098
Rimactane, 871
Rimantadine HCl, 913
Rimexolone, 1076
Riopan, 665
Risedronate Sodium, 179
Risperdal, 565
Risperidone, 565
Ritalin, 571
Ritalin-SR, 571
Ritonavir, 921
Ritonavir/Lopinavir, 930

Rivastigmine, 578
Rizatriptan Benzoate, 485
RMS, 423
Robinul, 669
Robitussin Cough Calmers,
    405
Robitussin Pediatric, 405
Rocephin, 741
Rofecoxib, 464
Roferon-A, 1095
Romazicon, 192
Ropinirole, 652
Rosiglitazone Maleate, 167
Rowasa, 706
Roxanol, 423
Roxanol 100, 423
Roxanol T, 423
Roxicodone, 424
Roxicodone Intensol, 424
Ru-Vert-M, 498
Rum-K, 15
Rythmol, 226

S

S2, 353
Sal-Tropine, 669
Salagen, 715
Salflex, 455
Salicylate Combinations, 455
Salicylates, 455
Salicylsalicyclic Acid, 455
Saline Laxatives, 693
Salmeterol, 353
Salmeterol/Fluticasone, 412
Salsalate, 455
Salsitab, 455
Saluron, 330
Sandimmune, 1024
Sandoglobulin, 983
Sani-Supp, 692
Sansert, 490
Saquinavir Mesylate, 919
Sarafem, 537
Scalpicin, 1045
Scopolamine HBr, 669
Scot-Tussin Allergy DM, 394
Scot-Tussin DM Cough
    Chasers, 405
Secobarbital Sodium, 592
Seconal Sodium Pul-
    vules, 592
Sectral, 255
Sedatives/Hypnotics,
    Barbiturate, 592
Sedatives/Hypnotics,
    Nonbarbiturate, 585

Selective Estrogen Receptor Modulator, 100
Selective Serotonin Reuptake Inhibitors, 537
Selegiline HCl, 650
Senna-Gen, 693
Sennosides, 693
Senokot, 693
Senokot-S Tablets, 693
SenokotXTRA, 693
Septra, 970
Septra DS, 970
Septra IV, 970
Serax, 509
Serentil, 553
Serevent, 353
Serevent Diskus, 353
Seromycin Pulvules, 880
Seroquel, 562
Serotonin 5-HT$_1$ Receptor Agonists, 485
Sertraline HCl, 537
Serutan, 693
Serzone, 535
Sibutramine, 420
Silace, 692
Silace-C, 693
Siladryl, 394
Sildenafil Citrate, 319
Silphen Cough, 406
Silphen DM, 405
Simvastatin, 306
Sinarest 12 Hour, 386
Sinemet, 645
Sinemet CR, 645
Sinequan, 519
Sinex, 386
Singulair, 410
Sinustop Pro, 386
Sirolimus, 1016
Skeletal Muscle Relaxants, 635
Skelid, 179
Slo-bid Gyrocaps, 365
Slo-Phyllin, 365
Slo-Phyllin Gyrocaps, 365
Slo-Salt-K, 20
Slow FE, 27
Slow-K, 15
Slow-Mag, 13
Smoking Deterrents, 657
Snaplets-FR Granules, 453
Sodium Ascorbate, 7
Sodium Bicarbonate,
  Antacids, 665
  Nutritionals, 22
Sodium Chloride, 20
  with Heparin, 69

Sodium Citrate, 665
Sodium Diuril, 330
Sodium Salicylate, 455
Sodium Thiosalicylate, 455
Sodium Thiosulfate, 185
Solfoton, 592
Solu-Cortef, 132
Solu-Medrol, 132
Sonata, 587
Sorbitrate, 205
Sotalol HCl, 255
Sparfloxacin, 781
Sparine, 553
Spec-T, 407
Spectracef, 740
Spectrobid, 719
Spironolactone, 343
Sporanox, 857
SSRIs, see Selective Serotonin Reuptake Inhibitors
St. Joseph Adult Chewable Aspirin, 455
St. Joseph Aspirin-Free Fever Reducer for Children, 453
St. Joseph Aspirin-Free for Children, 453
St. Joseph Cough Suppressant, 405
Starlix, 145
Stavudine, 944
Stelazine, 554
Stool Softener, 692
Stool Softener DC, 692
Streptomycin Sulfate,
  Aminoglycosides, Parenteral, 832
  Antituberculosis Agents, 882
Sublimaze, 423
Succimer, 185
Sucralfate, 668
Sucrets 4-Hour Cough, 405
Sucrets Cough Control, 405
Sudafed, 386
Sudafed 12 Hour Caplets, 386
Sudafed, Children's, 386
Sudex, 386
Sufenta, 424
Sufentanil Citrate, 424
Sular, 241
Sulbactam Sodium and Ampicillin, 719
Sulfadiazine, 864
Sulfamethizole, 864
Sulfamethoxazole, 864

Sulfamethoxazole/ Trimethoprim, 970
Sulfasalazine,
  Antirheumatic Agents, 477
  GI, 710
Sulfisoxazole,
  Miscellaneous Anti-infectives, 973
  Sulfonamides, 864
Sulfonamides, 864
Sulfonylureas, 156
Sulindac, 464
Sumatriptan Succinate, 485
Sumycin 250, 804
Sumycin 500, 804
SunKist Vitamin C, 7
Suppress, 405
Suprax, 740
Surfak Liquigels, 692
Surmontil, 519
Sustaire, 365
Sustiva, 966
Syllact, 693
Symadine, 649
Symmetrel,
  Antiparkinson Agents, 649
  Antiviral Agents, 905
Sympathomimetics, 353
Synalar, 1044
Synthetic Conjugated Estrogens, A, 91
Synthroid, 172
Syrup of Ipecac, 186
Systemic Anti-infective Agents, 717

T

T-Gen, 501
T-Phyl, 365
T/Scalp, 1045
Tac-3, 133
Tacrine HCl, 576
Tacrolimus,
  Immunosuppressives, 1013
  Topical, 1054
Tagamet, 674
Tagamet HB, 674
Talacen Caplets, 447
Talwin, 445
Talwin Compound Caplets, 447
Talwin NX, 445
Tambocor, 228
Tamiflu, 916
Tamoxifen Citrate, 1093
Tamsulosin HCl, 283
Tao, 811

Tapazole, 177
Tavist, 394
Tazicef, 740
Tazidime, 740
Tazobactam and
    Piperacillin, 720
Tebamide, 501
Tegretol, 621
Tegretol-XR, 621
Telmisartan, 298
Temazepam, 589
Temovate, 1044
Tempra Drops, 453
Ten-K, 15
Tenofovir Disoproxil
    Fumarate, 933
Tenormin, 255
Tensilon, 185
Tenuate, 420
Tenuate Dospan, 420
Tequin, 781
Terazosin, 283
Terbinafine HCl, 862
Terbutaline, 353
Terramycin, 804
Terramycin IM, 804
Tessalon Perles, 406
Testoderm, 122
Testoderm TTS, 122
Testoderm with Adhesive,
    122
Testopel, 122
Testosterone Cypionate (in
    Oil), 122
Testosterone Enanthate (in
    Oil), 122
Testosterone Gel, 122
Testosterone, Long-Acting,
    122
Testosterone Pellets, 122
Testosterone Transdermal
    System, 122
Testred, 122
Tetanus Immune Globulin,
    987
Tetracyclic Compounds, 525
Tetracycline HCl, 804
Tetracyclines, 804
Tetrahydroaminoacridine,
    576
Tetrahydrozoline, 386
Teveten, 298
Texacort, 1045
THA, 576
Thalitone, 330
Theo-24, 365
Theo-Dur, 365
Theo-X, 365

Theochron, 365
Theoclear L.A., 365
Theolair, 365
Theolair-SR, 365
Theophylline, 365
Theophylline and Dextrose,
    365
Theospan SR, 365
Theovent, 365
Therevac-Plus, 693
Therevac-SB, 693
Thiazides and Related
    Diuretics, 330
Thiazolidinediones, 167
Thiethylperazine, 494
Thioridazine HCl, 553
Thiosulfil Forte, 864
Thiothixene, 554
Thioxanthene Derivatives,
    554
Thorazine,
    Antiemetic/Antivertigo
        Agents, 494
    Antipsychotics, 553
Thorazine Spansules,
    Antiemetic/Antivertigo
        Agents, 494
    Antipsychotics, 553
Thyroid Dessicated, 172
Thyroid Drugs, 172
Thyroid Hormones, 172
Thyroid USP, 172
Thyrolar, 172
Tiagabine HCl, 625
Tiazac, 241
Ticar, 720
Ticarcillin and Clavulanate
    Potassium, 720
Ticarcillin Disodium, 720
Ticlid, 56
Ticlopidine HCl, 56
Ticon, 501
Tigan, 501
Tilade, 384
Tiludronate Sodium, 179
Timentin, 720
Timolol Maleate,
    Ophthalmics, 1066
    Systemic, 255
Timoptic, 1066
Timoptic-XE, 1066
Tinzaparin, 63
TMP-SMZ, 970
TOBI, 832
Tobramycin, 1080
Tobramycin Sulfate, 832
Tobrex, 1080
Tocainide HCl, 225

Tofranil, 519
Tofranil-PM, 519
Tolazamide, 156
Tolbutamide, 156
Tolectin 200, 464
Tolectin 600, 464
Tolectin DS, 464
Tolinase, 156
Tolmetin Sodium, 464
Tolterodine Tartrate, 327
Tonocard, 225
Topamax, 627
Topical Corticosteroids, 1044
Topical Drugs,
    Miscellaneous, 1049
Topical Immunomodulators,
    1053
Topical Ophthalmics, 1059
Topicort, 1044
Topiramate, 627
Toprol XL, 255
Toradol, 463
Torecan, 494
Tornalate, 353
Torsemide, 336
Totacillin, 719
Tramadol HCl, 451
Trandate, 269
Trandolapril, 290
Trans-Retinoic Acid, 1049
Tranxene, 509
Tranxene-SD, 509
Tranxene-SD Half Strength,
    509
Tranxene-T, 605
Tranylcypromine, 545
Travatan, 1074
Travoprost, 1074
Trazodone HCl, 528
Trecator-SC, 879
Tretinoin, 1049
Tri-K, 16
Tri-Levlen, 106
Tri-Nasal, 390
Tri-Norinyl, 106
Triamcinolone,
    Adrenal Cortical Steroids,
        133
    Intranasal Steroids, 390
    Respiratory Inhalants, 371
Triamcinolone Acetonide,
    Systemic, 133
    Topicals, 1045
Triamcinolone Diacetate, 133
Triamcinolone
    Hexacetonide, 133
Triaminic AM Decongestant
    Formula, 386

Triamolone 40, 133
Triamonide 40, 133
Triamterene, 345
Triazolam, 589
Triban, 501
Tricalcium Phosphate, 9
Trichlormethiazide, 330
Tricor, 312
Tricosal, 455
Tricyclic Compounds, 519
Tridate Bowel Cleansing
    System, 693
Tridesilon, 1044
Tridihexethyl Chloride, 669
Tridil, 205
Trifluoperazine, 554
Trifluorothymidine, 1085
Triflupromazine,
    Antiemetic/Antivertigo
        Agents, 494
    Antipsychotics, 553
Trifluridine, 1085
Trihexyphenidyl HCl, 642
Trilafon,
    Antiemetic/Antivertigo
        Agents, 494
    Antipsychotics, 553
Trileptal, 631
Trilisate, 455
Trimazide, 501
Trimethobenzamide HCl,
    501
Trimethoprim/Sulfa-
    methoxazole, 970
Trimetrexate Glucuronate,
    977
Trimipramine Maleate, 519
Trimox, 719
Trimox Pediatric Drops, 719
Triostat, 172
Tripelennamine HCl, 395
Triphasic Oral
    Contraceptives, 106
Triphasil, 106
Triptone Caplets, 500
Trivora-28, 106
Trizivir, 958
Trocal, 405
Troleandomycin, 811
Trovafloxacin Mesylate, 781
Trovan, 781
Truphylline, 364
Trusopt, 1072
Tuinal 100 mg Pulvules, 592
Tuinal 200 mg Pulvules, 592
Tums 500, 9
Tums E-X, Extra Strength,
    665

Tums Ultra, 665
Tusstat,
    Antihistamines, 394
    Antitussives, 406
Twin-K, 16
Tylenol, 453
Tylenol Children's, 453
Tylenol Extended Relief, 453
Tylenol Extra Strength, 453
Tylenol Infants' Drops, 453
Tylenol Junior Strength, 453
Tylenol Regular Strength
    Tablets, 453
Tyzine, 386
Tyzine Pediatric Drops, 386

U

U-Cort, 1045
Ultiva, 424
Ultralente, 149
Ultram, 451
Ultravate, 1045
Unasyn, 719
Uni-Dur, 365
Unifiber, 693
Unipen, 719
Uniphyl, 365
Univasc, 290
Unoprostone Isopropyl, 1074
Urinary Acidifiers, 186
Urinary Alkalinizers, 186
Urispas, 325
Uro-Mag,
    Antacids, 665
    Minerals/Electrolytes, 13
Urobak, 864
Uticort, 1044

V

Vaccines,
    Bacterial, 993
    Viral, 998
Vagifem, 91
Vaginal Estrogens, 98
Valacyclovir HCl, 903
Valcyte, 895
Valdecoxib, 464
Valergen 20, 91
Valergen 40, 91
Valganciclovir, 895
Valisone, 1044
Valium,
    Antianxiety Agents, 509
    Anticonvulsants, 606
    Skeletal Muscle Relaxants,
        636

Valproic Acid and
    Derivatives, 615
Valsartan, 298
Valtrex, 903
Vancenase, 390
Vancenase AQ, 390
Vancenase Pockethaler, 390
Vanceril, 371
Vanceril Double Strength,
    371
Vancocin, 822
Vancoled, 822
Vancomycin, 822
Vantin, 740
Vaqta, 1002
Varicella Virus Vaccine, 1003
Varicella-Zoster Immune
    Globulin (Human), 989
Varivax, 1003
Vascor, 241
Vasopressors Used in Shock,
    253
Vasotec, 289
Vasotec I.V., 289
Veetids, 720
Veetids '250', 720
Velosef, 741
Velosulin BR, 148
Venlafaxine, 532
Venofer, 33
Venoglobulin-S, 983
Ventolin, 353
Ventolin Nebules, 353
Verapamil HCl, 241
Verelan, 241
Vergon, 498
Vertab, 500
Vesprin,
    Antiemetic/Antivertigo
        Agents, 494
    Antipsychotics, 553
Vexol, 1076
Viagra, 319
Vibra-Tabs, 804
Vibramycin, 804
Vibramycin IV, 804
Vicks Cough Silencers, 407
Vicks Dry Hacking Cough,
    405
Vicks Formula 44 Cough
    Control Discs, 407
Vicks Inhaler, 386
Vicks Sinex 12-Hour, 386
Vicks Vatronol, 386
Vidarabine, 1084
Videx, 935
Videx EC, 935
Vioxx, 464

Vira-A, 1084
Viracept, 926
Viral Vaccines, 998
Viramune, 962
Virazole, 908
Viread, 933
Virilon, 122
Virilon IM, 122
Viroptic, 1085
Visken, 255
Vistaril,
    Antianxiety Agents, 515
    Antihistamines, 395
Vita-C, 7
Vitamin A Acid, 1049
Vitamin B$_{12}$, 39
Vitamin C, 7
Vitamin K,
    Antidotes, 185
    Blood Modifiers, 42
Vitamins, 7
Vivactil, 519
Vivelle, 91
Volmax, 353
Voltaren, 463
Voltaren-XR, 463
VZIG, 989

W

Warfarin Sodium, 73
Welchol, 304
Wellbutrin, 529
Wellbutrin SR, 529
Westcort, 1045
Women's Gentle Laxative,
    692

Wycillin, 720
Wymox, 719

X

X-Prep Bowel Evacuant
    Kit-1, 693
X-Prep Bowel Kit-2, 693
X-Prep Liquid, 693
Xalatan, 1074
Xanax, 509
Xanthine Derivatives, 364
Xenical, 686
Xopenex, 353
Xylocaine HCl IV for
    Cardiac Arrhythmias,
    222
Xylometazoline, 386

Y

Yasmin, 106

Z

Zafirlukast, 408
Zagam, 781
Zalcitabine, 947
Zaleplon, 587
Zanamivir, 915
Zantac, 674
Zantac 75, 674
Zantac EFFERdose, 674
Zantac GELdose, 674
Zantryl, 420
Zaroxolyn, 330
Zebeta, 255

Zefazone, 740
Zerit, 944
Zestril, 289
Zetran, 636
Ziagen, 954
Zidovudine, 951
Zidovudine/Lamivudine, 957
Zileuton, 409
Zinacef, 741
Ziprasidone HCl, 565
Zithromax, 811
Zocor, 306
Zofran, 503
Zofran ODT, 503
Zoledronic, 179
Zolicef, 740
Zolmitriptan, 485
Zoloft, 537
Zolpidem Tartrate, 585
Zometa, 179
Zomig, 485
Zomig ZMT, 485
Zonegran, 603
Zonisamide, 603
ZORprin, 455
Zostrix, 1051
Zostrix-HP, 1051
Zosyn, 720
Zovia, 106
Zovirax, 898
Zyban, 660
Zyflo, 409
Zyloprim, 480
Zyprexa, 562
Zyprexa Zydis, 562
Zyrtec, 394
Zyvox, 825